Wardlaw's
Perspectives in Nutrition, Eighth Edition

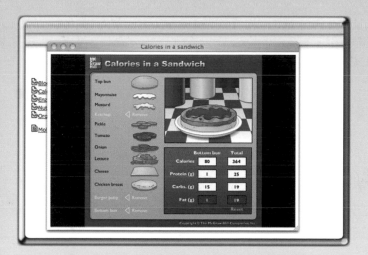

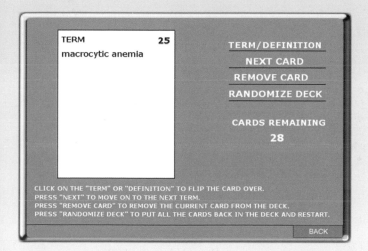

ON TRACK . . .

Check out the study tools that best suit your learning style. A variety of interactivities and quizzes keep you motivated and on track to master key concepts.

- **Animations** Access to approximately 75 animations helps you visualize key nutrition concepts and processes. Each animation is accompanied by a quiz to help you test your comprehension.

- **Test Yourself** Prepare for exams by taking a chapter quiz at the *Perspectives in Nutrition,* Eighth Edition ARIS site. Use the quiz questions and accompanying feedback for incorrect answers to help you gauge your mastery of the chapter content. You can even e-mail your quiz results to your professor!

- **Learning Activities** Helpful and engaging learning experiences await you at the *Perspectives in Nutrition,* Eighth Edition ARIS site. In addition to quizzes and animations, you can study nutrition terminology with flashcards, and you can use links to reliable websites to help you complete assignments.

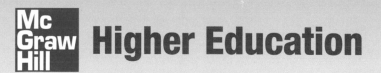

WARDLAW'S
Perspectives in
NUTRITION

EIGHTH EDITION

Carol Byrd-Bredbenner, Ph.D., R.D.
Rutgers, The State University of New Jersey

Donna Beshgetoor, Ph.D.
San Diego State University

Gaile Moe, Ph.D., R.D.
Seattle Pacific University

Jacqueline Berning, Ph.D., R.D.
University of Colorado at Colorado Springs

 Higher Education

Boston   Burr Ridge, IL   Dubuque, IA   New York   San Francisco   St. Louis
Bangkok   Bogotá   Caracas   Kuala Lumpur   Lisbon   London   Madrid   Mexico City
Milan   Montreal   New Delhi   Santiago   Seoul   Singapore   Sydney   Taipei   Toronto

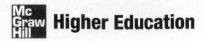

WARDLAW'S PERSPECTIVES IN NUTRITION, EIGHTH EDITION

Published by McGraw-Hill, a business unit of The McGraw-Hill Companies, Inc., 1221 Avenue of the Americas, New York, NY 10020. Copyright © 2009 by The McGraw-Hill Companies, Inc. All rights reserved. Previous editions © 2007, 2004, 2002, 1999, 1996, 1993 and 1990. No part of this publication may be reproduced or distributed in any form or by any means, or stored in a database or retrieval system, without the prior written consent of The McGraw-Hill Companies, Inc., including, but not limited to, in any network or other electronic storage or transmission, or broadcast for distance learning.

Some ancillaries, including electronic and print components, may not be available to customers outside the United States.

 This book is printed on recycled, acid-free paper containing 10% postconsumer waste.

1 2 3 4 5 6 7 8 9 0 QPD/QPD 0 9 8

ISBN 978–0–07–296999–3
MHID 0–07–296999–7

Publisher: *Michelle Watnick*
Executive Editor: *Colin H. Wheatley*
Director of Development: *Kristine Tibbetts*
Senior Developmental Editor: *Lynne M. Meyers*
Project Manager: *April R. Southwood*
Senior Production Supervisor: *Kara Kudronowicz*
Senior Media Project Manager: *Tammy Juran*
Manager, Creative Services: *Michelle D. Whitaker*
Cover/Interior Designer: *Greg Nettles/Squarecrow Design*
(USE) Cover Image: *© Brand X Pictures/PunchStock RF*
Senior Photo Research Coordinator: *John C. Leland*
Photo Research: *Mary Reeg*
Compositor: *S4Carlisle Publishing Services*
Typeface: *10/12 Galliard*
Printer: *Quebecor World Dubuque, IA*

The credits section for this book begins on page C-1 and is considered an extension of the copyright page.

Library of Congress Cataloging-in-Publication Data

Wardlaw's perspectives in nutrition / Carol Byrd-Bredbenner ... [et al.]. -- 8th ed.
    p. cm.
  Previously published as: Wardlaw, Gordon M. Perspectives in nutrition, c2007.
  Includes index.
  ISBN 978–0–07–296999–3 --- ISBN 0–07–296999–7 (hard copy : alk. paper) 1. Nutrition. I. Byrd-Bredbenner, Carol. II. Wardlaw, Gordon M. Perspectives in nutrition.
  QP141.W38 2009
  612.3--dc22
                                                                    2008010733

Brief Contents

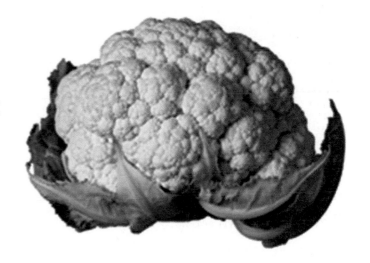

Contents

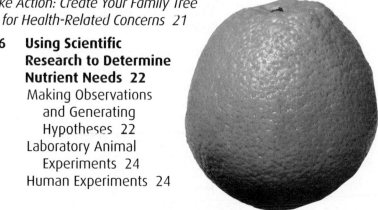

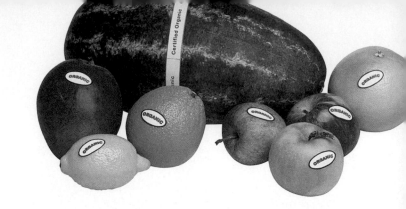

Part 2 Energy-Yielding Nutrients and Alcohol

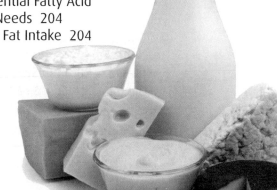

Part 3   Metabolism and Energy Balance

9 ENERGY METABOLISM 280

10 ENERGY BALANCE, WEIGHT CONTROL, AND EATING DISORDERS 312

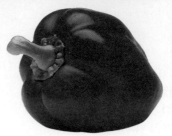
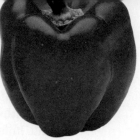

14 WATER AND MAJOR MINERALS 482

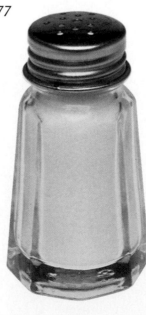

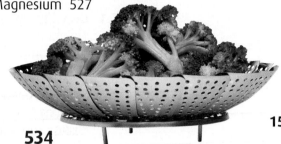
Part 5 Nutrition Applications in the Life Cycle

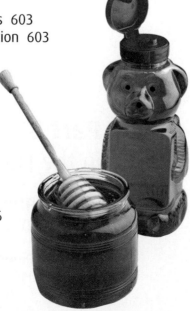

17   NUTRITION DURING THE GROWING YEARS 612

Appendixes

Meet the New Author Team

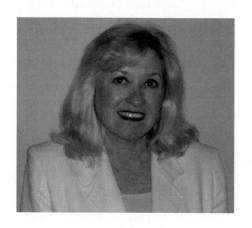

Carol Byrd-Bredbenner, PhD, RD, FADA, received her doctorate from Pennsylvania State University. Currently, she is Professor in the Nutritional Sciences Department at Rutgers, The State University of New Jersey. She teaches a wide range of undergraduate and graduate nutrition courses. Her research interests focus on investigating environmental factors that affect dietary choices and health outcomes. Dr. Byrd-Bredbenner has authored numerous nutrition texts, journal articles, and computer software packages. She has received teaching awards from the American Dietetic Association, Society for Nutrition Education, and U.S. Department of Agriculture. In 2007, she received the American Dietetic Association's Anita Owen Award for Innovative Nutrition Education Programs. She also was a Fellow of the United Nations, World Health Organization at the WHO Collaborating Center for Nutrition Education, University of Athens, Greece. She enjoys exploring food and culinary customs, traveling, diving, and gardening.

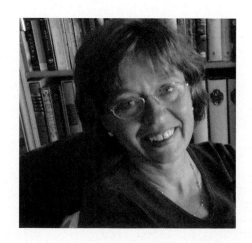

Gaile L. Moe, PhD, RD, earned a doctorate in nutritional sciences at the University of Washington. She is a registered dietitian who has worked in clinical nutrition, research, and management, as well as education. She is currently Associate Professor and Director of the Didactic Program in Dietetics at Seattle Pacific University. She has published in peer-reviewed journals in the areas of nutrition and cancer and media reporting of nutrition research. Gaile enjoys swimming, cycling, walking, and hiking, along with learning about culinary traditions, food, and food policy.

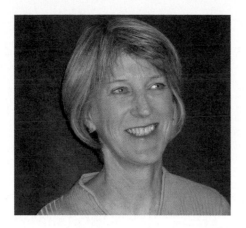

Donna Beshgetoor, PhD, earned her doctorate in nutrition and physiological chemistry from the University of California–Davis. She is currently an Associate Professor at San Diego State University (SDSU) where she teaches introductory and clinical nutrition to undergraduate and graduate students in the School of Exercise and Nutritional Science and the Global Health Program in the School of Public Health at San Diego State University (SDSU). She has been recognized by SDSU as a "Most Influential Associate Professor" and an "Outstanding Student Mentor." Her research and journal publications focus on nutritional risk assessment in master athletes and individuals with chronic diseases. Prior to her university appointment, Dr. Beshgetoor worked as a corporate wellness director and a clinical dietitian. She is an active member of the American Society of Nutrition (ASN) and the American College of Sports Medicine (ACSM). She enjoys music, hiking, cycling, beach walks, windsurfing and time with family, friends, and Taz.

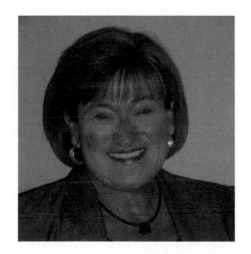

Jacqueline R. Berning, PhD, RD, CSSD, earned her doctorate in nutrition from Colorado State University in Fort Collins, Colorado. She is currently Associate Professor and Chair of the Biology Department at the University of Colorado at Colorado Springs, where she has won numerous teaching awards. Jackie is published in the area of sports dietetics and is currently the sports dietitian for the Denver Broncos Football Club and the Cleveland Indians Baseball Club. She is active in the American Dietetic Association (ADA), where she serves as a member of the Program Planning Committee for Food and Nutrition Conference and Exposition and is a committee member for the development of standards of practice for sports dietitians. Additionally, she served 6 years as an ADA spokesperson and is a former chair of the Sports, Cardiovascular, and Wellness Nutritionists dietetics practice group. Jackie enjoys walking, hiking, gardening, and watching her 2 athletic sons compete.

Welcome to the Eighth Edition of Wardlaw's *Perspectives in Nutrition*

Gordon Wardlaw's *Perspectives in Nutrition* has the richly deserved reputation of providing an accurate, current, in-depth, and thoughtful introduction to the dynamic field of nutrition that is unparalleled by any other textbook. As the new author team on the eighth edition, we have endeavored to enrich this edition for both students and instructors. (See p. xvi, *Meet the New Author Team,* to learn more about us.) Our passion for nutrition, genuine desire to promote student learning, and commitment to scientific accuracy, coupled with constructive comments from instructors and students, guided us in this effort. Our primary goal has been to maintain the strengths and philosophy that have been the hallmark of this book yet enhance the accessibility of the science content and the application of materials for today's students.

Our Intended Audience

This textbook was developed with nutrition and health science majors in mind. The chemistry, biochemistry, and physiology presented in the text assume that students have had at least some college-level science. Because this course often attracts students from a broad range of majors, we have been careful to include examples and explanations that are relevant to them and to include sufficient scientific background to make the science accessible to them. The appendices are provided for students who wish to learn more or need assistance with the science involved in human physiology, chemistry, and metabolism.

To better bridge the span of differing science backgrounds and to enhance student interest and achievement of course objectives, we reorganized the presentation of material within chapters to flow seamlessly from concrete to abstract learning. In chapters focusing on nutrients, for example, concrete concepts, such as food sources of the nutrients and recommended intakes, are introduced early in the chapter to create a framework for more abstract concepts, such as functions, digestion, and absorption.

What Makes the Eighth Edition Special:

- Enhanced Accessibility
- Improved Personal Focus and Applications
- Assessment and Evaluation of Learning

xviii

Enhanced Accessibility

Accurate, Current Science Presented in an Engaging Manner

This edition continues the tradition of presenting scientific content that is reliable, accurate, and up-to-date. It also retains the in-depth coverage students need to fully understand and appreciate the role of nutrition in overall health and to build the scientific knowledge base needed to pursue health-related careers or simply live healthier lives. To enhance these strengths and promote greater student comprehension, new research findings and peer-reviewed references were incorporated and artwork was enhanced to further complement discussions. The presentation of complex concepts was scrutinized in an effort to increase clarity through the use of clear, streamlined, precise, and student-friendly language. Timely and intriguing examples, illustrative analogies, clinical insights, and historical notes were added to make the text enjoyable and interesting to students and instructors alike.

Logical Organization, Flexible Sequencing

This new edition addresses the curricular realities of today's college coursework by organizing and consolidating the content into 5 main parts and 18 chapters. This reorganization presents the core content in a thorough yet manageable fashion. To give instructors even greater flexibility in tailoring reading assignments to course requirements and cross-referencing lectures to the book, this edition numbers each major section in chapters. If, for example, an instructor plans to address only part of a chapter on a certain day, he or she can direct students to focus on just those sections.

- **Part 1,** *Nutrition Basics,* has a new addition: Chapter 3, *The Food Supply.* Consumer-related issues, such as food safety, food additives, organic foods, biotechnology, and hunger, draw many students to nutrition. However, numerous instructors told us they can seldom fit these chapters into their crowded course content and wanted innovative strategies for incorporating these vital concepts. In response, we thoughtfully trimmed and sharply focused the content of the food safety and world nutrition chapters of the previous edition and moved the content forward in the textbook, where it logically sets the stage for further study of nutrition.

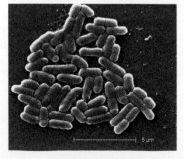 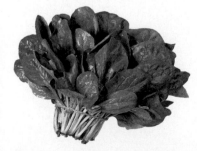

- **Part 2, *Energy-Yielding Nutrients and Alcohol,*** includes a fully updated presentation of each macronutrient and alcohol. Chapters address food sources, absorption, transport, and functions of each macronutrient. A complete discussion of the effects of alcohol is included in the alcohol chapter (Ch. 8).

- **Part 3, Metabolism and Energy Balance,** now contains Chapter 9, *Energy Metabolism.* This change was made to respond to the question many instructors ask "When should energy metabolism be taught, before or after the macronutrients?" Having taught it both ways, we came to the conclusion that our students more easily mastered metabolism after they had studied the macronutrients and alcohol and had built the critical foundational knowledge needed to grasp the abstract concepts of metabolism. We were careful to thoroughly address the topics of energy metabolism, so that instructors who prefer to cover it before macronutrients and alcohol have the flexibility to do so. Part 3 also addresses energy balance, weight control, and eating disorders (Ch. 10) and nutrition, exercise, and sports (Ch. 11). The discussion of eating disorders, which are primarily psychological conditions with nutritional ramifications, was streamlined and merged into Chapter 10. Chapter 11 allows students to understand how the principles of metabolism relate to athletic performance and how physical activity pairs with dietary practices to prevent and treat obesity and related diseases.

- **Part 4, *Vitamins and Minerals,*** addresses the food sources, requirements, absorption, transport, storage, excretion, functions, and effects of deficient and excessive intakes of micronutrients. Links between these nutrients and a variety of medical conditions are highlighted.

- **Part 5, *Nutrition Applications in the Life Cycle,*** applies the information from earlier parts to demonstrate the vital role of nutrition throughout the life span.

Attractive, Accurate Artwork

More than 1000 drawings, photographs, and tables in the text were critically analyzed to identify how each could be enhanced and refined to help students more easily master complex scientific concepts.

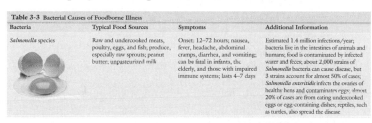

- Photographs were added to many tables to promote interest and retention of information. Many photographs were updated or replaced to inspire student inquiry and comprehension.

Table 3-3 Bacterial Causes of Foodborne Illness			
Bacteria	**Typical Food Sources**	**Symptoms**	**Additional Information**
Salmonella species	Raw and undercooked meats, poultry, eggs, and fish; produce, especially raw sprouts; peanut butter; unpasteurized milk	Onset: 12–72 hours; nausea, fever, headache, abdominal cramps, diarrhea, and vomiting; can be fatal in infants, the elderly, and those with impaired immune systems; lasts 4–7 days	Estimated 1.4 million infections/year; bacteria live in the intestines of animals and humans; food is contaminated by infected water and feces; about 2,000 strains of *Salmonella* bacteria can cause disease, but 3 strains account for almost 50% of cases; *Salmonella enteritidis* infects the ovaries of healthy hens and contaminates eggs; almost 20% of cases are from eating undercooked eggs or egg-containing dishes; reptiles, such as turtles, also spread the disease

- Many of existing illustrations were redesigned to use brighter colors and a more attractive, contemporary style. Others were fine-tuned to make them clearer and easier to follow. Navigational aids were added to many illustrations to show where a function occurs and to put it in perspective of the whole body.

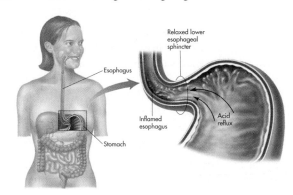

- Coordinated color schemes and drawing styles were introduced to keep presentations consistent and strengthen the educational value of the artwork. Color-coding and directional arrows added to energy metabolism figures make it easier to follow events and reinforce the interrelationships among nutrients and their metabolites.

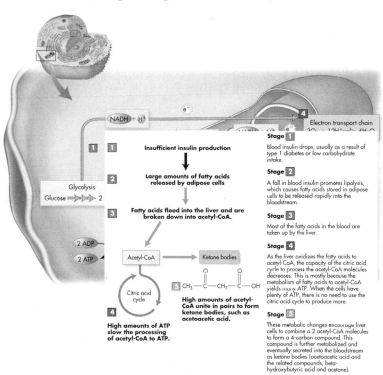

- Process descriptions within many figures were moved from the legend into the body of the figure. This pairing of the action and explanation walks students step-by-step through the process and increases the teaching effectiveness of these figures.

Finally, a careful comparison of artwork with its corresponding written text was done to ensure that they were completely coordinated and consistent. The final result is a striking new visual program that holds readers' attention and supports the goals of clarity, ease of comprehension, and critical thinking. The attractive new layout and design of this edition is clean, bright, and inviting. This creative presentation of the material is geared toward engaging today's visually oriented students.

Improved Personal Focus and Applications

Applying Nutrition on a Personal Level

A key objective in nearly all introductory courses is for students to be able to apply their new knowledge of nutrition to their own lives. Practical applications clearly linked to nutritional science concepts are woven throughout each chapter to help students apply their knowledge to improving and maintaining their own health and that of others for whom they are responsible, such as future patients or offspring. Examples of features that help students draw relationships from nutrition concepts to their own lives include

- Updated **case studies** showcase realistic scenarios and thought-provoking questions.

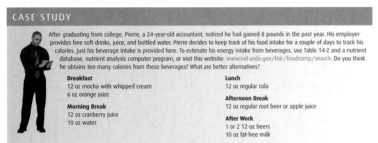

CASE STUDY

After graduating from college, Pierre, a 24-year-old accountant, noticed he had gained 8 pounds in the past year. His employer provides free soft drinks, juice, and bottled water. Pierre decides to keep track of his food intake for a couple of days to track his calories. Just his beverage intake is provided here. To estimate his energy intake from beverages, use Table 14-2 and a nutrient database, nutrient analysis computer program, or visit this website: www.nal.usda.gov/fnic/foodcomp/search. Do you think he obtains too many calories from these beverages? What are better alternatives?

Breakfast
12 oz mocha with whipped cream
6 oz orange juice

Morning Break
12 oz cranberry juice
10 oz water

Lunch
12 oz regular cola

Afternoon Break
12 oz regular root beer or apple juice

After Work
1 or 2 12-oz beers
10 oz fat-free milk

- Two *Take Action* features in each chapter (many are new) allow students to examine their own diets and health issues.

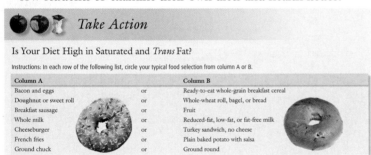

Take Action

Is Your Diet High in Saturated and *Trans* Fat?

Instructions: In each row of the following list, circle your typical food selection from column A or B.

Column A		Column B
Bacon and eggs	or	Ready-to-eat whole-grain breakfast cereal
Doughnut or sweet roll	or	Whole-wheat roll, bagel, or bread
Breakfast sausage	or	Fruit
Whole milk	or	Reduced-fat, low-fat, or fat-free milk
Cheeseburger	or	Turkey sandwich, no cheese
French fries	or	Plain baked potato with salsa
Ground chuck	or	Ground round

Stimulating Pedagogy

The pedagogical elements that support student learning and application were retained, updated, or enhanced to make nutritional science even more readable, accessible, and achievable for today's students. The following elements are just some of the tutorial aids designed to challenge students to organize their thinking, focus their studying, synthesize information, think critically, and apply concepts to everyday situations.

- The former *Expert Opinion* feature, now called *Expert Perspective from the Field,* emphasizes cutting-edge topics and demonstrates how emerging, and sometimes controversial, research results affect nutrition knowledge and practice.

Expert Perspective *from the Field*

Organic Foods and Local Food Systems

Nutrition, agriculture, access to food and water, food processing and preparation, public policy, personal health, and environmental quality are all interrelated. When these relationships are out of balance and practices are not sustainable, the quality, quantity, and future of our food and water supplies may be negatively affected. Concern about these interrelationships, as well as environmental quality and personal health, may affect food choices. For example,

directly from them. Visiting farmers' markets, food co-ops, Community Supported Agriculture (CSA) farms, or Cooperative Extension System websites can help consumers learn which foods are produced locally. Many CSA farms rely on volunteers during the growing season—this may provide those with limited budgets an opportunity to access high-quality, fresh food. To save money, she also recommends buying fresh food when it is in season.

- New *Medical Perspective* features highlight the role of nutrition in the prevention and treatment of diseases. These topics will be especially interesting to students planning careers in dietetics or health-related fields.

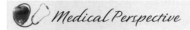

Medical Perspective

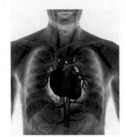

Cardiovascular Disease (CVD)

Cardiovascular disease (CVD) is the major killer of North Americans. Each year, about 500,000 people die of CVD in the United States, about 60% more than die of cancer. The figure rises to almost 1 million if strokes and other circulatory diseases are included. About 1.5 million people in the United States each year have a heart attack. The overall male-to-female ratio for heart disease is about 2:1. Women generally lag about 10 years behind men in developing the disease. Still, it eventually kills more women than any other disease—twice as many as cancer. And, for each person in North America who dies of CVD, 20 more (over 13 million people) have symptoms of the disease.

High-fat diets, especially those rich in saturated and *trans* fats, increase the risk of CVD. (Recall that the vascular system includes the blood, heart, arteries, and veins.) The symptoms develop over many years and often do not become obvious until old age. Nonetheless, autopsies of those under 20 years of age have shown that many already had atherosclerotic plaque in their arteries.

- New *Global Perspective* features emphasize concepts related to critical health and nutrition issues around the world. These timely features, sprinkled judiciously throughout the book, also aim to engage students with thought-provoking challenges.

 Global Perspective

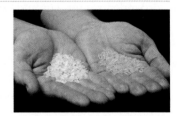

Vitamin A Deficiency

In many parts of the developing world, vitamin A deficiency is a major public health concern (Fig. 12-8). Recent estimates indicate that 100 to 140 million children worldwide suffer from vitamin A deficiency. Women of childbearing years also are at increased risk of deficiency, especially in impoverished areas of Africa and Southeast Asia. In many of these areas, where HIV infection also is prevalent, vitamin A deficiency in pregnancy increases the likelihood of the transmission of HIV to the developing fetus and increases the risk of maternal mortality. Approximately 600,000 women die each year from pregnancy- and childbirth-related causes. Many of these deaths result from complications secondary to poor vitamin A and overall nutritional status.[11]

- Each major heading in the chapter is now numbered and cross-referenced to the end-of-chapter summary to make it easy to locate and prioritize important concepts.

Assessment and Evaluation of Learning

One of our primary goals as nutrition educators is to ensure that our students leave our courses with a meaningful understanding of the nutrition principles and concepts they need to advance their education and improve their diets and health. Determining how well we have met this goal requires assessment, on both the student level and the instructor level. To this end, we have integrated a number of assessment tools that will allow students and instructors alike to measure their success.

- Because many colleges and universities are beginning to implement **student learning outcomes** as a way to measure student achievement, we have introduced student learning outcomes at the beginning of each chapter. They have been crafted to clearly delineate for students the competencies they are expected to master in that chapter. The following are the broader, course-wide student learning outcomes, on which the chapter level objectives are based:
  1. Identify functions and sources of nutrients.
  2. Demonstrate basic knowledge of digestion, absorption, and metabolism.
  3. Apply current dietary guidelines and nutrition recommendations.

STUDENT LEARNING OUTCOMES

After studying this chapter, you will be able to

1. Explain the differences among metabolism, catabolism, and anabolism.

2. Describe aerobic and anaerobic metabolism of glucose.

3. Illustrate how energy is extracted from glucose, fatty acids, amino acids, and alcohol using metabolic pathways, such as glycolysis, beta-oxidation, the citric acid cycle, and the electron transport system.

5. Identify the conditions that lead to ketogenesis and its importance in survival during fasting.

6. Describe the process of gluconeogenesis.

7. Discuss how the body metabolizes alcohol.

8. Compare the fate of energy from macronutrients during the fed and fasted states.

9. Describe common inborn errors of metabolism.

4. Analyze and evaluate nutrition information scientifically.

5. Relate roles of nutrients in good health, optimal fitness, and prevention and treatment of diseases.

6. Summarize basic concepts of nutrition throughout the life cycle.

7. Evaluate a personal diet record using a nutrient database.

- The online test bank questions that accompany the chapters of this text have been correlated to individual student learning outcomes. This will help instructors identify which concepts students have mastered and those that may require additional reinforcement. The test items were developed by the authors and are used in their courses.

- New **Knowledge Check** questions appear after each major section to encourage students to self-assess their understanding of key concepts before proceeding to the next section.

- Chapters now conclude with reformatted **Study Questions** (multiple-choice and true/false, with answer key) to provide students with a practice test to assess their mastery and build self-confidence.

CRITICAL	THINKING

According to a recent poll, about one-quarter of Americans favor the introduction of GM foods into our food supply, whereas nearly half are opposed to this.[74] Further, 75% acknowledge that they know little about GM foods. Do you think the public should know more about GM foods? If they did know more, do you think that this would change their opinions about introducing such foods into the food supply? Do you think Americans would be surprised to know the extent to which GM corn and soybeans are used?

- **Critical Thinking** questions in the margins challenge students to link key nutrition concepts with real-life situations. These questions also provide a springboard for provocative classroom discussions.

Chapter-by-Chapter Updates

Chapter 1, *The Science of Nutrition*

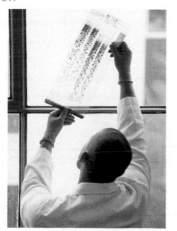

- New concepts included are zoochemicals, the state of the American diet, and modern influences on food choices.

- In response to a rapidly growing research base, coverage of the role of genetics in health and nutrition has been expanded.

- Section on nutrition research methods has been updated to promote greater understanding of the scientific basis of nutrition.

Chapter 2, *Tools of a Healthy Diet*

- Specific applications for each dietary guidance tool (i.e., DRIs/RDAs, Daily Values, nutrient databases, Dietary Guidelines, MyPyramid) enhance student understanding.

- Section on the nutrient composition of food has been added.

- Nutrient content claims table has been redesigned.

- Putting MyPyramid into practice menus have been updated and enhanced with photographs.

Chapter 3, *The Food Supply*

- This new chapter streamlines the material formerly presented in Chapters 19 and 20 in the previous edition. It was moved forward in the text to respond to growing interest in food issues as they impact health and nutritional status.

- Updated information is provided on domestic and international food security, malnutrition and health, food and nutrition assistance programs, organic foods, food additives, biotechnology, meat and milk from cloned animals, prions and mad cow disease, environmental contaminants (e.g., lead, pesticides), and food and water safety.

- New *Take Action* encourages students to assess the availability of organic foods where they normally shop.

- Updated food and water pathogens information has been reorganized into tables that summarize foodborne illnesses, typical foods source, prevalence, and symptoms.

- New table summarizes the functions and examples of common food additives.

- *Global Perspective* on traveler's diarrhea has been added.

- *Expert Perspective from the Field* on organic foods and local food systems has been added.

Chapter 4, *Human Digestion and Absorption*

- New overview of all major body systems provides a foundation for study of the nutrients.

- New organization addresses the entire process of digestion and absorption sequentially.

- New *Global Perspective* explores the causes of diarrheal disease and its relationship to malnutrition in developing countries.

- New *Expert Perspective from the Field* addresses gluten intolerance disorders that are being diagnosed at an increasing rate.

- New tables summarize important digestive and absorption topics, such as hormonal regulation, gallstone formation, heartburn and ulcer prevention, and food intolerances.

- Chapter was expanded to address food intolerances and intestinal gas.

- New figures more clearly illustrate GI tract anatomy and physiology.

Chapter 5, *Carbohydrates*

- New figures depict sources and health benefits of soluble and insoluble fiber.

- Table of sweetener sources is updated.
- Table of practical ways (at the supermarket, in the kitchen, and at the table) to reduce sugar intake has been added.

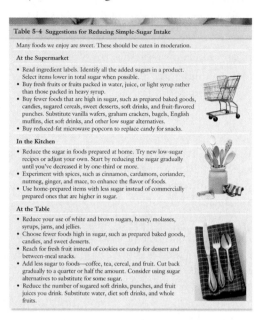

- New *Take Action* activities to estimate fiber intakes have been added.
- Discussion on health concerns related to carbohydrates is updated.
- New *Medical Perspective* on diabetes reflects the latest diagnostic criteria and treatments.

Chapter 6, *Lipids*

- Major concepts in the chapter have been reorganized for better flow and understanding.
- New, color-coded, "talking" drawings of polyunsaturated, monounsaturated, and saturated fat structures facilitate the understanding of students with little chemistry background.
- Section on health concerns related to fat has been added.
- Revised *Take Action* assesses heart disease risk.
- *Medical Perspective* on cardiovascular disease has been added.
- Tables on the 10-year cardiovascular disease risks for men and women have been added.
- *Expert Perspective from the Field* on the nutritional value of nuts has been updated.

Chapter 7, *Proteins*

- Focus on vegetarian diets has been updated, with a new discussion on issues related to children.
- New *Expert Perspective from the Field* explores the role of nutrition in immune function.
- New discussion of food allergies has been incorporated into the chapter.
- *Take Action* activity on planning a vegan diet has been added.

- New *Critical Thinking* activities reinforce key issues regarding protein intake.
- Table on the limiting amino acids in food has been added.
- Table on the protein content of sample menus has been added.

Chapter 8, *Alcohol*

- Updated tables include the alcoholic beverages commonly consumed by college-age students and the signs and symptoms of alcohol poisoning.
- New table summarizes the 3 main pathways for alcohol metabolism.
- New figure illustrates how sex, body weight, and the number of drinks consumed affect the degree of impairment.
- Section on the effects of alcohol consumption during pregnancy and breastfeeding has been added.
- New drawings graphically depict the effect of alcohol use on the liver.
- Statistics on alcohol use have been updated.

Chapter 9, *Energy Metabolism*

- Chapter now follows macronutrient and alcohol chapters to more seamlessly build on the foundation provided by these chapters and to enable students with limited science backgrounds to more fully grasp energy metabolism concepts. This resequencing also streamlines the macronutrient chapters by reducing repetition.
- Attractive new, color-coded figures more clearly convey metabolic pathways. "Talking" figures move systematically through metabolic pathways, explaining key steps in the sequence they occur.

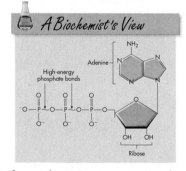

- Chemical structures are identified with a *Biochemist's View* icon to focus student attention and make it easier for instructors to indicate whether students need to learn structures.
- Step-by-step process artwork for each major energy metabolism pathway has been added.
- New summary table describes the major pathways and where metabolism takes place in the cell.
- Section on the metabolics of feasting and fasting has been added.
- Alcohol metabolism and inborn errors of metabolism (e.g., PKU) are now included.

Chapter 10, *Energy Balance, Weight Control, and Eating Disorders*

- By bringing together what were two separate chapters, this chapter eliminates repetition and helps instructors cover key concepts more efficiently.

- Streamlined eating disorder section focuses on the physiological effects of the eating disorder, treatments, and nutritional therapies.
- Body composition techniques have been updated.
- Fad diets and weight control treatments have been updated.
- New *Expert Perspective from the Field* focuses on the growing controversy related to the use of high fructose corn syrup.
- *Medical Perspective* on professional help for weight control has been added.

Chapter 11, *Nutrition, Exercise, and Sports*

- Characteristics of a good fitness program have been added.
- More comprehensive approach to fitness, energy sources for muscles, fluid replacement, and ergogenic aids is presented.
- Discussion of relationships between energy substrates being utilized and intensity of exercise has been enhanced.
- Section on the use of muscle glycogen versus blood glucose as a fuel for exercise has been updated.
- Tables on fuel use estimates based on percent VO_{2max}, muscle fiber types, and athletic dietary regimens have been added.
- Updated section on sports nutrition focuses on nutrition and performance, pre- and post-exercise meals, recovery nutrition, and fluid replacement and hydration.

Chapter 12, *Fat-Soluble Vitamins*

- Comparison of general characteristics of fat- and water-soluble vitamins has been updated and enhanced.
- New, attractive, color-coded bar graphs depict typical, standardized servings of common food sources of each nutrient in relation to recommended intakes. Nutrient values are based on the lastest USDA nutrient composition data.
- New *Expert Perspective from the Field* highlights the increasing evidence of insufficient vitamin D intakes and the related health concerns.
- New *Global Perspective* addresses the problem of vitamin A deficiency throughout the developing world.
- Information on the functions of fat-soluble vitamins has been updated.

Chapter 13, *Water-Soluble Vitamins*

- New tables summarize how to preserve vitamins in foods, as well as water-soluble vitamins and their respective coenzymes.
- New figures show whole-grain components, the role of NAD^+/NADH in glycolysis and the citric acid cycle, the signs of vitamin deficiency diseases, and the roles of vitamin B-12 and folate in homocysteine and methionine metabolism.
- Navigational tools have been added to figures to illustrate where each vitamin is involved in metabolism.
- New photos illustrate health conditions caused by vitamin deficiencies.
- Current information on the role of vitamin B-6 in treating carpal tunnel syndrome, PMS, and nausea in pregnancy has been added.
- Data on neural tube defects and folic acid fortification of the food supply have been added.
- Review of the efficacy of vitamin B-12, folic acid, and vitamin B-6 supplementation in reducing coronary heart disease and improving cognitive function has been updated.

Chapter 14, *Water and Major Minerals*

- Navigational tools have been added to figures to show the location of the organs involved in water balance in the body.
- New tables list the electrolytes in intracellular and extracellular fluids, the energy content of beverages, and ideas for reducing sodium intake.
- New figures illustrate the variability in calcium bioavailability and compare osteoporotic and normal bone.
- New *Global Perspective* addresses water quality and its effect on

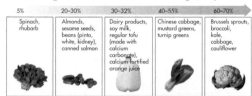

health.

- Discussion of the role of caffeine on fluid balance has been enhanced.
- New *Medical Perspective* on osteoporosis has been added.
- New *Medical Perspective* on hypertension features information from the "Seventh Report of the Joint National Committee on Prevention, Detection, Evaluation and Treatment of High Blood Pressure" and describes the DASH diet.
- New *Case Study* highlights the importance of beverages to the overall energy intake of the diet.
- *Take Action* presents new screening tool for calculating calcium intake.

Chapter 15, *Trace Minerals*

- Discussion on the metabolism of iron has been updated.
- New table depicts the stages of iron deficiency.
- New table summarizes recommendations for the ultra trace minerals.
- New *Global Perspective* focuses on the International Micronutrient Initiative project.
- *Medical Perspective* on the relationship between diet, nutrients, and cancer has been added.

Chapter 16, *Nutritional Aspects of Pregnancy and Breastfeeding*

- New tables describe the potential effects of calorie and nutrient deficiencies on the embryo and fetus, as well as maternal factors that increase risk of nutrient deficiencies and poor pregnancy outcome.
- New table summarizes the benefits of breastfeeding for the mother.
- *Expert Perspective from the Field* on folate fortification and neural tube defects has been added.
- *Medical Perspective* on nutrition-related physiological changes of concern during pregnancy has been added.
- New *Global Nutrition Perspective* discusses pregnancy and malnutrition.
- Discussion of neural tube defects has been enhanced.

Chapter 17, *Nutrition during the Growing Years*

- New table summarizes the benefits of breastfeeding for infants.
- Discussion of tracking growth, the impact of nutrition on normal growth patterns, and nutrition-related health issues in infancy, childhood, and adolescence has been enhanced.
- New table summarizes physical and eating skills, hunger and fullness cues, and appropriate food textures for children 0 to 24 months of age.
- USDA children's activity pyramid has been added.

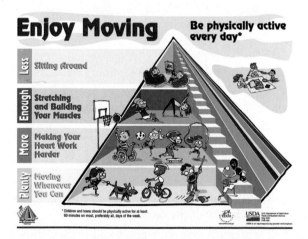

- Discussion of nutrition-related problems of the growing years has been expanded and reformatted as a *Medical Perspective*.

Chapter 18, *Nutrition during the Adult Years*

- Discussion of the effects of nutrition and lifestyle on the aging process and compression of mortality has been enhanced.
- Coverage of nutrition programs for seniors has been expanded.
- Enhanced *Take Action* helps students identify lifestyle, environmental, and dietary changes they need to make to improve their health and compress mortality.
- Discussion on how physiological and physical changes affect nutrient needs during the adult years has been updated.

- Enhanced complementary and alternative medicine practices section has been reformatted into a *Medical Perspective*.

Appendices

The appendices have been reordered to supplement knowledge of human physiology and chemistry, enhanced by adding *CDC Growth Charts* and *Caffeine Content of Foods and Beverages*, and updated with the latest *Dietary Advice for Canadians*, current values for *Fatty Acids, Including Omega-3 Fatty Acids, in Foods*, and current websites for *Sources of Nutrition Information*.

Acknowledgments

We offer a hearty and profound thank you to the many individuals who have supported and guided us along the way.

To our loved ones: Without your patience, understanding, assistance, and encouragement, this work would not have been possible.

To our wonderful students—past, present, and future: The lessons you have taught us over the years have enlightened us and sustained our desire to provide newer, better opportunities to help you successfully launch your careers and promote healthful lifelong living.

To our amazing team at McGraw-Hill: Thank you to the entire McGraw-Hill Higher Education Division. Executive Editor Colin Wheatley and Senior Developmental Editor Lynne Meyers—we thank you most of all for your confidence in us! We deeply appreciate your endless encouragement and patience as you expertly shepherded us along the way. A special thanks to Editor-in-Chief Martin Lange, Publisher Michelle Watnick, and Marketing Manager Tami Petsche and the entire marketing team. Sincere thanks to Project Manager April Southwood for keeping production on track and Copy Editor Debra DeBord for her meticulous attention to detail. We also thank Photo Editor John Leland, Photo Researcher Mary Reeg, Asset Acquisitions Editor Jill Braaten, and the many talented illustrators and photographers for their expert assistance.

Thank You, Reviewers, Contributors, and Symposium Participants

To our conscientious, dedicated expert reviewers and instructors: Thank you for sharing your insightful and constructive comments with us. We truly appreciate the time you committed to reviewing this book and discussing your thoughts about and goals for this course. We especially appreciate the assistance provided by Angie Tagtow, Cynthia Kupper, Stephanie Atkinson, Maureen Story, Penny Kris-Etherton, Wahida Karmally, Robert P. Heaney, and Judi Adams, those who shared their expertise in compiling the *Expert Perspective from the Field* features. Your suggestions and contributions clearly reflect dedication to excellence in teaching and student learning and were invaluable to this edition.

Laurie Allen
University of North Carolina, Greensboro

Alex Anderson
The University of Georgia

Keryn Bickman-Morris
Arizona State University

Carmen Boyd
Missouri State University

Linda Brady
University of Minnesota

Alyssa Brown
San Juan College

Georgia Brown
Southern University

Danielle Carbonaro
University of Cincinnati

Lakshmi N. Chilukuri
University of California, San Diego

Susan S. Chou
American River College

Deborah Cohen
Southeast Missouri State University

Julie Collins
Eastern Oklahoma State College

Linda A. Costarella
Lake Washington Technical College

Jeannette Davidson
Bradley University

Maggi Dorsett
Butte College

Sara Ducey
Montgomery College

Karen J. Gabrielsen
Everett Community College

Margaret L. Gunther
Palomar Community College

Kimberly Heidal
East Carolina University

Tawni Holmes
University of Central Oklahoma

Georgette Howell
Montgomery County Community College

Janine Jensen
Tulsa Community College

Elizabeth A. Kirk
University of Washington and Bostyr University

Allen Knehans
University of Oklahoma

Dale A. Larson
Johnson County Community College

Robert D. Lee
Central Michigan University

Linda Lolkus
Indiana University Purdue University, Fort Wayne

Susan McDonald
Western Iowa Technical Community College

Allison Miner
Prince George's Community College

Amy Miracle
University of Nevada, Las Vegas

Maria Montamagni
College of the Sequoias

Megan Murphy
Southwest Tennessee Community College

Anna M. Page
Johnson County Community College

Sarah Panarello
Yakima Valley Community College

Wanda Ragland
Macomb Community College

Scott Reaves
California Polytechnic State University

Maureen Reidenauer
Camden County College

Judy Sargent
Texas Christian University

Tiffany Schlinke
University of Central Oklahoma

Dana Sherman
Ozarks Technical Community College

Tammy Stephenson
University of Kentucky, Lexington

Leeann Sticker
Northwestern State University

Kathy Timperman
West Virginia University

Richard E. Trout
Oklahoma City Community College

Priya Venkatesan
Pasadena City College

Special Contributors to the Eighth Edition

James Bailey
University of Tennessee, Knoxville

Eugene Fenster
Longview Community College

Thunder Jalili
University of Utah

Kathy Munoz
Humboldt State University

William Proulx
State University of New York at Oneonta

Jon Story
Purdue University

An Invitation to Students and Instructors

Nutrition profoundly affects all of our lives every day. For the authors, as well as many other educators, researchers, and clinicians, this is the compelling reason for devoting our careers to this dynamic field. The rapid pace of nutrition research and provocative (and sometimes controversial) findings challenges us all to stay abreast of the latest research and understand its implications for health. We invite you to share with us topics that you believe deserve greater or less attention in the next edition.

To your health!

Carol Byrd-Bredbenner
Gaile Moe
Donna Beshgetoor
Jacqueline Berning

Teaching and Learning Supplements

McGraw-Hill offers various tools and technology products to support *Perspectives in Nutrition*. Instructors can obtain teaching aids by calling the McGraw-Hill Customer Service Department at 1–800–338–3987, visiting our nutrition catalog at www.mhhe.com, or contacting their local McGraw-Hill sales representative.

ARIS Course Management and Text Website

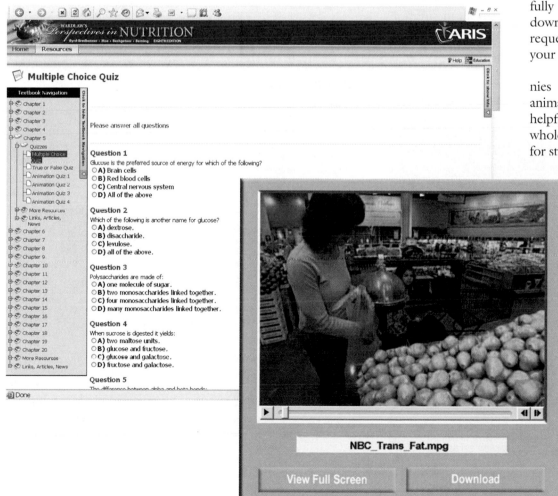

McGraw-Hill's **ARIS**—*Assessment, Review, and Instruction System*—is a complete electronic homework and course management system. Instructors can create and share course materials and assignments with colleagues with a few clicks of the mouse. Instructors can edit questions, import their own content, and create announcements and due dates for assignments. ARIS has automatic grading and reporting of easy-to-assign generated homework, quizzing, and testing. Once a student is registered in the course, all student activity within McGraw-Hill's ARIS website is automatically recorded and available to the instructor through a fully integrated grade book that can be downloaded to Excel. To access ARIS, request registration information from your McGraw-Hill sales representative.

The ARIS website that accompanies *Perspectives in Nutrition* includes animations, videos, practice quizzes, helpful Internet links, and more—a whole semester's worth of study help for students. Instructors will find a complete electronic homework and course management system where they can create and share course materials and assignments with colleagues in just a few clicks of the mouse. Instructors also can edit questions, import their own content, and create announcements and/or due dates for assignments. ARIS offers automatic grading and reporting of easy-to-assign homework, quizzing, and testing.

Check out www.aris.mhhe.com, select your subject and text-book, and start benefiting today!

Presentation Center—Complete Set of Electronic Book Images and Assets for Instructors

Build instructional materials wherever, whenever, and however you want! Accessed from your textbook's ARIS website, **Presentation Center** is an online digital library containing photos, artwork, animations, and other media types that can be used to create customized lectures, visually enhanced tests and quizzes, compelling course websites, or attractive printed support materials. All assets are copyrighted by McGraw-Hill Higher Education but can be used by instructors for classroom purposes. The visual resources in this collection include

- **Art.** Full-color digital files of all illustrations in the book can be readily incorporated into lecture presentations, exams, or custom-made classroom materials. In addition, all files are pre-inserted into PowerPoint slides for ease of lecture preparation.

- **Photos.** The photo collection contains digital files of photographs from the text, which can be reproduced for multiple classroom uses.

- **Tables.** Every table that appears in the text has been saved in electronic form for use in classroom presentations and/or quizzes.

- **Animations.** Numerous full-color animations illustrating important processes also are provided. Harness the visual impact of concepts in motion by importing these files into classroom presentations or online course materials.

- **Videos.** Enliven lectures with short video selections that highlight nutrition topics in the news.

Also residing on your textbook's ARIS website are

- **PowerPoint lecture outlines.** Ready-made presentations that combine art, animations, and lecture notes are provided for each chapter of the text.

- **PowerPoint slides.** For instructors who prefer to create their lectures from scratch, all illustrations, photos, and tables are pre-inserted by chapter into blank PowerPoint slides.

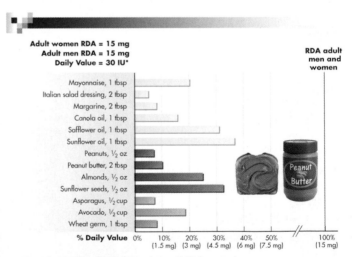

A computerized test bank that uses testing software to quickly create customized exams is available. The user-friendly program allows instructors to search for questions by topic or format, edit existing questions or add new ones, and scramble questions for multiple versions of the same test. Word files of the test bank questions are provided for instructors who prefer to work outside the test-generator software.

e-Instruction with CPS

The Classroom Performance System (CPS) is an interactive system that allows the instructor to administer in-class questions electronically. Students answer questions via handheld remote control keypads (clickers), and their individual responses are logged into a grade book. Aggregated responses can be displayed in graphical form. Using this immediate feedback, the instructor can quickly determine if students understand the lecture topic or if more clarification is needed. CPS promotes student participation, class productivity, and individual student confidence and accountability.

Electronic Books

If you, or your students, are ready for an alternative version of the traditional textbook, McGraw-Hill now offers innovative and inexpensive electronic textbooks. By purchasing E-books from McGraw-Hill, students can save as much as 50% on selected titles.

E-books from McGraw-Hill will help students study smarter and quickly find the information they need while saving money. **Contact your McGraw-Hill sales representative to discuss E-book packaging options.**

NutritionCalc Plus 3.0

CD (Windows only) ISBN: 007-332865-0
Online ISBN: 007-337552-7
NutritionCalc Plus 3.0 is a suite of powerful dietary self-assessment tools available on CD and online. This newest release features approximately 27,000 foods from the ESHA Research nutrient database and a new, user-friendly interface that makes creating a personal diet analysis even easier. Users now have the ability to add up to 3 profiles and

to create their own recipes. The program functions are supported by detailed Help documents and helpful cautionary notes that warn the user of possible entry errors.

Course Delivery Systems

In addition to McGraw-Hill's ARIS course management options, instructors can also design and control their course content with help from our partners WebCT, Blackboard, Top-Class, and eCollege. Course cartridges containing website content, online testing, and powerful student tracking features are readily available for use within these or any other HTML-based course management platforms.

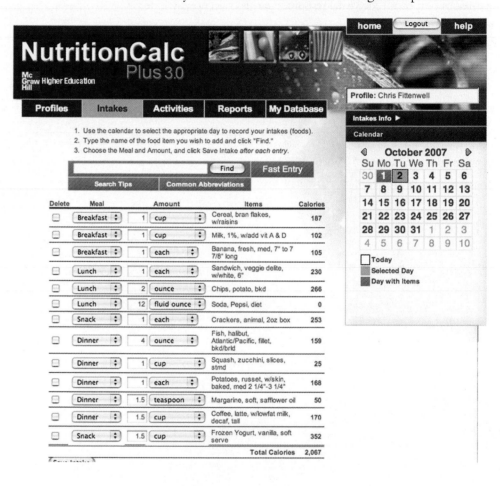

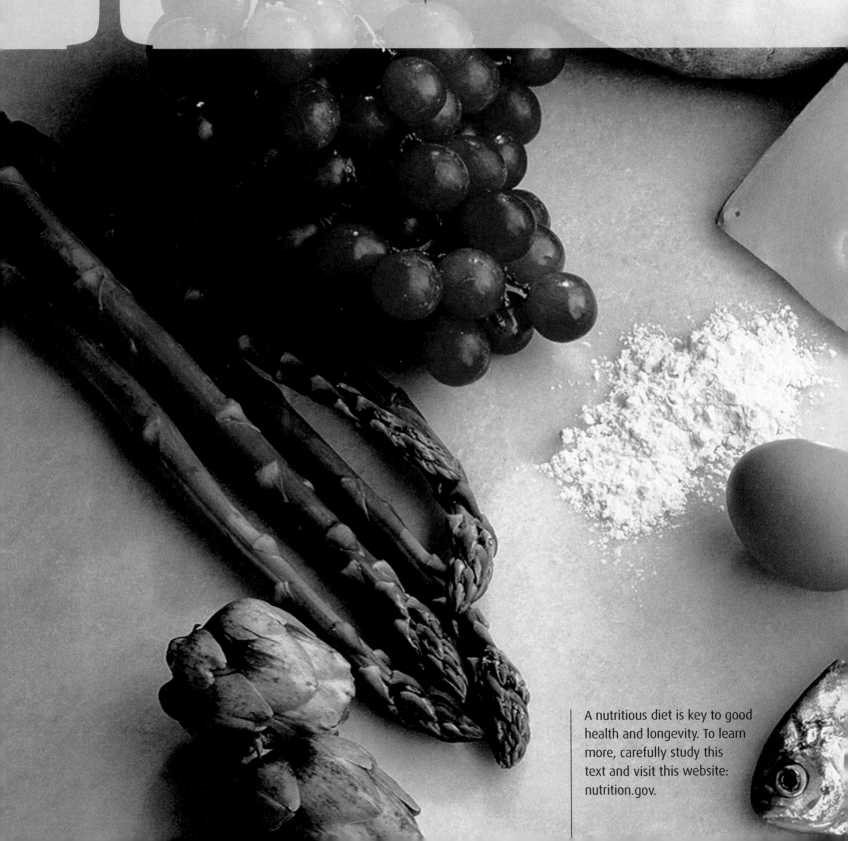

The Science of Nutrition

A nutritious diet is key to good health and longevity. To learn more, carefully study this text and visit this website: nutrition.gov.

STUDENT LEARNING OUTCOMES

After studying this chapter, you will be able to:

1. Define the terms *nutrition, carbohydrates, proteins, lipids (fats and oils), vitamins, minerals, water,* and *calories.*

2. Use the physiological fuel values of energy-yielding nutrients to determine the total energy content (calories) in a food or diet.

3. Describe the major characteristics of the North American diet and the food behaviors that often need improvement.

4. Describe the factors that affect our food choices.

5. Discuss the components and limitations of nutritional assessment.

6. List the attributes of a healthful lifestyle that are consistent with the *Healthy People 2010* goals.

7. Identify diet and lifestyle factors that contribute to the leading causes of death in North America.

8. Describe the role of genetics in the development of nutrition-related diseases.

9. Explain how the scientific method is used in developing hypotheses and theories in the field of nutrition.

10. Identify reliable sources of nutrition information.

In our lifetimes, we will eat about 60 tons of food served at 70,000 meals and countless snacks. Research over the last 50 years has shown that the foods we eat have a profound impact on our health and longevity. A healthy diet—especially one rich in fruits and vegetables—coupled with frequent exercise can prevent *and* treat many age-related diseases.[1] In contrast, eating a poor diet and getting too little exercise are **risk factors** for many common life-threatening chronic diseases, such as cardiovascular (heart) disease, diabetes, and certain forms of cancer.[2,3] Another diet-related problem, drinking too much alcohol, can impair nutritional status and is associated with liver disease, some forms of cancer, accidents, and suicides. As you can see in the chart (Fig. 1-1), diet plays a role in the development of most of the leading causes of death in the United States. The combination of poor diet and too little physical activity is indirectly the second leading cause of death. In addition, obesity is considered the second leading cause of preventable death (smoking is the first).[4]

3

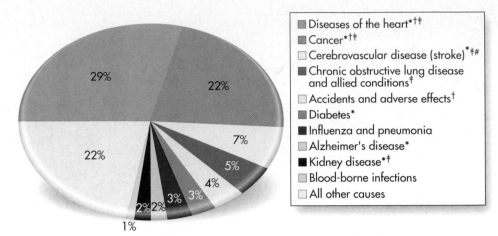

Figure 1-1 **Leading causes of death in the United States. The major health problems in North America are largely caused by a poor diet, excessive energy intake, and not enough physical activity.**

From Centers for Disease Control and Prevention, National Vital Statistics Report. Canadian statistics are quite similar.

* Causes of death in which diet plays a part
† Causes of death in which excessive alcohol consumption plays a part
‡ Causes of death in which tobacco use plays a part
\# Diseases of the heart and cerebrovascular disease are included in the more global term *cardiovascular disease.*

We live longer than our ancestors did, so preventing age-related diseases is more important now than ever before. Today, many people want to know more about how nutritious dietary choices can bring the goal of a long, healthy life within reach.[5] They may wonder what the best dietary choices are, how nutrients contribute to health, or if multivitamin and mineral supplements are needed. How can people know if they are eating too much saturated fat, *trans* fat, or cholesterol? Why are carbohydrates important? Is it possible to get too much protein? Is the food supply safe to eat? Would a vegetarian diet lead to better health? This book, beginning with this chapter, will help you build the nutrition knowledge base needed to answer these questions (and many more!) and apply this knowledge to safeguard your health, as well as the health of others.

As you begin your study of nutrition, keep in mind that this field of study draws heavily on chemistry, biology, and other sciences. For the greatest understanding of nutrition principles, you may want to review human physiology (Appendix A), basic chemistry concepts (Appendix B), and the metric system (Appendix L).

1.1 Nutrition Overview

The American Medical Association defines **nutrition** as the "science of food; the nutrients and the substances therein; their action, interaction, and balance in relation to health and disease; and the process by which the organism (e.g., human body) ingests, digests, absorbs, transports, utilizes, and excretes food substances." Food provides the nutrients needed to fuel, build, and maintain all body cells.

Nutrients

▶ Bold terms in the book are defined in the Glossary. Bold terms also are defined in the text and/or chapter margin when first presented.

You probably are already familiar with the terms *carbohydrates, lipids (fats and oils), proteins, vitamins,* and *minerals* (Table 1-1). These, plus water, make up the 6 classes of nutrients in food. **Nutrients** are substances essential for health that the body cannot make or makes in quantities too small to support health.

Table 1-1 Essential Nutrients in the Human Diet and Their Classes*

Energy-Yielding Nutrients

Carbohydrate	Lipids (Fats and Oils)	Protein (Amino Acids)
Glucose (or a carbohydrate that yields glucose)	Linoleic acid (omega-6) a-Linolenic acid (omega-3)	Histidine Isoleucine Leucine Lysine Methionine Phenylalanine Threonine Tryptophan Valine

Non-Energy Yielding Nutrients

	Vitamins			Minerals		
Water-Soluble	Fat-Soluble	Major	Trace	Some Questionable Minerals	Water
Thiamin	A	Calcium	Chromium	Arsenic	Water
Riboflavin	D	Chloride	Copper	Boron	
Niacin	E	Magnesium	Fluoride	Nickel	
Pantothenic acid	K	Phosphorus	Iodide	Silicon	
Biotin		Potassium	Iron	Vanadium	
B-6		Sodium	Manganese		
B-12		Sulfur	Molybdenum		
Folate			Selenium		
C			Zinc		

*This table includes nutrients that the current *Dietary Reference Intakes* and related publications list for humans. Some disagreement exists over the questionable minerals and certain other minerals not listed. Fiber could be added to the list of essential substances, but it is not a nutrient (See Chapter 5). The vitamin-like compound choline plays essential roles in the body but is not listed under the vitamin category at this time. Alcohol is a source of energy but is not an essential nutrient.

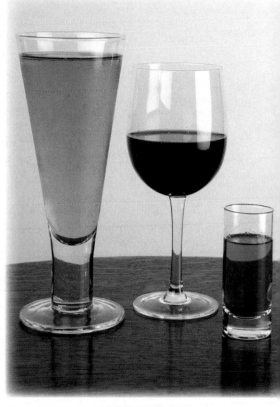

Alcoholic beverages are rich in energy, but alcohol is not an essential nutrient.

To be considered an essential nutrient, a substance must have these characteristics:

1. It has a specific biological function.
2. Removing it from the diet leads to a decline in human biological function, such as the normal functions of the blood cells or nervous system.
3. Adding the omitted substance back to the diet before permanent damage occurs restores to normal those aspects of human biological function impaired by its absence.

Nutrients can be assigned to 3 functional categories: (1) those that primarily provide energy (typically expressed in kilocalories [kcal]); (2) those that are important for growth and development (and later maintenance); and (3) those that keep body functions running smoothly. Some overlap exists among these groupings. The energy-yielding nutrients and water make up a major portion of most foods.[6]

Provide Energy	Promote Growth and Development	Regulate Body Processes
Most carbohydrates	Proteins	Proteins
Proteins	Lipids	Some lipids
Most lipids (fats and oils)	Some vitamins	Some vitamins
	Some minerals	Some minerals
	Water	Water

Because carbohydrates, proteins, lipids, and water are needed in large amounts, they are called **macronutrients**. In contrast, vitamins and minerals are needed in such small amounts in the diet that they are called **micronutrients**. Let's now look more closely at the classes of nutrients.

Carbohydrates

Carbohydrates are composed mainly of the **elements** carbon, hydrogen, and oxygen. Fruits, vegetables, and grains are the primary dietary sources of carbohydrate. The main types of carbohydrates are simple and complex. Small carbohydrate structures are called sugars or **simple carbohydrates**—table sugar (sucrose) and blood sugar (glucose) are examples. Some sugars, such as glucose, can chemically bond together to form large carbohydrates, called polysaccharides or **complex carbohydrates** (Fig. 1-2). Examples of complex carbohydrates include the starch in grains and the glycogen stored in our muscles. Fiber is another type of complex carbohydrate that forms the structure of plants.

Glucose, which the body can produce from simple carbohydrates and starch, is a major source of energy in most cells. It and most other carbohydrates provide an average of 4 calories per gram (kcal/g).[7] (Fiber provides little energy because it cannot be broken down by digestive processes.) When too little carbohydrate is eaten to supply sufficient glucose, the body is forced to make glucose from proteins. (Chapter 5 focuses on carbohydrates.)

macronutrient Nutrient needed in gram quantities in the diet.

micronutrient Nutrient needed in milligram or microgram quantities in the diet.

element Substance that cannot be separated into simpler substances by chemical processes. Common elements in nutrition include carbon, oxygen, hydrogen, nitrogen, calcium, phosphorus, and iron.

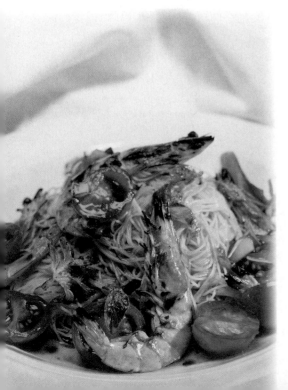
Many foods are rich sources of nutrients that we recognize today as essential for health.

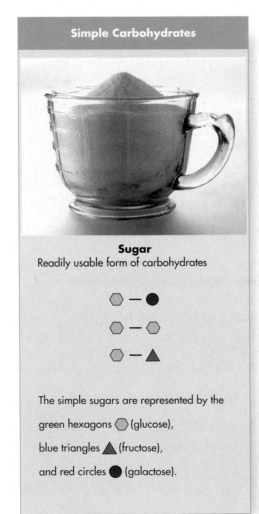
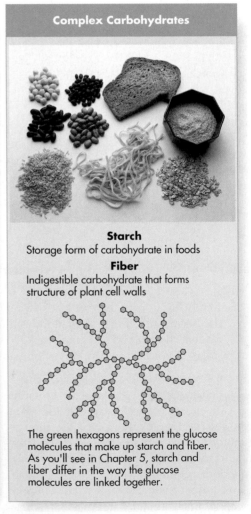

Simple Carbohydrates	Complex Carbohydrates
Sugar Readily usable form of carbohydrates	**Starch** Storage form of carbohydrate in foods **Fiber** Indigestible carbohydrate that forms structure of plant cell walls
The simple sugars are represented by the green hexagons ⬡ (glucose), blue triangles ▲ (fructose), and red circles ● (galactose).	The green hexagons represent the glucose molecules that make up starch and fiber. As you'll see in Chapter 5, starch and fiber differ in the way the glucose molecules are linked together.

Figure 1-2 Two views of carbohydrates—chemical and dietary perspectives.

Lipids

Like carbohydrates, lipids (e.g., fats, oils, and cholesterol) are composed mostly of the elements carbon, hydrogen, and oxygen (Fig. 1-3). Note that the term *fats* refers to lipids that are solid at room temperature, whereas oils are those that are liquid at room temperature. Because they contain fewer oxygen **atoms**, lipids yield more energy per gram than carbohydrates—on average, 9 calories per gram. (See Chapter 9 for more details concerning the reason for the high energy yield of lipids.) Lipids are insoluble in water but can dissolve in certain organic solvents (e.g., ether and benzene).

The lipid type called a **triglyceride** is the major form of fat in foods and a key energy source for the body. Triglycerides are also the major form of energy stored in the body.[6] They are composed of 3 fatty acids attached to a glycerol **molecule**. **Fatty acids** are long chains of carbon flanked by hydrogen with an acid group attached to the end opposite glycerol.

Most lipids can be separated into 2 basic types—saturated and unsaturated—based on the chemical structure of their dominant fatty acids. This difference helps determine whether a lipid is solid or liquid at room temperature, as well as its effect on health. Although almost all foods contain a variety of saturated and unsaturated fatty acids, plant oils tend to contain mostly unsaturated fatty acids, which make them liquid at room temperature. Many animal fats are rich in saturated fatty acids, which make them solid at room temperature. Unsaturated fats tend to be healthier than saturated fats—saturated fat raises blood cholesterol, which can clog arteries and eventually lead to cardiovascular disease.

Two specific unsaturated fatty acids—linoleic acid and alpha-linolenic acid—are essential nutrients. They must be supplied by our diets. These essential fatty acids have many roles, including being structural components of cell walls and helping regulate blood pressure and nerve transmissions. A few tablespoons of vegetable oil daily and eating fish at least twice weekly supply sufficient amounts of essential fatty acids.[7]

Some foods also contain *trans* fatty acids—unsaturated fats that have been processed to change their structure from the more typical *cis* form to the *trans* form (see Chapter 6). These are found primarily in deep-fried foods (e.g., doughnuts and french fries), baked snack foods (e.g., cookies and crackers), and solid fats (e.g., stick margarine and shortening). Large amounts of *trans* fats in the diet pose health risks, so, like saturated fat, their intake should be minimized.[7] (Chapter 6 focuses on lipids.)

Proteins

Proteins, like carbohydrates and fats, are composed of the elements carbon, oxygen, and hydrogen (Fig. 1-4). Proteins also contain another element—nitrogen. Proteins are the main structural material in the body. For example, they constitute a major part of bone and muscle; they also are important components in blood, cell membranes, **enzymes**, and immune factors.[7] Proteins can provide energy for the body—on average, 4 calories per gram; however, the body typically uses little protein to meet its daily energy needs.

Proteins are formed by the bonding together of amino acids. Twenty common amino acids are found in food; 9 of these are essential nutrients for adults, and 1 additional amino acid is essential for infants. (Chapter 7 focuses on proteins.)

Vitamins

Vitamins have a wide variety of chemical structures and can contain the elements carbon, hydrogen, nitrogen, oxygen, phosphorus, sulfur, and others. The main function of vitamins is to enable many **chemical reactions** to occur in the body. Some of these reactions help release the energy trapped in carbohydrates, lipids, and proteins. Vitamins themselves provide no usable energy for the body.[6]

The 13 vitamins are divided into 2 groups. Fat-soluble vitamins (vitamins A, D, E, and K) dissolve in fat. Vitamin C and the B-vitamins (thiamin, riboflavin, niacin, vitamin B-6, pantothenic acid, biotin, folate, and vitamin B-12) are water-soluble vitamins. The vitamin groups often act quite differently. For example, cooking is more likely to destroy water-soluble vitamins than fat-soluble vitamins. Water-soluble vitamins are excreted from

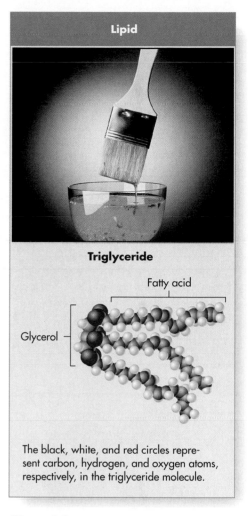

Lipid

Triglyceride

Fatty acid

Glycerol

The black, white, and red circles represent carbon, hydrogen, and oxygen atoms, respectively, in the triglyceride molecule.

Figure 1-3 **Chemical and dietary views of lipids.**

atom Smallest unit of an element that still has all of the properties of the element. An atom contains protons, neutrons, and electrons.

molecule Atoms linked (bonded) together; the smallest part of a compound that still has all the properties of the compound.

compound Atoms of 2 or more elements bonded together in specific proportions.

enzyme Compound that speeds the rate of a chemical process but is not altered by the process. Almost all enzymes are proteins.

chemical reaction Interaction between 2 chemicals that changes both chemicals.

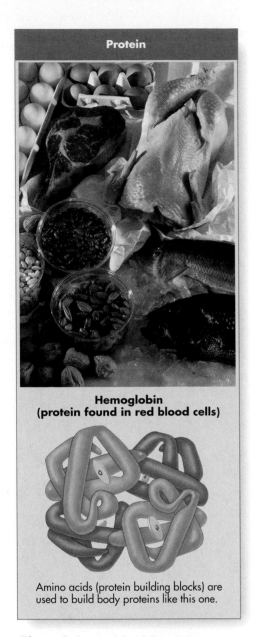

Protein

Hemoglobin
(protein found in red blood cells)

Amino acids (protein building blocks) are used to build body proteins like this one.

Figure 1-4 Chemical and dietary views of protein.

---

metabolism Chemical processes in the body that provide energy in useful forms and sustain vital activities.

Foods rich in phytochemicals are sometimes referred to as functional foods. A functional food provides health benefits beyond those supplied by the traditional nutrients it contains. A tomato contains the phytochemical lycopene; thus, it can be called a functional food. You may hear this term more from the food industry in the future.

---

the body much more readily than fat-soluble vitamins. As a result, fat-soluble vitamins, especially vitamin A, are much more likely to accumulate in excessive amounts in the body, which then can cause toxicity. (Vitamins are the focus of Chapters 11 and 12.)

Minerals

The nutrients discussed so far are all complex organic compounds, whereas minerals are structurally very simple, inorganic substances. The chemical structure of an **organic compound** contains carbon atoms bonded to hydrogen atoms, whereas an **inorganic substance** generally does not. In this case, the term *organic* is not related to the farming practices that produce organic foods (these are described in Chapter 3).

Minerals typically function in the body as groups of one or more of the same atoms (e.g., sodium or potassium) or as parts of mineral combinations, such as the calcium and phosphorus-containing compound called hydroxyapatite, found in bones. Because they are elements, minerals are not destroyed during cooking. (However, they can leak into cooking water and get discarded if that water is not consumed.) Minerals yield no energy for the body but are required for normal body function. For instance, minerals play key roles in the nervous system, skeletal system, and water balance.[6]

Minerals are divided into 2 groups: major minerals and trace minerals. Major minerals are needed daily in gram amounts. Sodium, potassium, chloride, calcium, and phosphorus are examples of major minerals. Trace minerals are those that we need in amounts of less than 100 mg daily. Examples of trace minerals are iron, zinc, copper, and selenium. (Minerals are the focus of Chapters 14 and 15.)

Water

Water is the sixth class of nutrients. Although sometimes overlooked as a nutrient, water is the macronutrient needed in the largest quantity. Water (H_2O) has numerous vital functions in the body. It acts as a solvent and lubricant and is a medium for transporting nutrients to cells. It also helps regulate body temperature. Beverages, as well as many foods, supply water. The body even makes some water as a by-product of **metabolism**.[6] (Water is examined in detail in Chapter 14.)

Phytochemicals and Zoochemicals

Phytochemicals (plant components in fruits, vegetables, legumes, and whole grains) and **zoochemicals** (components in animals) are physiologically active compounds. They are not considered essential nutrients in the diet. Still, many of these substances provide significant health benefits.[8] For instance, numerous studies show reduced cancer risk among people who regularly consume fruits and vegetables. Researchers surmise that some phytochemicals in fruits and vegetables block the development of cancer (see Chapter 15).[9, 10] Some phytochemicals and zoochemicals also have been linked to a reduced risk of cardiovascular disease. It will likely take many years for scientists to unravel the important effects of the myriad of phytochemicals and zoochemicals in foods. Current multivitamin and mineral supplements contain few or none of these beneficial chemicals. Thus, nutrition and health experts suggest that a diet rich in fruits, vegetables, legumes, and whole-grain breads and cereals is the most reliable way to obtain the potential benefits of phytochemicals.[11] In addition, foods of animal origin, such as fatty fish, can provide the beneficial zoochemical omega-3 fatty acids (see Chapter 6), and fermented dairy products provide probiotics (see Chapter 4). Table 1-2 lists some phytochemicals under study with their common food sources.

Table 1-2 Examples of Phytochemical Compounds under Study[6]

Phytochemical	Food Sources
Allyl sulfides/organosulfides	Garlic, onions, leeks
Saponins	Garlic, onions, licorice, legumes
Carotenoids (e.g., lycopene)	Orange, red, yellow fruits and vegetables (egg yolks are a source as well)
Monoterpenes	Oranges, lemons, grapefruit
Capsaicin	Chili peppers
Lignans	Flaxseed, berries, whole grains
Indoles	Cruciferous vegetables (broccoli, cabbage, kale)
Isothiocyanates	Cruciferous vegetables, especially broccoli
Phytosterols	Soybeans, other legumes, cucumbers, other fruits and vegetables
Flavonoids	Citrus fruit, onions, apples, grapes, red wine, tea, chocolate, tomatoes
Isoflavones	Soybeans, other legumes
Catechins	Tea
Ellagic acid	Strawberries, raspberries, grapes, apples, bananas, nuts
Anthocyanosides	Red, blue, and purple plants (eggplant, blueberries)
Fructooligosaccharides	Onions, bananas, oranges (small amounts)
Resveratrol	Grapes, peanuts, red wine

Some related compounds, zoochemicals, under study are found in animal products, such as sphingolipids (meat and dairy products) and conjugated linoleic acid (meat and cheese). These compounds are not phytochemicals per se because they are not from plant sources, but they have been shown to have health benefits.

Knowledge Check

1. What are the 6 classes of nutrients?
2. What characteristics do the macronutrients share?
3. How are vitamins categorized?
4. How are minerals different from carbohydrates, fat, protein, and vitamins?

1.2 Energy Sources and Uses

Humans obtain the energy needed to perform body functions and do work from carbohydrates, fats, and proteins. Alcohol is also a source of energy, supplying about 7 calories per gram. It is not considered an essential nutrient, however, because alcohol has no required function. After digesting and absorbing energy-producing nutrients, the body transforms the energy trapped in carbohydrate, protein, fat, and alcohol into other forms of energy in order to do the following:[6]

- Build new compounds
- Perform muscular movements
- Promote nerve transmissions
- Maintain **ion** balance within cells

(See Chapter 4 for more on digestion and absorption. Chapter 9 describes how energy is released from chemical bonds and then used by body cells to support the processes just described.)

ion Atom with an unequal number of electrons (negative charges) and protons (positive charges). Negative ions have more electrons than protons; positive ions have more protons than electrons.

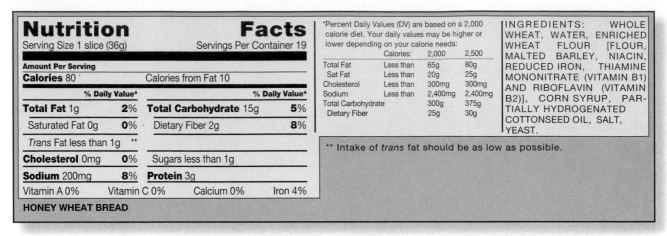

Nutrition	**Facts**
Serving Size 1 slice (36g)	Servings Per Container 19

Amount Per Serving

Calories 80		Calories from Fat 10	
	% Daily Value*		**% Daily Value***
Total Fat 1g	2%	**Total Carbohydrate** 15g	5%
Saturated Fat 0g	0%	Dietary Fiber 2g	8%
Trans Fat less than 1g	**		
Cholesterol 0mg	0%	Sugars less than 1g	
Sodium 200mg	8%	**Protein** 3g	
Vitamin A 0%	Vitamin C 0%	Calcium 0%	Iron 4%

HONEY WHEAT BREAD

*Percent Daily Values (DV) are based on a 2,000 calorie diet. Your daily values may be higher or lower depending on your calorie needs:

		Calories:	2,000	2,500
Total Fat	Less than		65g	80g
Sat Fat	Less than		20g	25g
Cholesterol	Less than		300mg	300mg
Sodium	Less than		2,400mg	2,400mg
Total Carbohydrate			300g	375g
Dietary Fiber			25g	30g

INGREDIENTS: WHOLE WHEAT, WATER, ENRICHED WHEAT FLOUR [FLOUR, MALTED BARLEY, NIACIN, REDUCED IRON, THIAMINE MONONITRATE (VITAMIN B1) AND RIBOFLAVIN (VITAMIN B2)], CORN SYRUP, PARTIALLY HYDROGENATED COTTONSEED OIL, SALT, YEAST.

** Intake of *trans* fat should be as low as possible.

Figure 1-5 Use the nutrient values on the Nutrition Facts label to calculate the energy content of a food. Based on carbohydrate, fat, and protein content, a serving of this food (honey wheat bread) contains 81 kcal ([15 × 4] [1 × 9] [3 × 4] = 81). The label lists 80 because Nutrition Facts labels round values.

Physiological fuel values.

Carbohydrate
4 kcal per gram

Protein
4 kcal per gram

Energy sources for body functions

Alcohol
7 kcal per gram

Fat
9 kcal per gram

▶ Many scientific journals express energy content of food as kilojoules (kJ), rather than calories. A mass of 1 gram moving at a velocity of 1 meter/second possesses the energy of 1 joule (J); 1000 J = 1 kJ. Heat and work are two forms of energy; thus, measurements expressed in terms of kilocalories (a heat measure) are interchangeable with measurements expressed in terms of kilojoules (a work measure): 1 kcal = 4.18 kJ.

Calorie is often the term used to express the amount of energy in foods. Technically, a **calorie** is the amount of heat energy it takes to raise the temperature of 1 gram of water 1 degree Celsius (1°C). Because a calorie is such a tiny measure of heat, food energy is more accurately expressed in terms of the kilocalorie (kcal), which equals 1000 calories. (If the *c* in calories is capitalized, this also signifies kilocalories.) A kilocalorie is the amount of heat energy it takes to raise the temperature of 1000 g (1 liter) of water 1°C. In everyday usage, the word *calorie* (without a capital *c*) also is used to mean kilocalorie. Thus, the term *calorie* and its abbreviation, *kcal,* are used throughout this book. Any values given on food labels in calories are actually in kilocalories (Fig. 1-5).

The calories in food can be measured using a bomb calorimeter (see Chapter 10). Or, they can be estimated by multiplying the amount of carbohydrates, proteins, lipids, and alcohol in a food by their physiological fuel values. The **physiological fuel values** are 4, 9, 4, and 7 for carbohydrate, fat, protein, and alcohol, respectively. These values are adjusted to account for the extent to which foods can be digested and substances (e.g., waxes and fibers) that humans cannot digest. Thus, they should be considered estimates.

Physiological fuel values can be used to determine the calories in food. Consider these foods:

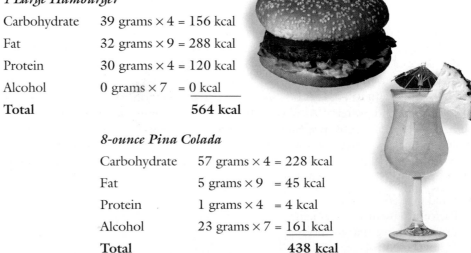

1 Large Hamburger

Carbohydrate	39 grams × 4	= 156 kcal
Fat	32 grams × 9	= 288 kcal
Protein	30 grams × 4	= 120 kcal
Alcohol	0 grams × 7	= 0 kcal
Total		**564 kcal**

8-ounce Pina Colada

Carbohydrate	57 grams × 4	= 228 kcal
Fat	5 grams × 9	= 45 kcal
Protein	1 grams × 4	= 4 kcal
Alcohol	23 grams × 7	= 161 kcal
Total		**438 kcal**

These values also can be used to determine the portion of total energy intake that carbohydrate, fat, protein, and alcohol provide to your diet. Assume that one day you consume 283 g of carbohydrates, 60 g of fat, 75 g of protein, and 9 g of alcohol. This consumption yields a total of 2035 kcal ([283 × 4] + [60 × 9] + [75 × 4] + [9 × 7] = 2035). The percentage of your total energy intake derived from each nutrient can then be determined:

$$\% \text{ of energy intake as carbohydrate} = (283 \times 4) / 2035 = 0.57 \times 100 = 57\%$$

$$\% \text{ of energy intake as fat} = (60 \times 9) / 2035 = 0.27 \times 100 = 27\%$$

$$\% \text{ of energy intake as protein} = (75 \times 4) / 2035 = 0.14 \times 100 = 14\%$$

$$\% \text{ of energy intake as alcohol} = (9 \times 7) / 2035 = 0.03 \times 100 = 3\%$$

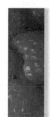

Knowledge Check

1. What does the term *calorie* mean?
2. How do calories, kilocalories, and kilojoules differ?
3. How many calories are in a food that has 8 g carbohydrate, 2 g alcohol, 4 g fat, and 2 g protein?

1.3 The North American Diet

Large surveys are conducted in the United States and Canada to determine what people are eating. The U.S. government uses the National Health and Nutrition Examination Survey (NHANES) administered by the U.S. Department of Health and Human Services. In Canada, this information is gathered by Health Canada in conjunction with Agriculture and Agrifood Canada. Results from these surveys and others show that North American adults consume, on average, 16% of their energy intake as proteins, 50% as carbohydrates, and 33% as fats. These percentages are estimates and vary slightly from year to year and to some extent from person to person. Although these percentages fall within a healthy range[12] (see Chapter 2), many people are eating more than they need to maintain a healthy weight.[12, 13]

Animal sources, such as meat, seafood, dairy products, and eggs, supply about two-thirds of the protein intake for most North Americans; plant sources provide only about a third. In many other parts of the world, it is just the opposite: plant proteins—from rice, beans, corn, and other vegetables—dominate protein intake. About half the carbohydrate in North American diets comes from simple carbohydrates (sugars); the other half comes from starches (e.g., pastas, breads, and potatoes). Most North Americans need to reduce sugar intake and increase intake of starch and fiber. Because approximately 60% of dietary fat comes from animal sources and only 40% from plant sources, many North Americans are consuming far more saturated fat and cholesterol than is recommended.

These surveys also indicate that most of us could improve our diets by focusing on rich food sources of vitamin A, vitamin E, iron, and calcium and reducing our intake of sodium. Nutrient intake varies in some demographic groups, which means these individuals need to pay special attention to certain nutrients. For example, older adults often get too little vitamin D and women of childbearing years frequently have inadequate iron intake.

In terms of food, many North Americans could improve their nutrient intake by moderating intake of sugared soft drinks and fatty foods and eating more fruits, vegetables, whole-grain breads, and reduced-fat dairy products. Vitamin and mineral supplements also can help meet nutrient needs but, as you'll see in Chapter 12, they cannot fully make up for a poor diet in all respects.[14]

Increasing vegetable intake, such as a daily salad, is one strategy to boost intake of important nutrients.

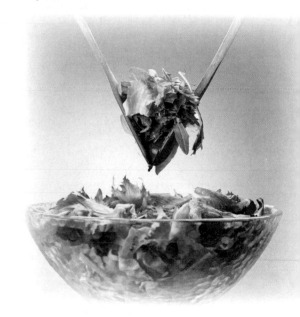

What Influences Our Food Choices?

Although we have to eat to obtain the nutrients needed to survive, many factors other than health and nutrition affect food choices. Daily food intake is a complicated mix of the need to satisfy **hunger** (physical need for food) and social and psychological

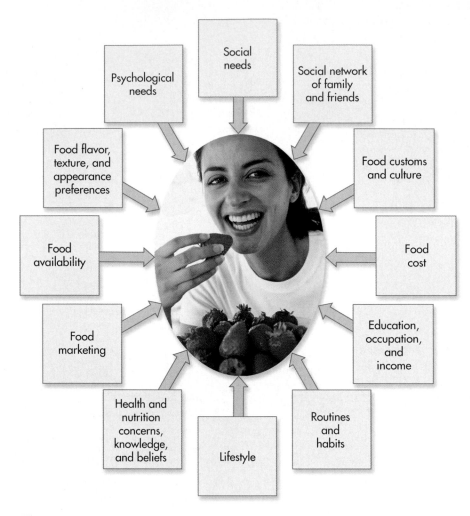

Figure 1-6 Food choices are affected by many factors. Which have the greatest impact on your food choices?

needs (Fig. 1-6).[15, 16] In areas of the world where food is plentiful and fairly easy to access (e.g., the U.S., Canada, Europe, Australia, and Japan), the food selected to meet our needs is largely guided by **appetite**—the desire to eat certain foods and reject others. Appetite and food choice depend on many factors.

- *Food flavor, texture, and appearance preferences*—for many people, these are the most important factors affecting food choices. Creating more flavorful foods that are both healthy and profitable is a major focus of the food industry.
- *Culture* (knowledge, beliefs, religion, and traditions shared by a group of people) teaches individuals which foods are considered proper or appropriate to eat and which are not. For example, many people in North America believe it is proper to eat beef; however, people in some cultures never consider eating beef. Some cultures savor foods such as blood, mice, and insects—even though these foods are packed with nutrients and safe to eat, few people in North America feel they are proper to eat. Early experiences with people, places, and situations influence lifelong food choices. Many aspects of ethnic diet patterns begin when our parents introduce us to foods as children.
- *Lifestyle* includes the way we spend our resources and assign priorities. People with very busy lives often have limited time and energy to buy and prepare foods, so they opt for convenience or fast food. For some, it may be more important to spend extra time working rather than making it a priority to exercise and eat healthfully.
- *Routines and habits* related to food and eating affect what as well as when we eat. Most of us eat primarily from a core group of foods—only about 100 basic items account for 75% of a person's total food intake.
- *Food cost* is important, but it plays only a moderate role in food choices for many of us because food is relatively inexpensive in North America. In fact, we spend only about 10% of after-tax income on food.
- *Environment* includes your surroundings and experiences. In North America, the environment is filled with opportunities to obtain affordable, delicious, high-calorie food—vending machines, bake sales, food courts in shopping areas, and candy displays in bookstores—and encourages (via marketing) the consumption of these foods. Experiences with friends, family, and others also can influence food choices.
- *Food marketing* is any type of action a company takes to create a desire in consumers to buy its food; *advertising* is one type of food marketing. The food industry in the United States spends well over $34 billion annually on advertising. Some of this advertising is helpful, such as when it promotes the importance of calcium and fiber intake. However, the food industry more frequently advertises fast food, highly sweetened cereals, cookies, cakes, and pastries because such products generate the greatest profits.
- *Health and nutrition concerns, knowledge, and beliefs* also can affect food choices. Those most concerned about health and who have the greatest nutrition knowledge tend to be well-educated, middle-income professionals. The same people are generally health-oriented, have active lifestyles, and work hard to keep their bodies at a healthy weight.

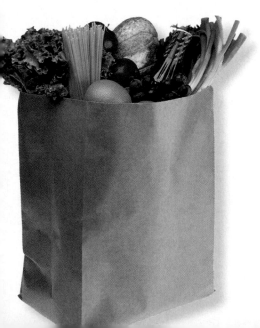

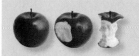

Take Action

Why You Eat What You Do

Choose 1 day of the week that is typical of your eating pattern. List all the foods and drinks you consume for 24 hours. Using the factors that influence food choices discussed in Section 1.3, indicate why you consumed each item. Note that there can be more than one reason for choosing a particular food or drink.

Now ask yourself: What was the most frequent reason for eating or drinking? To what extent are health or nutrition concerns the reason for your food choices? Should you make these reasons higher priorities?

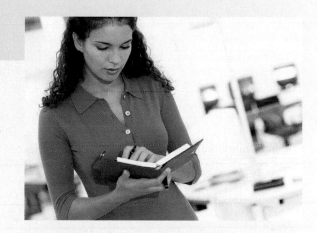

Knowledge Check

1. What type of food provides most of the protein in the diets of North Americans?
2. Which types of carbohydrates do most North Americans need to increase in their diets?
3. Which vitamins and minerals do many North Americans need to increase in their diets?
4. What factors affect food choices?

1.4 Nutritional Health Status

In a well-nourished person, the total daily intake of protein, fat, and carbohydrate weighs about 450 g (about 1 pound). In contrast, the typical daily mineral intake weighs about 20 g (about 4 teaspoons) and the daily vitamin intake weighs less than 300 mg (1/15th of a teaspoon). These nutrients can come from a variety of sources—fruits, vegetables, meats, dairy products, or other foods. Our body cells are not concerned with which food supplied a nutrient—what is important, however, is that each nutrient be available in the amounts needed for the body to function normally.

The body's nutritional health is determined by the sum of its status with respect to each nutrient. There are 3 general categories of nutritional status: desirable nutrition, undernutrition, and overnutrition. The common term *malnutrition* can refer to either overnutrition or undernutrition, neither of which is conducive to good health.

Optimal, or **desirable**, **nutritional status** for a particular nutrient is the state in which the body tissues have enough of the nutrient to support normal functions, as well as to build and maintain surplus stores that can be used in times of increased need.[17] A desirable nutritional state can be achieved by obtaining essential nutrients from a variety of foods.

Undernutrition occurs when nutrient intake does not meet nutrient needs, causing surplus stores to be used. Once nutrient stores are depleted and tissue concentrations of an essential nutrient fall sufficiently low, the body's metabolic processes eventually slow down or even stop. The early stage of a nutrient deficiency is termed **subclinical** because there are no overt signs or symptoms that can be detected or diagnosed.

Table 1-3 Nutritional Status Using Iron as an Example

Condition	Signs and Symptoms Related to Iron
Undernutrition: nutrient intake does not meet needs	Decline in iron-related compounds in the blood, which reduces the ability of the red blood cells to carry oxygen to body tissues and, in turn, causes fatigue on exertion, poor body temperature regulation, and eventually pale complexion
Desirable nutrition: nutrient intake supports body function and permits storage of nutrients to be used in times of increased need	Adequate liver stores of iron, adequate blood levels of iron-related compounds, and normal functioning of red blood cells
Overnutrition: nutrient intake exceeds needs	Excess liver stores, which damage liver cells

Table 1-4 Sample of Nutrition-Related Objectives from *Healthy People 2010*

	Target	Current Estimate
Increase the proportion of adults who are at a healthy weight.	60%	35%
Reduce the proportion of adults who are obese.	15%	23%
Increase the proportion of persons age 2 years and older who consume at least 2 daily servings of fruit.	75%	28%
Increase the proportion of persons age 2 years and older who consume at least 3 daily servings of vegetables, with at least one-third being dark green or deep yellow vegetables.	50%	3%
Increase the proportion of persons age 2 years and older who consume at least 6 daily servings of grain products, with at least 3 being whole grains.	50%	7%
Increase the proportion of persons age 2 years and older who consume less than 10% of energy intake from saturated fat.	75%	36%
Increase the proportion of persons age 2 years and older who consume 6 g or less of salt daily.	65%	5%
Increase the proportion of persons age 2 years and older who meet dietary recommendations for calcium.	75%	46%
Reduce iron deficiency among young children and females of childbearing age.	6%	10%

Note: Related objectives include those addressing osteoporosis, various forms of cancer, diabetes, food allergies, cardiovascular disease, low birth weight, nutrition during pregnancy, breastfeeding, eating disorders, physical activity, and alcohol use.

If a deficiency becomes severe, **clinical** signs and symptoms eventually develop and become outwardly apparent.[17] A **sign** is a feature that can be observed, such as flaky skin. A **symptom** is a change in body function that is not necessarily apparent to a health-care provider, such as feeling tired or achy. Table 1-3 describes the signs and symptoms associated with iron status.

Consumption of more nutrients than the body needs can lead to **overnutrition**. In the short run—for instance, a week or so—overnutrition may cause only a few symptoms, such as intestinal distress from excessive fiber intake. If an excess intake continues, the levels of some nutrients in the body may increase to toxic amounts.[17] For example, too much vitamin A can have negative effects, particularly in children, pregnant women, and older adults. The most common type of overnutrition in industrialized nations—excess intake of energy-yielding nutrients—often leads to obesity. Obesity, in turn, can lead to other serious chronic diseases, such as type 2 diabetes and certain forms of cancer.

Health Objectives for the United States for the Year 2010

Health promotion and disease prevention have been public health strategies in the United States and Canada since the late 1970s. One part of this strategy is *Healthy People 2010*, a report issued in 2000 by the U.S. Department of Health and Human Services, Public Health Service.[18] This report set health promotion and disease prevention goals for the year 2010—many of these goals have nutrition-related objectives (see Table 1-4 for examples). The main objective of *Healthy People 2010* is to promote healthful lifestyles that reduce preventable death and disability. Minority groups are a particular focus of *Healthy People 2010* programs because overall health status currently lags in these population groups, especially with respect to hypertension, type 2 diabetes, and obesity.

Assessing Nutritional Status

A nutritional assessment can help determine how nutritionally fit you are (Table 1-5). Generally, assessments are performed by a physician, often with the aid of a registered dietitian.[19]

Table 1-5 Conducting an Evaluation of Nutritional Health

Factors	Examples
Background	**Medical history** (e.g., current and past diseases and surgeries, body weight history, current medications) **Family medical history**
Nutritional	**Anthropometric assessment** (e.g., height, weight, skinfold thickness, arm muscle circumference) **Biochemical (laboratory) assessment** (e.g., compounds in blood and urine) **Clinical assessment** (e.g., physical examination of skin, eyes, and tongue; ability to walk) **Dietary assessment** (e.g., usual food intake, food allergies, supplements used) **Environmental assessment** (e.g., education and economic background, marital status, housing condition)

Assessments include an analysis of numerous background factors known to affect health. For example, many diseases have a genetic component, so family history plays an important role in determining nutritional and health status. Another background factor is a person's own medical history, especially for any health conditions, diseases, or treatments that could hinder nutrient absorptive processes or the use of a nutrient.

In addition to background factors, parameters that complete the picture of nutritional status are anthropometric, biochemical, clinical, dietary, and environmental assessments. **Anthropometric assessment** involves measuring various aspects of the body, including height, weight (and weight changes), body circumferences (e.g., waist, hips, arm), and skinfold thickness (an indicator of body fatness). Anthropometric measurements are easy to obtain and are generally reliable.

Biochemical assessments include the measurement of the concentrations of nutrients and nutrient by-products in the blood, urine, and feces and of specific blood enzyme activities.[17] For example, in Chapter 13 you will learn that the status of the vitamin thiamin is measured, in part, by determining the activity of an enzyme called transketolase used to metabolize glucose. To test for this, cells (e.g., red blood cells) are broken open and thiamin is added to see how it affects the rate of the transketolase enzyme activity.

During a **clinical assessment**, health-care providers search for any physical evidence of diet-related diseases (e.g., high blood pressure, skin conditions). The health-care provider tends to focus the clinical assessment on potential problem areas identified from the dietary assessment. **Dietary assessment** examines how often a person eats certain types of foods (called a food frequency); the types of foods eaten over a long period of time, perhaps as far back as childhood (called a food history); and typical intake, such as foods eaten in the last 24 hours or several days (e.g., a 24-hour recall or a 3-day recall). Finally, an **environmental assessment** (based on background data) provides information on the person's education and economic background. This information is important because people who have inadequate education, income, and housing and/or live alone often have a greater risk of poor health. Those with limited education may have a reduced ability to follow instructions given by health-care providers and/or incomes that hinder their ability to purchase, store, and prepare nutritious food. Taken together, these 5 parameters form the ABCDEs of nutritional assessment: anthropometric, biochemical, clinical, dietary, and environmental (Fig. 1-7).

Limitations of Nutritional Assessment

Nutritional assessments can be helpful in improving one's health. However, it is important to recognize the limitations of these assessments. First, many signs and symptoms

► A practical example using the ABCDEs for evaluating nutritional state can be illustrated in a person who chronically abuses alcohol. On evaluation, the physician notes the following:

Anthropometric: Low weight-for-height, recent 10-lb weight loss, muscle wasting in the upper body

Biochemical: Low amounts of the vitamins thiamin and folate in the blood

Clinical: Psychological confusion, skin sores, and uncoordinated movement

Dietary: Consumed mostly alcohol-fortified wine and hamburgers for the last week

Environmental: Currently residing in a homeless shelter, $35.00 in his wallet, unemployed

Assessment: This person needs professional medical attention, including nutrient repletion.

CRITICAL THINKING

Ying loves to eat hamburgers, fries, and lots of pizza with double amounts of cheese. He rarely eats any vegetables and fruits but, instead, snacks on cookies and ice cream. He insists that he has no problems with his health, is rarely ill, and doesn't see how his diet could cause him any health risks. How would you explain to Ying that, despite his current good health, his diet could predispose him to future health problems?

For suggested answers to the Critical Thinking questions in this and every chapter, see the website for this book: www.mhhe.com/ wardlawpers8.

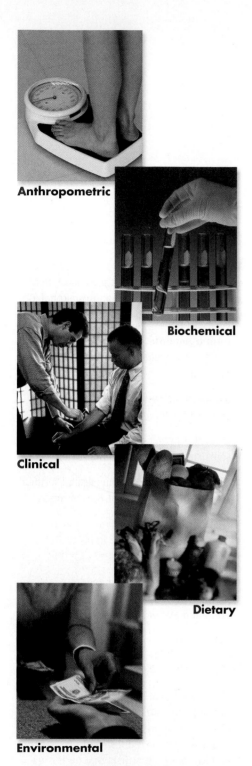

Anthropometric

Biochemical

Clinical

Dietary

Environmental

Figure 1-7 The ABCDEs of nutritional assessment: Anthropometric, Biochemical, Clinical, Dietary, and Environmental status.

of nutritional deficiencies—diarrhea, skin conditions, and fatigue—are not very specific. They may be caused by poor nutrition or by other factors unrelated to nutrition. Second, it can take a long time for the signs and symptoms of nutritional deficiencies to develop and, because they can be vague, it is often difficult to establish a link between an individual's current diet and his or her nutritional status.

Third, a long time may elapse between the initial development of poor nutritional health and the first clinical evidence of a problem. For instance, a diet high in saturated fat often increases blood cholesterol, but it does not produce any clinical evidence for years. Nonetheless, the cholesterol is building up in blood vessels and may lead to a heart attack. Another example of a serious nutrition-related health condition with symptoms that often don't appear until later in life is low bone density (osteoporosis) resulting from insufficient calcium intake that may have begun in the teen years. Currently, a great deal of nutrition research is trying to identify better methods for detecting nutrition-related problems early—before they damage the body.

Importance of Being Concerned about Your Nutritional Status

Regardless of the limitations of nutritional assessment, people who focus on maintaining desirable nutritional health are apt to enjoy a long, vigorous life and are less likely to develop health problems, such as those in Figure 1-8. In fact, a recent study found that women who followed a healthy lifestyle experienced an 80% reduction in risk of heart attacks, compared with women without such healthy practices.[4] Here is what these healthy women did:

- Consumed a healthy diet that was varied, rich in fiber, and low in animal fat and *trans* fat and that included some fish
- Avoided becoming overweight
- Regularly drank a small amount of alcohol
- Exercised for at least 30 minutes daily
- Did not smoke

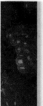

Knowledge Check

1. What is the difference between a sign and a symptom?
2. How does undernutrition differ from overnutrition?
3. What are the ABCDEs of nutritional assessment?
4. What are 3 limitations of nutritional assessment?

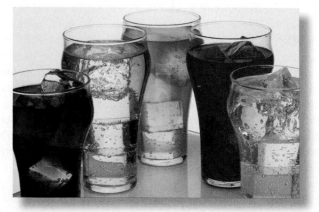

Soft drinks account for about 10% of the energy intake of teenagers in North America and, in turn, contribute to generally poor calcium intakes seen in this age group. Consuming insufficient calcium increases their risk of osteoporosis in future years.

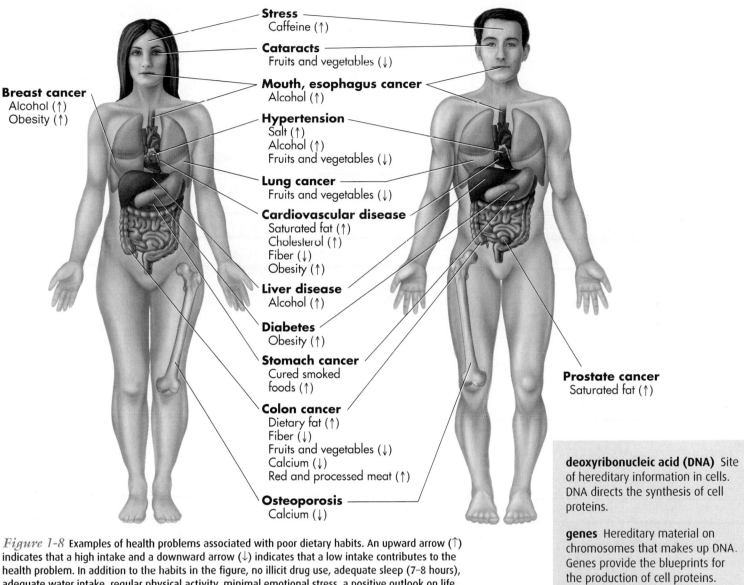

Stress
Caffeine (↑)

Cataracts
Fruits and vegetables (↓)

Mouth, esophagus cancer
Alcohol (↑)

Breast cancer
Alcohol (↑)
Obesity (↑)

Hypertension
Salt (↑)
Alcohol (↑)
Fruits and vegetables (↓)

Lung cancer
Fruits and vegetables (↓)

Cardiovascular disease
Saturated fat (↑)
Cholesterol (↑)
Fiber (↓)
Obesity (↑)

Liver disease
Alcohol (↑)

Diabetes
Obesity (↑)

Stomach cancer
Cured smoked
foods (↑)

Colon cancer
Dietary fat (↑)
Fiber (↓)
Fruits and vegetables (↓)
Calcium (↓)
Red and processed meat (↑)

Osteoporosis
Calcium (↓)

Prostate cancer
Saturated fat (↑)

Figure 1-8 Examples of health problems associated with poor dietary habits. An upward arrow (↑) indicates that a high intake and a downward arrow (↓) indicates that a low intake contributes to the health problem. In addition to the habits in the figure, no illicit drug use, adequate sleep (7–8 hours), adequate water intake, regular physical activity, minimal emotional stress, a positive outlook on life, and close friendships provide a more complete approach to good health. Also important is regular consultation with health-care professionals—early diagnosis is especially useful for controlling the damaging effects of many diseases.

deoxyribonucleic acid (DNA) Site of hereditary information in cells. DNA directs the synthesis of cell proteins.

genes Hereditary material on chromosomes that makes up DNA. Genes provide the blueprints for the production of cell proteins.

The major health problems in North America are largely caused by a poor diet, excessive energy intake, and not enough physical activity.

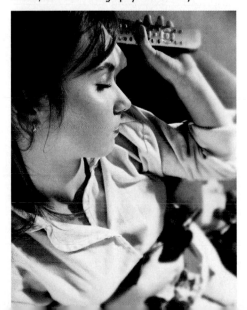

1.5 Genetics and Nutrition

In addition to lifestyle and diet, genetic endowment also affects almost every medical condition. During digestion, the nutrients supplied by food are broken down, absorbed into the bloodstream, and transported to cells. There, genetic material, called **deoxyribonucleic acid (DNA)**, inside the nucleus of the cells directs how the body uses the nutrients consumed. As you can see in Figure 1-9, foods and humans contain the same nutrients, but the proportions differ—**genes** in body cells dictate the type and amount of nutrients in food that will be transformed and reassembled into body structures and compounds.

Genes direct the growth, development, and maintenance of cells and, ultimately, of the entire organism. Genes contain the codes that control the expression of individual traits, such as height, eye color, and susceptibility to many diseases. An individual's genetic risk of a given disease is an important factor, although often not the only factor, in determining whether he or she develops that disease.

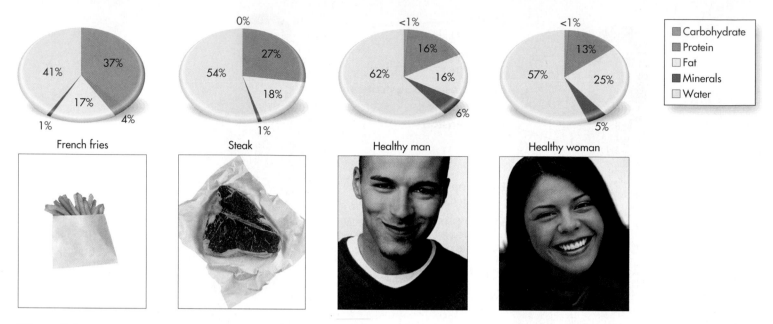

French fries   Steak   Healthy man   Healthy woman

Legend:
- Carbohydrate
- Protein
- Fat
- Minerals
- Water

Figure 1-9 Proportions of nutrients in the human body, compared with those in typical foods—animal or vegetable. Note that the amount of vitamins found in the body is extremely small and, so, is not shown.

mutation Change in the chemistry of a gene that is perpetuated in subsequent divisions of the cell where it occurred; a change in the sequence of the DNA.

risk factor Hereditary characteristic or lifestyle behavior (e.g., dietary habits, smoking) that increases the chances of developing a disease.

Genes are present on DNA—a double helix. The cell nucleus contains most of the DNA in the body.

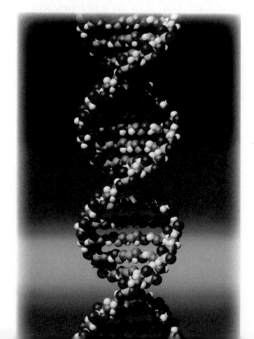

Each year, new links between specific genes and diseases are reported. It is likely that soon it will be relatively easy to screen a person's DNA for genes that increase the risk of disease. Currently, there are about 600 tests that can determine whether a person has a genetic **mutation** that increases the risk of certain illnesses. For example, a woman can be tested for a mutation in certain genes that elevates her chances of developing breast cancer.

Nutritional Diseases with a Genetic Link

Most chronic nutrition-related diseases (e.g., diabetes, cancer, osteoporosis, cardiovascular disease, hypertension, obesity, and cancer) are influenced by interactions among genetic, nutritional, and other lifestyle factors. Studies of families, including those with twins and adoptees, provide strong support for the effect of genetics in these disorders. In fact, family history is considered one of the most important **risk factors** in the development of many nutrition-related diseases.[20]

For example, both of the common types of diabetes, certain cancers (e.g., colon, prostate, and breast cancer), and osteoporosis have genetic links. In addition, about 1 in every 500 people in North America has a defective gene that greatly delays cholesterol removal from the bloodstream—this defective gene increases the risk of cardiovascular disease. Another example is hypertension (high blood pressure). Numerous North Americans are very sensitive to salt intake. When these salt-sensitive individuals consume too much salt, their blood pressure climbs above the desirable range. The fact that more of these people are African-American than white suggests that at least some cases of hypertension have a genetic component. Obesity also has genetic links. A variety of genes (likely 250 or more) are involved in the regulation of body weight.

Although some individuals may be genetically predisposed to chronic disease, whether they actually develop the disease depends on lifestyle choices and environmental factors that influence the disease.[21] It's important to realize that predisposition to chronic disease is not the same type of genetic characteristic as being born with blue eyes or larger ears. With chronic disease, heredity is not necessarily destiny—individuals can exert some control over the expression of their genetic potential. For instance, those with a predisposition to premature heart disease can take steps to delay its onset by eating a nutritious diet, getting regular exercise, keeping weight under control, and getting medical treatment to lower blood cholesterol levels and control blood pressure. Likewise, those who

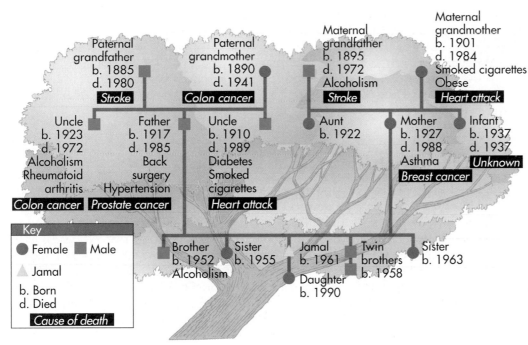

Paternal
grandfather
b. 1885
d. 1980
Stroke

Paternal
grandmother
b. 1890
d. 1941
Colon cancer

Maternal
grandfather
b. 1895
d. 1972
Alcoholism
Stroke

Maternal
grandmother
b. 1901
d. 1984
Smoked cigarettes
Obese
Heart attack

Uncle
b. 1923
d. 1972
Alcoholism
Rheumatoid
arthritis
Colon cancer

Father
b. 1917
d. 1985
Back
surgery
Hypertension
Prostate cancer

Uncle
b. 1910
d. 1989
Diabetes
Smoked
cigarettes
Heart attack

Aunt
b. 1922

Mother
b. 1927
d. 1988
Asthma
Breast cancer

Infant
b. 1937
d. 1937
Unknown

Key
● Female ■ Male
▲ Jamal
b. Born
d. Died
Cause of death

Brother
b. 1952
Alcoholism

Sister
b. 1955

Jamal
b. 1961

Daughter
b. 1990

Twin
brothers
b. 1958

Sister
b. 1963

Figure 1-10 Example of a family tree for Jamal. If a person is deceased, the cause of death is shown. In addition to causes of death, medical conditions family members experienced are noted.

did not inherit the potential for heart disease put themselves at risk of this disease by becoming obese, smoking, abusing alcohol, and not getting medical treatment to keep blood cholesterol, blood pressure, and type 2 diabetes under control.

Your Genetic Profile

By recognizing your potential for developing a particular disease, you can avoid behaviors that contribute to it. For example, women with a family history of breast cancer should avoid becoming obese, minimize alcohol use, and get mammograms regularly. In general, the more relatives with a genetically transmitted disease and the more closely they are related to you, the greater your risk. One way to assess your risk is to create a family tree of illnesses and deaths (a genogram) by compiling a few key facts on your primary relatives: siblings, parents, aunts, uncles, and grandparents (Fig. 1-10).

High-risk conditions include having more than one first-degree relative (i.e., one's parents, siblings, and offspring) with a specific disease, especially if the disease occurred before age 50 to 60 years.[20] In the family in Figure 1-10, prostate cancer killed Jamal's father. Knowing this, his physician likely would recommend that he be tested for prostate cancer more frequently or starting at an earlier age than men without a family history of the disease. Because their mother died of breast cancer, his sisters' doctor may recommend they consider having their first regular mammograms at a younger age than typical, as well as adopting other preventive practices. Heart attack and stroke also are common in the family, so all the children should adopt a lifestyle that minimizes the risk of developing these conditions, such as moderating their intake of animal fat and sodium. Colon cancer is evident in the family, which makes it important for them to have careful screening throughout life.

Gene Therapy

Scientists are currently developing therapies to correct the damaged DNA that causes some genetic disorders. Typically, scientists isolate normal DNA, package it into a molecular delivery vehicle (usually a disabled **virus**), and inject it into the cells affected

CRITICAL THINKING

Wesley notices that at family gatherings his parents, uncles, aunts, and older siblings tend to be overweight. His father has had a heart attack, as has one of his aunts. Two of his uncles died before the age of 60 from diabetes. His grandfather died of prostate cancer. Wesley wonders if he is destined to become obese and develop heart disease, cancer, or diabetes. What advice would you give to Wesley?

virus Smallest known type of infectious agent, many of which cause disease in humans. They do not metabolize, grow, or move by themselves. They reproduce by the aid of a living cellular host. Viruses are essentially a piece of genetic material surrounded by a coat of protein.

by the disease—such as liver cells. Inside the cell, the normal genetic material begins functioning and restores the cells to normal. Scientists hope that gene therapy applications can be used in the future to treat many diseases, especially those that are inherited. Although there has been some success with gene therapy, there are still many obstacles to overcome before gene therapy can become an effective treatment. Currently, the U.S. Food and Drug Administration (FDA) has not approved the sale of any human gene therapies.

Genetic Testing

▶ These websites can help you gather more information about genetic conditions and testing.

www.geneticalliance.org

www.kumc.edu/gec/support

cancernet.nci.nih.gov/p_genetics.html

www.nhgri.nih.gov

www.faseb.org/genetics

vector.cshl.org

www.ncgr.org

In recent years, scientists have developed ways of testing a person's genes for the likelihood of developing certain diseases. Genetic tests are especially valuable for families afflicted by certain illnesses. In addition, they can help people who are healthy now predict the illnesses they will probably develop.[6] Advance knowledge that a disease is likely to develop may provide opportunities to replace genes that encourage diseases, such as cancer and Alzheimer's, with those that do not. Advance knowledge also could help couples attempting to have children make more informed choices (e.g., consider alternatives, such as adoption) and help health-care providers develop health and nutrition care plans that delay the onset of the disease. Additionally, this knowledge could help health-care providers diagnose diseases earlier and more accurately and prescribe individualized medical and nutrition therapies, instead of giving the same treatment to all patients with the same disease. It is likely that many medications may be more appropriate in people with certain genetic traits.

Given the limit on resources presently allocated to medical care in North America, it is not possible to identify all the people at genetic risk of the major chronic diseases and other health problems. In addition, in many cases, genetic susceptibility does not necessarily guarantee development of the disease. And, in almost all cases, there is no way to cure a specific gene alteration—only the health problems that result can be treated. Researchers also are concerned that people who are found to have genetic alterations that increase disease risk may face job and medical insurance discrimination. Testing positive also could lead to unnecessary radical treatment. As well, a seemingly hopeless diagnosis could result in depression when a cure is out of reach.[22,23] Thus, the wisdom of genetic testing is an open question. Perhaps preventive measures and careful scrutiny of the specific genetically linked diseases using one's family tree would suffice.

Some experts recommend that anyone considering genetic testing first undergo genetic counseling. Genetic counselors are trained to analyze family history and evaluate the risk of developing or passing along an inherited disease. They also can help determine whether testing is worth the time and effort because genetic tests are primarily for people whose family history puts them at especially high risk of having a genetic defect. Genetic counselors can be found by contacting a local hospital or nearby university-affiliated hospital or medical school.

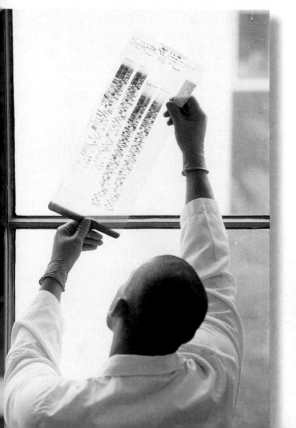

Genetic analysis for disease susceptibility will be more common in the future as the genes that increase the risk of developing various diseases are isolated and decoded.

In the final analysis, would you want to know if you were at risk of a specific disease that a genetic test could point out? If so, ask your physician about the possibility and wisdom of testing you for the genetically linked diseases in your family tree. Also, be aware that, throughout this book, discussions will point out how to avoid "controllable" risk factors that contribute to the development of genetically linked nutrition-related diseases present in your family.

Knowledge Check

1. What is the role of genes?
2. What are 3 chronic nutrition-related diseases with a genetic link?
3. What is a genogram?

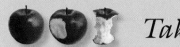

Take Action

Create Your Family Tree for Health-Related Concerns

Adapt this diagram to your own family tree. Under each heading, list year born, year died (if applicable), major diseases that developed during the person's lifetime, and cause of death (if applicable). Figure 1-10 provides an example.

Note that you are likely to be at risk of developing any diseases listed. Creating a plan for preventing such diseases when possible, especially those that developed in your family members before age 50 to 60 years, is advised. Check out the website www.hhs.gov/familyhistory for more information on using a family tree in health-related evaluations. Speak with your health-care provider about any concerns arising from this activity.

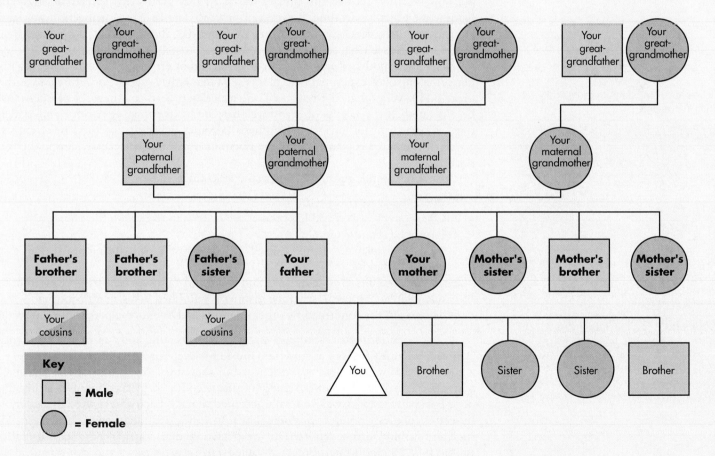

CASE STUDY

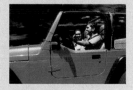

While Allen was driving to campus last week, he heard a radio advertisement for a nutrient supplement containing a plant substance that was discovered recently. It supposedly gives people more energy and helps them cope with the stress of daily life. This advertisement caught Allen's attention because he has been feeling run-down lately. He is taking a full course load and has been working 30 hours a week at a local restaurant. Allen doesn't have a lot of extra money to spare. Still, he likes to try new things, and this recent breakthrough sounded almost too good to be true. After searching for more information on the Internet, he discovered that the recommended dose would cost $60 per month. Because Allen is looking for some help with his low energy level, he decides to order a 30-day supply. Does this extra expense make sense to you?

1.6 Using Scientific Research to Determine Nutrient Needs

How do we know what we know about nutrition? How has this knowledge been gained? In a word, research. Like other sciences, the research that sets the foundation for nutrition has developed through the use of the scientific method—a testing procedure designed to uncover facts and detect and eliminate error. The first step is the observation of a natural phenomenon. Scientists then suggest possible explanations, called **hypotheses**, about the causes of the phenomenon. Distinguishing a true cause-and-effect relationship from mere coincidence can be difficult. For instance, early in the 20th century, many people in orphanages, prisons, and mental hospitals suffered from the disease pellagra, which suggested this disease was caused by germs that spread among people living close together. In time, however, it became clear that this connection was simply coincidental—the real cause of pellagra is a poor diet that contains too little of the B-vitamin niacin (see Chapter 13).

To test hypotheses and eliminate coincidental or erroneous explanations, scientists perform controlled experiments to gather data that either support or refute a hypothesis (Fig. 1-11). Very often, the results of one experiment lead to a new set of questions to be answered. If the results of many well-designed experiments provide valid evidence that supports a hypothesis, the hypothesis becomes generally accepted by scientists as a well-documented explanation for the phenomenon and is called a scientific theory or scientific law.

Sound scientific research requires the following:

1. Phenomena are observed.
2. Questions are asked and hypotheses are generated to explain the phenomena.
3. Research is conducted.
4. Incorrect explanations are rejected and the most likely explanation is used as the basis for a model.
5. Research results are scrutinized and evaluated by other scientists. Research conducted in an unbiased, scientific manner is published in a scientific journal.
6. The results are confirmed by other scientists and by more experiments and studies.

The scientific method requires an open, curious mind and a questioning, skeptical attitude. Scientists (as well as students) must not accept proposed hypotheses until they are supported by considerable evidence, and they must reject hypotheses that fail to pass critical analysis. A recent example of this need for skepticism involves stomach ulcers. For many years, it was generally accepted that stomach ulcers were caused mostly by a stressful lifestyle and a poor diet. Then, in 1983, Australian physicians, Barry Marshall and Robin Warren, reported in a respected medical journal that ulcers usually are caused by a common microorganism called *Helicobacter pylori* and can be cured with antibiotics. At first, other physicians were skeptical about this finding and continued to prescribe medications, such as antacids, that reduce stomach acid. As more studies were published, however, and patients were cured of ulcers using antibiotics, the medical profession eventually accepted the findings. (Marshall and Warren were even given the Nobel Prize for Medicine in 2005 for this discovery.) Scientific theories, laws, and discoveries always should be subjected to challenge and change.

Making Observations and Generating Hypotheses

Historical observations have provided clues to important relationships in nutrition science. In the 15th and 16th centuries, for example, many European sailors on long voyages developed the often fatal disease scurvy. A British naval surgeon, Lind, observed that the diet eaten while at sea differed from usual diets. In specific, few fruits and vegetables

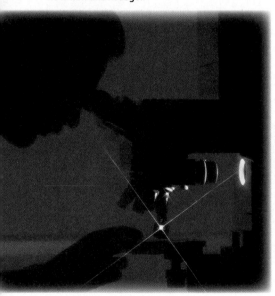

Careful research contributes to scientifically valid nutrition knowledge.

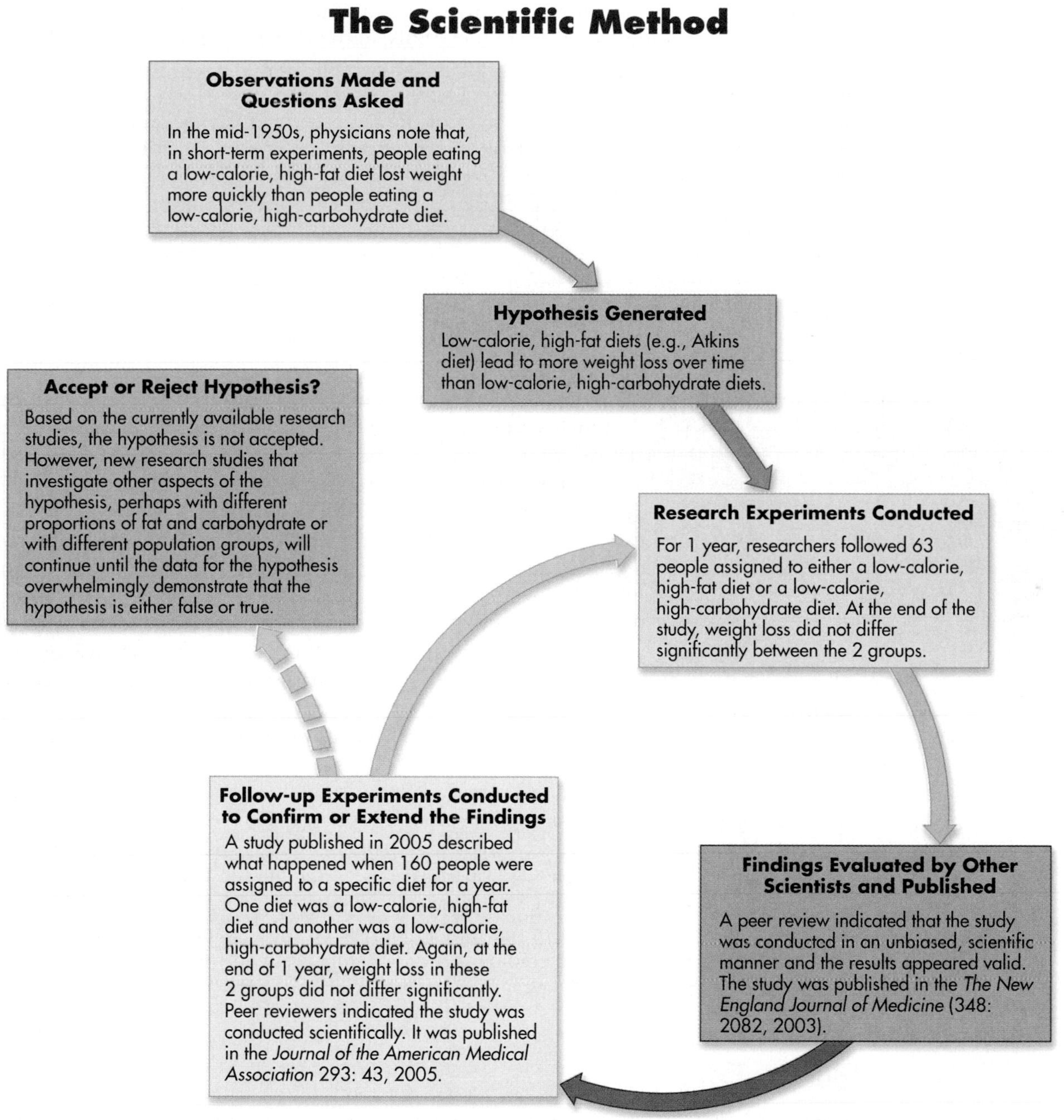

The Scientific Method

Observations Made and Questions Asked

In the mid-1950s, physicians note that, in short-term experiments, people eating a low-calorie, high-fat diet lost weight more quickly than people eating a low-calorie, high-carbohydrate diet.

Hypothesis Generated

Low-calorie, high-fat diets (e.g., Atkins diet) lead to more weight loss over time than low-calorie, high-carbohydrate diets.

Accept or Reject Hypothesis?

Based on the currently available research studies, the hypothesis is not accepted. However, new research studies that investigate other aspects of the hypothesis, perhaps with different proportions of fat and carbohydrate or with different population groups, will continue until the data for the hypothesis overwhelmingly demonstrate that the hypothesis is either false or true.

Research Experiments Conducted

For 1 year, researchers followed 63 people assigned to either a low-calorie, high-fat diet or a low-calorie, high-carbohydrate diet. At the end of the study, weight loss did not differ significantly between the 2 groups.

Follow-up Experiments Conducted to Confirm or Extend the Findings

A study published in 2005 described what happened when 160 people were assigned to a specific diet for a year. One diet was a low-calorie, high-fat diet and another was a low-calorie, high-carbohydrate diet. Again, at the end of 1 year, weight loss in these 2 groups did not differ significantly. Peer reviewers indicated the study was conducted scientifically. It was published in the *Journal of the American Medical Association* 293: 43, 2005.

Findings Evaluated by Other Scientists and Published

A peer review indicated that the study was conducted in an unbiased, scientific manner and the results appeared valid. The study was published in the *The New England Journal of Medicine* (348: 2082, 2003).

Figure 1-11 This example shows how the scientific method was used to test a hypothesis about the effects of low-calorie, high-fat diets on weight loss. Scientists consistently follow these steps when testing all types of hypotheses. Scientists do not accept a nutrition or another scientific hypothesis until it has been thoroughly tested using the scientific method.

were available while onboard ships. He hypothesized that a missing dietary component caused scurvy. He set up an experiment in which he supplied sailors with a ration of salt water, vinegar, cider, citrus juice, or other liquid. The results of this experiment indicated that citrus (lemons, limes) prevented and cured scurvy. After this, British sailors were given a ration of lime juice, earning them the nickname "limeys." About 200 years later, science had advanced to the point that researchers were able to identify vitamin C as the component in citrus juice that prevents and cures scurvy.

Observations of differences in dietary and disease patterns among various populations also have suggested important relationships in nutrition science. If one group tends to develop a certain disease but another group does not, scientists can speculate about how diet causes this difference. The study of diseases in populations, called

epidemiology, ultimately forms the basis for many laboratory studies. An example of the use of epidemiology occurred in the 1920s, in the United States, when Goldberger noticed that residents in mental institutions—but not their caretakers—suffered from pellagra. He reasoned that, if pellagra were an infectious disease, both groups would suffer from it. Because they did not, he hypothesized that pellagra was caused by a dietary deficiency. The controlled experiments he conducted found that yeast and high-protein foods can cure pellagra if it is not in its final stage. These research results indicated that pellagra is caused by a deficiency of a component present in these foods. Eventually, this component was found to be niacin.

Laboratory Animal Experiments

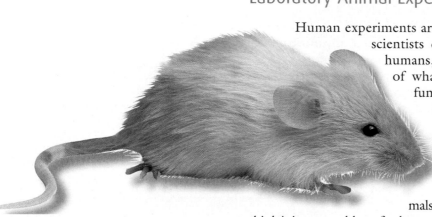

Human experiments are the most convincing to scientists; however, when scientists cannot test their hypotheses in experiments with humans, they often use laboratory animals. In fact, much of what is known about human nutritional needs and functions has been generated from laboratory animal experiments.

Experiments may be conducted with laboratory animals when the study would be unethical to conduct with humans. Although some people argue that laboratory animal experiments also are unethical, most believe that the careful, humane use of animals is an acceptable alternative. For example, most people think it is reasonable to feed rats a low-copper diet to study the importance of this mineral in the formation of blood vessels. Almost everyone, however, would object to a similar study in infants.

The use of laboratory animal experiments to study the role of nutrition in human diseases depends on the availability of an **animal model**—a disease in laboratory animals that closely mimics a human disease. For example, in the early 1900s, scientists showed that thiamin (a B-vitamin) cures a beriberi-like disease in chickens. As a result, chickens could be used to study this vitamin deficiency disease. If no animal model is available and human experiments are ruled out, scientific knowledge often cannot advance beyond what can be learned from epidemiological studies. Most human chronic diseases do not occur in laboratory animals.

Research using laboratory animals contributes to knowledge of nutrition.

Human Experiments

Before any research study can be conducted with humans (or laboratory animals), researchers must obtain approval from the research review board at their university or company. The review board approves only studies that have a valid experimental protocol, are expected to produce important knowledge, and treat study participants fairly and ethically. The review board also assesses the risks and benefits of the potential treatment to study participants. In human studies, the review board also requires researchers to inform the participants of the study's purpose, procedures, known risks, and benefits, so that they can make informed decisions about whether to participate. This process, called informed consent, is the voluntary, documented confirmation of the participants' agreement to participate in the study.

A variety of experimental approaches are used to test research hypotheses in humans. **Migrant studies,** for example, look at changes in the health of people who move from one country to another. **Cohort studies** start with a healthy population and follow it, looking for the development of disease. Other experimental approaches are case-control and double-blind studies.

Case-Control Study

In a case-control study, scientists compare individuals who have the condition in question ("cases"), such as lung cancer, with individuals who do not have the condition ("controls"). The strongest case-control studies compare groups that are matched for other major characteristics (e.g., age, race, and gender) not being studied. You can think of a case-control study as a "mini" epidemiological study. This type of study may identify factors other than the disease being studied, such as fruit and vegetable intake, that differ between the groups, thereby providing researchers with clues about the cause, progression, and prevention of the disease. However, without a controlled experiment, researchers cannot definitely claim cause and effect.[24]

Double-Blind Study

An important approach for more definitive testing of hypotheses is a controlled experiment using a blinded protocol. In a double-blind study, one group of participants—the experimental group—follows a specific protocol (e.g., receives a treatment, such as consuming a certain food or nutrient) while the participants in a corresponding control group follow their usual habits. The control group also usually receives a **placebo** (fake treatment). The placebo camouflages who is in the experimental group and who is in the control group. Study participants are assigned randomly to the control or experimental group, such as by the flip of a coin. Scientists then observe both groups over time to identify any changes that occur in the experimental and the control groups. Sometimes individuals are used as their own control: first they are observed for a period of time while they follow their usual habits. Then, they follow the experimental protocol and their responses are observed.

Two features of a double-blind study help reduce the risk of bias (prejudice), which can easily affect the outcome of an experiment. First, during the course of the experiment, neither the study participants nor the researchers know who is getting the real treatment (experimental group) and who is getting the placebo (control group). An independent third party holds the key to the study group assignment and the data until the study is completed. Second, the expected effects of the experimental protocol are not disclosed to the participants or researchers collecting the data until after the entire study is completed. These features reduce the possibility that the researchers will misperceive or overemphasize changes they hoped to see in the participants to prove a certain hypothesis they believe is true or will unconsciously ignore or minimize the importance of changes that disprove their hypothesis. These features also reduce the chance that study participants begin to feel better simply because they are involved in a research study or are receiving a new treatment, a phenomenon called the **placebo effect**. Double-blind studies improve the chances that any differences observed between the experimental and control groups really are due to the experimental treatment. Sometimes only a single-blind study protocol is possible—in this case, only the study participants are kept uninformed about which participants are assigned to the experimental and control groups. Conducting blinded studies in nutrition is very challenging because it is difficult to create placebo foods and menus.

A recent example illustrates the need to test hypotheses based on epidemiological observations in double-blind studies.[24] Epidemiologists using primarily case-control studies found that smokers who regularly consumed fruits and vegetables had a lower risk of lung cancer than smokers who ate few of these foods. Some scientists proposed that it was the beta-carotene (a yellow-orange pigment that is a precursor to vitamin A) present in many fruits and vegetables that reduced the lung damage caused by tobacco smoke that leads to lung cancer. However, in double-blind studies involving heavy smokers, the risk of lung cancer was found to be higher in those who took beta-carotene supplements than in those who did not. Some researchers criticized these studies, arguing that the beta-carotene was given too late in the

placebo A fake treatment (such as a sham medicine, supplement, or procedure) that seems like the experimental treatment. It is used to disguise whether a study participant is in the experimental or control group.

placebo effect *Placebo* is derived from a Latin word that means "I shall please." The placebo effect occurs when control group participants experience changes that cannot be explained by the action of the placebo they received. These changes may be linked to a reduction in stress and anxiety, hope that the treatment is working, or a desire to help the researchers achieve their goals. Overall, it is critical for researchers to take the placebo effect into consideration when interpreting research results.

▶ For a list of more nutrition- and health-related peer-reviewed journals, see Appendix L.

▶ These are examples of websites that provide reliable health and nutrition information.

www.healthfinder.gov

www.nutrition.gov

www.eatright.org

www.webmd.com.

peer-reviewed journal Journal that publishes research only after 2 or more researchers who were not part of the study agree that the study was carefully designed and executed and the results are presented in an unbiased, objective manner. Thus, the research has been approved by peers of the research team.

CRITICAL THINKING

For thousands of years, early humans consumed a diet rich in vegetable products and low in animal products. These diets were generally lower in fat and higher in dietary fiber than modern diets. Do the differences in human diets throughout history necessarily tell us which diet is better—that of early humans or of modern humans? If not, what is a more reliable way to pursue this question of potential diet superiority?

smokers' lives to prevent lung cancer, but even these critics did not suspect that the supplement would increase cancer risk. Soon after these results were reported, the U.S. federal agency supporting other large studies of beta-carotene supplements halted the research, stating that these supplements are ineffective in preventing lung cancer. Although it appears that beta-carotene does not protect against lung cancer, other components in fruits and vegetables might offer protection and may become the focus of future studies.

Overall, health and nutrition advice provided by family, friends, and other well-meaning individuals cannot be accepted as valid until studied in a rigorous, scientific manner.[24] Until that is done, it isn't possible to know whether a substance or procedure is truly effective. When people say, "I get fewer colds now that I take vitamin C," they overlook the facts that many cold symptoms disappear quickly with no treatment, that they want the supplement to work, and that the apparent curative effect of vitamin C or any other remedy is often coincidental rather than causal. Failure to understand the scientific method, as well as the accepted standards of evidence and current limitations of science, leads many people to believe erroneous information about health, nutrition, and disease. Using remedies that are not supported by credible scientific evidence can damage health and delay treatment that could preserve health.

Peer Review of Experimental Results

Once an experiment is complete, scientists summarize the findings and seek to publish the results in scientific journals. Generally, before such results are published in scientific journals, they are critically reviewed by other scientists familiar with the subject. The objective of this peer review is to ensure that only the most unbiased, objective findings from carefully designed and executed research studies are published.

Peer review is an important step because most scientific research is funded by the government, nonprofit foundations, drug companies, and other private industries—all of which have strong expectations about research outcomes. In theory, the scientists conducting research studies will be fair in evaluating their results and will not be influenced by the funding agency. Peer review helps ensure that the researchers are as objective as possible. This then helps ensure that the results published in **peer-reviewed journals**, such as the *American Journal of Clinical Nutrition, New England Journal of Medicine,* and *Journal of the American Dietetic Association,* are much more reliable than those found in popular magazines or promoted on television talk shows.

Press releases from reputable journals and major universities are the main sources for the information presented in the popular media. Unfortunately, these press releases often oversimplify study findings, which may get misinterpreted or overextended in the popular press. Thus, when you hear or see a report that cites a journal, it is best to review the journal article, so that you can judge for yourself whether the research findings are valid.

Follow-Up Studies

Even when a study has followed a well-designed protocol and the results have been published in a peer-reviewed journal, one experiment is never enough to prove a particular hypothesis or provide a basis for nutrition recommendations. Rather, the results obtained in one laboratory must be confirmed by experiments conducted in other laboratories and possibly under varying circumstances. Only then can we really trust and use the results. The more lines of evidence available to support a hypothesis or idea, the more likely it is to be true (Fig. 1-12). It is important to avoid rushing to accept new ideas as fact or incorporating them into your health habits until they are proved by several lines of evidence.[25]

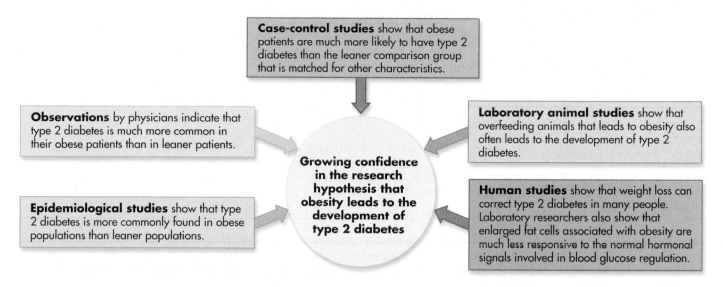

Figure 1-12 Data from a variety of sources can come together to support a research hypothesis. This diagram shows how various types of research data support the hypothesis that obesity leads to the development of type 2 diabetes (see Chapter 5).

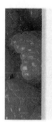

Knowledge Check

1. What elements are required for scientific research to be considered valid?
2. What is the difference between single- and double-blind studies?
3. What is an animal model?
4. What is a peer-reviewed journal?

1.7 Evaluating Nutrition Claims, Products, and Advice

Nutrition claims often appear in media stories and in advertisements. Sometimes it is difficult to discern whether the claims are true. The following suggestions can help you make healthful and logical nutrition decisions.[22]

1. Apply the basic principles of nutrition, as outlined in this book, to any nutrition claim. Do you note any inconsistencies?
2. Be wary if the answer is yes to any of the following questions about a health-related nutrition claim:
   - Are only advantages discussed and possible disadvantages ignored?
   - Is this a new or "secret" scientific breakthrough?
   - Are claims made about "curing" disease?
   - Do the claims sound too good to be true?
   - Is extreme bias against the medical community or traditional medical treatments evident? Physicians as a group strive to cure diseases in their patients using proven techniques—they do not ignore reliable cures.
3. Examine the scientific credentials of the individual, organization, or publication making the nutrition claim. Usually, a reputable author is one whose educational background or present employer is affiliated with a nationally recognized university, research institute, or medical center that offers programs or courses in nutrition, medicine, or closely related fields.

▶ These websites can help you evaluate ongoing nutrition and health claims.

www.acsh.org

www.quackwatch.com

dietary-supplements.info.nih.gov

www.fda.gov

www.eatright.org

Appendix L also lists many reputable sources of nutrition advice for your use.

▶ *10 Red Flags That Signal Poor Nutrition Advice*

1. Promise of a quick fix
2. Dire warnings of dangers from a single product or regimen
3. Claims that sound too good to be true
4. Simplistic conclusions drawn from a complex study
5. Recommendations based on a single study
6. Dramatic statements that are refuted by reputable scientific organizations
7. Lists of "good" and "bad" foods
8. Recommendations made to help sell a product
9. Recommendations based on studies published without peer review
10. Recommendations from studies that ignore differences among individuals or groups

4. If research is cited to support a claim, note the size and duration of any study. The larger the study and the longer it went on, the more dependable its findings. Also consider the type of study: epidemiology versus case-control versus blinded. Keep in mind that "contributes to," "is linked to," or "is associated with" does not mean "causes." Do reliable, peer-reviewed journal articles support the claims? Beware of testimonials about personal experience, disreputable publication sources, dramatic results (rarely true), and lack of evidence from supporting studies conducted by other scientists.

5. Be wary of press conferences and other hype regarding the latest findings. Much of this will not survive rigorous scientific evaluation.

Buying Nutrition-Related Products

Popular nutrition-related products claim to increase muscle growth, enhance sexuality, boost energy, reduce body fat, increase strength, supply missing nutrients, increase longevity, and even improve brain function. Although many of us are willing to try these products and believe they can cause the miraculous effects advertised, few of these products have been thoroughly evaluated by reputable scientists. They may not be effective, and the amount and potency of the product may not match what is on the package.

A cautious approach to nutrition-related products is important because of sweeping changes in U.S. law in 1994. The Dietary Supplement Health and Education Act (DSHEA) of 1994 classified vitamins, minerals, amino acids, and herbal remedies as "foods," effectively restraining the U.S. Food and Drug Administration (FDA) from regulating them as rigorously as food additives and drugs. According to this act, rather than the manufacturer having to prove a dietary supplement is safe, the FDA must prove it is unsafe before preventing its sale. In contrast, the safety of food additives and drugs must be rigorously demonstrated before the FDA allows them to be sold (see Chapter 3).

Currently, a product labeled as a dietary supplement (or an herbal product) can be marketed in the United States without FDA approval if there is a history of its use or other evidence that it is reasonably safe when used under the conditions indicated in its labeling. (Note that the FDA can act if the product turns out to be dangerous, as with the ban on the sale of the supplement ephedra after numerous deaths.) It is important to note that the "evidence" used to support a claim often is vague or unsubstantiated. Given its budget and regulatory constraints, the FDA is able to challenge only a few of these claims. Some other means for challenging these claims are now emerging. For example, the Federal Trade Commission (FTC), which is responsible for ensuring that advertising is not deceptive, may investigate dubious claims made in advertisements. In addition, the supplement industry itself is trying to develop self-policing procedures.

To protect your health, it is important to scrutinize nutrition-related product labels carefully and check with reputable sources to be certain there is scientific proof that the product is likely to perform as described on the label. Be especially skeptical of using the product for purposes not stated on the label—a product is unlikely to perform a function that is not specifically stated on its label or package insert (legally part of the label). The labels on dietary supplements and herbal products are allowed to claim that general well-being results from consumption of the ingredients, to explain how the product provides a benefit related to a classic nutrient deficiency disease, and to describe how a nutrient affects human body structure or function (called structure/function claims). Structure/function claim examples include "maintains bone health" and "improves blood circulation." The labels of products bearing such claims also must prominently display a disclaimer regarding a lack of FDA review (Fig. 1-13). Despite this warning, many consumers mistakenly assume that the FDA has carefully evaluated the products.

Figure 1-13 The FDA requires this highlighted disclaimer to appear on supplement labels.

Supplement Facts

Serving Size 1 Softgel

Each Softgel Contains	% DV
Ginseng Extract *(Panax ginseng)* (root) 100 mg (Standardized to 4% Ginsenosides)	*

*Daily Value (DV) not established.

INGREDIENTS: Gelatin, Soybean Oil, Panax Ginseng Extract, Vegetable Oil, Lecithin, Palm Oil, Glycerin, Sorbitol, Yellow Beeswax, Hydrogenated Coconut Oil, Titanium Dioxide, Yellow 5, Blue 1, Red 40, Green 3, Chlorophyll.

DIST. BY NUTRA ASSOC., INC.
4411 WHITE POINT RD., SPRING CITY, IL 12345

Suggested use: Adults- 1 to 2 capsules daily taken with a full glass of water, or as a tea, add one to two capsules to a cup of hot water.

When you need to perform your best, take ginseng.

This statement has not been evaluated by the Food and Drug Administration. This product is not intended to diagnose, treat, cure, or prevent disease.

Getting Nutrition-Related Advice

For those who feel they need to improve their diet and health, a safe approach is to consult a physician or registered dietitian (R.D.) before purchasing dietary supplements.[19, 23] A person with the credentials "R.D." after his or her name ("R.D.N." also is used in Canada) has completed a rigorous baccalaureate degree program approved by the American Dietetic Association, has performed at least 900 hours of supervised professional practice, and has passed a registration examination. Registered dietitians are trained to provide scientifically valid nutrition advice. To find a registered dietitian, visit the websites of the American Dietetic Association (www.eatright.org) or Dietitians of Canada (www.dietitians.ca), consult the telephone directory, contact the local dietetic association, or call the dietary department of a local hospital.

When you meet with a nutrition professional, you should expect that he or she will do the following:

- Ask questions about your medical history, lifestyle, and current eating habits
- Formulate a diet plan tailored to your needs, as opposed to simply tearing a form from a tablet that could apply to almost anyone
- Schedule follow-up visits to track your progress, answer any questions, and help keep you motivated
- Involve family members in the diet plan, when appropriate
- Consult directly with your physician and readily refer you back to your physician for those health problems a nutrition professional is not trained to treat

Be skeptical of health practitioners who prescribe very large doses of vitamin, mineral, or protein supplements for everyone.

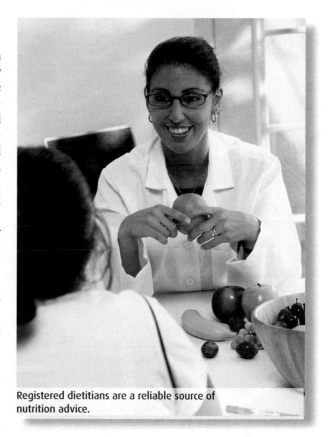
Registered dietitians are a reliable source of nutrition advice.

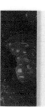
Knowledge Check

1. What are 5 tips for determining whether nutrition claims are true?
2. Why does DSHEA make it wise to be cautious about dietary supplements?
3. What should you expect when you meet with a nutrition professional?

CASE STUDY FOLLOW-UP

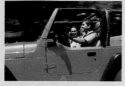

Allen should be cautious about taking any supplement, especially one advertised as a "recent breakthrough." There likely have not been enough studies of the supplement to confirm its effectiveness. Also, as you have read, dietary supplements are not closely regulated by the FDA; a general phrase, such as "increases energy," is considered a structure/function claim and such product labeling does not require prior approval by the FDA. Furthermore, the FDA will not have evaluated either the safety or the effectiveness of such a product. Even harmful dietary supplements are difficult for the FDA to recall. There is also a chance that the supplement contains little or none of the advertised ingredient. Unfortunately, Allen will find all this out the hard way and will be out $60. His hard-earned money would be better spent on a nutritious diet and a medical checkup at the student health center. All consumers need to be cautious about nutrition information, especially regarding dietary supplements marketed as cure-alls and breakthroughs—let the buyer beware!

Summary

1.1 *Nutrition* is defined as the "science of food; the nutrients and the substances therein; their action, interaction, and balance in relation to health and disease; and the process by which the organism (e.g., human body) ingests, digests, absorbs, transports, utilizes, and excretes food substances." Nutrients are substances essential for health that the body cannot make or makes in quantities too small to support health. Nutrients primarily provide energy, support growth and development, and/or keep body functions running smoothly. Carbohydrates, proteins, lipids, and water are macronutrients. Vitamins and minerals are micronutrients. Phytochemicals are plant components and zoochemicals are components in animals that may provide significant health benefits.

1.2 Humans obtain the energy needed to perform body functions and do work from carbohydrates, fats, and proteins. Alcohol also provides energy but is not considered an essential nutrient. A kilocalorie is the amount of heat energy it takes to raise the temperature of 1000 g (1 liter) of water 1°C. The physiological fuel values are 4, 9, 4, and 7 for carbohydrate, fat, protein, and alcohol, respectively.

1.3 North American adults consume, on average, 16% of their energy intake as proteins, 50% as carbohydrates, and 33% as fats. Animal sources, such as meat, seafood, dairy products, and eggs, are the main protein sources for North Americans. About half the carbohydrate in North American diets comes from simple carbohydrates; the other half comes from starches. Many North Americans are consuming more saturated fat, cholesterol, and sodium and less vitamin A, vitamin E, iron, and calcium than recommended. Daily food intake satisfies hunger (physical need for food) and social and emotional needs. Appetite and food choice depend on many factors.

1.4 Nutritional health is determined by the sum of the status of each nutrient. Optimal, or desirable, nutritional status for a nutrient is the state in which body tissues have enough of the nutrient to support normal functions and to build and maintain surplus stores. Undernutrition occurs when nutrient intake does not meet needs, causing surplus stores to be used. The consumption of more nutrients than needed leads to overnutrition. *Healthy People 2010* set health promotion and disease prevention goals, many of which promote desirable nutrition that supports healthful lifestyles and reduces preventable death and disability. A nutritional assessment considers background factors, as well as anthropometric, biochemical, clinical, dietary, and environmental assessments.

1.5 Genetic endowment affects almost every medical condition. Genes direct the growth, development, and maintenance of cells and, ultimately, of the entire organism. Most chronic nutrition-related diseases are influenced by genetic, nutritional, and lifestyle factors. Although some individuals may be genetically predisposed to chronic disease, the actual development of the disease depends on lifestyle and environmental factors. Scientists are currently developing therapies to correct some genetic disorders. Experts recommend that anyone considering genetic testing first undergo genetic counseling.

1.6 Research that creates the foundation for nutrition has developed through the use of the scientific method. To test hypotheses and eliminate coincidental or erroneous hypotheses, scientists perform controlled experiments. The scientific method requires an open, curious mind and a questioning, skeptical attitude. Scientists must not accept hypotheses until they are supported by considerable research evidence. Scientific theories, laws, and discoveries always should be subjected to challenge and change. Experimental approaches used to test research hypotheses in humans include migrant, cohort, case-control, and blinded studies. Once an experiment is complete, scientists summarize the findings and seek to publish the results in a scientific, peer-reviewed journal. The objective of peer review is to ensure that only the most unbiased, objective findings from carefully designed and executed research studies are published.

1.7 Nutrition claims often appear in media stories and in advertisements. It can be difficult to discern whether the claims are true. A cautious approach to nutrition-related claims and products is important. The Dietary Supplement Health and Education Act classified vitamins, minerals, amino acids, and herbal remedies as "foods," effectively restraining the FDA from regulating them as rigorously as food additives and drugs. When selecting nutrition-related products, carefully scrutinize product labels. For those who feel they need to improve their diet and health, a safe approach is to consult a physician or registered dietitian before purchasing dietary supplements.

Study Questions

1. Which nutrient does not provide energy?
   a. carbohydrates
   b. vitamins
   c. protein
   d. lipids

2. Which element is found in protein but is not found in carbohydrates and lipids?
   a. nitrogen
   b. carbon
   c. hydrogen
   d. oxygen

3. How many calories per gram are supplied by fats and oils?
   a. 9
   b. 4
   c. 5
   d. 7

4. A kilocalorie is the amount of heat energy it takes to raise the temperature of 1 gram of water 1 degree Celsius (1°C).
   a. true
   b. false

5. How many calories are in a food that contains 12 g carbohydrate, 3 g alcohol, 0 g fat, and 3 g protein?
   a. 112
   b. 81
   c. 75
   c. 124

6. Animal sources, such as meat, seafood, dairy products, and eggs, supply about two-thirds of the protein intake for most people around the world.
   a. true
   b. false

7. Foods are selected based mainly on _____.
   a. hunger
   b. appetite
   c. custom
   d. cost

8. Anthropometric assessment involves measuring _____.
   a. blood pressure
   b. enzyme activity
   c. skinfold thickness
   d. all of the above

9. Clinical assessment involves measuring _____.
   a. concentrations of nutrients in the blood
   b. nutrient content in the diet
   c. body circumferences
   d. education and economic levels

10. Genes direct the growth, development, and maintenance of cells.
    a. true
    b. false

11. Which disease has a genetic link?
    a. diabetes
    b. osteoporosis
    c. cancer
    d. all of the above

12. The risk of developing a specific genetic disease is high if you have 2 or more first-degree relatives with the disease, especially if the disease occurred before age 50 to 60 years.
    a. true
    b. false

13. Which type of study examines disease in populations?
    a. epidemiology
    b. double-blind studies
    c. single-blind studies
    d. animal modeling

14. Which type of study follows a healthy population, looking for the development of diseases?
    a. cohort study
    b. case-control study
    c. migrant study
    d. double-blind study

15. Which statement is false about the Dietary Supplement Health and Education Act (DSHEA)?
    a. DSHEA classified vitamins as foods.
    b. DSHEA causes the FDA to regulate herbal supplements as rigorously as it does drugs.
    c. DSHEA effectively restrains the FDA from regulating mineral supplements.
    d. DSHEA requires the FDA to prove a dietary supplement is unsafe before preventing its sale.

Answer Key: 1-b; 2-a; 3-a; 4-b; 5-b; 6-b; 7-b; 8-c; 9-a; 10-a; 11-d; 12-a; 13-a; 14-a; 15-b

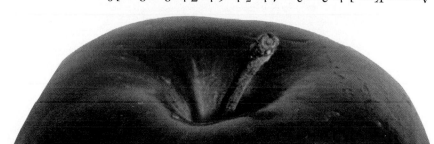

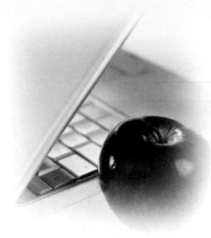

Websites

To learn more about the topics covered in this chapter, visit these websites.

Reliable Health and Nutrition Information

www.healthfinder.gov

www.nutrition.gov

www.eatright.org

www.webmd.com

Nutrition and Health Claims Evaluation

www.acsh.org

www.quackwatch.com

dietary-supplements.info.nih.gov

www.fda.gov

www.eatright.org

Genetics

genomics.energy.gov/

www.hhs.gov/familyhistory

www.geneticalliance.org

www.kumc.edu/gec/support

cancernet.nci.nih.gov/p_genetics.html

www.nhgri.nih.gov

www.faseb.org/genetics

vector.cshl.org

www.ncgr.org

For more websites, see Appendix L.

References

1. ADA Reports. Position of the American Dietetic Association and Dietitians of Canada: Nutrition and women's health. *J Am Diet Assoc.* 2004; 104:984.

2. Lee S and others. Trends in diet quality for coronary heart disease prevention between 1980–1982 and 2000–2002: The Minnesota Heart Survey. *J Am Diet Assoc.* 2007; 107:213.

3. Mokdad AH and others. Actual causes of death in the United States, 2000. *JAMA.* 2004; 291:1238.

4. Olshansky SJ and others. A potential decline in life expectancy in the United States in the 21st century. *New Eng J Med* 2005; 352:1138.

5. Lubin F and others. Lifestyle and ethnicity play a role in all-cause mortality. *J Nutr.* 2003; 133:1180.

6. Gropper SS and others. *Advanced nutrition and human metabolism.* 4th ed. Belmont, CA: Thomson Wadsworth; 2005.

7. Food and Nutrition Board. *Dietary Reference Intakes for energy, carbohydrate, fiber, fat, fatty acids, cholesterol, protein, and amino acids.* Washington, DC: Food and Nutrition Board; 2002.

8. ADA Reports. Position of the American Dietetic Association: Functional foods. *J Am Diet Assoc.* 2004; 104:814.

9. Milner JA. Molecular targets for bioactive food components. *J Nutr.* 2004; 134:2492S.

10. Neto CC. Cranberry and blueberry: Evidence for protective effects against cancer and vascular diseases. *Molecular Nutr Food Res.* 2007; 51:652.

11. Hasler C. Functional foods: Benefits, concerns, and challenges—A position paper from the American Council on Science and Health. *J Nutr.* 2002; 132:3772.

12. Institute of Medicine. *Dietary Reference Intakes for energy, carbohydrate, fiber, fat, fatty acids, cholesterol, protein, and amino acids (macronutrients).* Washington, DC: National Academies Press; 2005.

13. Maurer Abbot J, Byrd Bredbenner C. The state of the American diet. How can we cope? *Topics Clin Nutr.* 2007; 3:202.

14. ADA Reports. Position of the American Dietetic Association: Total diet approach to communicating food and nutrition information. *J Am Diet Assoc.* 2007; 107:1224.

15. Tholin S and others. Genetic and environmental influences on eating behavior: The Swedish Young Male Twins Study. *Am J Clin Nutr.* 2005; 81:564.

16. Wetter AC and others. How and why do individuals make food and physical activity choices? *Nutr Rev.* 2001; 59:S11.

17. Cordain L and others. Origins and evolution of the Western diet: Health implications for the 21st century. *Am J Clin Nutr.* 2005; 81:341.

18. Healthy People 2010 targets healthy diet and healthy weight as critical goals. *J Am Diet Assoc.* 2000; 100:300.

19. Roles of registered dietitians and dietetic technicians in health promotion and disease prevention. *J Am Diet Assoc.* 2006; 106:1875.

20. Wattendorf DJ, Hadley DW. Family history: The three-generation pedigree. *Am Fam Phys.* 2005; 72:441.

21. Genuis, SJ. Our genes are not our destiny: incorporating molecular medicine into clinical practice. *J Eval Clin Pract.* 2008; 14:94.

22. Guttmacher AF, Collins FC. Realizing the promise of genomics in biomedical research. *JAMA.* 2005; 294:1399.

23. Reilly, PR and Debusk, RM. Ethical and legal issues in nutritional genomics. *J Am Diet Assoc.* 2008; 108:36.

24. Making sense of medical news. *Consumer Reports on Health.* 2005; May:8.

25. ADA Reports. Position of the American Dietetic Association: Food and nutrition misinformation. *J Am Diet Assoc.* 2006; 106:601.

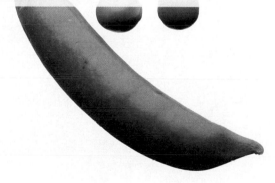

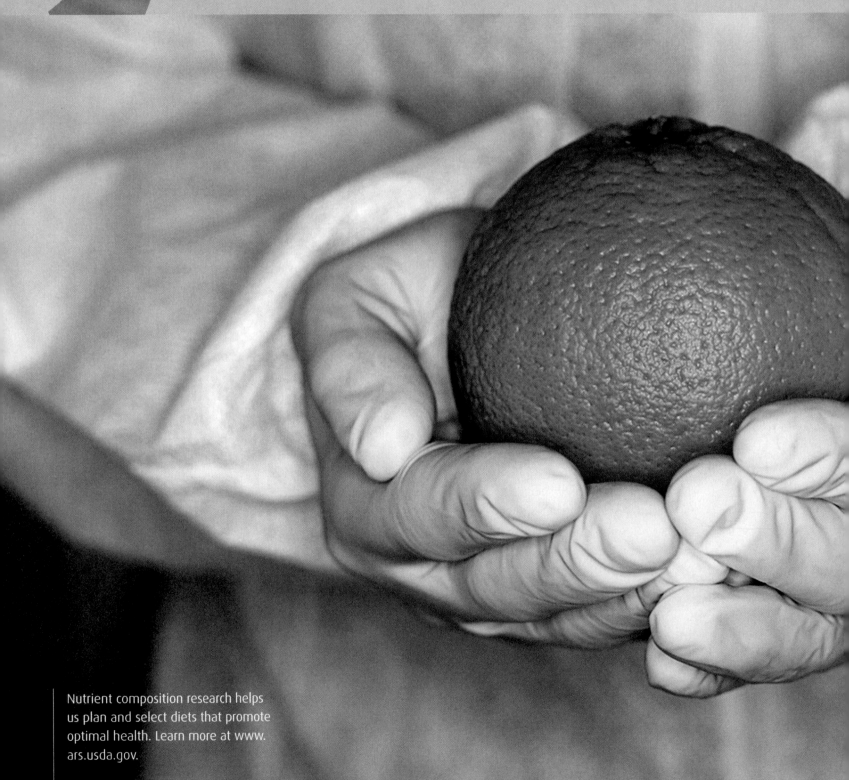

2 Tools of a Healthy Diet

Nutrient composition research helps us plan and select diets that promote optimal health. Learn more at www.ars.usda.gov.

STUDENT LEARNING OUTCOMES

After studying this chapter, you will be able to

1. Explain the purpose of the Recommended Dietary Allowances (RDAs) and relate them to the other standards included in the Dietary Reference Intakes.

2. Compare the Daily Values to the Dietary Reference Intakes and explain how they are used on Nutrition Facts panels.

3. Describe Nutrition Facts panels and the claims permitted on food packages.

4. Describe the uses and limitations of the data in nutrient databases.

5. Discuss the 2005 Dietary Guidelines for Americans and the diseases they are designed to prevent or minimize.

6. Discuss the MyPyramid food groupings and plan a diet using this tool.

7. Develop a healthy eating plan based on the concepts of variety, balance, moderation, nutrient density, and energy density.

Nutrition is a popular topic in the media. News stories often highlight up-to-the-minute research results. Magazine articles, websites, and books tout the "latest" way to lose weight or improve your diet. Deciding whether to incorporate advice given by the media can be a challenge. Relying on peer-reviewed research and recommendations by experts can help you decide whether to follow any of this nutrition advice. There also are a number of other useful tools based on nutrition research and assessment methods that can assist you in deciding what advice to follow as well as in planning a dietary pattern that helps you live as healthfully as possible now while minimizing the risk of developing nutrition-related diseases later on.

One tool for planning diets that support overall health is the Dietary Reference Intakes—they provide guidance on the quantities of nutrients that are most likely to result in optimal health. Using Daily Values, food labels, nutrient databases, nutrient density, and energy density also can help facilitate efforts to identify foods that contain the array of nutrients needed in the amounts recommended. The Dietary Guidelines outline key steps that support good health and reduce risk of chronic, nutrition-related diseases. Finally, MyPyramid is a handy tool you can use to create a dietary pattern that promotes excellent health and lets you eat foods you enjoy.

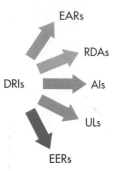

The DRIs are composed of Estimated Average Requirements (EARs), Recommended Dietary Allowances (RDAs), Adequate Intakes (AIs), Tolerable Upper Intake Levels (Upper Levels, or ULs), and Estimated Energy Requirements (EERs).

Dietary Reference Intakes (DRIs) Term used to encompass nutrient recommendations made by the Food and Nutrition Board of the National Academy of Sciences. These include RDAs, EARs, AIs, EERs, and ULs.

Estimated Average Requirements (EARs) Nutrient intake amounts estimated to meet the needs of 50% of the individuals in a specific life stage.

A key to healthy living is gaining a firm knowledge of these basic diet planning tools. With this understanding, you'll know why scientists believe that optimal nutritional health can be accomplished by doing what you've heard many times before: eat a balanced diet, consume a variety of foods, moderate the amount you eat, and stay physically active.

2.1 Dietary Reference Intakes (DRIs)

When many young men were rejected from military service in World War II because of the effects of poor nutrition on their health, scientists realized the need for dietary intake recommendations. As a result, in 1941, a group of scientists formed the Food and Nutrition Board with the purpose of reviewing existing research and establishing the first official dietary standards. These standards were designed to evaluate nutrient intakes of large populations and to plan agricultural production.[1] Since they were first published in 1943, these standards have been periodically reviewed and updated to reflect the latest scientific research.

The latest recommendations from the Food and Nutrition Board are called Dietary Reference Intakes (DRIs).[2] The DRIs apply to people in both the United States and Canada because scientists from both countries worked together to establish them. The DRIs include 5 sets of standards: Estimated Average Requirements (EARs), Recommended Dietary Allowances (RDAs), Adequate Intakes (AIs), Tolerable Upper Intake Levels (Upper Levels, or ULs), and Estimated Energy Requirements (EERs) (see the inside covers of this textbook).[1] DRIs are set for almost 40 nutrients. Although not a DRI, Adequate Macronutrient Distribution Ranges (AMDRs) were established for guidance on intake levels of carbohydrates, protein, and fat to help reduce the risk of nutrition-related chronic diseases.[3-5] As you can see from charts on the inside covers of this book, the DRIs differ by life stage (i.e., age group; by gender after age 9 years; pregnancy, lactation). All of the recommendations should be applied to dietary intake averaged over a number of days, not a single day.

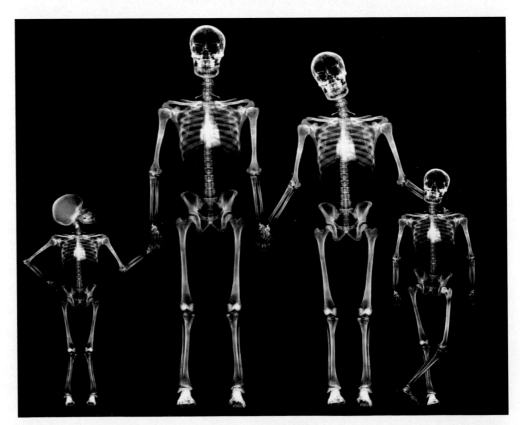

DRIs vary by life stage because nutrient needs differ with age and, after age 9 years by gender. Pregnancy and lactation also affect nutrient needs; thus, there is a set of DRIs specially designed for these women.

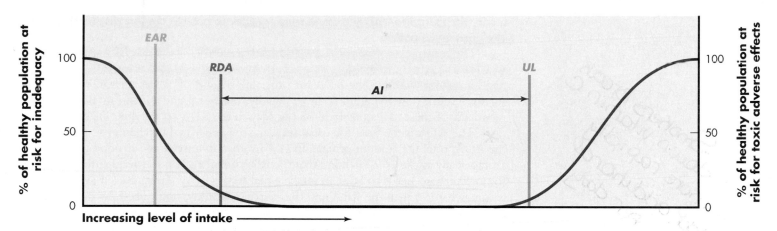

Figure 2-1 This figure shows the relationship of the Dietary Reference Intakes (DRIs) to each other and the percent of the population covered by each.

Estimated Average Requirement (EAR): 50% of healthy North Americans would have an inadequate intake if they consumed the EAR, whereas 50% would have their needs met.

Recommended Dietary Allowance (RDA): 2 to 3% of healthy North Americans would have an inadequate intake if they met the RDA, whereas 97 to 98% would have their needs met.

Upper Level (UL): highest nutrient intake level that is likely to pose no risks of adverse health effects in almost all healthy individuals. At intakes above the UL, the margin of safety to protect against adverse effects is reduced. At intakes between the RDA and UL (Upper Level), the risk of either an inadequate diet or adverse effects from the nutrient is close to 0%.

Adequate Intake (AI): set for some nutrients instead of an RDA, lies somewhere between the RDA and UL. Thus, the AI should cover the needs of more than 97 to 98% of individuals.

Estimated Average Requirements (EARs)

Estimated Average Requirements (EARs) are daily nutrient intake amounts that are estimated to meet the needs of half of the people in a certain life stage (Fig. 2-1). EARs are set for 17 nutrients. An EAR for a nutrient is set only when the Food and Nutrition Board agrees that there is an accurate method for measuring whether intake is adequate. These measures, called functional markers, typically evaluate the activity of an enzyme in the body or the ability of a cell or an organ to maintain normal physiological function.[1] If no measurable functional marker is available, an EAR cannot be set, which is the case for the mineral calcium. Each EAR is adjusted to account for the amount of the nutrient that passes through the digestive tract unabsorbed. Because EARs meet the needs of only 50% of those in a life stage, they can be used to evaluate only the adequacy of diets of groups, not of individuals.[1] Specific EARs are listed in Appendix J.

To illustrate how EARs are determined, let's take a look at vitamin C. The amount of vitamin C needed daily to prevent scurvy is about 10 mg. However, as you will learn in Chapter 13, vitamin C has other functions as well, including some related to the immune system (see Appendix A for details on the immune system). In fact, the concentration of vitamin C in one component of the immune system—notably, white blood cells (specifically, neutrophils)—can be used as a functional marker for vitamin C. The Food and Nutrition Board concluded that nearly maximal saturation of these white blood cells with vitamin C is the best functional marker for optimal vitamin C status. It takes a daily vitamin C intake of about 75 mg for men and 60 mg for women to nearly saturate these white blood cells. These average amounts became the EARs for young adult men and women.

Recommended Dietary Allowances (RDAs)

Recommended Dietary Allowances (RDAs) are daily nutrient intake amounts sufficient to meet the needs of nearly all individuals (97 to 98%) in a life stage (see the inside covers). RDAs are based on a multiple of the EARs (generally, the RDA = EAR × 1.2). Because of this relationship, an RDA can be set only for nutrients that have an EAR. (Recall that a measurable functional marker is required to set an EAR.) An additional consideration

★ important ★

Recommended Dietary Allowance (RDA) Nutrient intake amount sufficient to meet the needs of 97 to 98% of the individuals in a specific life stage.

Adequate Intake (AI) Nutrient intake amount set for any nutrient for which insufficient research is available to establish an RDA. AIs are based on estimates of intakes that appear to maintain a defined nutritional state in a specific life stage.

Tolerable Upper Intake Level (UL) Maximum chronic daily intake level of a nutrient that is unlikely to cause adverse health effects in almost all people in a specific life stage.

Estimated Energy Requirement (EER) Estimate of the energy (kcal) intake needed to match the energy use of an average person in a specific life stage.

Adequate Macronutrient Distribution Range (AMDR) Range of macronutrient intake, as percent of energy, associated with reduced risk of chronic diseases while providing for recommended intake of essential nutrients.

made when setting an RDA is the nutrient's ability to prevent chronic disease rather than just prevent deficiency.[1]

For example, to determine the RDA for vitamin C, its EAR (75 mg for men and 60 mg for women) was multiplied by 1.2. In this case, the RDA was set at 90 mg for men and 75 mg for women. The RDA for other life-stage groups was set similarly. Because smokers break down vitamin C more rapidly, the Food and Nutrition Board recommended that these individuals add 35 mg/day to the RDA set for their life stage.

The RDA is the goal for usual intake. To assess whether vitamin C intake meets the RDA, total the amount of vitamin C consumed in a week and divide by 7 to get an average daily intake. Keep in mind that the RDA is higher than the average human needs, so not everyone needs to have an intake equal to the RDA. Thus, even if average intake is somewhat less than the RDA and the person is healthy, one's need for this vitamin is probably less than the RDA. As a general rule, however, the further intake regularly drops below the RDA—particularly as it drops below the EAR—the greater the risk of developing a nutrient deficiency.[1]

Adequate Intakes (AIs)

Adequate Intakes (AIs) are daily intake amounts set for nutrients for which there are insufficient research data to establish an EAR (see the inside covers). AIs are based on observed or experimentally determined estimates of the average nutrient intake that appears to maintain a defined nutritional state (e.g., bone health) in a specific life-stage group.[1] In determining the AI for a nutrient, it is expected that the amount exceeds the RDA for that nutrient, if an RDA were known. Thus, the AI should cover the needs of more than 97 to 98% of the individuals in a specific life-stage group. The actual degree to which the AI exceeds the RDA likely differs among the various nutrients and life-stage groups. Like the RDA, the AI can be used as the goal for usual intake of that nutrient by an individual. Currently, essential fatty acids, fiber, and 9 vitamins and minerals, including some B-vitamins, vitamin D, the vitamin-like compound choline, calcium, and fluoride, have AIs.

Tolerable Upper Intake Levels (Upper Levels, or ULs)

Tolerable Upper Intake Levels, or Upper Levels (ULs), are the maximum daily intake amounts of nutrients that are not likely to cause adverse health effects in almost all individuals (97 to 98%) in a life-stage group (see the inside covers).[1] The amount applies to chronic daily use and is set to protect even those who are very susceptible in the healthy general population. For example, the UL for vitamin C is 2000 mg/day. Intakes greater than this amount can cause diarrhea and inflammation of the stomach lining.

The UL for most nutrients is based on the combined intake of food, water, supplements, and fortified foods. The exceptions are the vitamin niacin and the minerals magnesium, zinc, and nickel—the UL for each refers only to nonfood sources, such as medicines and supplements. This is because niacin, magnesium, zinc, or nickel toxicity from food sources is unlikely.

The UL is not a nutrient intake goal; instead, it is a ceiling below which nutrient intake should remain. Still, for most individuals, there is a margin of safety above the UL before any adverse effects are likely to occur. Too little information is available to set a UL for all nutrients, but this does not mean that toxicity from these nutrients is impossible. Plus, there is no clear-cut evidence that intakes above the RDA or AI confer any additional health benefits for most of us.

Estimated Energy Requirements (EERs)

RDAs and Adequate Intakes for nutrients are set high enough to meet the needs of almost all healthy individuals. In contrast, Estimated Energy Require-

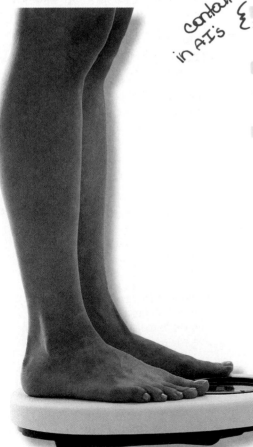

Although Estimated Energy Requirements (EERs) provide a guide for energy needs, the best estimate of energy need is the amount needed to maintain a healthy weight.

ments (EERs) are set at the average daily energy (calorie) need for each life-stage group. Unlike most vitamins and minerals, energy (carbohydrate, fat, protein, alcohol) consumed in amounts above that needed is not excreted but is stored as body fat. Thus, to promote healthy weight a more conservative standard is to set EERs rather than RDAs and AIs.[5] Overall, EERs are estimates because energy needs depend on energy expenditure and, in some cases, the energy needed to support growth or human milk production. For most adults, the best estimate of energy need is the amount required to achieve and maintain a healthy weight (see Chapter 10 for details).

human milk production.

Maintains. weight.

Adequate Macronutrient Distribution Ranges (AMDRs)

In addition to EERs, the Food and Nutrition Board also established Adequate Macronutrient Distribution Ranges (AMDRs) for intake of carbohydrate, protein, fat, and essential fatty acids (see inside covers). For each macronutrient, the AMDRs provide a range of intake, as a percent of energy, associated with good health and a reduced risk of chronic diseases while providing for recommended intakes of essential nutrients. The AMDRs complement the DRIs.[1] For example, the AMDR for fat is 20 to 35% of calories. For an average energy intake of 2000 kcal/day, this is equal to 400 to 700 kcal per day from fat. To translate this to grams of fat per day, divide by 9 kcal/g. Thus, a healthy amount of fat for a 2000-kcal diet is 44 to 78 g fat/day.

Appropriate Uses of the DRIs

The DRIs are intended mainly for diet planning (Table 2-1). Specifically, a diet plan should aim to meet any RDAs or AIs set. Finally, when planning diets, it is important not to exceed the upper level for a nutrient (Fig. 2-2).[1,6] Keep in mind also that DRIs apply to healthy people—none are necessarily appropriate amounts for undernourished individuals or those with diseases that require higher intakes. This concept will be covered in Chapters 12 through 15.

(Breakdown)

Table 2-1	Putting the DRIs for Nutrient Needs to Use
RDA	**Recommended Dietary Allowance.** Use to evaluate current intake for a specific nutrient. The farther intake strays above or below this value, the greater the likelihood a person will develop nutrition-related problems.
AI	**Adequate Intake.** Use to evaluate current intake for a specific nutrient, realizing that an AI implies that further research is required before scientists can establish a more definitive intake amount needed to set an RDA.
UL	**Upper Level.** Use to evaluate the highest amount of daily nutrient intake that is unlikely to cause adverse health effects in the long run. This value applies to chronic use and is set to protect even very susceptible people in the healthy general population. As intake rises higher than the UL, the potential for adverse effects generally increases.
EER	**Estimated Energy Requirement.** Use to estimate energy needs according to height, weight, gender, age, and physical activity pattern.
AMDR	**Adequate Macronutrient Distribution Range.** Use to determine whether percent of calories from each macronutrient falls within suggested range. The greater the discrepancy with AMDR, the greater the risk for nutrition-related chronic diseases.

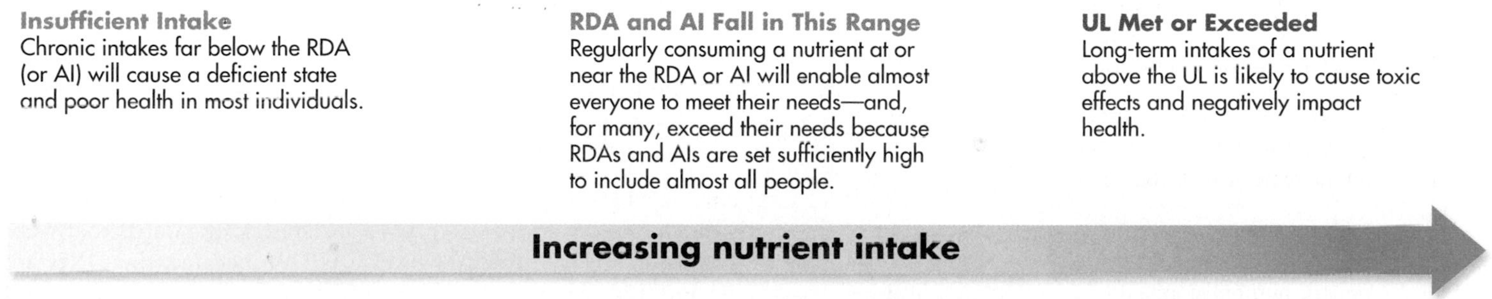

Insufficient Intake
Chronic intakes far below the RDA (or AI) will cause a deficient state and poor health in most individuals.

RDA and AI Fall in This Range
Regularly consuming a nutrient at or near the RDA or AI will enable almost everyone to meet their needs—and, for many, exceed their needs because RDAs and AIs are set sufficiently high to include almost all people.

UL Met or Exceeded
Long-term intakes of a nutrient above the UL is likely to cause toxic effects and negatively impact health.

Increasing nutrient intake

Figure 2-2 Think of the nutrient standards that are part of DRIs as points along a line ranging from an insufficient intake to a healthy intake level to an excessive intake.

Putting the DRIs into Action to Determine the Nutrient Density of Foods

[handwritten: higher the density the better the food source.]

Nutrient density has gained acceptance in recent years as a tool for assessing the nutritional quality of an individual food.[7] To determine the **nutrient density** of a food, divide the amount of a nutrient (protein, vitamin, mineral) in a serving of the food by your daily recommended intake (e.g., RDA, AI). Next, divide the calories in a serving of the food by your daily calorie need (EER). Then, compare these values—a food is said to be nutrient dense if it provides a greater contribution to your nutrient need than calorie need. The higher a food's nutrient density, the better it is as a source for a particular nutrient. For example, the 70 mg of vitamin C and 65 calories provided by an orange supplies 108% of the RDA for a teenage girl (65 mg vitamin C) and only 4% of her 1800 daily calorie need. It is considered a nutrient-dense food for vitamin C. In contrast, the 52 mg of calcium in an orange provides only 4% of the teenage girl's calcium RDA (1300 mg).

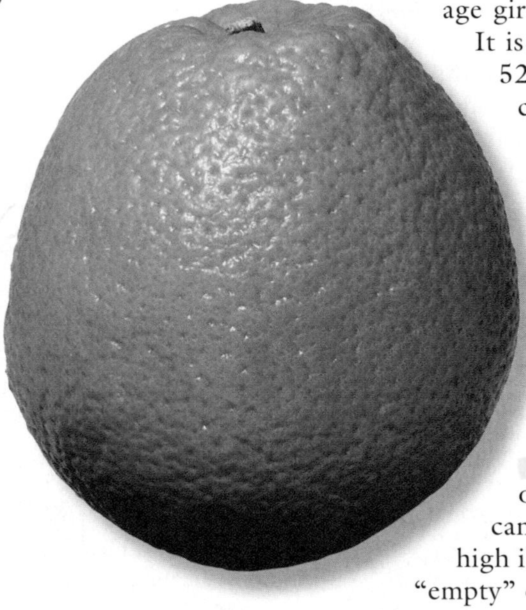

On a nutrient-by-nutrient basis, comparing the nutrient density of different foods is an easy way to identify the more nutritious choice.[8] It's more difficult to obtain an overall picture of nutritional quality. Some experts recommend averaging the nutrient density for key nutrients and comparing the average with the percent of daily calorie need provided. For example, as Figure 2-3 shows, an average of the nutrients in the fat-free milk is about 15% and supplies only 4% of calories, whereas the nutrients in the cola average approximately 0 while supplying 5% of calories. The fat-free milk is much more nutrient dense than a sugared soft drink for many nutrients. Sugared soft drinks and other foods that are not nutrient dense (e.g., chips, cookies, and candy) are often called **empty-calorie foods** because they tend to be high in sugar and/or fat but few other nutrients—that is, the calories are "empty" of nutrients.

*[handwritten: key term *]*

*[handwritten: Good Ques for chap Test *]*

Knowledge Check

1. Which dietary standard is set based on Estimated Average Requirements (EARs)?
2. Which dietary standard is set when an Estimated Average Requirement (EAR) cannot be set?
3. Which of the Dietary Reference Intakes (DRIs) is set at the maximum daily intake amount?

▶ **DV = RDI + DRV**

Daily Value (DV): Generic nutrient standard used on Nutrition Facts labels; it comprises both Reference Daily Intakes (RDIs) and Daily Reference Values (DRVs).

Reference Daily Intakes (RDIs): Part of the DV; generic nutrient standard set for vitamins and minerals (except sodium and potassium).

Daily Reference Values (DRVs): Part of the DV; generic nutrient standard set for energy-producing nutrients (fat, carbohydrate, protein, fiber), cholesterol, sodium, and potassium.

 ## 2.2 Daily Values (DVs)

The Nutrition Facts panel on a food label compares the amount of nutrients in the food with a set of standards called Daily Values (DVs). DVs are generic standards that were developed by the U.S. Food and Drug Administration (FDA) because the DRIs are age- and gender-specific and it isn't practical to have different food labels for men and women or for teens and adults.

DVs have been set for 4 groups: infants, toddlers, pregnant or lactating women, and people over 4 years of age. The DVs that appear on all food labels—except

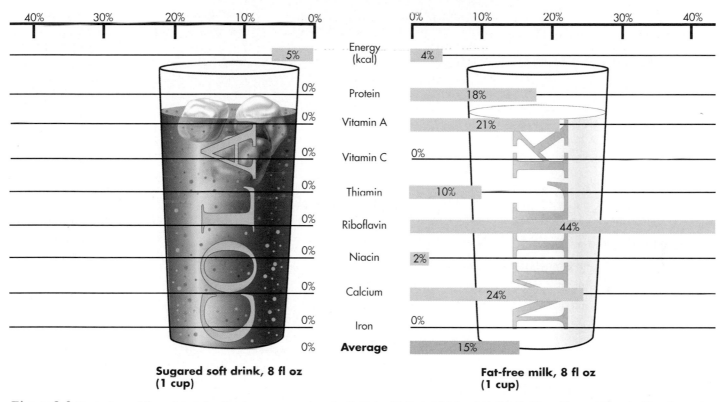

Percent Contribution to Adolescent Female RDAs

	Sugared soft drink, 8 fl oz (1 cup)	Fat-free milk, 8 fl oz (1 cup)
Energy (kcal)	5%	4%
Protein	0%	18%
Vitamin A	0%	21%
Vitamin C	0%	0%
Thiamin	0%	10%
Riboflavin	0%	44%
Niacin	0%	2%
Calcium	0%	24%
Iron	0%	0%
Average	0%	15%

Figure 2-3 Comparison of the nutrient density of a sugar-sweetened soft drink with that of fat-free (skim) milk. The milk provides a significantly greater contribution to nutrient intake per calorie than the soft drink. Compare the lengths of the bars indicating vitamin or mineral contribution with the bar that represents energy content. For the soft drink, no nutrient surpasses energy content. Fat-free milk, in contrast, has longer nutrient bars for protein, vitamin A, the vitamins thiamin and riboflavin, and calcium.

those specially marketed to infants, toddlers, or pregnant or lactating women—are those set for people over age 4 years. This book will focus on the DVs for those over age 4 years.

The DVs are based on 2 sets of dietary standards: Reference Daily Intakes and Daily Reference Values. These terms—*Reference Daily Intakes* and *Daily Reference Values*—do not appear on food labels. Instead, the term *Daily Value* is used to represent the combination of these 2 sets of dietary standards. Table 2-2 displays the DVs. Even though the term *DV* is used on Nutrition Facts panels, it is important for nutrition and health professionals to understand how Reference Daily Intakes and Daily Reference Values differ.

▶ Canada also has a set of Daily Values for use on food labels (see Appendix D).

Reference Daily Intakes (RDIs)

Reference Daily Intakes (RDIs) are set for vitamins and most minerals—these nutrients all have established nutrient standards, such as RDAs. RDI values for people over age 4 years tend to be set at the highest value for any life-stage group in the 1968 edition of the RDAs. Consider iron—in 1968, adult women and adolescents had the highest iron RDA (i.e., 18 mg/day). The iron RDI for people over age 4 years was set at this value. The RDI values currently in use are generally slightly higher than current RDAs and related nutrient standards (see Table 2-2). Many nutrition experts believe the RDIs should be revised to reflect the latest nutrient standards.[9]

Table 2-2 Comparison of Daily Values with Current RDAs and Other Nutrient Standards

Dietary Constituent	Unit of Measure[1]	Current Daily Values for People over 4 Years of Age	RDA or Other Dietary Standard	
			Males 19–30 Years Old	Females 19–30 Years Old
Daily Reference Values (DRVs)				
Total fat	g	30% kcal	—	—
Saturated fatty acids	g	10% kcal	—	—
Protein	g	10% kcal	56	46
Cholesterol	mg	<300	—	—
Carbohydrate	g	60% kcal	130	130
Fiber	g	11.5g/1000 kcal	38	25
Sodium[2]	mg	<2400	1500	1500
Potassium	mg	3500	4700	4700
Reference Daily Intakes (RDIs)				
Vitamin A	µg Retinol Activity Equivalents	1000	900	700
Vitamin D	International units (µg)	400 (10)	200 (5)	200 (5)
Vitamin E	International units (mg)	30 (14–20)	22–33 (15)	22–33 (15)
Vitamin K	µg	80	120	90
Vitamin C	mg	60	90	75
Folate	µg	400	400	400
Thiamin	mg	1.5	1.2	1.1
Riboflavin	mg	1.7	1.3	1.1
Niacin	mg	20	16	14
Vitamin B-6	mg	2	1.3	1.3
Vitamin B-12	µg	6	2.4	2.4
Biotin	mg (µg)	0.3 (300)	0.03 (30)	0.03 (30)
Pantothenic acid	mg	10	5	5
Calcium	mg	1000	1000	1000
Phosphorus	mg	1000	700	700
Iodide	µg	150	150	150
Iron	mg	18	8	18
Magnesium	mg	400	400	310
Copper	mg	2	0.9	0.9
Zinc	mg	15	11	8
Chloride[2]	mg	3400	2300	2300
Manganese	mg	2	2.3	1.8
Selenium	µg	70	55	55
Chromium	µg	120	35	25
Molybdenum	µg	75	45	45

[1]Abbreviations: g = gram; mg = milligram; µg = microgram.
[2]The considerably higher Daily Values for sodium and chloride allow for greater diet flexibility, but the extra amounts are not needed to maintain health.

Daily Reference Values (DRVs)

Daily Reference Values (DRVs) are standards for energy-producing nutrients (fat, saturated fat, carbohydrate, protein, fiber), cholesterol, sodium, and potassium. Many of these nutrients do not have an established RDA or other nutrient standard (e.g., total fat, saturated fat, carbohydrate).

The DRVs for the energy-producing nutrients are based on daily calorie intake. The FDA selected 2000 calories as the reference for calculating percent DVs for energy-producing nutrients, although larger food packages can display values for both a 2000- and a 2500-calorie diet. Regardless of the calorie level used, the DRVs for energy-producing nutrients are always calculated like this:

- Fat is set at 30% of calories.
- Saturated fat is set at 10% of calories.
- Carbohydrate is set at 60% of calories.
- Protein is set at 10% of calories.
- Fiber is set at 11.5 g of fiber per 1000 calories.

Note that the values for sodium, potassium, and cholesterol, as well as the vitamins and minerals that have RDIs, do not vary with calorie intake.

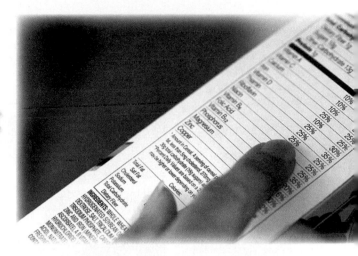

Use the Nutrition Facts panel to learn more about the nutrient content of the foods you eat. Nutrient content is expressed as a % Daily Value. Canadian food laws and related food labels have a slightly different format (see Appendix D).

Putting the Daily Values into Action on Nutrition Facts Panels

With few exceptions, information related to the Daily Values is found on almost every food and beverage sold in the supermarket today. Their labels include the product name, name and address of the manufacturer, amount of product in the package, ingredients listed in descending order by weight, ingredients that are common allergens[10] (milk, eggs, fish, shellfish, peanuts, tree nuts, wheat, and soy; see Chapter 7 for details), and a Nutrition Facts panel. The Nutrition Facts panel lists the amounts of certain food components and reports many of them as % Daily Value. This required labeling is monitored in North America by government agencies, such as the FDA in the United States.

As you can see in Figure 2-4, Nutrition Facts panels present information for a single serving of food. Serving sizes are specified by the FDA so that they are consistent among similar foods. This means that all brands of ice cream, for example, must use the same serving size on their label. The serving sizes on Nutrition Facts panels are based on typical serving sizes eaten by Americans; as a result, they may differ from the serving sizes recommended by MyPyramid (see Section 2.5).

The following components must be listed on most Nutrition Facts panels: total calories (kcal), calories from fat, total fat, saturated fat, *trans* fat, cholesterol, sodium, total carbohydrate, fiber, sugars, protein, vitamin A, vitamin C, calcium, and iron. Labels of food that contain few nutrients, such as candy and soft drinks, may omit some nutrients. In addition to the components required on Nutrition Facts panels, manufacturers can choose to list other nutrients, such as polyunsaturated fat or potassium. Manufacturers are required to include a nutrient on the Nutrition Facts panel if they make a claim about its health benefits (see Claims on Food Labels later in this chapter) or if the food is fortified with that nutrient.

Notice in Figure 2-4 that the amount of fats, cholesterol, sodium, carbohydrates, and protein in a food is given in grams or milligrams. Most of these nutrients also are given as % Daily Value, as are vitamins and other minerals. Because protein deficiency is not a public health concern in the United States, listing % Daily Value for protein is not mandatory on foods for people over 4 years of age. If the % Daily Value is given on a label, the FDA requires that the product be analyzed for protein quality (see Chapter 7). This procedure is expensive and time

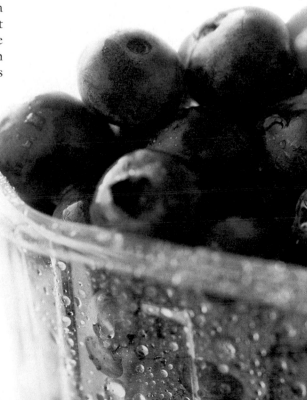

Fresh fruits, vegetables, fish, meats, and poultry are not required to have Nutrition Facts panels. However, many grocers distribute leaflets or display posters or notebooks that include Nutrition Facts panels for these foods. Nutrition Fact panels on fresh meat products likely will be required in the coming years. Examples of these posters are available at www.cfsan.fda/~dms/nutinfo.html

Figure 2-4 Food packages must list product name, name and address of the manufacturer, amount of product in the package, and ingredients. The Nutrition Facts panel is required on virtually all packaged food products. The % Daily Value listed on the label is the percent of the amount of a nutrient needed daily that is provided by a single serving of the product.

Serving size

Serving size is listed in household units (and grams). Pay careful attention to serving size to know how many servings you are eating: e.g., if you eat double the serving size, you must double the % Daily Values and calories.

Servings per container

The number of servings of the size given in the serving size above that are in one package of the food

% Daily Value

This shows how a single serving compares to the DV. Recall that the DVs for fat, saturated fat, cholesterol, protein, and fiber are based on a 2000-calorie diet.

Sugars DV

There is no % Daily Value for sugars. Limiting intake is the best advice.

Protein DV

% Daily Value for protein is generally not included due to expensive testing required to determine protein quality.

Daily Value Footnote

This footnote appears on many labels. It is omitted when there is too little space on the label to print it. The footnote reports the DVs used to compute the % Daily Value for a 2000- and 2500-calorie diet.

Nutrient claims, such as "*Good source,*" and health claims, such as "*Reduce the risk of osteoporosis,*" must follow legal definitions.

Nutrients

These nutrients must appears on most labels. Labels of foods that contain few nutrients, such as candy and soft drinks, may omit some nutrients. Some manufacturers list more nutrients. Other nutrients must be listed if manufacturers make a claim about them or if the food is fortified with them.

Name and address of the food manufacturer

Ingredients are listed in descending order by weight.

A Quick Guide to Nutrient Sources

% Daily Value

20% or more = *Rich source*
10%–19% = *Good source*

MICROMAC
Macaroni and Cheese ®

Good Source of Calcium

A diet rich in calcium may reduce the risk of osteoporosis

Quick Foods
191 Toronto St
Mitchell, ON
M2K1A3
PO box 1435

Nutrition Facts
Serving Size 1 Pouch (61g)
Servings Per Container 6

Amount Per Serving

Calories 250	Calories from Fat 70

	% Daily Value*
Total Fat 7g	**11%**
Saturated Fat 2.5g	**13%**
Trans Fat 1g	**
Cholesterol 5mg	**2%**
Sodium 400mg	**16%**
Total Carbohydrate 38g	**13%**
Dietary Fiber <1g	**3%**
Sugars 6g	
Protein 7g	

Vitamin A 0% • Vitamin C 10%
Calcium 12% • Iron 8%

*Percent Daily Values are based on a 2,000 calorie diet. Your daily values may be higher or lower depending on your calorie needs:

	Calories:	2,000	2,500
Total Fat	Less than	65g	80g
Sat Fat	Less than	20g	25g
Cholest	Less than	300mg	300mg
Sodium	Less than	2,400mg	2,400mg
Total Carb		300g	375g
Fiber		25g	30g

Calories per gram:

Fat 9 • Carbohydrate 4 • Protein 4

**Intake should be as low as possible.

INGREDIENTS:ENRICHED MACARONI PRODUCT (DURUM WHEAT FLOUR, GLYCERYL MONO-STEARATE, SALT, NIACIN, FERROUS SULPHATE, THIAMIN MONONITRATE (VITAMIN B1), RIBOFLAVIN (VITAMIN B2), FOLIC ACID), CHEESE SAUCE MIX (WHEY, PARTIALLY HYDROGENATED SOYBEAN OIL, MALTODEXTRIN, WHEY PROTEIN CONCENTRATE, CORN SYRUP SOLIDS, SALT, MILKFAT, SUGAR, SODIUM, NATURAL FLAVOR, CITRIC ACID, MONOSODIUM GLUTAMATE, MODIFIED FOOD STARCH, LACTIC ACID, YELLOW 5.

consuming; thus, many companies opt not to list % Daily Value for protein. However, labels on food for infants and children under 4 years of age must include the % Daily Value for protein, as must labels on any food carrying a claim about protein content.

Recall that all of the values shown on Nutrition Facts panels are for a single serving of the food. Thus, to determine the total amount of calories or a nutrient in more than 1 serving, the value on the label must be multiplied by the number of servings consumed. For instance, let's say you ate the entire box of MicroMac shown in Figure 2-4—that would be 6 servings. The entire package would provide 1500 calories (250 kcal per serving × 6 servings per container = 1500 calories), 78% of total carbohydrate (13% per serving × 6 servings per container = 78%), 36 grams of sugar, and so on.

You can use the DVs to determine how a particular food fits in an overall diet (Fig. 2-5). If, for example, a single food provides 50% of the DV for fat, then it is a good idea to either select a different food that is lower in fat or be sure other choices that day are low in fat. The DVs also can help you determine how close your overall diet comes to meeting recommendations. For instance, if you consume 2000 calories per day, your total fat intake for the day should be 65 g or less. If you consume 10 g of fat at breakfast, you have 55 grams, or 85%, of your DV for fat left for the rest of the day. If you eat more or less than 2000 calories per

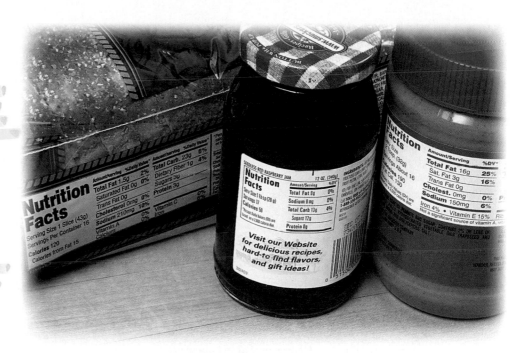

The nutrition information on the Nutrition Facts panels on these products can be combined to determine the nutrient intake for a peanut butter and jelly sandwich.

day, you can still use the Nutrition Facts panel. For example, if you consume only 1600 calories per day, the total percentage of DV you eat for fat, saturated fat, carbohydrate, protein, and fiber should add up to 80% DV because 1600/2000 = 0.8, or 80%. If you eat 3000 calories daily, the total percentage of DV you eat of fat, saturated fat, carbohydrate, protein, and fiber in all the foods you eat in 1 day can add up to 150% DV because 3000/2000 = 1.5, or 150%. Remember, you need to make adjustments only for the nutrients that are based on calorie intake: carbohydrate, protein, fat, saturated fat, and fiber. For nutrients not based on calorie intake, such as vitamin A and cholesterol, just add percentage of DVs in all the foods you eat to determine how close your diet comes to meeting recommendations.

As you may have noticed, the nutrients listed on Nutrition Facts panels tend to be the ones of greatest health concern in North America. Many people eat too much fat, saturated fat, *trans* fat, cholesterol, sodium, and sugar. Many also are concerned that they don't get enough fiber, calcium, iron, vitamin A, and vitamin C. Thus, for the best health, most people should aim to keep their intake of the following nutrients at or below 100% Daily Value: total fat, saturated fat, cholesterol, and sodium. Most people also should plan their diets to achieve 100% of the DV for fiber, vitamin A, vitamin C, iron, and calcium.

Nutrition Facts panels often include a footnote that shows the intake recommendations for dietary components such as fat, saturated fat, cholesterol, sodium, carbohydrate, and fiber. The amounts listed are for a 2000-calorie diet and, when package space allows, a 2500-calorie diet. This footnote helps label readers see how the DVs are calculated for these nutrients.

▶ As you saw in Figure 1-12 (Chapter 1), the labels on nutrient and herbal supplements have a different layout than those on foods. These labels include a "Supplement Facts" heading.

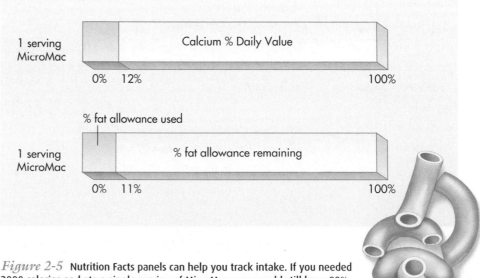

Figure 2-5 Nutrition Facts panels can help you track intake. If you needed 2000 calories and ate a single serving of MicroMac, you would still have 89% Daily Value of your fat allowance left. In addition, you would have met 12% Daily Value for calcium.

▶ Canada has established a set of health claims for nutrition labels (see Appendix D).

▶ Claims on foods fall into these categories:
- Nutrient content claims—closely regulated by the FDA
- Health claims—closely regulated by the FDA
- Preliminary health claims—regulated by the FDA but there is only limited scientific evidence for the claim
- Structure/function claims—not FDA approved; manufacturer is responsible for their accuracy

Claims on Food Labels

As a marketing tool directed toward health-conscious consumers, food manufacturers like to assert that some of their products have certain nutrient levels or health benefits. After reviewing hundreds of comments on the proposed rule allowing nutrient and health claims, the FDA, which has legal oversight for most food products, decided to permit certain specific claims. Although these claims must comply with FDA regulations, you can use Daily Value information on Nutrition Facts panels to verify nutrient content and health claims made on food packages.[11]

Nutrient content claims are those that describe the nutrients in a food. Examples are "low in fat," "rich in vitamin A," and "zero calories."

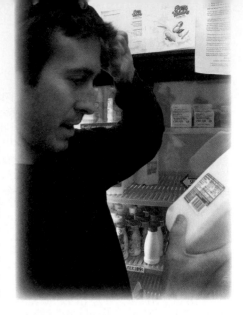

Nutrition Facts panels can help you locate foods that will provide a nutrient-rich diet.

Table 2-3 Summary of Nutrient Claims on Food Labels

Calories	
Calorie free	Less than 5 kcal per serving
Low calorie	40 kcal or less per serving (if the serving is small,* per 50 g of the food)
Reduced or fewer calories	At least 25% less kcal per serving than reference food
Light or lite	50% less fat if half or more of the food's kcal are from fat; 50% less fat or 33% less kcal if less than half of the food's kcal are from fat
Total Fat	
Fat free	Less than 0.5 g fat per serving
Low fat	3 g or less per serving (if the serving is small, per 50 g of the food)
Reduced or less fat	At least 25% less per serving than reference food
Lean	Seafood, poultry, or meat with less than 10 g total fat, 4.5 g or less saturated fat, and less than 95 mg cholesterol per reference amount
Extra lean	Seafood, poultry, or meat with less than 5 g total fat, less than 2 g saturated fat, and less than 95 mg cholesterol per reference amount
Saturated Fat	
Saturated fat free	Less than 0.5 g saturated fat and less than 0.5 g *trans* fatty acids per serving
Low saturated fat	1 g or less per serving and 15% or less of kcal from saturated fat
Reduced or less saturated fat	At least 25% less per serving than reference food
Cholesterol	
Cholesterol free	Less than 2 mg cholesterol and 2 g or less saturated fat per serving
Low cholesterol	20 mg or less cholesterol and 2 g or less saturated fat per serving (if the serving is small, per 50 g of the food)
	Reduced or less cholesterol. At least 25% less cholesterol per serving than reference food and 2 g or less saturated fat
Sugar	
Sugar free	Less than 0.5 g per serving
No added sugar or without added sugar	No sugars or sugar-containing ingredient (e.g., jam, applesauce) added during processing or packing
Reduced sugar	At least 25% less sugar per serving than reference food

All nutrient content claims must comply with regulations set by the FDA. Table 2-3 summarizes the legal definitions of nutrient content claims permitted to appear on food packages. For example, if a product claims to be "low sodium," it must have 140 mg or less of sodium per serving.

Health claims describe a relationship between a disease and a nutrient, food, or food constituent.[12] All permitted health claims have significant scientific agreement that they are true. All health claims must use a *may* or *might* qualifier in the statement. The following are permitted health claims.

- A diet with enough calcium may reduce risk of osteoporosis.
- A diet low in total fat may reduce risk of some cancers.
- A diet low in saturated fat and cholesterol may reduce risk of cardiovascular disease (typically referred to as *heart disease* on the label).
- A diet low in saturated fat and cholesterol that also includes 25 g/day of soy protein may reduce risk of cardiovascular disease. The statement "one serving of (food name) provides _____ g of soy protein" must also appear as part of the health claim.
- Fatty acids from oils present in fish may reduce risk of cardiovascular disease.

Sodium	
Sodium free or salt free	Less than 5 mg per serving
Very low sodium	35 mg or less per serving (if the serving is small, per 50 g of the food)
Low sodium	140 mg or less per serving (if the serving is small, per 50 g of the food)
Light (for sodium reduced products)	If food meets definition of low calorie and low fat, and sodium is reduced by at least 50%
Light in sodium	At least 50% less per serving than reference food
Reduced or less sodium	At least 25% less per serving than reference food
Lightly salted	At least 50% less sodium than normally added to reference food; if it doesn't meet definition of low sodium, this must be stated on the label
No salt added, unsalted	If not sodium free, must declare "This Is Not a Sodium Free Food"
Fiber	
Any claim	If food is not low in total fat, must state total fat in conjunction with fiber claim
Other Claims	
High, rich in, or excellent source	20% or more of the DV per reference amount; may be used to describe protein, vitamins, minerals, dietary fiber, or potassium; may not be used for total carbohydrate
Good source, contains, or provides	10 to 19% of the DV per reference amount; may be used to describe protein, vitamins, minerals, dietary fiber, or potassium; may not be used for total carbohydrate
More, added, extra, or plus	10% or more of the DV per reference amount; may be used for vitamins, minerals, protein, dietary fiber, and potassium
High-potency	May be used to describe individual vitamins or minerals present at 100% or more of the DV per reference amount
Fortified or enriched	Vitamins and/or minerals added to the product in amounts in at least 10% above levels normally present in food; *enriched* generally refers to replacing nutrients lost in processing, whereas *fortified* refers to adding nutrients not originally present in the specific food
Healthy	Varies with food type; generally is a food that is low fat and low saturated fat, has no more than 480 to 600 mg of sodium or 95 mg of cholesterol per serving, and provides at least 10% of the DV for vitamin A, vitamin C, protein, calcium, iron, or fiber
Light or lite	Used with calories and sodium (see above); also may be used to describe texture and color, as long as the label explains the intent—for example, *light brown sugar* and *light and fluffy*

*Small serving size or small reference amount = reference amount of 30 g or less or 2 tbsp or less.

- Margarines containing plant stanols and sterols may reduce risk of cardiovascular disease (see Chapter 6).
- A diet low in sodium and high in potassium may reduce risk of hypertension and stroke.
- A diet adequate in the synthetic form of the B-vitamin folate (i.e., folic acid) may reduce risk of neural tube defects (a type of birth defect) (see Chapter 13).
- The use of sugarless gum may reduce risk of tooth decay, especially when compared with foods high in sugars and starches.
- A diet rich in fruits and vegetables may reduce risk of some cancers.
- A diet rich in fiber-containing grain products, fruits, and/or vegetables may reduce risk of some cancers.
- A diet rich in fruits, vegetables, and/or grain products that contain fiber may reduce risk of cardiovascular disease. Oats (oatmeal, oat bran, and oat flour) and **psyllium** are fiber-rich ingredients that can be singled out in reducing the risk of cardiovascular disease, as long as the statement also says the diet should also be low in saturated fat and cholesterol.
- A diet rich in whole-grain foods and/or other plant foods as well as low in total fat, saturated fat, and cholesterol may reduce risk of cardiovascular disease and certain cancers.

psyllium Type of dietary fiber found in the seeds of the plantago plant.

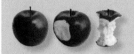

Take Action

Applying the Nutrition Facts Label to Your Daily Food Choices

Imagine that you are at the supermarket, looking for a quick meal before a busy evening. In the frozen food section, you find 2 brands of frozen cheese manicotti (see labels *a* and *b*). Which of the 2 brands would you choose? What information on the Nutrition Facts labels contributed to this decision?

Nutrition Facts

Serving Size 1 Package (260g)
Servings Per Container 1

Amount Per Serving

Calories 390 — Calories from Fat 160

	% Daily Value*
Total Fat 18g	27%
Saturated Fat 9g	45%
Trans Fat 2g	**
Cholesterol 45mg	14%
Sodium 880mg	36%
Total Carbohydrate 38g	13%
Dietary Fiber 4g	15%
Sugars 12g	
Protein 17g	

Vitamin A 10% • Vitamin C 4%

Calcium 40% • Iron 8%

*Percent Daily Values are based on a 2,000 calorie diet. Your daily values may be higher or lower depending on your calorie needs:

	Calories:	2,000	2,500
Total Fat	Less than	65g	80g
Sat Fat	Less than	20g	25g
Cholesterol	Less than	300mg	300mg
Sodium	Less than	2,400mg	2,400mg
Total Carbohydrate		300g	375g
Dietary Fiber		25g	30g

Calories per gram:
Fat 9 • Carbohydrate 4 • Protein 4

**Intake of *trans* fat should be as low as possible.

(a)

Nutrition Facts

Serving Size 1 Package (260g)
Servings Per Container 1

Amount Per Serving

Calories 230 — Calories from Fat 35

	% Daily Value*
Total Fat 4g	6%
Saturated Fat 2g	10%
Trans Fat 1g	**
Cholesterol 15mg	4%
Sodium 590mg	24%
Total Carbohydrate 28g	9%
Dietary Fiber 3g	12%
Sugars 10g	
Protein 19g	

Vitamin A 10% • Vitamin C 10%

Calcium 35% • Iron 4%

*Percent Daily Values are based on a 2,000 calorie diet. Your daily values may be higher or lower depending on your calorie needs:

	Calories:	2,000	2,500
Total Fat	Less than	65g	80g
Sat Fat	Less than	20g	25g
Cholesterol	Less than	300mg	300mg
Sodium	Less than	2,400mg	2,400mg
Potassium		3,500mg	3,500mg
Total Carbohydrate		300g	375g
Dietary Fiber		25g	30g

Calories per gram:
Fat 9 • Carbohydrate 4 • Protein 4

**Intake of *trans* fat should be as low as possible.

(b)

Only food products that meet the following requirements can bear a health claim. First, the food must be a "good source" (before any fortification) of fiber, protein, vitamin A, vitamin C, calcium, or iron—it must provide at least 10% of the Daily Value for 1 or more of these nutrients. Second, a single serving of the food cannot contain more than 13 g of fat, 4 g of saturated fat, 60 mg of cholesterol, or 480 mg of sodium. If a food exceeds any one of these requirements, no health claim can be made for it despite its other nutritional qualities. For example, even though whole milk is high in calcium, its label can't make a health claim about calcium and a reduced risk of osteoporosis because whole milk contains 5 g of saturated fat per serving. Third, the product must meet criteria specific to the health claim being made. For example, a health claim regarding fat and cancer can be made only if the product contains 3 g or less of fat per serving, which is the standard for low-fat foods.

In December 2002, the FDA began permitting **preliminary health claims** based on incomplete scientific evidence as long as the label qualified it with a disclaimer such as "this evidence is not conclusive" and the food meets the definition of being healthy (see Table 2-3).[12] So far, few preliminary health claims have appeared on food packages (nuts, such as walnuts, and fish have been some of the first examples).

Recall from Chapter 1 that another type of claim, structure/function claim, can appear on food labels. **Structure/function claims** describe how a nutrient affects human body structure or function, such as "iron builds strong blood." They do not focus on disease risk reduction, as health claims do. The FDA does not approve or authorize structure/function claims; however, manufacturers are responsible for ensuring that these claims are accurate and not misleading.

▶ To learn more about nutrient content claims, visit

www.cfsan.fda.gov.

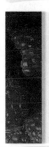

Knowledge Check

1. How do Reference Daily Intakes and Daily Reference Values differ?
2. Which nutrients on Nutrition Facts panels should most people aim to keep below 100% Daily Value?
3. What requirements must a food meet before a health claim can be made about it?

2.3 Nutrient Composition of Foods

Nutrient databases make it possible to estimate quickly the amount of calories and many nutrients in the foods we eat. With this information, it is possible to see how closely intake matches dietary standards, such as the RDA and DV. These databases also can be used to determine the nutrient density and energy density of foods.

The data in nutrient databases are the results of thousands of analytical chemistry studies conducted in laboratories around the world. They are easy to use; however, generating the data requires years of research to develop laboratory methods that produce accurate and reliable data and years more to analyze samples of many different foods and then construct the data tables. Keep in mind that there are many nutrients, and all require a unique laboratory analysis method. To get an idea of the enormity of this task, multiply the number of nutrients by all the different foods (plant and animal species) people eat. As you might guess, countless foods have not been analyzed yet and some nutrients have been measured in only a limited number of foods.

Nutrient values in the databases are average amounts found in the analyzed samples of the food. Currently, these values cannot account for the many factors that affect nutrient levels in food we eat, factors such as farming conditions (e.g., soil type, fertilizers, weather, season, geographic region, genetic differences in plant varieties and animal breeds, and animal feed), maturity and ripeness of plants when harvested, food processing, shipping conditions, storage time, and cooking processes. For instance, the vitamin C content of an orange is influenced by where it was grown, the variety of the orange, and how ripe it was when picked. It also is affected by how long it took to get the orange to the store where you bought it, the temperature of the truck that delivered it there, and how long it stayed in your refrigerator before you ate it. Nutrient databases also cannot account for how nutrients are handled in the body—as you'll see in later chapters, the ability to absorb nutrients, especially minerals, can be affected by factors such as medications, compounds in foods, and digestive disorders.

The variations in nutrient content do not mean that nutrient databases are unreliable or that you cannot depend on food to supply nutrients in amounts that support optimal health. But it is wise to view nutrient databases as tools that approximate nutrient intake, rather than precise measurements. Even with these limitations, nutrient databases are important tools for estimating calories and nutrients.

Putting Nutrient Databases into Action to Determine Energy Density and Dietary Intake

Nutrient databases can be used in many ways, including calculating a food's energy density. **Energy density** is determined by comparing a food's calorie content per gram weight of the food. Energy-dense foods are high in calories but weigh very little. Examples include nuts, cookies, most fried foods, and snack foods. For example, there are more than 5.5 kcal in 1 gram of bacon. Foods low in energy density contain large amounts of water, which makes them weigh a lot, but contain few calories (keep in mind that water is calorie-free). Low-energy-dense foods include fruits, vegetables, and any other food that incorporates lots of water during cooking, such as stews, casseroles, and oatmeal (Table 2-4). Lettuce, for instance, has about 0.1 calorie in a gram. As you'll see in Chapter 10, foods that are low in energy density help a person feel full, whereas foods with high energy density must be eaten in greater amounts in order to contribute to fullness.[7, 13] Thus, low-energy-dense foods can help keep calorie intake under control.[14, 15] And foods with high energy density can help people with poor appetites, such as some older people, maintain or gain weight.

You also can use nutrient databases to find out the amounts of nutrients and calories you consume. This involves locating a food you ate and noting the quantity of each

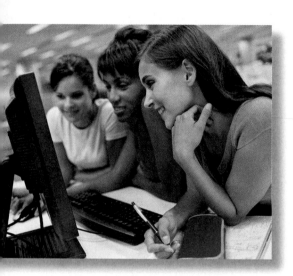

Computerized nutrient data tables provide a quick and easy way to discover just how nutrient and energy dense the foods you eat are. Visit this website: **www.nal.usda.gov/fnic/foodcomp/search**.

Table 2-4 Energy Density of Common Foods (Listed in Relative Order)

Very Low Energy Density (Less Than 0.6 kcal/g)	Low Energy Density (0.6 to 1.5 kcal/g)	Medium Energy Density (1.5 to 4 kcal/g)	High Energy Density (Greater Than 4 kcal/g)
Lettuce	Whole milk	Eggs	Graham crackers
Tomatoes	Oatmeal	Ham	Fat-free sandwich cookies
Strawberries	Cottage cheese	Pumpkin pie	Chocolate
Broccoli	Beans	Whole-wheat bread	Chocolate chip cookies
Salsa	Bananas	Bagels	Tortilla chips
Grapefruit	Broiled fish	White bread	Bacon
Fat-free milk	Non-fat yogurt	Raisins	Potato chips
Carrots	Ready-to-eat breakfast cereals with 1% low-fat milk	Cream cheese	Peanuts
Vegetable soup	Plain baked potato	Cake with frosting	Peanut butter
	Cooked rice	Pretzels	Mayonnaise
	Spaghetti noodles	Rice cakes	Butter or margarine
			Vegetables oils

Data adopted from Rolls B, Barnett RA: *Volumetrics*. New York: HarperCollins, 2000.

nutrient. If you ate more or less than the serving size stated, you will need to adjust the values. For instance, if you ate 4 ounces of cheese and the database values are for 2 ounces, you'll need to double the values in the table. Because not every food has been analyzed, you may need to select a food that is similar to the one you actually ate. If you ate Roquefort cheese or Bob's Pizza, for example, you may need to use the values for blue cheese or Tom's Pizza. Many combination foods (e.g., tuna salad, bean burritos) may not be included in the tables; for these foods, you will need to identify the ingredients used, estimate the amounts in the recipe (e.g., 2 oz tuna, 2 tbsp mayonnaise), and look up the nutrient values for each ingredient. Becoming aware of the amounts of nutrients and calories in the foods you eat can help you improve the healthfulness of your diet.

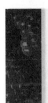

Knowledge Check

1. What are some factors that affect nutrient levels in food?
2. What is energy density?
3. What are some examples of high energy-density and low energy-density foods?

 ## 2.4 Dietary Guidelines for Americans

The diets of many people in the United States and Canada are too high in calories, fat, saturated fat, *trans* fat, cholesterol, sugar, salt, and alcohol.[16] Many consume insufficient amounts of whole grains, fruits, and vegetables. These dietary patterns put many of us at risk of major chronic "killer" diseases, such as cardiovascular disease, cancer, and alcoholism. In response to concerns about the prevalence of these killer disease patterns, every 5 years since 1980, the U.S. Department of Agriculture (USDA) and U.S. Department of Health and Human Services (DHHS) publish the Dietary Guidelines for Americans (Dietary Guidelines for short).

The Dietary Guidelines are the foundation of the U.S. government's nutrition policy and education. They reflect what scientific experts believe is the most accurate and up-to-date scientific knowledge about nutritious diets, physical activity, and related healthy lifestyle choices. The Dietary Guidelines are designed to meet nutrient needs while reducing the risk of obesity, hypertension, cardiovascular disease, type 2 diabetes, alcoholism, and foodborne illness. The Dietary Guidelines also guide government nutrition programs, research, food labeling, and nutrition education and promotion. For example, the Dietary Guidelines provide the scientific basis for the design of federal nutrition assistance programs, such as the USDA's school breakfast and lunch programs, the Food Stamp Program, and the WIC Program (Supplemental Food Program for Women, Infants and Children). In addition, MyPyramid is based on the recommendations of the Dietary Guidelines (see the next section in this chapter).

A basic premise of the Dietary Guidelines is that nutrient needs should be met primarily by consuming foods.[17] Foods provide an array of nutrients and other compounds that may have beneficial effects on health. In certain cases, fortified foods and dietary supplements may be useful sources of one or more nutrients that otherwise might be consumed in less than recommended amounts. These practices are especially important for people whose typical food choices lead to a diet that cannot meet nutrient recommendations, such as for calcium. However, dietary supplements are not a substitute for a healthful diet.

The latest Dietary Guidelines for Americans (2005) have 41 key recommendations, of which 23 are for people aged 2 years and older and 18 are for special population groups, such as pregnant women and older adults. The Dietary Guidelines recommendations are grouped into the 9 general topics shown in Figure 2-6.

For helpful consumer publications related to the 2005 Dietary Guidelines for Americans, visit www.healthierus.gov/dietaryguidelines.

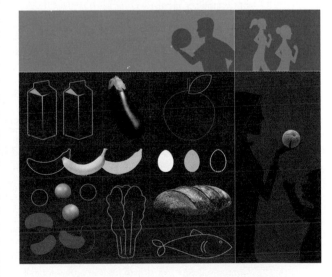

Dietary Guidelines
for Americans
2005

U.S. Department of Health and Human Services
U.S. Department of Agriculture
www.healthierus.gov/dietaryguidelines

Figure 2-6 Key recommendations within each general topic from the latest Dietary Guidelines for Americans.

ADEQUATE NUTRIENTS WITHIN ENERGY NEEDS

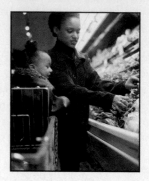

- Consume a variety of nutrient-dense foods and beverages within and among the basic food groups while choosing foods that limit the intake of saturated and *trans* fats, cholesterol, added sugars, salt, and alcohol.

- Meet recommended intakes within energy needs by adopting a balanced eating pattern, such as MyPyramid or the DASH diet (see chapter 14).

Key Recommendations for Specific Population Groups

- *People over age 50.* Consume vitamin B-12 in its crystalline form (i.e., fortified foods or supplements).

- *Women of childbearing age who may become pregnant.* Eat foods high in iron from animal products and/or consume iron-rich plant foods or iron-fortified foods with an enhancer of iron absorption, such as vitamin C–rich foods.

- *Women of childbearing age who may become pregnant and those in the first few months of pregnancy.* Consume adequate amount of the synthetic form of the B vitamin folate (i.e., folic acid) daily (from fortified foods or supplements) in addition to food forms of folate found in a varied diet.

- *Older adults, people with dark skin, and people exposed to insufficient ultraviolet band radiation (i.e., sunlight).* Consume extra vitamin D from vitamin D–fortified foods and/or supplements.

WEIGHT MANAGEMENT

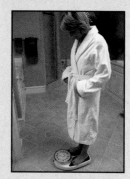

- To maintain body weight in a healthy range, balance calorie intake from foods and beverages with energy expended.

- To prevent gradual weight gain over time, make small decreases in calorie intake from food and beverages and increase physical activity.

Key Recommendations for Specific Population Groups

- *Those who need to lose weight.* Aim for a slow, steady weight loss by decreasing calorie intake while maintaining an adequate nutrient intake and increasing physical activity.

- *Overweight children.* Reduce the rate of body weight gain while allowing for growth and development. Consult a health-care provider before placing a child on a weight-reduction diet.

- *Pregnant women.* Ensure appropriate weight gain as specified by a health-care provider.

- *Breastfeeding women.* Moderate weight reduction is safe and does not compromise weight gain of the breastfeeding infant.

- *Overweight adults and overweight children with chronic diseases and/or on medication.* Consult a health-care provider about weight-loss strategies prior to starting a weight-reduction program to ensure appropriate management of other health conditions.

FOOD GROUPS TO ENCOURAGE

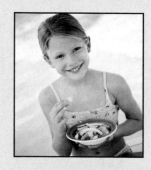

- Consume a sufficient amount of fruits and vegetables while staying within calorie needs. Two cups of fruit and 2½ cups of vegetables per day are recommended for a reference 2000-kcal intake, with higher or lower amounts depending on one's calorie needs.

- Choose a variety of fruits and vegetables each day. In particular, select from all 5 vegetable subgroups (dark green vegetables, orange vegetables, legumes, starchy vegetables, and other vegetables) several times a week.

- Consume 3 or more ounce-equivalents of whole-grain products per day, with the rest of the recommended grains coming from enriched or whole-grain products. In general, at least half the grains should come from whole grains.

- Consume 3 cups per day of fat-free or low-fat milk or equivalent milk products.

Key Recommendations for Specific Population Groups

- *Children and adolescents.* Consume whole-grain products often; at least half the grains should be whole grains. Children 2 to 8 years should consume 2 cups per day of fat-free or low-fat milk or equivalent milk products. Children 9 years of age and older should consume 3 cups per day of fat-free or low-fat milk or equivalent milk products.

Figure 2-6 Continued

PHYSICAL ACTIVITY

- Engage in regular physical activity and reduce sedentary activities to promote health, psychological well-being, and a healthy body weight.

- To reduce the risk for chronic disease in adulthood: engage in at least 30 minutes of moderate-intensity physical activity, above usual activity, at work or home on most days of the week.

- For most people, greater health benefits can be obtained by engaging in physical activity of more vigorous intensity or longer duration.

- To help manage body weight and prevent gradual, unhealthy body weight gain in adulthood: engage in approximately 60 minutes of moderate- to vigorous-intensity activity on most days of the week while not exceeding energy intake needs.

- To sustain weight loss in adulthood: participate in at least 60 to 90 minutes of daily moderate-intensity physical activity while not exceeding calorie needs. Some people (men over 40 years of age and women over 50 years of age) may need to consult with a health-care provider before participating in this level of activity.

- Achieve physical fitness by including cardiovascular conditioning, stretching exercises for flexibility, and resistance exercises or calisthenics for muscle strength and endurance.

Key Recommendations for Specific Population Groups

- *Children and adolescents.* Engage in at least 60 minutes of physical activity on most, preferably all, days of the week.

- *Pregnant women.* In the absence of medical complications, incorporate 30 minutes or more of moderate-intensity physical activity on most, if not all, days of the week. Avoid activities with a high risk of falling or abdominal trauma.

- *Breastfeeding women.* Be aware that neither acute nor regular exercise adversely affects the mother's ability to breastfeed successfully.

- *Older adults.* Participate in regular physical activity to reduce functional declines associated with aging and to achieve the other benefits of physical activity identified for all adults.

SODIUM AND POTASSIUM

- Consume less than 2300 mg of sodium per day (approximately 1 tsp of salt).

- Choose and prepare foods with little salt. At the same time, consume potassium-rich foods, such as fruits and vegetables.

Key Recommendations for Specific Population Groups

- *Individuals with hypertension, blacks, and middle-aged and older adults.* Aim to consume no more than 1500 mg of sodium per day, and meet the potassium recommendation (4700 mg per day) with food.

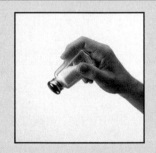

ALCOHOLIC BEVERAGES

- Those who choose to drink alcoholic beverages should do so sensibly and in moderation—defined as the consumption of up to 1 drink per day for women and up to 2 drinks per day for men (12 oz of a regular beer, 5 oz of wine, or $1\frac{1}{2}$ oz of 80–proof distilled spirits count as 1 drink).

- Alcoholic beverages should not be consumed by some individuals, including those who cannot restrict their alcohol intake, women of childbearing age who may become pregnant, pregnant and lactating women, children and adolescents, individuals taking medications that can interact with alcohol, and those with specific medical conditions.

- Alcoholic beverages should be avoided by individuals engaging in activities that require attention, skill, or coordination, such as driving or operating machinery.

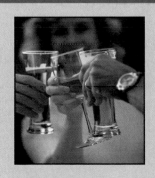

Figure 2-6 Continued

FATS

- Consume less than 10% of calories from saturated fatty acids and less than 300 mg per day of cholesterol, and keep *trans* fatty acid consumption as low as possible.

- Keep total fat intake between 20 and 35% of calorie intake, with most fats coming from sources of polyunsaturated and monounsaturated fatty acids, such as fish, nuts, and vegetable oils.

- When selecting and preparing meat, poultry, dry beans, and milk or milk products, make choices that are lean, low-fat, or fat-free.

- Limit intake of fats and oils high in saturated and/or *trans* fatty acids, and choose products low in such fats and oils.

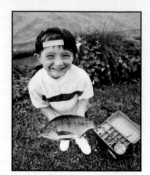

Key Recommendations for Specific Population Groups

- *Children and adolescents.* Keep total fat intake between 30 and 35% of calorie intake for children 2 to 3 years of age and between 25 and 35% of calorie intake for children and adolescents 4 to 18 years of age, with most fats coming from sources of polyunsaturated and monounsaturated fatty acids, such as fish, nuts, and vegetable oils.

FOOD SAFETY

To Avoid Microbial Foodborne Illness

- Clean hands, food contact surfaces, and fruits and vegetables. Meat and poultry should *not* be washed or rinsed to avoid spreading bacteria to other foods.

- Separate raw, cooked, and ready-to-eat foods while shopping, preparing, and storing foods.

- Cook foods to a safe temperature to kill microorganisms.

- Chill (refrigerate) perishable food promptly and defrost foods safely.

- Avoid raw (unpasteurized) milk or any products made from unpasteurized milk, raw or partially cooked eggs or foods containing raw eggs, and raw or undercooked meat and poultry, unpasteurized juices, and raw sprouts.

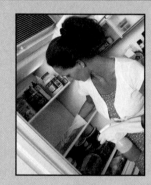

Key Recommendations for Specific Population Groups

- *Infants and young children, pregnant women, older adults, and those who are immunocompromised.* Do not eat or drink raw (unpasteurized) milk or any products made from unpasteurized milk, raw or partially cooked eggs or foods containing raw eggs, raw or undercooked meat and poultry, raw or undercooked fish or shellfish, unpasteurized juices, and raw sprouts.

- *Pregnant women, older adults, and those who are immunocompromised.* Eat only certain deli meats and frankfurters that have been reheated to steaming hot.

CARBOHYDRATES

- Choose fiber-rich fruits, vegetables, and whole grains often.

- Choose and prepare foods and beverages with little added sugars or caloric sweeteners, such as amounts suggested by MyPyramid.

- Reduce the incidence of dental caries by practicing good oral hygiene and consuming sugar- and starch-containing foods and beverages less frequently.

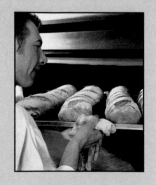

Other scientific groups, such as the American Heart Association, American Cancer Society, Canadian Ministries of Health, and World Health Organization also have issued dietary recommendations. All are consistent with the spirit of the Dietary Guidelines for Americans. These scientific groups, like the Dietary Guidelines, encourage people to modify their eating behavior in ways that are both healthful and pleasurable.

Putting the Dietary Guidelines in Action

The Dietary Guidelines can be easily incorporated into our diets.[18, 19] Table 2-5 provides a variety of easy-to-implement suggestions that can improve any diet.[20] Despite popular

▶ The American Dietetic Association suggests 5 basic principles with regard to diet and health:
- Be realistic; make small changes over time.
- Be adventurous; try new foods regularly.
- Be flexible; balance some sweet and fatty foods with physical activity.
- Be sensible; include favorite foods in smaller portions.
- Be active; include physical activity in daily life.

Table 2-5 Recommended Diet Changes Based on the Dietary Guidelines

If You Usually Eat This,	Try This Instead.	Benefit
White bread	Whole-wheat bread	• Higher nutrient density • More fiber
Sugary breakfast cereal	Low-sugar, high-fiber cereal with fresh fruit	• Higher nutrient density • More fiber • More phytochemicals
Cheeseburger with french fries	Hamburger and baked beans	• Less saturated fat and *trans* fat • Less cholesterol • More fiber • More phytochemicals
Potato salad	Three-bean salad	• More fiber • More phytochemicals
Doughnuts	Bran muffin or bagel with light cream cheese	• More fiber • Less fat
Regular soft drinks	Diet soft drinks	• Fewer kcal • Less sugar
Fruit canned in syrup	Fresh or frozen fruit Fruit canned in water or juice	• Less sugar • Fewer kcal
Boiled vegetables	Steamed or sauteed vegetables	• Higher nutrient density due to reduced loss of water-soluble vitamins
Canned vegetables	Fresh or frozen vegetables Low-sodium canned vegetables	• Lower in sodium
Fried meats	Broiled meats	• Less saturated fat
Fatty meats, such as ribs or bacon	Lean meats, such as ground round, chicken, or fish	• Less saturated fat
Whole milk	Low-fat or fat-free milk	• Less saturated fat • Fewer kcal • More calcium
Ice cream	Frozen yogurt	• Less saturated fat • Fewer kcal
Mayonnaise or sour cream salad dressing	Oil and vinegar dressings or light creamy dressings	• Less saturated fat • Less cholesterol • Fewer kcal
Cookies	Air-popped popcorn with minimal margarine or butter	• Less *trans* fat • Fewer kcal
Heavily salted foods	Foods flavored primarily with herbs, spices, lemon juice	• Less sodium
Chips	Pretzels	• Less fat

CRITICAL THINKING

Shannon has grown up eating the typical American diet. Having recently read and heard many media reports about the relationship between nutrition and health, she is beginning to look critically at her diet and is considering making changes. However, she doesn't know where to begin. What advice would you give her?

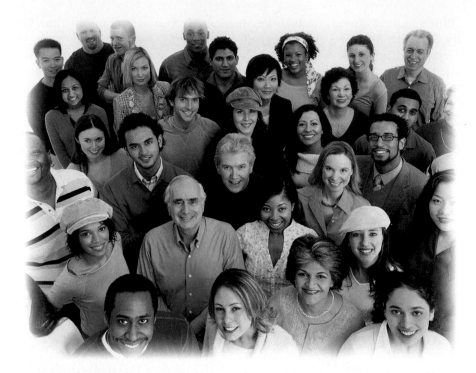

For practical reasons, nutrition recommendations, such as the Dietary Reference Intakes, Daily Values, Dietary Guidelines, and MyPyramid, are made on a population-wide basis. The key to making these recommendations work for you is considering your personal health status and then applying the recommendations to your diet and lifestyle.

misconceptions, the healthy diet recommended by the Dietary Guidelines is not especially expensive. Fruits, vegetables, and low-fat and fat-free milk often are similar in price to the chips, cookies, and sugared soft drinks they should replace. Plus, there are many lower-cost options, including canned and frozen fruits and vegetables and non-fat dry milk.

When applying the Dietary Guidelines to yourself, start by taking into account your current health status and family history for specific diseases. Then, identify specific changes you need to make and develop a plan for incorporating the changes into your lifestyle. MyPyramid can help you design a nutritious diet that meets your needs. When your plan is ready, make a couple of changes. As changes become part of your usual routine, add another change. Continue making changes until your diet is healthful and reflects the Dietary Guidelines.

When making changes, it is a good idea to see whether they are effective. Keep in mind that results of dietary changes sometimes take a while to occur. Also, note that sometimes changes don't result in the outcome you anticipated. Some people, for instance, who eat a diet low in saturated fat may not see a decrease in blood cholesterol because of genetic background.[21] If the changes are not leading to the health improvements you anticipated, it is a good idea to see a registered dietitian or physician.

CASE STUDY

Andy is like many other college students. He grew up on a quick bowl of cereal and milk for breakfast and a hamburger, fries, and cola for lunch, either in the school cafeteria or at a local fast-food restaurant. At dinner, he generally avoided eating any salad or vegetables, and by 9 PM he was deep into bags of chips and cookies. Andy has taken these habits to college. He prefers coffee for breakfast and possibly a chocolate bar. Lunch is still mainly a hamburger, fries, and cola, but pizza and tacos now alternate more frequently than when he was in high school. What dietary advice do you think Andy needs? Start with his positive habits and then provide some constructive criticism based on what you now know.

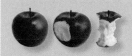 *Take Action*

Are You Putting the Dietary Guidelines into Practice?

The advice provided by the 2005 Dietary Guidelines for Americans can help you determine the healthfulness of your diet and identify changes to make. This checklist includes the major points to consider. How closely are you following the basic intent of the Dietary Guidelines?

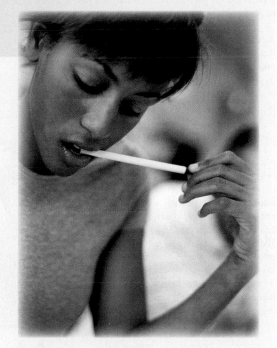

Yes   No

Do you consume a variety of nutrient-dense foods and beverages within and among the basic food groups of MyPyramid?

Do you choose foods that limit the intake of

Yes	No	
		Saturated fat?
		Trans fats?
		Cholesterol?
		Added sugars?
		Salt?
		Alcohol (if used)?

Do you emphasize in your food choices

Yes	No	
		Vegetables?
		Fruits?
		Legumes (beans)?
		Whole-grain breads and cereals?
		Fat-free or low-fat milk or equivalent milk products?

Do you keep your body weight in a healthy range by balancing energy intake from foods and beverages with energy expended?

Do you engage in at least 30 minutes of moderate-intensity physical activity (above usual activity) at work or home on most days of the week?

Do you wash your hands, food contact surfaces, and fruits and vegetables before preparation?

Do you cook foods to a safe temperature to kill harmful microorganisms?

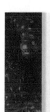 *Knowledge Check*

1. Which government agencies published the Dietary Guidelines for Americans?
2. What are the 9 Dietary Guidelines?
3. What are the specific Dietary Guidelines for carbohydrates?

 ## 2.5 MyPyramid

Since the early 20th century, researchers have worked to translate the science of nutrition into practical terms, so that consumers could estimate whether their nutritional needs were being met. A plan with 7 food groups, based on foods traditionally eaten by North Americans, was one of the first formats designed by the USDA. Daily food choices were to include items from each group. This plan was simplified in the mid-1950s to a 4 food

▶ Appendix D contains the Canadian Food Guide to Healthy Eating.

Figure 2-7 MyPyramid symbolizes a personalized approach to healthy eating and physical activity. The symbol has been developed to remind consumers to make healthy food choices and to be active every day.

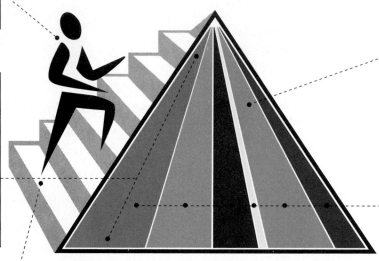

Activity
Activity is represented by the steps and the person climbing them, as a reminder of the importance of daily physical activity.

Moderation
Moderation is represented by the narrowing of each food group from bottom to top. The wider base stands for foods with little or no solid fats or added sugars. These should be selected more often. The narrower top area stands for foods containing more added sugars and solid fats. The more active you are, the more of these foods can fit into your diet.

Personalization
Personalization is shown by the person on the steps, the slogan, and the website. Find the kinds and amounts of food to eat each day at MyPyramid.gov.

Proportionality
Proportionality is shown by the different widths of the food group bands. The widths suggest how much food a person should choose from each group. The widths are just a general guide, not exact proportions. Check the website for how much is right for you.

Variety
Variety is symbolized by the 6 color bands representing the 5 food groups of the Pyramid and oils. This illustrates that foods from all groups are needed each day for good health.

Gradual Improvement
Gradual improvement is encouraged by the slogan. It suggests that individuals can benefit from taking small steps to improve their diet and lifestyle each day.

MyPyramid.gov
STEPS TO A HEALTHIER YOU

| Grains | Vegetables | Fruits | Oils | Milk | Meat & Beans |

▶ Some research suggests that increasing variety in a diet can lead to overeating. Thus, as you include a wide variety of foods in your diet, pay attention to total energy intake as well.

group plan: milk, meat, fruit and vegetable, and bread and cereal groups. In 1992, this plan was depicted using a pyramid shape.

When the 2005 Dietary Guidelines for Americans was released, the food group plan was revised once again and is currently called MyPyramid, Steps to a Healthier You (Fig. 2-7). Its goal is to provide advice that will help consumers live longer, better, and healthier lives.

MyPyramid was carefully designed to depict the key elements of a healthy diet and lifestyle.

* *Variety:* From left to right, the colorful triangles making up MyPyramid represent grains, vegetables, fruits, oils, milk, and meat and beans. All foods are included in MyPyramid because any food can be part of a nutritious diet—the key, though, is to choose mostly nutrient-dense foods. Eating nutrient-dense foods is especially important for people who tend not to eat a lot of food. This includes some older people and those following weight-loss diets.

* *Proportionality:* The widths of the triangles suggest how much food a person should choose from each group. The triangles are wider for grains, vegetables, and fruits because these groups should form the bulk of one's diet. The narrowest triangle is for oils, indicating these should be eaten sparingly. All the widths are just a general guide, however, and not exact proportions.

* *Moderation*: Notice how the triangles within MyPyramid are wider at the bottom than the top. The wider base represents the most-nutrient-dense foods—that is, those with little or no added fat or sugars. Less-nutrient-dense foods, such as those with added fats (e.g., fries in the vegetable group) or added sugar (e.g., ice cream in the

CRITICAL THINKING

Margit would benefit from more variety in her diet. What are some practical tips she can use to increase her fruit and vegetable intake?

	Energy Intake Range (kcal)		
Children	Sedentary	→	Active
2–3 years	1000	→	1400
Females			
4–8 years	1200	→	1800
9–13	1600	→	2200
14–18	1800	→	2400
19–30	2000	→	2400
31–50	1800	→	2200
51+	1600	→	2200
Males			
4–8 years	1400	→	2000
9–13	1800	→	2600
14–18	2200	→	3200
19–30	2400	→	3000
31–50	2200	→	3000
51+	2000	→	2800

Sedentary means a lifestyle that includes only the light physical activity associated with typical day-to-day life.

Active means a lifestyle that includes physical activity equivalent to walking more than 3 miles per day at 3 to 4 miles per hour in addition to the light physical activity associated with typical day-to-day life.

Figure 2-8 Levels of energy needs provided by MyPyramid.

▶ Special versions of MyPyramid are available for pregnant and lactating women,[25] as well as older adults.[26]

milk group), would appear nearer the narrowing point of MyPyramid. The narrowing triangles are a reminder that less-nutrient-dense foods should constitute a smaller amount of the diet than more-nutrient-dense foods.

- *Personalization:* By including separate pyramids based on the levels of energy needs ranging from 1000 to 3200 kcal/day (Fig. 2-8), MyPyramid provides a more individualized approach to improving diet and lifestyle than did previous food guides.[22] These energy needs mostly account for the recommended amounts of nutrient-dense foods, as well as a few for discretionary calories (last row of Table 2-6). **Discretionary calories** are those left after meeting nutrient needs with nutrient-dense foods. They can be used for any type of food, including those that contain added sugars, solid fat, or alcohol. For most of us, very few discretionary calories are available in daily diet

Table 2-6 MyPyramid Recommendations for Daily Amounts of Foods to Consume from the Food Groups Based on Energy Needs

Energy Intake	1000	1200	1400	1600	1800	2000	2200	2400	2600	2800	3000	3200
Fruits	1 c	1 c	1.5 c	1.5 c	1.5 c	2 c	2 c	2 c	2 c	2.5 c	2.5 c	2.5 c
Vegetables[1,2]	1 c	1.5 c	1.5 c	2 c	2.5 c	2.5 c	3 c	3 c	3.5 c	3.5 c	4 c	4 c
Grains[3]	3 oz-eq	4 oz-eq	5 oz-eq	5 oz-eq	6 oz-eq	6 oz-eq	7 oz-eq	8 oz-eq	9 oz-eq	10 oz-eq	10 oz-eq	10 oz-eq
Meat & Beans[2]	2 oz-eq	3 oz-eq	4 oz-eq	5 oz-eq	5 oz-eq	5.5 oz-eq	6 oz-eq	6.5 oz-eq	6.5 oz-eq	7 oz-eq	7 oz-eq	7 oz-eq
Milk[4]	2 c	2 c	2 c	3 c	3 c	3 c	3 c	3 c	3 c	3 c	3 c	3 c
Oils[5]	3 tsp	4 tsp	4 tsp	5 tsp	5 tsp	6 tsp	6 tsp	7 tsp	8 tsp	8 tsp	10 tsp	11 tsp
Discretionary calorie allowance[6]	165[7]	171[7]	171[7]	132	195	267	290	362	410	426	512	648

Abbreviations: c = cup or cups; oz-eq = ounces or equivalent; tsp = teaspoon.

[1]Vegetables are divided into 5 subgroups (dark green vegetables, orange vegetables, legumes, starchy vegetables, and other vegetables). Over a week's time a variety of vegetables should be eaten, especially green and orange vegetables.

[2]Dry beans and peas can be counted *either* as vegetables (dry beans and peas subgroup) *or* in the meat & beans group.

[3]At least half of these servings should be whole-grain varieties.

[4]Most servings should be fat-free or low-fat.

[5]Limit solid fats such as butter, stick margarine, shortening, and meat fat as well as foods that contain these.

[6]*Discretionary calories* refers to food choices with added sugars, solid fat, or alcohol.

[7]The amount of discretionary kcalories is higher for 1000- to 1400-kcal diets than for a 1600-kcal diet because the diets with less energy are intended for children 2 to 8 years of age. Adults typically need at least 1600 kcal daily.

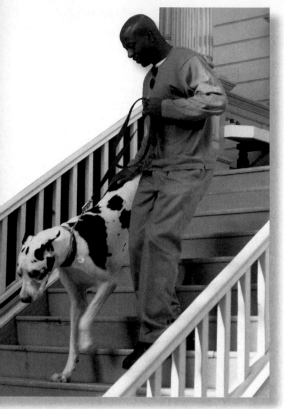

What about physical activity? Walking, gardening, briskly pushing a baby stroller, climbing stairs, playing soccer, and dancing the night away are all good examples of being physically active.

▶ There are no "good" or "bad" foods—to make all foods fit into a nutritious dietary pattern and reduce the risk of many chronic diseases, balance, variety, and moderation are needed.

▶ The Exchange System is another menu-planning tool. It organizes foods based on energy, protein, carbohydrate, and fat content. The result is a framework for designing diets, especially for the treatment of diabetes. For more information on the Exchange System, see Appendix E.

planning. To benefit more fully from the individualized advice, visit the website www.MyPyramid.gov.

- *Physical activity:* This element was not previously found in food guides. The figure climbing the stairs is a visual reminder to be more physically active.
- *Gradual improvement:* The title, Steps to a Healthier You, suggests that individuals can benefit from making gradual changes to improve their diet and lifestyle.

An innovative aspect of MyPyramid is the interactive technology found at the www.MyPyramid.gov website. The programs there help consumers use MyPyramid and personalize it to their life stage. One program at this website, *MyPyramid Plan,* provides a quick estimate of what and how much food a person should eat from the different food groups based on age, gender, and activity level. The *MyPyramid Tracker* program provides detailed information on diet quality and physical activity status by comparing all foods a person eats and all the exercise completed in 1 day to the MyPyramid recommendations. There are over 8000 foods and 600 activities included in *MyPyramid Tracker.* Nutrition and physical activity messages are based on the need to maintain current weight or lose weight. Another program, *Inside the Pyramid,* provides in-depth information for every food group, including recommended daily intake amounts expressed in commonly used measures, such as cups and ounces, with examples and everyday tips. The section also includes recommendations for choosing healthy oils, discretionary calories, and physical activity. The *Steps to a Healthier Weight* program provides tips and resources on nutrient-dense food choices, portion sizes, and physical activity. MyPyramid Menu Planner helps you plan food choices to meet MyPyramid goals.

Table 2-7 MyPyramid Food Serving Sizes

Grains Group	
1-ounce equivalent =	1 slice of bread
	1 cup of ready-to-eat breakfast cereal
	½ cup of cooked cereal, rice, or pasta
Vegetable Group	
1 cup =	1 cup of raw or cooked vegetables
	1 cup of vegetable juice
	2 cups of raw leafy greens
Fruits Group	
1 cup =	1 cup of fruit
	1 cup of 100% fruit juice
	½ cup of dried fruit
Milk Group	
1 cup =	1 cup of milk or yogurt
	1½ ounces of natural cheese
	2 ounces of processed cheese
Meat & Beans Group	
1-ounce equivalent =	1 ounce of meat, poultry, or fish
	1 egg
	1 tablespoon of peanut butter
	¼ cup of cooked dry beans
	½ ounce of nuts or seeds
Oils	
1 teaspoon of vegetable or fish oil	
1 teaspoon of oil-rich foods (e.g., mayonnaise and soft margarine).	

Putting MyPyramid into Action

To put MyPyramid into action, begin by estimating your energy needs (see Fig. 2-8 or visit **www.MyPyramid.gov**). Next, use Table 2-6 to discover how your energy needs correspond to the recommended number of servings from each food group. The servings are based on the sizes listed in Table 2-7.

When planning menus using MyPyramid, keep these points in mind:

1. MyPyramid applies only to people age 2 years and older.
2. No one food is required for good nutrition. Every food supplies some nutrients but provides insufficient amounts of at least 1 essential nutrient.
3. No one food group provides all essential nutrients in adequate amounts (Table 2-8). Each food group makes an important, distinctive contribution to nutritional intake.
4. The foods within a group may vary widely with respect to nutrients and energy content. For example, the energy content of 3 ounces of baked potato is 98 calories, whereas that of 3 ounces of potato chips is 470 calories.
5. To keep calories under control, pay close attention to the serving size of each choice when following MyPyramid. Figure 2-9 provides a convenient guide to estimating portion sizes. Note that serving sizes listed for 1 serving in a MyPyramid group are often less than individuals typically serve themselves or the sizes of portions served in many restaurants.[23, 24]
6. Variety is the key to getting the array of nutrients offered by each food group. Variety starts with including foods from every food group and then continues by consuming a variety of different foods within each group. The nutritional adequacy of diets planned using MyPyramid depends greatly on the selection of a variety of foods (Table 2-9).

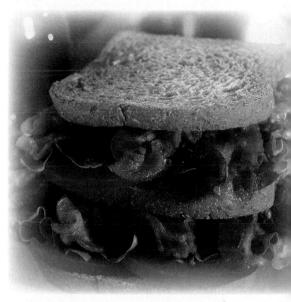

Typical restaurant portions contain numerous servings from the individual groups in MyPyramid.

Table 2-8 Nutrient Contributions of Groups in the MyPyramid Food Guide Plan

Food Category — **Major Nutrient Contributions**

Milk	Meat & Beans	Fruits	Vegetables	Grains	Oils
Calcium	Protein	Carbohydrate	Carbohydrate	Carbohydrate	Fat
Phosphorus	Thiamin	Vitamin A	Vitamin A	Thiamin[3]	Essential fatty acids
Carbohydrate	Riboflavin	Vitamin C	Vitamin C	Riboflavin[3]	Vitamin E
Protein	Niacin	Folate	Folate	Niacin[3]	
Riboflavin	Vitamin B-6	Magnesium	Magnesium	Folate[3]	
Vitamin D	Folate[1]	Potassium	Potassium	Magnesium[4]	
Magnesium	Vitamin B-12[2]	Fiber	Fiber	Iron[3]	
Zinc	Phosphorus			Zinc[4]	
	Magnesium[1]			Fiber[4]	
	Iron				
	Zinc				

[1]Primarily in plant protein sources.
[2]Only in animal foods.
[3]If enriched or whole-grain.
[4]Whole grains.

Figure 2-9 A golf ball, tennis ball, deck of cards, and baseball are standard-size objects that make convenient guides for judging MyPyramid serving sizes. Your hand provides an additional handy guide (for the greatest accuracy, compare your fist with a baseball and adjust the following guides accordingly).

Fist = 1 cup
Thumb = 1 oz of cheese
Thumb tip to first joint = 1 tsp
Palm of hand = 3 oz
Handful = 1 or 2 oz of a snack food

 2 tbsp salad dressing, peanut butter, margarine, etc.

 Baked potato
Small/medium fruit
Ground or chopped food
Bagel
English muffin

 3 oz meat, poultry, or fish

 Large apple or orange
1 cup ready-to-eat breakfast cereal

Portion sizes

= **2 tbsp measure**   = **½ to ⅔ cup measure**   = **½ to ¾ cup**   = **1 cup**

Table 2-9 Putting MyPyramid into Practice

Breakfast

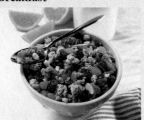

1 orange	Fruits
¾ cup low-fat granola	Grains
topped with 2 tbsp dried cranberries	Fruits
1 cup non-fat milk	Milk
Optional: coffee or tea	

Lunch

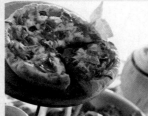

8-inch pizza	Grains
¼ cup chopped vegetables	Vegetables
topped with 2 oz low-fat cheese	Milk
2 cups green salad	Vegetables
topped with ¾ oz nuts	Meat & Beans
5 tsp salad dressing	Oils
Optional: diet soft drink or iced tea	

Study Break Snack

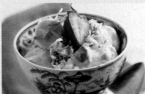

1 cup non-fat yogurt	Milk
topped with ½ cup fresh fruit	Fruit

Dinner

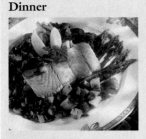

3.5 oz salmon	Meat & Beans
½ cup asparagus	Vegetables
1¼ cups salsa (½ cup fresh fruit and	Fruits
¾ cup vegetables)	Vegetables
Sparkling water	

Late-Night Snack

3 small chocolate chip cookies as discretionary calories

Nutrient Breakdown
Calories: 1800
Carbohydrate: 56% of kcal
Protein: 18% of kcal
Fat: 26% of kcal

Here are some points that will help you choose the most nutritious diet.

- *Grains group:* Make at least half of your grain choices those that are whole-grain. Whole-grain varieties of breads, cereals, rice, and pasta have the greatest array of nutrients and more fiber than other foods in this group. A daily serving of a whole-grain, ready-to-eat breakfast cereal is an excellent choice because the vitamins and minerals typically added to it, along with fiber it naturally contains, help fill in potential nutrient gaps. Although cakes, pies, cookies, and pastries are made from grains, these foods are higher in calories, fat, and sugar and lower in fiber, vitamins, and minerals than other foods in this group. The most nutritious diets limit the number of grain products with added fat or sugar.
- *Vegetables group:* Variety within the vegetables group (Table 2-10) is especially important because different types of vegetables are rich in different nutrients and phytochemicals (see Table 1-2 in Chapter 1). For instance, dark green vegetables (e.g., kale, bok choy) tend to be good sources of iron, calcium, folic acid, and vitamins A and C. Vegetables with orange flesh (e.g., carrots, acorn squash) are rich in beta-carotene, the precursor to vitamin A. Starchy vegetables (e.g., corn) provide B-vitamins and carbohydrates. Legumes (dried beans and peas) are also in the meat and beans group because they are rich in protein. Other vegetables, including celery, onions, and radishes, provide a wide array of phytochemicals, vitamins, and minerals. It is important to eat a variety of vegetables each week from all 5 vegetable subgroups.
- *Fruit group:* Like vegetables, fruits also vary in the nutrients and phytochemicals they contain. To be sure you get the fiber that fruits have to offer, keep the amount of fruit juice to less than half of total fruit intake. Select 100% fruit juice—punches,

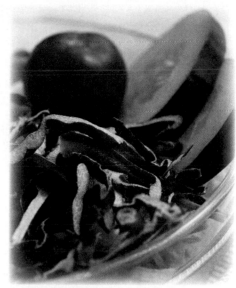

Vegetables are a rich source of nutrients and phytochemicals.

Table 2-10 Vegetable Subgroup Recommendations per Week*

Life Span Group	Dark Green Vegetables	Orange Vegetables	Dry Beans and Peas	Starchy Vegetables	Other Vegetables
Children					
2–3 years old	1 cup	½ cup	½ cup	1½ cups	4 cups
4–8 years old	1½ cups	1 cup	1 cup	2½ cups	4½ cups
Girls					
9–13 years old	2 cups	1½ cups	2½ cups	2½ cups	5 ½ cups
14–18 years old	3 cups	2 cups	3 cups	3 cups	6½ cups
Boys					
9–13 years old	3 cups	2 cups	3 cups	3 cups	6½ cups
14–18 years old	3 cups	2 cups	3 cups	6 cups	7 cups
Women					
19–30 years old	3 cups	2 cups	3 cups	3 cups	6½ cups
31–50 years old	3 cups	2 cups	3 cups	3 cups	6½ cups
51+ years old	2 cups	1½ cups	2½ cups	2½ cups	5½ cups
Men					
19–30 years old	3 cups	2 cups	3 cups	6 cups	7 cups
31–50 years old	3 cups	2 cups	3 cups	6 cups	7 cups
51+ years old	3 cups	2 cups	3 cups	3 cups	6½ cups

* It is not necessary to eat vegetables from each subgroup daily; however, over a week they should be varied, as shown in this table.

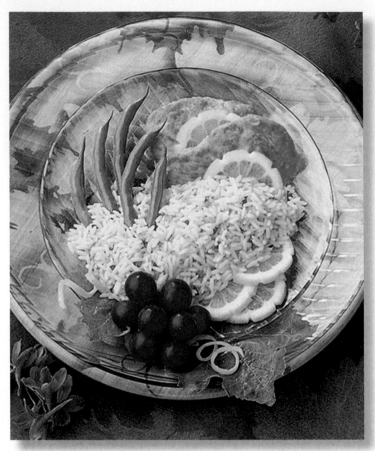

Choosing a variety of foods every day helps meet all of your nutrient needs.

ades, fruit-flavored soft drinks, and most fruit drinks contain little or no juice but do have substantial amounts of added sugar and do not count toward fruit servings.

- *Milk group:* Choose primarily low-fat and fat-free items from the milk group, such as part skim cheese, fat-free milk, and low-fat yogurt. These foods contain all the nutrients in other milk products, except they are lower in fat, saturated fat, and cholesterol. In addition, go easy on milk desserts (e.g., pudding, ice cream) and chocolate milk because of the added sugar. By reducing energy intake in this way, you free up calories that can be used to select more items from other food groups.

- *Meat and beans group:* Keep meat serving sizes under control— many people eat far more meat than is considered healthful. Except for beans and fish, most foods in this group are high in fat. Meat, poultry, seafood, and eggs also supply cholesterol. When selecting foods from the meat and beans group, focus on seafood, lean meat, poultry without skin, and beans—these foods are lower in fat than others in this group. To further reduce fat, avoid fried foods and trim away any fat you see on meat. Include protein-rich plant foods, such as beans and nuts, at least several times a week because many are rich in vitamins (e.g., vitamin E), minerals (e.g., magnesium), and fiber and contain less saturated fat than meat.

- *Oils:* Oils are the fats from fish and plants that are liquid at room temperature. Include some plant oils on a daily basis, such as those in salad dressing and olive oil, and eat fish at least twice a week. Oils supply you with health-promoting fats, called essential fatty acids (see Chapter 6).

Remember, eating a balanced diet means choosing foods from every food group in the recommended amounts. Variety means eating many different foods from each food group. Variety makes meals more interesting and helps ensure that a diet contains sufficient nutrients. For example, carrots—a rich source of a pigment that forms vitamin A in our bodies—may be your favorite vegetable; however, if you choose carrots every day as your only vegetable source, you may miss out on other important vitamins supplied by vegetables. This concept is true for all groups of foods.

Moderation means keeping portion sizes under control, so that you can eat a balanced and varied diet without consuming more calories, fat, cholesterol, sugar, and sodium than you need. Moderation only requires some simple planning and doesn't have to mean deprivation and misery. For example, if you eat a food that is relatively high in fat, salt, and energy, such as a bacon cheeseburger, it is a good idea to choose foods the rest of the day that are less concentrated sources of these nutrients, such as fruits and salad greens. Moderation doesn't mean completely giving up foods you enjoy. If you prefer reduced-fat milk to non-fat milk, decrease the fat in other foods you eat. You could use low-fat salad dressings, choose a baked potato instead of french fries, or opt for jam instead of butter on toast. You also could choose smaller servings of high-fat or high-sugar foods you enjoy, such as regular soft drinks or chocolate. Overall, it's best to strive for moderate serving sizes of some foods (rather than eliminate these foods altogether) and include mostly nutrient-dense foods.

▶ For more suggestions on how to increase fruit, vegetable, and phytochemical intake, visit
www.5aday.com
5aday.nci.nih.gov

Rating Your Current Diet

Regularly comparing your daily food intake with MyPyramid recommendations for your age, gender, and physical activity level is a relatively simple way to evaluate your overall diet. The diets of many adults don't match the recommendations—many eat too few

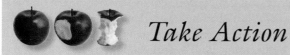

Take Action

Does Your Diet Meet MyPyramid Recommendations?

In the accompanying chart, list all the foods you ate in the past 24 hours. For each food, indicate how many servings it contributes to each group based on the amount you ate (see Table 2-7 for serving sizes). Note that many of your food choices may contribute to more than 1 group. For example, toast with soft margarine contributes to the grains group and oils group. After entering all the values, add the number of servings consumed in each group. Finally, compare your total in each food group with the recommended number of servings shown in Table 2-6 or at the www.MyPyramid.gov website. Enter a minus sign (–) if your total falls below the recommendation, a zero (0) if it matches the recommendation, or a plus sign (+) if it exceeds the recommendation.

Food or Beverage	Amount Eaten	Milk	Meat & Beans	Fruits	Vegetables	Grains	Oils
Group Totals							
Recommended Servings							
Shortages in Numbers of Servings							

► A meal consisting of a bean burrito, a lettuce and tomato salad with oil and vinegar dressing, a glass of milk, and an apple covers all groups.

servings of whole grains, vegetables, fruits, and milk products and go overboard on meat and oil intake. Knowing how your diet stacks up can help you determine which nutrients likely are lacking and how you can take steps to improve. For example, if you do not consume enough servings from the milk group, your calcium intake is most likely too low, so you'll need to find calcium-rich foods you enjoy, such as calcium-fortified orange juice or non-fat yogurt.

Customizing MyPyramid to accommodate your own food habits may seem a daunting task now, but it is not difficult once you start using it. The *MyTracker* program at the www.MyPyramid.gov website is easy to use and can help you follow your progress. Implementing even small diet and exercise changes can have positive results. Better health will likely follow as you strive to meet your nutrient needs and balance physical activity and energy intake. In addition, the guidance from the 2005 Dietary Guidelines for Americans regarding alcohol and sodium intake and safe food preparation can help you incorporate other important changes to safeguard your health.

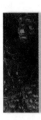

Knowledge Check

1. How does MyPyramid depict variety and proportionality?
2. What are discretionary calories?
3. What types of vegetables should be selected over a week's time?

CASE STUDY FOLLOW-UP

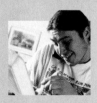

The most positive aspect of Andy's diet is that it contains adequate protein, zinc, and iron because it is rich in animal protein. On the downside, his diet is low in calcium, some B-vitamins (such as folate), and vitamin C. This is because it is low in dairy products, fruits, and vegetables. It is also low in many of the phytochemical substances discussed in Chapter 1. In addition, his fiber intake is low because fast-food restaurants primarily use refined-grain products rather than whole-grain products. His diet is likely excessive in fat and sugar, too.

He could alternate between tacos and bean burritos to gain the benefits of plant proteins in his diet. He could choose a low-fat granola bar instead of the candy bar for breakfast, or he could take the time to eat a bowl of whole-grain breakfast cereal with low-fat or fat-free milk to increase fiber and calcium intake. He also could order milk at least half the time at his restaurant visits and substitute diet soft drinks for the regular variety. This would help moderate his sugar intake. Overall, Andy could improve his intake of fruits, vegetables, and dairy products if he focused more on variety in food choice and balance among the food groups.

Summary

2.1 The Dietary Reference Intakes (DRIs) differ by life stage and include Estimated Average Requirements (EARs), Recommended Dietary Allowances (RDAs), Adequate Intakes (AIs), Tolerable Upper Intake Levels (Upper Levels, or ULs), and Estimated Energy Requirements (EERs). EARs are daily nutrient intake amounts estimated to meet the needs of half of the people in a life stage. EARs are set only if a method exists for accurately measuring whether intake is adequate. RDAs are daily nutrient intake amounts sufficient to meet the needs of nearly all individuals (97 to 98%) in a life stage. RDAs are based on a multiple of the EAR. AIs are daily intake amounts set for nutrients for which there are insufficient data to establish an EAR. AIs should cover the needs of virtually all individuals in a specific life stage. ULs are the maximum daily intake amount of a nutrient that is not likely to cause adverse health effects in almost everyone. EERs are average daily energy needs. For each macronutrient, the Adequate Macronutrient Distribution Ranges (AMDRs) provide a range of recommended intake, as a percent of energy. DRIs are intended mainly for diet planning. Nutrient density is a tool for assessing the nutritional quality of individual foods.

2.2 Daily Values (DVs) are generic standards developed by the FDA for Nutrition Facts panels. DVs are based on Reference Daily Intakes and Daily Reference Values. Nutrition Facts panels present information for a single serving of food using serving sizes specified by the FDA. These components must be listed on most Nutrition Facts panels: total calories (kcal), calories from fat, total fat, saturated fat, *trans* fat, cholesterol, sodium, total carbohydrate, fiber, sugars, protein, vitamin A, vitamin C, calcium, and iron. Food labels may include nutrient content claims, health claims, preliminary health claims, and structure/function claims.

2.3 Nutrient databases make it possible to estimate quickly the amount of calories and many nutrients in the foods we eat. The data in nutrient databases are the results of thousands of analytical chemistry studies. Nutrient values in the nutrient databases are average amounts found in the analyzed samples of the food. It is wise to view nutrient composition databases as tools that approximate nutrient intake, rather than precise measurements. Energy density is determined by comparing a food's calorie content with the weight of food.

2.4 The Dietary Guidelines are the foundation of the U.S. government's nutrition policy and education. They reflect what experts believe is the most accurate and up-to-date scientific knowledge about nutritious diets, physical activity, and related lifestyle choices. Dietary Guideline recommendations are grouped into 9 topics: adequate nutrients within energy, weight management, physical activity, food groups to encourage, fats, carbohydrates, sodium and potassium, alcoholic beverages, and food safety.

2.5 The goal of MyPyramid, Steps to a Healthier You, is to provide advice that helps consumers live longer, better, and healthier lives. MyPyramid was designed to depict elements that form the basis of a healthy diet and lifestyle: variety, proportionality, moderation, personalization, physical activity, and gradual improvement. The nutritional adequacy of diets planned using MyPyramid depend on selecting a variety of foods, including grains, vegetables, fruits, milk, meat and beans, and oils. A balanced diet includes foods from every food group in the recommended amounts. Variety means eating many different foods from each food group. Moderation means keeping portions sizes under control

Study Questions

1. Which dietary standard is set at a level that meets the needs of practically all healthy people?
   a. RDA ✓
   b. DRI
   c. UL
   d. EER

2. Which dietary standard is set at a level that meets the needs of about half of all healthy people?
   a. RDA   d. EER
   b. AI   e. both c and d
   c. EAR

3. Daily Reference Values are standards established for Nutrition Facts panels for energy-producing nutrients—cholesterol, sodium, and potassium.
   a. true
   b. false

4. Most people should aim to keep intake of which nutrient at or below 100% Daily Value?
   a. total fat   c. vitamin A
   b. fiber   d. calcium

5. Foods that are a "good source" of a nutrient must contain at least _____ % Daily Value of that nutrient.
   a. 5
   b. 10
   c. 25
   d. 50

6. Which factor affects nutrient levels in food?
   a. food processing
   b. plant variety
   c. ripeness when harvested
   d. all of the above

7. A food's energy density is determined by comparing its calorie content with the weight of food.
   a. true
   b. false

8. The FDA publishes the Dietary Guidelines for Americans.
   a. true
   b. false

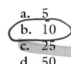

9. Which is true about the Dietary Guidelines for Americans?

    a. They are the foundation of the U.S. government's nutrition policy.
    b. They are designed to reduce the risk of obesity and hypertension.
    c. They guide government programs, such as the USDA's school lunch program.
    d. All of the above are true.

10. Which food group is missing from this meal: cheese sandwich, macaroni salad, and orange juice?

    a. milk group
    b. vegetable group
    c. fruit group
    d. meat and beans group
    e. b and d
    f. a, b, and c

11. MyPyramid recommends that at least 75% of the foods from the grain group should be whole grains.

    a. true
    b. false

12. Which key element that forms the basis of a healthy diet and lifestyle is not depicted by MyPyramid?

    a. variety
    b. moderation
    c. proportionality
    d. physical activity
    e. All of the above are depicted.

13. Which type of vegetables (e.g., kale, bok choy) tend to be good sources of iron, calcium, folic acid, and vitamins A and C?

    a. starch vegetables
    b. legumes
    c. vegetables with orange flesh
    d. dark green vegetables
    e. all of the above

Answer Key: 1-a; 2-c; 3-a; 4-a; 5-b; 6-d; 7-a; 8-b; 9-d; 10-e; 11-b; 12-c; 13-d

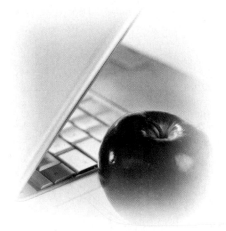

Websites

To learn more about the topics covered in this chapter, visit these websites.

fnic.nal.usda.gov

www.cfsan.fda.gov/label.html

www.nal.usda.gov/fnic/foodcomp/search

www.health.gov/dietaryguidelines/dga2005/document

www.MyPyramid.gov

www.fruitsandveggiesmorematters.org

5aday.nci.nih.gov

www.cnpp.usda.gov

References

1. Yates A. Dietary Reference Intakes: Rationale and applications. In: Shils M and others, eds., *Modern nutrition in health and disease*. 10th ed. Philadelphia: Lippincott Williams & Wilkins; 2006.

2. Murphy S and others. Using the Dietary Reference Intakes to assess intakes of groups: Pitfalls to avoid. *J Am Diet Assoc*. 2006;106:1550.

3. Barr S. Introduction to Dietary Reference Intakes. *Appl Physio Nutr Metab*. 2006;31:61.

4. Food and Nutrition Board. *Dietary Reference Intakes: Guiding principles for nutrition labeling and fortification*. Washington, DC: National Academies Press; 2003.

5. Institute of Medicine. *Dietary Reference Intakes for energy, carbohydrate, fiber, fat, fatty acids, cholesterol, protein, and amino acids (macronutrients)*. Washington, DC: National Academies Press; 2005.

6. Barr S and others: Planning diets for individuals using the Dietary Reference Intakes. *Nutr Rev*. 2003;61:352.

7. Pennington J and others. Practice paper of the American Dietetic Association: Nutrient density: Meeting nutrient goals within calorie needs. *J Am Diet Assoc*. 2007;107:860.

8. Kolodinsky J and others. Knowledge of current dietary guidelines and food choice by college students: Better eaters

have higher knowledge of dietary guidance. *J Am Diet Assoc.* 2007;107:1409.

9. Yates A. Which Dietary Reference Intake is best suited to serve as the basis for nutrition labeling for daily values? *J Nutr.* 2006;136:2457.

10. Food Allergen Labeling and Consumer Protection Act of 2004, Public Law 108-282; 2004.

11. van Trijp HC and others. Consumer perceptions of nutrition and health claims. *Appetite.* 2007;48:305.

12. Liebman B. Which ones can you believe? *Nutr Action Health Letter.* 2003;30(5):1.

13. Ledikwe J and others. Dietary energy density is associated with energy intake and weight status in US adults. *Am J Clin Nutr.* 2006;83:1362.

14. Fisher J and others. Effects of portion size and energy density on young children's intake at a meal. *Am J Clin Nutr.* 2007;86:174.

15. Ledikwe J and others. Low-energy-density diets are associated with high diet quality in adults in the United States. *J Am Diet Assoc.* 2006;106:1172.

16. Maurer Abbot J, Byrd-Bredbenner C. The state of the American diet. How can we cope? *Top Clin Nutr.* 2007;3:202.

17. Revised Dietary Guidelines to help Americans live better lives. *FDA Consumer.* 2005;March-April:18.

18. ADA Reports. Position of the American Dietetic Association: Total diet approach to communicating food and nutrition information. *J Am Diet Assoc.* 2007;107:1224.

19. Smitasiri S and others. Beyond recommendations: Implementing food-based dietary guidelines for healthier populations. *Food Nutr Bull.* 2007;28:S141.

20. Rebuilding the pyramid. *Tufts University Health & Nutrition Letter.* 2005;June:1.

21. Go V and others. Nutrient-gene interaction: Metabolic genotype-phenotype relationship. *J Nutr.* 2005;135:3016S.

22. Krebs-Smith S and others. How does MyPyramid compare to other population-based recommendations for controlling chronic disease? *J Am Diet Assoc.* 2007;107:830.

23. Young L, Nestle M. Expanding portion sizes in the US marketplace: Implications for nutrition counseling. *J Am Diet Assoc.* 2003;103:231.

24. Schwartz J, Byrd-Bredbenner C. Portion distortion: Typical portion sizes selected by young adults. *J Am Diet Assoc.* 2006;106:1412.

25. USDA. MyPyramid for Pregnancy and Breastfeeding. 2008; www.mypyramid.gov.

26. Lichtenstein AH and others. Modified MyPyramid for older adults. *J Nutr.* 2008; 138:5.

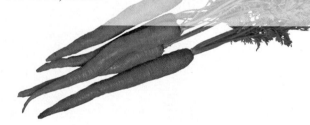

3 The Food Supply

Both synthetic and natural flavor additives are used to make foods more appealing. This orchid produces vanilla beans and is the source of natural vanilla flavor. Learn more at www.foodsafety.gov and unitproj. library.ucla.edu/biomed/spice.

STUDENT LEARNING OUTCOMES

After studying this chapter, you will be able to:

1. Compare food security and food insecurity and identify the factors that contribute to each.

2. Discuss the effects of hunger and malnutrition and their impact on children.

3. Describe U.S. government programs designed to increase food security.

4. Describe organic food production, its regulation, and its potential benefits.

5. Discuss the current and potential uses of genetically modified foods, along with concerns related to safety.

6. Explain how food preservation and processing methods affect food availability.

7. Describe the role of food additives in the food supply, along with how they are regulated.

8. List the major causes of foodborne and waterborne illnesses in the U.S. and describe how consumers can reduce the risk of these illnesses.

9. Describe common environmental contaminants (heavy metals, industrial chemicals, pesticides, and antibiotics), their potential harmful effects, and how to reduce exposure to them.

A bountiful, varied, nutritious, and safe food supply is available to many individuals, especially those in developed countries. For example, most Americans have ready access to generous food supplies—each of the 34,000 supermarkets in the United States sells 45,000 or more foods. In addition to purchases from food stores, Americans are buying more ready-to-eat food than ever from restaurants, cafeterias, vending machines, and the like. Despite ample food supplies and the efforts of private and government programs that aim to help at-risk individuals obtain enough healthy foods, malnutrition and poor health from poor diets still plague people throughout the world, especially in developing countries.

Food preservation and processing methods (e.g., refrigeration, canning, and irradiation) and food additives, along with varied food production practices (e.g., conventional and organic farming and biotechnology), continue to expand the variety and availability of the food supply. These processing and production methods offer many benefits; however, there are still concerns about the safety of the food and water supply. For example, common foods, such as fresh produce, peanut butter, and ground beef, sometimes are contaminated with harmful bacteria that cause foodborne illness. The safety of and need for pesticides, antibiotic use in food animals (animals intended for consumption), the biotechnology processes that genetically modify plants and animals, and the food additives we see listed on food labels continue to be debated. In this chapter, you'll learn more about the complex issues of food access, food constituents, and food safety and some steps that you can take to keep food safe in your home.

71

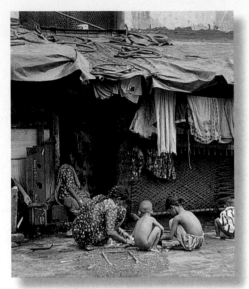

Poverty aggravates the problem of hunger in the developing world.

▶ In the 1940s, a group of researchers, led by Dr. Ancel Keys, examined the effects of undernutrition on 32 healthy male volunteers. They ate an average of about 1800 calories daily for 6 months. During this time, the men lost an average of 24% of their body weight; experienced fatigue, muscle soreness, irritability, intolerance to cold, and hunger; exhibited lack of ambition, self-discipline, and concentration; and were often moody, apathetic, and depressed. Their heart rate and muscle tone decreased and they retained abnormal amounts of fluid in their bodies. When the men were permitted to eat normally again, feelings of recurrent hunger and fatigue persisted, even after 12 weeks of rehabilitation. Full recovery required about 18 months. This study tells us much about the general state of undernourished adults worldwide.[73]

 # 3.1 Food Availability and Access

Good nutritional status and health for each of us requires access to a safe and healthy food supply. Worldwide, agriculture produces enough food to provide each person with 2720 kcal/day—more than enough to meet the energy requirements of each of the nearly 7 billion persons on earth. Even with this abundance, almost 1 in 8 (about 854 million) people are unable to access enough food to lead active, healthy lives—that is, they are **food insecure**. Another 2 billion people suffer from micronutrient (vitamin and mineral) deficiencies. The serious problems of food insecurity and malnutrition exist in virtually every nation. They are most common in the developing world, especially sub-Saharan Africa, Latin America, the Caribbean, and parts of Asia. Nearly all people suffering from food insecurity, hunger, or malnutrition are poor.

According to the Food and Agriculture Organization (FAO) of the United Nations, the problems of malnutrition (including too much food) and hunger account for over half of the world's disease burden.[1] Overnutrition that results in overweight and obesity is the primary problem in industrialized countries, such as the United States, Canada, and the countries of Western Europe. However, overnutrition also is becoming a problem in developing countries—for example, more than half of the adults in Mexico are now overweight or obese.[2, 3] As developing countries become westernized, their diets contain more meat, dairy, sugar, fat, and processed foods and fewer grains and vegetables. This phenomenon, known as the "nutrition transition," poses new challenges for nutritionists and other health-care providers in developing countries; however, undernutrition from lack of food and nutrient-poor diets remains the most pressing nutritional problem in these countries.

Health Consequences of Food Insecurity

When individuals don't get enough to eat or have access to only a few foods, problems related to hunger and malnutrition arise. The United Nations estimates that adults require a minimum of 2100 kcal per day to support a normal, healthy life (children require less). When energy intake falls below needs, a variety of problems arise—physical and mental activity declines; growth slows or ceases altogether; muscle and fat wasting occurs; the immune system weakens, increasing susceptibility to disease; and death rates rise (Fig. 3-1). The consequences of micronutrient deficiencies can be equally devastating. For example, in developing countries vitamin A deficiency causes blindness in over 250,000 children per

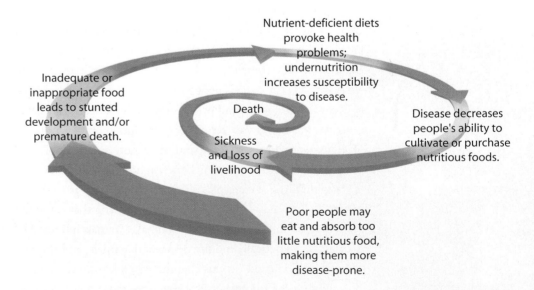

Figure 3-1 The downward spiral of poverty and illness can ultimately end in death (based on World Food Program graphic).

year and makes children more vulnerable to common diseases, such as measles and respiratory infections. Iodine deficiency is the world's leading cause of preventable mental retardation and brain damage. (See Chapters 12 through 15 for more details on micronutrient deficiencies.)

Food insecurity in westernized countries, although not as widespread and profound as that in developing countries, contributes to serious health and nutritional problems for millions of people.[4] For instance, in the U.S. those who are food insecure often eat fewer servings of nutrient-dense foods, such as vegetables, milk, and meat, and consume poorer-quality diets in general. These nutrient-poor diets can impair physical and mental health status. Food insecure children report more stomachaches, headaches, and colds[5, 6] and may not grow normally.[7] Behavioral problems in school, lower educational achievement, higher rates of depression and suicidal symptoms, and increased levels of psychological distress also have been linked to food insecurity.[5, 8, 9] Parents may compromise their own diets to allow children to have better diets.[10] Food insecure adults have a higher risk of chronic diseases, such as diabetes, and poorer management of these diseases.[11, 12]

In the U.S. food insecurity and poverty also are linked with obesity, particularly in women, perhaps because food insecurity predisposes individuals to overeating when food is more plentiful or because mostly inexpensive, high-energy-density foods are purchased.[13-16] In fact, many low-nutrient-density foods cost less than foods that are more nutrient dense, which means that food insecure individuals often get enough (or too many) calories without meeting some vitamin and mineral needs.[7, 8, 15]

Food Insecurity and Malnutrition in the United States

Since 1995, the United States Department of Agriculture (USDA) has monitored the food security of U.S. households. Although the U.S. has one of the world's most abundant, nutritious, and affordable food supplies, currently 11% (12.6 million) of households are not able to obtain enough food at times during the year—they are food insecure.[17] According to the USDA, in a **food secure** household, food needs are met all of the time. Food insecure households in the U.S. are those in which the quality, variety, and/or desirability of the diet is reduced and there is difficulty at times providing enough food for everyone in the household. With very low food security, households report multiple indications of disrupted eating patterns and reduced food

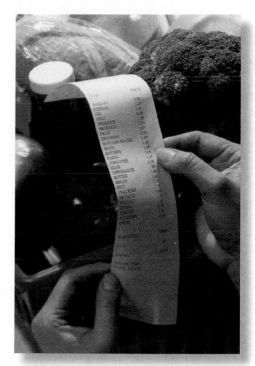

Fresh produce may be too expensive for some low-income families.

▶ A comparison between soft drinks and milk demonstrates the cost disparity between low- and high-nutrient-dense foods. Recently advertised prices for generic supermarket brand soda and milk were 99 cents for a dozen 12-oz cans (total: 144 oz) of the soft drink and $3.69 for a gallon (128 oz) of fat-free milk. The soft drink is just 6 cents for 8 oz, but the milk is 23 cents for the same amount. The milk costs 383% more than the soda.

Food insecurity is part of the North American landscape. A safety net of programs exists, but it is porous.

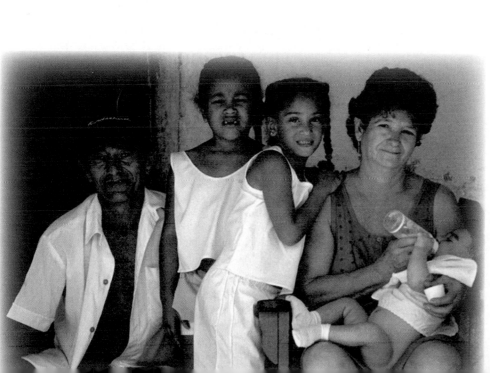

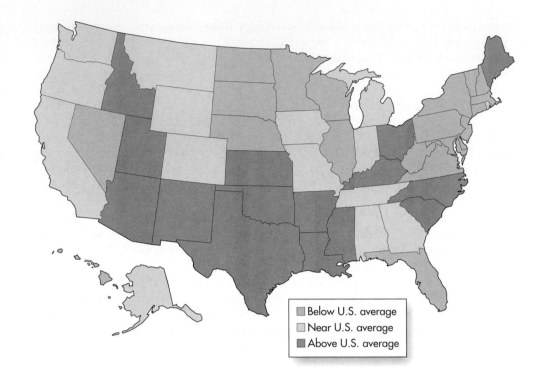

Figure 3-2 **Food insecurity in the United States, average 2004–2006.**

Source: USDA, Economic Research Service.

▶ One goal of *Healthy People 2010* is to increase food security among U.S. households from the current 89% to 94%. Another goal aims to lower the incidence of growth retardation among low-income children ages 5 and under from the baseline of 8% to 5%.

> **poverty guidelines** Preferred term for the federal poverty level; income level calculated each year by the U.S. Census Bureau. Guidelines are used to determine eligibility for many federal food and nutrition assistance programs.

▶ The federal minimum wage of $5.85 per hour is due to increase to $7.25 per hour in 2009. A full-time worker earning $7.25 per hour makes $15,080 per year. If this person is the sole wage earner in the family, they will live below the federal poverty guideline. If that family's rent is $700 per month, $8400 of the $15,080 goes to housing, leaving just $6680 for all other family expenses, including food, in the year.

intake. About a third of food insecure households fall into this category.[18] Figure 3-2 shows how food security varies by state in the U.S.

Food insecurity is closely linked to poverty. In the U.S., about 37 million people (12% of the population)—more than a third of whom are children—live at or below the **poverty guidelines**, currently estimated at $20,650 for a family of 4.[19] Poverty rates are even greater for children living in single-parent households and for certain racial and ethnic groups. Currently, 25% of African-Americans and Native Americans and 22% of Hispanics live in poverty, compared with approximately 9% of Asians and Caucasians. Low-paying jobs and unemployment, coupled with a lack of health-care benefits, high housing costs, family break-ups, and catastrophic illness, contribute to economic hardship and poverty.

Programs to Increase Food Security in the United States

Since the 1930s, the U.S. government has provided food assistance to individuals and families in need. Today, the 15 food and nutrition assistance programs administered by the USDA account for about 60% of the total USDA budget.[20] Food and nutrition assistance programs increase access to food and help reduce food insecurity. However, not everyone in need of assistance receives it—individuals may not know about the programs, may find the application process too difficult, may not have transportation to the program site, or may feel uncomfortable about participating. The following are the largest government assistance programs; the websites of these programs are listed at the end of the chapter.

- *Food Stamp Program.* The Food Stamp Program (FSP) is regarded as the cornerstone of the food assistance programs. It provides monthly benefits in the form of an Electronic Benefit Transfer card, which works like a debit card. The average benefit per person is $93 per month. About 1 in 11 persons in the United States participates in the program.[20] Benefits can be used to purchase food, as well as seeds to grow food; they cannot be used to buy tobacco, alcoholic beverages, and non-edible products. Food Stamp Nutrition Education, intended to help FSP participants make healthier food choices, is available in almost all states.

- *Special Supplemental Nutrition Program for Women, Infants, and Children (WIC).* This program provides low-income pregnant, breastfeeding, and post-partum women, infants, and children up to age 5 who are at nutritional risk with vouchers to purchase specific nutrient-dense foods. These individuals also receive nutrition education and referrals to health-care and social services. Currently, about 75% of WIC participants are infants and children.

- *National School Lunch Program.* This program helps schools provide nutritious lunches to children, thereby helping them concentrate and learn. About 60% of children at participating schools take part in the program. The program subsidizes lunches by providing schools with cash and food. All children can participate, but children from families with qualifying incomes receive either free or reduced-price lunches, which must meet federal nutrition guidelines. Summer food service programs operate in some locations across the country to meet the need for food assistance during the summer break.

- *School Breakfast Program.* This program began in response to concerns about children attending school hungry. It operates similarly to the National School Lunch Program. Breakfasts must meet federal nutrition guidelines.

- *Child and Adult Care Food Program.* Reimbursement is provided to eligible child-care and nonresidential adult day-care centers that provide meals and snacks. Like the School Lunch and School Breakfast Programs, the meals must meet certain nutrition criteria.

- *Programs for seniors.* The Older Americans Act provides funding for nutrition programs targeted at older adults. Many communities offer congregate meal programs (often lunch served daily at a variety of sites in a community) and home-delivered meals—popularly known as Meals on Wheels. Meals must meet nutrition guidelines and are available at little or no cost. Senior Farmers' Market Nutrition Programs also are available in many states.

- *Food distribution programs.* Commodity foods are agricultural products purchased by the government. They typically include canned foods (fruits, vegetables, juices, meat, tuna), dry food (ready-to-eat cereal, non-fat dry milk, beans, dehydrated potatoes, pasta, rice, infant cereal), and limited amounts of fresh foods, such as cheese, fruits, and vegetables. These programs distribute commodity foods and provide nutrition assistance to low-income households, emergency feeding programs, disaster relief programs, Indian reservations, and older adults. Many food banks and pantries distribute commodity foods to their clients.

In addition to the government programs, many private programs provide food assistance to individuals at food banks and pantries, soup kitchens, and homeless shelters. Each year, about 27 million people in the U.S. obtain food from these programs.[21] The programs rely on support from individuals, faith-based organizations, businesses, foundations, and grants. Many of these programs greatly depend on volunteer workers.

The largest contributor of food to these emergency food programs is America's Second Harvest. This organization distributes food it receives from private and corporate donations and government commodities to large regional food banks, which then distribute to individual food pantries, soup kitchens, and shelters. In 2006, America's Second Harvest provided 2.16 billion pounds of food to 29,700 food pantries, 5600 soup kitchens, and 4100 emergency shelters.[22] Table 3-1 lists some ways individuals can help fight hunger.

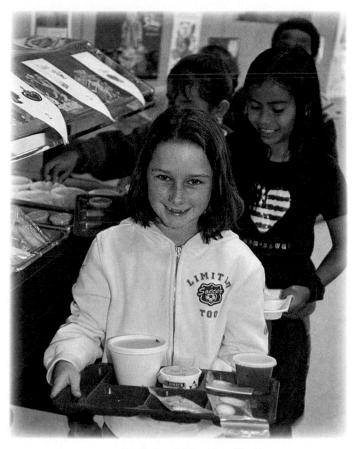

The National School Breakfast Program serves 9.8 million students per day.

▶ One of the many challenges faced by food banks and pantries is the lack of culturally appropriate foods. For example, providing dehydrated mashed potatoes or non-fat dry milk to a Chinese family unaccustomed to these foods may do little to help them meet their nutritional needs.

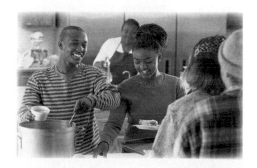

Food pantries and soup kitchens are important sources of nutrients for a growing number of people in the United States. Consider volunteering some of your time at a local program.

Table 3-1 Ways Individuals Can Help Fight Hunger in Their Communities

- Donate food—high-protein foods (e.g., tuna and peanut butter), baby food, and culturally appropriate foods are often in high demand.
- Start or participate in a campus or community program that targets hunger.
- Organize or work at a food drive.
- Donate money to organizations that fight hunger and food insecurity.
- Volunteer at a local food bank or pantry.
- Advocate for hunger programs by writing letters to newspapers, contacting state and national legislators, or joining an organization that advocates politically for hungry people.
- Attend events targeted at food security.
- Stay informed about hunger and food-security-related issues.
- Pay special attention to World Food Day, October 16 each year.

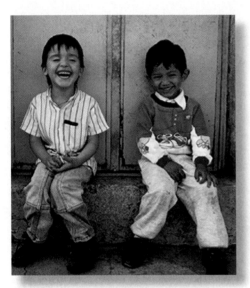

Insufficient calories, protein, zinc, and other nutrients limit the growth of children worldwide. About 30% of children in developing countries show evidence of poor growth rates.

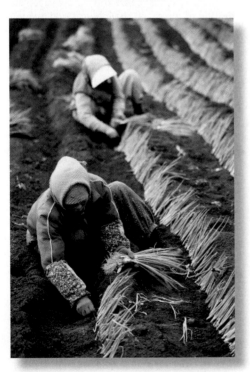

Food security is fostered by communities raising and distributing locally grown food.

Food Insecurity and Malnutrition in the Developing World

In developing countries, the most obvious form of undernutrition is a lack of energy-producing nutrients (fat, carbohydrate, protein). The most common micronutrient deficiencies are iron, vitamin A, and iodine deficiencies.

Undernutrition disproportionately affects young children and women. Every year, more than 5.5 million preschool children (or about 12 children every minute) in the developing world die of causes related to undernutrition.[23] About a quarter of the world's children are underweight and almost a third have stunted growth.[24] Such children are more likely to suffer from infectious diseases and to have problems learning. Many women have access to less food than men in the household because some social customs dictate that women eat last. When a woman is poorly nourished, her developing fetus or breastfed infant also may suffer malnutrition.

Many hungry people in developing countries live in rural areas where they are unemployed or work as **subsistence farmers**—those who can grow food only for their families, with not enough extra to sell for an income. Farming is difficult in many regions because of poor-quality farmland; lack of fertilizer, seeds, and farming equipment; and water availability (drought or flooding). The poor health caused by food insecurity limits farmers' physical capabilities and ability to work. Natural disasters, war, and political unrest make the situation worse and can trigger food shortages and famine. Famine disrupts every aspect of life: rates of disease and death increase, jobs disappear, poverty worsens, crime increases, civil wars may erupt or intensify, and government corruption may plague relief efforts. Many people who migrate to cities in hopes of finding work live in crowded, extremely poor-quality, unsafe housing and lack access to clean water, sufficient food, and medical care.

Most experts agree that reducing malnutrition depends on economic development to reduce poverty. Agricultural development is especially important because most poor people live in rural areas.[25] With agricultural improvements, households can grow more crops, eat healthier diets, and earn an income from the extra food and crops they grow. Increasing agricultural productivity is costly and complex, though, and requires infrastructure (e.g., roads, irrigation, electricity, and banks), agricultural research, education, and health. Improvements in health, especially by eliminating micronutrient deficiencies, providing clean food and water, and offering family planning methods, are critical because economic growth requires healthy people who are able to work, learn, and make improvements.

At the September 2000 United Nations Millennium Summit, the world's leaders agreed upon a goal to reduce extreme poverty and hunger by half. Some progress has been made toward this goal—hunger and poverty are decreasing throughout much of Asia and hunger is declining in Latin America. However, hunger and poverty are on the increase in sub-Saharan Africa and in Eastern Europe, although to a lesser extent.[26]

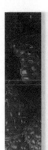

Knowledge Check

1. What are the causes of food insecurity?
2. What are the effects of food insecurity and malnutrition?
3. How does food insecurity and hunger in developing countries differ from what is seen in the U.S.?
4. What are some of the federal food and nutrition programs? Which of these programs serve children?

3.2 Food Production

Agriculture, the production of food and livestock, has supplied humans with food for millennia. At one time, nearly everyone was involved in food production. Only about 1 in 3 people around the globe and far fewer in the U.S. (less than 1%), is now involved in farming. Today, numerous advances in agricultural sciences are affecting our food supply; of particular note are organic food production and biotechnology.

Organic Foods

Organic foods are increasingly available in supermarkets, specialty stores, farmers' markets, and restaurants. Consumers can select organic fruits, vegetables, grains, dairy products, meats, eggs, and many processed foods, including sauces and condiments, breakfast cereals, cookies, and snack chips. Interest in personal and environmental health has contributed to the increasing availability and sales of organic foods. Despite this rapid growth, less than 3% of foods sold are organic.[27] Organic foods, because they often cost more to grow and produce, are typically more expensive than comparable conventional foods.

The term **organic** refers to the way agricultural products are produced. Organic production relies on farming practices such as **biological pest management**, composting, manure applications, and crop rotation to maintain healthy soil, water, crops, and animals. Synthetic pesticides, fertilizers, and hormones; antibiotics; sewage sludge (used as fertilizer); genetic engineering; and irradiation are not permitted in the production of organic foods (pesticides, antibiotics, and genetic engineering are discussed later in the chapter). Additionally, organic meat, poultry, eggs, and dairy products must come from animals allowed to graze outdoors and fed only organic feed.[28]

The Organic Foods Production Act of 1990 established standards for the production of foods that bear the USDA organic seal. Foods labeled and marketed as organic must be grown on farms that are certified by the USDA as following all of the rules established in the 1990 act. Foods made from multiple ingredients (e.g., breakfast cereal) labeled as organic must have at least 95% of their ingredients (by weight) meet organic standards. The term "made with organic" can be used if at least 70% of the ingredients are organic. Small organic producers and farmers with sales less than $5000 per year are exempt from the certification regulation. Some farmers use organic production methods but choose not to be USDA certified. Their foods cannot be labeled as organic, but many of these farmers market and sell to those seeking organic foods.

Organic Foods and Health

Consumers may choose to eat organic foods to reduce their pesticide intake, to protect the environment, and to improve the nutritional quality of their diets. Those who

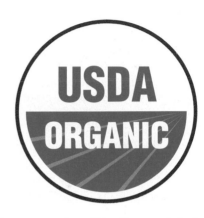

The USDA organic seal identifies organic foods grown on USDA-certified organic farms.

biological pest management Control of agricultural pests by using natural predators, parasites, or pathogens. For example, ladybugs can be used to control an aphid infestation.

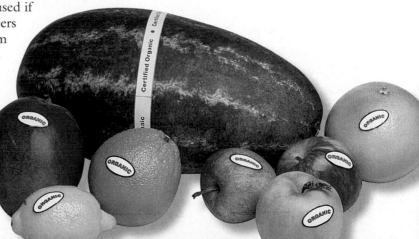

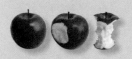

sustainable agriculture Agricultural system that provides a secure living for farm families; maintains the natural environment and resources; supports the rural community; and offers respect and fair treatment to all involved, from farm workers to consumers to the animals raised for food.

CRITICAL THINKING

Stephanie, a college sophomore, is adamant about eating only organic foods. She frequently states that conventionally grown and processed foods are unhealthy, full of harmful chemicals, and almost nutrient-free. Knowing that you are studying nutrition, Stephanie discusses her beliefs with you and asks for your opinion. What are some ways you might respond to her?

consume organic produce do ingest lesser amounts of pesticides (only 1 in 4 organically grown fruits and vegetables contains pesticides and in lower amounts than conventional produce), but it's still not known whether or how this affects the health of most consumers. However, organic foods may be a wise choice for young children because pesticide residues may pose a greater risk to them. Consumers also may opt for organic foods to encourage environmentally friendly **sustainable agriculture** practices.

Most studies do not show that organic foods have higher amounts of vitamins and minerals.[29] However, researchers have found that, in some cases, organic fruits and vegetables contain more vitamin C and antioxidants that help protect cells against damage.[29-31] At this point, it's not possible to recommend organic foods over conventional foods based on nutrient content—both can meet nutritional needs. A healthy dose of common sense also is important—an "organic" label does not change a less healthy food into a more healthy food. Organic potato chips have the same calorie and fat content as conventional potato chips.

One concern raised about organic foods is that food safety may be jeopardized because animal manures used for fertilizers might cause more pathogen contamination of food. However, research does not show that certified organic food has higher contamination with bacterial pathogens.[32] Consumers should wash or scrub all produce—organic as well as conventional—under running water.

Take Action

A Closer Look at Organic Foods

Visit one or more supermarkets to see what organic foods are available. Note your findings below.

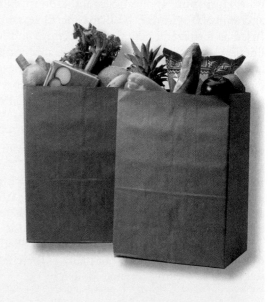

	Available	Not Available
Meat		
Poultry		
Milk		
Eggs		
Cheese		
Lettuce		
Apples		
Bananas		
Broccoli		
Other produce		
Breakfast cereal		
Snack chips		
Crackers		
Bread		
Pasta		
Beer		

Do you currently purchase organic foods? Why or why not?

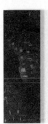

Knowledge Check

1. What substances and practices are not allowed in organic food production?
2. What are the potential advantages and disadvantages of eating organic foods?

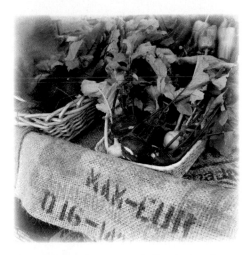

Farmers' markets are a good place to shop for organic foods.

Biotechnology—Genetically Modified Foods

Traditional biotechnology is almost as old as agriculture. The first farmer to improve his stock by selectively breeding the best bull with the best cows was implementing biotechnology in a simple sense. By the 1930s, biotechnology had made possible the selective breeding of better plant hybrids. As a result, corn production in the United States quickly doubled. Through similar methods, agricultural wheat was crossed with wild grasses to confer more desirable properties, such as greater yield, increased resistance to mildew and bacterial diseases, and tolerance to salt and adverse climatic conditions.

Development of the biotechnology processes now known as genetic engineering or modification, allowed scientists to directly alter the genetic makeup of an organism. Using **recombinant DNA technology,** scientists can transfer a gene that confers a specific trait, such as disease resistance, from almost any plant, animal, or microorganism into another (Fig. 3-3). The resulting organism is commonly referred to as a genetically modified food (GM food), a genetically engineered food (GE food), or a transgenic plant or animal. (A term in previous use, *genetically modified organism, or GMO,* is no longer recommended.) A GM food differs from the original food by only 1 or 2 genes (plants contain thousands of genes). Compared with traditional breeding, this process allows access to a wider gene pool and the faster and more accurate transfer of genes. Note, however, that developing a transgenic plant often takes years of careful research because it can be very difficult to identify the specific genes associated with desired traits.

recombinant DNA technology Test tube technology that rearranges DNA sequences in an organism by cutting the DNA, adding or deleting a DNA sequence, and rejoining DNA molecules using a series of enzymes.

GM Foods

Genetic engineering is widely used in agriculture. The U.S. grows more than 50% of such crops, and the developing countries of Argentina, Brazil, India, and China account for almost all the rest.[33] Soybeans, corn, and cotton are the main GM crops in the U.S.; others include papayas, canola, and squash.[34] Currently, biotechnology is used primarily to improve the control of pests, weeds, and plant diseases. Farmers growing crops genetically modified to be tolerant to herbicides (weed killers) can apply herbicides without harming the crop itself. This helps increase crop yield, decrease use of the most toxic herbicides (but with a higher use of lower-toxicity herbicides), and reduce tilling to decrease weeds; less tilling can reduce soil erosion and save fuel.[33] About 90% of all soybeans planted in the U.S. are herbicide tolerant. To aid pest control, the gene for a protein made by the soil bacterium *Bacillus thuringiensis*, Bt, was introduced into corn. The Bt protein is a naturally occurring pesticide that kills caterpillars, a major threat to corn. Before Bt corn was introduced, farmers often applied toxic pesticides to protect corn. Today, almost 75% of the U.S. corn crop is genetically modified. GM potatoes can produce a beetle-killing toxin in their leaves, and genetic engineering created resistance (much like a vaccine) against a devastating virus common in papayas; over half of all papayas are genetically engineered.

There are currently no genetically modified animals on the market, but scientists have developed many such animals. GM salmon, developed several years ago as an efficient food source for people, can grow to 7 times their normal size; however, these fish have not been approved for commercial production. In one study, wild salmon grown with the transgenic salmon in

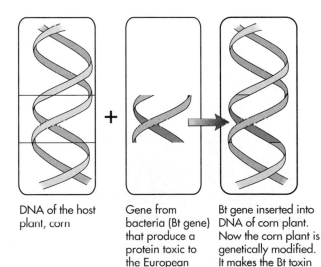

DNA of the host plant, corn

Gene from bacteria (Bt gene) that produce a protein toxic to the European corn borer

Bt gene inserted into DNA of corn plant. Now the corn plant is genetically modified. It makes the Bt toxin and, so, is resistant to the European corn borer.

Figure 3-3 In this diagram, a gene from the bacterium *Bacillus thuringiensis* (Bt) is spliced into the DNA of a host corn plant. The corn plant, now referred to as a GM plant, is resistant to the European corn borer.

▶ One very successful application of genetic engineering is the production of insulin, a drug used to treat diabetes. Genetically engineered insulin, known as humulin, was approved by the FDA in 1982. It is produced by introducing the human gene for insulin into *E. coli* bacteria and letting the bacteria grow in the laboratory and produce insulin. Today, almost all insulin produced in the United States is made this way.

▶ Golden rice was first developed with the daffodil beta-carotene gene spliced into rice. Although this was successful, the beta-carotene content of the rice was too low to have a positive impact on nutritional status. Scientists then switched to using the beta-carotene gene from corn. This GM rice has a much higher amount of beta-carotene.

Over 90% of the soybeans in the marketplace are genetically modified.

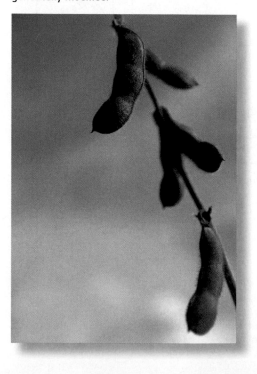

an experimental setting did not survive when food supplies were low.[35] This study raised concern about the release of transgenic fish into the ocean and about the compatibility of wild species with transgenic species.

Another agricultural application of biotechnology is the use of recombinant bovine growth hormone (rBGH) (also called recombinant bovine somatotropin, rBST), approved by the Food and Drug Administration (FDA) in 1993, to increase milk production in dairy cows. Bovine growth hormone is a protein, normally produced in the pituitary gland of cows, that triggers the production of another protein, insulin-like growth factor, which in turn stimulates milk production. Concerns about the use of rBGH relate to animal health, especially mastitis (inflammation of cow udders), which may require extra use of antibiotics.[36] Although there is evidence that elevated insulin-like growth factor is associated with certain cancers in humans,[36] there is no evidence that drinking milk is associated with these cancers. The FDA allows farmers who do not use rBGH in their dairy herds to indicate this on milk labels. U.S. organic food regulations do not permit the use of rBGH in organic milk, nor is it approved for use in Canada and Europe.

Chymosin, also known as rennin, is the enzyme used to make cheese from milk. Traditionally, chymosin was harvested from the stomach of calves, an expensive process. Now almost all chymosin is produced by genetically engineered bacteria or yeast. Chymosin produced in this manner has the advantage of being much purer than that extracted from calves.

GM Foods of the Future A variety of new GM foods are under study. Some of these, like those currently grown in the U.S., are designed to help farmers grow foods more easily and to increase yields. Others are being developed to withstand harsh growing conditions, such as drought, extreme cold, and salty soil. Still others are designed to provide more direct benefits to consumers. These include fresh produce with extended shelf lives and more nutrient-dense foods. For example, rice with increased levels of beta-carotene, a yellow-orange compound that can be converted to vitamin A in the body, is in development. This "golden rice" may help improve nutritional status in regions where low vitamin A intakes are a problem. Vegetable oils with a more "heart-healthy" profile are being developed, along with peanuts, soybeans, wheat, eggs, and milk that no longer cause allergic reactions in susceptible individuals.[37]

Many scientists believe that biotechnology has great potential to help reduce hunger and malnutrition[33, 37] by improving agricultural yields, allowing crops to grow in poor-quality soil, increasing vitamin levels in foods, and decreasing environmental degradation by reducing the use of agricultural chemicals. However, there are some obstacles to its use. One frequently cited barrier concerns the ability of poor farmers to access this technology.[33, 38] Biotechnology research often is conducted by large corporations that patent their products and sell them to farmers at higher prices than conventional seed. Poor farmers who cannot afford the seeds may suffer economic losses. One positive development is that researchers at public universities are developing a variety of GM crops—the problem has been that these researchers haven't been able to readily get them tested and into use.[38] Another closely related concern is that most of the crops developed by corporations (corn, cotton, soybeans) tend to have industrial uses, whereas far less research has focused on foods that are the dietary staples of millions of people, such as rice, wheat, yams, chickpeas, and peanuts.[33]

Regulation of GM Foods In the U.S., GM foods are regulated by the FDA, USDA, and Environmental Protection Agency (EPA).[39] The FDA's role is to ensure that the food is safe for humans and animals to eat (e.g., no toxins or allergens are present). It is the responsibility of the USDA to make sure GM crops are safe to grow. The EPA ensures that pesticides introduced into foods (e.g., Bt corn) are safe for consumption and for the environment. Companies with a new GM plant to release to the marketplace enter into a consultation process with the FDA to ensure its safety. Although the process is not mandatory, the FDA has evaluated all GM foods on the market and has found them safe to eat. Critics contend that this process should be required instead of voluntary and should be more stringent.

Labeling for GM foods or those with GM ingredients is not required in the U.S.; however, some countries, including New Zealand, Australia, Japan, South Korea, and many European countries, do require this information on food labels. The FDA contends that such labeling is not required because GM foods are not tangibly different from foods that are not genetically modified. Many critics of GM food disagree, arguing that consumers have a right to information about the food they consume. Because corn (to make sweeteners and oil) and soybeans (to make vegetable oil) are so widely used in the U.S. food supply and are fed to cattle, most people have consumed GM foods.

Safety of GM Foods Consumers often question if the benefits of GM foods outweigh their risks. Concerns about food and environmental safety include the following:

• The addition of allergens, such as those in peanuts, eggs, milk, wheat, and shellfish, to GM foods that previously did not contain them. Evidence of allergen contamination was seen in one instance in soybeans but, in more than 10 years of the use of GM crops, there has been no evidence of any harmful reactions or effects in humans. The FDA examines all GM products and will enforce labeling requirements regarding potential allergens that may be present in food altered by biotechnology.

• The possibility of "gene flow" from GM crops to plants not intended for modification. One result of this hybridization might be the development of "superweeds" resistant to herbicides and insecticides.

• The development of Bt-resistant insects. This is of particular concern to organic farmers who, although they do not grow GM crops, apply the *Bacillus thuringiensis* bacteria to crops as a biological pest-management method. Bt resistance also may lead to increased pesticide use by nonorganic farmers.

• The loss of genetic diversity. If GM crops are widely adopted, the use of local indigenous conventional seeds may decline and these plants may disappear.

• Insufficient regulation and oversight of GM plants and animals. Some argue that more rigorous regulation, testing, and oversight are needed to assure safety and benefits for consumers.

Still other concerns relate to ways the technology might be used in the future: the transfer of animal (even human) genes into plants, the genetic engineering of animals to create new species, and the bioengineering of plants to produce medications (known as **biopharming**). Biopharming is not yet approved as a way to manufacture medications in the U.S.; one concern is that biopharmed crops might mix with crops intended for food, thus exposing many people to a potentially harmful medication. Other fears relate to unknowns, such as how widespread use of GM crops might affect both the agricultural system and the overall ecosystem. Some fear that scientists know too little about how genes function to ensure benefits and safety. Many consumers, especially in countries where food is abundant, question the need for GM crops and believe that they benefit mainly large-scale farmers and the corporations that have developed the technology.

Meat and Milk from Cloned Animals

In 1997, the famous sheep Dolly introduced the world to animal **cloning**—the process of making genetically identical animals by nonsexual reproduction. Because the DNA is not altered, cloned animals are not genetically modified. Cloning is done by extracting the genetic material from a donor adult cell and transferring it to an egg that has had its own genetic material removed. The cloned embryo that results is transferred to the uterus of a female, where it continues to grow and develop until birth.[40] The biological process of cloning is not new—plants have been cloned for centuries. Growing a new plant from the leaf of another is an example of plant cloning. Some animals, such as worms and frogs, can clone on their own, a process called parthenogenesis.

Some ranchers and farmers are interested in cloning as a way to reproduce their best-growing, best milk-producing, or best egg-laying animal for economic gain. After several years of study, the FDA announced in 2008 that it had determined that both meat and milk from cattle, swine, and goats are safe to eat.[40] However, these foods cannot

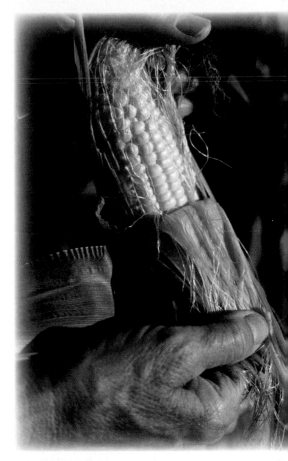

Both traditional plant breeding and biotechnology have produced high-yielding and disease-resistant plant varieties, such as with corn.

CRITICAL THINKING

According to a recent poll, about one-quarter of Americans favor the introduction of GM foods into our food supply, whereas nearly half are opposed to this.[74] Further, 75% acknowledge that they know little about GM foods. Do you think the public should know more about GM foods? If they did know more, do you think that this would change their opinions about introducing such foods into the food supply? Do you think Americans would be surprised to know the extent to which GM corn and soybeans are used?

Food Preservation Methods

Methods That Decrease Water Content to Deter Microbial Growth

Drying (raisins)

Salting (salted fish)

Sugaring (candied fruit)

Smoking (smoked fish)

Methods That Increase Acidity or Alcohol to Deter Microbial Growth

Fermentation and pickling (e.g., sauerkraut, kimchi, pickles, cheese, yogurt, wine)

Methods That Use Heat to Eradicate or Reduce Number of Microbes

Pasteurization (milk)

Sterilization (aseptic cartons of milk, soup)

Canning (beef stew)

Methods That Slow Rate of Microbial Growth

Refrigeration (eggs)

Freezing (meat)

Methods That Inhibit Microbial Growth

Food additives: chemical preservatives (sodium nitrate in cured meat)

Irradiation (raspberries)

To help keep processed food, such as potato chips and bagged salad greens, fresh longer, they are packed in airtight bags, which are then filled with nitrogen.

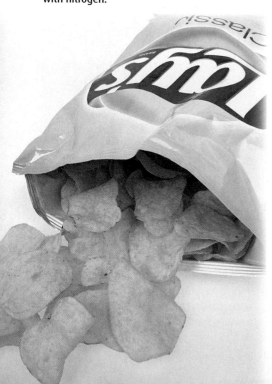

enter the marketplace until the USDA gives its approval. Although meat and milk from cloned animals appear safe for human consumption, many consumers are uncomfortable with cloning for religious and ethical reasons, and others question the need to add food produced from cloned animals to the food supply.

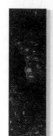

Knowledge Check

1. What is the main use of GM crops today?
2. What is Bt corn? How is it produced?
3. What is golden rice? How might it help improve nutritional status in the future?
4. How are GM foods regulated in the U.S.?
5. What are at least 3 objections related to using GM foods?

 3.3 Food Preservation and Processing

The vast majority of foods we purchase have been preserved or processed—frozen, refrigerated, canned, dehydrated, or milled, to name a few methods. Food preservation methods extend a food's shelf life by slowing the rate at which microorganisms (e.g., bacteria, mold, yeast) and enzymes in food cause spoilage. Food preservation permits a wide variety of good-quality, nutritious, and safe foods to be available year round. The oldest food preservation methods, some in use for thousands of years, are drying, salting, sugaring, smoking, and fermenting. Over the last 200 years, scientific discoveries and technological innovations have added pasteurization, sterilization, canning, aseptic processing, refrigeration, freezing, nitrogen packing, food irradiation, and preservative food additives to the list of food preservation techniques.

Food Irradiation

Food irradiation, sometimes known as cold or electronic pasteurization, is one of the newest food preservation methods. It uses radiant energy from gamma rays, X rays, or electron beams to extend the shelf life of food and to control the growth of insects and pathogens (bacteria, fungi, parasites) in foods.[41] Foods are exposed to controlled doses of radiant energy, which essentially pass through the food. Just as an airport scanner or dental X rays do not make your luggage or teeth radioactive, irradiated food is not radioactive. The history of food irradiation goes back nearly a century and includes scientific research, evaluation, and testing. Irradiated foods are safe in the opinion of the FDA and many other health authorities, including the American Academy of Pediatrics.[41]

Foods approved for irradiation in the U.S. include fresh meat and poultry, wheat and wheat powder, white potatoes, spices and dry vegetable seasonings, fresh shell eggs, and fresh produce.[42] Irradiated food, except for dried seasonings, must be labeled with the international food irradiation symbol, the Radura, and a statement that the product has been treated by irradiation. Although the demand for irradiated foods is still low in the U.S., other countries, including Canada, Japan, Italy, and Mexico, use food irradiation technology widely. Barriers to its use in the U.S. include consumers' lack of familiarity with the technology, the potentially higher cost of irradiated foods, and concerns about the taste and safety of irradiated foods.[43]

Food Additives

Food additives, especially those that help preserve and flavor foods (e.g., salt, vinegar, and alcohol), have been used for thousands of years. However, until the 20th century, food production and safety were not regulated, and harmful substances were sometimes added to foods. In the 1800s, toxic minerals (arsenic, lead, mercury) were used to color foods such as candies, pickles, meat, and even milk. Flour was diluted with chalk or limestone and preserved with borax, a substance commonly used to kill ants. Concern about such dangerous practices led Harvey Wiley, the chief chemist at the USDA, to test the safety of food additives. He enlisted the help of the "poison squad," a group of human volunteers who ate foods with high amounts of additives (fortunately, none of the volunteers suffered lasting ill effects). Wiley's work led to the first federal law regulating food, The Pure Food and Drugs Act of 1906.

Today, the FDA regulates over 3000 food additives. **Food additives** are substances added to foods to produce a desired effect, such as a longer shelf life (preservative), greater nutritional value, or a more appealing color. As the demand for convenient, time-saving prepared foods has increased, so have the need for and use of food additives. Many foods are prepared at large, central processing plants, transported long distances, and then held in warehouses for some time before purchase. Food additives can help keep foods appetizing, fresh, nutritious, and safe. Consider a typical lunch menu of a hamburger, cucumber salad with dressing, and lemonade. The hamburger bun is enriched with nutrient additives and contains a preservative to keep it fresh. The cucumber skin may be waxed to extend its shelf life and may contain an infinitesimal amount of pesticide residue, which technically is an additive. The dressing contains an emulsifier additive to keep it from separating and a preservative to keep it from spoiling. The convenient lemonade mix consists of additives (sweeteners, flavors, and colors) dissolved in water.

Intentional vs. Incidental Food Additives

All food additives are classified as either intentional or incidental. Intentional food additives are purposely added to achieve a goal, such as keeping a food fresh or enhancing its flavor. These additives are listed on food ingredient labels. Incidental additives, also called indirect additives, are not intentionally added but become part of a food through some aspect of food production, processing, packaging, transport, or storage. They have no function in finished products. One example is benzene, a carcinogen found in very small amounts in some beverages. It forms when benzoate salts (preservatives) and vitamin C react. The small amount in beverages is not thought to be a risk for consumers.[44] Another example is acrylamide, a neurotoxin and possible carcinogen, which forms when high-carbohydrate foods, such as potato chips and french fries, are fried. Research to determine if acrylamide in food poses a risk is ongoing. Pesticide residues on produce are another example of an incidental additive.

Synthetic vs. Natural Additives

Although most food additives are synthetic compounds, this does not make them inherently less safe than natural compounds. The toxicity of a substance is determined by its effects in the body, not whether it is synthesized in a laboratory or a plant. The dose of the substance also is critical. Even a common substance, such as table salt, can cause illness or even death when ingested in large amounts. Further, many plants contain natural toxins that are even more potent and prevalent than the additives intentionally added to foods. Some cancer researchers suggest that we ingest at least 10,000 times more (by weight) natural toxins produced by plants than synthetic additives or pesticides.[45] (Natural toxins are discussed later in this chapter.)

Uses of Food Additives

Intentional food additives are used to (1) improve freshness and safety, (2) enhance or maintain nutritional value, (3) enhance or maintain color and flavor, and (4) contribute to functional characteristics, such as the texture and acidity of a food. Examples of additives in each of these categories appear in Table 3-2. In the U.S., regulations do not permit

radiation Energy that is emitted from a center in all directions. Various forms of radiation energy include X rays, microwaves, and ultraviolet rays from the sun.

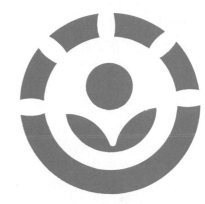

This Radura symbol indicates that a foods has been irradiated.

▶ Many additives are ingredients you know, such as sodium chloride (salt), sucrose (table sugar), and sodium bicarbonate (baking soda). The complete list of food additives is in the FDA database "Everything Added to Foods in the US." Visit vm.cfsan.fda.gov/~dms/eafus.html.

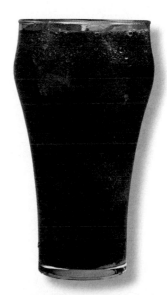

Many soft drinks contain several intentional food additives, including colors, flavors, and sweeteners.

Table 3-2 Functions and Examples of Common Food Additives

Type of Food Additive	Examples of Additives	Examples of Uses
Improve Freshness and Safety		
Antimicrobial Agents	Sodium benzoate Sorbic acid Calcium propionate	Inhibit growth of molds, fungi, and bacteria in beverages, baked goods, jams, jellies, salad dressings, processed meats
Antioxidants	Butylated hydroxyanisole (BHA) Butylated hydroxytoulene (BHT) Ascorbic acid Erythorbic acid Alpha-tocopherol Sulfites	Control adverse effects of oxygen and/or prevent fats from spoiling; used in breakfast cereals, chewing gums, nuts, processed meats. Prevent light-colored foods (sliced potatoes, white wine, fruit) from discoloring
Curing Agents	Sodium nitrate Sodium nitrite	Prevent growth of *Clostridium botulinum* in bacon, ham, salami, hot dogs, and other cured meats Contribute to pink color of cured meats
Acidic Agents	Acetic acid, ascorbic acid, phosphoric acid, lactic acid	Add tartness and inhibit growth of microorganisms in foods such as beverages, salad dressings, candies, frozen desserts, salsas, pickles, and processed meats
Alter Nutritional Value		
Replace nutrients lost in processing (enrichment); add nutrients (fortification)	Vitamins, minerals, protein	Vitamins A and D in milk Thiamin, riboflavin, niacin, folic acid, iron in cereal and grain products Iodine in salt
Alternative Sweeteners	aspartame, saccharin	Saccharin in soft drinks
Fat Replacers	olestra, salatrim	Fried snack foods
Enhance Flavor or Color		
Flavors and Spices	Salts, sugars, herbs, spices, flavors	Grape flavor in popsicles
Flavor Enhancers	Monosodium glutamate (MSG) Guanosine monophosphate (GMP)	Enhance existing flavor or contribute savory flavor to foods, such as soups, rice, and noodle mixes
Color Additives	Beta-carotene, annatto, beet coloring, cochineal, caramel coloring	Natural colors or humanmade counterparts of natural color derivatives used in many foods; exempt from FDA certification
Certifiable Color Additives	FD&C Blue #1, FD&C Blue #2, FD&C Green #3, FD&C Red #3, FD&C Red #40, FD&C Yellow #5, FD&C Yellow #6, Citrus Red #2	The only humanmade dyes currently certified by the FDA for use in foods; found in a variety of foods
Enhance Functional Characteristics		
Emulsifiers	Egg yolks, soy lecithin, mono- and diglycerides	Salad dressings, peanut butter, frozen desserts, baking mixes, margarine
Anticaking Agents	Calcium silicate, ammonium citrate, magnesium stearate	Keep foods, especially powdered mixes, free-flowing
Humectants	Glycerol, sorbitol	Retain moisture, flavor, and texture in foods, such as marshmallows, soft candies, energy bars
Stabilizers, Thickeners	Pectin, gums (guar, carrageenan, xanthan), gelatin	Add creaminess and thickness to foods, such as frozen desserts, yogurt, dairy products, salad dressings, pudding, gelatin mixes
Enzymes	Lactase, rennet, chymosin, pectinase	Act on proteins, fats, or carbohydrates in foods. Lactase makes milk more digestible; rennet and chymosin are required for cheese-making; pectinase improves the clarity of some jellies and fruit juices.
Leavening Agents	Yeast, baking soda, baking powder	Contribute leavening gases (mainly CO_2) to improve texture of baked products, such as breads, cookies, cakes, baking mixes

food additives to be used to hide defective food ingredients or poor product quality (as they were earlier in history), to deceive customers, or to replace good manufacturing practices.

Flavors and flavor enhancers are the largest and most commonly used groups of additives—nearly 2000 are approved. In most food products, flavors and flavor enhancers are used in small amounts. (Some flavors are so potent that a single drop could flavor the entire contents of an Olympic-size swimming pool.) Additives such as salt, sugar, corn syrup, citric acid, baking soda, vegetable colors, and spices are among the most commonly used.

Regulation and Safety of Food Additives

The responsibility for the safety of food additives lies with the FDA, as set out by the 1958 Food Additives Amendment of the Food, Drug, and Cosmetics Act. Another amendment, enacted in 1960, specifies regulations for color additives. These laws require food manufacturers to obtain FDA approval for an additive before using it in food. They also require manufacturers to be responsible for testing and proving the safety of an additive.

Prior-Sanctioned Substances and the GRAS List The 1958 Food Additives Amendment exempted 2 groups of substances from the food additive regulation process. All substances that the FDA or USDA determined were safe for use in specific foods prior to this amendment were designated **prior-sanctioned substances.** Examples of prior-sanctioned substances are sodium nitrite and potassium nitrite, used to preserve luncheon meats. A second category of substances excluded from the food additive regulation process are substances **Generally Recognized As Safe (GRAS)** by experts, based on the substances' extensive history of use in food before 1958 or by published scientific evidence. Salt, sugar, spices, vitamins, and monosodium glutamate are classified as GRAS substances, along with several hundred other substances.

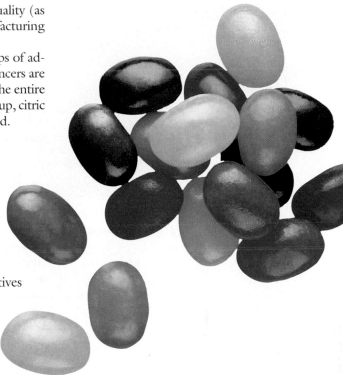

Color additives make some foods more desirable.

Since 1958, some substances on the GRAS list have been reviewed and some have been deleted from the list and the food supply. One example is safrole, a natural flavoring once used in root beer. Many certified color additives have been removed because of evidence of cancer and organ damage. Most chemicals on the GRAS list have not been reviewed (e.g., vanilla, salt, vinegar), primarily because of expense and their long histories of use coupled with lack of evidence for toxicity.

Food Additive Safety Tests Intentional food additives are tested under FDA scrutiny for safety on at least 2 animal species, usually rats and mice. Scientists determine the highest dose of the additive that produces *no observable effects* in the animals. This dose, the **no-observable-effect level (NOEL),** is proportionately much higher than humans would ever encounter in food. The amount of an additive permitted in food is the NOEL divided by at least 100—this establishes a very large margin of safety to ensure that the food additive will cause no harmful health effects in humans.

One important exception applies to the testing of food additives. The Delaney Clause in the 1958 Food Additive Amendments prohibits the use of any food additive shown to cause cancer in humans or animals at any dose. However, incidental food additives that may cause cancer are treated differently. The FDA cannot simply ban various industrial chemicals, pesticide residues, and natural mold toxins from foods because they are not purposely added to foods. However, the FDA does set an acceptable level for these substances. Basically, an incidental additive cannot contribute to more than 1 cancer case during the lifetimes of 1 million people. If a higher risk exists, the amount of the compound in a food must be reduced until the guideline is met.

New Food Additive Approval Today, before a new additive can be used in foods, the FDA must approve it. Manufacturers must offer proof from rigorous tests that show the additive will accomplish its intended purpose in a food, that it is safe, and that it is to be used in no greater amounts than needed to achieve its purpose. Manufacturers also must give the FDA information about how the additive is manufactured and the laboratory

▶ These 2 brands of tortilla chips differ greatly in their use of food additives:

Brand 1

Whole corn, vegetable oil, salt, cheddar cheese, maltodextrin, wheat flour, whey, monosodium glutamate, buttermilk solids, Romano cheese from cow's milk, whey protein concentrate, onion powder, partially hydrogenated soybean and cottonseed oils, corn flour, disodium phosphate, lactose, natural and artificial flavor, tomato powder, spices, lactic acid, artificial color (including yellow 6, yellow 5, and red 40), citric acid, sugar, garlic powder, red and green bell pepper powder, sodium caseinate, disodium inosinate, disodium guanylate, nonfat milk solids, whey protein isolate, corn syrup solids.

Brand 2

Organic stone ground blue corn with a trace of lime, organic vegetable oil, sea salt.

methods used to detect and measure the amount in foods. Two of the newer additives approved for use in the food supply include the artificial sweetener sucralose (sold as Splenda®) and the fat substitute olestra (sold as Olean®).

Concerns about Food Additives Many people continue to wonder about the long-term safety of some food additives. Of course, many food additives on the GRAS list have not been adequately tested. It also is possible that new, more sensitive research methods will reveal that currently permitted additives are not as safe as they are currently believed to be. Alternately, newer scientific techniques may indicate that some non-permitted substances are safer than currently thought. Recall that the scientific method requires us to challenge current knowledge and reassess our thinking when credible new findings are presented.

Food additives that may be of concern to some include aspartame, sodium nitrite, sodium nitrate, and artificial colors. For example, one study indicated that rats exposed throughout their life spans to the artificial sweetener aspartame had a higher risk of cancer.[46] Some consumers report dizziness and headaches after consuming it, but scientific studies do not support that it causes these effects. Sodium nitrate and sodium nitrite, added to cured meats to prevent growth of the deadly bacterium *Clostridium botulinum*, can be converted to carcinogenic nitrosamines in the stomach. Adding ascorbic acid or erythorbic acid to cured meats limits nitrosamine production. Many deem the benefit of minimizing deadly botulism infections greater than the small risk of nitrosamine formation. Some artificial colors have been reported to cause allergic-type reactions in children; others have been linked to cancer in animals. If credible future research confirms these effects, the amount permitted in food might be reduced or banned altogether. On the other hand, a banned additive might once again be permitted. For instance, cyclamate was banned in the U.S. and other countries when some research indicated it was a carcinogen. However, when a number of subsequent studies found no cancer risk, dozens of countries, including Canada, once again permitted it as a food additive. It is possible that the FDA will reapprove cyclamate in the future.

A few food additives cause adverse symptoms in sensitive individuals. Sulfites, a group of sulfur-based chemicals, are used as antioxidants and preservatives in foods. About 1 in 100 persons, particularly those with asthma, experiences shortness of breath or gastrointestinal symptoms after ingesting sulfites. Because of this, the use of sulfites is prohibited on salad bars and other raw vegetables. However, sulfites are found in a variety of foods, such as frozen or dehydrated potatoes, wine, and beer. Food labels indicate their presence. Monosodium glutamate, a flavor enhancer, also can cause problems; some individuals report flushing, chest pain, dizziness, rapid heartbeat, high blood pressure, headache, and/or nausea after consuming monosodium glutamate.

Many food producers are making foods with fewer additives to meet consumer preferences for **natural foods**—those free of food colors and synthetic substances. Reading ingredient lists will help you identify foods with fewer additives. Also, keep in mind that the more processed a food is, the more additives it is likely to contain. Many prepackaged, precooked, frozen, canned, and instant foods, mixes, and snack foods contain additives. To lower your intake of additives, read food labels and eat fewer highly processed foods. Although no evidence shows that limiting additives will make you healthier, replacing highly processed foods with fruits, vegetables, whole grains, meats, and dairy products is a healthy practice.

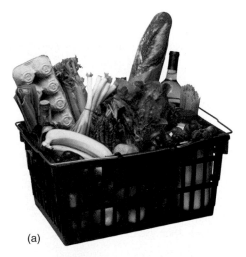

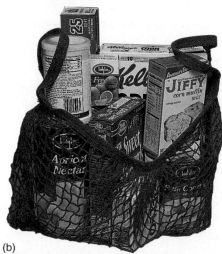

Cured meats derive their pink color from nitrates and nitrites.

(a)

(b)

Depending on food choices, a diet can be either (*a*) essentially devoid of food additives or (*b*) high in food additives.

Knowledge Check

1. How do food preservation methods preserve foods and decrease spoilage?
2. How can irradiated foods be identified?
3. How do intentional food additives differ from incidental food additives?
4. What are GRAS food additives?
5. What are the broad functions of intentional food additives?

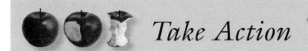 *Take Action*

A Closer Look at Food Additives

Evaluate the food label of a food item, either one in the supermarket or one you have available.

1. Write out the list of ingredients.

2. Identify the ingredients that you think are food additives.

3. Based on the information available in this chapter, what are the functions and relative safety of these food additives?

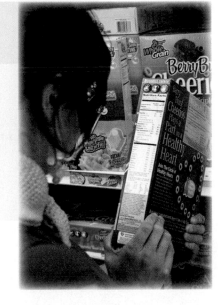

 ## 3.4 Food and Water Safety

In addition to having access to abundant, varied, and nutritious foods, we must have safe food and water supplies to support good health. Scientific knowledge of the pathogens in food and of safe food handling practices, technological developments (e.g., refrigeration, water purification, and milk pasteurization), and laws and regulations have greatly improved the safety of the food and water supplies and have contributed to a steep decline in foodborne and waterborne illness.

Scientists and health authorities agree that North Americans enjoy relatively safe water and food supplies. Nonetheless, pathogens and certain chemicals in foods and water still pose a health risk. Thus, the nutritional and health benefits of food and water must be balanced against related hazards. The next 3 sections of the chapter examine these hazards and how you can minimize your exposure.

Foodborne Illness

Foodborne illness caused by microbial pathogens remains a significant public health problem in the 21st century, so much so that it is one of the priorities in the *Healthy People 2010* initiative. According to the U.S. Centers for Disease Control and Prevention, foodborne pathogens cause about 76 million illnesses, 325,000 hospitalizations, and 5000 deaths in the United States each year.[47] The World Health Organization (WHO) estimates that, in developed nations, a third of the population has a foodborne illness event yearly, accounting for about 20 million deaths.[48] Foodborne illnesses are expensive—in the U.S. each year, the costs of lost productivity are estimated at $9 billion and hospital costs are more than $3 billion, not including the cost of the chronic, long-term consequences of some types of foodborne illness.

The importance of foodborne illness as a current health concern is underscored by the increasing numbers of at-risk individuals—in the U.S., one-quarter of the population is at increased risk of foodborne illness. At-risk individuals include those with weakened immune systems due to disease, pharmaceutical, or radiological treatments (e.g., HIV/AIDS, transplant and cancer patients); pregnant women and their fetuses; lactating mothers; infants and young children; and elderly persons. Others who may be at disproportionately greater risk are those living in institutional settings and homeless persons.

Most cases of foodborne illness go undiagnosed because the symptoms are mild enough that the ill persons do not seek medical care. These symptoms typically include gastrointestinal effects, such as nausea, vomiting, diarrhea, and intestinal cramping. However, some bouts of foodborne

foodborne illness Sickness caused by the ingestion of food containing pathogenic microorganisms or toxins made by these pathogens.

Food contaminated in a central plant can go on to produce illness in people in surrounding states or even across the nation. In the case of juices, shown here, it is important that they are pasteurized to reduce the risk of foodborne illness.

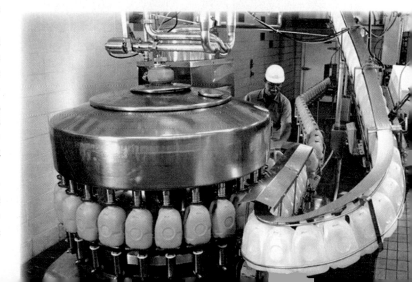

▶ To find information about the microbial pathogens in food and water, visit www.cdc.gov/DiseasesConditions.

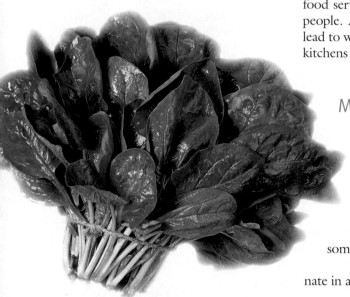

Spinach, lettuce, unpasteurized milk and juice, and undercooked ground beef have been implicated in outbreaks of *E. coli* 0157:H7.

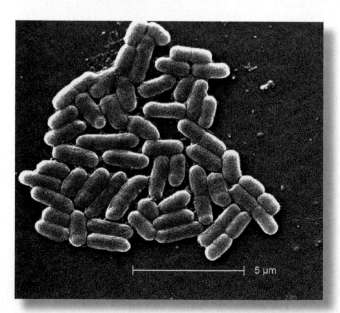

Most types of *Escherichia coli* are not dangerous, but *E. coli* 0157:H7 is the leading cause of bloody diarrhea in the United States. In children and the elderly, it can cause kidney failure and death.

illness, especially when coupled with ongoing health problems, are lengthy and lead to food allergies, seizures, blood poisoning (from microorganisms or their toxins in the bloodstream), chronic complications (e.g., arthritis), and even death.

Our food system affects the spread of foodborne illness. Most of the food we eat is grown on large farms far from our homes and is transported either to supermarkets, where we buy it fresh, or to food processing plants, where it is cleaned, prepared, and packaged before shipment to warehouses and then on to grocery stores. Large-scale production means that, if contamination occurs at any point, many people can be affected. This was evident in an outbreak associated with fresh, bagged spinach that was contaminated with the *Escherichia coli* bacterium; the spinach was shipped to 25 states and caused 200 cases of food poisoning, 100 hospitalizations, and 4 deaths.[49] Similarly, food mishandling in food service establishments, such as cafeterias and restaurants, can cause illness in many people. Although mishandling by food processors and food service establishments can lead to widespread problems, it is important to remember that food mishandling in home kitchens also is a cause of foodborne illness.

Microbial Pathogens

The greatest health risk from food and water today is contamination by bacteria and viruses and, to a lesser extent, by various forms of fungi and parasites. Foodborne illness occurs when microorganisms either directly infect the cells of the gastrointestinal tract, and sometimes other organs in the body, or secrete a toxin into food, which harms us when we eat it (called food intoxication). Unlike foodborne infections, live pathogens need not be present in food for a foodborne intoxication to occur. Toxin-producing bacteria need only to have, at some point, infused the food with their toxin.

Most of the pathogenic bacteria and viruses that cause foodborne illness originate in an infected human or animal and reach food by these fairly well defined routes:

- *Contamination by feces.* Many foodborne illness causing bacteria and viruses are excreted profusely in the feces of infected humans and animals. In countries with inadequate sanitation, the water used for drinking, cooking, washing produce and dishes, irrigating crops, and fishing is frequently contaminated with sewage and is a major source of illness. In the U.S. and other industrialized countries, fecal contamination usually occurs when food is handled by a person who has come in contact with feces or sewage (as in using the bathroom or changing diapers) and has not thoroughly washed his or her hands. Insects, such as houseflies, also may carry bacteria from sewage to food. Foodborne illnesses that are acquired from fecal matter in one of these ways are said to be transmitted by the fecal-oral route.

- *Contamination by an infected individual.* Some pathogenic bacteria and viruses can be transferred to food directly by an infected individual. For example, a food handler who has an open wound or who coughs or sneezes onto food may contaminate the food. Pets also may be a source of foodborne pathogens that can contaminate food via the unwashed hands of food preparers.

- *Cross-contamination.* Cross-contamination occurs when an uncontaminated food touches a pathogen-contaminated food or any object, such as a plate, knife, or cutting board, that has come in contact with contaminated food. For instance, let's say a person cuts up a raw chicken contaminated with pathogenic bacteria and then chops lettuce for a salad. When the person is cutting the chicken, the cutting board, the knife, and the food preparer's hands become contaminated with bacteria. If these items are not thoroughly washed before the person chops the lettuce, it will be cross-contaminated with bacteria. Although the bacteria on the chicken will be killed with cooking, the lettuce is not cooked and can cause foodborne illness.

Bacteria

Bacteria are single-cell organisms found in the food we eat, the water we drink, and the air we breathe. They live in our intestines, on our skin, in our refrigerators, and on kitchen countertops. Luckily, most are harmless, but a few are pathogenic and can cause illness. Any food can transmit pathogenic bacteria; however, the most common sources are meats, poultry, eggs, fish, shellfish, dairy products, and fresh produce.

Table 3-3 lists many of the bacteria that cause foodborne illness and describes typical food sources and the symptoms of the illnesses they cause. *Salmonella, Campylobacter,* and *Escherichia coli* cause most bacterial foodborne illness in the U.S.[50] Others, such as *Clostridium botulinum* and *Listeria monocytogenes,* cause fewer cases but are more likely to result in serious illness and death. In developing countries, pathogens such as *Vibrio cholerae* are more important.

To proliferate, bacteria require nutrients, water, and warmth. Most grow best in **danger zone** temperatures of 41° to 135°F (5° to 57°C) (Fig. 3-4). Pathogenic bacteria typically do not multiply when food is held at temperatures above 135°F (57°C) or stored at safe refrigeration temperatures, 32° to 40°F (0° to 4.4°C). One important exception is *Listeria* bacteria, which can multiply at refrigeration temperatures. Also note that high temperatures can kill toxin-producing bacteria, but any toxin produced in the food will not be inactivated by high temperatures. Most pathogenic bacteria also require oxygen for growth, but *Clostridium botulinum* and *Clostridium perfringens* grow only in anaerobic (oxygen-free) environments, such as those found in tightly sealed cans and jars. Food acidity can affect bacterial growth, too. Although most bacteria do not grow well in acidic environments, some, such as disease-causing *E. coli,* can grow in acidic foods, such as fruit juice.

As you can see, different types of pathogenic bacteria can thrive in a variety of environmental conditions. Some can even survive in harsh environmental conditions (e.g., dry conditions or very hot or cold temperatures) through spore formation. In the spore

▶ The temperature range for the danger zone is listed by some sources as 41 to 140°F (5 to 60°C). The FDA has lowered the upper end of the range to 135°F (57°C) because the risk posed by holding food between 135 and 140°F (57 and 60°C) is minimal.

▶ In a recent 6-month period, more than 45 million pounds of hot dogs, luncheon meats, and other ready-to-eat meat products were recalled because of contamination with potentially deadly *Listeria* bacteria. Because of the likelihood of serious harm to their fetuses, pregnant women are advised to avoid these foods or heat them until they are 165°F (75°C).

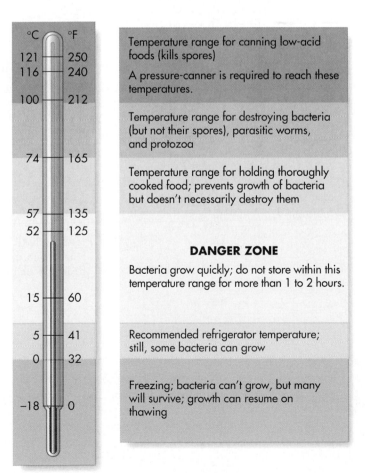

Figure 3-4 **Effects of temperature on microbes that cause foodborne illness.**

Table 3-3 Bacterial Causes of Foodborne Illness

Bacteria	Typical Food Sources	Symptoms	Additional Information
Salmonella species	Raw and undercooked meats, poultry, eggs, and fish; produce, especially raw sprouts; peanut butter; unpasteurized milk	Onset: 12–72 hours; nausea, fever, headache, abdominal cramps, diarrhea, and vomiting; can be fatal in infants, the elderly, and those with impaired immune systems; lasts 4–7 days	Estimated 1.4 million infections/year; bacteria live in the intestines of animals and humans; food is contaminated by infected water and feces; about 2,000 strains of *Salmonella* bacteria can cause disease, but 3 strains account for almost 50% of cases; *Salmonella enteritidis* infects the ovaries of healthy hens and contaminates eggs; almost 20% of cases are from eating undercooked eggs or egg-containing dishes; reptiles, such as turtles, also spread the disease
Campylobacter jejuni	Raw and undercooked meat and poultry (more than half of raw poultry in the U.S. is contaminated), unpasteurized milk, contaminated water	Onset: 2–5 days; muscle pain, abdominal cramping, diarrhea (sometimes bloody), fever; lasts 2–7 days	Estimated 1 million infections/year; produces a toxin that destroys intestinal mucosal surfaces; can cause Guillain-Barré syndrome, a rare neurological disorder that causes paralysis
Escherichia coli (0157:H7 and other strains)	Undercooked ground beef; produce—lettuce, spinach, sprouts; unpasteurized juice and milk	Onset: 1—8 days; bloody diarrhea, abdominal cramps; in children under age 5 and the elderly, hemolytic uremic syndrome (HUS) is a serious complication; red blood cells are destroyed and kidneys fail; can be fatal; lasts 5–10 days	Leading cause of bloody diarrhea in the U.S.; estimated 73,000 cases/year; lives in the intestine of healthy cattle; cattle and cattle manure are chief sources; illness caused by a powerful toxin made by the bacteria; petting zoos, lakes, and swimming pools can contain pathogenic *E. coli*
Shigella species	Fecal/oral transmission; water supplies, produce, and other foods contaminated by infected food handlers with poor hygiene	Onset: 1–3 days; abdominal cramps, fever, diarrhea (often bloody); lasts 5–7 days	Estimated 448,000 cases/year; humans and primates are the only sources; common in day-care centers and custodial institutions from poor hygiene; traveler's diarrhea often caused by *Shigella dysenteriae*
Staphylococcus aureus	Ham, poultry, egg salads, cream-filled pastries, custards, whipped cream	Onset: 1–6 hours; diarrhea, vomiting, nausea, abdominal cramps; lasts 1–3 days	Bacteria on skin and nasal passages of up to 25% of people; can be passed to foods; multiplies rapidly when contaminated foods are held for extended time at room temperature; illness caused by a heat-resistant toxin that cannot be destroyed by cooking

Table 3-3 Continued

Bacteria	Typical Food Sources	Symptoms	Additional Information
Clostridium perfringens	Beef, poultry, gravy, Mexican food	Onset: 8–24 hours; abdominal pain and diarrhea, usually mild; can be more serious in elderly or ill persons; lasts 1 day or less	Estimated 10,000 cases/year; anaerobic bacteria widespread in soil and water; multiplies rapidly in prepared foods, such as meats, casseroles, and gravies, held for extended time at room temperature
Listeria monocytogenes	Unpasteurized milk and soft cheeses, raw meats, uncooked vegetables, ready-to-eat deli meats and hotdogs, refrigerated smoked fish	Onset: 9–48 hours for early symptoms, 14–42 days for severe symptoms; fever, muscle aches, headache, vomiting; can spread to nervous system, resulting in stiff neck, confusion, loss of balance, or convulsion; can cause premature birth and stillbirth	Estimated 2500 cases with 500 fatalities/year; widespread in soil and water and can be carried in healthy animals; grows at refrigeration temperatures; about one-third of cases occur during pregnancy; high-risk persons should avoid uncooked deli meats, soft cheeses (e.g., feta, Brie, and Camembert), blue-veined cheeses, Mexican-style cheeses (e.g., queso blanco made from unpasteurized milk), refrigerated meat spreads or pates, uncooked refrigerated smoked fish
Clostridium botulinum	Incorrectly home-canned vegetables, meats, and fish; incorrectly canned commercial foods; herb-infused oils; bottled garlic; potatoes baked in foil and held at room temperature; honey	Onset: 18–36 hours but can be 6 hours to 10 days; neurological symptoms—double and blurred vision, drooping eyelids, slurred speech, difficulty swallowing, muscle weakness, and paralysis of face, arms, respiratory muscles, trunk, and legs; can be fatal; lasts days to weeks	Estimated 100 cases/year; caused by a neurotoxin; *C. botulinum* grows only in the absence of air in non-acidic foods; incorrect home canning causes most botulism, but in 2007 commercially canned chili sauce caused an outbreak; honey can contain botulism spores and should not be given to infants younger than 1 year of age
Vibrio	*V. parahemolyticus:* raw and undercooked shellfish, especially oysters	Onset: 24 hours; watery diarrhea, nausea, vomiting, fever, chills; lasts 3 days	Found in coastal waters; more infections in summer; number of infections hard to determine because it is difficult to isolate in the lab
	V. vulnificus: raw and undercooked shellfish, especially oysters	Onset: 1–2 days; vomiting, diarrhea, abdominal pain; in more severe cases, bloodstream infection with fever, chills, decreased blood pressure, blistering skin lesions; lasts 3 or more days	Estimated 95 cases/year; found in coastal waters; more infections in summer; those with impaired immune systems and liver disease at higher risk of infection; fatality rate of 50% with bloodstream infection
	V. cholerae: contaminated water and food, human carriers	Onset: 2–3 days; severe, dehydrating diarrhea, vomiting; dehydration, cardiovascular collapse, and death can occur	Occurs mainly in countries without adequate water purification and sewage treatment
Yersinia enterocolitica	Raw or undercooked pork, particularly pork intestines (chitterlings); tofu; water; unpasteurized milk	Onset: 4–7 days; fever, abdominal pain, diarrhea (often bloody); lasts 1–3 weeks or longer	Yersinosis most common in children under age 5 years; relatively rare; bacteria live mainly in pigs but can be found in other animals

CRITICAL THINKING

Recognizing that José is taking a nutrition class, his roommate asks him, "What is more risky: the bacteria that can be present in food or the additives listed on the label of my favorite cookie?" How should José respond? On what information should he base his conclusions?

state, bacteria can remain viable for months or years—then, when environmental conditions improve, they begin proliferating. For example, uncooked rice contains little water, which prevents bacterial growth. When you add water and cook it, especially if you leave it sitting on the kitchen counter (danger zone temperatures) instead of refrigerating it, you provide a hospitable environment (moisture, nutrients, warmth) for disease-causing bacteria and their spores to multiply rapidly. (Measures to prevent bacterial and other foodborne illness are described later in this chapter.)

Viruses

Viruses, like bacteria, are widely dispersed in nature. Unlike bacteria, however, viruses can reproduce only after invading body cells, such as those that line the intestines. Thus, the key to preventing foodborne viral illnesses is to use sanitary food preparation practices to keep viruses from contaminating food and to cook food thoroughly to kill any that have found their way into food via contamination from infected food handlers, other foods, and feces.

Table 3-4 describes the 2 most common viral causes of foodborne illness and describes typical food sources and symptoms of the illnesses they cause. Noroviruses are thought to account for many foodborne illnesses—if you have had the "stomach flu," you may well have experienced a norovirus infection. There are many reports of norovirus outbreaks on cruise ships, in hotels and restaurants, and even in hospitals.[51] Rotaviruses, a type of norovirus, are an important cause of diarrhea in children (see Chapter 4). Hepatitis A virus causes liver disease and is spread by contaminated food or water.

Raw shellfish, especially bivalves (e.g., oysters and clams), present a particular risk related to foodborne viral disease. These animals filter feed, a process that concentrates viruses, bacteria, and toxins present in the water as it is filtered for food. Adequate cooking of shellfish will kill viruses and bacteria, but toxins may not be affected. It's important to buy shellfish from reliable sources who have harvested these foods from safe areas.

Table 3-4 Viral Causes of Foodborne Illness

Viruses	Typical Food Sources	Symptoms	Additional Information
Norovirus (Norwalk and Norwalk-like viruses), human rotavirus	Foods prepared by infected food handlers; shellfish from contaminated waters; vegetables and fruits contaminated during growing, harvesting, and processing	Onset: 1–2 days; "stomach flu"—severe diarrhea, nausea, vomiting, stomach cramping, low-grade fever, chills, muscle aches; lasts 1–2 days or longer	Viruses found in stool and vomit of infected persons; food handlers can contaminate foods or work surfaces; noroviruses are very infectious—as few as 10–100 particles can lead to infection; workers with norovirus symptoms should not work until 2 or 3 days after they feel better
Hepatitis A virus	Foods prepared by infected food handlers, especially uncooked foods or those handled after cooking, such as sandwiches, pastries, and salads; shellfish from contaminated waters; vegetables and fruits contaminated during growing, harvesting, and processing	Onset: 15–50 days; anorexia, diarrhea, fever, jaundice, dark urine, fatigue; may cause liver damage and death; lasts several weeks up to 6 months	Infected food handlers contaminate food and transmit the disease to dozens of persons; children and young adults are more susceptible; a vaccine is available, decreasing the number of infections dramatically; immunoglobulin given within 1 week to those exposed to hepatitis A virus can also decrease infection

Avian bird flu, a serious influenza caused by a virus found in wild birds, can spread to domestic poultry flocks. However, it is important to know that the Centers for Disease Control and Prevention (CDC) states that avian bird flu is not a foodborne illness. It is of great concern because it can cross the species barrier and be transmitted to humans who handle the infected birds. Outbreaks in poultry and humans have occurred in Asia, the Near East, Europe, and North America. Eradicating infected flocks is the chief way of controlling an outbreak. There is no scientific evidence that the influenza is contracted through consuming poultry or eggs. Further, the safe handling and cooking of poultry and eggs eliminates the virus.[52]

Parasites

Parasites live in or on another organism, known as the host, from which they absorb nutrients. Humans may serve as a host to parasites. These tiny ravagers rob millions of people around the globe of their health and, in some cases, their lives. Those hardest hit live in tropical countries where poor sanitation fosters the growth of parasites. However, epidemiologists report that parasitic infections seem to be on the increase in the U.S. and other industrialized countries.[53] For example, in 1993 a *Cryptosporidium* outbreak involving more than 400,000 people occurred in Milwaukee due to contamination of the water supply. *Cyclospora* outbreaks have occurred from the ingestion of raspberries.

The more than 80 foodborne parasites known to affect humans include mainly **protozoa** (one-celled animals), such as *Cryptosporidium* and *Cyclospora,* and **helminths,** such as tapeworms and the roundworm *Trichinella spiralis*. Table 3-5 describes common parasites and typical food sources and symptoms of the illnesses they cause. Parasitic infections spread via person-to-person contact and contaminated food, water, and soil.

Prions

A very rare, but fatal, brain disease in humans has been linked to a similar fatal disease in cattle widely known as mad cow disease. More formally known as bovine spongiform encephalopathy (BSE), it is caused by an infectious protein particle called a **prion**, found mainly in the brain and spinal cord. An epidemic of BSE in the mid-1980s in the United

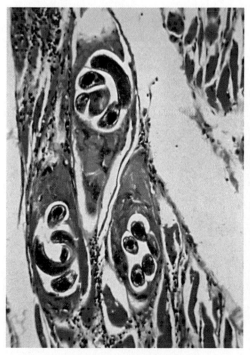

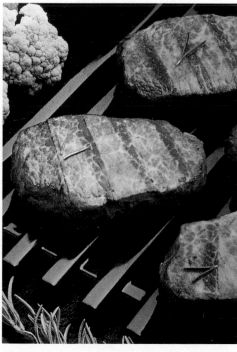

(a) Muscle tissue with *Trinchinella spiralis* roundworm cysts. Eating meat that contains *Trichinella* cysts causes the disease trichinosis. (b) Grill pork to an internal temperature of 160°F (72°C). This eliminates the risk of trichinosis and produces a desirable product. Trichinosis cases from pork are rare today because of more sanitary hog feeding practices.

(a)   (b)

Table 3-5 Parasitic Causes of Foodborne Illness

Parasite	Typical Food Sources	Symptoms	Additional Information
Trichinella spiralis	Pork, wild game	Onset: weeks to months; GI symptoms followed by muscle weakness, fluid retention in the face, fever, flulike symptoms	The number of trichinosis infections has decreased greatly because pigs are now less likely to harbor this parasite; cooking pork to 160°F (72°C) will kill *trichinella*, as will freezing it for 3 days at −4°F (−20°C)
Anisakis	Raw or undercooked fish	Onset: 12 hours or less; violent stomach pain, nausea, vomiting	Caused by eating the larvae of roundworms; the infection is more common where raw fish is routinely consumed
Tapeworms	Raw beef, pork, and fish	Abdominal discomfort, diarrhea	
Toxoplasma gondii	Raw or undercooked meat, unwashed fruits and vegetables	Onset: 5–20 days; most people are asymptomatic; those with symptoms have fever, headache, sore muscles, diarrhea; can be fatal to the fetus of pregnant women	Parasite is spread to humans from animals, including cats, the main reservoir of the disease; humans acquire the disease from ingesting contaminated meat or from fecal contamination from handling cat litter
Cyclospora cayetanensis	Water, contaminated food	Onset: 1 week; watery diarrhea, vomiting, muscle aches, fatigue, anorexia, weight loss; lasts 10–12 weeks	Most common in tropical and subtropical areas, but since 1990 about a dozen outbreaks, affecting 3600 people, have occurred in the U.S. and Canada
Cryptosporidium	Water, contaminated food	Onset: 2–10 days; watery diarrhea, abdominal pain, fever, nausea, vomiting, weight loss; those with impaired immune systems become more ill; lasts 1–2 weeks in otherwise healthy persons	Outbreaks occur worldwide; the largest U.S. outbreak was in 1993 in Milwaukee, with more than 443,000 persons affected; also can be spread in water parks and community swimming pools

CASE STUDY

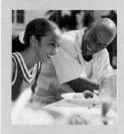

Aaron and his wife attended an international potluck on a warm July afternoon. Their contribution was Argentine beef, a stewlike dish. They followed the recipe and the cooking time carefully, removed the dish from the oven at 1 P.M., and kept it warm by wrapping the pan in a towel. They drove to the party and set the dish out on the buffet table at 3 P.M. Dinner was to be served at 4 P.M., but the guests were enjoying themselves so much that no one began to eat until 6 P.M. Aaron made sure he sampled the Argentine beef they had prepared, but his wife did not. He also had some salads, garlic bread, and a sweet coconut dessert. The couple returned home at 11 P.M. and went to bed. At 2 A.M., Aaron knew something was wrong. He had severe abdominal pain and had to make a mad dash to the toilet. He spent most of the next 3 hours in the bathroom with diarrhea. By dawn, the diarrhea had subsided and he was feeling better. He ate a light breakfast and felt fine by noon. It's very likely that Aaron contracted foodborne illness from the Argentine beef. What precautions for avoiding foodborne illness were ignored by Aaron and the rest of the people at the party? How might this case study be rewritten to substantially reduce the risk of foodborne illness?

Kingdom (UK), followed by the discovery of a similar fatal brain disease in humans, now known as variant Creutzfeldt-Jakob disease (vCJD), focused attention on the relationship between the diseases. Both BSE and vCJD are chronic, degenerative brain and nerve disorders for which there is no known cure.[54, 55]

Scientists determined that BSE is spread through cattle feed, which at that time contained by-products (e.g., brain, spinal cord, intestines) from sheep infected with scrapie, a disease like BSE. Scientists now believe that vCJD is similarly transmitted to humans by the consumption of beef from BSE-afflicted cattle. The risk of developing vCJD is very low—it is estimated that 1 case develops for every 10 billion servings of beef in a BSE-affected country (about 97% of all reported BSE cases are from the UK; only 16 cases have been discovered in the U.S. and Canada).[55] Only about 200 cases of vCJD have been reported worldwide, most from the UK and only 4 from the U.S. and Canada.[54]

Even when heated to high temperatures, prions remain infective. Thus, many countries, including the UK, the U.S., and Canada, have programs to prevent BSE-infected meat from entering the food supply. In the U.S., this program includes banning imports from countries where BSE is reported, prohibiting the use of animal by-products in cattle feed, monitoring and testing cattle for BSE, and banning the use of cattle parts that might contain prion particles (eyes, brain, spinal cord, intestines) in human foods.[55] Cattle suspected of having BSE are destroyed. Milk and other dairy products do not pose any risk of transmitting vCJD. At this point, it's safe to conclude that the risk of acquiring vCJD from eating beef is negligible in the U.S. Even for travelers to countries where BSE rates are higher, the CDC believes that the risk is extremely low—almost zero.[54] Of course, travelers who wish to reduce their risk even more can choose to avoid beef.

Toxins

A number of toxins produced by molds, algae, and plants can cause serious illness (Table 3-6). **Molds** are a type of fungus that can be scattered by the wind or carried by animals. Molds grow best in moist, dark places where air circulates. When conditions are right, the mold grows by sending rootlike "threads" deep into the food it lives on and forming endospores on the outside of the food. These endospores give mold its fuzzy, colorful look and are the form in which the mold travels to new locations. The foods most likely to mold in U.S. homes are cheese, breads, and fresh produce.

Thousands of types of mold grow on foods. Most just alter the color, texture, taste, and/or odor of foods, making them unpalatable and inedible. Some destroy crops and shorten the length of time a food will remain fresh and safe to eat. Others cause allergies or respiratory problems. A few fungi produce toxins known as **mycotoxins** (*myco* means mold), which cause blood diseases, nervous system disorders, and kidney and liver damage. The most important mycotoxins are aflatoxin, ergot, and those produced by the *Fusaria* fungi. Liver cancer–causing **aflatoxin** is produced by a mold that attacks peanuts,

Table 3-6 Toxins in Food

Toxin	Typical Food Sources	Symptoms	Additional Information
Mycotoxins			
Aflatoxin (from *Apergillus flavus* and *Aspergillus parasiticus*)	Corn, peanuts, rice, wheat, spice, nuts, especially when these foods are stressed due to drought or disease	Acute toxicity: liver damage or failure, malnutrition, malaise, impaired immune function; can be fatal. Chronic toxicity: vomiting, abdominal pain, liver failure, liver cancer; can be fatal	Aflatoxin B-1 is the most common fungal toxin to contaminate grains and nuts. It causes significant crop losses around the world and disease when consumed by humans.
Ergot (from *Claviceps purpurea*)	Improperly stored grains, especially rye	Hallucinations, spontaneous abortion, severely constricted blood flow to limbs (which can lead to gangrene), tingling and burning sensations, involuntary muscle twitching and contractions	Ergot poisoning is thought to be the cause of the odd physical behaviors attributed to women tried at the Salem witch trials.
Algae Toxins			
Ciguatera toxin	Tropical and subtropical fish (e.g., amberjack, barracuda, grouper, hogfish, moray eels, snapper, scorpion fish, surgeonfish, triggerfish) that have ingested toxin-producing algae	Onset: 6 hours; nausea, vomiting, neurological symptoms (weakness, temperature reversal—hot feels cold and vice versa); symptoms can last days, months, or years	The number of cases is not known.
Shellfish poisoning (paralytic, diarrheic, neurotoxic, and amnesic)	Mussels, cockles, clams, scallops, oysters, crabs, lobster	*Paralytic* onset: 15 minutes to 10 hours; numb and tingling skin, respiratory paralysis, death. *Diarrheic* onset: few minutes to a few hours; nausea, vomiting, diarrhea, abdominal pain, chills, headache, fever. *Neurotoxic* onset: 30 minutes to 3 hours; tingling and numbness of mouth and throat, muscle aches, dizziness, reversal of sensations of hot and cold, diarrhea, vomiting. *Amnesic* onset: 24 to 48 hours. Vomiting, diarrhea, abdominal pain, confusion, memory loss, disorientation, seizure, coma	It is associated with red tide algal blooms. The toxin accumulates in the shellfish. It is common in both the Pacific and Atlantic oceans
Scombroid Poisoning	Scombridae family (tunas and mackerels) and related fish (bluefish, mahi-mahi, amberjacks)	Onset: 2 to several hours; rash, diarrhea, flushing, sweating, headache, vomiting, difficulty breathing; symptoms resolve quickly	Bacterial decomposition of fish results in histamine production, which causes symptoms.
Tetrodotoxin	Pufferfish (fugu) liver	Onset: 20 minutes to 3 hours; mouth numbness, headache, nausea, diarrhea, vomiting, paralysis	Fugu is a traditional delicacy in Japan, where chefs must be licensed to prepare and serve this fish.

Table 3-6 Continued.

Toxin	Typical Food Sources	Symptoms	Additional Information
Plant Toxins			
Safrole	Sassafras, mace, nutmeg	Cancer when consumed in high doses	It was previously used as a food additive but is now banned.
Solanine	Potato sprouts, green spots on potato skins	Onset: 8–12 hours; nausea, diarrhea, vomiting, hallucinations, loss of sensation, paralysis	It can be prevented by storing potatoes in a dark area and discarding the sprouts, the peel, bruised or cut areas, and any green-tinged spots.
Mushroom toxins	Some mushrooms species, such as amanita	Stomach upset, dizziness, hallucinations, and other neurological symptoms; more lethal varieties can cause liver and kidney failure, coma, and death	Illness is almost always caused by wild mushrooms picked by nonexperts.
Herbal teas	Teas containing senna or comfrey	Onset: depends on dose; diarrhea and liver damage	Teas are used in folk medicines and are not considered safe for internal use.
Lectins	Raw or undercooked legumes, usually kidney beans	Onset: 1–3 hours; nausea, vomiting, abdominal pain, diarrhea	As few as 4 or 5 raw beans can cause symptoms. Outbreaks have occurred when beans were insufficiently cooked in crockpots and casseroles.

tree nuts (e.g., walnuts and pecans), corn, and oilseeds (e.g., cottonseed). Ergot is produced by a dark purple mold that grows on inappropriately stored grains, especially rye. Several types of *Fusaria* fungi can grow on grains stored for long periods and produce deadly mycotoxins.

Mycotoxins are rarely a problem in most industrialized nations because food production practices are designed to minimize mold growth. In addition, food producers and government inspectors closely monitor foods to detect molds and destroy any foods found to contain them. Unfortunately, mycotoxin poisonings are frequent in other parts of the world. For example, in Kenya in 2004 an aflatoxin poisoning caused liver damage in many people and many deaths.

Hunting wild mushrooms should be left to experts. Many varieties contain deadly toxins.

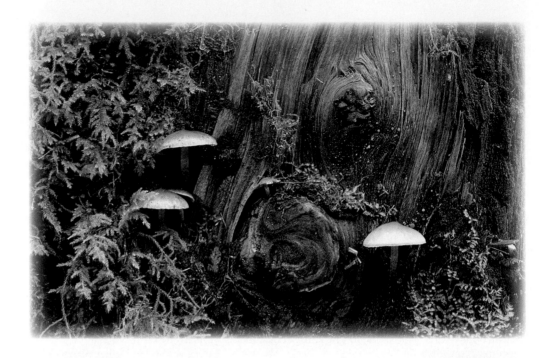

Toxin-containing algae ingested by some fish and shellfish also can cause foodborne disease. One example is the **ciguatera** toxin found in some large tropical and subtropical fish. Another example is **shellfish poisoning** caused by shellfish harvested from waters experiencing an algae population explosion called a red tide (sometimes the algae are so thick they color the water red). The fish and shellfish are not harmed by the toxins and the toxins are not destroyed by cooking or freezing. To avoid ciguatera, do not eat large fish that may contain this toxin; instead, choose the smaller specimens and don't eat fish heads or organs where toxins concentrate. The only protection against shellfish poisoning is to avoid shellfish from affected waters until nature thins the algae population. Both the U.S. and Canada quarantine waters experiencing an algae surge and prohibit shellfish harvesting until the shellfish are safe. However, some countries are not as rigid in their regulations regarding shellfish and red tides.

Scombroid poisoning is caused by eating certain fish left at room temperature for several hours after being caught. The toxin is not destroyed by freezing or cooking but can be prevented by refrigerating or freezing the fish immediately after they're caught.

Foods contain a variety of **natural toxins** that can cause illness (see Table 3-6) but, in actuality, rarely do.[56] For instance, licorice contains a natural toxicant that can elevate blood pressure and cause heart failure. There is cyanide in lima beans and almonds. Nutmeg, bananas, and some herbal teas contain substances that can cause hallucinations. Plants produce and concentrate toxins to compete with their neighbors and protect themselves from plant-eating molds, bacteria, insects, and other predators, including people. When stressed by environmental conditions or damaged, plants tend to produce even greater quantities of toxins. An example is the stress caused by incorrect storage on the production of **solanine**, a powerful, narcotic-like toxin produced by potatoes. The amount produced is normally small, but it increases when potatoes sprout and when they are stored in a brightly lit place.

Humans have coped with natural toxins for thousands of years by learning to avoid some of them and to limit intake of others. Farmers know potatoes must be stored in the dark, so that solanine won't be synthesized. Cooking limits the potency of certain natural toxins. Spices are used in such small amounts that health risks from any toxins are unlikely to result. Another important way to cope with these toxins is to eat a wide variety of foods to minimize the chance that any single toxin is eaten in amounts that exceed the body's ability to detoxify it. Natural toxins are so widespread in foods that it would be unrealistic to try to avoid them totally—and doing so would likely limit food choices so severely that nutrient deficiency diseases would occur. Nevertheless, it's important to remember that some potentially harmful chemicals in foods occur naturally.

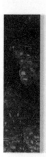

Water Safety

The U.S. water supply ranks among the safest in the world. Nearly all of the water we consume comes to us from the faucets in our homes, schools, and offices; most of it is from a public water supply (also known as a municipal water supply). The water provided by public water systems comes from either underground aquifers or surface water, such as lakes, rivers, and steams. About 15% of consumers get their water from private sources, typically wells. Bottled water is another increasingly popular source of water. Many consumers are attracted to the perceived health value or taste of bottled water. This popularity now brings in $10 billion per year to the bottled water industry.

Public water supplies are regulated by the EPA.[57] Under the Safe Drinking Water Act, all public drinking water suppliers are required to rigorously test for contaminants, such as bacteria, various chemicals, and toxic metals (e.g., lead and arsenic) and submit test results to the EPA. However, the actual delivery and safety of water are under the jurisdiction of the more than 54,000 local municipal water departments in the United States. These departments pipe water from its source to a treatment center, treat it, and then pipe it to customers. Water treatments vary, depending on the source water, but all water is disinfected, usually with a chlorine-based chemical. The addition of such chemicals has raised concern that drinking water may increase rectal and bladder cancer risk, although there is currently no conclusive proof. If chlorine in tap water does increase cancer risk, it is likely extremely small (perhaps 2 cases of cancer per 1 million people).

Private water supplies, such as wells, are not regulated by the EPA. Water from these sources should be tested for coliforms, nitrates, dissolved solids, and pH. Local health departments usually can give advice on such testing and on keeping well water safe.

Bottled waters vary, depending on the source, in mineral content, carbonation, and additives. All bottled waters must list the source of the water on the label. This source can include wells, spas, springs, geysers, and quite often the public water supply. The FDA has set definitions for the terms used on labels, such as *artesian water, distilled water, purified water, spring water,* and *mineral water.* For example, spring water must come from an underground spring. Some bottled water contains minerals, such as calcium, magnesium, and potassium, that are either naturally occurring or added by the water company to give the water a better taste. The water is carbonated when carbon dioxide gas naturally occurs in the water source (called naturally sparkling water) or is added during bottling. Additives such as flavors and vitamins also are common.

Bottled waters are regulated by the FDA, which sets high standards for their purity. It periodically collects and analyzes samples, but not to the extent that municipal water supplies are monitored. Water that is bottled in a sanitary manner and kept in a sealed container has an indefinite shelf life, so no expiration date is required. However, some states require expiration dates as a guide for freshness.

Threats to Safe Water

There are numerous threats to the safety of our drinking water—agricultural runoff (animal waste, pesticides, fertilizer), inappropriate disposal of chemicals, municipal solid waste (contains bacteria, viruses, nitrates, synthetic detergents, household chemicals) leaking

▶ To find information about the purity of the water provided by municipal water departments, visit www.EPA.gov/water.

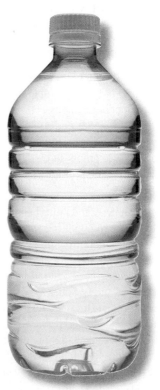

Bottled water is a convenient but relatively expensive source of water. In most cases, tap water is just as healthy a choice to meet water needs.

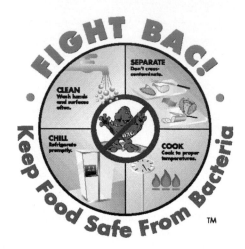

into waterways, inadequate treatment of human wastes, and pollution from boats and ships (contains solvents, gas, detergents, raw sewage), to name just a few. This makes regular testing of the water supply critical.

The EPA requires that the public be notified if water contamination is a danger to public health. For instance, nitrate contamination that may come from fertilizer runoff is particularly dangerous to infants because it prevents oxygen from circulating in the body. As related earlier, *Cryptosporidium* can contaminate water supplies (it is not affected by chlorination). Boiling tap water for a minimum of a minute is the best way to kill *Cryptosporidium*. Alternatively, individuals can purchase a water filter that screens out this parasite.

Fortunately, water contamination that poses a danger to health is rare. There are about 30 drinking water–related outbreaks each year, affecting fewer than 3000 people.[58] Two-thirds of the outbreaks are related to microbial pathogens, with most of these being bacteria. About half of the 30 outbreaks are from non-EPA–regulated water sources— well and bottled waters.

Knowledge Check

1. Which government agencies regulate drinking water?
2. How can you determine if your municipal drinking water is safe?
3. What are 3 threats to public water supply systems?

3.5 Preventing Foodborne and Waterborne Illnesses

Safe food and water supplies require a "farm to fork" approach. Those who grow our food, along with processors, distributors, and consumers, all have responsibilities for food and water safety. Several government agencies regulate and coordinate these efforts, monitor food and water, conduct research, enforce wholesomeness and quality standards and laws, and educate consumers (Table 3-7).

To do their part, consumers need to know how to handle food safely at home. In general, foodborne illness prevention focuses on using good personal and kitchen hygiene; handling food safely by using appropriate thawing, cooking, chilling, and storage procedures; and knowing which foods pose extra risk to those more susceptible to foodborne illness.

Select and Purchase Foods Carefully

- Don't use food from damaged cans or jars that leak, bulge, or are severely dented or cracked. Don't taste food that smells or looks odd. Discard canned foods that spurt liquid when the can is opened; the deadly botulism toxin may be present.
- When food shopping, place perishable foods, such as milk, eggs, and raw meat, poultry, and seafood, in your cart last and keep them separate from other foods in the cart, so that they don't contaminate them. Placing them in separate plastic bags prevents cross-contamination.
- Take groceries home promptly and refrigerate or freeze perishable foods right away. Leaving them in a warm car allows pathogens to grow.

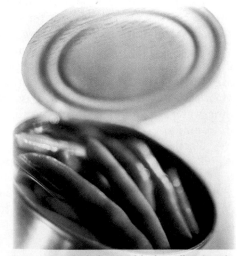
Inspect cans for bulges and foul-smelling liquid as signs of the presence of the botulism toxin.

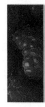 A website coordinating the U.S. efforts on food safety is www.foodsafety.gov. Other useful websites are www.ama-assn.org/ama/pub/category/1948.html and www.homefoodsafety.org.

▶ The Fight Bac! Program (check out www.fightbac.org) has 4 simple rules for preventing foodborne illness.
1. Clean. Wash hands and surfaces often.
2. Separate. Don't cross-contaminate.
3. Cook. Cook to proper temperatures.
4. Chill. Refrigerate promptly.

▶ Hazard Analysis and Critical Control Point, or HACCP (pronounced HAS-sip), was developed more than 30 years ago as a food safety system for astronauts. Today, it is widely used by food processors to ensure food safety. Some food service establishments, such as restaurants and cafeterias, have adopted it too. The goal of the HACCP system is to identify potential problems *before* they happen and thereby prevent food safety problems. To learn more, visit www.FoodSafety.gov.

▶ As the old adage says, when in doubt, throw the food out!

Table 3-7 U.S. Agencies Responsible for Monitoring the Food Supply

Agency Name	Responsibilities	Methods	How to Contact
United States Department of Agriculture (USDA)	• Enforces wholesomeness and quality standards for grains and produce (while in the field), meat, poultry, milk, eggs, and egg products	• Conducts inspections • Monitors imported meat and poultry • Administers "Safe Handling Label"	www.usda.gov/fsis or www.nal.usda.gov/fnicfoodborne/foodborne.htm or call 1-800-535-4555
Bureau of Alcohol, Tobacco, and Firearms and Explosives (ATF)	• Enforces laws on alcoholic beverages	• Conducts inspections	www.atf.treas.gov
Environmental Protection Agency (EPA)	• Regulates pesticides • Establishes water quality standards	• Approves all U.S. pesticides • Sets pesticide residue limits in food	www.epa.gov
Food and Drug Administration (FDA)	• Ensures safety and wholesomeness of all foods in interstate commerce (except meat, poultry, and processed egg products) • Regulates seafood • Controls product labels	• Conducts inspections • Conducts food sample studies • Sets standards for specific foods	www.fda.gov or call 1-800-FDA-4010
Centers for Disease Control and Prevention (CDC)	• Promotes food safety	• Responds to emergencies concerning foodborne illness • Surveys and studies environmental health problems • Conducts research about foodborne illness • Directs/enforces quarantines • Conducts national programs for prevention and control of foodborne and other diseases	www.cdc.gov
National Marine Fisheries Service or NOAA Fisheries	• Monitors domestic and international conservation and management of living marine resources	• Conducts voluntary seafood inspection program • Can use mark to show federal inspection	www.nmfs.noaa.gov
State and local governments	• Promote milk safety • Monitor food industry within their borders	• Conduct inspections of food-related establishments	Government pages of telephone book or Internet

• Use the sell-by, use-by, and expiration dates found on many food products. *Sell-by* is the last date a retailer can sell the product so that it still maintains its quality with normal use in the home. *Use-by* (also called the freshness date) indicates when quality may start to decline, although the product will still be safe to eat. Expiration dates, found on foods such as infant formulas, are the last dates foods should be eaten.

Avoid Unsafe Food and Water

• Avoid eating foods likely to be contaminated with pathogens, including raw sprouts and raw or undercooked meat, fish, shellfish, poultry, and eggs.
• Drink only milk and juice that have been pasteurized.
• If at increased risk of foodborne illness, avoid soft cheeses, cold deli salads, and cold smoked fish, and heat hot dogs and deli meats to 165°F (75°C) before consumption.
• Use only purified water for drinking, cooking, and washing food and food preparation equipment. If you have a well, test it for pathogens.

CRITICAL THINKING

Ahmed wants to buy a cutting board for his new kitchen. He's been looking at all the possibilities: glass, plastic, and wood. How would you advise him, so that he can minimize the risk of foodborne illness?

▶ Safe Refrigeration Storage

Food	Use Within
Raw meat	
Ground beef, poultry, fish	1–2 days
Steaks, chops, roasts	3–5 days
Bacon	1 week
Hot dogs	2 weeks
Cooked meat, poultry, casseroles, soups	3–5 days
Tuna, egg, ham, chicken, or macaroni salads	3–5 days
Fresh eggs in shell	3–5 weeks
Hard-cooked eggs	1 week

Find more information at fightbac.org.

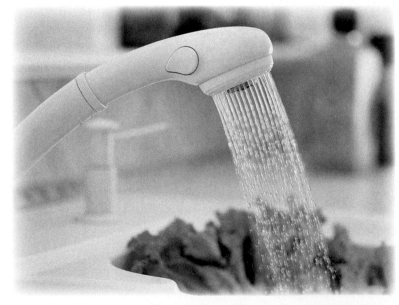

Wash fresh fruits and vegetables under running water to remove bacteria and soil. Special antibacterial washing products are not necessary.

Practice Good Personal Hygiene

- Thoroughly wash hands for 20 seconds with warm, soapy water after using the bathroom, changing diapers, playing with pets, coughing, sneezing, or smoking. Also wash them before and after handling food, especially if you have touched unwashed produce or raw meat, fish, poultry, and eggs. Plain soap works as well as antibacterial soaps—just be sure to wash frequently and thoroughly.
- Cover any cuts, burns, sores, or infected areas when preparing foods. This helps keep bacteria (often *Staphylococcus*) from wounds out of food.
- Avoid preparing food when sick with diarrhea.

Keep a Clean Kitchen

- Prevent cross-contamination by cleaning counters, cutting boards, dishes, and other equipment thoroughly before and after use. Wash them with hot, soapy water or in the dishwasher. They also can be sanitized with a dilute solution of bleach. Regularly cleaning surfaces and equipment with a dilute bleach solution (1 part bleach to 10 parts water) helps reduce the risk of cross-contamination.
- Replace sponges and wash kitchen towels frequently. (Microwaving wet sponges for 2 minutes helps kill bacteria.)
- Cutting boards should be made of non-porous, smooth material, such as hard plastic, marble, glass, or hardwood (oak, maple). Bacteria are hard to remove from porous or deeply scratched cutting boards.

Handle Food Safely

- Wash fresh fruits and vegetables under running water just prior to eating them to remove bacteria, soil, and pesticides.
- Scrub firm produce, such as melons and cucumbers, under running water with a brush before slicing them. (Bacteria on the skin can contaminate the inside of produce when it is cut.)
- Discard soft or liquid foods (e.g., jam, syrups) that are moldy. If a firm-textured food has molded, trim off a large area around the mold and at least 1 inch below the mold. Prevent mold growth by storing food at cold temperatures and using food promptly.
- Be aware of how long foods have been in your refrigerator. Freezing keeps foods safe indefinitely, but quality deteriorates if they are kept too long.
    - Store raw meats and poultry below other foods in the refrigerator to prevent cross-contamination by drippings from leaky packages.
    - Be careful not to recontaminate cooked food with raw meat or juices on hands, cutting boards, or dirty equipment. For example, when grilling burgers, don't put cooked burgers on the same plate that was used to carry the raw patties out to the grill.
    - For outdoor cooking, cook food completely at the picnic site, with no partial cooking in advance.

Keep Foods Out of the Danger Zone and Cook Foods Appropriately

- Never thaw foods on the counter. Thaw foods in the refrigerator, under cold running water, or in a microwave oven. Cook foods immediately after thawing in the microwave because cooking may have begun, putting the food temperature in the danger zone (41° to 135°F [5° to 57°C]).
- Use a refrigerator thermometer to assure your refrigerator operates at a safe temperature range (32° to 40°F [0° to 4.4°C]).

- Marinate food in the refrigerator.
- Cook food to a safe internal temperature. Don't rely on how the food looks—use a food thermometer. Cook to at least the minimum temperatures shown in Figure 3-5.
- Cook eggs until yolks and whites are firm, not runny. *Salmonella* bacteria may survive in sunny-side up or over-easy eggs. Avoid homemade ice cream, eggnog, mayonnaise, and other foods made with unpasteurized raw eggs.
- Avoid eating raw animal products. Raw fish dishes, such as sushi, can be eaten safely by most people who are not at increased risk of foodborne illness if the dish is made with very fresh fish that has been commercially frozen (freezing helps eliminate parasites) and purchased from a reputable establishment.
- Cook stuffing separately from poultry or stuff immediately before cooking and cook to 165°F (74°C). Immediately after cooking, transfer the stuffing to a clean bowl.
- Once a food is cooked, consume it right away, or refrigerate or freeze it within 2 hours. In hot weather (90°F [32°C] and above), refrigerate it within 1 hour.
- Cool foods in shallow pans (not deep containers) to provide a large surface area for rapid cooling.
- Reheat leftovers thoroughly to 165°F (74°C).

Safe Handling Instructions

This product was prepared from inspected and passed meat and/or poultry. Some food products may contain bacteria that could cause illness if the product is mishandled or cooked improperly. For your protection, follow these safe handling instructions.

Keep refrigerated or frozen. Thaw in refrigerator or microwave.

Keep raw meat and poultry separate from other foods. Wash working surfaces (including cutting boards), utensils, and hands after touching raw meat or poultry.

Cook thoroughly.

Keep hot foods hot. Refrigerate leftovers immediately or discard.

▶ The USDA answers questions about the safe use of animal products (800-535-4555, 10 A.M. to 4 P.M. weekdays, Eastern time).

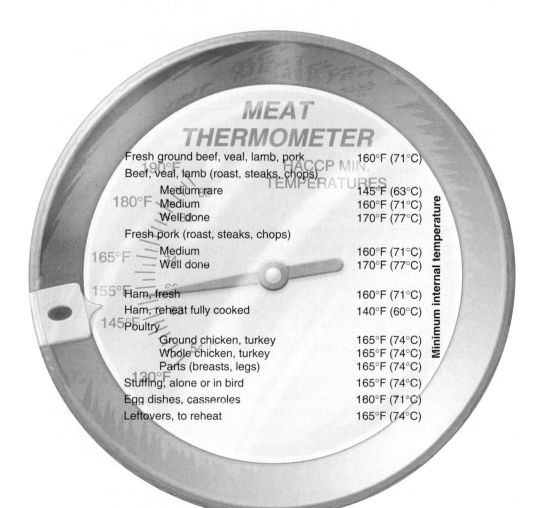

Figure 3-5 Minimum internal temperatures for cooking or reheating foods.

MEAT THERMOMETER HACCP MIN. TEMPERATURES	Minimum internal temperature
Fresh ground beef, veal, lamb, pork	160°F (71°C)
Beef, veal, lamb (roast, steaks, chops)	
Medium rare	145°F (63°C)
Medium	160°F (71°C)
Well done	170°F (77°C)
Fresh pork (roast, steaks, chops)	
Medium	160°F (71°C)
Well done	170°F (77°C)
Ham, fresh	160°F (71°C)
Ham, reheat fully cooked	140°F (60°C)
Poultry	
Ground chicken, turkey	165°F (74°C)
Whole chicken, turkey	165°F (74°C)
Parts (breasts, legs)	165°F (74°C)
Stuffing, alone or in bird	165°F (74°C)
Egg dishes, casseroles	160°F (71°C)
Leftovers, to reheat	165°F (74°C)

CASE STUDY FOLLOW-UP

Although the dish was cooked thoroughly, it was held at an unsafe temperature from the time it was removed from the oven at 1:00 P.M. until it was served at 6:00 P.M. This 5-hour time span greatly exceeded the maximum time of 2 hours at room temperature for a cooked food. This allowed the growth of a foodborne illness–causing pathogen. Ideally, this product should have been transported on ice in a cooler to the party, refrigerated at the party, and then reheated to 165°F (74°C) before serving at 6:00 P.M. Overall, it is risky to leave perishable items, such as meat, fish, poultry, eggs, and dairy products, at room temperature for more than 2 hours.

Global Perspective

Traveler's Diarrhea

Traveler's diarrhea afflicts 30 to 50% of those who travel to areas that tend to be hot and lack advanced water treatment systems and refrigeration, such as most of Central and South America, Africa, Asia, and the Middle East. Traveler's diarrhea usually occurs abruptly and lasts for 3 to 4 days, but it can go longer.[61] According to the Centers for Disease Control and Prevention, most traveler's diarrhea is caused by bacterial infections, especially *Enterotoxigenic Escherichia coli,* spread through contaminated food and water. The following guidelines can help reduce the risk of traveler's diarrhea.

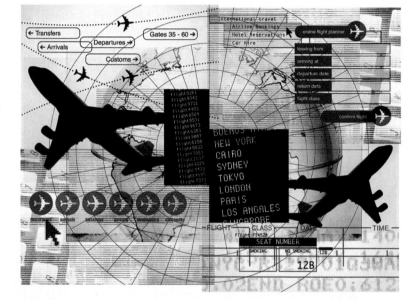

- Eat foods that are freshly cooked and served piping hot.
- Avoid food from street vendors and buffets.
- Avoid salads and raw fruits and vegetables.
- Avoid raw or undercooked meat and seafood.
- Avoid tap water and beverages reconstituted with tap water (including ice and possibly fruit juice and milk).
- Bottled and sealed beverages, including soft drinks, water, beer, and wine are generally safe.
- Beverages made with boiled water, such as coffee and tea, are generally safe.
- Travelers also can treat tap water by boiling, chemical disinfection, or filtering. To learn how, visit wwwn.cdc.gov/travel/default.aspx.

Even when following these guidelines, traveler's diarrhea can be hard to avoid. Pepto-Bismol®, an over-the-counter drug used to treat indigestion, can reduce traveler's diarrhea substantially when it is taken throughout the stay. However, before traveling to a high-risk area, it is wise to consult with a physician about using any medication, getting needed vaccinations, and taking other health precautions.

▶ A phrase familiar to those traveling to developing countries is "boil it, peel it, or don't eat it." Of course, this advice is simplistic—many foods that may be safe to eat can't be boiled or peeled.

▶ For more health advice, visit the CDC website for travelers: www.cdc.gov/ncidod/dpd/travel.htm.

3.6 Environmental Contaminants in Foods

In addition to pathogens and natural toxins, a number of environmental toxins can contaminate food and cause health problems. Common environmental contaminants include heavy metals (lead, mercury), industrial chemicals (dioxins, polychlorinated biphenyls), and agricultural chemicals (pesticides, antibiotics).

Lead

Lead can damage every organ system in the body—especially the nervous system and kidneys—and it impairs the synthesis of hemoglobin, the oxygen-carrying protein in the blood. Lead is particularly toxic to the developing nervous system of children; even low amounts in the body can lower IQ, cause behavior disorders, and impair coordination. It also can impair growth and hearing and predispose children to high blood pressure and kidney disease later in life. About 2% of children ages 1 to 5 years in the U.S. have dangerously high blood lead levels.[59] In developing countries, many more children are affected.

To avoid ingesting lead, people living in homes built before 1986, when federal law banned lead pipes and solder, should let cold water run a minute or so before using it. This practice lets lead that leached into the water while it sat in the pipes go down the drain. Also, hot tap water in these homes should not be used for preparing food because lead leaches more easily into hot water than cold. A plumber can install a filter that helps remove lead and/or treat the pipes with compounds that prevent lead leaching. In homes built before 1978, chances are great that lead-based paint was used—it is the most common culprit in lead poisoning cases. This paint isn't dangerous if it is intact; the danger occurs when it deteriorates and deposits a powdery dust on home furnishings, floors, and lawns. This dust gets on hands, which can then transfer it to food. Keeping hands clean and washing objects that may be placed in the mouth can help reduce exposure. Also, never serve or store foods or beverages in lead-containing containers (e.g., leaded crystal, pottery, and older or imported dishes).

Other documented lead sources include certain candies from Mexico, vegetables grown in contaminated soils, mineral supplements, herbal remedies, and toys painted with lead-containing paints. (Children often place toys in their mouths, making them particularly dangerous.) In one study, 20% of the herbal remedies tested contained dangerous levels of lead, mercury, and/or arsenic.[60] Lead is no longer used in food cans in the U.S., but food cans from other countries may contain lead.

Preventing lead poisoning is best done by removing lead from the environment. Good nutrition plays a role, too. Children with iron deficiency absorb more iron and lead, so preventing iron deficiency (see Chapter 15) may help limit lead absorption.[62]

▶ For more information about lead, visit www.epa.gov/lead or call the National Lead Information Center and Clearinghouse at 1-800-424-LEAD.

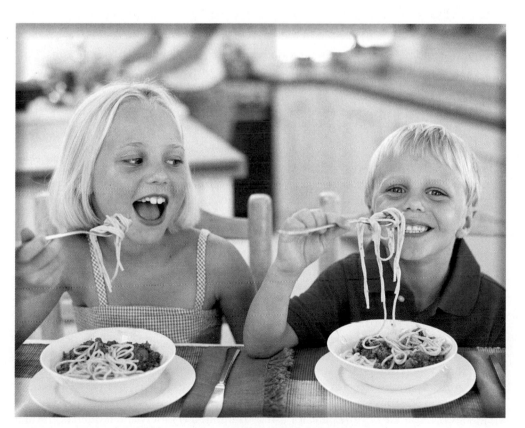

Eating a healthy diet with plenty of iron may help prevent lead poisoning in children.

Dioxins

▶ For information on fish contamination with dioxins, mercury, and PCBs, visit www. epa.gov/waterscience/fish/.

Dioxins (chlorine and benzene-containing chemicals) are by-products of industrial processes (bleaching paper, pesticide manufacture) and the incineration of waste products; they increase the risk of cancer. They also cause liver and nerve damage and may have adverse effects on reproduction and increase the risk of type 2 diabetes mellitus. Exposure is primarily from dioxin-contaminated food and inhalation of contaminated air. Food sources are animal fats (where dioxins tend to accumulate) and fish from dioxin-contaminated waterways. The EPA recommends absolutely no consumption of some fish species and the fish from certain waterways. Eating commercially caught fish is usually safe because these fish come from a variety of sources and most of these rivers, streams, and lakes are not contaminated. Eating a variety of fish, not just one species, also is a good idea.

Mercury

Mercury is abundant in the environment; in aquatic environments, bacteria convert mercury to the neurotoxin methylmercury. The FDA first limited the amount of mercury in foods in 1969, after 120 people in Japan became ill from eating mercury-contaminated fish. Birth defects in the offspring of some of these people also were traced to mercury exposure. Methylmercury can cause nerve damage, fatigue, and poor learning. As with dioxins, fish are the primary source of the toxic chemical. Most at risk are children and pregnant and breastfeeding women—the FDA and EPA suggest that these individuals limit their exposure to mercury by following these guidelines:

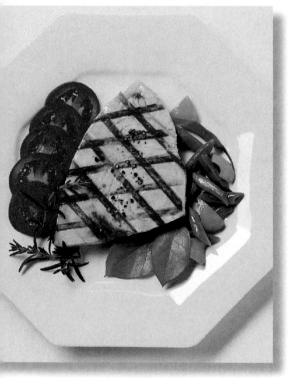

Swordfish is a common source of mercury in our diets. Children and pregnant and lactating women should avoid swordfish and other fish that contain high levels of mercury.

- Do not eat shark, swordfish, king mackerel, or tilefish because they contain high levels of mercury. (Large fish concentrate mercury in their tissues.)

- Limit albacore (white) tuna to 6 ounces or 1 meal per week because it is higher in mercury.

- Limit the intake of fish containing less mercury (e.g., shrimp, canned light tuna, pollock, salmon, and catfish) to 12 ounces per week or no more than 2 meals per week. Children should have smaller portions.

- Check the EPA advisories for the mercury content of fish from local waterways. If no advice is available, eat 1 fish meal per week from these sources, but don't eat any other fish that week.

These guidelines are controversial, however. Fish is an important source of fatty acids that promote brain and nervous system development in fetuses and infants. Ongoing research suggests that the benefits from these fatty acids outweigh the risk of mercury from fish.[63] As scientists learn more about the risks and benefits of eating fish, these guidelines may be relaxed to encourage fish intake.

Polychlorinated Biphenyls (PCBs)

Polychlorinated biphenyls (PCBs) were widely used for years in a variety of industrial products. They were linked to liver tumors and reproductive problems in animals and are no longer produced. However, they do not degrade quickly and can still be detected in the environment. The FDA has established limits for PCBs in susceptible foods and in paper used for food-packaging material. The most significant food source of PCB residues is fish, primarily freshwater fish, such as fish from the Great Lakes and bottom-feeding freshwater species from waters in other industrial areas, such as the Hudson River Valley in New York. Again, a key guideline for fish consumption is variety and moderation when local sources have the potential for contamination.

Pesticides

Pesticides, products used to eliminate pests, include insecticides, herbicides (weed killers), fungicides, and rodenticides. Farmers have used them since the 1940s to limit crop-damaging pests and thereby increase agricultural production. Pesticides also can help improve the appearance of fruits and vegetables. For example, a fungicide helps prevent apple scab fungus, which makes apples look unappealing (and less likely to sell), but the fruit is still tasty and nutritious. Fungicides also help prevent carcinogenic aflatoxin from forming on some crops.

The EPA permits the use of about 10,000 pesticides, containing over 1000 active ingredients. This amounts to about 1.2 billion pounds of pesticides (about half are herbicides) being used each year in the U.S., with much of this being applied to agricultural crops. However, pesticide use is not limited to agriculture—many pesticides are used in homes, businesses, schools, and health-care facilities for insect and rodent control. Pesticides also are widely applied to lawns, golf courses, and home gardens.

The 2 major classes of pesticides are synthetic pesticides and biopesticides. Many of the earliest synthetic pesticides were persistent chemicals—they did not break down easily and remained in water, soil, and plants for decades, thus posing a risk to the animals and humans who ingested contaminated water and plants. Many of these early pesticides have been banned. The synthetic compounds in use today break down much more quickly (they are less persistent), but they also are more powerful chemicals. Organophosphates, carbamates, organochlorine insecticides, and pyrethroid pesticides are the main classes of synthetic pesticides.[64]

Three types of biopesticides were developed to provide safer pesticide alternatives. The first type consists of microbial pesticides, such as the soil bacterium *Bacillus thuringiensis* (Bt), which produces proteins that are toxic to various insects. The second type is plants that are genetically modified to produce their own pesticides, such as the Bt protein. The third type is biochemical pesticides that don't directly kill an organism but limit its reproduction or growth.

A number of problems are associated with pesticide use. One is that the organisms intended for elimination can become resistant to the pesticide action. This means that either more of the pesticide must be applied or a new pesticide must be used. Another problem is pesticide drift; once a pesticide is applied to a field, it can be carried by wind currents to non-target sites. Pesticides that remain in the soil may be taken up by non-target organisms or enter groundwater and aquatic habitats. Each of these paths is a route to the food chain. Still another problem is the unintended effects; pesticides can harm non-target species, such as frogs, fish, and beneficial insects (e.g., bees); decrease biological diversity by acting on the lower levels of the food chain; have harmful effects on water quality; disrupt natural wildlife habitats; damage soil and the nutrients in it; and contribute to erosion.

Regulating Pesticides

The EPA, FDA, and USDA share responsibility for regulating pesticides. The EPA is responsible for determining that a pesticide is beneficial and will not pose unreasonable health or environmental risks. The EPA sets limits on how much of a pesticide may be used on food during growth and processing and how much can remain on the food you buy—this is known as pesticide tolerance. Because children are thought to be more vulnerable to any adverse effects of pesticides,[65] the Food Quality Protection Act of 1996 requires the EPA to consider children's pesticide exposure from foods they normally eat, such as apples and apple juice, potatoes, sugar, eggs, chicken, and beef.

The FDA and USDA are jointly responsible for testing foods for pesticides and enforcing the EPA pesticide tolerances. A 2006 USDA report indicated that 73% of fresh fruits and vegetables, 49% of grains, 8% of pork, and 99% of dairy products had detectable pesticide residues. The dairy product residues were almost all from persistent pesticides no longer allowed. Overall, 34% of the samples had no detectable pesticides, 30% had a single residue only, and 36% had 2 or more, but only 0.2% had residues exceeding tolerances.[66] The low level of residues that exceeded tolerance confirms that farmers are using pesticides according to EPA regulations.

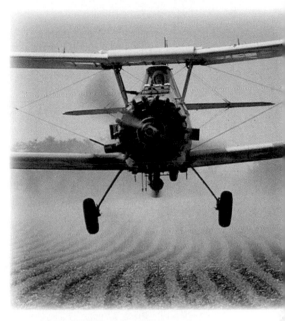

Pesticide use poses a risk-versus-benefit question. Each side has points that deserve to be considered. Rural communities, where exposure is more direct, experience the greatest short-term risk.

Common Types of Pesticides

Organophosphates: compounds toxic to the nervous system of insects and animals; in fact, some were used in World War II as nerve agents; they usually are not persistent in the environment[64]

Carbamates: compounds that act similarly to the organophosphates but are less toxic

Organochlorine insecticides: commonly used in the past, but many (e.g., DDT and chlordane) have been removed from the market due to their health and environmental effects and their persistence

Pyrethroid pesticides: compounds that mimic naturally occurring pesticides found in chrysanthemums, some of which are toxic to the nervous system

► The environmental damage caused by the pesticide DDT (dichlorodiphenyltrichloroethane) was chronicled by Rachel Carson in her book *Silent Spring*, published in 1962. DDT was widely used around the world because it increased crop yields and was inexpensive. But scientists soon learned that DDT and its metabolites are toxic to humans and animals, especially young fish and birds, and that it persists for years in the environment. DDT can no longer be used in the U.S. and many other countries, but it is still used in some developing countries to kill malaria-carrying mosquitoes.

Minimizing Exposure to Pesticides

There is no doubt that pesticides are toxic. Their purpose, after all, is to eliminate pests. Accidental pesticide poisonings occur each year, often related to careless use or storage of these chemicals. Studies also link people who work with pesticides, such as farmers and those who apply pesticides for a living, with higher rates of asthma, Parkinson's disease (a neurological disorder), prostate cancer, leukemia, and other cancers.[67, 68] However, there is much less certainty about the effects of long-term exposure to much lower doses, such as occurs when we eat our usual diets. In this regard, infants (including before birth) and children deserve special attention.[64, 65, 69] Young animals exposed to chemicals such as pesticides can experience damage to their developing reproductive, nervous, and immune systems. Risk may increase in young children because they often consume relatively higher doses of pesticides, when their lower body weight is considered. Infants and young children also may not metabolize the pesticides as readily as adults because the liver, the main organ that breaks down drugs and toxins for excretion, is still immature.[64]

Even though government agencies work to keep pesticide residues in food to a minimum, consumers should take steps to minimize their exposure. The EPA recommends washing and peeling fruits and vegetables and trimming away fat in meat (where pesticides may accumulate), along with selecting a variety of foods. Although these measures cannot eliminate all pesticide residues, the fear of pesticides should not deter consumers from eating fruits and vegetables. These foods provide an abundance of important vitamins, minerals, and phytochemicals; eating a *variety* of them is key to meeting nutrient needs and will reduce the likelihood of exposure to a single pesticide.

Certified organic foods are grown without synthetic pesticides and can further minimize exposure to pesticides. However, these foods may contain very small amounts of pesticide residues because of background contamination (pesticides persisting in soil and water) and pesticide drift from nearby conventional farms. One study of 23 school-aged children showed that eating an organic diet can decrease exposure to pesticides.[70] After the children consumed an organic diet for 5 days, organophospate pesticides disappeared from their urine.

Antibiotics

Farmers can give low-dose antibiotics to food animals to promote animal growth and prevent disease. One estimate is that 60 to 80% of all antibiotics produced in the U.S. are used for this purpose.[71] Many of these antibiotics are the same medications used to treat human infections. Scientists are concerned that this practice fosters the growth and spread of antibiotic-resistant bacteria strains in the animals (and, thus, foodborne illness in humans), as well as in the water, soil, and air around large-scale feeding areas.[72] The development of antibiotic-resistant bacteria is a major public health concern. Infections from antibiotic-resistant bacteria are very difficult to treat and, further, the arsenal of antibiotics available to health-care providers is limited. This issue is currently receiving considerable attention by scientists in the field. Note that the use of antibiotics is prohibited in organically produced animals.

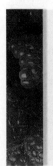

Knowledge Check

1. What are the sources of lead in the diet?
2. Which environmental contaminants are likely to be found in fish? Where can you find out if fish caught from lakes, rivers, and streams in your area are safe to eat?
3. What is a pesticide tolerance?
4. What methods can you use to reduce the amount of pesticides you ingest?

Expert Perspective *from the Field*

Organic Foods and Local Food Systems

Nutrition, agriculture, access to food and water, food processing and preparation, public policy, personal health, and environmental quality are all interrelated. When these relationships are out of balance and practices are not sustainable, the quality, quantity, and future of our food and water supplies may be negatively affected. Concern about these interrelationships, as well as environmental quality and personal health, may affect food choices. For example, consumers are increasingly choosing organic foods because of personal and environmental health concerns.

According to Angie Tagtow,* a registered dietitian and sustainable food systems advocate, the most important reason for eating organic fruits and vegetables is to decrease exposure to pesticide residues. By consuming organic meat, dairy, and eggs, she notes, consumers avoid the antibiotics and synthetic hormones commonly used in conventional farming. Another benefit is that animals that are certified organic often are treated humanely and have access to pasture. Tagtow's own concerns about health and the environment have led her to seek locally grown organic food. The benefits of local food systems, where local farmers and producers grow and sell foods to local consumers, may include increased biodiversity of farm products, increased access to fresh food, decreased impact on the environment, and greater community economic development.[75]

Tagtow states that her vision of an ideal food system is one that provides food that is

- *Healthy*—food that has optimal nutritional value, is free of preservatives and additives, and does not promote the development of diet-related chronic diseases
- *Green*—food production that has no or low environmental impact, keeps ecosystems in balance, uses minimal nonrenewable energy (e.g., oil and coal), and recycles wastes
- *Fair*—food production that does not exploit anyone or anything, enables farmers to earn enough income to be economically self-sufficient, keeps local food systems economically sound, and contributes to the overall economic development of communities
- *Affordable and accessible*—food that is safe, nutritious, produced in a sustainable manner, and equally and regularly available to everyone

When asked for advice on how those with a limited budget can incorporate organically grown foods in their diets, Tagtow recommended identifying local organic farmers and buying fruits, vegetables, dairy, eggs, or meat directly from them. Visiting farmers' markets, food co-ops, Community Supported Agriculture (CSA) farms, or Cooperative Extension System websites can help consumers learn which foods are produced locally. Many CSA farms rely on volunteers during the growing season—this may provide those with limited budgets an opportunity to access high-quality, fresh food. To save money, she also recommends buying fresh food when it is in season.

Consumers who find it too costly to buy all organic foods may want to focus on specific foods. For instance, Tagtow pointed out that the foods with the highest pesticide residues are apples, peaches, bell peppers, celery, nectarines, strawberries, cherries, lettuce, imported grapes, and pears—consumers concerned about pesticide residues may want to choose organic versions of these foods whenever they can. To learn more about local food systems and organic foods, visit the Leopold Center at www.leopold.iastate.edu/index.htm; The Organic Center at www.organic-center.org/; Local Harvest at www.localharvest.org/; and the Organic Farming Research Foundation at ofrf.org/index.html.

Angie Tagtow, MS, RD, LD, is a 2008–2009 Food and Society Policy Fellow, the owner of Environmental Nutrition Solutions, the managing editor of the Journal of Hunger & Environmental Nutrition, a member of the American Dietetic Association's Sustainable Food System Task Force, past chair of the Hunger and Environmental Nutrition Dietetic Practice Group of the American Dietetic Association, and a member of the Leopold Center for Sustainable Agriculture Regional Food System Working Group.

Summary

3.1 Food insecurity and hunger occur in virtually every country. About 1 in 8 people worldwide do not get enough food to meet their requirements. Food insecurity is linked to poverty. Food insecure people tend to have poorer diets and suffer more health problems. Children without enough food do not grow normally and are more likely to suffer diseases and death. In the U.S., the USDA monitors food insecurity. About 11% of U.S. households are food insecure, with a third of these having very low food security. The Food Stamp Program is the most important food assistance program offered by the U.S. government. Other programs include WIC and the National School Lunch and Breakfast Programs. Emergency food programs also play an important role for food insecure people.

3.2 Organic foods are grown in ways that promote healthy soils, waterways, crops, and animals. Many substances and processes cannot be applied to organic foods. The USDA certifies foods as organic. Organic foods contain fewer pesticides but their nutritional value may not differ from conventionally grown food. Genetically modified (GM) foods have new or modified genes to produce a plant, an animal, or another organism with a new trait. The most common GM foods in the U.S. are soybeans, corn, and cotton altered either to be herbicide resistant or to produce their own pesticides. Other GM applications are used to increase milk production and to produce chymosin for cheese making. GM foods are regulated by the FDA, USDA, and EPA. Labeling of GM foods is not required. Many concerns have been voiced about GM foods, including the safety of these foods for people and the environment.

3.3 Food spoilage results from microorganism and enzyme action. Food preservation methods stop or slow the rate of spoilage. Food irradiation is approved for some foods. Irradiated foods are not radioactive. Food additives are regulated by the FDA. Some food additives are considered GRAS and have not had formal testing. New food additives must be carefully tested by the manufacturer and evaluated by the FDA. Over 3000 food additives are approved for use in the U.S. Intentional food additives are used for a specific purpose, whereas incidental food additives become a part of food because of some aspect of production. Some people are concerned about the safety of food additives; however, no evidence shows that limiting additives will make you healthier. To lower your intake of additives, read food labels and eat fewer highly processed foods.

3.4 Foodborne pathogens are a significant cause of illness and death in the U.S. People more at risk are infants, children, the elderly, people with certain diseases, pregnant women, and those who have weakened immune systems. Foodborne illness usually causes gastrointestinal effects, but

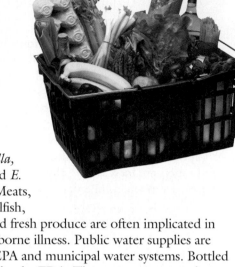

it can have more serious lasting effects. Over 250 pathogens, including viruses, bacteria, parasites, and toxins, can cause foodborne illness, but most are caused by bacteria (*Salmonella*, *Campylobacter*, and *E. coli*) and viruses. Meats, poultry, eggs, shellfish, dairy products, and fresh produce are often implicated in outbreaks of foodborne illness. Public water supplies are regulated by the EPA and municipal water systems. Bottled water is regulated by the FDA. There are numerous threats to safe water, but water contamination that poses a danger to health is rare.

3.5 Several government agencies, including the USDA, FDA, and CDC, are responsible for coordinating food safety efforts, but everyone has a responsibility for keeping food safe to eat. The risk of foodborne illness can be reduced by using good personal and kitchen hygiene, handling food safely, and avoiding foods that present extra risk. Washing hands, preventing cross-contamination, washing produce, keeping foods out of danger zone temperatures, and cooking meat, poultry, eggs, fish, and casseroles to the safe temperatures are especially important. Cooked foods should be either consumed right away or refrigerated within 2 hours. Traveler's diarrhea is common in visitors to developing countries. Following guidelines about water and produce consumption can help reduce the likelihood of contracting it.

3.6 Environmental contaminants in food include lead, mercury, industrial contaminants (e.g., dioxins and polychlorinated biphenyls [PCBs]), and pesticides. Lead can damage the developing nervous system; children are most at risk. Iron-deficient children may be at more risk of lead toxicity. Dioxins can contaminate food, especially fish. They are carcinogens and cause liver and nerve damage. Mercury also is found in fish, especially shark, swordfish, king mackerel, and tilefish. The FDA and EPA recommend that children and pregnant and breastfeeding women limit their exposure to high-mercury fish. PCBs can be found in fish, too. Farmers use pesticides to increase agricultural productivity. Pesticides are regulated by the EPA, USDA, and FDA. Pesticides in foods are a special concern for young children. The widespread use of antibiotics in animal feed is a concern because they foster the growth of antibiotic-resistant bacteria.

Study Questions

1. Which of the following is a sign of malnutrition caused by insufficient food and nutrient intake?
    a. stunting (shortness for age)
    b. wasting (loss of fat and muscle tissue)
    c. vitamin and mineral deficiencies, especially vitamin A, iron, and iodine
    d. all of the above

2. About _____ of U.S. households are food insecure.
    a. 20%   c. 4%
    b. 11%   d. 1%

3. The Food Stamp Program benefits _____.
    a. only low-income women, infants, and children
    b. poor households that meet eligibility guidelines
    c. food banks and pantries in communities across the country
    d. seniors in adult day-care settings

4. Populations disproportionately affected by hunger and malnutrition include _____.
    a. preschool children and women
    b. working adults
    c. teenagers
    d. all of the above

5. Which of the following statements about organic foods is *not* true?
    a. They are more nutritious than conventionally raised foods.
    b. Synthetic fertilizers, pesticides, antibiotics, synthetic hormones, and sewage sludge are prohibited in their production.
    c. A food labeled organic must have 95% of its ingredients by weight meet organic standards.
    d. The USDA is responsible for organic certification of farms and foods.

6. The main use of genetically modified foods in the U.S. food supply is to _____.
    a. improve nutritional quality by the production of additional amounts of beta-carotene
    b. eliminate potential allergens by altering the proteins synthesized in the plant or animal
    c. produce pharmaceutical products in an inexpensive way
    d. improve pest control and weed management and protect crops against diseases

7. In the U.S., food labels must indicate the presence of genetically modified ingredients.
    a. true   b. false

8. Which of the following statements about food irradiation is true?
    a. Irradiated food is radioactive.
    b. Irradiation can be used to destroy pathogens in food, such as *Salmonella* bacteria.
    c. All foods in the U.S. legally can be irradiated.
    d. Irradiation is used in only 2 countries around the world.

9. Food additive use and safety are regulated mainly by the _____.
    a. FDA   c. CDC
    b. USDA   d. EPA

10. Which of the following pathogens cause the most foodborne illness in the U.S.?
    a. Hepatitis A, *Clostridium botulinum*, *Listeria monocytogenes*, and *Staphylococcus aureus*
    b. *Campylobacter jejuni, Cryptosporidium, Aspergillus,* and *Clostridium botulinum*
    c. *Cryptosporidium,* hepatitis A, *Clostridium perfringens,* and *Salmonella*
    d. *Salmonella, Campylobacter jejuni, E. coli* 0157:H7, and noroviruses

11. Aflatoxin is produced by a mold that grows most often on _____.
    a. cheese
    b. bread products
    c. peanuts and corn
    d. fruit and other produce

12. The temperature danger zone is _____.
    a. 41° to 135°F (5° to 57°C)
    b. 32° to 40°F (0° to 4°C)
    c. 120° to 160°F (48° to 71°C)
    d. 0° to 212°F (0° to 100°C)

13. Thawing foods, such as chicken, on the counter overnight is a safe food handling practice.
    a. true   b. false

14. Which of the following statements about pesticides is *not* true?
    a. Organic foods sometimes contain very low amounts of pesticides.
    b. Some pesticides may persist in the environment for many years.
    c. Washing produce removes all pesticide residues.
    d. The EPA regulates the type and amount of pesticides that may be applied to food.

15. The food most likely to contain mercury, dioxins, or PCBs is _____.
    a. water from plumbing in older homes
    b. vegetables and fruits grown with pesticides
    c. fish from rivers, streams, and lakes
    d. milk from transgenic dairy cattle

Answer Key: 1-d; 2-b; 3-b; 4-a; 5-a; 6-d; 7-b; 8-b; 9-a; 10-d; 11-c; 12-a; 13-b; 14-c; 15-c

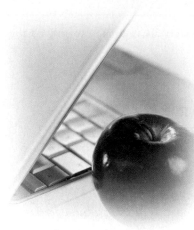

Websites

To learn more about the topics covered in this chapter, visit these websites.

Major USDA Food Assistance Programs

Food Stamp Program

www.fns.usda.gov/fsp

Special Supplemental Nutrition Program for Women, Infants, and Children (WIC)

www.fns.usda.gov/wic

National School Lunch Program

www.fns.usda.gov/cnd/lunch

National School Breakfast Program

www.fns.usda.gov/cnd/breakfast

Child and Adult Care Food Programs

www.fns.usda.gov/cnd/Care/default.htm

America's Second Harvest

www.secondharvest.org

Food Additives

vm.cfsan.fda.gov/~dms/eafus.html

Water Safety

www.EPA.gov/water

Food Safety

www.foodsafety.gov

www.ama-assn.org/ama/pub/category/1948.html

www.homefoodsafety.org

www.fightbac.org

www.cdc.gov/ncidod/dpd/travel.htm

www.epa.gov/waterscience/fish

Government Agencies

www.cdc.gov

www.usda.gov/fsis

www.nal.usda.gov

www.atf.treas.gov

www.epa.gov

www.fda.gov

www.nmfs.noaa.gov

References

1. Food and Agriculture Organization of the United Nations. *The state of food insecurity in the world.* Rome, Italy: 2006.

2. Popkin B. The world is fat. *Scientific Am.* 2007;297(3):88.

3. Prentice AM. The emerging epidemic of obesity in developing countries. *Int. J. Epidemiol.* 2006;35:93.

4. Hampton T. Food insecurity harms health, well-being of millions in the United States. *JAMA.* 2007;298:1851.

5. Alaimo K and others. Food insufficiency and American school-aged children's cognitive, academic and psychosocial development. *Pediatrics.* 2001;108:44.

6. Cook J and others. Child food insecurity increases risks posed by household food insecurity to young children's health. *J. Nutr.* 2006;136:1073.

7. Kaiser L, Townsend M. Food insecurity among US children: Implications for nutrition and health. *Top Clin Nutr.* 2005;20:313.

8. American Dietetic Association. Position of the American Dietetic Association: Food insecurity and hunger in the United States. *J Am Diet Assoc.* 2006;106:446.

9. Connell C and others. Children's experiences of food insecurity can assist in understanding its effect on their well-being. *J Nutr.* 2005;135:1683.

10. McIntyre L and others. Do low-income mothers compromise their nutrition to feed their children? *Can Med Assoc J.* 2003;168:686.

11. Biros M and others. The prevalence and perceived health consequences of hunger in emergency department patient populations. *Acad Emerg Med.* 2005;12:310.

12. Holben D, Pheley A. Obesity and diabetes are greater in food insecure households in rural Appalachian Ohio. *Prev Chronic Dis [serial online].* 2006; July.

13. Drewnowski A, Specter S. Poverty and obesity: The role of energy density and energy costs. *Am J Clin Nutr.* 2004;79:6.

14. Miech R and others. Trends in the association of poverty with overweight among US adolescents, 1971–2004. *JAMA.* 2006;295:2385.

15. Olson C. Food insecurity in women: A recipe for unhealthy trade-offs. *Top Clin Nutr.* 2005;20:321.

16. Wilde PE, Peterman JN. Individual weight change is associated with household food security status. *J Nutr.* 2006;136:1395.

17. United States Department of Agriculture ERS. Food security in the United States: Hunger and food security. 2006; www.ers.usda.gov/Briefing/FoodSecurity/labels.htm.

18. Nord M and others. *Household food security in the United States, 2005.* Washington, DC: United States Department of Agriculture, Economic Research Service; 2007.

19. United States Department of Health and Human Services. The 2007 HHS poverty guidelines. 2007; aspe.hhs.gov/poverty/07poverty.shtml.

20. Economic Research Service, United States Department of Agriculture. *The food assistance landscape annual report.* 2006; www.ers.usda.gov/publicationseib6-4.

21. America's Second Harvest. The almanac of hunger and poverty in America. 2007; www.secondharvest.org/learn_about_hunger/hunger_almanac_2007.html.

22. America's Second Harvest. Hunger in America. 2006; www.hungerinamerica.org.

23. Caulfield LE and others. Undernutrition as an underlying cause of child deaths associated with diarrhea, pneumonia, malaria, and measles. *Am J Clin Nutr.* 2004;80:193.

24. United Nations Children's Fund (UNICEF). The state of the world's children, 2007: Women and children, the double dividend of gender equality. www.unicef.org/sowc07.

25. Pinstrup-Andersen P, Cheng F. Still hungry. *Scientific Am.* 2007;297(3):96.

26. United Nations. UN millennium development goals, 2007; www.un.org/millenniumgoals.

27. Organic Trade Association. Market trends. 2007; www.ota.com/organic/mt.html.

28. Agriculture Market Service, United States Department of Agriculture. National Organic Program; 2008. www.ams.usda.gov/NOP/indexIE.htm.

29. Williamson CS. Is organic food better for our health? *Nutr Bulletin.* 2007;32(2):104.

30. Amodio M and others. A comparative study of composition and postharvest performance of organically and conventionally grown kiwifruits. *J Sci Food Agric.* 2007;87:1228.

31. Mitchell AE and others. Ten-year comparison of the influence of organic and conventional crop management practices on the content of flavonoids in tomatoes. *J Agric Food Chem.* 2007;55:6154.

32. Mukherjee A and others. Preharvest evaluation of coliforms, *Escherichia coli, Salmonella,* and *Escherichia coli 0157:H7* in organic and conventional produce grown by Minnesota farmers. *J Food Protection.* 2004;67:894.

33. Raney T, Prabhu P. Sowing a gene revolution. *Scientific Am.* 2007;297(3):104.

34. Fernandez-Cornejo J, Caswell M. *The first decade of genetically engineered crops in the United States.* Washington, DC: United States Department of Agriculture; 2006.

35. Devlin RH and others. Population effects of growth hormone transgenic coho salmon depend on food availability and genotype by environment interactions. *Proc National Acad Sci.* 2004;101:9303.

36. Gray TW. Dairy dilemma. Ban on rBGH use by Tillamook sparks conflict. *Rural Cooperatives;* 2006:4.

37. James C. *Brief 35: Global status of commercialized biotech/ GM crops: 2006;* Ithaca, NY: International Service for the Acquisition of Agri-biotech Applications; 2006.

38. Cohen J. Poorer nations turn to publicly developed GM crops. *Nature Biotech.* 2005;23:27.

39. The National Biological Information Infrastructure. United States Regulatory Agencies Unified Biotechnology Website. usbiotechreg.nbii.gov. 2008.

40. U.S. Food and Drug Administration, Center for Veterinary medicine. CVM and animal cloning. 2008; www.fda.gov/cvm/cloning.htm. 2008.

41. Osterholm M, Norgan A. The role of food irradiation in food safety. *New Eng J Med.* 2004;350.

42. United States Department of Agriculture Food Safety and Inspection Service. Irradiation and food safety. Answers to frequently asked questions. 2005; www.fsis.usda.gov/Fact_Sheets/Irradiation_and_Food_Safety/index.asp.

43. Hoefer D and others. Knowledge, attitude and practice of the use of irradiated meat among respondents to the FoodNet Population Survey in Connecticut and New York. *J Food Protection.* 2006;69:2441.

44. United States Food and Drug Administration Office for Food Safety and Applied Nutrition. Data on benzene in soft drinks and other beverages. 2007; www.cfsan.fda.gov/~dms/benzdata.html.

45. Ames B and others. Ranking possible carcinogenic hazards. *Science.* 1987;236:271.

46. Soffriti M and others. Life-span exposure to low doses of aspartame beginning during prenatal life increases cancer effects in human. *Environ Health Perspect.* 2007;115:1293.

47. Mead P and others. Food-related illness and death in the United States. *Emerging Infectious Diseases.* 1999;5:607.

48. World Health Organization. Food safety and foodborne illness, fact sheet no 237. 2007; www.who.int/mediacentre/factsheets/fs237/en.

49. Calvin L. Spinach forces reassessment of food safety practices. *Amber Waves.* 2007;5(3):25.

50. Centers for Disease Control and Prevention. Foodborne illness; 2005. www.cdc.gov/ncidod/dbmd/diseaseinfo/foodborneinfections_g.htm.

51. Johnston C and others. Outbreak management and implications of a nosocomial norovirus outbreak *Clinical Infectious Diseases.* 2007;45:534.

52. Centers for Disease Control and Prevention. Avian influenza (bird flu). 2007; www.cdc.gov/flu/avian.

53. Karanis P and others. Waterborne transmission of protozoan parasites: A worldwide review of outbreaks and lessons learnt. *J Water Health.* 2007;5(1):1.

54. Centers for Disease Control and Prevention. vCJD (variant Creutzfeldt-Jakob disease). 2007; www.cdc.gov/ncidod/dvrd/vcjd/factsheet_nvcjd.htm.

55. Centers for Disease Control and Prevention. BSE (bovine spongiform encephalopathy, or mad cow disease). 2007; www.cdc.gov/ncidod/dvrd/bse/index.htm.

56. Taylor SL. Food additives, contaminants and natural toxicants. In: Shils M and others, eds. *Modern nutrition in health and disease.* 10th ed. Baltimore: Lippincott Williams & Wilkins; 2006:1809.

57. Environmental Protection Agency. Drinking water. 2007; www.epa.gov/ebtpages/watedrinkingwater.html.

58. Liang J and others. Surveillance for waterborne disease and outbreaks associated with drinking water and water not intended for drinking: United States, 2003–2004. *MMWR.* 2006;55(SS12):31.

59. Meyer PA and others. Surveillance for elevated blood lead levels among children: United States, 1997–2001. *MMWR.* 2003;52(SS10):1.

60. Saper RB and others. Heavy metal content of Ayurvedic herbal medicine products. *JAMA.* 2004;292:2868.

61. Tuteja, AK and others. Development of functional diarrhea, constipation, irritable bowel syndrome, and dyspepsia during and after traveling outside the USA, *Digest Dis Sci.* 2008;53:271.

62. Zimmermann MB and others. Iron fortification reduces blood lead levels in children in Bangalore, India. *Pediatrics.* 2006;117:2014.

63. Mozaffarian D, Rimm EB. Fish intake, contaminants and human health. *JAMA.* 2006;296:1885.

64. Environmental Protection Agency. Pesticides; 2007. www.epa.gov/pesticides.

65. National Research Council. *Pesticides in the diets of infants and children.* Washington, DC: National Academy Press; 1993.

66. United States Department of Agriculture. Pesticide Data Program—Progress report. 2006; www.ams.usda.gov/science/pdp.

67. Agricultural Health Study. Publications. 2007; aghealth.org/publications.html.

68. Sanbourn M and others. *Pesticides literature review: Systematic review of pesticides human health effects.* Ontario, Canada: Ontario College of Physicians; 2004.

69. Grandjean P and others. The Faroes statement: Human health effects of developmental exposure to chemicals in our environment. *Basic Clin Pharmacol Tox.* 2007;102:73.

70. Lu C and others. Organic diets significantly lower children's exposure to organophosphorus pesticides. *Environ Health Perspect.* 2006;114:260.

71. Mellon M and others. Hogging it: Estimates of antimicrobial abuse in livestock. 2001; www.ucsusa.org/food_and_environment/antibiotics_and_food/hogging-it-estimates-of-antimicrobial-abuse-in-livestock.html.

72. Sapkota AR and others. What do we feed to food-production animals? A review of animal feed ingredients and their potential impacts on human health. *Environ Health Perspect.* 2007;115:663.

73. Keys A. *The biology of human starvation.* Minneapolis: University of Minnesota Press; 1950.

74. Pew Initiative on Food and Biotechnology. Public sentiment about genetically modified food. 2006; www.pewtrusts.org/news_room_ektid32802.aspx.

75. Swenson D. The economic impact of fruit and vegetable production in Iowa. 2006; www.leopold.iastate.edu/pubs/staff/health/health.htm.

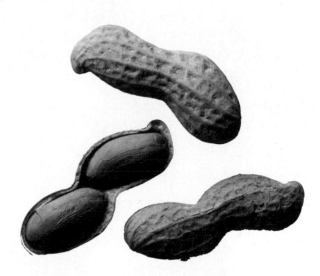

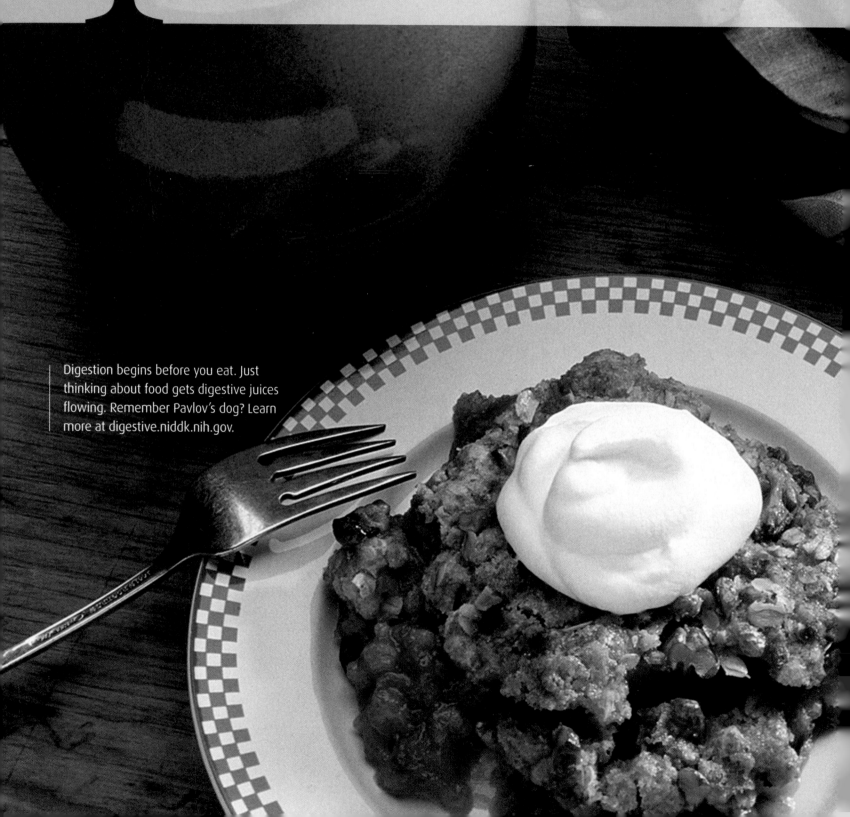

4 *Human Digestion and Absorption*

Digestion begins before you eat. Just thinking about food gets digestive juices flowing. Remember Pavlov's dog? Learn more at digestive.niddk.nih.gov.

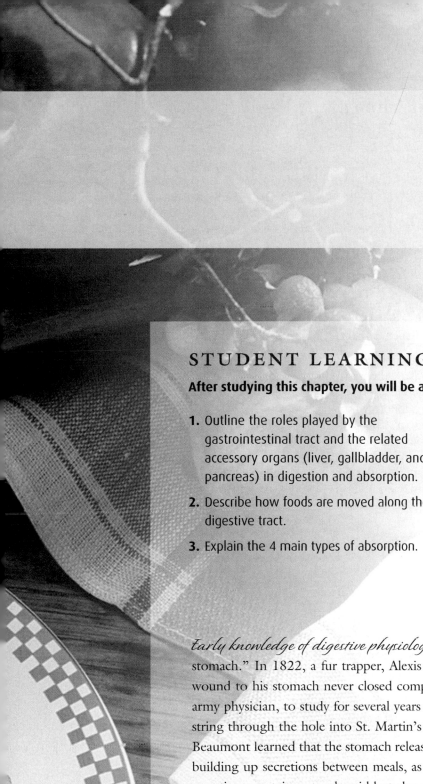

STUDENT LEARNING OUTCOMES

After studying this chapter, you will be able to:

1. Outline the roles played by the gastrointestinal tract and the related accessory organs (liver, gallbladder, and pancreas) in digestion and absorption.

2. Describe how foods are moved along the digestive tract.

3. Explain the 4 main types of absorption.

4. Identify the key enzymes and hormones involved in digestion and absorption and their functions.

5. Identify major nutrition-related gastrointestinal diseases and disorders and typical approaches to prevention and treatment.

6. Explain why diarrhea represents a serious health challenge to infants and young children around the world.

Early knowledge of digestive physiology came from a surprising source—"the man with a hole in his stomach." In 1822, a fur trapper, Alexis St. Martin, was accidentally hit by a shotgun blast. The blast wound to his stomach never closed completely, allowing an opportunity for William Beaumont, a U.S. army physician, to study for several years how foods are digested. For example, he lowered food tied to string through the hole into St. Martin's stomach and then periodically removed it to observe changes. Beaumont learned that the stomach releases its secretions in response to food in the stomach, rather than building up secretions between meals, as was commonly believed. He also discovered that the stomach secretions contain not only acid but also a substance that allows meat to be digested. We now know this substance as the digestive enzyme pepsin. Beaumont also observed that, when his subject was distressed or angry, digestion was impaired. Throughout his life, St. Martin remained in poor health, but he lived almost 60 years after the shooting accident.

Since the time of Beaumont and St. Martin, scientists have continued to study how the digestive system functions and the many digestive system disorders and diseases. This chapter will explore the processes of digestion and absorption and the related aspects of human physiology that support nutritional health. You will become acquainted with the basic anatomy (structure) and physiology (function) of the digestive system. You also will learn the causes of some common digestive system disorders, along with ways to prevent and treat them.

4.1 Organization of the Human Body

The cell is the smallest functional unit of the human body. (Appendix A reviews the parts of a cell.) The body's 10 trillion cells have the ability to grow; take in (absorb) substances, including nutrients; use energy; synthesize and secrete new compounds; and excrete waste. Cellular processes and chemical reactions, which occur constantly in every living cell, require a continuous supply of energy in the form of dietary carbohydrate, protein, and fat. Almost all cells need oxygen to transform the energy in nutrients into the form the body can use—**adenosine triphosphate (ATP)** (see Chapter 9 for more on ATP). Cells also need water, building supplies (e.g., amino acids and minerals), and chemical regulators (e.g., vitamins). Of course, adequately supplying all nutrients to the body's cells begins with a healthful diet.

Cells of the same type join together to form tissue (Fig. 4-1). **Tissue** is made of groups of similar cells working together to perform a specific task. Humans are composed of 4 primary types of tissue: epithelial, connective, muscle, and nervous.

- **Epithelial tissue** is composed of cells that cover surfaces outside and inside the body. The skin and linings of the gastrointestinal (GI) tract are examples. Epithelial cells absorb nutrients, secrete important substances, and excrete waste.
- **Connective tissue** supports and protects the body by holding structures (e.g., cells and cell parts) together, stores fat, and produces blood cells. Tendons, cartilage, and parts of bone, arteries, and veins are made of connective tissue.
- **Muscle tissue** can contract and relax and is designed to permit movement.
- **Nervous tissue,** found in the brain and spinal cord, transmits nerve impulses from one part of the body to another.

adenosine triphosphate (ATP) Chemical that supplies energy for many cellular processes and reactions.

1 **Chemical level.** Atoms combine to form molecules.

2 **Cell level.** Molecules form organelles, such as the nucleus and mitochondria, which make up cells.

3 **Tissue level.** Similar cells and surrounding materials make up tissues.

4 **Organ level.** Different tissues combine to form organs, such as the stomach.

5 **Organ system level.** Organs such as the stomach and intestines make up an organ system.

6 **Organism level.** Organ systems make up an organism.

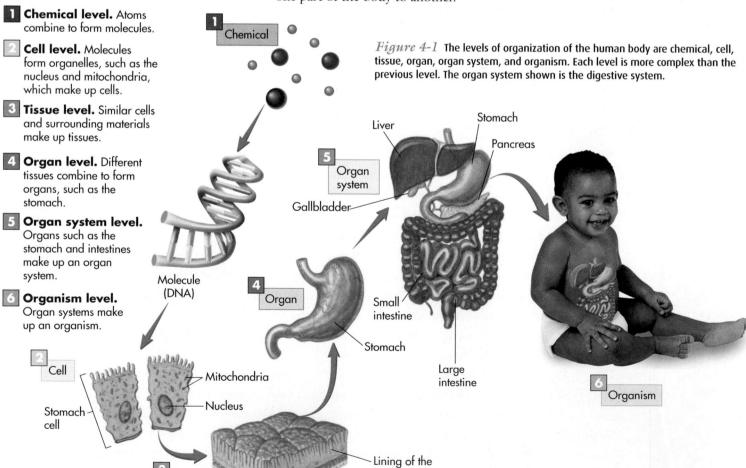

Figure 4-1 The levels of organization of the human body are chemical, cell, tissue, organ, organ system, and organism. Each level is more complex than the previous level. The organ system shown is the digestive system.

Tissues combine in a specific way to form structures, known as **organs,** which perform specific functions. All organs play a role in nutritional health, and nutrient intake affects how well each organ functions. An **organ system** is formed when several organs work together to perform a specific function. For example, the digestive system includes the GI tract (mouth, esophagus, stomach, small intestine, and large intestine, which terminates with the rectum and anus), liver, pancreas, and gallbladder (Fig. 4-2). The coordinated work of all organ systems allows the entire body to function normally. Table 4-1 summarizes the components and functions of the body's organ systems.

The primary theme of human nutrition is to understand how nutrients affect different cells, tissues, organs, organ systems, and, finally, overall health. This chapter focuses on the digestive system. Learning how the digestive system makes nutrients in foods available to body organs, tissues, and cells is critical to understanding human nutrition.

Knowledge Check

1. What is the form of energy that can be used by almost all cells?
2. How do the 4 types of tissue differ?
3. What are the organs that make up the digestive system?

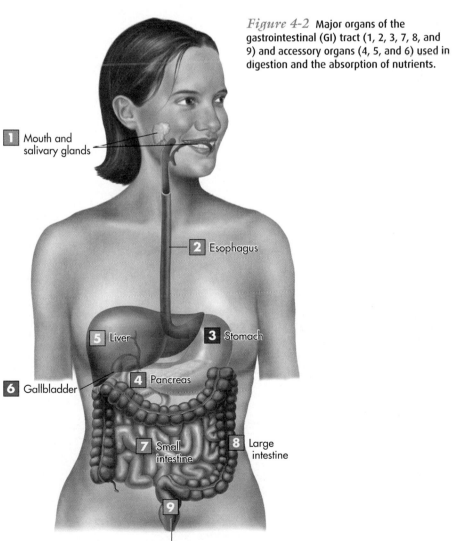

Figure 4-2 Major organs of the gastrointestinal (GI) tract (1, 2, 3, 7, 8, and 9) and accessory organs (4, 5, and 6) used in digestion and the absorption of nutrients.

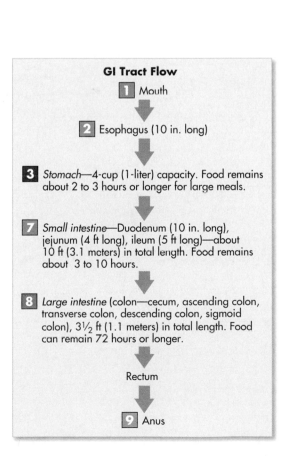

GI Tract Flow

1 Mouth

2 Esophagus (10 in. long)

3 *Stomach*—4-cup (1-liter) capacity. Food remains about 2 to 3 hours or longer for large meals.

7 *Small intestine*—Duodenum (10 in. long), jejunum (4 ft long), ileum (5 ft long)—about 10 ft (3.1 meters) in total length. Food remains about 3 to 10 hours.

8 *Large intestine* (colon—cecum, ascending colon, transverse colon, descending colon, sigmoid colon), $3\frac{1}{2}$ ft (1.1 meters) in total length. Food can remain 72 hours or longer.

Rectum

9 Anus

Table 4-1 Organ Systems of the Body

System	Major Components	Functions Related to Nutrition
Digestive	Mouth, esophagus, stomach, intestines, and accessory organs (liver, gallbladder, and pancreas)	Performs the mechanical and chemical processes of digestion, absorption of nutrients, metabolizing of nutrients (especially the liver), and elimination of wastes
Circulatory	Cardiovascular: Heart, blood vessels, and blood Lymphatic: Lymphatic vessels, lymph nodes, and other lymph organs	Transports nutrients, waste products, gases (oxygen, carbon dioxide), and hormones throughout the body; plays a role in the immune response and regulation of body temperature system, removes foreign substances from the blood and lymph and combats disease
Immune	White blood cells, lymphatic vessels and lymph nodes, spleen, thymus gland, and other lymph tissues	Provides defense against foreign invaders
Nervous	Brain, spinal cord, nerves, and sensory receptors	Detects sensation, controls movements, controls physiological and intellectual functions
Endocrine	Endocrine glands, such as the pituitary, thyroid, and adrenal glands	Regulates metabolism, growth, reproduction, and many other functions by producing and releasing hormones
Urinary	Kidneys, urinary bladder, and the ducts that carry urine	Removes waste products from the blood and regulates blood acid-base (pH) balance, overall chemical balance, and water balance

Table 4-1 Continued

System	Major Components	Functions Related to Nutrition
Integumentary	Skin, hair, nails, and sweat glands	Protects other organ systems, regulates body temperature, prevents water loss, and produces a substance that converts to vitamin D on sun exposure
Skeletal	Bones, cartilage, ligaments, and joints	Protects, supports, and allows body movement, produces blood cells, and stores minerals
Muscular	Smooth, cardiac, and skeletal muscle	Produces body movement, maintains posture, and produces body heat
Respiratory	Lungs and respiratory passages	Exchanges gases (oxygen and carbon dioxide) between the blood and the air and regulates blood acid-base (pH) balance
Reproductive	Gonads (ovaries and testes) and genitals	Performs the processes of reproduction and influences sexual functions and behaviors

The cardiovascular and lymphatic organ systems together make up the circulatory system and so contribute to circulatory functions in the body. The lymphatic system is part of the immune system. The endocrine and nervous organ systems contribute to the regulatory functions. The digestive, urinary, integumentary, and respiratory organ systems contribute to the excretory functions, whereas the muscular and skeletal organ systems contribute to storage abilities in the body.

4.2 Digestive System Overview

Digestion, the process of breaking down foods into a form the body can use, and **absorption**, the uptake of nutrients from the GI tract into either the blood or the lymph, are accomplished by the digestive system. Figure 4-3 provides an overview of the functions of the organs of the digestive system. About 29 cups (7 liters) of fluid containing water, mucus, acid, digestive enzymes, bile, and hormones are secreted into the GI tract each day to assist with the processes of digestion and absorption. All of the nutrients—proteins, fats, carbohydrates, vitamins, minerals, and water—are readily digested and absorbed along the GI tract. And, at the end of the GI tract, the excretion of waste matter occurs in a convenient, voluntary process. Like many other processes, such as breathing and the beating of the heart, digestion and absorption are carefully controlled by hormones and the nervous system.

Figure 4-3 Physiology of the GI tract. Many organs cooperate in a regulated fashion to allow the digestion and absorption of nutrients in foods.

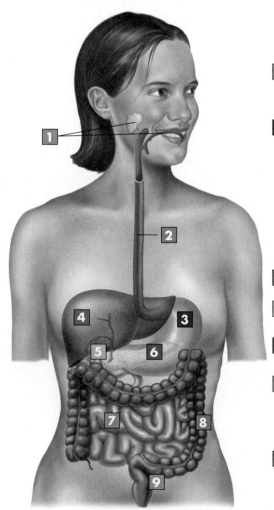

Organ	Digestive Functions
1 Mouth and salivary glands	Chew food
	Perceive taste
	Moisten food with saliva
	Lubricate food with mucus
	Release starch-digesting (amylase) enzyme
	Initiate swallowing reflex
2 Esophagus	Lubricate with mucus
	Move food to stomach by peristaltic waves (swallowing)
3 Stomach	Store, mix, dissolve, and continue digestion of food
	Dissolve food particles with secretions
	Kill microorganisms with acid
	Release protein-digesting (pepsin) enzyme
	Lubricate and protect stomach surface with mucus
	Regulate emptying of dissolved food into small intestine
	Produce intrinsic factor for vitamin B-12 absorption
4 Liver	Produce bile to aid fat digestion and absorption
5 Gallbladder	Store, concentrate, and later release bile into the small intestine
6 Pancreas	Secrete sodium bicarbonate and enzymes for digesting carbohydrate, fat, and protein
7 Small intestine	Mix and propel contents
	Lubricate with mucus
	Digest and absorb most substances using enzymes made by the pancreas and small intestine
8 Large intestine	Mix and propel contents
	Absorb sodium, potassium, and water
	House bacteria
	Lubricate with mucus
	Synthesize some vitamins and short-chain fatty acids
	Form feces
9 Rectum	Hold feces and expel via the anus, which is the opening to the outside of the body

In addition to its main functions of digestion and absorption, the GI tract also serves as a barrier to the entry of harmful bacteria into the body. Further, healthy bacteria in the large intestine help keep pathogenic (disease-causing) bacteria under control. They also synthesize nutrients, such as vitamin K and biotin, along with short-chain fatty acids that can serve as an energy source for the large intestine.

Anatomy of the GI Tract

The GI tract, also known as the **alimentary canal**, is a long, hollow, muscular tube that extends almost 15 feet from mouth to anus. Nutrients must pass through the wall of this tube to be absorbed into the body. The wall consists of 4 layers (Fig. 4-4):

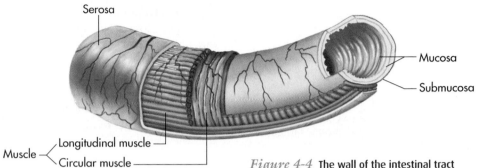

Figure 4-4 **The wall of the intestinal tract consists of 4 layers: mucosa, submucosa, muscle, and serosa.**

- **Mucosa**, the innermost layer, is lined with epithelial cells and glands. The mucosa is not smooth and in some areas has tiny, fingerlike structures that project into the GI tract **lumen** (the hollow area inside the tube) and trap nutrients.
- **Submucosa**, the second layer, consists of loose connective tissue, glands, blood vessels, and nerves. The blood vessels carry substances, including nutrients, both to and from the GI tract.
- **Muscle**, the next layer, occurs as double layers in most parts of the GI tract: an inner layer of circular smooth muscle that encircles the tube and an outer layer of longitudinal muscle fibers that runs up and down the tube. These muscles move food forward through the GI tract. The stomach has a third layer of muscle fiber that runs diagonally around it.
- **Serosa**, the outermost layer, protects the GI tract. The serosa secretes fluid that cushions the GI tract and reduces friction as it and other organs move.

Along the GI tract are **sphincters,** ringlike muscles that open and close like valves to control the flow of the contents (Fig. 4-5). The sphincters prevent food from moving through the GI tract too quickly. This allows food in the GI tract to be mixed thoroughly with digestive system secretions. The sphincters also help with GI **motility** (the propulsion of food through the GI tract).

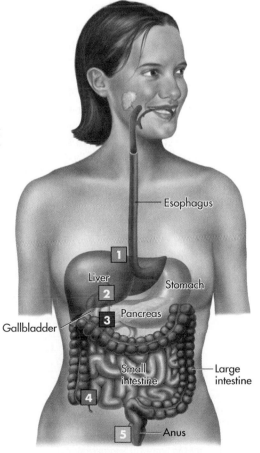

	Sphincter	Function
1	Lower esophageal sphincter	Prevent backflow (reflux) of stomach contents into the esophagus
2	Pyloric sphincter	Control the flow of stomach contents into the small intestine
3	Sphincter of Oddi	Control the flow of bile from common bile duct into the small intestine
4	Ileocecal sphincter	Prevent the contents of the large intestine from reentering the small intestine
5	Anal sphincters	Prevent defecation until person desires to do so

Figure 4-5 **Sphincters of the GI tract. These ringlike muscles control the flow of contents through the GI tract. They open and close in response to stimuli from nerves, hormones, hormonelike compounds, and pressure that builds up around the sphincters.**

▶ Hunger pangs are strong, somewhat uncomfortable peristaltic contractions that usually occur several hours after the last meal.

fecal matter Substances discharged from the bowel during defecation, including undigested food residue, dead GI tract cells, mucus, and bacteria; also called feces.

hydrolysis reaction Chemical reaction that breaks down a compound by adding water. One product receives a hydrogen ion (H^+); the other product receives a hydroxyl ion (OH^-). Hydrolytic enzymes break down compounds using water in this manner.

▶ The naming system for many enzymes is quite simple. The first part of the enzyme name usually indicates the target and is followed by the suffix *-ase*. For instance, sucrase is the enzyme that digests the sugar sucrose; similarly, lactase digests lactose.

▶ In cystic fibrosis, an inherited genetic disease, excess production of thick, sticky mucus may prevent pancreatic enzymes from reaching the small intestine. This results in malabsorption of nutrients, physical discomfort, and serious malnutrition if not treated. An affected person may be prescribed replacement enzymes, which are taken right before eating. Usually, these are coated to protect the enzymes from destruction by acid in the stomach.

GI Motility: Mixing and Propulsion

Food is mixed with digestive secretions and propelled down the GI tract by a process called peristalsis. A snake swallowing its prey graphically illustrates the process. Recall that most of the GI tract has 2 layers of muscles—circular and longitudinal. **Peristalsis** consists of a coordinated wave of contraction (squeezing and shortening) and relaxation of these muscles (Fig. 4-6). This process begins in the esophagus as 2 waves of muscle action closely following each other. The thickest and strongest muscles of the GI tract are in the stomach, where 3 opposing muscle layers (to allow for more complete mixing and churning) contract as often as 3 times per minute after a meal to mix food with gastric juices.

The most frequent peristalsis takes place in the small intestine, where contractions occur about every 4 to 5 seconds. The small intestine also experiences segmental contractions (segmentation), which move the intestinal contents back and forth, causing the contents to break apart and mix with digestive juices. The large intestine has comparatively sluggish peristaltic waves. These lead to occasional **mass movements,** which are peristaltic waves that simultaneously coordinate contractions over a widespread area of the large intestine. Mass movements propel **fecal matter** from one part of the large intestine to the next and finally into the rectum for elimination.

Digestive System Secretions

Throughout the GI tract, many secretions that aid in digestion are released. Digestive tract secretions include saliva, mucus, hydrochloric acid, digestive enzymes, hormones, bicarbonate, and bile (Table 4-2).

Saliva, from salivary glands in the mouth, moistens food and begins the process of digestion. Mucus and digestive enzymes are secreted in the mouth, stomach, and small intestine and by the pancreas. **Mucus** is a thick fluid that protects body cells and lubricates digesting food to help it move smoothly along the GI tract. **Digestive enzymes** are protein molecules that speed up digestion by catalyzing chemical reactions. Catalysis brings certain molecules close together and then creates a favorable environment for the chemical reaction. (Appendix B provides details on enzyme action.) Digestive enzymes catalyze chemical reactions known as **hydrolysis reactions**. In these reactions, water (*hydro-*) breaks apart (*-lysis*) molecules that are too large to pass though the GI tract wall. Hydrolysis reactions eventually yield simple molecules that are small enough to be absorbed through the intestinal wall. For example, sucrose (table sugar) is unabsorbable because it is too large to pass through the GI tract wall. In Figure 4-7, you can see how a molecule of the sugar sucrose is hydrolyzed to form the smaller glucose and fructose molecules, both of which can be absorbed through the intestinal wall.

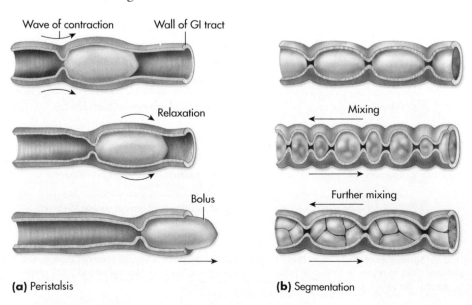

Figure 4-6 Peristalsis and segmentation. (*a*) Peristalsis is a coordinated wave of contraction and relaxation that moves the bolus (chewed food) ahead of the wave through the GI tract toward the anus. (*b*) Segmentation is a back-and-forth action in the small intestine that breaks apart the bolus into increasingly smaller pieces and mixes them with digestive juices.

(a) Peristalsis

(b) Segmentation

Digestive enzymes aid mostly in the breakdown of carbohydrates, proteins, and fats. Each enzyme usually acts on one specific substance; for example, an enzyme that recognizes sucrose ignores lactose (milk sugar). Notice in Figure 4-7 that the sucrase enzyme hydrolyzes sucrose.

The mouth and the stomach make a few digestive enzymes. Most, however, are synthesized by the pancreas and small intestine (Chapters 5, 6, and 7 review these enzymes in detail). The pancreas adjusts its enzyme production to match the macronutrient content of the diet. Increased protein intake results in an increase in protein-digesting enzymes. Diets high in fat and low in carbohydrate lead to increased production of fat-digesting enzymes.

Inadequate amounts of digestive enzymes may be produced when the small intestine or the pancreas is diseased. This scarcity can result in incomplete digestion and limited absorption. If food is not completely digested, bacteria in the large intestine convert some of it into gases and acids. The gases often distend (bloat) the abdomen. In addition, the feces look foamy and greasy because of trapped gases and the presence of undigested fat.

Some digestive enzymes not only digest food but also can digest the GI tract itself! For this reason, nerves and hormones tightly control enzyme release. Four **hormones** that play key roles in digestion are gastrin, secretin, cholecystokinin (CCK), and gastric inhibitory peptide. The functions of these hormones, as well as those of hydrochloric acid, bicarbonate, and bile, are described later in the chapter in Sections 4.4 and 4.5.

Table 4-2 Important Secretions of the Digestive System

Secretion	Site of Production	Function
Saliva	Mouth	Contributes to starch digestion, lubrication, swallowing
Mucus	Mouth, stomach, small and large intestines	Protects GI tract cells, lubricates digesting food
Enzymes (amylases, lipases, proteases)	Mouth, stomach, small intestine, pancreas	Promotes digestion of carbohydrates, fats, and protein into forms small enough for absorption
Acid (HCl)	Stomach	Promotes digestion of protein, destroys microorganisms, increases solubility of minerals
Bile	Liver (stored in gallbladder)	Aids in fat digestion (emulsifies fat)
Bicarbonate	Pancreas, small intestine	Neutralizes stomach acid when it reaches small intestine
Hormones	Stomach, small intestine	Regulates digestion and absorption

hormone Chemical messenger produced in one tissue that subsequently acts on cells or tissues in another part of the body.

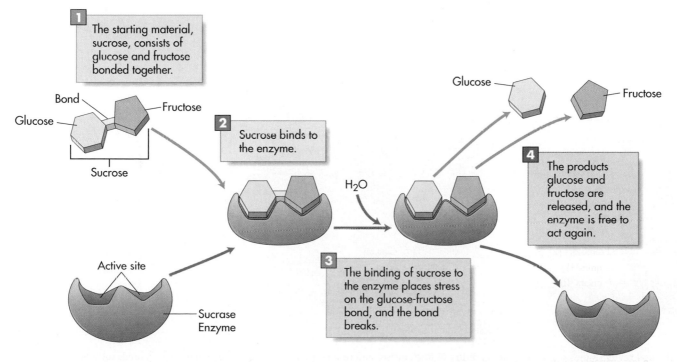

1 The starting material, sucrose, consists of glucose and fructose bonded together.

Bond
Fructose
Glucose
Sucrose

Glucose
Fructose

2 Sucrose binds to the enzyme.

H_2O

4 The products glucose and fructose are released, and the enzyme is free to act again.

Active site

3 The binding of sucrose to the enzyme places stress on the glucose-fructose bond, and the bond breaks.

Sucrase Enzyme

Figure 4-7 A model of enzyme action. The enzyme sucrase splits the sugar sucrose into two simpler sugars; glucose and fructose. [Note that sometimes energy input is needed to make reactions occur.]

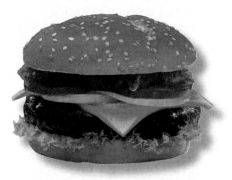

The GI tract digests the foods eaten. Despite what you may have heard, the order in which foods are eaten has no effect on digestive processes.

Knowledge Check

1. What is the difference between digestion and absorption?
2. What are the 4 layers of the GI tract?
3. How are the contents of the GI tract propelled along its length?
4. What are the main secretions of the GI tract?
5. What is the function of enzymes in digestion?

 ## 4.3 Moving through the GI Tract: Mouth and Esophagus

Before we eat a bite of most foods, the work of digestion has already started. Food preparation, such as cooking, marinating, pounding, and dicing, often begins the process. Starch granules in food swell as they soak up water during cooking, making them much easier to digest. Cooking also softens tough connective tissues in meats and fibrous tissue of plants, such as that in broccoli stalks. As a result, the food is easier to chew, swallow, and break down during digestion.

In the body, digestion begins in the mouth, or oral cavity (Fig. 4-8). The teeth tear and grind solid food into smaller pieces, which increases the surface area exposed to saliva. During chewing, the tongue presses morsels of food against the hard palate and helps mix the food with saliva. The food is now referred to as a **bolus**.

The salivary glands produce about 4 cups (1 liter) of saliva each day. **Saliva** is a dilute, watery fluid that contains several substances, including mucus to lubricate the bolus and hold it together; **lysozyme** to kill bacteria; and **amylase** to break down starch into simple sugars. However, food remains in the mouth such a short time that only about 5% of the starch gets broken down by salivary amylase. Lingual lipase, also released from salivary glands, is a fat-digesting enzyme that is produced mainly during infancy. Saliva also helps prevent tooth decay because it contains antibacterial agents, minerals to repair teeth, and substances that neutralize acid.

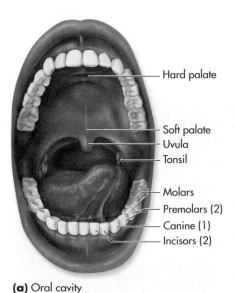

(a) Oral cavity

Hard palate
Soft palate
Uvula
Tonsil
Molars
Premolars (2)
Canine (1)
Incisors (2)

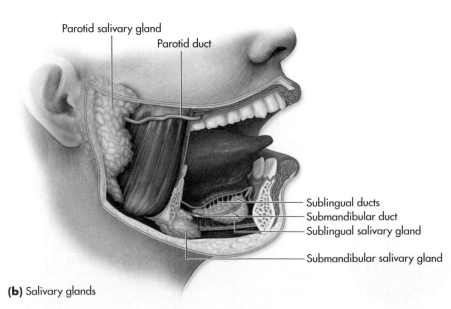

(b) Salivary glands

Parotid salivary gland
Parotid duct
Sublingual ducts
Submandibular duct
Sublingual salivary gland
Submandibular salivary gland

Figure 4-8 (*a*) The oral cavity (mouth) is the beginning of the GI tract. Incisor and canine (pointed) teeth are useful in tearing food, such as from a chicken leg. Molars (flat teeth) are used to grind food into smaller pieces. (*b*) The salivary glands near the oral cavity produce saliva to aid in swallowing and digesting food.

Taste and Smell

Saliva enhances our perception of the flavor of foods by dissolving the taste-forming compounds in foods. Taste buds, found on the tongue and soft palate, contain cells that interact with taste compounds in foods. Taste cells can detect each of the following 5 basic taste sensations,[1] but sensitivity to a particular taste may be more pronounced on certain areas of the tongue.

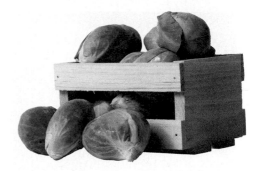

Cabbage contains bitter compounds. The ability to taste these compounds depends on one's genetic background.

- Salty, from metal ions, such as sodium (Na^+)
- Sour, from acids (think about how sour—and acidic—a lemon is)
- Sweet, from organic compounds such as sugars
- Bitter, from a diverse group of compounds, including caffeine and quinine, and numerous other compounds in vegetables and fruits; many bitter compounds are toxic, but others are beneficial phytochemicals and have antioxidant and cancer-protecting activity[2]
- Umami, a savory, brothy, or meaty taste[3] from amino acids, primarily glutamate; foods such as mushrooms, cooked tomatoes, Parmesan cheese, and seaweed cause the umami taste sensation, and the seasoning monosodium glutamate (MSG) often is added to processed and restaurant foods to enhance the umami sensation

The sense of taste is enhanced by input from approximately 6 million **olfactory** (sense of smell) cells in the nose, which are stimulated when we chew. Thus, it makes perfect sense that, when our noses are congested, even strong-tasting foods have little taste. A variety of diseases and drugs, as well as the effects of aging, can alter taste and smell sensations. Taste perception also is affected by human genetic variation in both taste and olfactory sensations. The ability to detect bitter substances—such as in broccoli or cabbage—is one example.

Swallowing

Swallowing moves food from the mouth into the esophagus, the 10-inch-long muscular tube that extends to the stomach (Fig. 4-9). At its entrance is the **epiglottis**, a valvelike flap of tissue that prevents food from lodging in the **trachea** (windpipe). When food is swallowed, it drops onto the epiglottis, which then covers the **larynx** (the

▶ When we talk about liking the taste of a food, we mean we like its flavor. That's because taste along with smell and the physical effect caused by food textures and certain chemicals in foods (such as capsaicin in chili peppers) combine to create flavor sensations.

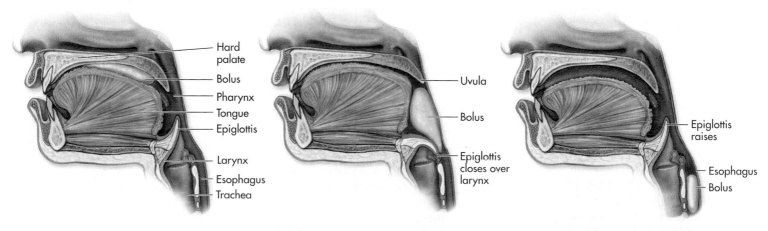

(a) Bolus of food is pushed by tongue against hard palate and then moves toward pharynx.

(b) As bolus moves into pharynx, epiglottis closes over larynx.

(c) Esophageal muscle contractions push bolus toward stomach. Epiglottis then returns to its normal position.

Figure 4-9 The process of swallowing. Swallowing occurs as the food bolus is forced (*a*) into the pharynx (throat) from the oral cavity, (*b*) through the pharynx, and (*c*) into the esophagus on the way to the stomach. Choking occurs when the bolus becomes lodged in the trachea (windpipe), blocking air to the lungs, instead of passing into the esophagus.

opening of the trachea). Breathing automatically stops. These involuntary responses ensure that swallowed food, aided by peristalsis of the esophagus and gravity, travels down the esophagus, not into the trachea. Small pieces of food that enter the trachea may end up in the lungs and cause a serious infection. Larger pieces of food entering the trachea may cause choking (the victim is not able to speak or breathe). A series of steps to treat such a person is called the Heimlich maneuver (see www.heimlichinstitute.org for details).

Knowledge Check

1. What substances are found in saliva?
2. What are the 5 basic taste sensations?
3. How does the swallowing process prevent food from entering the trachea?

 ## 4.4 Moving through the GI Tract: Stomach

The entry of food into the stomach is through the lower esophageal sphincter (sometimes called the cardiac sphincter due to its proximity to the heart), located between the esophagus and the stomach (Fig. 4-10). It prevents backflow (**reflux**) of the highly acidic stomach contents into the esophagus. If the sphincter malfunctions, causing reflux, the pain commonly known as **heartburn** occurs.

The stomach is essentially a holding and mixing tank. The average adult stomach holds about 2 ounces (50 ml) when empty and expands to 4 to 6 cups (1–1.5 liters) after a typical meal, but it can hold up to 16 cups (4 liters) when extremely full. Little digestion occurs in the stomach and only water, a few forms of fats, and about 20% of any alcohol consumed can be absorbed there.

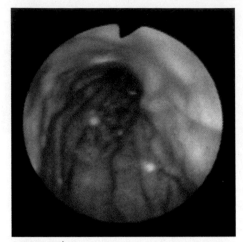

(a) Normal

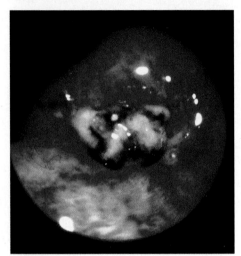

(b) Peptic ulcer

Figure 4-10 The esophagus can be seen opening into the stomach. (*a*) A healthy gastric mucosa; the small white spots are reflections of light. (*b*) A bleeding peptic ulcer. An ulcer is a small erosion of the top layer of cells. A peptic ulcer typically has an oval shape and yellow-white color. Here the yellowish floor of the ulcer is partially obscured by black blood clots, and fresh blood is visible around the margin of the ulcer.

▶ Another term to describe the stomach is *gastric.*

▶ Individuals with heartburn often take a class of drugs that suppress HCl production in the stomach. These medications may increase the risk of bone fractures. The lack of HCl may decrease the stomach's ability to dissolve calcium, thereby limiting the intestine's ability to absorb calcium.[30]

Each day, the stomach secretes about 8 cups (2 liters) of "gastric juice" that aids the digestive process. These secretions include a very strong acid, called hydrochloric acid (HCl) (Figs. 4-11 and 4-12), from the **parietal cells; pepsinogen,** an inactive protein-digesting enzyme; and gastric lipase from the **chief cells. Gastrin,** a hormone made in the stomach, controls the release of HCl and pepsinogen. Gastrin is secreted when we eat or think about eating. As a meal progresses, gastrin secretions decline, causing the release of HCl and pepsinogen to taper off.

The HCl produced by the stomach is very important. It inactivates the biological activity of ingested proteins, such as certain plant and animal hormones. This prevents them from affecting human functions. HCl also destroys most harmful bacteria and viruses (**pathogens**) in foods; dissolves dietary minerals (e.g., calcium), so that they can be more easily absorbed; and converts pepsinogen into the active protein-digesting enzyme **pepsin.**

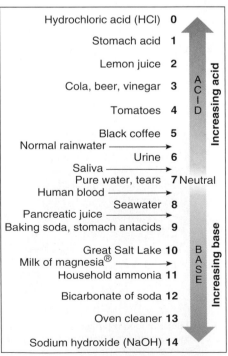

Substance	pH
Hydrochloric acid (HCl)	0
Stomach acid	1
Lemon juice	2
Cola, beer, vinegar	3
Tomatoes	4
Black coffee	5
Normal rainwater →	
Urine	6
Saliva →	
Pure water, tears	7 Neutral
Human blood →	
Seawater	8
Pancreatic juice →	
Baking soda, stomach antacids	9
Great Salt Lake	10
Milk of magnesia® →	
Household ammonia	11
Bicarbonate of soda	12
Oven cleaner	13
Sodium hydroxide (NaOH)	14

ACID — Increasing acid

BASE — Increasing base

Figure 4-11 The pH of various substances. The pH scale ranges from 0 (most acidic) to 14 (most basic).

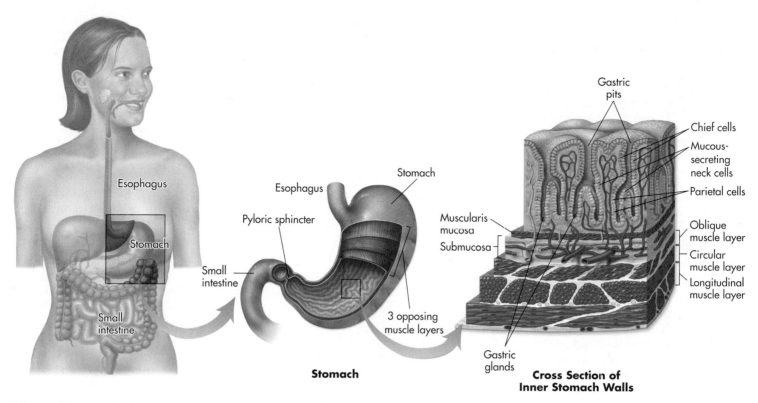

Figure 4-12 **Physiology of the stomach.** Surface mucous cells produce mucus for protection from stomach acid and enzymes. Parietal cells produce the hydrochloric acid (HCl) and chief cells produce the enzymes. Mucous neck cells, scattered among the cells in the gastric pits, also produce mucus.

The stomach also secretes mucus from mucous cells found on the gastric mucosa. Mucus lubricates and protects the stomach from being digested by HCl and pepsin. Mucus production relies on the presence of hormonelike compounds called **prostaglandins.** Heavy use of aspirin and other **non-steroidal anti-inflammatory drugs** (e.g., ibuprofen, naproxen) can damage the stomach wall because they inhibit prostaglandin production. The reduced mucous barrier in the stomach means stomach acid may damage the stomach wall.

Contraction of the 3 muscle layers in the stomach thoroughly mixes food with gastric secretions. Mixing transforms solid food into **chyme** (pronounced kime), a soupy, acidic mixture. The **pyloric sphincter,** located between the stomach and the duodenum (the first part of the small intestine), controls the flow of chyme into the small intestine. Only 1 teaspoon of chyme is released at a time into the small intestine. **Gastric inhibitory peptide**, a hormone, helps slow the release of chyme into the small intestine, giving the small intestine time to neutralize the acid and digest the nutrients. The pyloric sphincter also prevents the backflow of bile into the stomach (bile, discussed later in the chapter, can damage the stomach lining). It typically takes 1 to 4 hours for meals to move out of the stomach into the small intestine; less time is needed when meals are mostly liquid, more time when meals are large and high in fat.

Another important function of the stomach is the production of a substance called intrinsic factor (IF). This substance is required for the absorption of vitamin B-12 in the small intestine (discussed further in Chapter 13).

nonsteroidal anti-inflammatory drugs (NSAIDS) Class of medications that reduce inflammation, fever, and pain but are not steroids. Aspirin, ibuprofen (Advil®), and naproxen (Aleve®) are some examples.

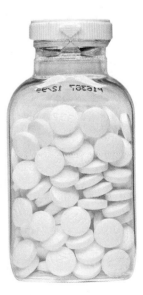

The heavy use of aspirin, an NSAID, may result in ulcer formation.

Knowledge Check

1. How do HCl and the enzyme pepsin aid in digestion?
2. What is the function of the sphincters located between the esophagus and stomach and between the stomach and small intestine?
3. What is the function of HCl?

enterocytes Specialized absorptive cells in the villi of the small intestine.

glycocalyx Projections of proteins on microvilli. They contain enzymes to digest protein and carbohydrate.

 ## 4.5 Moving through the GI Tract: Small Intestine and Accessory Organs

The small intestine is the major site of digestion and absorption of food. It is coiled below the stomach in the abdomen (Fig. 4-13). The small intestine is divided into 3 sections: the first part, the **duodenum,** is about 10 inches (25 cm) long; the middle segment, the **jejunum,** is about 4 feet (122 cm) long; and the last section, the **ileum,** is about 5 feet (152 cm) long. The small intestine is considered small because of its narrow, 1-inch (2.5-cm) diameter, not its length.

The interior of the small intestine has circular folds and fingerlike projections (**villi** and **microvilli**) that increase its surface area 600 times over that of a smooth tube. This large surface area contributes to the thoroughness and efficiency of digestion and absorption. The **circular folds** make the chyme flow slowly, following a spiral path as it travels through the small intestine. Slow spiraling completely mixes the chyme with digestive juices and brings it in contact with the villi that extend into the lumen (Fig. 4-14). Villi are lined with goblet cells that make mucus, **endocrine cells** that produce hormones and hormonelike substances, and cells that produce digestive enzymes and absorb nutrients (**enterocytes**). Each enterocyte has a **brush border** made up of **microvilli** that are covered with the digestive enzyme–containing **glycocalyx.** The villi and microvilli make the small intestine interior look fuzzy, like terrycloth or velvet (Fig. 4-15).

Most digestion in the small intestine occurs in the duodenum and upper part of the jejunum and requires many secretions from the small intestine itself, as well as the pancreas, liver, and gallbladder. Table 4-2 reviews these secretions and their functions. Each day, the small intestine secretes about 6 cups (1.5 liters) of mucus, enzyme, and hormone-containing fluid. Enzymes produced in the small intestine, also known as brush border enzymes, are responsible for the chemical digestion of the macronutrients. They typically complete the last steps of digestion, resulting in compounds that are small enough to be absorbed.

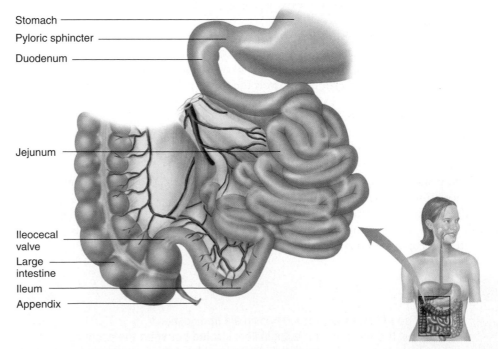

Stomach
Pyloric sphincter
Duodenum
Jejunum
Ileocecal valve
Large intestine
Ileum
Appendix

Figure 4-13 The small intestine and beginning of the large intestine. The 3 parts of the small intestine are the duodenum, jejunum, and ileum. Notice the smaller diameter of the small intestine, compared with the large intestine.

Figure 4-14 Organization of the small intestine. The small intestine has several structural levels. Because of the circular folds in the intestinal wall, the villi "fingers" that project into the intestine, and the microvilli (brush border) on each absorptive cell that makes up the villi, the surface area for absorption is up to 600 times that of a smooth tube.

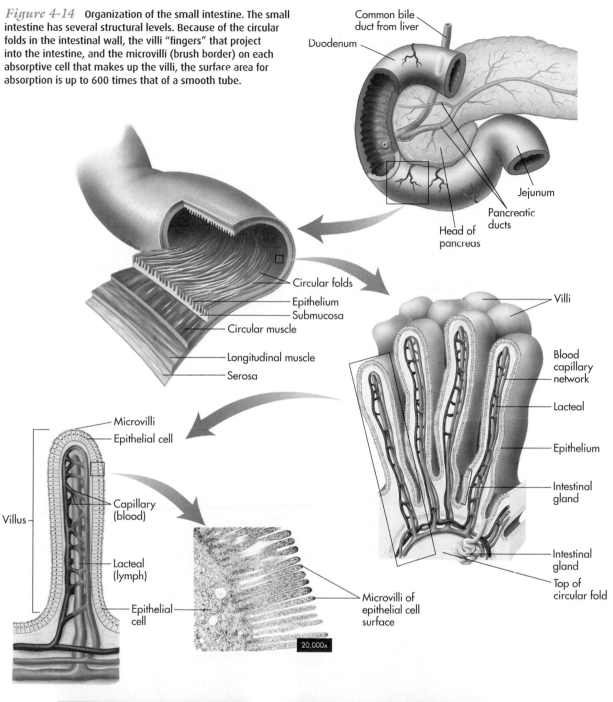

Common bile duct from liver

Duodenum

Jejunum

Pancreatic ducts

Head of pancreas

Circular folds

Epithelium

Submucosa

Circular muscle

Longitudinal muscle

Serosa

Villi

Blood capillary network

Lacteal

Epithelium

Intestinal gland

Intestinal gland

Top of circular fold

Microvilli

Epithelial cell

Villus

Capillary (blood)

Lacteal (lymph)

Epithelial cell

Microvilli of epithelial cell surface

20,000x

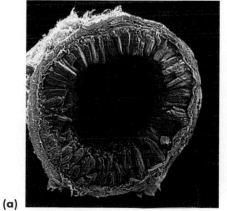

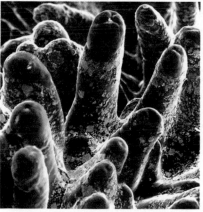

(a)

(b)

Figure 4-15 (*a*) Cross section of the small intestine shows the villi that project into the lumen. Each villus is about 1 mm high. (*b*) The millions of villi in the small intestine increase the surface area for absorption of nutrients.

enterohepatic circulation Continual recycling of compounds between the small intestine and the liver. Bile is one example of a recycled compound.

Liver, Gallbladder, and Pancreas

The liver, gallbladder, and pancreas, known as the accessory organs of the digestive system, work with the small intestine but are not a physical part of it. Secretions from these organs are delivered through the common bile duct and the pancreatic duct. These ducts come together at the sphincter of Oddi (also called the hepatopancreatic sphincter) and empty into the duodenum (Fig. 4-16).

The liver provides **bile,** a cholesterol-containing yellow-green fluid that aids in fat digestion and absorption by emulsifying fat. That is, it disperses fat into many tiny droplets, known as micelles, that are suspended in water. The liver secretes about 2 to 4 cups (500 to 1000 ml) of bile per day. Bile released into the duodenum is reabsorbed in the last section of the small intestine (ileum) and returned to the liver. During a meal, bile is recirculated 2 or more times. This system of bile recycling is called **enterohepatic circulation**. A small amount of bile is not reabsorbed and is excreted in feces—this is the body's only way to excrete cholesterol, one of the components of bile. Bile is stored in the gallbladder until needed.

The pancreas produces about 5 to 6 cups (1.5 liters) of pancreatic juice per day. This juice is an alkaline (basic) mixture of **sodium bicarbonate ($NaHCO_3$)** and enzymes. The sodium bicarbonate neutralizes the acidic chyme arriving from the stomach, thereby protecting the small intestine from damage by acid. Digestive enzymes from the pancreas include pancreatic amylase (to digest starch), pancreatic **lipase** (to digest fat), and several **proteases** (to digest protein). Pancreatic enzymes break large macronutrient molecules into smaller subunits.

Gastrointestinal Hormones—a Key to Orchestrating Digestion

The remarkable work of the digestive system requires the careful regulation and coordination of several processes, including the production and release of hormones throughout the length of the GI tract. Four hormones, part of the endocrine system, play key

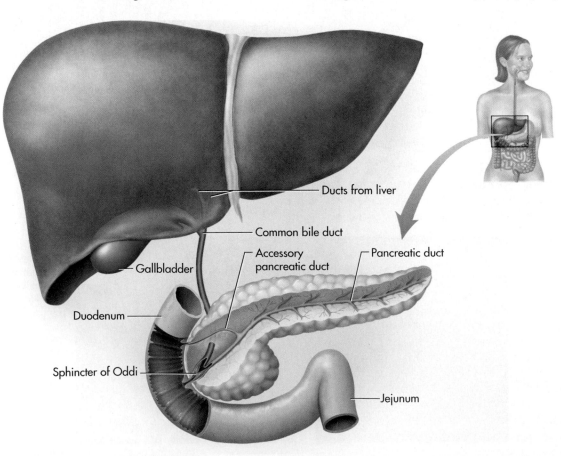

Figure 4-16 The common bile duct from the liver and gallbladder and the pancreatic duct join together at the sphincter of Oddi to deliver bile, pancreatic enzymes, and bicarbonate to the duodenum.

Ducts from liver

Common bile duct

Accessory pancreatic duct

Pancreatic duct

Gallbladder

Duodenum

Sphincter of Oddi

Jejunum

Table 4-3 Major Regulatory Hormones of the GI tract

Hormone	Released By	Function
Gastrin	Stomach and duodenum in response to food reaching the stomach	Triggers the stomach to release HCl and pepsinogen; stimulates gastric and intestinal motility
Cholecystokinin (CCK)	Small intestine in response to presence of dietary fat in chyme	Stimulates release of pancreatic enzymes and release of bile from the gallbladder
Secretin	Small intestine in response to acidic chyme	Stimulates release of pancreatic bicarbonate
Gastric inhibitory peptide	Small intestine as digestion progresses	Signals the stomach to limit release of gastric juices and slows gastric motility

roles in this regulation: gastrin, **secretin, cholecystokinin (CCK),** and gastric inhibitory peptide (Table 4-3). To illustrate their functions, let's follow a turkey sandwich through the digestive system.

1. As you eat a turkey sandwich (or even just think about it), gastrin is produced by cells in the stomach. Gastrin signals other stomach cells to release HCl and pepsinogen (for protein digestion). After thorough mixing, the turkey sandwich, now chyme, is released in small amounts into the small intestine.
2. As chyme flows out of the stomach into the small intestine, gastrin production slows and the small intestine secretes secretin and CCK. Both hormones trigger the release of enzyme- and bicarbonate-containing pancreatic juices that digest carbohydrate, fat, and protein and reduce the acidity of the intestinal contents. Fat in the small intestine (from the mayonnaise and the turkey) further stimulates the secretion of CCK by the small intestine. CCK promotes contraction of the gallbladder, which releases the bile (for fat digestion) that is stored there. Relaxation of the sphincter of Oddi allows bile and pancreatic juices to flow into the small intestine. CCK also slows GI motility to give digestive enzymes from the small intestine and pancreas enough time to do their work.
3. The sandwich becomes progressively digested and absorbed. The small intestine now releases gastric inhibitory peptide. This hormone, as its name suggests, signals the stomach to slow motility and decrease the release of gastric juice.

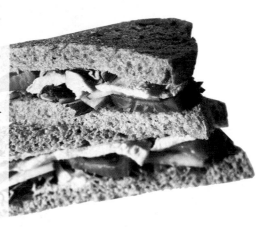

Many other hormones and hormonelike compounds, such as vasoactive intestinal peptide, bombesin, substance P, and somatostatin, also play important roles in regulating the digestive system. The cells that synthesize these compounds are located throughout the GI tract and in the brain and pancreas.

Absorption in the Small Intestine

The absorptive cells of the small intestine originate in open-ended pits (called crypts) located at the base of the villi. The absorptive cells migrate from the crypts to the villi. As they migrate, absorptive cells mature and their absorptive capabilities increase. By the time they reach the tips of the villi, they are partially destroyed by digestive enzymes and are shed into the lumen. The body's entire supply of absorptive cells is replaced every 2 to 5 days.

The digestive capabilities and health of the small intestine rapidly deteriorate during a nutrient deficiency or in semi-starvation. This is because cells that are constantly broken down and replaced, such as absorptive cells, are particularly dependent on a constant supply of nutrients. These nutrients are provided by the diet, as well as from broken-down cell parts that are recycled.

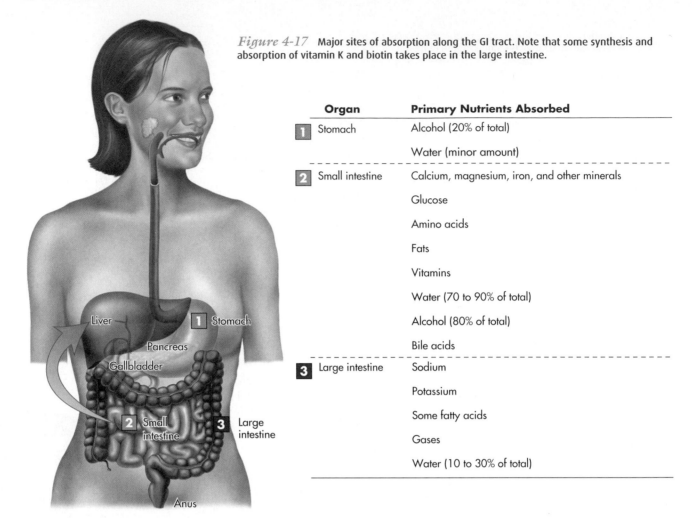

Figure 4-17 Major sites of absorption along the GI tract. Note that some synthesis and absorption of vitamin K and biotin takes place in the large intestine.

	Organ	Primary Nutrients Absorbed
1	Stomach	Alcohol (20% of total)
		Water (minor amount)
2	Small intestine	Calcium, magnesium, iron, and other minerals
		Glucose
		Amino acids
		Fats
		Vitamins
		Water (70 to 90% of total)
		Alcohol (80% of total)
		Bile acids
3	Large intestine	Sodium
		Potassium
		Some fatty acids
		Gases
		Water (10 to 30% of total)

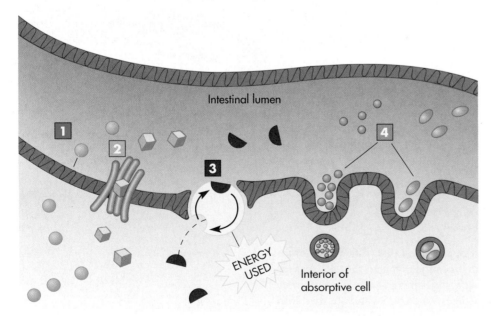

Figure 4-18 Nutrient absorption relies on 4 major absorptive processes. **1** Passive diffusion (in green) is diffusion of nutrients across the absorptive cell membranes. **2** Facilitated diffusion (in blue) uses a carrier protein to move nutrients down a concentration gradient. **3** Active absorption (in red) involves a carrier protein as well as energy to move nutrients (against a concentration gradient) into absorptive cells. **4** Phagocytosis and pinocytosis (in gray and orange) are forms of active transport in which the absorptive cell membrane forms an in vagination that engulfs a nutrient to bring it into the cell.

Virtually all nutrients are absorbed in the small intestine (Fig. 4-17). The small intestine absorbs about 95% of the food energy in protein, carbohydrate, fat, and alcohol. Nutrients move from the lumen of the small intestine into the absorptive cells in the ways illustrated in Figure 4-18.

- **Passive diffusion:** When the concentration of a nutrient is higher in the lumen of the small intestine than in the absorptive cells, the difference in concentration moves the nutrient into the absorptive cells by diffusion. Fats, water, and some minerals are absorbed by passive diffusion.

- **Facilitated diffusion:** A higher concentration of a nutrient in the lumen than in the absorptive cells is not enough to move some nutrients into the absorptive cells. They need carrier proteins to shuttle them from the lumen into absorptive cells. For instance, the sugar fructose is absorbed by facilitated diffusion.

- **Active absorption:** In addition to the need for a carrier protein, some nutrients also require energy (ATP) for absorption. Active absorption (also known as active transport) allows the cell to concentrate nutrients on either side of the cell membrane. For example, amino acids and some sugars, such as glucose, are actively absorbed.

- **Endocytosis (phagocytosis and pinocytosis):** In this type of active absorption, absorptive cells engulf compounds (phagocytosis) or liquids (pinocytosis) In both these processes, an absorptive cell forms an invagination in its cell membrane that engulfs the particles or fluid to form a vesicle. The vesicle is finally pinched off from the cell membrane and brought into the cell. This process allows immune substances (large protein particles) in human breast milk to be absorbed by infants.

Knowledge Check

1. What are the 3 sections of the small intestine?
2. Where is bile synthesized and what is its function?
3. What is the role of the pancreas in digestion? Which type of absorption requires energy?

Global Perspective

Diarrhea in Infants and Children

Diarrhea is rarely considered a serious threat to young children in countries such as the United States and Canada. However, in developing countries, diarrhea is a leading killer of children—it is responsible for 1 of every 7 deaths in children less than age 5 years. That's more than 1.5 million young children every year! In fact, more children die from diarrhea each year in developing countries than from malaria, measles, and HIV/AIDS combined.[4]

Diarrhea in young children is typically caused by pathogenic microorganisms—viruses, bacteria, and parasites—found in water, food, and human secretions and feces. One of the most common causes of severe diarrhea in young children around the world is rotavirus.[5] Scientists believe that rotavirus infects virtually all children between the ages of 3 months and 5 years. Each year, it kills an estimated 610,000 children worldwide.[5] Rotavirus, like many other microbial pathogens, replicates rapidly in the epithelial cells of the intestinal mucosa. Toxins produced by the virus cause the epithelial cells to slough off faster than they can be replaced. Fluid and **electrolytes,** which normally would have been absorbed in the intestine, are excreted rapidly. Infants and young children can become dangerously dehydrated. Death occurs if fluids are not replaced.

Being well-nourished helps lowers the risk of developing diarrhea. Breastfeeding also can prevent diarrhea in young children. Unfortunately, malnutrition afflicts many children in developing countries. In parts of Asia and Africa, more than 40% of preschool children are malnourished.[6] Malnutrition increases susceptibility to diarrhea in several ways. When a child is malnourished, the mucosa of the intestine can become thin, damaged, and leaky—this allows pathogens to invade more easily.[6] Additionally, immune function declines in malnourished children. Moreover, repeated bouts of diarrhea can make malnutrition even worse due to decreased food intake and poor absorption during illness.

To prevent severe illness and death, it is vital that children with diarrhea receive electrolytes and water in an oral solution.[7] This therapy is known as oral rehydration salts and oral rehydration therapy. This oral solution can be made by dissolving small amounts of electrolytes (sodium, chloride, and potassium) and the sugar glucose in water.[7] This simple recipe has helped decrease the number of diarrhea-related deaths from 4.5 million in 1979 to 1.5 million today. Supplemental zinc (an essential mineral) may be useful in treating and preventing diarrhea.[6] Children treated with supplemental zinc are less likely to suffer from diarrhea and, if they do have diarrhea, it is less severe. Another promising advance in the prevention of diarrhea is the development of a vaccine for rotavirus, which may be available in the next few years.[5]

Life-threatening diarrhea can be successfully treated in many cases. Equally important is the prevention of diarrhea. In many developing countries, the keys to prevention are improved sanitation that keeps food and water pathogen-free and the ready availability of affordable, nutritious foods that promote good health. Unfortunately, access to these basic needs is limited for many.

Diarrhea and infection ↑ → Food intake ↓ → Absorption ↓ → Malnutrition ↑ → Protection from mucosal wall ↓ → Immune function ↓ → Diarrhea and infection ↑

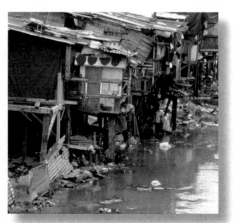

electrolytes Compounds that separate into ions in water and, in turn, are able to conduct an electrical current. These include sodium, chloride, and potassium.

🍑 4.6 Moving Nutrients around the Body: Circulatory Systems

Nutrients absorbed in the small intestine are delivered to one of the body's 2 circulatory systems: the cardiovascular (blood) system and the **lymphatic system** (Fig. 4-19). The choice of system used to transport nutrients is based primarily on whether the nutrients are water- or fat-soluble.

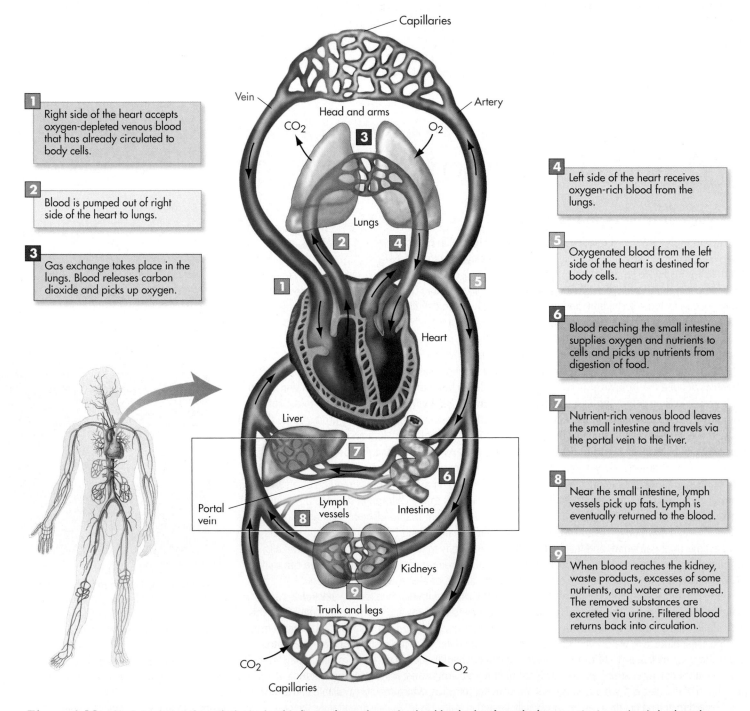

1 Right side of the heart accepts oxygen-depleted venous blood that has already circulated to body cells.

2 Blood is pumped out of right side of the heart to lungs.

3 Gas exchange takes place in the lungs. Blood releases carbon dioxide and picks up oxygen.

4 Left side of the heart receives oxygen-rich blood from the lungs.

5 Oxygenated blood from the left side of the heart is destined for body cells.

6 Blood reaching the small intestine supplies oxygen and nutrients to cells and picks up nutrients from digestion of food.

7 Nutrient-rich venous blood leaves the small intestine and travels via the portal vein to the liver.

8 Near the small intestine, lymph vessels pick up fats. Lymph is eventually returned to the blood.

9 When blood reaches the kidney, waste products, excesses of some nutrients, and water are removed. The removed substances are excreted via urine. Filtered blood returns back into circulation.

Figure 4-19 Blood circulation through the body. This figure shows the paths that blood takes from the heart to the lungs (1–3), back to the heart (4), and through the rest of the body (5–9). The reddish-orange color indicates blood that is richer in oxygen; blue is for blood carrying more carbon dioxide. Keep in mind that arteries and veins go to all parts of the body. Pay particular attention to sites 7 and 8. These sites are key parts of the process of nutrient absorption.

Cardiovascular System

The cardiovascular system includes the heart, blood vessels (arteries, capillaries, veins), and blood. Water-soluble nutrients (proteins, carbohydrates, **short- and medium-chain fatty acids,** B-vitamins, and vitamin C) are transported by the cardiovascular system. These nutrients are absorbed directly into the bloodstream in the **capillary** beds inside the villi (see Fig. 4-14). Blood flows from the capillary beds and collects in the large **portal vein,** which leads directly to the liver. This direct path allows the liver to process absorbed nutrients before they enter the general circulation. Blood leaving the liver, rich with nutrients from the GI tract and oxygen from the lungs, travels to all body cells. The cells take in the nutrients and oxygen from the blood, use them, then release carbon dioxide and other waste products into the blood. The waste products circulate to the lungs and kidney, where they are excreted.

short-chain fatty acid Fatty acid that contains fewer than 6 carbon atoms.

medium-chain fatty acid Fatty acid that contains 6 to 10 carbon atoms.

capillary Smallest blood vessel; the major site for the exchange of substances between the blood and the tissues.

portal vein Large vein leaving from the intestine and stomach. It connects to the liver.

Lymphatic System

The lymphatic system contains lymph, which flows throughout the body in lymphatic vessels, which are similar to veins. Unlike blood, lymph is not pumped through the vessels. Instead, it slowly flows as muscles contract and squeeze the lymphatic vessels.

The lymphatic system provides an alternative route into the bloodstream for large molecules that cannot be absorbed by the capillary beds. Fat-soluble nutrients (most fats and the fat-soluble vitamins A, D, E, and K) and large particles (e.g., large proteins that escape from the bloodstream) are transported in lymph. Lymph, usually a clear, colorless fluid, looks milky when it leaves the small intestine because of its fat content. Special lymphatic vessels (**lacteals**) in the villi transport nutrients to larger lymphatic vessels that connect to the thoracic duct. The thoracic duct extends from the abdomen to the neck, where it connects to the bloodstream at a large vein called the left subclavian vein. Once in the blood, nutrients originally absorbed by the lymphatic system are transported to body tissues in the cardiovascular system.

Knowledge Check

1. What are 3 nutrients that are transported by the cardiovascular system?
2. What are 3 nutrients that are transported first in the lymphatic system?
3. Which organ first receives nutrients from the cardiovascular system?
4. Why is diarrhea life-threatening for many young children in developing countries?

 4.7 Moving through the GI Tract: Large Intestine

The small intestine empties into the large intestine through the sphincter between the ileum and the colon (**ileocecal valve**). After digestion and absorption in the small intestine, normally only water, some minerals, and undigested food fibers and starches are left. About 5% of carbohydrate, protein, and fat escapes absorption in the small intestine.

The large intestine, so called because its 2½-inch (6-cm) lumen diameter is larger than that of the small intestine, is about 5 feet (1.5 meters) long. It has 3 main parts: the colon, rectum, and anus (Fig. 4-20). The colon, the largest portion of the large intestine, has 5 sections: **cecum, ascending colon, transverse colon, descending colon**, and **sigmoid colon**.

The large intestine performs 3 main functions. It houses bacterial flora that keep the GI tract healthy; it absorbs water and electrolytes, such as sodium and potassium; and it forms and expels feces.

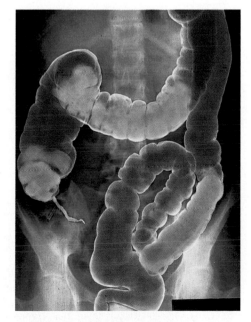

A radiograph of the large intestine.

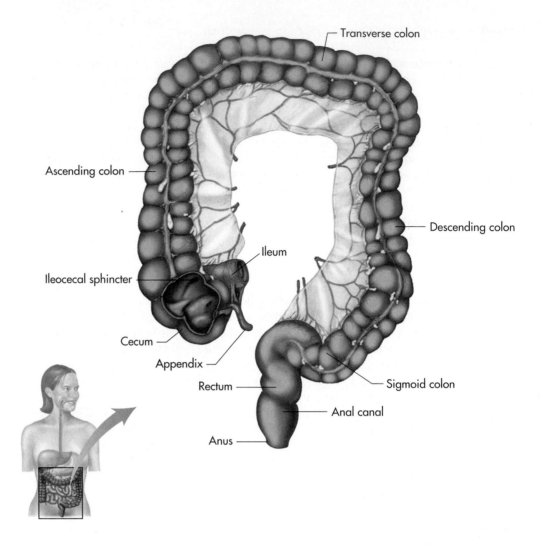

Figure 4-20 The parts of the colon: cecum ascending colon, transverse colon, descending colon, and sigmoid colon.

Bacterial Flora

The large intestine is home to over 400 species of bacteria, collectively numbering more than 100 trillion microbial cells, or more than 10 times the number of cells in the human body! Some of the bacteria are beneficial but others are pathogenic. The ileocecal valve prevents these bacteria from migrating into the small intestine (where they could disrupt normal function and compete with the body for nutrients).

Beneficial bacteria keep the growth of pathogenic bacteria under control. Antibiotic treatment, radiation therapy, surgery, and some diseases often reduce the number of beneficial bacteria cells, which can allow pathogenic bacteria to multiply quickly. Disrupting the normal balance between beneficial and pathogenic bacteria can cause conditions such as vomiting, diarrhea, and dehydration.

Beneficial bacteria also synthesize vitamin K and the B-vitamin biotin, aid lactose digestion, and ferment (digest) some of the fibers and starches not digested in the small intestine. **Fermentation** creates short-chain fatty acids that can be absorbed and used as an energy source in the colon.[8] Nutrition scientists are studying how fiber, beneficial intestinal bacteria, and short-chain fatty acids may prevent diseases such as irritable bowel syndrome, colon cancer, and inflammatory bowel disease.[9] Intestinal bacteria also produce gas, or **flatus,** discussed later in this chapter.

Probiotics and Prebiotics

One proposed strategy for achieving a healthy balance of intestinal bacteria is the consumption of probiotics and prebiotics. **Probiotics** are live microorganisms that provide

fermentation Breakdown of large organic compounds into smaller compounds, especially organic acids. The breakdown is often by anaerobic bacteria.

health benefits when they are consumed in sufficient amounts.[10] Probiotics are found in fermented foods, such as yogurt and miso (fermented soybean paste), and are sold in capsules and powders. Probiotic bacteria usually are *Lactobacilli* or *Bifidobacteria*.

Probiotic bacteria are thought to colonize in the large intestine and provide certain health benefits. For instance, probiotics may help prevent and treat diarrhea, prevent food allergies and colon cancer, and treat irritable bowel syndrome and inflammatory bowel disease.[11] However, this research is not conclusive. Probiotics are difficult to study because of the many types and doses of microorganisms available to test. Most studies have had relatively few participants and short treatment durations. Currently, the best evidence is that probiotics can help prevent and treat diarrhea in children. Probiotics also can help treat antibiotic-associated diarrhea and prevent the travelers' diarrhea that afflicts many individuals traveling to less developed nations.[11]

Prebiotics are non-digestible carbohydrates that promote the growth of beneficial bacteria in the large intestine.[12] One example is **inulin**, a carbohydrate made of several units of fructose (a sugar). Inulin is found in many foods, including chicory, wheat, onions, garlic, asparagus, and bananas. Inulin and other related compounds, such as **fructans,** are added to some processed foods to add texture, bulk, and potential health benefits. Another prebiotic is **resistant starch,** found in whole grains and some fruits. Resistant starch resists the action of digestive enzymes in the small intestine; thus, bacteria in the large intestine can ferment it. Prebiotics fermented in the large intestine produce short-chain fatty acids and other organic acids. In studies of prebiotics, participants typically ingest 10 to 20 grams per day; such large amounts can cause flatulence, bloating, and other GI distress. As with probiotics, the research that prebiotics improve health is not yet conclusive.

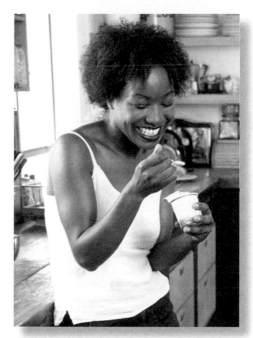

Yogurt is a convenient source of probiotic bacteria, which contribute to GI tract health.

Absorption of Water and Electrolytes

The GI tract receives a total of 10 liters of water (3 liters from the diet and 7 liters from intestinal secretions) per day. The small intestine absorbs about 90% of the water and the large intestine completes the job. Just 1% (less than ½ cup, or 100 ml) of the water in the GI tract remains in excreted feces. The large intestine also is the main site where electrolytes, especially sodium and potassium, are absorbed (see Fig. 4-17). Electrolyte absorption occurs mostly in the first half of the large intestine.

Defecation of Feces

It takes 12 to 24 hours for the residue of a meal to travel through the large intestine. By the time the contents have passed through the first two-thirds of its length, a semisolid mass has been formed. This mass remains in the large intestine until peristaltic waves and mass movements, usually greatest following the consumption of a meal, push it into the rectum. Feces in the rectum are a powerful stimulation for **defecation**, the expulsion of feces. This process involves muscular reflexes in the sigmoid colon and rectum, as well as relaxation of the internal and external anal sphincters. Only the external sphincter is under voluntary control. Once toilet-trained, a person can determine when to relax the sphincter for defecation, as well as when to keep it constricted.

When excreted, feces are normally about 75% water and 25% solids. The solids are primarily indigestible plant fibers, tough connective tissue from animal foods, and bacteria from the large intestine. During episodes of diarrhea, the percentage of water in feces rises.

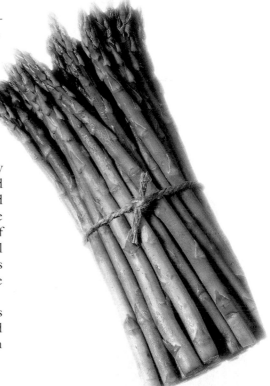

Inulin, a prebiotic, is found in asparagus.

Knowledge Check

1. What are the 3 main functions of the large intestine?
2. What are some of the beneficial actions of bacteria in the large intestine?
3. What is the difference between a prebiotic and a probiotic? Where can they be found in the diet?

▶ Lactose intolerance and diverticulosis are two other common GI tract disorders (these are discussed in Chapter 5).

4.8 When Digestive Processes Go Awry

The fine-tuned organ system we call the digestive system can develop problems. Knowing about common problems can help you avoid or lessen them.

Heartburn and Gastroesophageal Reflux Disease

About half of U.S. adults occasionally experience **heartburn** (acid indigestion). Heartburn has nothing to do with the heart; it occurs when stomach acid backs up into the esophagus (Fig. 4-21), causing a burning sensation or sour taste in the back of the mouth. Heartburn occurs after a large or high-fat meal. Experiencing heartburn 2 or more times per week may signal the more serious **gastroesophageal reflux disease (GERD).**[13] GERD occurs when the lower esophageal sphincter relaxes and lets stomach contents backflow into the esophagus. (Normally, this sphincter relaxes only with swallowing.) Not everyone with GERD has heartburn—other symptoms include hoarseness, trouble swallowing, coughing, gagging, and nausea. In addition to the uncomfortable physical symptoms of GERD, more serious complications can occur. These include weight loss, ulceration, bleeding in the esophagus, **anemia**, and a higher risk of cancer of the esophagus.

Heartburn and GERD can occur in infants and children, too, usually due to an immature digestive system. It can cause frequent spitting up, or vomiting, and coughing. Most children outgrow this by 1 year of age.[13]

The cause of GERD is not known, but factors that may contribute to it include **hiatal hernia**, alcohol use, overweight, smoking, and even pregnancy. Studies have shown that obesity slows stomach emptying and relaxes the lower esophageal sphincter.[14] Foods such as citrus fruits, chocolate, caffeinated drinks (e.g., coffee), fatty and fried foods, garlic, onion, spicy foods, and tomato-based foods (e.g., spaghetti sauce and pizza) may increase reflux.

Heartburn and GERD are treated with both lifestyle modification and medications.[13, 15] Lifestyle change recommendations include eating small meals instead of large ones, avoiding foods that cause reflux, waiting several hours before lying down after eating (remaining upright limits reflux), losing weight, stopping smoking, and limiting alcohol intake. The following medications are used to treat GERD:

- Antacids (Tums®, Maalox®) are over-the-counter medications that neutralize stomach acid. Excessive intake of those that contain magnesium can cause diarrhea and those that contain aluminum may cause constipation.

- H$_2$ blockers (cimetidine [Tagamet®] and famotidine [Pepcid AC®]) block the increase of stomach acid production caused by histamine. Histamine, a breakdown product of the amino acid histidine, stimulates acid secretion by the stomach and has many other effects on the body. H$_2$ blockers are available in both prescription and less potent, non-prescription forms.

- Proton pump inhibitors (esomeprazole [Nexium®] and lansoprazole [Prevacid®]) are the most potent acid-suppressing medications. They inhibit the ability of gastric cells to secrete hydrogen ions and make acid. Low doses of this class of medication also are available without prescription, such as omeprazole (Prilosec-OTC®).

Surgery to strengthen the lower esophageal sphincter may be needed when lifestyle modifications and medications do not work.

anemia Decreased oxygen-carrying capacity of the blood. It occurs for many reasons, including blood loss.

hiatal hernia Protrusion of part of the stomach upward through the diaphragm into the chest cavity.

Figure 4-21 **Heartburn results from stomach acid refluxing into the esophagus.**

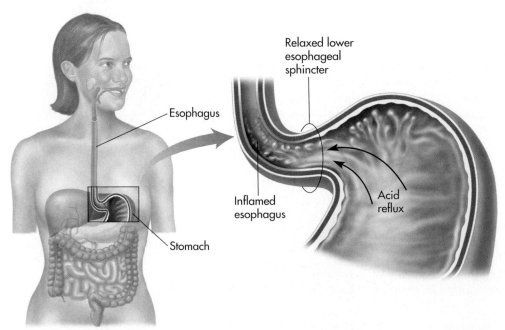

Esophagus

Stomach

Relaxed lower esophageal sphincter

Inflamed esophagus

Acid reflux

Ulcers

An **ulcer** is a very small (usually no larger than a pencil eraser) erosion of the top layer of cells in the stomach or duodenum (Fig. 4-22). The general term for this condition is **peptic ulcer**. About 20 million North Americans develop ulcers during their lifetimes.[16] Ulcers in younger people tend to develop in the small intestine, whereas in older people they occur in the stomach.

The leading cause of peptic ulcer disease is an acid-resistant bacterial infection (*Helicobacter pylori* [*H. pylori*]), but ulcer disease also is associated with the heavy use of aspirin and other NSAID medications,[17] alcohol use, and smoking. Disorders that cause excessive stomach acid production also can cause ulcers. Spicy foods and stress do not cause ulcers, although stress may make individuals more susceptible to the effects of *H. pylori* infection.

Being infected with *H. pylori* does not necessarily lead to an ulcer. In fact, over half of people over the age of 60 are infected with *H. pylori* and most do not have an ulcer.[17] *H. pylori* cause an ulcer by weakening the mucus coating that protects the stomach and duodenum. This allows HCl and digestive juices to attack and erode stomach and duodenal cells. *H. pylori* itself also irritates these cells. Recall that aspirin and other NSAID medications can cause ulcers by suppressing the synthesis of prostaglandins, compounds that promote the formation of the protective mucus.

The most common symptom of an ulcer is a gnawing or burning pain in the stomach region between meals or during the night. This pain often can be relieved by eating or taking antacids. Other less common symptoms are nausea, vomiting, loss of appetite, and weight loss.[17] The primary complications of ulcers are bleeding and perforation. Slow bleeding eventually can cause anemia and fatigue. Rapid bleeding makes the feces tarry and black from the digested blood, or the person may vomit what looks like coffee grounds. Perforated ulcers (those that eat through the stomach or intestinal wall) allow chyme to escape and enter the abdomen, where it may cause a major infection that can be deadly. It is important to pay attention to the early warning signs of an ulcer.

In the past, "bland" diets that include large amounts of milk and cream—the so-called Sippy diet—were used to treat ulcers. Clinicians now know that milk and cream are among the worst foods a person with an ulcer can eat. The calcium in these foods stimulates the stomach to produce HCl and actually inhibits ulcer healing.

Today, a combination of approaches is used for ulcer therapy (Table 4-4).[16, 17] Those infected with *H. pylori* are treated with antibiotics and either proton pump inhibitors or an H$_2$ blocker to suppress acid production. Bismuth subsalicylate (a component of Pepto-Bismol®) is taken to protect the stomach lining from acid. Most people (80 to 95%) treated with these drugs heal their ulcers. Not smoking and limiting NSAID use are important, too. A dietary recommendation is to avoid foods that increase ulcer symptoms.

Gallstones

Gallstones, a frequent cause of illness and surgery, affect 10 to 20% of U.S. adults. The stones develop in the gallbladder when substances in the bile—mainly cholesterol (80% of gallstones) and bile

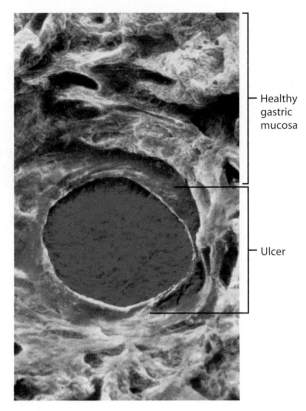

Figure 4-22 **Close-up of a stomach ulcer. Without treatment, eventual perforation of the stomach is possible.**

Healthy gastric mucosa

Ulcer

Table 4-4 Recommendations to Prevent Ulcers and Heartburn from Occurring or Recurring

Ulcers

1. Stop smoking if you smoke.
2. Avoid large doses of aspirin, ibuprofen, and other NSAID compounds unless a physician advises otherwise. For people who must use these medications, the FDA has approved taking an NSAID along with a medication that reduces gastric damage.
3. Limit intake of coffee, tea, and alcohol (especially wine), if this helps.
4. Limit consumption of pepper, chili powder, and other strong spices, if this helps.
5. Eat nutritious meals on a regular schedule; include enough fiber (see Chapter 5 for sources of fiber).
6. Chew foods well.
7. Lose weight if you are currently overweight.

Heartburn

1. Follow ulcer prevention recommendations.
2. Wait about 2 hours after a meal before lying down.
3. Don't overeat. Eat smaller meals that are low in fat.
4. Elevate the head of the bed at least 6 inches.

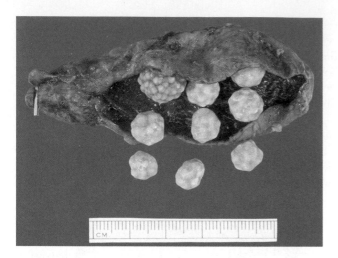

Figure 4-23   Gallbladder and gallstones after surgical removal from the body. Size and composition of the stones vary from one case to another.

pigments (20%)—form crystal-like particles. Gallstones can be as small as a grain of sand or as large as a golf ball (Fig. 4-23). Gallstone formation is related to slow gallbladder motility and bile composition. Too little bile and phospholipids and too much cholesterol allow cholesterol to crystallize into stones. Factors that increase the risk of gallstone formation are listed in Table 4-5.[18, 19]

Preventing gallstones includes maintaining a healthy weight, especially for women. Avoiding rapid weight loss, choosing plant instead of animal protein, eating a high-fiber diet, and using unsaturated fats, such as olive oil, may help prevent stone formation, too.[20] Regular physical activity also is important.

Most individuals with gallstones do not have symptoms; stones are usually detected during an examination for another illness. Symptoms can include intermittent pain in the right upper abdomen, pain between the shoulder blades or near the right shoulder, nausea, vomiting, gas, and bloating. Gallstone "attacks" occur when stones block the bile ducts and stop the free flow of bile. Attacks may last from 20 minutes to several hours.

Surgical removal of the gallbladder is the most common treatment for gallstones (500,000 surgeries per year in the U.S.).[21] Fortunately, removal of the gallbladder does not have serious consequences. Instead of being stored in the gallbladder, bile flows directly from the liver through the bile pancreatic duct to the small intestine.

Food Intolerances

Food intolerances are caused by an individual's inability to digest certain food components, usually due to low amounts of specific enzymes. Generally, large amounts of an offending food are required to produce the symptoms of food intolerance. Note that food allergies and food intolerances are not the same. Food allergies cause an immune response as a result of exposure to certain food proteins (allergens) (see Chapter 7).

Food intolerances afflict many individuals. Symptoms vary widely, depending on the cause of the food intolerance. Common causes include

- Deficiencies in digestive enzymes, such as lactase (see Chapter 5)
- Sensitivities to food components, such as gluten (see Expert Perspective from the Field)
- Certain synthetic compounds added to foods, such as food-coloring agents, sulfites, and monosodium glutamate (MSG). The food coloring tartrazine, for instance, may cause airway spasms, itching, and reddening skin in some people. Sulfites, which of-

Table 4-5 Factors Associated with Gallstone Formation
• High-calorie, low-fiber diets
• Prolonged fasting
• Obesity—especially excess abdominal fat
• Rapid weight loss (more than 3 lb per week)
• Type 2 diabetes
• High blood lipids
• Sedentary lifestyle
• Some medications, especially estrogen replacement therapy and birth control pills
• Female gender
• Pregnancy
• Increasing age
• Family history of gallstones
• Ethnicity—especially Native Americans and Mexican-Americans

ten are added to protect the color of wine, dried foods (fruit, potatoes, soup mixes), and salad greens, may cause flushing, airway spasms, and a drop in blood pressure in susceptible people. MSG, a flavor enhancer frequently added to restaurant and processed foods, may increase blood pressure and cause numbness, sweating, vomiting, and headache in certain people.

- Residues of medications (e.g., antibiotics) and other chemicals used in the production of livestock and crops, as well as insect parts not removed during processing (see Chapter 3)
- Toxic contaminants, such as mold or bacteria (see Chapter 3)

Intestinal Gas

Everyone has gas. In fact, we produce about 1 to 4 pints of gas each day and pass gas about 14 times a day, although there is considerable variability from one person to the next.[24] Gas is eliminated by burping and passing it through the rectum. Intestinal gas (also known as **flatulence**) is a mixture of carbon dioxide, oxygen, nitrogen, hydrogen, methane, and small amounts of sulfur-containing gas. The sulfur is responsible for the unpleasant odor associated with flatulence. Large quantities of intestinal gas can cause bloating and abdominal pain.

Gas comes from swallowed air and the breakdown of undigested carbohydrates by bacteria in the large intestine. The bacteria produce gas as they metabolize carbohydrate. Some people are particularly sensitive to certain carbohydrates (Table 4-6), whereas others can eat them with little problem. Enzyme preparations, such as Beano®, and lactase may help prevent gas by limiting the amount of undigested carbohydrate available to the bacteria in the large intestine. The enzyme in Beano® breaks down raffinose and other similar carbohydrates, whereas the lactase enzyme digests the lactose in milk. Eating fewer gas-forming foods also can help reduce intestinal gas. A "trial and error" approach is usually required.

Constipation

Constipation is defined as difficult or infrequent (fewer than 3 times per week) bowel movements. Slow movement of fecal material through the large intestine causes constipation. As fluid is increasingly absorbed during the extended time the feces stay in the large intestine, they become dry and hard. Constipation is commonly reported by older adults because the colon becomes more sluggish as we age.

Constipation is caused by many factors. It may occur when people regularly ignore normal urges to defecate for long periods. Constipation also can result from conditions such as diabetes mellitus, irritable bowel syndrome, and depression.[25] Pregnant women frequently experience constipation because hormones released in pregnancy slow GI motility. Antacids, antidepressants, and calcium and iron supplements are examples of medications that can cause constipation. Low-fiber diets also contribute to constipation.

Eating foods with plenty of fiber, such as whole-grain breads and cereals, beans, fruits, and

Table 4-6 Carbohydrates That May Contribute to Intestinal Gas Formation

Carbohydrate	Description and Food Sources
Raffinose and stachyose	Complex sugars found in beans and vegetables, such as cabbage, Brussels sprouts, and broccoli, that are poorly absorbed
Lactose	Sugar found in milk and milk products; (lactose intolerance is discussed in Chapter 5)
Fructose	Sugar found in fruit, onions, artichoke, and wheat
Sorbitol	Sugar alcohol that is poorly absorbed, found in many fruits (apples, pears, prunes), and used to sweeten some sugar-free products
Starches	Some of the starch found in potatoes, corn, noodles, and wheat that is not fully digested
Fiber	Soluble fiber found in beans, oat bran, and fruits

Expert Perspective *from the Field*

Celiac Disease

A recent National Institutes of Health panel has drawn attention to celiac disease, an immune-mediated disorder that affects primarily the gastrointestinal tract. Celiac disease, sometimes known as gluten intolerance, is caused by a physiological response to a protein called *gluten*, found in wheat and related grains, such as rye, barley, spelt, and triticale. In persons with celiac disease, these proteins damage the villi of the small intestine, causing the villi to flatten. In many persons with celiac disease, damage to the villi results in the malabsorption of nutrients. Currently, health experts believe that celiac disease results from both genetic and immunological factors.

Celiac disease is common—approximately 1 in 133 people (3 million) in the U.S. is thought to have celiac disease. Most of these individuals are not yet diagnosed. Further, according to Cynthia Kupper,* executive director of the Gluten Intolerance Group of North America and a celiac disease sufferer, 2 to 3 times more people do not meet the diagnostic criteria for celiac disease but are sensitive to gluten and experience health improvements when gluten is eliminated from their diets.

Celiac disease can affect a number of body systems. Classic symptoms of celiac disease include intestinal gas, bloating, diarrhea, constipation, abdominal pain, and weight loss or gain. Non-gastrointestinal symptoms include anemia, early bone disease, autoimmune diseases (e.g., type 1 diabetes and thyroid disease), fatigue, slower than normal growth in children, ataxia (impaired coordination) and other neurological conditions, a skin condition called dermatitis herpetiformis, and infertility.

Although there is research underway to develop drug therapies, currently the only treatment is a lifetime of eating a gluten-free diet.[27] A healthy diet that includes all food groups is important. However, the only foods consumed from the grain group should be those that are gluten-free, such as corn, rice, and buckwheat. A registered dietitian can help a person plan a healthy gluten-free diet. Kupper has pointed out that food labels can help consumers avoid foods with ingredients that contain gluten. The recently passed Food Allergy Labeling and Consumer Protection Act has made it especially easy to identify foods that contain wheat. To further assist those following a gluten-free diet, the FDA is considering whether to allow food manufacturers to indicate voluntarily which food products are gluten-free.

Those with a gluten intolerance disorder who consume gluten risk experiencing the symptoms of this health condition in the short term. In the long term, untreated celiac disease may lead to weight loss, diarrhea, anemia, headaches, and muscle pain. In addition, without treatment, there is an increased risk of aggressive GI tract cancers and associated health conditions related to malabsorption and malnutrition.

Kupper recommends that those who have symptoms of gluten intolerance should not try to treat the symptoms themselves because they might be caused by another condition, such as **Crohn's disease** or **colitis**. Also, following a gluten-free diet is challenging and can be expensive. Kupper notes that it's best to get a diagnosis from a physician. Blood tests for celiac disease are accurate, and a small intestinal biopsy can confirm the condition. To learn more about celiac disease, visit the websites listed at the end of the chapter.

* *The Gluten Intolerance Group of North America reviews scientific research and translates it into practical information to help individuals with gluten intolerance disorders manage their diseases. Ms. Kupper often provides expert input to the food industry and government agencies, such as the National Institutes of Health (NIH) and the FDA.*

People with gluten intolerance should avoid foods, such as bread, that are made with wheat.

Crohn's disease Inflammatory disease of the GI tract that often reduces the absorptive capacity of the small intestine. Family history is a major risk factor.

Colitis Inflammation of the colon that can lead to ulcers (ulcerative colitis).

vegetables, and drinking more fluid help treat typical cases of mild constipation.[26] The recommended fiber intake for most adults is 25 to 35 grams per day. Fiber stimulates peristalsis by drawing water into the large intestine and helping form bulky, soft feces. The bulky fecal material stretches the peristaltic muscles; the muscles respond by constricting, causing the feces to be propelled forward.

People with constipation may need to develop more regular bowel habits—setting the same time each day for a bowel movement (usually on awakening or shortly after a meal) can help train the large intestine to respond routinely. Additionally, relaxation and daily exercise promote regular bowel movements.

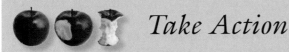

Take Action

Investigate Over-the-Counter Medications for Treating Common GI Tract Problems

Visit your local pharmacy and check out the medications on sale for treating indigestion, heartburn, constipation, diarrhea, and hemorrhoids. Select a category and compare 4 brands for the following characteristics.

Characteristic	Brand 1	Brand 2	Brand 3	Brand 4
1. Price				
2. Usual daily dose				
3. Active ingredients				
4. Warning to users				
5. Advice as to when to see a physician				

Write a critique of your discoveries about these products, and summarize what you would say about their safety and effectiveness.

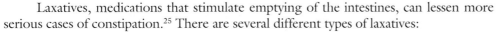

Laxatives, medications that stimulate emptying of the intestines, can lessen more serious cases of constipation.[25] There are several different types of laxatives:

- Bulk-forming laxatives (Metamucil® and Citrucel®) contain different types of fiber (e.g., psyllium fiber, methylcellulose). Like fiber in food, bulk-forming laxatives draw water into the intestine and increase fecal volume.
- Osmotic laxatives (Milk of Magnesia®) keep fluid in the intestine, which helps keep the fecal matter soft and bulky.
- Stimulant laxatives (Dulcolax® and ExLax®) agitate intestinal nerves to stimulate the peristaltic muscles.
- Stool softeners (Colace®) allow water to enter the bowel more readily.
- Lubricant laxatives (mineral oil) are not recommended because they may block absorption of fat-soluble vitamins.

For most people, bulk-forming laxatives are the safest to use. The regular use of laxatives, especially stimulant laxatives, may lead to dependence and damage the intestine. Consult a physician before using laxatives longer than a week.

Physicians infrequently treat more severe cases of constipation with an **enema**. An enema is the insertion of fluid into the rectum and colon via the anus. The fluid stimulates the bowel and the liquid and feces are expelled. Some alternative health practitioners advocate the use of enemas to remove toxins from the colon and the body, but there is little evidence that this practice is beneficial.

Diarrhea

Diarrhea, loose, watery stools occurring more than 3 times per day, is a common GI tract problem. It usually lasts only a few days and goes away on its own. Most cases of diarrhea result from bacterial or viral infection, often from contaminated food or water (see Chapter 3). These infections cause the intestinal tract to secrete fluid instead of absorbing it. Diarrhea also can be caused by parasites, food intolerances, medications (e.g., magnesium-containing antacids and certain antibiotics), intestinal diseases, and irritable bowel syndrome. Consuming substances that are not readily absorbed, such as the sugar alcohol sorbitol found in sugarless gum and candy, can cause diarrhea as well

▶ You may have heard that taking laxatives after overeating prevents the body from storing the excess calories as body fat. This erroneous and dangerous idea has gained popularity among some fad dieters. Laxatives may cause you to feel less full temporarily because they speed up the emptying of the large intestine and increase fluid loss. Most laxatives, however, do not speed the passage of food through the small intestine, where most digestion and most nutrient absorption take place. As a result, laxatives won't prevent fat gain from excess energy intake.

CRITICAL THINKING

Joci is considering going on a new diet that emphasizes eating only fruits before noon, meat at lunchtime, and starch and vegetables at dinner. In addition, the diet recommends "cleansing" the intestines with laxatives and enemas every other week. What reasons would you give Joci to steer clear of this regimen? What are some possible harmful effects?

(see Chapter 5). When ingested in large amounts, unabsorbed substances draw excess water into the intestine, causing diarrhea.

The treatment of diarrhea generally requires consuming plenty of fluid (beverages, soups, broths) to replace lost fluid and electrolytes. Prompt treatment is vital for infants and older people because they are more susceptible to the effects of dehydration associated with diarrhea. Most infants and children with diarrhea can be treated at home. Special fluids, such as Pedialyte®, can be given for fluid and electrolyte replacement. Most children can continue to eat a normal diet. A health-care provider should evaluate children with diarrhea who are less than 6 months of age or who have blood in the stool, frequent vomiting, high fever, and signs of dehydration (fewer than 6 wet diapers per day; weight loss; extreme thirst; or dry, sticky mouth).[28] Diarrhea in adults that lasts more than 3 days, especially if accompanied by fever, blood in the stool, or severe abdominal pain, also warrants investigation by a health-care provider. When recovering from diarrhea, it is best to avoid greasy, high-fiber, and very sweet foods because these can aggravate diarrhea.

Irritable Bowel Syndrome

About 10 to 15% of the U.S. population suffers from irritable bowel syndrome (IBS).[22, 23] This disorder is more common in women than in men. IBS symptoms include irregular bowel function (diarrhea, constipation, or alternating episodes of both), abdominal pain, and abdominal distension. The irregular bowel function is thought to be caused by abnormal intestinal motility; the abdominal pain is caused by a decreased pain threshold for abdominal distension. Even a minor amount of abdominal bloating that most people would not sense may cause pain in those with IBS. The abdominal pain is often relieved by a bowel movement. IBS symptoms may be mild or very severe. Although IBS often requires medical care, it does not increase the risk of other serious digestive problems or cancer.

The cause of IBS is not known; factors that may play a role include stress and dietary intolerances. Diagnosis of IBS should be made by a physician. Referral to a registered dietitian can be beneficial because many patients experience improvement with dietary changes. Therapy may include increases in high-fiber foods and the consumption of probiotics (currently being studied). Diets that restrict high-fat foods, dairy products, wheat, citrus, caffeine, corn, and gas-forming foods, such as legumes and certain fruits and vegetables (e.g., grapes, raisins, cherries, cantaloupe, cabbage, beans, and broccoli), also may help. Consuming low-fat and frequent, small meals may help because fat and large meals can trigger intestinal contractions. Other treatment strategies include stress reduction, psychological counseling, and antidepressant medications. Medications that restore normal intestinal motility and stop diarrhea may be prescribed. Some patients seek relief with alternative therapies, such as peppermint oil and ginger.[23] The website www.ibsgroup.org provides further information.

Hemorrhoids

Hemorrhoids, also called piles, are swollen veins of the rectum and anus (like varicose veins in the legs). The blood vessels in this area are subject to intense pressure, especially during bowel movements. Obesity, prolonged sitting, and violent coughing or sneezing add stress to the vessels. Many pregnant women also develop hemorrhoids (see Chapter 16). Hemorrhoids develop unnoticed until a strained bowel movement triggers symptoms, which may include itching, pain, and bleeding.

Itching is caused by moisture, swelling, or other irritation in the anal canal (an approximately 2-inch-long section between the rectum and anus). Pain, if present, is usually a steady ache. Bleeding from a hemorrhoid may appear in the toilet as a bright red streak in the feces. The sensation of a mass in the anal canal after a bowel movement is a symptom of an internal hemorrhoid that protrudes through the anus.

Anyone can develop a hemorrhoid—about half of adults over age 50 do.[29] Pressure from prolonged sitting or exertion is often enough to bring on symptoms, although diet, lifestyle, and possibly heredity play a role. For example, a low-fiber diet

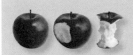

Take Action

Are You Taking Care of Your Digestive Tract?

All of us need to think about the health of our digestive tracts. To protect our GI tracts, there are symptoms we need to notice and habits we need to practice. Now that you know some basics about how your digestive system functions, use the following questionnaire to assess the health of your digestive tract. Section 4.8, When Digestive Systems Go Awry, can help you understand why these habits are important to examine. Answer each question yes or no.

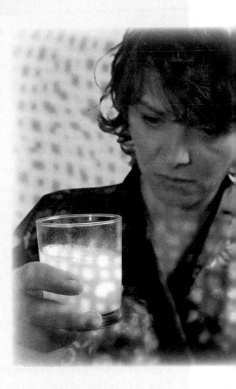

Yes	No	1.	Are you currently experiencing greater than normal stress and tension?
Yes	No	2.	Do you have a family history of digestive tract problems (e.g., ulcers, hemorrhoids, acid indigestion, constipation, lactose intolerance)?
Yes	No	3.	Do you feel pain in your stomach region about 2 hours after eating?
Yes	No	4.	Do you smoke cigarettes?
Yes	No	5.	Do you take aspirin frequently?
Yes	No	6.	Do you have heartburn at least once per week?
Yes	No	7.	Do you commonly lie down after eating a large meal?
Yes	No	8.	Do you drink alcoholic beverages more than 2 or 3 times per day?
Yes	No	9.	Do you experience abdominal pain, bloating, and gas about 30 minutes to 2 hours after consuming milk products?
Yes	No	10.	Do you often have to strain while having a bowel movement?
Yes	No	11.	Do you consume less than 9 cups (women) to 13 cups (men) of a combination of water and other fluids per day?
Yes	No	12.	Do you perform physical activity (e.g., jog, swim, walk briskly, row, stair climb) less than 30 minutes on fewer than 5 days of the week?
Yes	No	13.	Do you eat a diet relatively low in fiber (significant fiber is found in whole fruits, vegetables, legumes, nuts, seeds, whole-grain breads, and whole-grain cereals)?
Yes	No	14.	Do you frequently have diarrhea?
Yes	No	15.	Do you frequently use laxatives or antacids?

Interpretation

If you answered yes to more than 8 questions, your habits and symptoms may put you at risk of digestive tract problems. Take particular note of the habits to which you answered yes. Consider trying to cooperate more with your digestive tract.

can lead to hemorrhoids as a result of constipation and straining during bowel movements. If you think you have a hemorrhoid, you should consult your physician. Rectal bleeding, although usually caused by hemorrhoids, may also indicate other problems, such as cancer.

A physician may suggest a variety of self-care measures for hemorrhoids. Pain can be reduced by applying warm, soft compresses or sitting in a tub of warm water for 15 to 20 minutes. Dietary recommendations are the same as those for treating mild constipation, emphasizing the need to exercise every day and consume adequate fiber (25 to 35 grams daily) and fluid. Over-the-counter remedies, such as Preparation H®, offer relief of symptoms. Some hemorrhoids require procedures usually done in a surgeon's office to eliminate the hemorrhoids.

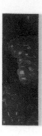

Knowledge Check

1. Which foods or eating practices may increase the risk of heartburn?
2. What is the most common cause of peptic ulcers?
3. What are 2 nutritional factors that can increase the risk of gallstones?
4. What are 3 factors that increase the chances of developing constipation?

Summary

4.1 The cell is the basic structural unit of the human body. Cells join together to make up tissues. The 4 primary types of tissues are epithelial, connective, muscle, and nervous. Tissues unite to form organs and organs work together as an organ system.

4.2 The gastrointestinal (GI) tract includes the mouth, esophagus, stomach, small intestine, and large intestine (colon, rectum, and anus). Sphincters along the GI tract control the flow of digesting food. The accessory organs (liver, gallbladder, and pancreas) are an important part of the digestive system. Movement through the GI tract is mainly through muscular contractions known as peristalsis. GI contents are mixed with segmental contractions. Enzymes are specialized protein molecules that speed up digestion by catalyzing chemical reactions. Most digestive enzymes are synthesized in the small intestine and pancreas. A lack of digestive enzymes can result in poor digestion, poor absorption, malnutrition, and weight loss.

4.3 The mouth chews food to break it into smaller parts and increase its surface area, which enhances enzyme activity. Amylase produced by salivary glands digests a small amount of starch. Chewed food mixed with saliva is called a bolus. When swallowing is initiated, the epiglottis covers the trachea to prevent food from entering it. Peristalsis moves food down the esophagus. There are 5 basic taste sensations perceived by taste cells found on taste buds in the mouth, especially the tongue. Genetic variability affects the ability to taste bitter compounds. The sense of smell contributes greatly to flavor perceptions.

4.4 The lower esophageal sphincter protects the esophagus from the backflow of acidic stomach contents. When this sphincter does not work normally, heartburn and GERD may occur. Stomach cells produce gastric juice (HCl, pepsinogen, mucus, and intrinsic factor). Pepsin (from pepsinogen) starts the digestion of protein. Mixing of food and gastric juice results in the production of chyme, the liquid substance released in small amounts into the small intestine.

4.5 The small intestine has 3 sections: duodenum, jejunum, and ileum. Most digestion occurs in the small intestine. Secretions from the liver, gallbladder, and pancreas are released into the small intestine. These secretions contain enzymes, bile, and sodium bicarbonate. Villi in the small intestine greatly increase its surface area, which enhances absorption. Villi are lined by enterocytes that release enzymes. Enterocytes are constantly broken down and replaced. Diseases, such as celiac disease, damage the villi and enterocytes. The liver, gallbladder, and pancreas aid digestion and absorption. The liver produces bile, which is stored in the gallbladder and used to emulsify fat. Pancreatic juices contain the alkaline sodium bicarbonate and digestive enzymes. Bile and pancreatic juice are released into the small intestine via the pancreatic bile duct. Most nutrients are absorbed primarily in the small intestine. There are 4 main types of absorption: passive diffusion, facilitated diffusion, active absorption, and endocytosis. Hormones regulate digestion and absorption. The 4 major GI-regulating hormones are gastrin, cholecystokinin, secretin, and gastric inhibitory peptide.

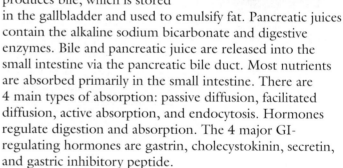

4.6 Nutrients absorbed into the absorptive cells are transported in the body via either the cardiovascular or the lymphatic circulation. Water-soluble nutrients entering the cardiovascular system from absorptive cells travel via the portal vein to the liver, then to the general circulation and body tissues. Fat-soluble and large particles enter the lymphatic system from absorptive cells. Lymphatic vessels drain into the thoracic duct that releases its contents to the bloodstream.

4.7 The large intestine is the last part of the GI tract. It houses many species of beneficial and pathogenic bacteria, absorbs water and electrolytes, and forms and eliminates feces. GI contents entering the large intestine are mainly water, some minerals, fiber, and some starch. Carbohydrates (fiber and starch) can be digested to some extent by bacteria in the large intestine and form short-chain fatty acids, which serve as an energy source for the large intestine and may help prevent and treat diseases. Bacteria in the large intestine also produce intestinal gas. Probiotics are live microorganisms found in fermented foods and supplements. They may promote intestinal health, such as preventing diarrhea in children. Prebiotics are nondigestible carbohydrates that promote the growth of beneficial bacteria in the large intestine. It takes 12 to 24 hours for contents to pass through the large intestine. Feces defecated through

the rectum contain about 75% water and 25% solids—indigestible plant fibers, tough connective tissues from animal foods, and bacteria.

4.8 Common digestive disorders include heartburn, GERD, peptic ulcers, gallstones, constipation, diarrhea, irritable bowel syndrome, and hemorrhoids. These disorders often can be prevented or treated with healthy nutrition and lifestyle habits.

Study Questions

1. What is the smallest functional unit of the human body?
   a. organ
   b. organ system
   c. cell
   d. epithelial tissue

2. Most digestive enzymes are produced in the _____.
   a. mouth and esophagus
   b. esophagus and stomach
   c. small intestine and pancreas
   d. liver and gallbladder

3. The coordinated squeezing and shortening of the muscles of the GI tract is called _____.
   a. enzyme hydrolysis
   b. peristalsis
   c. olfaction
   d. diarrhea

4. Which part of the digestive system normally houses large numbers of bacteria?
   a. large intestine
   b. small intestine
   c. stomach
   d. pancreas

5. The main role of the stomach in digestion and absorption is to _____.
   a. absorb proteins and carbohydrates
   b. digest fats
   c. mix ingested foods to form chyme
   d. produce enzymes that digest carbohydrates and fats

6. Villi are found mainly in the _____.
   a. large intestine
   b. small intestine
   c. esophagus
   d. stomach

7. Which of the following is known to prevent or treat diarrhea in developing countries?
   a. oral rehydration therapy
   b. supplemental zinc
   c. prevention of malnutrition
   d. all of the above

8. The _____ both empty their contents into the small intestine via the sphincter of Oddi.
   a. stomach and gallbladder
   b. pancreas and stomach
   c. liver and pancreas
   d. pancreas and small intestine

9. Fat-soluble vitamins are absorbed directly into the cardiovascular system.
   a. true
   b. false

10. _____ are absorbed in the large intestine.
    a. Vitamins and minerals
    b. Vitamins and water
    c. Fatty acids and minerals
    d. Water and electrolytes

11. Probiotics may be most useful in treating _____.

   a. constipation
   b. diarrhea in children
   c. celiac disease
   d. food intolerance

12. Which of the following digestive disorders is caused by the bacterium *Helicobacter pylori*?

   a. excessive intestinal gas
   b. constipation
   c. diarrhea
   d. peptic ulcer

13. Irritable bowel syndrome (IBS) is caused by bacterial pathogens.

   a. true
   b. false

14. A good way to treat mild constipation is to consume 25 to 35 grams of fiber each day.

   a. true
   b. false

15. Match each secretion with the organ that produces it. Some organs may be selected more than once.

   hydrochloric acid   a. pancreas
   sodium bicarbonate   b. liver
   bile   c. stomach
   CCK   d. small intestine
   lipase

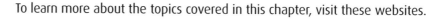

Answer Key: 1-c; 2-c; 3-b; 4-a; 5-c; 6-b; 7-d; 8-c; 9-b; 10-d; 11-b; 12-d; 13-b; 14-a; 15 hydrochloric acid—stomach; sodium bicarbonate—pancreas; bile—liver; CCK—small intestine; lipase—pancreas and small intestine.

Websites

To learn more about the topics covered in this chapter, visit these websites.

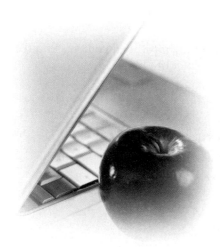

Digestion

digestive.niddk.nih.gov

www.acg.gi.org

www.healthfinder.org

www.heimlichinstitute.org

Irritable Bowel Syndrome

www.ibsgroup.org

Celiac Disease and Gluten Sensitivities

www.celiachealth.org

digestive.niddk.nih.gov/ddiseases/pubs/celiac/index.htm

consensus.nih.gov/2004/2004CeliacDisease118html.htm

www.celiac.nih.gov

www.gluten.net

www.celiac.org

www.celiac.com

www.celiaccenter.org

www.bidmc.harvard.edu/display.asp?node_id=5449

www.celiacdiseasecenter.columbia.edu/CF-HOME.htm

celiaccenter.ucsd.edu

References

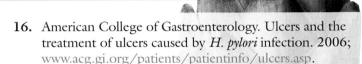

1. Smith D, Margolskee RF. Making sense of taste. *Scientific Am.* 2001;284:32.

2. Drewnowski A, Gomez-Carneros C. Bitter taste, phytonutrients, and the consumer: A review. *Am J Clin Nutr.* 2000;72:1424.

3. Le Coutre J. Taste: The metabolic sense. *Food Tech.* 2003;57:34.

4. Muller O, Krawinkel M. Malnutrition and health in developing countries. *Can Med Assoc J.* 2005;173.

5. Glass RI. New hope for defeating rotavirus. *Scientific Am.* 2006;294:46.

6. Brown KH. Diarrhea and malnutrition. *J Nutr.* 2003;133.

7. United Nations Children's Fund/World Health Organization. *Clinical management of acute diarrhea*: World Health Organization; 2004. WHO/FCH/CAH/04.7.

8. Food and Nutrition Board, Institute of Medicine. *Dietary Reference Intakes for energy, carbohydrate, fiber, fat, fatty acids, cholesterol, protein and amino acids.* Washington DC: National Academy Press; 2005.

9. Liong M. Probiotics: A critical review of their potential role as antihypertensives, immune modulators, hypocholesterolemics, and perimenopausal treatments. *Nutr Rev.* 2007;65:316.

10. Report of a Joint FAO/WHO Working Group. *Guidelines for the evaluation of probiotics in food.* London, Ontario, Canada: FAO/WHO; 2002.

11. Santosa S and others. Probiotics and their potential health claims. *Nutr Rev.* 2006;64:265.

12. Guarner F. Inulin and oligofructose: Impact on intestinal diseases and disorders. *Br J Nutr.* 2005;93(Suppl 1):S61.

13. National Digestive Diseases Information Clearinghouse. Heartburn, hiatal hernia and gastroesophageal reflux disease. *Digestive Diseases.* 2003; digestive.niddk.nih.gov/ddiseases/pubs/gerd/index.htm.

14. Hampel H and others. Meta-analysis: Obesity and the risk for gastroesophageal reflux disease and its complications. *Ann Internal Med.* 2005;143:199.

15. Smith L. Updated ACG guidelines for diagnosis and treatment of GERD. *Am Family Physician.* 2005;71:2376.

16. American College of Gastroenterology. Ulcers and the treatment of ulcers caused by *H. pylori* infection. 2006; www.acg.gi.org/patients/patientinfo/ulcers.asp.

17. National Digestive Diseases Information Clearinghouse. *H. pylori* and peptic ulcer. *Digestive Diseases.* 2004; digestive.niddk.nih.gov/ddiseases/pubs/hpylori/index.htm.

18. Portincaso P and others. Cholesterol gallstone disease. *Lancet.* 2006;368:230.

19. Bellows CF and others. Management of gallstones. *Am Family Physician.* 2005;72.

20. Tsai C-J and others. Dietary protein and the risk of cholecystectomy in a cohort of US women: The Nurses Health Study. *Am J Epi.* 2004;160:11.

21. National Digestive Diseases Information Clearinghouse. Gallstones. 2004; digestive.niddk.nih.gov/ddiseases/pubs/gallstones/index.htm.

22. Mertz M. Irritable bowel syndrome. *New Eng J Med.* 2003;349:2136–2146.

23. Moynihan NT and others. How do you spell relief for irritable bowel syndrome? *J Fam Pract.* 2008;57:100.

24. National Digestive Diseases Information Clearinghouse. Gas in the digestive tract. *Digestive Diseases.* March 2004; digestive.niddk.nih.gov/ddiseases/pubs/gas/index.htm.

25. Hsieh C. Treatment of constipation in older adults. *Am Family Physician.* 2005;72.

26. Muller-Lisser S and others. Myths and misconceptions about constipation. *Am J Gastroenterology.* 2005;100.

27. Niewinski, M.M. Advances in celiac disease and gluten-free diet. *J Am Diet Assoc.* 2008;108:661.

28. American Academy of Pediatrics. Children's health topics: Gastroenterology and hepatology. 2007; www.aap.org/healthtopics/gastroenterology.cfm.

29. Harvard Medical Center. Hemorrhoids and what to do about them. *Harvard Women's Health Watch.* July:2004:4.

30. Yang Y and others. Long-term proton pump inhibitor therapy and risk of hip fracture *JAMA.* 2006;296:2947.

5

Carbohydrates

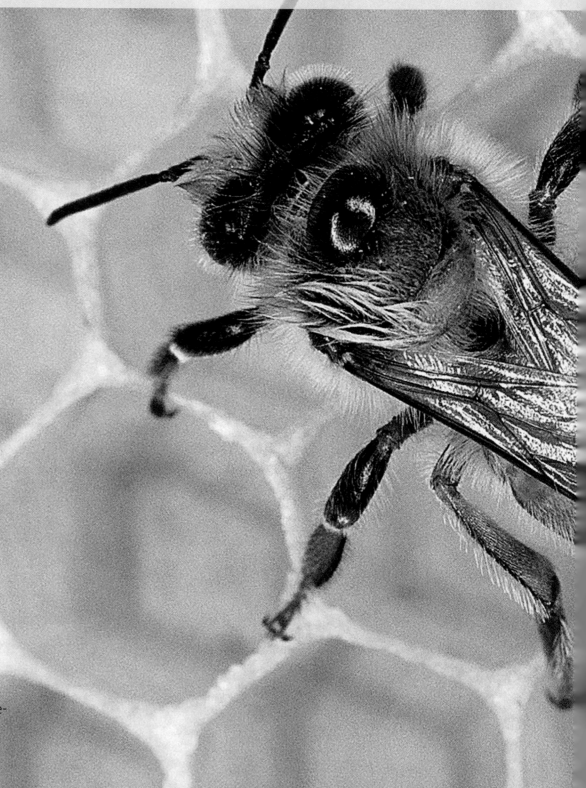

Honey is one of the few carbohydrate-rich foods provided by an animal. To learn more, visit www.honey.com.

STUDENT LEARNING OUTCOMES

After studying this chapter, you will be able to

1. Identify the major types of carbohydrates and give examples of food sources for each.

2. List alternative sweeteners that can be used to reduce sugar intake.

3. Describe recommendations for carbohydrate intake and health risks caused by low or excessive intakes.

4. List the functions of carbohydrates in the body.

5. Explain how carbohydrates are digested and absorbed.

6. Identify the cause of, effects of, and dietary treatment for lactose intolerance.

7. Describe the regulation of blood glucose, conditions caused by blood glucose imbalance, types of diabetes, and dietary treatments for diabetes.

8. Describe dietary measures to reduce the risk of developing type 2 diabetes.

Fruits, vegetables, dairy products, cereals, breads, pasta, and desserts—all of these supply carbohydrates (i.e., sugar, starch, and fiber). Maybe you've avoided many of these foods in an attempt to lose weight or "bulk up" with muscle. Unfortunately, the benefits of carbohydrates are frequently misunderstood.[1] People often mistakenly think carbohydrate-rich foods are fattening or cause diabetes. However, high-carbohydrate foods—especially fiber-rich foods, such as fruits, vegetables, legumes, and whole-grain breads and cereals—provide essential nutrients and should constitute about 45 to 65% of our daily energy intake.[2] They also add interest to our diets—consider the vivid colors of fruits and vegetables, the crunchiness of cereals, and the delicious flavors of desserts.

Carbohydrates are a primary fuel source for cells, especially the cells of the central nervous system and red blood cells.[3] Muscle cells also rely on carbohydrates to fuel intense physical activity. Yielding an average of 4 kcal/g, carbohydrates are a readily available fuel for all cells in the form of glucose (a sugar) in the blood and glycogen (a starch) in the liver and muscles. Glycogen can be broken down to glucose and released into the blood to maintain blood glucose levels when the diet does not supply enough. Regular intake of carbohydrate is important because glycogen stores in the liver and muscles are exhausted in about 18 hours if no carbohydrate is consumed.[3] After that point, the body is forced to produce glucose from protein or to use fat as the primary source of energy; as you will learn later in this chapter, this eventually leads to health problems.

Figure 5-1 Food sources of carbohydrates.

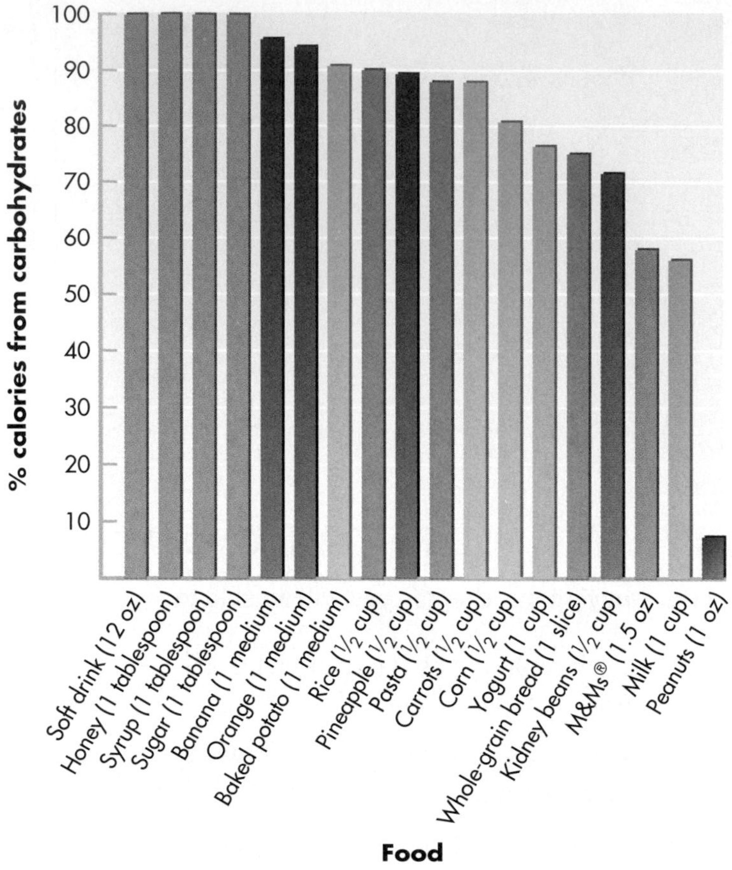

% calories from carbohydrates

Food categories (x-axis):
Soft drink (12 oz), Honey (1 tablespoon), Syrup (1 tablespoon), Sugar (1 tablespoon), Banana (1 medium), Orange (1 medium), Baked potato (1 medium), Rice (½ cup), Pineapple (½ cup), Pasta (½ cup), Carrots (½ cup), Corn (½ cup), Yogurt (1 cup), Whole-grain bread (1 slice), Kidney beans (½ cup), M&Ms® (1.5 oz), Milk (1 cup), Peanuts (1 oz)

Food

---

monosaccharide Class of single sugars that are not broken down further during digestion.

disaccharide Class of sugars formed by the chemical bonding of 2 monosaccharides.

polysaccharide Class of complex carbohydrates containing many glucose units, from 10 to 1000 or more.

---

6 carbon dioxide (CO_2) + 6 water (H_2O)

Sun

Energy →

Glucose ($C_6H_{12}O_6$) + 6 oxygen (O_2)

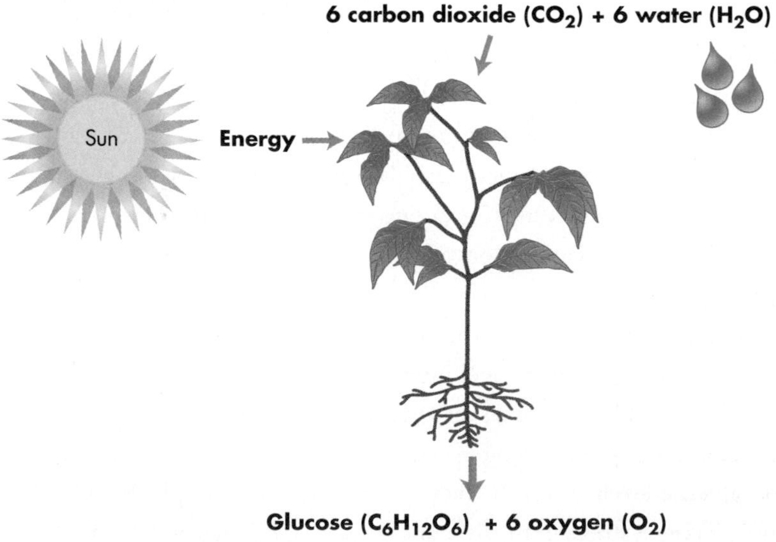

Figure 5-2 A summary of photosynthesis. Plants use carbon dioxide, water, and energy to produce glucose. Glucose is then stored in the leaves but also can undergo further metabolism to form starch and fiber in the plant. With the addition of nitrogen from the soil or air, glucose also can be transformed into protein.

5.1 Structures of Carbohydrates

The carbohydrate family includes sugar, starch, and fiber (Fig. 5-1). Most forms of carbohydrates are composed of carbon, hydrogen, and oxygen. Plants are the main source of carbohydrates. During **photosynthesis**, plants produce glucose by using carbon and oxygen from carbon dioxide in the air, hydrogen from water, and energy from the sun (Fig. 5-2). Plants either store the glucose or transform it into starch, fiber, fat, or protein.

The general formula for carbohydrates is $(CH_2O)n$, where *n* represents the number of times the formula is repeated. For example, the chemical formula for glucose is $C_6H_{12}O_6$ or $(CH_2O)_6$. The simpler forms of carbohydrates are called **monosaccharides** and **disaccharides**. Monosaccharides are single sugars with the general formula of $(CH_2O)_6$. Disaccharides are double sugars, made of 2 monosaccharide sugars, with the general formula of $(CH_2O)_{12}$. The more complex forms of carbohydrates (i.e., glycogen, starch, and fiber) are called **polysaccharides** and typically contain many glucose molecules linked together.

Monosaccharides: Glucose, Fructose, Galactose, Sugar Alcohols, and Pentoses

The common monosaccharides (*mono* means one; *saccharide* means sugar) are glucose, fructose, and galactose. The structures of these monosaccharides are shown in Figure 5-3. No-

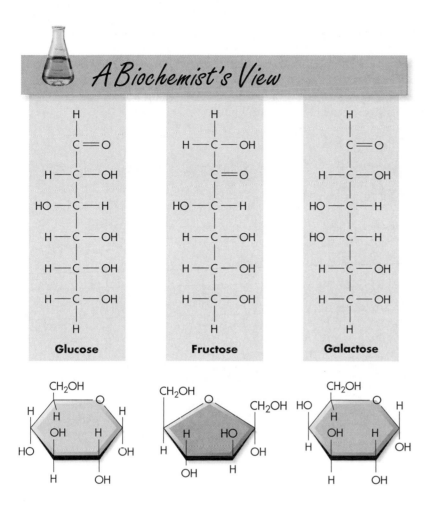

A Biochemist's View

Glucose

Fructose

Galactose

Figure 5-3 The 6-carbon monosaccharides—glucose, fructose, and galactose—shown in the linear form and in their most common form—as a ring (each corner represents a carbon atom unless otherwise indicated). Being familiar with the chemical structures makes it easier to understand how sugars are interrelated, combined, digested, metabolized, and synthesized.

tice that each of the monosaccharides contains 6 carbon, 12 hydrogen, and 6 oxygen molecules, but in slightly different configurations. Because each is a 6-carbon sugar, it is classified as a **hexose** (*hex* means 6; *ose* refers to sugar or carbohydrate).

Glucose is the most abundant monosaccharide, although we eat very little of it as a monosaccharide. Much of the glucose in our diets is linked together with additional sugars to form disaccharides or polysaccharides. In the body, glucose is sometimes called "blood sugar."

The monosaccharide **fructose** is found in fruits, vegetables, honey (which is about 50% fructose and 50% glucose), and high-fructose corn syrup. Because **high-fructose corn syrup** is sweeter and less expensive than table sugar, it is used to sweeten many food products, especially beverages. The presence of fructose in these products makes it a common sugar in our diets. In most North American diets, fructose accounts for about 8 to 10% of total energy intake.

Galactose is the third major monosaccharide of nutritional importance. A comparison of the structure of this sugar with that of glucose shows that they are almost identical (see Fig. 5-3). Galactose usually is not found free in nature in large quantities. Instead, it combines with glucose to form a disaccharide called **lactose**, which is found in milk and other dairy products.

The sugar alcohols, which are derivatives of monosaccharides, include sorbitol, mannitol, and xylitol. These are used primarily as sweeteners in sugarless gum and dietetic foods.

The additional monosaccharides found in nature are ribose and deoxyribose. These are classified as "pentoses" because they contain 5 carbons (*penta* means 5). Although these sugars are needed in only small quantities in the diet, they are very important in the body because they are an essential part of the cell's genetic material. Ribose is part of ribonucleic acid (RNA), and deoxyribose is part of deoxynucleic acid (DNA).

glucose Most abundant monosaccharide; also called dextrose.

fructose Monosaccharide found in fruits and honey; also called levulose.

galactose Monosaccharide found most abundantly as a part of lactose (milk sugar).

Simple Forms of Carbohydrates

Monosaccharides: glucose, fructose, galactose

Disaccharides: sucrose, lactose, maltose

Complex Forms of Carbohydrates

Oligosaccharides: raffinose, stachyose

Polysaccharides: starches (amylose and amylopectin), glycogen, fiber

Disaccharides: Maltose, Sucrose, and Lactose

condensation reaction Chemical reaction in which 2 molecules bond to form a larger molecule by releasing water.

Carbohydrates containing 2 monosaccharides are called disaccharides (*di* means 2). The linking of 2 monosaccharides occurs in a **condensation reaction.** During this reaction, 1 molecule of water is formed (and released) by taking a hydroxyl group (OH) from 1 sugar and a hydrogen (H) from the other sugar (Fig. 5-4).

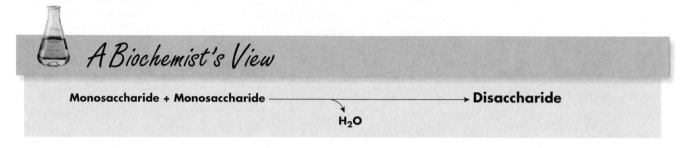

Figure 5-4 Two monosaccharides combine to form a disaccharide.

• Maltose is made up of 2 glucose molecules.
• Sucrose, or common table sugar, is made up of glucose and fructose.
• Lactose, or milk sugar, is made up of glucose and galactose. Note that lactose contains a different type of bond (beta, or β) than maltose and sucrose (alpha, or α); this type of bond makes it difficult for individuals who produce little of the enzyme lactase to digest lactose.

One carbon on each monosaccharide participating in the condensation reaction chemically bonds with a single oxygen. Two forms of this C—O—C bond exist in nature: **alpha (α) bonds** and **beta (β) bonds**. As shown in Figure 5-4, maltose and sucrose contain the alpha form, whereas lactose contains the beta form. Many carbohydrates contain long chains of glucose with the individual monosaccharides bonded together by either alpha or beta bonds.

Beta bonds differ from alpha bonds in that they cannot be easily broken down by digestive enzymes for absorption in the small intestine. Thus, foods that contain saccharide molecules linked together by beta bonds (e.g., in milk and dietary fiber) are often difficult or impossible for individuals to digest because they lack the enzymes necessary for breaking beta bonds apart.

The disaccharide **maltose** contains 2 glucose molecules joined by an alpha bond. When seeds sprout, they produce enzymes that break down polysaccharides stored in the seed to sugars such as maltose and glucose. These sugars provide the energy for the plant to grow. Malting, the first step in the production of alcoholic beverages, such as beer, lets grain seeds sprout. Few other food products and beverages contain maltose. In fact, most of the maltose that we ultimately digest in the small intestine is produced when we break down longer-chain polysaccharides.

Sucrose, common table sugar, is composed of glucose and fructose linked by an alpha bond. Large amounts of sucrose are found naturally in plants, such as sugar cane, sugar beets, and maple tree sap. The sucrose from these sources may be purified to various degrees. Brown, white, and powdered sugars are common forms of sucrose sold in grocery stores.

Lactose, the primary sugar in milk and milk products, consists of glucose joined to galactose by a beta bond. As discussed later in this chapter, many people are unable to digest large amounts of lactose because they don't produce enough of the enzyme lactase, which is needed to break this beta bond. This can cause intestinal gas, bloating, cramping, and discomfort as the unabsorbed lactose is metabolized into acids and gases by bacteria in the large intestine.[4]

Many terms are used to refer to monosaccharides and disaccharides and products containing these sugars. Monosaccharides and disaccharides often are referred to as *simple sugars* because they contain only 1 or 2 sugar units. Food labels combine all the sugars either naturally present in food products or added during their manufacture into one category, listing them as "sugars."[1]

Oligosaccharides: Raffinose and Stachyose

Oligosaccharides are complex carbohydrates that contain 3 to 10 single sugar units (*oligo* means few). Two oligosaccharides of nutritional importance are **raffinose** and **stachyose**, which are found in onions, cabbage, broccoli, whole wheat, and legumes, such as kidney beans and soybeans. Oligosaccharides cannot be broken down by our digestive enzymes. Thus, when we eat foods with raffinose and stachyose, these oligosaccharides pass undigested into the large intestine, where bacteria metabolize them, producing gas and other by-products.[3]

Although many people have no symptoms after eating legumes, others experience unpleasant side effects from intestinal gas. An enzyme preparation, such as Beano®, can help prevent these side effects if taken right before a meal. This enzyme preparation works in the digestive tract to break down many of the indigestible oligosaccharides.

Polysaccharides: Starch, Glycogen, and Fiber

Polysaccharides are complex carbohydrates that often contain hundreds to thousands of glucose molecules. The polysaccharides include some that are digestible, such as starch, and some that are largely indigestible, such as fiber. The digestibility of these polysaccharides is mainly determined by whether the glucose units are linked together by alpha or beta bonds.[3]

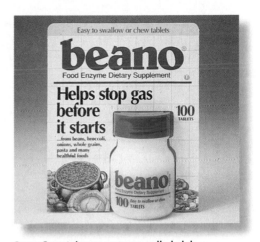

Beano® contains an enzyme, called alpha-galactosidase, that can break apart the bonds in oligosaccharides. This helps reduce the intestinal gas produced when beans and other legumes are eaten.

CRITICAL THINKING

Jason enjoys Mexican food, especially with a generous portion of black or pinto beans. However, he often develops gas and intestinal cramps after these meals. His friends suggest that he try using a product called Beano® to reduce his symptoms. How might it help Jason?

raffinose Indigestible oligosaccharide made of 3 monosaccharides (galactose-glucose-fructose).

stachyose Indigestible oligosaccharide made of 4 monosaccharides (galactose-galactose-glucose-fructose).

starch Complex carbohydrate made of multiple units of glucose attached together in a form that the body can digest.

fiber Complex carbohydrate in foods of plant origin that is made of multiple units of glucose attached together in a form that cannot be broken down by digestive processes in the stomach or small intestine.

glycogen Branched-chain polysaccharide in the liver and muscles; the primary storage form of glucose (and carbohydrate) in animals.

A Biochemist's View

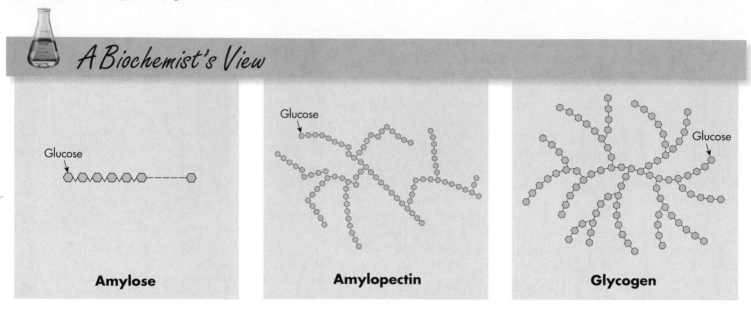

Figure 5-5 Digestible polysaccharides. Amylose and amylopectin are the storage form of glucose in plants. Glycogen is the storage form of glucose in animals.

Digestible Polysaccharides: Starch and Glycogen

Starch, the major digestible polysaccharide in our diets, is the storage form of glucose in plants. There are 2 types of plant starch—**amylose** and **amylopectin**—both of which are a source of energy for plants and for animals that eat plants.[5] Amylose and amylopectin are found in potatoes, beans, breads, pasta, rice, and other starchy products, typically in a ratio of about 1:4.

Amylose and amylopectin contain many glucose units linked by alpha bonds. The primary difference is that amylose is a straight-chain molecule, whereas amylopectin is highly branched (Fig. 5-5). Cooking increases the digestibility of these starches by making them more soluble in water and, thus, more available for attack by digestive enzymes. The enzymes act only at the ends of the glucose chains. Therefore, the more numerous the branches in a starch, the more sites (ends) available for enzyme action. This explains why the alpha bonds in amylopectin are digested more rapidly than those in amylose. In the body, this causes blood glucose levels to increase more quickly after digesting amylopectin than amylose.

The properties of amylopectin and amylose make them useful in food manufacturing. The branches in amylopectin allow it to retain water to form a very stable starch gel. Thus, food manufacturers commonly use starches rich in amylopectin to thicken sauces and gravies. Amylopectin also is used in many frozen foods because it remains stable over a wide temperature range. Amylose-rich molecules can be bonded to one another to produce **modified food starch,** a thickener used in baby foods, salad dressings, and instant puddings.

Glycogen, the storage form of carbohydrate in humans and animals, also contains many glucose units linked together with alpha bonds. The structure of glycogen is similar to that of amylopectin, but it is even more highly branched. As with amylopectin, the branched structure of glycogen allows it to be broken down quickly by enzymes in the body cells where it is stored.[5]

Liver and muscles cells are the major storage sites for glycogen. The amount stored in these cells is influenced by the amount of carbohydrate in the diet. Although the amount of glycogen that can be stored is limited, glycogen storage is extremely important.[3] The approximately 400 kcal of glycogen stored in the liver can be converted into blood glucose to supply the body with energy, whereas the 1400 kcal of glycogen stored in muscles supply glucose for muscle use, especially during high-intensity and endurance exercise. (See Chapter 11 for a detailed discussion of carbohydrate use during physical activity.)

Indigestible Polysaccharides: Dietary and Functional Fiber

Folklore surrounding fiber, or "roughage," has been a part of American culture since the 1800s, when a minister named Sylvester Graham traveled up and down the East Coast, extolling the virtues of fiber. He left us a legacy—the graham cracker. Although today's gra-

As some vegetables age, their sugars are converted to starches, making them taste less sweet.

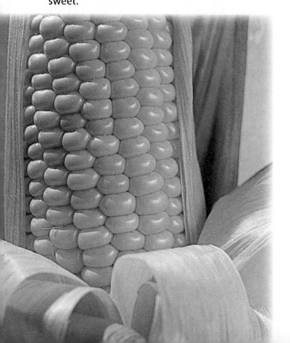

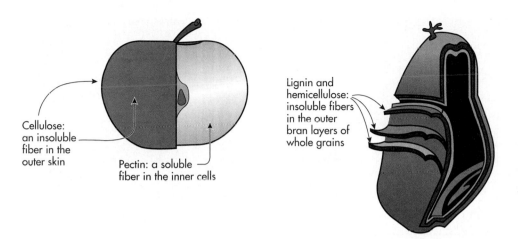

Cellulose: an insoluble fiber in the outer skin

Lignin and hemicellulose: insoluble fibers in the outer bran layers of whole grains

Pectin: a soluble fiber in the inner cells

Figure 5-6 Types of dietary fiber. The skin of an apple consists of the insoluble fiber cellulose, which provides structure for the fruit. The soluble fiber pectin "glues" the fruit cells together. The outside covering of a wheat kernel is made of layers of bran—insoluble fibers.

ham cracker bears little resemblance to the whole-grain product he promoted, present-day scientific evidence supports this early promotion of fiber as part of a healthy diet.

Total fiber (or just the term *fiber*) refers to the **dietary fiber** that occurs naturally in foods, as well as the **functional fiber** (fiber that provides health benefits) that may be added to food.[2] Currently, Nutrition Facts labels include only dietary fiber and do not reflect any added functional fiber.

Fibers are composed primarily of the non-starch polysaccharides **cellulose, hemicelluloses, pectins, gums,** and **mucilages.** The lignins are the only non-carbohydrate components of dietary fibers. Unlike the digestible polysaccharides that contain alpha bonds, the monosaccharide units in fibers are linked by beta bonds. As noted earlier, monosaccharide molecules joined by beta bonds are not broken down by human digestive enzymes. Thus, these undigested fibers pass through the small intestine into the large intestine, where bacteria metabolize some and form short-chain fatty acids and gas. These short-chain fatty acids provide fuel for cells in the large intestine and enhance intestinal health.[6] Pectins, gums, and mucilages are most readily digested by the intestinal bacteria, yielding about 1.5 to 2.5 kcal/g. Cellulose, hemicellulose, and lignins are more resistant to being broken down by bacteria. The body tends to adapt over time to a high-fiber intake, leading to fewer symptoms of bloating, gas, and discomfort.

Cellulose, hemicelluloses, and lignins form the structural part of the plant cell wall in vegetables and whole grains. Bran layers form the outer covering of all seeds; thus, whole grains (those in which the bran and outer layers have not been removed in processing) are good sources of fibers (Fig. 5-6). Because of their chemical structure, these fibers do not dissolve in water. Therefore, they are often referred to as **insoluble fibers**.

In contrast to the insoluble fibers, pectins, gums, mucilages, and some hemicelluloses dissolve easily in water and are classified as **soluble fibers**. In water, they become viscous (gel-like) in consistency. This property makes them useful for thickening jams, jelly, yogurt, and other food products. They also occur naturally inside and around plant cells in oat bran, many fruits, legumes, and psyllium.

The physical properties of soluble and insoluble fibers have health benefits when the fibers are consumed in adequate quantities (Fig. 5-7). For example, soluble fibers have been shown to lower blood cholesterol levels and blood glucose levels, thereby reducing risks of cardiovascular disease and diabetes.[7] Insoluble fibers decrease intestinal transit time, thus reducing risks of constipation, diverticular disease, and colon cancer.[8-11] The health benefits of fiber are discussed in detail later in the chapter.

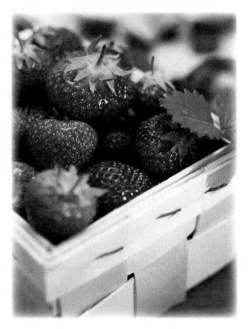

Fruit is a good source of dietary fiber.

insoluble fibers Fibers that are not easily dissolved in water or metabolized by bacteria in the large intestine; includes cellulose, some hemicelluloses, and lignins.

soluble fibers Fibers that dissolve in water and can be metabolized (fermented) by bacteria in the large intestine; includes pectin, gums, and mucilages; also called viscous fibers.

▶ The Food and Nutrition Board has recommended that the terms *soluble* and *insoluble fibers* gradually be replaced by other terms, such as *viscosity* and *fermentability*, which more clearly describe the properties of fibers. The actual terms used may change as scientific knowledge expands.

Knowledge Check

1. Which sugars are classified as monosaccharides? As disaccharides?
2. Why are foods that contain saccharide units linked by beta bonds difficult to digest?
3. What types of carbohydrates are classified as polysaccharides?

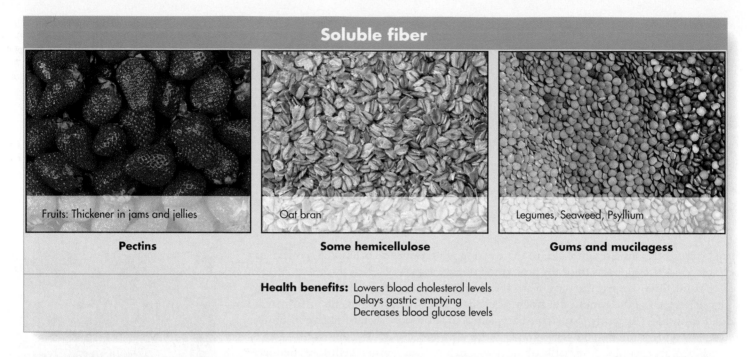

Soluble fiber

Fruits: Thickener in jams and jellies

Pectins

Oat bran

Some hemicellulose

Legumes, Seaweed, Psyllium

Gums and mucilagess

Health benefits: Lowers blood cholesterol levels
Delays gastric emptying
Decreases blood glucose levels

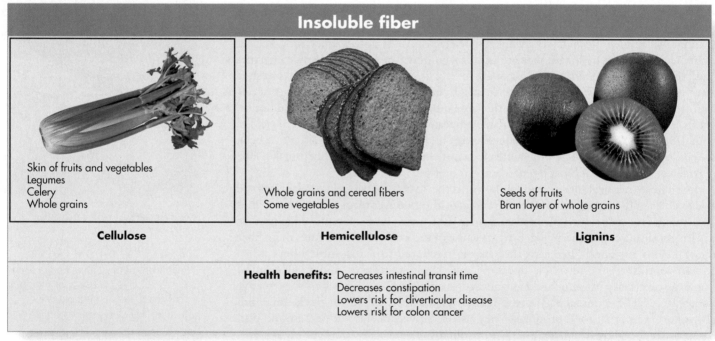

Insoluble fiber

Skin of fruits and vegetables
Legumes
Celery
Whole grains

Cellulose

Whole grains and cereal fibers
Some vegetables

Hemicellulose

Seeds of fruits
Bran layer of whole grains

Lignins

Health benefits: Decreases intestinal transit time
Decreases constipation
Lowers risk for diverticular disease
Lowers risk for colon cancer

Figure 5-7 **Soluble and insoluble fibers.** Fibers can be classified as either soluble or insoluble based on their properties. Soluble fibers dissolve in water, whereas insoluble fibers do not dissolve in water.

5.2 Carbohydrates in Foods

Carbohydrates are found in a wide variety of foods. Foods such as table sugar, jam, jelly, fruit, fruit juices, soft drinks, baked potatoes, rice, pasta, cereals, and breads are predominantly carbohydrates. Other foods, such as dried beans, lentils, corn, peas, and dairy products (milk and yogurt), also are good sources of carbohydrate, although they contribute protein, and in some cases fat, to our diets as well. Foods with little or no carbohydrate include meats, fish, poultry, eggs, vegetable oils, butter, and margarine.

Starch

Starches contribute much of the carbohydrate in our diets. Recall that plants store glucose as polysaccharides in the form of starches. Thus, plant-based foods, such as legumes, tubers, and the grains (wheat, rye, corn, oats, barley, and rice) used to make breads, cereals, and pasta, are the best sources of starch. A diet rich in these starches provides ample carbohydrate, as well as many micronutrients.

Fiber

Fiber can be found in many of the same foods as starch, so a diet rich in grains, legumes, and tubers also can provide significant amounts of dietary fiber (especially insoluble cellulose, hemicellulose, and lignins). Because much of the fiber in whole grains is found in the outer layers, which are removed in processing, highly processed grains are low in fiber. Soluble fibers (pectin, gums, mucilages) are found in the skins and flesh of many fruits and berries; as thickeners and stabilizers in jams, yogurts, sauces, and fillings; and in products that contain psyllium and seaweed.

For individuals who have difficulties consuming adequate dietary fiber, fiber is available as a supplement or as an additive to certain foods (functional fiber). In this way, individuals with relatively low dietary fiber intakes can still obtain the health benefits of fiber.

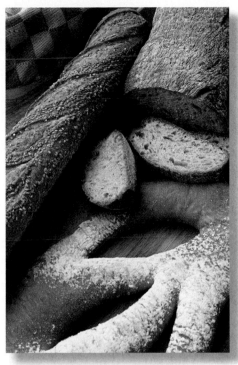

Breads are a rich source of carbohydrate.

Nutritive Sweeteners

The various substances that impart sweetness to foods fall into 2 broad classes: nutritive sweeteners, which can be metabolized to yield energy, and alternative sweeteners, which provide no food energy (Table 5-1). The sweetness of sucrose (table sugar) makes it the benchmark against which all other sweeteners are measured. As shown in Figure 5-8, the alternative sweeteners are much sweeter on a per gram basis than the nutritive sweeteners.[1]

The monosaccharides (glucose, fructose, and galactose) and disaccharides (sucrose, lactose, and maltose) are classified as nutritive sweeteners (Table 5-2).[1] Sucrose is obtained from sugar cane and sugar beet plants. Most of the sucrose and the other sugars we eat comes from foods and beverages to which sugar has been added during processing and/or manufacturing. The major sources are soft drinks, candy, cakes, cookies, pies, fruit drinks, and dairy desserts, such as ice cream. The more processed the food, generally the higher its simple sugar content. The rest of the sugar in our diets is present naturally in foods, such as fruits and juices.

A nutritive sweetener used frequently by the food industry is high-fructose corn syrup. High-fructose corn syrup is made by treating cornstarch with acid and enzymes to break down much of the starch into glucose. Then some of the glucose is converted by enzymes into fructose. The final syrup is about 55% fructose, although it can range from 40 to 90% fructose. High-fructose corn syrup is similar in sweetness to sucrose, but it is much cheaper to use in food products. High-fructose corn syrup is used in soft drinks, candies, jam, jelly, and desserts (e.g., packaged cookies).[1]

Table 5-1 Typical Sources of Sweeteners

Type of Sweetener	Typical Sources
Sugars	
Lactose	Dairy products
Maltose	Sprouted seeds, some alcoholic beverages
Glucose	Corn syrup, honey
Sucrose	Table sugar, most sweets
Invert sugar[1]	Some candies, honey
Fructose	Fruit, honey, some soft drinks, corn syrup
Sugar Alcohols	
Sorbitol	Sugarless candies, sugarless gum
Mannitol	Sugarless candies
Xylitol	Sugarless gum
Alternative Sweeteners	
Tagatose (Naturlose®)	Ready-to-eat cereals, diet soft drinks, health bars, frozen yogurt, fat-free ice cream, candies, frosting, sugarless gum
Cyclamate	Not currently in use in the U.S. but available in Canada
Aspartame (Equal®)	Diet soft drinks, diet fruit drinks, sugarless gum, powdered diet sweetener
Acesulfame-K (Sunette®)	Sugarless gum, diet drink mixes, powdered diet sweeteners, puddings, gelatin desserts
Saccharin (Sweet 'n Low®)	Diet soft drinks
Sucralose (Splenda®)	Diet soft drinks, tabletop use, sugarless gum, jams, frozen desserts
Neotame	Tabletop sweetener, baked goods, frozen desserts, diet soft drinks, jams and jellies

[1]Sucrose broken down into glucose and fructose.

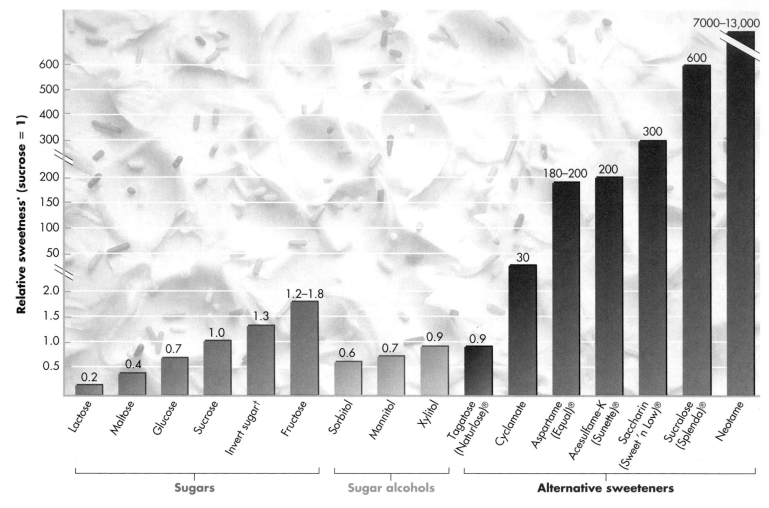

Figure 5-8 Sweetness of sugars and alternative sweeteners compared with sucrose.

* On a per gram basis
† Sucrose broken down into glucose and fructose

Table 5-2 Names of Nutritive Sweeteners Used in Foods

Sugar	Honey
Sucrose	Corn syrup or sweeteners
Brown sugar	High-fructose corn syrup
Confectioner's sugar (powdered sugar)	Molasses
Turbinado sugar	Date sugar
Invert sugar	Maple syrup
Glucose	Dextrin
Sorbitol	Dextrose
Levulose	Fructose
Polydextrose	Maltose
Lactose	Caramel
Mannitol	Fruit sugar

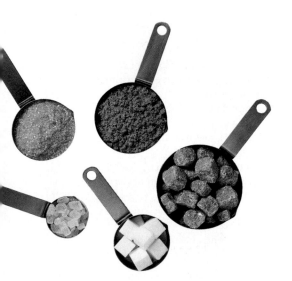

There are many forms of sugar in our diets.

Sugar Alcohols

The sugar alcohols, **sorbitol**, **mannitol**, and **xylitol**, are nutritive sweeteners used in sugarless gum and candies. Sugar alcohols are not readily metabolized by bacteria in the mouth and thus do not promote dental caries as readily as do sugars such as sucrose. Sugar alcohols do contribute energy (about 1.5–3 kcal/g), but they are absorbed and metabolized to glucose more slowly than sugars. In large quantities, sugar alcohols can cause diarrhea, so labels must include this warning.

Sugar alcohols are listed individually on ingredient labels if only 1 sugar alcohol is used in a product; they are grouped together under the heading "sugar alcohols" if 2 or more are used. The calories listed on Nutrition Facts labels account for the calories in each sugar alcohol in the food products.

Alternative Sweeteners

Alternative (or artificial or non-nutritive) sweeteners provide non-caloric or very-low-calorie sugar substitutes for people with diabetes and those trying to lose (or control) body weight. Alternative sweeteners include **saccharin, cyclamate, aspartame, neotame, sucralose, acesulfame-K,** and **tagatose**.[1] Alternative sweeteners yield little or no energy when consumed in amounts typically used in food products and do not promote dental caries. All but cyclamate are currently available in the U.S. Cyclamate was banned for use in the U.S. in 1970, although it has never been conclusively proved to cause health problems when used appropriately. Cyclamate is used in Canada as a tabletop sweetener and as a sweetener in certain medications.

The safety of sweeteners is determined by the FDA and is indicated by an **Acceptable Daily Intake (ADI)** guideline. The ADI is the amount of alternative sweetener considered safe for daily use over one's lifetime. ADIs are based on studies in laboratory animals and are set at a level 100 times less than the level at which no harmful effects were noted in animal studies. Alternative sweeteners can be used safely by adults and children. Although general use is considered safe during pregnancy, pregnant women may want to discuss this issue with their health-care providers.[1]

Saccharin

The oldest alternative sweetener, saccharin is approximately 300 times sweeter than sucrose. Saccharin was once thought to pose a risk of bladder cancer based on studies using laboratory animals. It is no longer listed as a potential cause of cancer in humans because the earlier research is now considered weak and inconclusive.[1] The FDA has set the ADI for saccharin at 5 mg/kg body weight per day. For a 154-pound (70-kg) adult, this equates to approximately 3 12-ounce diet soft drinks or 7 packets of the sweetener (as in Sweet 'n Low®) daily. Saccharin is used as a tabletop sweetener and in a variety of foods and beverages. It is not useful in cooking because heating causes it to develop a bitter taste.

Aspartame

Aspartame is used throughout the world to sweeten beverages, gelatin desserts, chewing gum, cookies, and toppings and fillings of prepared bakery goods. Aspartame breaks down when heated and loses its sweetness when foods are cooked or heated. Nutra-Sweet® and Equal® are brand names for aspartame.

Although aspartame yields about 4 kcal/g (the same calories as sucrose), it is 180 to 200 times sweeter than sucrose. Thus, because only a small amount of aspartame is needed to sweeten a food or beverage, it does not contribute calories to foods. The ADI for aspartame for an adult is 50 mg/kg body weight/day. This is equivalent to about 14 cans of diet soft drink or about 80 packets of Equal®.

Scientific evidence has shown that the use of aspartame is safe for most individuals. However, the FDA has received reports of adverse reactions (headaches, dizziness, seizures, nausea, and other side effects) to aspartame. Although the percentage of people affected is very small, it is important for people who are sensitive to aspartame to avoid it. Those with the genetic disease phenylketonuria (PKU), which interferes with the metabolism of the amino acid phenylalanine, also should avoid aspartame because of its high phenylalanine content.

Neotame

Neotame is approved by the FDA for use as a general purpose sweetener in a wide variety of food products, such as baked goods, non-alcoholic beverages (including soft drinks), chewing gum, confections and frostings, frozen desserts, gelatins and puddings, jams and

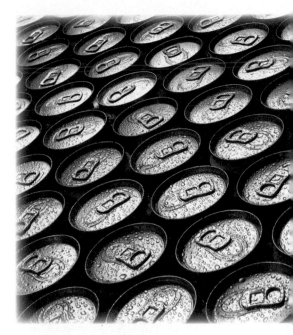
Soft drinks are common sources of sugars and alternative sweeteners.

Acceptable Daily Intake (ADI) Estimate of the amount of a sweetener that an individual can safely consume daily over a lifetime. ADIs are given as mg per kg of body weight per day.

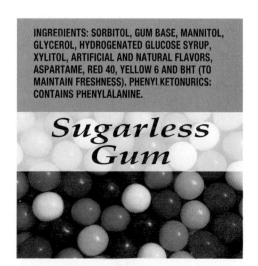
INGREDIENTS: SORBITOL, GUM BASE, MANNITOL, GLYCEROL, HYDROGENATED GLUCOSE SYRUP, XYLITOL, ARTIFICIAL AND NATURAL FLAVORS, ASPARTAME, RED 40, YELLOW 6 AND BHT (TO MAINTAIN FRESHNESS), PHENYLKETONURICS: CONTAINS PHENYLALANINE.

Sugarless Gum

Sugar alcohols and the alternative sweetener aspartame are used to sweeten this product. Note the warning for people with phenylketonuria (PKU) that this product is made with aspartame and, thus, contains phenylalanine.

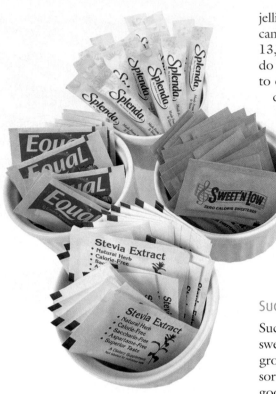

A variety of alternative sweeteners are available.

jellies, processed fruits and fruit juices, toppings, and syrups. Neotame is heat stable and can be used in cooking and as a tabletop sweetener. Neotame is approximately 7000 to 13,000 times sweeter than sucrose. Thus, the small amounts needed to sweeten products do not contribute calories. Although neotame also contains phenylalanine, its bonding to other amino acids differs from that of aspartame and prevents it from being broken down. Therefore, it does not cause a problem for individuals with PKU. The ADI for neotame is 2 mg/kg body weight/day.

Acesulfame-K

The alternative sweetener acesulfame-K (the *K* stands for potassium) is sold for use in the U.S. as Sunette®. Acesulfame-K is 200 times sweeter than sucrose. It contributes no energy to the diet because it is not digested by the body.[1] Acesulfame-K can be used in baking because it does not lose its sweetness when heated. In the U.S., it is currently approved for use in chewing gum, powdered drink mixes, gelatins, puddings, baked goods, tabletop sweeteners, candy, throat lozenges, yogurt, and non-dairy creamers. The ADI for acesulfame-K is 15 mg/kg body weight/day.

Sucralose

Sucralose, sold as Splenda®, is 600 times sweeter than sucrose. It is the only artificial sweetener made from sucrose. It is made by substituting 3 chlorines (Cl) for 3 hydroxyl groups (–OH) on sucrose.[1] This substitution prevents it from being digested and absorbed. Sucralose is used as a tabletop sweetener and in soft drinks, chewing gum, baked goods, syrups, gelatins, frozen dairy desserts (e.g., ice cream), jams, and processed fruits and fruit juices. Sucralose is heat stable; thus, it can be used in cooking and baking. The ADI for sucralose is 5 mg/kg body weight/day.

Tagatose

Tagatose, sold as Naturlose®, is an isomer of fructose. It is almost as sweet as sucrose and can be used in cooking and baking. Because it is poorly absorbed, tagatose yields only 1.5 kcal/g to the body. It has a prebiotic effect because it is fermented by bacteria in the large intestine (see Chapter 4). Tagatose is approved for use in ready-to-eat cereals, diet soft drinks, health bars, frozen yogurt, fat-free ice cream, soft and hard confectionary products, frosting, and chewing gum. It is metabolized like fructose, so individuals with disorders of fructose metabolism should avoid using it.

Stevia

Stevia is an alternative sweetener derived from a South American shrub. It is 100 to 300 times sweeter than sucrose but provides no energy. Although it has been used in teas and as a sweetener in Japan since the 1970s, the FDA has not approved its use in foods. Stevia can be purchased as a dietary supplement in natural and health food stores.[1] However, food processors cannot use it as a sweetener or an additive in food products.

Knowledge Check

1. Which foods are good sources of starch?
2. What contributes the greatest amount of sugar to our diets?
3. Which sugars are classified as non-nutritive sweeteners?

5.3 Recommended Intake of Carbohydrates

According to the RDA, adults need about 130 g/day of digestible carbohydrate to supply adequate glucose for the brain and central nervous system, without having to rely on partial replacement of glucose by ketone bodies as an energy source (see Section 5.4). The Food and Nutrition Board recommends that to provide for total body energy needs, carbohy-

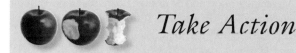

Take Action

Choose the Sandwich with the Most Fiber

Dietitians and personal nutritionists often are asked to assist clients with making healthier choices, especially when eating out. Your client has asked you to help him get more fiber in his lunch from the local deli. The sandwiches on the blackboard all provide about 350 kcal. The fiber content ranges from approximately 1 gram to 8 grams. Rank the sandwiches from the highest amount of fiber (1) to the lowest amount (6); then check your answers at the bottom of the page.

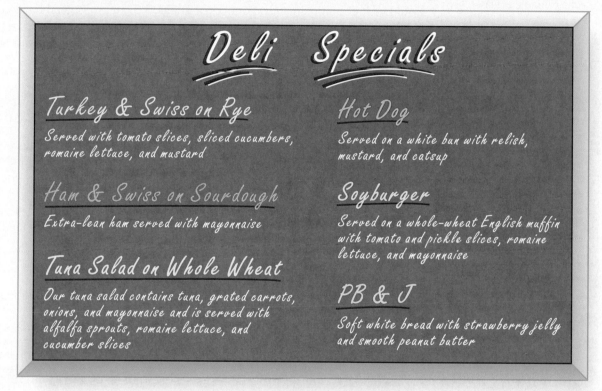

Deli Specials

Turkey & Swiss on Rye
Served with tomato slices, sliced cucumbers, romaine lettuce, and mustard

Ham & Swiss on Sourdough
Extra-lean ham served with mayonnaise

Tuna Salad on Whole Wheat
Our tuna salad contains tuna, grated carrots, onions, and mayonnaise and is served with alfalfa sprouts, romaine lettuce, and cucumber slices

Hot Dog
Served on a white bun with relish, mustard, and catsup

Soyburger
Served on a whole-wheat English muffin with tomato and pickle slices, romaine lettuce, and mayonnaise

PB & J
Soft white bread with strawberry jelly and smooth peanut butter

Answer Key

1. Soyburger: 7.5 g, 2. Tuna Salad on Whole Wheat: 7 g, 3. Turkey & Swiss on Rye: 4 g, 4. PB & J: 3 g, 5. Ham & Swiss on Sourdough: 1.5 g, 6. Hot Dog: 1 g

drate intake should be considerably higher, ranging from 45 to 65% of total energy intake.[2] However, not all diet programs follow the Food and Nutrition Board recommendations. Some diet programs (e.g., the Atkins™ and South Beach™ diets) promote very low carbohydrate intakes, whereas others (e.g., the Pritikin and Eat More, Weigh Less diets) promote very high carbohydrate intakes. Despite these differences in opinion, most scientists and non-scientists agree that carbohydrates in our diets should include mostly fiber-rich fruits, vegetables, and whole grains and little added sugars and caloric sweeteners.[2]

North Americans obtain about half of their energy intakes from carbohydrates. The leading carbohydrate sources for U.S. adults are white bread, soft drinks, cookies, cakes, doughnuts, sugars, syrups, jams, and potatoes. Worldwide, carbohydrates account for about 70 to 80% of all energy consumed, with much greater intakes of whole grains, fruits, vegetables, and legumes than is typical in North American diets.

The Dietary Guidelines for Americans recommend limiting added sugars to approximately 6% of total energy intake.[10] The World Health Organization suggests that sugars added to foods during processing and preparation ("added sugars") should provide no more than about 10% of

Increasing intake of vegetables is a healthful way to include carbohydrates in the diet.

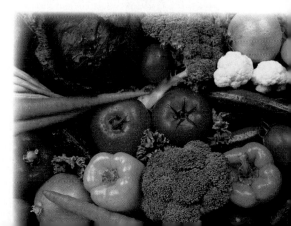

► *Healthy People 2010* set the following goals related to carbohydrate intake:

· Increase the proportion of persons age 2 years and older who consume at least 6 daily servings of grain products, with at least 3 being whole grains.
· Increase the proportion of persons age 2 years and older who consume at least 2 daily servings of fruit.
· Increase the proportion of persons age 2 years and older who consume at least 3 daily servings of vegetables, with at least one-third being dark green or orange vegetables.

total daily energy intake. The Institute of Medicine's Food and Nutrition Board set an upper limit of 25% of energy intake for added sugar consumption.[2] Based on a 2000-kcal diet, these guidelines correspond to approximately 12 teaspoons (50 grams) of sugars/day for 10% of energy intake and 30 teaspoons (125 grams) of simple sugars/day for 25% of energy intake.

The Adequate Intake for fiber is based on a goal of 14 g/1000 kcal consumed. For adults up to age 50 years, the Adequate Intake is set at 25 g for women and 38 g for men. After age 50, the Adequate Intake falls to 21 g/day and 30 g/day, respectively.[2] The Adequate Intake for fiber is aimed to reduce the risk of diverticular disease, cardiovascular disease, and other chronic diseases. The Daily Value used for fiber on food and supplement labels is 25 g for a 2000-kcal diet.

To plan a nutritious diet with ample sources of carbohydrate, your daily diet should include approximately 6 ounces of grains, 2.5 cups of vegetables, 2 cups of fruit, and 3 cups of milk. As a protein alternative to meat, include more dried beans and lentils in your diet to increase fiber and total carbohydrate intake. Table 5-3 shows a diet containing recommended intakes of carbohydrates.

Table 5-3 Sample Menus Containing 1600 kcal with 25 g of Fiber and 2000 kcal with 38 g of Fiber*

Menu	25 g Fiber			38 g Fiber		
	Serving Size	Carbohydrate Content (g)	Fiber Content (g)	Serving Size	Carbohydrate Content (g)	Fiber Content (g)
Breakfast						
Muesli cereal	1 cup	60	6	1 cup	60	6
Raspberries	½ cup	11	2	½ cup	11	2
Whole-wheat toast	1 slice	13	2	2 slices	26	4
Margarine	1 tsp	0	0	1 tsp	0	0
Orange juice	1 cup	28	0	1 cup	28	0
1% milk	1 cup	24	0	1 cup	24	0
Coffee	1 cup	0	0	1 cup	0	0
Lunch						
Bean and vegetable burrito	2 small	50	4.5	3 small	75	7
Guacamole	¼ cup	5	4	¼ cup	5	4
Monterey Jack cheese	1 oz	0	0	1 oz	0	0
Pear (with skin)	1	25	4	1	25	4
Carrot sticks	—	—	—	¾ cup	6	3
Sparkling water	2 cups	0	0	2 cups	0	0
Dinner						
Grilled chicken (no skin)	3 oz	0	0	3 oz	0	0
Salad	½ cup red cabbage ½ cup romaine ¼ cup peach slices	7	3	½ cup red cabbage ½ cup romaine 1 cup peach slices	19	6
Toasted almonds	—	—	—	½ oz	3	2
Fat-free salad dressing	2 tbsp.	0	0	2 tbsp.	0	0
1% milk	1 cup	24	0	1 cup	24	0
Total		247	25		306	38

*The overall diet is based on MyPyramid. Breakdown of approximate energy content: carbohydrate 58%; protein 12%; fat 30%.

Our Carbohydrate Intake

Carbohydrates supply about 50% of the energy intakes of adults in North America. Although the proportion of total energy provided by carbohydrates is in line with recommendations, the types of carbohydrates consumed are not. Added sugars account for almost 16% of total energy intake—nearly triple the 6% of total energy intake recommended by the Dietary Guidelines for Americans.[10] High sugar intakes are, in part, due to the popularity of sweetened beverages. Intake of the primary caloric sweetener used in these beverages (high-fructose corn syrup) adds, on average, over 300 calories daily to the diets of Americans age 2 years and older.[12] Table 5-4 provides suggestions for reducing sugar intake.

In contrast to high sugar intakes, the dietary fiber intakes of Americans fall well below the recommended 14 grams per 1000 calories. Throughout life, both males and females eat 25 to 50% less fiber than recommended. Insufficient fiber intake is due to low intakes of fruits and vegetables and high consumption levels of refined grains, such as pasta, corn chips, white rice, and white bread. Dietary surveys indicate that Americans age 2 and over eat only 1 fruit serving daily and only 1 serving or less of whole grain daily, usually in the form of breakfast cereals and yeast breads.[13]

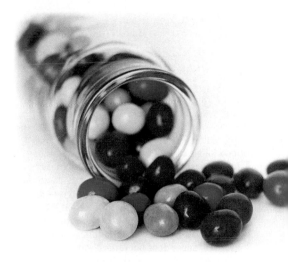

Many foods we enjoy contain simple sugars. To improve nutrient intake, limit the consumption of sweets.

Table 5-4 Suggestions for Reducing Simple-Sugar Intake

Many foods we enjoy are sweet. These should be eaten in moderation.

At the Supermarket

- Read ingredient labels. Identify all the added sugars in a product. Select items lower in total sugar when possible.
- Buy fresh fruits or fruits packed in water, juice, or light syrup rather than those packed in heavy syrup.
- Buy fewer foods that are high in sugar, such as prepared baked goods, candies, sugared cereals, sweet desserts, soft drinks, and fruit-flavored punches. Substitute vanilla wafers, graham crackers, bagels, English muffins, diet soft drinks, and other low sugar alternatives.
- Buy reduced-fat microwave popcorn to replace candy for snacks.

In the Kitchen

- Reduce the sugar in foods prepared at home. Try new low-sugar recipes or adjust your own. Start by reducing the sugar gradually until you've decreased it by one-third or more.
- Experiment with spices, such as cinnamon, cardamom, coriander, nutmeg, ginger, and mace, to enhance the flavor of foods.
- Use home-prepared items with less sugar instead of commercially prepared ones that are higher in sugar.

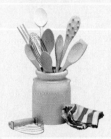

At the Table

- Reduce your use of white and brown sugars, honey, molasses, syrups, jams, and jellies.
- Choose fewer foods high in sugar, such as prepared baked goods, candies, and sweet desserts.
- Reach for fresh fruit instead of cookies or candy for dessert and between-meal snacks.
- Add less sugar to foods—coffee, tea, cereal, and fruit. Cut back gradually to a quarter or half the amount. Consider using sugar alternatives to substitute for some sugar.
- Reduce the number of sugared soft drinks, punches, and fruit juices you drink. Substitute water, diet soft drinks, and whole fruits.

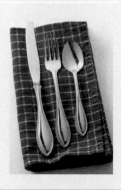

Many individuals lack knowledge about fiber-rich food sources and their benefits. Also, food ingredient labels can be confusing. For example, manufacturers list enriched white (refined) flour as "wheat flour" on food labels. Most people think that, if "wheat flour" or "wheat bread" is on the label, they are buying a whole-wheat product. However, if the label does not list "whole-wheat flour" first, the product is not truly whole-wheat bread and does not contain as much fiber as it could. Careful label reading is important

Figure 5-9 The Nutrition Facts panel on food labels can help us choose more nutritious foods. Based on the information from these panels, note which cereal is the better choice for breakfast. When choosing a breakfast cereal, it is generally wise to focus on those that are rich sources of fiber. Sugar content also can be used for evaluation. However, sometimes the value listed for sugar does not reflect added sugar but the addition of fruits, such as raisins.

Nutrition Facts

Serving Size: 1 cup (55g/2.0 oz.)
Servings Per Container: 10

Amount Per Serving	Cereal	Cereal with ½ Cup Vitamins A & D Skim Milk
Calories	170	210
Calories from Fat	10	10
	% Daily Value**	
Total Fat 1.0g*	2%	2%
Sat. Fat 0g	0%	0%
Trans Fat 0g		*
Cholesterol 0mg	0%	0%
Sodium 300mg	13%	15%
Potassium 340mg	10%	16%
Total Carbohydrate 43g	14%	16%
Dietary Fiber 7g	28%	28%
Sugars 16g		
Other Carbohydrate 20g		
Protein 4g		
Vitamin A	15%	20%
Vitamin C	20%	22%
Calcium	2%	15%
Iron	65%	65%
Vitamin D	10%	25%
Thiamin	25%	30%
Riboflavin	25%	35%
Niacin	25%	25%
Vitamin B$_6$	25%	25%
Folic acid	30%	30%
Vitamin B$_{12}$	25%	35%
Phosphorus	20%	30%
Magnesium	20%	25%
Zinc	25%	25%
Copper	10%	10%

*Amount in cereal. One half cup skim milk contributes an additional 40 calories, 65mg sodium, 6g total carbohydrate (6g sugars), and 4g protein.
**Percent Daily Values are based on a 2,000 calorie diet. Your daily values may be higher or lower depending on your calorie needs:

		Calories:	2,000	2,500
Total Fat	Less than		65g	80g
Sat Fat	Less than		20g	25g
Cholesterol	Less than		300mg	300mg
Sodium	Less than		2,400mg	2,400mg
Potassium			3,500mg	3,500mg
Total Carbohydrate			300g	375g
Dietary Fiber			25g	30g

Calories per gram:
Fat 9 • Carbohydrate 4 • Protein 4

*Intake of *trans* fat should be as low as possible.

Ingredients: Wheat bran with other parts of wheat, raisins, sugar, corn syrup, salt, malt flavoring, glycerin, iron, niacinamide, zinc oxide, pyridoxine hydrochloride (vitamin B$_6$), riboflavin (vitamin B$_2$), vitamin A palmitate, thiamin hydrochloride (vitamin B$_1$), folic acid, vitamin B$_{12}$, and vitamin D.

Nutrition Facts

Serving Size: ¾ Cup (30g)
Servings Per Package: About 17

Amount Per Serving	1 Cup Cereal	Cereal With ½ Cup Skim Milk
Calories	170	200
Calories from Fat	0	5
	%Daily Value**	
Total Fat 0g*	0%	1%
Saturated Fat 0g	0%	1%
Trans Fat 0g		*
Cholesterol 0mg	0%	1%
Sodium 60mg	2%	4%
Potassium 80mg	2%	8%
Total Carbohydrate 35g	9%	11%
Dietary Fiber 1g	4%	4%
Sugars 20g		
Other Carbohydrate 13g		
Protein 3g		
Vitamin A	25%	30%
Vitamin C	0%	2%
Calcium	0%	15%
Iron	10%	10%
Vitamin D	10%	20%
Thiamin	25%	25%
Riboflavin	25%	35%
Niacin	25%	25%
Vitamin B$_6$	25%	25%
Folic acid	25%	25%
Vitamin B$_{12}$	25%	30%
Phosphorus	4%	15%
Magnesium	4%	8%
Zinc	10%	10%
Copper	2%	2%

*Amount in Cereal. One-half cup skim milk contributes an additional 65mg sodium, 6g total carbohydrate (6g sugars), and 4g protein.
**Percent Daily Values are based on a 2,000 calorie diet. Your daily values may be higher or lower depending on your calorie needs:

		Calories:	2,000	2,500
Total Fat	Less than		65g	80g
Sat. Fat	Less than		20g	25g
Cholesterol	Less than		300mg	300mg
Sodium	Less than		2,400mg	2,400mg
Potassium			3,500mg	3,500mg
Total Carbohydrate			300g	375g
Dietary Fiber			25g	30g

Calories per gram:
Fat 9 • Carbohydrate 4 • Protein 4

*Intake of *trans* fat should be as low as possible.

Ingredients: Wheat, Sugar, Corn Syrup, Honey, Caramel Color, Partially Hydrogenated Soybean Oil, Salt, Ferric Phosphate, Niacinamide (Niacin), Zinc Oxide, Vitamin A (Palmitate), Pyridoxine Hydrochloride (Vitamin B6), Riboflavin, Thiamin Mononitrate, Folic Acid (Folate), Vitamin B12 and Vitamin D.

in the search for more fiber—especially for whole grains. Meeting fiber recommendations is possible if you include whole-wheat bread, fruits, vegetables, and legumes as a regular part of your diet. Eating a high-fiber cereal for breakfast is one easy way to increase your fiber intake (Fig. 5-9).[14] Use the Take Action activity to estimate the fiber content of your diet. What is *your* fiber score?

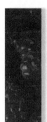

Knowledge Check

1. Why is the RDA for carbohydrate intake set at 130 g/day? Is this an optimal intake?
2. What is the Adequate Intake for dietary fiber?
3. Why are the dietary fiber intakes of many North Americans far below the recommended level?

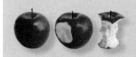

Take Action

Estimate Your Fiber Intake

To roughly estimate your daily fiber consumption, determine the number of servings that you ate yesterday from each food category listed here. Multiply the serving amount by the value listed and then add up the total amount of fiber.

Food	Servings	Grams
Vegetables		
(Serving size: 1 cup raw leafy greens or ½ cup other vegetables)	_____ × 2	_____
Fruits		
(Serving size: 1 whole fruit; ½ grapefruit; ½ cup berries or cubed fruit; ¼ cup dried fruit)	_____ × 2.5	_____
Beans, lentils, split peas		
(Serving size: ½ cup cooked)	_____ × 7	_____
Nuts, seeds		
(Serving size: ¼ cup; 2 tbsp peanut butter)	_____ × 2.5	_____
Whole grains		
(Serving size: 1 slice whole-wheat bread, ½ cup whole-wheat pasta, brown rice, or other whole grain; ½ each bran or whole-grain muffin)	_____ × 2.5	_____
Refined grains		
(Serving size: 1 slice bread; ½ cup pasta, rice, or other processed grains; ½ each refined bagels or muffins)	_____ × 1	_____
Breakfast cereals		
(Serving size: check package for serving size and amount of fiber per serving)	_____ × grams of fiber per serving	_____
Total grams of fiber =		_____

Adapted from Fiber: Strands of protection. *Consumer Reports on Health*, p. 1, August 1999.

How does your total fiber intake for yesterday compare with the general recommendation of 25 to 38 g of fiber per day for women and men, respectively? If you are not meeting your needs, how could you do so?

5.4 Functions of Carbohydrates in the Body

The digestible and indigestible carbohydrates in our diets have vital functions in our bodies.[3] These diverse functions are critical to normal metabolism and overall health.

Digestible Carbohydrates

Most of the digestible carbohydrates in our diets are broken down to glucose. As glucose, they provide a primary source of energy, spare protein from use as an energy source, and prevent ketosis.

Providing Energy

The main function of glucose is to act as a source of energy for body cells. In fact, red blood cells and cells of the central nervous system derive almost all of their energy from glucose. Glucose also fuels muscle cells and other body cells, although many of these cells rely on fatty acids to meet energy needs, especially during rest and light activity. Recall that glucose provides 4 kcal of energy per gram.

Sparing Protein from Use as an Energy Source

The amino acids that make up dietary protein are used to build body tissues and to perform other vital processes only when carbohydrate intake provides enough glucose for energy needs. If you do not consume enough carbohydrate to yield glucose, your body is forced to break down amino acids in your muscle tissue and other organs to make glucose. This process is termed **gluconeogenesis,** which means the production of new glucose (see Chapter 9 for details). However, when dietary carbohydrate intake is adequate to maintain blood glucose levels, protein is "spared" from use as energy. Generally, North Americans consume ample protein, so sparing protein is not an important role of carbohydrate in the diet. It does become important in some energy-reduced diets and in starvation. (Chapter 7 discusses the specific effects of starvation.)

Preventing Ketosis

A minimal intake of carbohydrates—at least 50 to 100 g/day—is necessary for the complete breakdown of fats to carbon dioxide (CO_2) and water (H_2O) in the body.[3] When carbohydrate intake falls below this level, the release of the hormone **insulin** decreases, resulting in the release of a large amount of fatty acids from adipose tissue to provide energy for body cells. These fatty acids travel in the bloodstream to the liver. The subsequent incomplete breakdown of these fatty acids in the liver results in the formation of acidic compounds called ketone bodies, or keto-acids, and a condition called ketosis, or ketoacidosis (see Chapter 9). Ketone bodies include acetoacetic acid and its derivatives.

Although the brain and other cells of the central nervous system normally cannot utilize energy from fats, these cells adapt to use ketones for energy when carbohydrate intake is inadequate. This is an important adaptive mechanism for survival during starvation.[3] If the brain could not use ketone bodies, the body would be forced to produce much more glucose from protein to support the brain's energy needs. The resulting breakdown of muscles, heart, and other organs to provide protein for gluconeogenesis would severely limit our ability to tolerate starvation.

Excessive ketone production also can occur in untreated diabetes. This is not usually the result of low carbohydrate intake, however. Diabetic ketosis develops when insulin production is inadequate or cells resist insulin action, thereby preventing glucose from entering body cells. Cells then rely on ketone bodies for energy. The accumulation of these ketones in the blood results in a more acidic pH. This condition, called diabetic ketoacidosis, is a very serious complication of untreated and poorly controlled diabetes.

gluconeogenesis Synthesis of new glucose by metabolic pathways in the cell. Amino acids derived from protein usually provide the carbons for this glucose.

insulin Hormone produced by beta cells of the pancreas. Among other processes, insulin increases the movement of glucose from the bloodstream into body cells, increases the synthesis of glycogen in the liver, and decreases the breakdown of fat (lipolysis).

Many low-carbohydrate/high-fat weight-reduction diets (e.g., the Atkins™ and South Beach™ diets) and fasting regimens promote ketosis as a beneficial state for successful weight loss. Ketosis can suppress one's appetite, resulting in a lower calorie intake. It also can cause increased loss of water from the body, which may be reflected in lower body weight. However, over time, ketosis can lead to serious consequences, such as dehydration, loss of lean body mass, and electrolyte imbalances. If severe, ketosis can cause coma and death..

Indigestible Carbohydrates

Although fiber is indigestible, it plays an important role in maintaining the integrity of the GI tract and overall health. Fiber helps prevent constipation and diverticular disease and enhances the management of body weight, blood glucose levels, and blood cholesterol levels.

Promoting Bowel Health

Fiber adds bulk to the feces, making bowel movements easier. When adequate fiber and fluid are consumed, the stool is large and soft because many types of plant fibers absorb water. The larger size stimulates the intestinal muscles, which aids elimination. Consequently, less force is necessary to expel the feces.

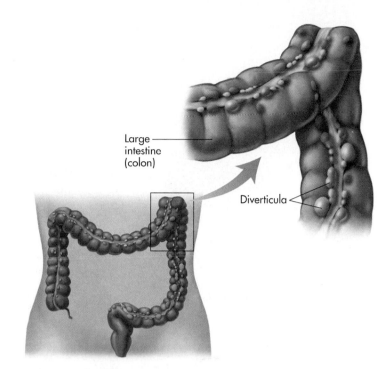

Figure 5-10 Diverticula in the large intestine. A low-fiber diet increases the risk of developing diverticula. About one-third of people over age 45 have this condition, whereas two-thirds of people over 85 do.

When too little fiber is eaten, the opposite can occur: the stool may be small and hard. Constipation may result, causing one to exert excessive force in the large intestine during defecation. Over time, excessive exertion can lead to the development of hemorrhoids. This high pressure from exertion also can cause parts of the large intestine wall to protrude through the surrounding bands of muscle, forming small pouches called **diverticula.**[15] Fibrous material, feces, and bacteria can become trapped in diverticula and lead to inflammation (Fig. 5-10).

Diverticular disease is asymptomatic (without noticeable symptoms) in about 80% of affected people. The asymptomatic form of this condition is called **diverticulosis.** If the diverticula become inflamed and symptomatic, the condition is known as **diverticulitis.** Intake of fiber then should be reduced to limit further bacterial activity and inflammation. Once the inflammation subsides, a high-fiber and high-fluid diet, along with regular physical activity, is advised to restore GI tract motility and reduce the risk of a future attack.[15]

Over the past 30 years, epidemiological studies have shown an association between increased fiber intake and decreased risk of colon cancer. However, more recently, scientists have questioned these findings.[8, 11] Current studies of diet and colon cancer are focusing on the potential preventive effects of increased intakes of fruits, vegetables, legumes, and whole-grain breads and cereals (rather than fiber per se); regular exercise; and adequate vitamin D, folate, magnesium, selenium, and calcium intakes. Overall, it appears that the potential cancer prevention benefits of a high-fiber diet are, for the most part, due to the nutrients that are commonly part of high-fiber foods, such as vitamins, minerals, and phytochemicals. Thus, it is more advisable to increase fiber intake using fiber-rich foods than to rely on fiber supplements.[8]

Reducing Obesity Risk

A diet high in fiber likely aids weight control and reduces the risk of developing obesity.[16] The bulky nature of high-fiber foods fills us up without yielding much energy. Fibrous foods also absorb water and expand in the GI tract, which may contribute to satiety, or a sense of fullness.

CRITICAL THINKING

Karla has a family history of colon cancer. What dietary advice would you give her to reduce her risk of developing colon cancer?

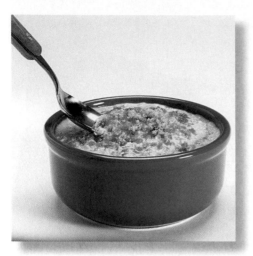

Because oatmeal is rich in soluble fiber, the FDA allows oatmeal package labels to list the benefits of oatmeal in lowering blood cholesterol as a part of a low-fat diet.

Enhancing Blood Glucose Control

When consumed in recommended amounts, soluble fibers slow glucose absorption from the small intestine and decrease insulin release from the pancreas. This contributes to better blood glucose regulation, which can be helpful in the treatment of diabetes. In fact, adults with low-fiber diets are more likely to develop diabetes than are those with high-fiber diets.[17, 18]

Reducing Cholesterol Absorption

A high intake of soluble fiber inhibits the absorption of cholesterol and the reabsorption of bile acids from the small intestine, thereby reducing the risk of cardiovascular disease and gallstones. The short-chain fatty acids resulting from bacterial degradation of soluble fiber in the large intestine also reduce cholesterol synthesis in the liver. Overall, a fiber-rich diet containing fruits, vegetables, legumes, and whole-grain breads and cereals is advocated as part of a strategy to reduce the risk of cardiovascular disease.[17, 19] Recall from Chapter 2 that the FDA has approved the claims that diets rich in whole-grain foods and other plant foods and low in total fat, saturated fat, and cholesterol may decrease the risk of cardiovascular disease and certain cancers.

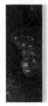

Knowledge Check

1. What are 3 functions of digestible carbohydrates?
2. How does carbohydrate spare protein from use as an energy source?
3. Why are indigestible carbohydrates an important component of our diets?

5.5 Carbohydrate Digestion and Absorption

The goal of carbohydrate digestion is to break down starch and sugars into monosaccharide units that are small enough to be absorbed. Food preparation can be viewed as the start of carbohydrate digestion because cooking softens the tough, fibrous tissues of vegetables, fruits, and grains. When starches are heated, the starch granules swell as they soak up water, making them much easier to digest. All these effects of cooking generally make these foods easier to chew, swallow, and break down during digestion.

Digestion

The enzymatic digestion of some carbohydrates begins in the mouth. Saliva contains an enzyme called salivary **amylase,** which mixes with starch containing amylose when the food is chewed. Amylase breaks down the starch into smaller polysaccharide and disaccharide units (Fig. 5-11). Because food is in the mouth for such a short amount of time, this phase of digestion is only a minor part of the overall digestive process.

When food reaches the stomach, the salivary enzyme is inactivated by the acidity of the stomach. Thus, the digestion of carbohydrate stops until it passes into the small intestine. In the small intestine, the polysaccharides in the food that were first acted on in the mouth now are digested further by pancreatic amylase. Disaccharides are digested to their monosaccharide units by specialized enzymes in the absorptive cells of the small intestine. The disaccharides include maltose from starch breakdown, lactose mainly from dairy products, and sucrose from sweetened foods. The enzyme **maltase** acts on maltose to produce 2 glucose molecules. **Sucrase** breaks down sucrose to produce glucose and fructose. **Lactase** digests lactose to produce glucose and galactose. Monosaccharides that occur in food (usually as glucose or fructose) do not require further digestion in the small intestine. The indigestible carbohydrates (dietary fibers and a small portion of starch in whole grains and some fruits, called resistant starch) cannot be broken down by the digestive enzymes of the small intestine. As discussed previously, they pass into the large intestine, where they are fermented by bacteria into acids and gases or are excreted in fecal waste.

Carbohydrates

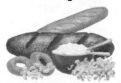

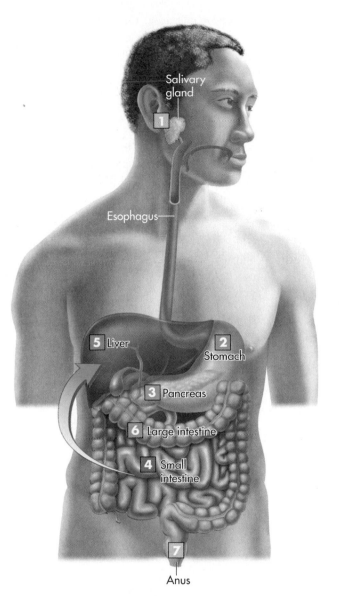

1 Mouth: Some starch is broken down to polysaccharide and disaccharide units by salivary amylase.

2 Stomach: Salivary amylase is inactivated by the acidity in the stomach. No further digestion occurs in the stomach.

3 Pancreas: Pancreatic amylase is secreted into the small intestine to break polysaccharides from starch into disaccharides.

4 Small intestine: Enzymes in the wall of the small intestine break down the disaccharides into monosaccharides.

5 The absorbed monosaccharides are transported to the liver by the portal vein.

6 Large intestine: Some soluble fiber is metabolized into acids and gases by bacteria in the large intestine.

7 Rectum and anus: Insoluble fiber escapes digestion and is excreted in feces.

Figure 5-11 Carbohydrate digestion and absorption. Enzymes made by the salivary glands, pancreas, and small intestine participate in the process of digestion. Most carbohydrate digestion and absorption take place in the small intestine (see Chapter 4 for details).

Intestinal diseases can interfere with the digestion of carbohydrates, such as lactose, and prevent their breakdown and absorption. When unabsorbed carbohydrates reach the large intestine, bacteria there digest them, producing acids and gases as by-products (see Fig. 5-11). If produced in large amounts, these gases can cause abdominal discomfort. People recovering from intestinal disorders, such as diarrhea, may need to avoid lactose for a few weeks or more because of temporary lactose maldigestion and malabsorption. A few weeks is often sufficient time for the small intestine to resume producing enough lactase enzyme to allow for more complete lactose digestion (see the later section on lactose intolerance).[4]

Absorption

With the exception of fructose, monosaccharides are absorbed by an active absorption process. Recall from Chapter 4 that this process requires a specific carrier and energy input for the substance to be taken up by the absorptive cells in the small intestine. Following digestion, glucose and galactose are pumped into the absorptive cells, along with sodium (Fig. 5-12). The ATP energy used in the process pumps sodium back out of the absorptive cell.

Fructose is taken up by the absorptive cells via facilitated diffusion. In this case, a carrier is used, but no energy input is needed. This absorptive process is slower than that of

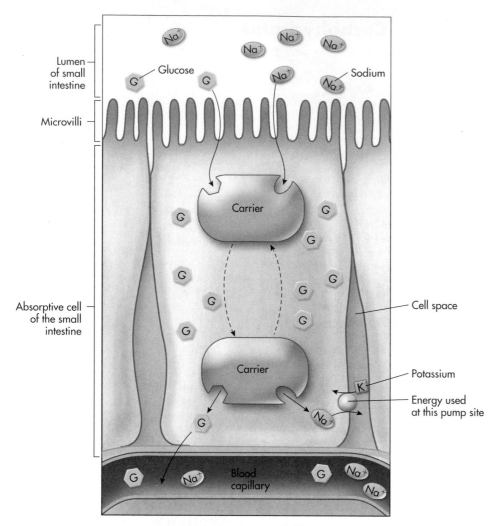

Figure 5-12 Active absorption of glucose in the absorptive cells that line the villi in the small intestine (see Figure 4-14 for a diagram of villi). Glucose and sodium pass across the absorptive cell membrane in a carrier-dependent, energy-requiring process. Once inside the absorptive cell, glucose can exit by facilitated diffusion and enter the bloodstream. Sodium is pumped out of the absorptive cell to maintain a low concentration in the absorptive cell and a high concentration in the extracellular fluid.

glucose or galactose. Once glucose, galactose, and fructose enter the intestinal cells, glucose and galactose remain in that form, whereas some fructose is converted to glucose. These monosaccharides are then transported via the portal vein to the liver. Within the liver, fructose and galactose are converted to glucose. Glucose is transported through the bloodstream for use by the cells of the body. If blood glucose levels are adequate to meet the energy needs of body cells, the liver stores additional glucose as glycogen. (Muscle cells also can store glycogen.) Although the liver's capacity to store glycogen is limited, glycogen storage provides an important reserve of energy to maintain blood glucose levels and cellular function. When carbohydrates are consumed in very high amounts, the glycogen storage capacity of the liver (and muscles) often is exceeded. The liver then converts the excess glucose to fat for storage in adipose tissue.

Knowledge Check

1. What is the goal of carbohydrate digestion?
2. Why do some individuals with intestinal diseases need to temporarily restrict their consumption of foods containing lactose?
3. How are monosaccharides absorbed?

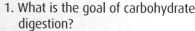 ## 5.6 Health Concerns Related to Carbohydrate Intake

As a part of a nutritious diet, adequate carbohydrate intake is important for maintaining health and decreasing the risk of chronic disease. However, as with many nutrients, excessive intakes of different forms of carbohydrate can be harmful to overall health. The following discussions will help you understand the benefits and risks of varied intakes of different types of carbohydrates.

Very High Fiber Diets

Adequate fiber intake provides many health benefits. However, very high intakes of fiber (i.e., above 50 to 60 g/day) can cause health risks. For example, high fiber consumption combined with low fluid intake can result in hard, dry stools that are painful to eliminate. Over time, this may cause hemorrhoids from increased exertion and pressure, as well as rectal bleeding. In severe cases, the combination of excess fiber and insufficient fluid may contribute to blockages in the intestine, requiring surgery.

Very high fiber diets also may decrease the absorption of certain minerals and increase the risk of deficiencies. This occurs because some minerals can bind to fiber, which prevents them from being absorbed. In countries where fiber intake is often greater than 60 g/day, deficiencies of zinc and iron have been reported.

High fiber diets can be of concern in young children, elderly persons, and malnourished individuals, all of whom may not eat adequate amounts of foods and nutrients. For these individuals, high fiber intakes may cause a sense of fullness and reduce their overall intake of foods, energy, and nutrients.

High Sugar Diets

For many Americans, sugars constitute a large part of their daily diets. In fact, on average, North Americans eat about 20 teaspoons (82 grams) of sugars daily. Recall that most of the sugar we eat comes from foods and beverages to which sugar has been added during processing and/or manufacturing. Major sources of added sugar are soft drinks, cakes, cookies, fruit punch, and dairy desserts, such as ice cream. Although sugars supply calories, they usually provide little else and often replace the intake of more nutritious foods. Children and adolescents are typically at greatest risk of overconsuming sugar and empty calories.[20] Dietary surveys indicate that many children and adolescents are drinking an excess of sugar-sweetened beverages and much less milk than ever before. Milk contains calcium and vitamin D, both of which are essential for bone health. Thus, replacing sugared drinks for milk can compromise bone development and health.

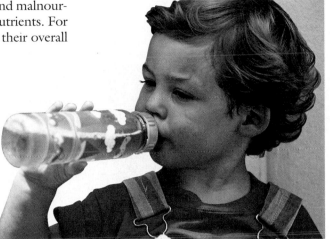

High carbohydrate beverages can contribute to tooth decay.

High intakes of sugars also can increase the risk of weight gain and obesity. (It is important to note, however, that, although obesity is a risk factor for type 2 diabetes, high sugar diets do not directly cause diabetes.)[21] The "supersizing" trend noted in food and beverage promotions is contributing to this concern. For example, in the 1950s, a typical soft drink serving was a 6.5-ounce bottle. Today, a 20-ounce bottle is a typical serving. This change alone contributes 170 extra calories of sugar to the diet. Drinking 1 bottle per day for a year would amount to 62,050 extra calories and a 17- to 18-pound (7.75–8.25 kg) weight gain.

The sugar in cakes, cookies, and ice cream also supplies extra energy, which promotes weight gain. Although dieters may be choosing more low-fat and fat-free snack products, these usually are made with substantial amounts of added sugar in order to produce a dessert with an acceptable taste and texture. The resulting product often is a high-calorie food that equals or even exceeds the energy content of the original high-fat food product it was designed to replace.

High intakes of sugar (especially fructose) have been associated with conditions that increase the risk of cardiovascular disease—namely, increased blood levels of triglycerides and LDL cholesterol and decreased levels of HDL cholesterol.[22] To date, scientists do not have enough evidence to conclude that increased sugar intake is a risk factor for cardiovascular disease. However, it is prudent to decrease intake of products sweetened with high-fructose corn syrup, the major source of excess fructose in our diets.

Diets high in sugar have been reported to cause hyperactivity in children. However, scientists have determined that hyperactivity and other behavioral problems are likely due to a variety of non-nutritional factors. Although eating a nutritious diet is important for a child's overall health and well-being, it will not prevent hyperactivity, behavioral problems, or learning disabilities.

High sugar diets increase the risk of developing dental caries (cavities).[23] Dental caries can develop when bacteria in the mouth metabolize sugars into acids (Fig. 5-13). The acids gradually dissolve the tooth enamel and the underlying structure, causing decay, discomfort, and even nerve damage. Sugar from any source can lead to caries. Sticky and gummy foods that are high in sugar and adhere to teeth, such as caramels, licorice, and gummy bears, are the most likely to promote dental caries. Starches that are readily fermented in the mouth, such as crackers and white bread, also increase the risk of dental caries. Sipping fruit juices, soft drinks, and milk throughout the day bathes

Figure 5-13 Dental caries. Bacteria in the mouth metabolize sugars in food and create acids that can dissolve tooth enamel. This leads to the development of caries. If the caries progress into the pulp cavity, damage to the nerve and pain are likely.

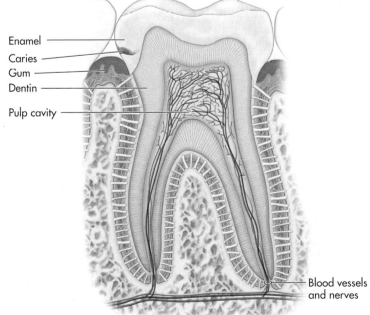

Enamel
Caries
Gum
Dentin
Pulp cavity
Blood vessels and nerves

the teeth in sugar and can increase the risk of caries.[23] Thus, parents should be cautioned against serving infants and young children these beverages to sip on between meals.

Lactose Intolerance

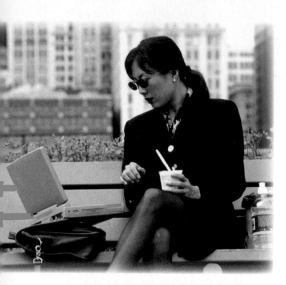

Yogurt helps those with lactose intolerance meet their calcium needs.

The amount of the enzyme lactase produced in the small intestine often begins to decrease after early childhood. The insufficiency of lactase, referred to as *primary* lactose intolerance, can cause symptoms of abdominal pain, bloating, gas, and diarrhea after consuming lactose, especially in large amounts. The bloating and gas are caused by the bacterial fermentation of undigested lactose in the large intestine. The undigested lactose also draws water into the large intestine, causing diarrhea.

Primary lactose intolerance may occur in up to 75% of the world's population. In North America, approximately 25% of adults show signs of decreased lactose digestion. Those who have Asian, African, or Latino/Hispanic backgrounds are more likely to experience lactose intolerance than Caucasians. Some people with primary lactose intolerance do not experience symptoms. In addition, many are able to consume moderate amounts of lactose with little or no intestinal discomfort because bacteria in the large intestine break down the lactose.[4] In fact, recent studies have shown that nearly all individuals with decreased lactase production can tolerate ½ to 1 cup of milk with meals. Hard cheese, yogurt, and acidophilus milk also are well tolerated because much of the lactose in these foods has been converted to lactic acid. Thus, it is unnecessary for many with lactose intolerance to greatly restrict their intakes of lactose-containing foods, such as milk and other dairy products.

Another type of lactose intolerance, called *secondary* lactose intolerance, occurs when conditions of the small intestine, such as Crohn's disease and severe diarrhea, damage the cells that produce lactase.[3] Secondary lactose intolerance also can cause gastrointestinal symptoms, but the symptoms are usually temporary and cease when the intestine recovers and lactase production normalizes.

Glucose Intolerance

hyperglycemia High blood glucose, above 126 mg/dl of blood on a fasting basis.

hypoglycemia Low blood glucose, below 50 mg/dl of blood.

Maintaining blood glucose within normal ranges is important for providing adequate glucose for body functions and for preventing the symptoms associated with changes in blood glucose levels. Abnormal regulation of blood glucose can lead to either **hyperglycemia** (high blood glucose) or **hypoglycemia** (low blood glucose). Hyperglycemia is a more common condition than hypoglycemia and is most commonly associated with diabetes (technically, *diabetes mellitus*) and Metabolic Syndrome.

Regulation of Blood Glucose

Under fasting conditions (several hours after eating), blood glucose normally varies between about 70 and 100 mg/dl of blood. A fasting blood glucose level above 126 mg/dl is classified as "diabetes." The symptoms of diabetes include hunger, thirst, frequent urination, and weight loss. When blood glucose falls below 50 mg/dl, the condition is classified as "hypoglycemia," and the person may experience hunger, shakiness, irritability, weakness, and headache as energy availability decreases.

The liver is important in controlling the amount of glucose in the bloodstream. As the first organ to screen the sugars absorbed from the small intestine, the liver helps de-

CASE STUDY

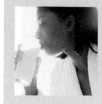

Myeshia, a 19-year-old female, recently read about the health benefits of calcium and decided to increase her intake of dairy products by drinking milk. Not long afterward, she experienced bloating, cramping, and gassiness. She suspected that the source of this discomfort was the milk she consumed, especially because her parents and sister had complained of the same problem. She wanted to determine if the milk was, in fact, the cause of her gastrointestinal discomfort, so the next day she substituted yogurt for the milk in her diet. Subsequently, she did not have any symptoms. What component of milk likely caused the problem? Why was she able to tolerate yogurt but not milk?

termine the amount of glucose that enters the bloodstream after a meal (see Fig. 5-11) and the amount that is stored as glycogen for later use.[3]

The pancreas also is important in blood glucose control. The pancreas releases small amounts of insulin as soon as a person starts to eat. Following carbohydrate digestion and absorption, blood glucose levels rise, signaling the pancreas to release large amounts of insulin. Insulin promotes increased glucose uptake by muscle, nerve, adipose, and other body cells. In addition, insulin promotes the storage of excess glucose as glycogen. These actions lower blood glucose to the normal fasting range within a few hours after a person eats.

Other hormones in the body counteract the effects of insulin. When a person has not eaten carbohydrates for a few hours, the amount of glucose in the blood is maintained by another pancreatic hormone, called glucagon. Glucagon is secreted in response to a decrease in blood glucose. It prompts the breakdown of glycogen in the liver and promotes gluconeogenesis, resulting in the release of glucose to the bloodstream and the normalization of blood glucose levels (Fig. 5-14).[3]

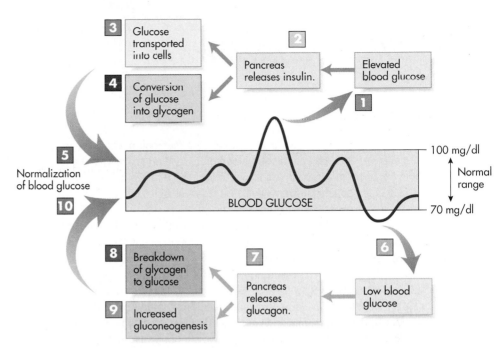

Figure 5-14 Regulation of blood glucose. Insulin and glucagon are key factors in controlling blood glucose. When blood glucose rises above the normal range ▮1, insulin is released ▮2 to lower it ▮3 and ▮4. Blood glucose then falls back into the normal range ▮5. When blood glucose falls below the normal range ▮6, glucagon is released ▮7, which has the opposite effect of insulin ▮8 and ▮9. This then restores blood glucose to the normal range ▮10. Other hormones, such as epinephrine, norepinephrine, cortisol, and growth hormone, also contribute to blood glucose regulation (see Table 5-5 for details).

The hormones epinephrine (adrenaline) and norepinephrine, from the adrenal glands, also trigger the breakdown of glycogen in the liver and result in glucose release into the bloodstream. These hormones are responsible for the "fight or flight" reaction. They are released in large amounts in response to a perceived threat, such as a car approaching head-on. The resulting rapid release of glucose into the bloodstream promotes quick mental and physical reactions. The hormones cortisol and growth hormone also help regulate blood glucose by decreasing glucose use by muscle (Table 5-5).

In essence, the actions of insulin on blood glucose are balanced by the actions of glucagon, epinephrine, norepinephrine, cortisol, and growth hormone. If hormonal balance is not maintained, such as during overproduction or underproduction of insulin or glucagon, major changes in blood glucose concentrations occur.[3] This system of checks and balances allows blood glucose to be maintained within fairly narrow ranges.

Table 5-5 Roles of Various Hormones in the Regulation of Blood Glucose

Hormone	Source	Target Organ or Tissue	Overall Effect on Organ or Tissue	Effect on Blood Glucose
Insulin	Pancreas	Liver, muscle, adipose tissue	Increases glucose uptake by muscles and adipose tissue, increases glycogen synthesis, suppresses gluconeogenesis	Decrease
Glucagon	Pancreas	Liver	Increases glycogen breakdown and release of glucose by the liver, increases gluconeogenesis	Increase
Epinephrine, norepinephrine	Adrenal glands	Liver, muscle	Increases glycogen breakdown and release of glucose by the liver, increases gluconeogenesis	Increase
Cortisol	Adrenal glands	Liver, muscle	Increases gluconeogenesis by the liver, decreases glucose use by muscles and other organs	Increase
Growth hormone	Pituitary gland	Liver, muscle, adipose tissue	Decreases glucose uptake by muscles, increases fat mobilization and utilization, increases glucose output by the liver	Increase

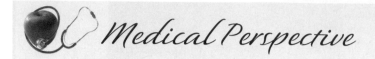

Medical Perspective

Diabetes Mellitus

As mentioned previously, an inability to regulate glucose metabolism can result in diabetes. Diagnosis of diabetes is based on a **fasting blood glucose level** above 126 mg/dl. Diabetes affects about 6% of North Americans and leads to over 200,000 deaths each year. An additional 15% of our population shows evidence of pre-diabetes (indicated by a borderline high blood glucose level between 100 and 126 mg/dl).

There are two major forms of diabetes: **type 1 diabetes** (formerly called insulin-dependent, or juvenile-onset diabetes) and **type 2 diabetes** (formerly called non-insulin-dependent, or adult-onset diabetes) (Table 5-6). The change in names to type 1 and type 2 diabetes stems from the fact that many with type 2 diabetes eventually must rely on insulin injections as a part of their treatment.[24] Approximately 90% of individuals with diabetes have type 2 diabetes.

In type 1 diabetes, individuals develop the classic symptoms of hyperglycemia (increased hunger, thirst, urination, and weight loss). However, in type 2 diabetes, 30 to 50% of individuals may not have any symptoms and are not aware that they have diabetes until diagnosed in routine health screening tests. Thus, new guidelines promote testing fasting blood glucose levels in adults over age 45 every 3 years to avoid missing cases and to prevent related morbidity and mortality.

A third form of diabetes is called gestational diabetes. Gestational diabetes occurs in approximately 7% of all pregnancies. It is usually treated with insulin and dietary modification, and it resolves after delivery of the baby. However, pregnant women who develop gestational diabetes are at high risk of developing type 2 diabetes later in life.[24]

fasting blood glucose Measurement of glucose levels in the blood taken after an 8- to 12-hour or overnight period without any food or caloric beverages (a fast).

type 1 diabetes Autoimmune disease causing failure of the pancreas to produce insulin and an inability to control blood glucose levels.

type 2 diabetes Progressive disease characterized by insulin resistance or loss of responsiveness of body cells to insulin, resulting in hyperglycemia.

▶ The classic symptoms of diabetes include polyuria (excessive urination), polydipsia (excessive thirst), and polyphagia (excessive hunger). No one symptom is diagnostic of diabetes. Other symptoms—such as unexplained weight loss, exhaustion, and blurred vision—may accompany these symptoms.[2]

▶ A common clinical method to determine a person's success in controlling blood glucose is to measure glycated (or glycosylated) hemoglobin (hemoglobin A1c). Over time, blood glucose attaches to (glycates) hemoglobin in red blood cells, especially when blood glucose remains elevated. Hemoglobin A1c values over 6.5 to 7% indicate poor blood glucose control.

Table 5-6 Comparison of Type 1 and Type 2 Diabetes

	Type 1 Diabetes	Type 2 Diabetes
Occurrence	5–10% of cases of diabetes	90% of cases of diabetes
Cause	Autoimmune attack on the pancreas	Insulin resistance
Risk Factors	Moderate genetic predisposition	Strong genetic predisposition Obesity and physical inactivity Ethnicity Metabolic Syndrome Pre-diabetes
Characteristics	Distinct symptoms (frequent thirst, hunger, and urination) Ketosis Weight loss	Mild symptoms, especially in early phases of the disease (fatigue and nighttime urination) Ketosis does not generally occur.
Treatment	Insulin Diet Exercise	Diet Exercise Oral medications to lower blood glucose Insulin (in advanced cases)
Complications	Cardiovascular disease Kidney disease Nerve disease Blindness Infections	Cardiovascular disease Kidney disease Nerve damage Blindness Infections
Monitoring	Blood glucose Urine ketones HbA1c*	Blood glucose HbA1c

*Hemoglobin A1c

CRITICAL THINKING

John and Mike are twins who like the same activities and foods. At a recent doctor's appointment, John was told that he has type 2 diabetes. He has been feeling good and has not noticed any changes in his health. He does not understand why he has diabetes and his brother does not and why he has not had any noticeable symptoms. How would you explain this to him?

Type 1 Diabetes

Although type 1 diabetes can occur at any age, it often begins in late childhood, between 8 and 12 years of age. The disease runs in families, suggesting a genetic link. Thus, children and siblings of those with diabetes are at increased risk. Most cases of type 1 diabetes begin as an autoimmune disorder that destroys the insulin-producing cells in the pancreas. As the pancreas loses its ability to synthesize insulin and thus regulate blood glucose levels, the clinical symptoms of the disease develop.

The onset of type 1 diabetes is associated with decreased release of insulin from the pancreas and increased blood glucose, especially after eating. When blood glucose exceeds the kidney's threshold for returning it to the bloodstream, the excess glucose ends up in the urine—hence the term *diabetes mellitus,* which means "flow of much urine" (*diabetes*) that is "sweet" (*mellitus*). Figure 5-15 shows a typical glucose tolerance curve observed in a patient with type 1 diabetes, after eating a test load of about 20 teaspoons (75 grams) of glucose.

Before 1921, if a person had type 1 diabetes, a high-fat, low-calorie diet was recommended. This approach was somewhat effective but resulted in poor growth in childhood and was difficult to follow. The isolation of insulin by Banting and Best in 1921, and the first use of it soon after by children, opened a new door in diabetes care.

Type 1 diabetes is treated by insulin therapy, either with injections several times per day or with an insulin pump. The pump dispenses insulin at a steady rate into the body, with greater amounts delivered after a meal. Dietary therapy includes

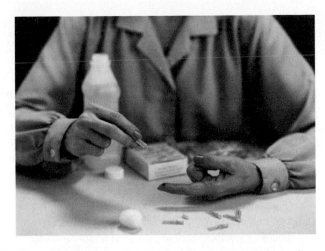

Checking blood glucose regularly is an important part of diabetes therapy.

3 regular meals and 1 or more snacks (including a bedtime snack), as well as a regulated ratio of carbohydrate:protein:fat to maximize insulin action and minimize swings in blood glucose.[25] The diet also should include ample fiber, supply energy in balance with expenditure, be low in saturated fats and cholesterol, and meet overall nutritional needs.

Carbohydrate counting and the diabetic exchange system are useful tools for balancing carbohydrate intake and improving blood glucose control while eating a wide selection of foods.[24] The carbohydrate counting method awards 1 point to approximately 12 to 15 g of carbohydrate. The exchange system is described in Appendix E.

Poorly controlled diabetes can lead to short-term and long-term health problems. The hormone imbalances that occur in people with uncontrolled type 1 diabetes lead to the breakdown of body fat for energy. Ketosis develops as fat is converted to ketone bodies. Ketones can increase to high levels in the blood, eventually ending up in the urine. Ketones also pull sodium and potassium ions with them into the urine, leading to dehydration, ion imbalance, coma, and even death. Treatment includes insulin and fluids, as well as sodium, potassium, and chloride.[24]

Over time, poorly controlled diabetes can cause degenerative conditions, such as blindness, cardiovascular disease, and kidney disease. Nerves also can deteriorate, resulting in decreased nerve stimulation throughout the body (called neuropathy). When this occurs in the intestinal tract, intermittent diarrhea and constipation result. Because of nerve deterioration in the arms, hands, legs, and feet, many people with diabetes lose the sensation of pain associated with injuries and infections. Without normal pain sensations, they often delay treatment. This delay, combined with an environment rich in glucose that readily supports bacterial growth, sets the stage for damage to and the death of tissues in the extremities, sometimes even leading to the need for amputation. Poorly controlled diabetes also contributes to a rapid buildup of fats in blood vessel walls, which increases the risk of cardiovascular disease.[24, 26]

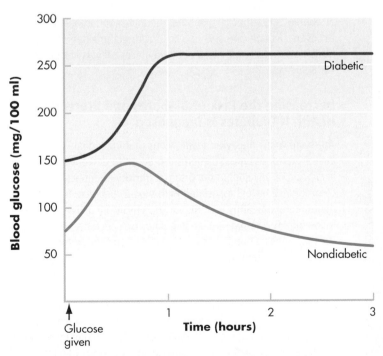

Figure 5-15 Glucose tolerance test. A comparison of blood glucose concentrations in untreated diabetic and healthy nondiabetic persons after consuming a 75-g test load of glucose.

(continued)

Medical Perspective, continued

The Diabetes Control and Complications Trial (DCCT) and other recent studies have shown that the development of diabetes-related cardiovascular disease and nerve damage can be delayed with aggressive treatment directed at keeping blood glucose within the normal range.[26, 27] The therapy poses some risks of its own, however, such as hypoglycemia, so it must be implemented under the close supervision of a physician.

A person with diabetes should work regularly with a physician and dietitian to monitor and adjust (when necessary) diet, medications, and physical activity. Physical activity enhances glucose uptake by muscles independent of insulin action, which in turn can lower blood glucose.[28] This outcome is beneficial, but people with diabetes need to be aware of their own blood glucose response to physical activity and plan appropriately to avoid hypoglycemia.

Type 2 Diabetes

Type 2 diabetes is a progressive disease characterized by insulin resistance or loss of responsiveness by body cells to insulin. As a result, glucose is not readily transferred into cells and builds in the bloodstream, causing hyperglycemia. In type 2 diabetes, insulin production may be low, normal, or at times even elevated. However, regardless of the amount of insulin produced, cells are less responsive to its actions.

Type 2 diabetes is the most common type, accounting for about 90% of the cases diagnosed in North America. Those over age 45 and with Latino/Hispanic, African, Asian, Native American, or Pacific Island backgrounds are at particular risk.[24] The number of people with type 2 diabetes is on the rise, primarily because of widespread inactivity and obesity in our population. There also has been a substantial increase in type 2 diabetes in children, mainly due to an increase in overweight in this population (coupled with limited physical activity). Type 2 diabetes is genetically linked, so

Regular exercise has a key role in decreasing the risk of type 2 diabetes. For individuals with type 2 diabetes, exercise also can be an important part of managing the disease.

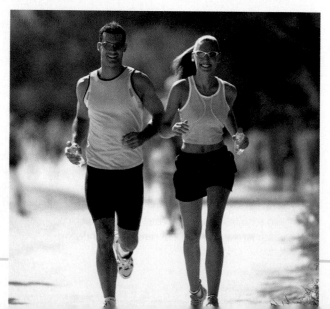

family history is a very important risk factor. Because of this genetic link, those with a family history should be careful to avoid other risk factors, such as obesity, inactivity, and diets rich in saturated fats, cholesterol, and high glycemic load foods.[29-32]

Treatments for type 2 diabetes are aimed at maintaining normal ranges of blood glucose through lifestyle modification and medication use. Adhering to a nutritious diet plan and a regular physical activity program is an important component of therapy. Consistent exercise and an energy-controlled, nutritious diet eaten at regular mealtimes promote a healthy body weight, enhance the uptake of glucose by muscle cells, lower blood lipids and cardiovascular risk, and help achieve normal blood sugar levels. For overweight or obese individuals, even a modest weight loss can improve blood glucose control.[33]

Many with type 2 diabetes need medications in addition to diet modification and regular activity to control blood glucose. Oral medications that reduce glucose production by the liver, increase insulin synthesis by the pancreas, slow intestinal absorption of glucose, or decrease cellular resistance to insulin are used by many with type 2 diabetes to regulate blood glucose.[34] However, when oral medications fail to normalize blood glucose levels, insulin injections are necessary.

Moderate amounts of alcohol (1 serving/day) can be allowed in the diets of those with both type 1 and type 2 diabetes. In fact, for some individuals, small amounts of alcohol may help increase HDL cholesterol and reduce cardiovascular disease risk. However, alcohol intake, especially without adequate food intake, can lead to severe hypoglycemia. Thus, those with diabetes need to use alcohol cautiously and monitor blood glucose levels closely to avoid hypoglycemia.

Decreasing the Risk of Diabetes and Protecting Health If Diabetes Is Diagnosed

There are many lifestyle modifications that individuals with an increased risk of type 2 diabetes can adopt to decrease their likelihood of developing the disease. Obesity and inactivity are common risk factors associated with type 2 diabetes.[21, 31, 33] Thus, maintaining a healthy weight, staying physically active, and following MyPyramid dietary guidelines can decrease diabetes risk. For those with a family history of diabetes and for women with a history of gestational diabetes, regular testing of fasting blood glucose levels or screening through glucose tolerance testing is an important part of personal health care.

Although diabetes is not yet a curable disease, it can be controlled through diet, exercise, and medications. Maintaining good glucose control is critical to prevent long-term diabetes-related complications of cardiovascular disease, renal disease, blindness, and nerve damage. Diabetes education, lifestyle modification, medication management, and self-monitoring of blood glucose levels are essential in maintaining overall health for those with all types of diabetes.

Metabolic Syndrome

Over 50 million American adults have a condition known as Metabolic Syndrome. **Metabolic Syndrome** is characterized by a group of factors that increase the risk of type 2 diabetes and cardiovascular disease, including insulin resistance or glucose intolerance (causing high blood glucose), abdominal obesity, high blood triglycerides and LDL cholesterol with low HDL cholesterol, elevated blood pressure, and increased inflammatory blood proteins (e.g., C-reactive protein) and higher concentrations of oxidized LDL cholesterol (see Chapter 6).[35,36] Metabolic Syndrome also is associated with overall obesity, physical inactivity, genetic predisposition, and aging.

To date, there are no fully established criteria for diagnosing Metabolic Syndrome. The American Heart Association and National Heart Lung and Blood Institute suggest that 3 or more of the following criteria be present for diagnosing Metabolic Syndrome: a waist circumference greater than 35 inches for women and 40 inches for men, a fasting triglyceride level above 150 mg/dl, blood HDL cholesterol below 40 mg/dl for men and below 50 mg/dl for women, elevated blood pressure above 130/85 mm Hg, and fasting blood glucose above 110 mg/dl. Lifestyle modification (focusing on weight loss, decreased dietary fat intake, and increased physical activity) is fundamental to decreasing the health risks associated with Metabolic Syndrome.

Hypoglycemia

Hypoglycemia, or low blood sugar, is a condition that can occur in people with or without diabetes. In those with diabetes, hypoglycemia can occur if they inject too much insulin, if they don't eat frequently enough, or if they exercise without eating additional carbohydrate.

In non-diabetics, 2 types of hypoglycemia have been reported: **reactive hypoglycemia** and **fasting hypoglycemia.** Reactive (or postprandial) hypoglycemia is caused by an exaggerated insulin response after eating. Symptoms of irritability, sweating, anxiety, weakness, headache, and confusion may develop 2 to 5 hours after a meal, especially one high in sugars. Fasting hypoglycemia is a condition of low blood glucose after fasting for 8 hours or more. However, it usually is caused by an underlying serious medical condition, such as cancer, liver disease, or renal disease, rather than by simply fasting.

The diagnosis of hypoglycemia requires the simultaneous presence of a blood glucose level below 50 mg/dl and classic hypoglycemic symptoms. Although healthy people may occasionally experience some hypoglycemic symptoms if they have not eaten for a prolonged period of time, this usually is not true hypoglycemia. However, these individuals also will benefit from the nutritional recommendations given to individuals diagnosed with hypoglycemia. Regular meals consisting of a balance of protein, fat, and low glycemic load carbohydrates, plus ample soluble fiber, help prevent hypoglycemia. Individuals also should substitute protein-containing snacks for those that contain mostly sugar and aim to spread carbohydrate intake throughout the day. Finally, limiting caffeine and alcohol intake can be beneficial in preventing symptoms of hypoglycemia.

▶ For more information on diabetes, consult this website: www.diabetes.org.

reactive hypoglycemia Low blood glucose that may follow a meal high in simple sugars, with corresponding symptoms of irritability, headache, nervousness, sweating, and confusion; also called postprandial hypoglycemia.

fasting hypoglycemia Low blood glucose that occurs after 8 hours or more of fasting.

glycemic index (GI) Blood glucose response of a given food, compared with a standard (typically, glucose or white bread).

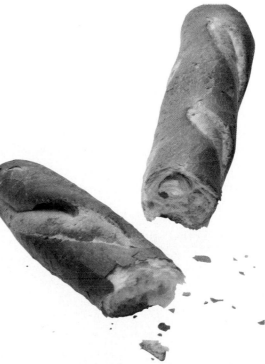

Glycemic Index and Glycemic Load

Our bodies react uniquely to different sources of carbohydrates. For example, a serving of high-fiber brown rice results in lower blood glucose levels, compared with the same-size serving of mashed potatoes. As researchers investigated the glucose response to various foods, they noted that it was not always as predicted. Thus, they developed 2 tools, the glycemic index and the glycemic load, to indicate how blood glucose responds to various foods[35] (Table 5-7).

The **glycemic index (GI)** is a ratio of the blood glucose response of a given food, compared with a standard (typically, glucose or white bread).[37] Glycemic index is influenced by a food's starch structure (amylose vs. amylopectin), fiber content, food processing, physical structure (small vs. large surface area), and temperature, as well as the amount of protein and fat in a meal. Foods with particularly high glycemic index values are potatoes, breads,

Table 5-7 Glycemic Index (GI) and Glycemic Load (GL) of Common Foods

Reference food glucose = 100

Low GI foods—below 55	Low GL foods—below 10
Intermediate GI foods—between 55 and 69	Intermediate GL foods—between 11 and 19
High GI foods—more than 70	High GL foods—more than 20

	Serving Size	Glycemic Index (GI)[1]	Carbohydrate (grams)	Glycemic Load (GL)
Pastas/Grains				
Brown rice	1 cup	55	46	25
White, short grain	1 cup	72	53	38
Vegetables				
Carrots, boiled	1 cup	49	16	8
Sweet corn	1 cup	55	39	21
Potato, baked	1 cup	85	57	48
Dairy Foods				
Milk, fat-free	1 cup	32	12	4
Yogurt, low-fat	1 cup	33	17	6
Ice cream	1 cup	61	31	19
Legumes				
Baked beans	1 cup	48	54	26
Kidney beans	1 cup	27	38	10
Lentils	1 cup	30	40	12
Sugars				
Honey	1 tsp	73	6	4
Sucrose	1 tsp	65	5	3
Lactose	1 tsp	46	5	2
Breads and Muffins				
Whole-wheat bread	1 slice	69	13	9
White bread	1 slice	70	10	7
Fruits				
Apple	1 medium	38	22	8
Banana	1 medium	55	29	16
Orange	1 medium	44	15	7
Peach	1 medium	42	11	5
Beverages				
Orange juice	1 cup	46	26	13
Gatorade	1 cup	78	15	12
Coca-Cola	1 cup	63	26	16
Snack Foods				
Potato chips	1 oz	54	15	8
Chocolate	1 oz	49	18	9
Jelly beans	1 oz	80	26	21

[1]Based on a comparison with glucose.

Source: Foster-Powell K and others. International table of glycemic index and glycemic load. *American Journal of Clinical Nutrition.* 2002; 76:5.

Gatorade, short-grain white rice, honey, and jelly beans. A major shortcoming of the glycemic index is that it is based on a serving of food that would provide 50 grams of carbohydrate. However, this amount of food may not reflect the amount typically consumed.

Glycemic load (GL) takes into account the glycemic index and the amount of carbohydrate consumed, so it better reflects a food's effect on blood glucose than does the glycemic index alone.[37] To calculate the glycemic load of a food, the number of grams of carbohydrate in 1 serving is multiplied by the food's glycemic index, then divided by 100 (because the glycemic index is a percentage). For example, vanilla wafers have a glycemic index of 77, and a serving of 5 cookies contains 15 g of carbohydrate. This yields a glycemic load of approximately 12.

$$(77 \times 15) / 100 = 12$$

Even though the glycemic index of vanilla wafers is considered high, the glycemic load calculation shows that the impact of this food on blood glucose levels is fairly low.

Why should we be concerned with the effects of various foods on blood glucose? Foods with a high glycemic load elicit an increased insulin response from the pancreas and a resulting drop in blood glucose. These dramatic fluctuations in blood glucose can cause short- and long-term consequences in individuals with diabetes.[38] Chronically high insulin output leads to many harmful effects on the body, such as high blood triglycerides, increased fat deposition in the adipose tissue, increased fat synthesis in the liver, and a more rapid return of hunger after a meal. Thus, increasing intakes of lower glycemic load foods is often recommended as a part of a healthful diet.[38] Because foods with a low glycemic load are often those that contain higher amounts of dietary fiber, increasing one's intake of these foods will, in turn, increase fiber intake and may help reduce risk of cardiovascular disease, Metabolic Syndrome, and certain cancers.[38, 39]

Use of the glycemic index and glycemic load remains somewhat controversial. Many researchers question their benefits. Nutritionally, neither tool indicates blood glucose responses when individual foods are eaten as a part of mixed meals. As most high glycemic foods are eaten in combination with low glycemic foods (e.g., rice cereals with milk, macaroni with cheese, bread with peanut butter), the glycemic index and glycemic load are often lower than the value given for these foods individually.

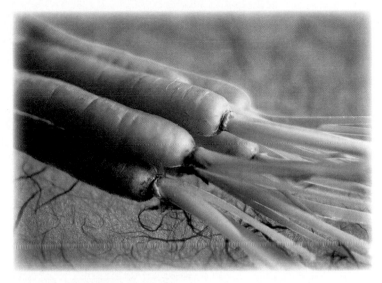
Carrots, criticized in the popular press for having a high glycemic index, actually contribute a low glycemic load to a diet.

glycemic load (GL) Amount of carbohydrate in a food multiplied by the glycemic index of that food. The result is then divided by 100.

▶ You might wonder why the glycemic index and glycemic load of white bread and whole-wheat bread are similar. This is because whole-wheat flour typically is ground so finely that it is quickly digested and absorbed. Thus, experts suggest we focus on more minimally processed grains, such as coarsely ground whole-wheat flour and steel-cut oats, to get the full benefits of these fiber sources in reducing blood glucose levels.

▶ A term you might see on food labels is *net carbs.* Although this term is not FDA-approved, sometimes it is used to describe the carbohydrates that increase blood glucose. Fiber and sugar alcohol content are subtracted from the total carbohydrate content to yield net carbs because they have a negligible effect on blood glucose.

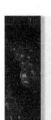
Knowledge Check

1. How do insulin and glucagon regulate blood glucose levels?
2. How does type 1 diabetes differ from type 2 diabetes?
3. What are the health-related risks associated with poorly controlled diabetes?
4. How does the glycemic index differ from the glycemic load?

CASE STUDY FOLLOW-UP

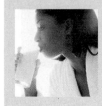
Myeshia suspected she had a problem with milk because, when she consumed it, she developed bloating and gas. She was successful in reducing these symptoms by replacing milk with yogurt. As you just learned, yogurt is tolerated better than milk by people with lactose intolerance because the bacteria that are present in yogurt digest much of the lactose. Note, however, that many people with lactose intolerance actually can consume small to moderate amounts of milk with few or no symptoms from the lactose present.

Summary

5.1 The general formula for carbohydrates is $(CH_2O)n$, where n represents the number of times the ratio is repeated. The common monosaccharides are glucose, fructose, and galactose. Sugar alcohols are derivatives of monosaccharides. Additional monosaccharides found in nature are ribose and deoxyribose. Carbohydrates containing 2 monosaccharides are called disaccharides. Disaccharides include maltose, sucrose, and lactose. Oligosaccharides are complex carbohydrates that contain 3 to 10 single sugar units. Polysaccharides are complex carbohydrates that often contain hundreds to thousands of glucose molecules. Digestible polysaccharides are starch and glycogen. Dietary and functional fibers are indigestible polysaccharides.

5.2 Carbohydrates are found in a wide variety of foods, including table sugar, jam, jelly, fruits, soft drinks, rice, pasta, cereals, breads, dried beans, lentils, corn, peas, and dairy products. Starches contribute much of the carbohydrate in our diets. A diet rich in grains, legumes, and tubers also can provide significant amounts of dietary fiber (especially insoluble cellulose, hemicellulose, and lignins). Substances that impart sweetness to foods fall into 2 broad classes: nutritive sweeteners, which can be metabolized to yield energy, and alternative sweeteners, which provide no food energy. The sugar alcohols, sorbitol, mannitol, and xylitol, are nutritive sweeteners used in sugarless gum and candies. Alternative (or artificial or non-nutritive) sweeteners provide non-caloric or very-low-calorie sugar substitutes.

5.3 Adults need about 130 g/day of digestible carbohydrate to supply adequate glucose for the brain and central nervous system, without having to rely on partial replacement of glucose by ketone bodies as an energy source. In North America, carbohydrates supply about 50% of energy intakes in adults. The Dietary Guidelines for Americans recommend limiting added sugars to approximately 6% of total energy intake. The Institute of Medicine's Food and Nutrition Board set an upper limit of 25% of energy intake for added sugar consumption. The Adequate Intake for fiber is based on a goal of 14 g/1000 kcal consumed. For adults up to age 50 years, the Adequate Intake is set at 25 g for women and 38 g for men. After age 50, the Adequate Intake falls to 21 g/day and 30 g/day, respectively. In North America, carbohydrates supply about 50% of the energy intakes of adults. Sugar intake tends to be higher than recommended and fiber intake lower than recommended.

5.4 Most of the digestible carbohydrates in our diets are broken down to glucose. As glucose, they provide a primary source of energy, spare protein for vital processes, and prevent ketosis. Fiber helps prevent constipation and diverticular disease and enhances the management of body weight, blood glucose levels, and blood cholesterol levels.

5.5 During digestion, starch and sugars are broken into monosaccharide units that are small enough to be absorbed. The enzymatic digestion of some carbohydrates begins in the mouth with the action of an enzyme called salivary amylase. Salivary enzyme is inactivated by the acidity of the stomach. In the small intestine, polysaccharides are digested further by pancreatic amylase and specialized enzymes in the absorptive cells of the small intestine. Glucose and galactose are absorbed by an active absorption process. Fructose is taken up by the absorptive cells via facilitated diffusion. Monosaccharides are transported via the portal vein to the liver. Within the liver, fructose and galactose are converted to glucose. Glucose is transported through the bloodstream for use by the cells of the body.

5.6 Adequate carbohydrate intake is important for maintaining health and decreasing the risk of chronic disease. Very high intakes of fiber (i.e., above 50 to 60 g/day) combined with low fluid intake can result in hard, dry stools that are painful to eliminate. Very high fiber intakes also may decrease the absorption of minerals. High intakes of sugars can displace more nutritious foods and increase the risk of weight gain, obesity, and dental caries. Lactose intolerance can cause symptoms of abdominal pain, bloating, gas, and diarrhea after consuming lactose, especially in large amounts. An inability to regulate glucose metabolism can result in diabetes. The major forms of diabetes are type 1 diabetes and type 2 diabetes. Type 1 diabetes often begins in late childhood and runs in families, suggesting a genetic link. The onset of type 1 diabetes is caused by insufficient insulin release by the pancreas, which results in increased blood glucose levels. Type 1 diabetes is treated by insulin and diet therapy. Poorly controlled diabetes can cause blindness, cardiovascular disease, kidney disease, and nerve deterioration. A person with diabetes should work regularly with a physician and dietitian to monitor and adjust diet, medications, and physical activity. Type 2 diabetes is a progressive disease characterized by insulin resistance or loss of responsiveness by body cells to insulin. As a result, glucose is not readily transferred into cells and builds up in the bloodstream, causing hyperglycemia. Treatments for type 2 diabetes are aimed at maintaining normal ranges of blood glucose through lifestyle modification and medication use. Glycemic index is a ratio of the blood glucose response of a given food, compared with a standard, such as white bread. Glycemic load takes into account the glycemic index and the amount of carbohydrate consumed.

Study Questions

1. Which of the following is a monosaccharide?

   a. lactose
   b. raffinose
   c. fructose
   d. maltose

2. Which of the following is classified as a digestible form of polysaccharide?

   a. cellulose
   b. raffinose
   c. lignin
   d. pectin

3. Carbohydrates are involved in all of the following functions *except* _____.

   a. providing energy
   b. preventing ketosis
   c. promoting bowel health
   d. promoting cell differentiation

4. Individuals with lactose intolerance have difficulty digesting milk products because they lack the enzyme needed to break apart the beta bond linkages.

   a. true
   b. false

5. The Adequate Intake for dietary fiber is set at 14 g/1000 kcal.

   a. true
   b. false

6. Which of the following sweeteners is classified as a non-nutritive sweetener?

   a. sorbitol
   b. honey
   c. aspartame
   d. mannitol

7. Which of the following is a poor source of dietary fiber?

   a. whole-grain oats
   b. fresh blueberries
   c. low-fat yogurt
   d. dried lentils

8. Which of the following is a good source of starch?

   a. citrus fruits
   b. dark leafy greens
   c. enriched grains
   d. barbequed chicken

9. Which of the following terms is used to describe an elevated blood sugar level?

   a. glucosuria
   b. hypoglycemia
   c. hyperlipidemia
   d. hyperglycemia

10. Which of the following is *not* a classic symptom of type 1 diabetes?

    a. polyuria
    b. polydipsia
    c. hunger
    d. rapid weight gain

11. Which of the following population groups is at lowest risk of diabetes?

    a. college athletes
    b. obese individuals
    c. individuals of Hispanic/Latino heritage
    d. adults over 45 years of age

12. High fiber diets can impair the absorption of minerals.

    a. true
    b. false

13. Which of the following is associated with low-fiber diets?

    a. diverticulosis
    b. dental caries
    c. diarrhea
    d. lactose intolerance

14. Diabetic exchanges and carbohydrate counting are effective ways for individuals with diabetes to monitor daily carbohydrate intake.

    a. true
    b. false

15. The glycemic index is a ratio of the blood glucose response of a given food, compared with a standard.

    a. true
    b. false

Answer Key: 1-c; 2-d; 3-d; 4-a; 5-a; 6-c; 7-c; 8-c; 9-d; 10-d; 11-a; 12-a; 13-a; 14-a; 15-a

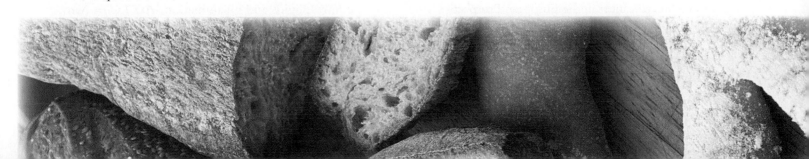

Websites

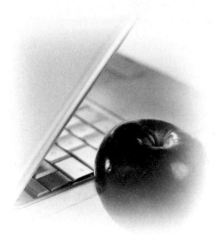

To learn more about the topics covered in this chapter, visit these websites.

www.ific.org

www.fda.gov/fdac/features/2006/406_sweeteners.html

www.diabetes.org

www.eatright.org

www.ada.org

www.ific.org

www.nidcr.nih.gov

www.niddk.nih.gov

www.healthfinder.gov

References

1. ADA Reports. Position of the American Dietetic Association. Use of nutritive and nonnutritive sweeteners. *J Am Diet Assoc.* 2004;104:225.

2. Food and Nutrition Board. *Dietary Reference Intakes for energy, carbohydrate, fiber, fat, fatty acids, cholesterol, protein, and amino acids.* Washington, DC: National Academy Press; 2002.

3. Keim NL and others. Carbohydrates. In: Shils ME and others, ed. *Modern nutrition in health and disease.* 10th ed. Philadelphia: Lippincott Williams & Wilkins; 2006.

4. Swagerty D and others. Lactose intolerance. *Am Fam Physician.* 2002;65:1845.

5. Mayes PA, Bender DA. Carbohydrates of physiological significance. In: Murray RK and others, ed. *Harper's illustrated biochemistry.* 26th ed. New York: Lange Medical Books/McGraw-Hill; 2005.

6. Murphy MM and others. Resistant starch intakes in the U.S., *J Am Diet Assoc.* 2008;108:67.

7. Schulze MB and others. Glycemic index, glycemic load, and dietary fiber intake and incidence of type 2 diabetes in younger and middle-aged women. *Am J Clin Nutr.* 2004;80:348.

8. Bingham S and others. Dietary fibre in food and protection against colorectal cancer in the European Prospective Investigation into Cancer and Nutrition (EPIC): An observational study. *Lancet.* 2004;36:1496.

9. Salzman H, Lillie D. Diverticular disease: Diagnosis and treatment. *Am Fam Physician.* 2005;72:1229.

10. U.S. Department of Health and Human Services and U.S. Department of Agriculture. *Dietary Guidelines for Americans.* 6th ed. Washington, DC: U.S. Government Printing Office; 2005.

11. Park Y and others. Dietary fiber intake and risk of colorectal cancer. *JAMA.* 2005;294:2849.

12. Bray GA, Nielsen SJ, Popkin BM. Consumption of high-fructose corn syrup in beverages may play a role in the epidemic of obesity. *Am J Clin Nutr.* 2004;79:537.

13. Serdula M and others. Trends in fruit and vegetable consumption among adults in the United States: Behavioral risk factor surveillance system, 1994–2000. *Am J Public Health.* 2004;94:1014.

14. Liu S and others. Is intake of breakfast cereals related to total and cause-specific mortality in men? *Am J Clin Nutr.* 2003;77:594.

15. Diverticular disease: The importance of getting enough fiber. *Mayo Clinic Health Letter.* 2005;23:1.

16. Koh-Banerjee P and others. Changes in wholegrain, bran, and cereal fiber consumption in relation to 8-y weight gain among men. *Am J Clin Nutr.* 2004;80:1237.

17. Jensen M and others. Whole grains, bran and germ in relation to homocysteine and markers of glycemic control, lipids and inflammation. *Am J Clin Nutr.* 2006;83:275.

18. Schulze M and others. Dietary pattern, inflammation, and incidence of type 2 diabetes in women. *Am J Clin Nutr.* 2005;82:675.

19. Jenkins D and others. Soluble fiber intake at a dose approved by the U.S. Food and Drug Administration for a claim of health benefits: Serum lipid risk factors for cardiovascular disease assessed in a randomized controlled crossover trial. *Am J Clin Nutr.* 2002;75:834.

20. James J and others. Preventing childhood obesity by reducing consumption of carbonated drinks: Cluster randomized controlled trial. *BMJ.* 2004;10:1136.

21. Schulze MB and others. Sugar-sweetened beverages, weight gain, and incidence of type 2 diabetes in young and middle-aged women. *JAMA.* 2004;292:927.

22. Fried SK, Rao SP. Sugars, hypertriglyceridemia and cardiovascular disease. *Am J Clin Nutr.* 2003;78:873S.

23. Sweeteners can sour your health. *Consumer Reports on Health.* 2005; January:8.

24. American Diabetes Association. Standards of care in diabetes. *Diabetes Care.* 2005;28:S36.

25. Diabetes. *Mayo Clinic Health Letter.* 2004;22 (Suppl).

26. Diabetes Control and Complications Trial/Epidemiology of Diabetes Interventions and Complications Research Study Group. Intensive diabetes treatment and cardiovascular disease in patients with type 1 diabetes. *N Engl J Med.* 2005;353:2643.

27. Tesfaye S and others. Vascular risk factors and diabetic neuropathy. *N Engl J Med.* 2005;352:341.

28. Klein S and others. Weight management through lifestyle modification for the prevention and management of type 2 diabetes. *Am J Clin Nutr.* 2004;80:257.

29. Tanasescu M and others. Dietary fat and cholesterol and the risk of cardiovascular disease among women with type 2 diabetes. *Am J Clin Nutr.* 2004;79:999.

30. Tirosh A and others. Normal fasting plasma glucose levels and type 2 diabetes in young men. *N Engl J Med.* 2005;353:1454.

31. Wang Y and others. Comparison of abdominal adiposity and overall obesity in predicting risk of type 2 diabetes in men. *Am J Clin Nutr.* 2005;81:555.

32. Weinstein AR and others. Relationship of physical activity versus body mass index with type 2 diabetes in women. *JAMA.* 2004;292:1188.

33. Hu G and others. Physical activity, body mass index, and risk of type 2 diabetes in patients with normal or impaired glucose regulation. *Arch Intern Med.* 2004;164:892.

34. Despres JP. Is visceral obesity the cause of the Metabolic Syndrome? *Ann Med.* 2006;38:52.

35. Wheeler, ML and Pi-Sunyer X, Carbohydrate Issues: Type and Amount. *J Am Diet Assoc.* 2008;108:S34.

36. Brand-Miller J. Glycemic load and chronic disease. *Nutr Rev.* 2003;61:S49.

37. Holvoet P and others. Association between circulating oxidized low-density lipoprotein and incidence of the Metabolic Syndrome. *JAMA.* 2008;299:2287.

38. Livesey G. Low glycemic diets and health: Implications for obesity. *Proc Nutr Soc.* 2005;64:105.

39. Ebbling CB and others. Effects of an ad libitum low-glycemic diet on cardiovascular risk factors in obese young adults. *Am J Clin Nutr.* 2005;81:976.

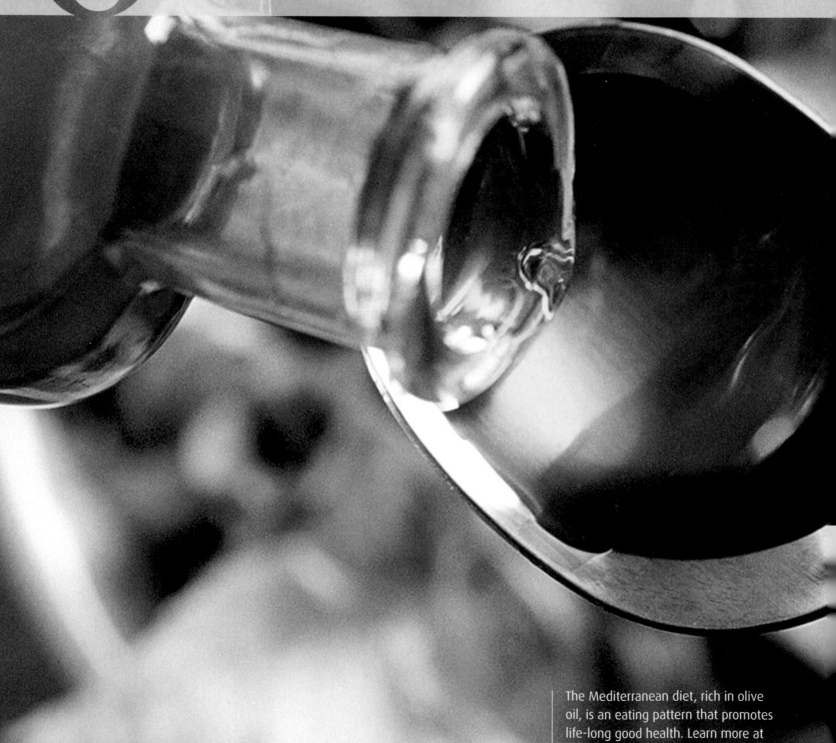

6 *lipids*

The Mediterranean diet, rich in olive oil, is an eating pattern that promotes life-long good health. Learn more at www.oldwayspt.org.

STUDENT LEARNING OUTCOMES

After studying this chapter, you will be able to

1. Explain the basic chemical structure of fatty acids and how they are named.

2. Describe the functions of triglycerides, fatty acids, phospholipids, and sterols in the body.

3. Classify and evaluate the different fatty acids based on their health benefits or consequences.

4. Identify food sources of triglycerides, fatty acids, phospholipids, and sterols.

5. Describe the recommended intake of lipids.

6. Identify strategies for modifying total fat, saturated fat, and *trans* fat intake.

7. Explain the digestion, absorption, and transport of lipids in the body.

8. Discuss health concerns related to dietary fat intake.

9. Describe dietary measures to reduce the risk of developing cardiovascular disease.

Fats (technically, lipids) give food a creamy, luscious mouthfeel. They also add a great deal of flavor to foods—think about the buttery taste of croissants or the savory flavor of beef. Nearly every food we eat contains at least some fat. The foods richest in fat are vegetable oil, margarine, butter, avocado, and nuts. All contain close to 100% of energy as fat. Many protein-rich foods, such as meat, cheese, and peanut butter, are high in fat, too. Cakes, pies, cookies, muffins, chocolate, ice cream, and snack foods, such as chips and crackers, also contain sizeable amounts of fat. In addition to providing flavor, texture, and energy, dietary fats supply fat-soluble vitamins (vitamins A, D, E, and K). Because they are more energy-dense than carbohydrates and proteins, lipids contribute to feeling full and satisfied (satiety) after eating a high-fat meal and may help you lengthen the time between meals. Fat in our bodies insulates the body and protects its organs from injuries. We also use it to make hormones.

As you can see, fats are essential for good health, so why do fats have such a bad reputation? It's because not all fats are created equal from a health perspective. Exploring the characteristics of the lipid family members will demystify this often misunderstood nutrient.

Figure 6-1 **Food sources of fat.**

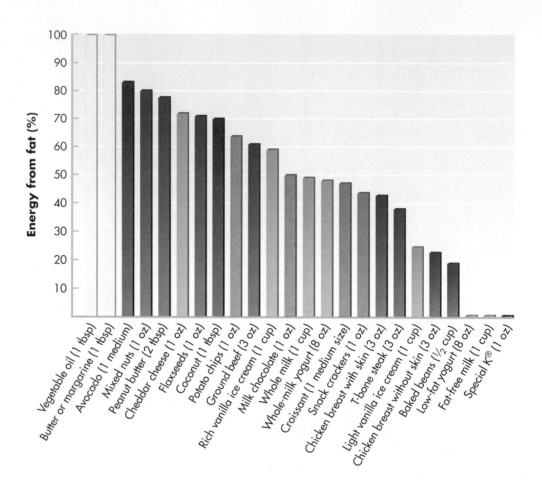

Types of Lipids

- Triglycerides
- Phospholipids
- Sterols

▶ Fat in foods has been considered the most satiating of all the macronutrients. However, recent studies show that protein and carbohydrate probably provide more satiety (gram for gram).[22] High-fat meals do provide satiety, but primarily because they are high in calories.

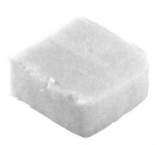

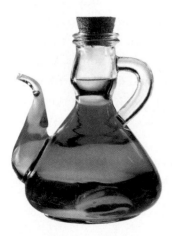

The term *fat* typically refers to lipids that are solid at room temperature. *Oil* refers to lipids that are liquid at room temperature.

6.1 Triglycerides

The word *lipid* conjures thoughts of butter, lard, olive oil, and margarine. We usually refer to lipids simply as *fats and oils;* however, the lipid family includes more than that—it includes triglycerides, phospholipids, and sterols. Although these diverse family members differ in their structures and functions, they all contain carbon, hydrogen, and oxygen and none of them dissolve in water. However, they do dissolve in organic solvents, such as chloroform, benzene, and ether. Think of oil and vinegar salad dressing. No matter how long or hard you shake the dressing, when you stop shaking, the vinegar and oil quickly separate into layers, with the oil floating on the vinegar. This insoluble property sets lipids apart from carbohydrates and proteins (Fig. 6-1).

Triglycerides are the most common type of lipid found in foods and in the body. About 95% of the fats we eat and 95% of the fat stored in the body are in the form of triglycerides.

Structure

Each triglyceride molecule consists of 3 fatty acids attached (bonded) to a glycerol, which serves as a backbone for the fatty acids (Fig. 6-2). A triglyceride is built by attaching a fatty acid to each of glycerol's 3 hydroxyl groups (-OH). The fatty acids can be all the same fatty acid or they can be different. One water molecule is released when each fatty acid bonds to glycerol. The process of attaching fatty acids to glycerol is called **esterification**. The release of fatty acids from glycerol is called **de-esterification.** Fatty acids released from the glycerol backbone are called **free fatty acids** to emphasize that they are unattached. A triglyceride that loses a fatty acid is a **diglyceride**. A **monoglyceride** results when 2 fatty acids are lost. The process of reattaching a fatty acid to glycerol that has lost a fatty acid is known as **re-esterification**.

Free fatty acids are long chains of carbons linked together and surrounded by hydrogens. The many kinds of free fatty acids have similar structures: long chains of carbon atoms linked together and surrounded by hydrogens. An acid (carboxyl) group is at one end of the chain, with a methyl group at the opposite end (Fig. 6-3). Their carbon chains can vary in 3 ways: the number of carbons in the chain, the extent to which the chain is saturated with hydrogen, and the shape of the chain (straight or bent).

Carbon Chain Length

Fatty acid chains usually have between 4 and 24 carbons. **Long chain fatty acids** have 12 or more carbon atoms. Fats from beef, pork, and lamb and most plant oils are long chain. Long chains of carbon atoms take the longest to digest and are transported via the lymphatic system. **Medium chain fatty acids** are 6 to10 carbons in length, are digested almost as rapidly as glucose, and are transported via the circulatory system. Coconut and palm oil are examples of medium-chain fatty acids. **Short chain fatty acids** are usually less than 6 carbons in length. The fat in dairy products, such as butter and whole milk, are short chain. They are rapidly digested and transported via the circulatory system.

Saturation

Fatty acids can be saturated, monounsaturated, or polyunsaturated. To understand saturation, it is important to note that, at a maximum, a carbon atom can form 4 chemical bonds, an oxygen atom can form 2 bonds, and a hydrogen atom can form only 1 bond. Each atom always tries to form the maximum number of bonds possible, but it cannot form more than the maximum.

Figure 6-3 shows a **saturated fatty acid (SFA)**. Notice that every carbon in the chain has formed the maximum of 4 bonds. Also note that each bond is formed with a separate atom (2 different carbons and 2 different hydrogens). It is a saturated fatty acid because all the bonds between the carbons are single connections and the other carbon bonds are filled with hydrogens. To understand this concept, picture a school bus with a child in every seat. The school bus is "saturated" with children—there are no empty seats on the bus.

A Biochemist's View

Building, Breaking Down, and Rebuilding Triglycerides
(Esterifying, De-esterifying, and Re-esterifying Fatty Acids)

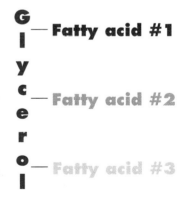

Triglycerides are built from a glycerol backbone and 3 fatty acids. As you can see, glycerol (in white) has 3 carbons in its chain. A triglyceride forms when each hydroxyl (-OH) group on the glycerol backbone bonds with the hydrogen atom from the acid (carboxyl) end of a fatty acid. The bond between a fatty acid and glycerol is called an ester bond. One molecule of water (H$_2$O) forms each time an ester bond forms (this is called esterification). Thus, when a diglyceride (2 fatty acids attached to a glycerol backbone) forms, 2 molecules of water form. Similarly, forming a triglyceride will generate 3 water molecules.

A molecule of water is used when a fatty acid breaks away from a glycerol backbone (called de-esterification). Reattaching the fatty acid to a glycerol backbone (called re-esterification) will produce a water molecule.

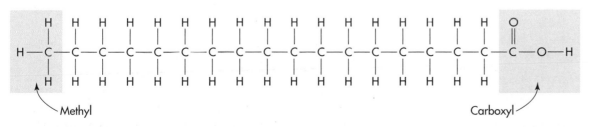

Figure 6-2 Triglycerides are made of 3 fatty acids attached to a glycerol backbone.

Figure 6-3 This fatty acid is saturated and is called stearic acid.

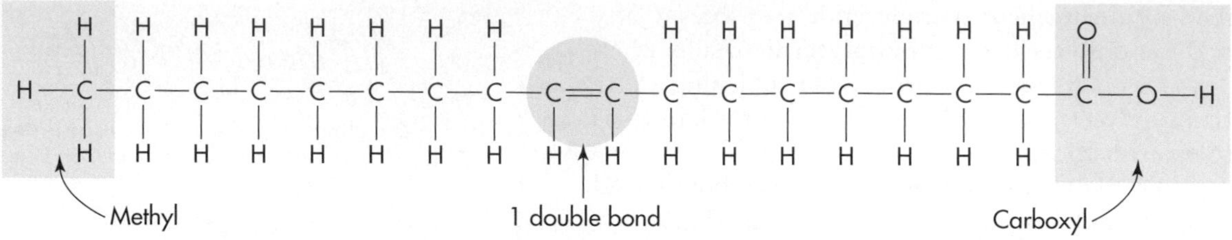

Figure 6-4 This fatty acid is monounsaturated and is called oleic acid.

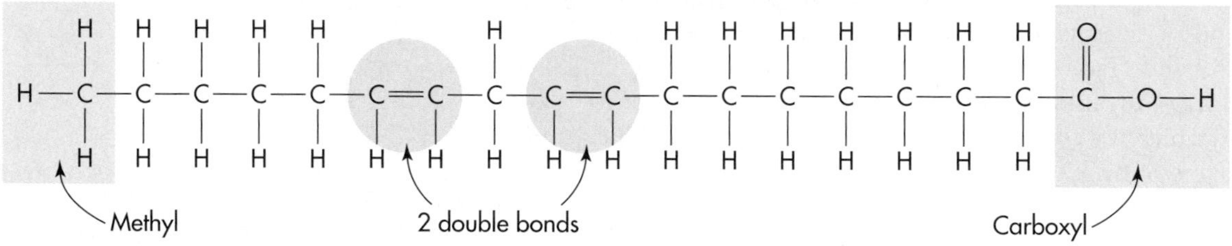

Figure 6-5 This fatty acid is polyunsaturated and is called linoleic acid.

► Chemists classify triglycerides as esters. Tri*acyl*glyceride is the chemical name for triglyceride. *Acyl* refers to a fatty acid that has lost its hydroxyl group (–OH). A fatty acid loses its hydroxyl group when it attaches to glycerol.

► Why are some fats solid at room temperature and others liquid? The fat's carbon chain shape and length determine this. Like crumpled paper, the kinked carbon chains of unsaturated fatty acids do not pack tightly together. This "loose" packing causes them to be soft or liquid at room temperature. In contrast, saturated fatty acids, with their straight carbon chain, like unfolded paper, pack tightly together. This tight packing helps them stay firm (not melt) at room temperature. However, the effect of the straight chain shape on saturated fats (but not unsaturated fats) can be overridden by chain length. That is, only saturated fatty acids with a long carbon chain, such as beef fat, are solid at room temperature. Medium and short chain saturated fats are soft or liquid at room temperature.

A **monounsaturated fatty acid (MUFA)** is shown in Figure 6-4. Notice how carbons 8 and 9 in the chain are each missing 1 hydrogen. These carbons formed a double bond between each other by each giving up 1 hydrogen. (Remember, carbons can form only 4 bonds.) Fatty acids that have 1 double bond in the carbon chain are called monounsaturated fatty acids. They have 1 (mono) location in the carbon chain that is not saturated with hydrogen. Using the school bus example, a MUFA is like having 1 empty seat.

A **polyunsaturated fatty acid (PUFA)** has at least 2 double bonds in its carbon chain (Fig. 6-5). If the school bus were a PUFA, it would have 2 or more empty seats.

Shape

The shape of the carbon chain varies with saturation. Saturated and *trans* fatty acids have straight carbon chains, and unsaturated *cis* fatty acids have bent or kinked carbon chains. In *cis* **fatty acids**, the hydrogens attached to the double-bonded carbons are on the same side of the carbon chain (see Fig. 6-5). In *trans* **fatty acids** (also called *trans* fats), the hydrogens attached to the double-bonded carbons zigzag back and forth across the carbon chain (Fig. 6-6). In Figure 6-7, notice how the *cis* fatty acid, which has the hydrogens next to the double bonds on the same side of the carbon chain, bends. The *trans* fatty acid, which has the hydrogens next to the double bonds on opposite sides of the carbon chain, is straight and resembles a saturated fatty acid.

Most unprocessed unsaturated fatty acids, such as oils freshly pressed from nuts and seeds, are in the *cis* form. *Trans* fatty acids are found mostly in the polyunsaturated oils modified by food manufacturers using a process called hydrogenation.

Hydrogenation adds hydrogen to the carbon chain of unsaturated fats. As the amount of added hydrogen increases, the unsaturated fat becomes more and more saturated (until it is totally saturated) and increasingly solid (Fig. 6-8). For instance, corn oil, which is polyunsaturated and liquid at room temperature, can be hydrogenated: a little to make squeeze margarine, some to make tub margarine, and a lot to make stick margarine.

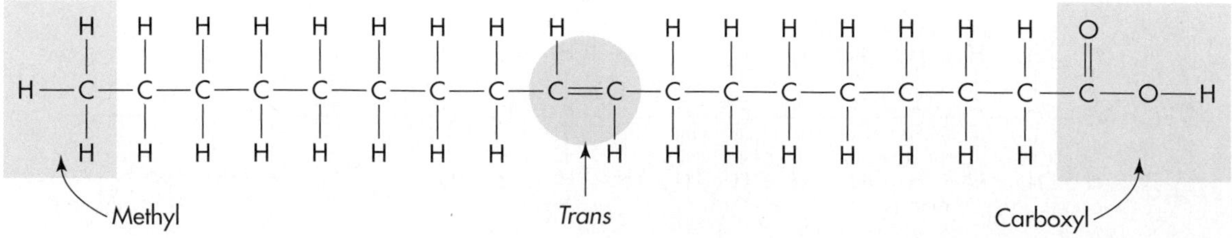

Figure 6-6 This monounsaturated fatty acid is a *trans* fat. It is called elaidic acid, which is the major *trans* fatty acid found in processed fats.

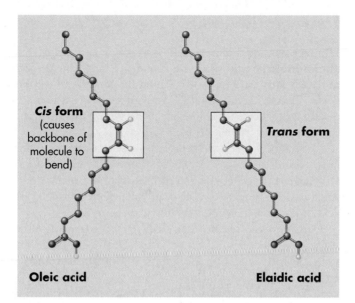

Figure 6-7 *Cis* and *trans* fatty acids. *Cis* fatty acids are more common in foods than *trans* fats. *Trans* fats are primarily found in foods containing hydrogenated fats, such as margarine, shortening, and deep fat–fried foods.

▶ Ball-and-stick models (e.g., Figure 6-7) show the spatial arrangement of atoms in a molecule. The blue balls are carbon, white hydrogen, and red oxygen. The lines between the balls represent bonds.

Hydrogenation is like putting children in some of the empty bus seats except, when the children are added to the bus, it changes the shape of the bus. The shape change occurs because hydrogenation creates *trans* fatty acids that have a straighter shape than *cis* fatty acids.

Naming Fatty Acids

Two systems are commonly used to name fatty acids. Both are based on the numbers of carbon atoms and the location of double bonds in a fatty acid's carbon chain. The omega (ω or n) system indicates where the first double bond closest to the methyl (omega) end of the chain occurs. For example, the fatty acid linoleic acid is named 18:2 ω6 (18:2 n6). This means that linoleic acid, shown on the right in Figure 6-9, has 18 carbons in its carbon chain and 2 double bonds, and the first double bond starts at the 6th carbon from the omega end (orange boxed area of Fig. 6-9). The delta (Δ) system describes fatty acids in relation to the carboxyl end of the carbon chain (blue boxed area of Fig. 6-9) and indicates the location of all double bonds. Thus, in the delta system, linoleic acid is written 18:2 $\Delta^{9,12}$. Whereas the scientific community uses both of these systems nearly equally, the popular media uses the omega system, as does this text.

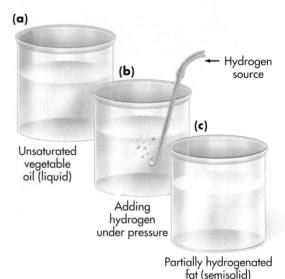

Figure 6-8 How liquid oils become solid fats. (*a*) Unsaturated fatty acids are present in liquid form. (*b*) Hydrogens are added (hydrogenation), changing some carbon-carbon double bonds to single bonds and producing some *trans* fatty acids. (*c*) The partially hydrogenated product is likely to be used in margarine or shortening or for deep-fat frying.

Omega-3 (alpha linolenic acid)

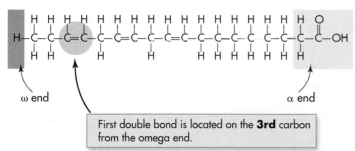

First double bond is located on the **3rd** carbon from the omega end.

Omega-6 (linolenic acid)

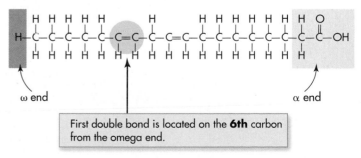

First double bond is located on the **6th** carbon from the omega end.

Figure 6-9 Omega-3 fatty acids have their first double bond 3 carbons in from the methyl (omega) end of the carbon chain. Likewise, omega-6 fatty acids have their first double bond 6 carbons in from the omega end. How would alpha-linolenic acid be named using the omega and delta system?

► Alpha is the first letter of the Greek alphabet and omega is the last letter. Alpha looks like this: α. Omega looks like this in Greek: ω. In English, a lowercase *n* is sometimes used in place of the Greek letter.

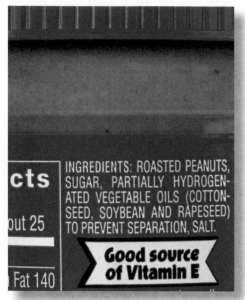

On food packages, hydrogenated fats appear in the ingredient list as partially hydrogenated fat or hydrogenated fat. Food manufacturers can call a food "*trans* fat free" if it contains 0.5 gram or less of *trans* fats.

Essential Fatty Acids

Humans can synthesize a wide variety of fatty acids, but we *cannot* make 2 PUFAs: **alpha-linolenic acid** (the major omega-3 fatty acid in food) and **linoleic acid** (the major omega-6 fatty acid in food). Alpha-linolenic acid and linoleic acid are **essential fatty acids (EFAs).** We must get EFAs from foods because our bodies are unable to synthesize essential fatty acids with a double bond before the 9th carbon in the chain, counting from the omega end (see Fig. 6-9).

The location of the double bond closest to the omega carbon (methyl end) of the fatty acid identifies the fatty acid's family. If the first double bond of a polyunsaturated fatty acid occurs after the 3rd carbon from the methyl end, it is called an omega–3 fatty acid (ω–3). If the first double bond occurs after the 6th carbon on a polyunsaturated fatty acid, it is called an omega–6 fatty acid (ω–6).

As you can see in Figure 6-10, the fatty acids eicosapentaenoic acid (EPA) and, subsequently, docosahexaenoic acid (DHA) are made from alpha-linolenic acid. Likewise, the fatty acids dihomo-gamma-linolenic acid and, subsequently, arachidonic acid are made from linoleic acid.

Different eicosanoids are produced from dihomo-gamma-linolenic acid, arachidonic acid, and eicosapentaenoic acid. **Eicosanoids** are hormonelike compounds, such as prostaglandins, prostacyclins, thromboxanes, leukotrienes, and lipoxins, that affect the body in the region where they are produced. (They are called *local* hormones because, unlike typical hormones, they are made *and* used in the same area of the body.)

Knowledge Check

1. What characteristics do all lipids have?
2. How do saturated, monounsaturated, and saturated fats differ?
3. What are the differences between *cis* and *trans* fats?
4. How do the omega and delta systems for naming fatty acids differ?
5. Why must essential fatty acids be provided by the diet?

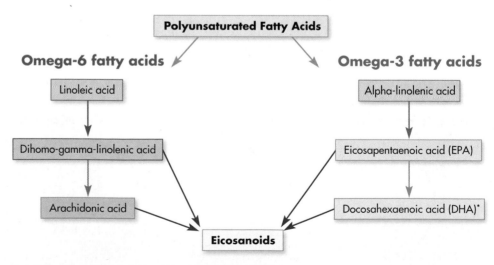

*Technically, DHA yields docosanoids, which are similar to eicosanoids.

Figure 6-10 The essential fatty acids alpha-linolenic acid and linoleic acids are used to make other important fatty acids.

6.2 Food Sources of Triglycerides

Almost all foods provide at least some triglycerides. Certain foods, such as animal fat and vegetable oils, are primarily triglycerides. Bakery items, snack foods, and dairy desserts also contain significant amounts of fat. In contrast, fat-free milk and yogurt, as well as many breakfast cereals and yeast breads, contain little or no fat. Other than coconut and avocados, fruits and vegetables are low in fat.

Table 6-1 lists the main sources of each type of fatty acid. For instance, fats from animal sources and tropical oils (coconut, palm, palm kernel) are rich in saturated fatty acids. Omega-3 fatty acid sources include cold-water fish (salmon, tuna, sardines, mackerel), walnuts, and flaxseed. Fish oil and flaxseed oil supplements are another source of omega-3 fatty acids.

Most triglyceride-rich foods contain a mixture of fatty acids. As you can see in Figure 6-11, butter contains saturated, monoun-saturated, and polyunsaturated fatty acids. Saturated fats are the predominant fatty acid in butter, so it is referred to as a saturated fat. Similarly, olive oil contains saturated, monounsaturated, and polyun-saturated fatty acids, but monounsaturated fat predominates. Thus, it is referred to as a monounsaturated fat.

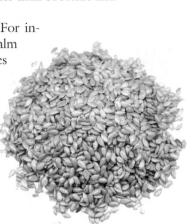

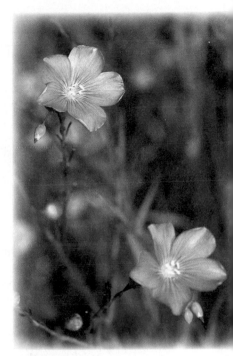

Flax is a common plant that produces seeds high in omega-3 fats. The seeds can be ground and used as a meal in baked goods. They also can be pressed to extract the oil, which is sold as a nutritional supplement.

Table 6-1 Main Sources of Fatty acids and Their State at Room Temperature

Type and Health Effects	Double Bonds	Main Sources	State at Room Temperature
Saturated Fatty Acids Increase blood levels of cholesterol	0		
Long Chain		Lard; fat in beef, pork, and lamb	Solid
Medium and Short Chain		Milk fat (butter), coconut oil, palm oil, palm kernel oil	Soft or liquid
Monounsaturated Fatty Acids Decrease blood levels of cholesterol	1	Olive oil, canola oil, peanut oil	Liquid
Polyunsaturated Fatty Acids Decrease blood levels of cholesterol	2 or more	Sunflower oil, corn oil, safflower oil, fish oil	Liquid
Essential Fatty Acids			
Omega 3: alpha-linolenic acid Reduces inflammation responses, blood clotting, and plasma triglycerides	3	Cold-water fish (salmon, tuna, sardines, mackerel), walnuts, flaxseed, hemp oil, canola oil, soybean oil	Liquid
Omega 6: Linoleic Acid Regulates blood pressure and increases blood clotting	2	Beef, poultry, safflower oil, sunflower oil, corn oil	Solid to liquid
Trans **Fatty Acids** Increase blood cholesterol more than saturated fat	Less than the PUFA used to make *trans* fat	Margarine (squeeze, tub, stick), shortening	Soft to very solid

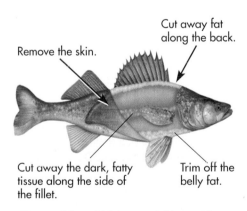

Remove the skin.

Cut away fat along the back.

Cut away the dark, fatty tissue along the side of the fillet.

Trim off the belly fat.

Cold-water fish are high in essential fatty acids, but are fish safe to eat? Some people worry about potential health risks related to fish and fish oil supplements, such as carcinogens (e.g., DDT, dieldrin, heptachlor, PCBs, dioxin) and toxins (e.g., methylmercury). Although these contaminants are present in low levels in fresh and salt water, they can be concentrated in fish. To minimize exposure, select small, non-predatory fish; vary the type of fish you eat; buy fish from reputable markets; and discard fatty portions of fish, where toxins concentrate. If you catch your own fish, always check local advisories to be sure that the water you plan to fish in is safe. You can call your local health department or visit your state government's website to learn about fishing advisories.

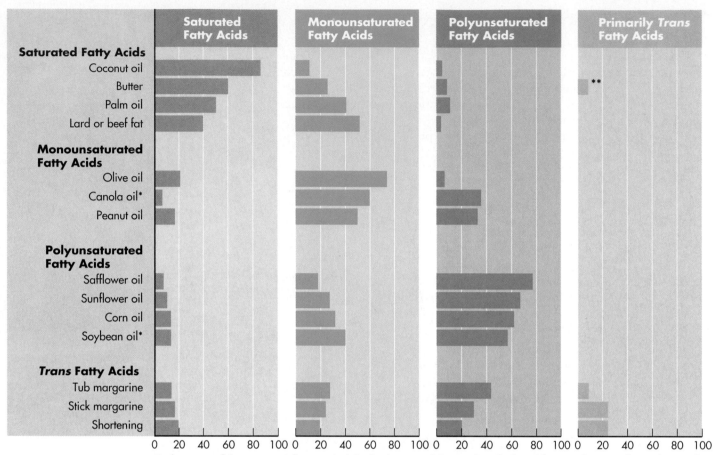

*Rich source of the omega-3 fatty acid alpha-linolenic acid (7% and 12% of total fatty acid content for soybean oil and canola oil, respectively).

**The natural *trans* fatty acids in butter are not harmful and may even have health-promoting properties, such as preventing certain forms of cancer.

Figure 6-11 Saturated, monounsaturated, polyunsaturated, and *trans* fatty acid composition of common fats and oils (expressed as % of all fatty acids in the product).

CRITICAL THINKING

Allison has decided to start eating a low-fat diet. She has mentioned to you that all she needs to do is add less butter, oil, or margarine to her foods and she will dramatically lower her fat intake. How can you explain to Allison that she needs to be aware of the hidden fats in her diet as well?

Hidden Fats

The fat in some foods is visible: butter on bread, mayonnaise in potato salad, and marbling in raw meat. In many foods, however, fat is hidden, as is the fat in whole milk, cheese, pastries, cookies, cake, hot dogs, crackers, french fries, and ice cream. Nutrition Facts labels can help you learn more about the quantity of fat in the foods you eat (Fig. 6-12).

Figure 6-12 Reading labels helps locate hidden fat. Who would think that wieners (hot dogs) can contain about 86% of energy content as fat? Looking at the hot dog itself does not suggest that almost all its energy content comes from fat, but the label shows otherwise. Do the math: 120 kcal from fat / 140 kcal = 0.86, or 86%.

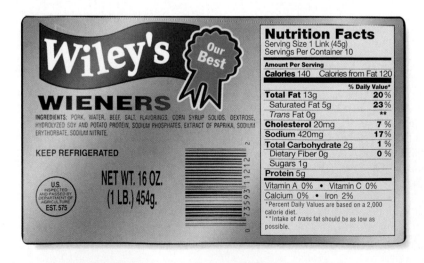

Fat Replacements

To help consumers trim their fat intake and still enjoy the mouthfeel sensations fat provides, food companies offer low-fat versions of many foods. To lower the fat in foods, manufacturers may replace some of the fat with water, protein (Dairy-Lo®), or forms of carbohydrates such as starch derivatives (Z-trim®), fiber (Maltrin®, Stellar™, Oatrim), and gums. Manufacturers also may use engineered fats, such as olestra (Olean®) and salatrim (Benefat®), that are made with fat and sucrose (table sugar) but that provide few or no calories because they cannot be digested and/or absorbed well.

So far, fat replacements have had little impact on our diets, partly because the currently approved forms are either not very versatile or not used extensively by manufacturers. In addition, fat replacements are not practical for use in the foods that provide the most fat in our diets—beef, cheese, whole milk, and pastries.[1]

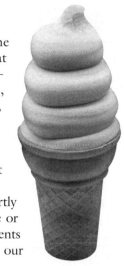

▶ Olestra binds fat-soluble vitamins and reduces their absorption. To compensate, the manufacturer adds these vitamins to foods containing olestra. At first, olestra was suspected of causing GI tract discomfort; however, careful research indicates this is not the case and warning labels on olestra-containing foods are no longer required.

▶ A "reduced-fat" food may not be lower in calories than its full-fat counterpart. That's because, when fat is removed from a product, something must be added—commonly, sugars—in its place.

Fat replacements, such as gum fiber, are often used in soft serve ice cream.

▶ Table 2-3 in Chapter 2 defines the fat claims that are permitted on food labels, such as "low-fat," "fat-free," and "reduced-fat."

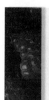

Knowledge Check

1. What are 3 sources of each type of fatty acid?
2. What are examples of foods that contain hidden fats?
3. What types of fat replacements are currently available?

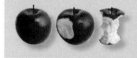

Take Action

Is Your Diet High in Saturated and *Trans* Fat?

Instructions: In each row of the following list, circle your typical food selection from column A or B.

Column A		Column B
Bacon and eggs	or	Ready-to-eat whole-grain breakfast cereal
Doughnut or sweet roll	or	Whole-wheat roll, bagel, or bread
Breakfast sausage	or	Fruit
Whole milk	or	Reduced-fat, low-fat, or fat-free milk
Cheeseburger	or	Turkey sandwich, no cheese
French fries	or	Plain baked potato with salsa
Ground chuck	or	Ground round
Soup with cream base	or	Soup with broth base
Macaroni and cheese	or	Macaroni with marinara sauce
Cream/fruit pie	or	Graham crackers
Cream-filled cookies	or	Granola bar
Ice cream	or	Frozen yogurt, sherbet, or reduced-fat ice cream
Butter or stick margarine	or	Vegetable oils or soft margarine in a tub

Interpretation

The foods listed in column A tend to be high in saturated fat, *trans* fatty acids, cholesterol, and total fat. Those in column B generally are low in these dietary components. If you want to help reduce your risk of cardiovascular disease, choose more foods from column B and fewer from column A.

6.3 Functions of Triglycerides

Triglycerides are important in many ways when it comes to your health. They are essential for optimal health, but high intakes, especially saturated and *trans* fat, and imbalances of EFAs can present health challenges.

Provide Energy

▶ A triglyceride's glycerol backbone can be used as a fuel for the nervous system. Another brain fuel that originates with triglycerides is ketones—compounds formed when fatty acids do not metabolize completely; large amounts of ketones form when carbohydrate (glucose) intake is restricted. (See Chapter 9.)

Triglycerides in food and body fat cells are a rich source of energy, with each gram providing about 9 calories. Triglycerides are the main fuel source for all body cells, except the nervous system and red blood cells. When you are resting or engaging in light physical activity, triglycerides provide 30 to 70% of the energy you burn. The exact amount depends on how well fed you are before exercise, how physically fit you are, and the intensity and duration of the exercise.

Provide Compact Energy Storage

Triglycerides are the body's main storage form of energy. Excess calories from carbohydrate, fat, protein, and alcohol all can be converted to fatty acids and then to triglycerides. Triglycerides make an excellent energy "savings account" because they are stable (don't react with other cell parts) and calorie-dense. Fat cells contain about 80% lipid and only 20% water and protein. Muscle cells also contain fat and protein but are 73% water. This difference means that the lipid-rich fat cells can deliver much more energy than the water-rich muscle cells. Another reason triglycerides make an excellent storage form of energy is that the amount we can store is nearly limitless. A single adipose (fat) cell can increase in weight about 50 times. When adipose cells are maxed out with fat, new fat cells can form. Although it is important to have some body fat stores, very small and large stores can pose numerous health risks. (Chapter 10 discusses the health issues associated with underweight, overweight, and obesity.)

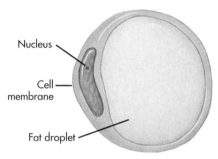

Nucleus

Cell membrane

Fat droplet

Adipose cell

Insulate and Protect the Body

The insulating layer of fat just beneath the skin (called subcutaneous fat) is made mostly of triglycerides. By insulating the body, subcutaneous fat helps keep body temperature at a constant level. Visceral fat is packed around some organs—kidneys, for example—to

When at rest or during light activity, the body uses mostly fatty acids for fuel.

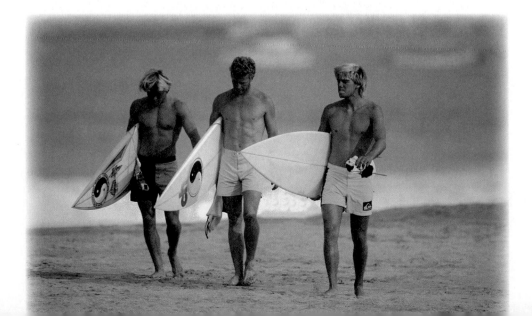

cushion them and keep them from jostling around and getting injured. We usually do not notice the insulating function of subcutaneous fat because we wear clothes and add more when needed. However, people who are starving lose most of their body fat and, as a result, feel chilled even when the environment is warm.

Aid Fat-Soluble Vitamin Absorption and Transport

Fats found in food carry fat-soluble vitamins (vitamins A, D, E, and K) to the small intestine. Once there, dietary fat assists in the absorption of these vitamins. Fat-soluble vitamins are transported in the bloodstream in the same manner as dietary fat (see Chapter 4). Those who eat an extremely low-fat diet, use mineral oil as a laxative, take certain medications (e.g., the weight-loss medication orlistat), consume large quantities of the fat replacer olestra, or have diseases that affect fat absorption (e.g., cystic fibrosis) may be unable to absorb sufficient amounts of fat-soluble vitamins.

Essential Fatty Acid Functions

Essential fatty acids, along with phospholipids and cholesterol, are important structural components of cell walls. They also keep the cell wall fluid and flexible, so that substances can flow into and out of the cell. The omega-3 fatty acid docosahexaenoic acid (DHA) is needed during fetal life and infancy for normal development and function of the retina (the part of the eye that senses light). Starting in the first few weeks of embryonic life, DHA is vital for normal development and maturation of the nervous system. Throughout life, DHA helps regulate nerve transmission and communication.

Eicosanoids, which are made from essential fatty acids, have over 100 different actions, such as regulating blood pressure, blood clotting, sleep/wake cycles, body temperature, inflammation or hypersensitivity reactions (e.g., asthma), stomach secretions, labor during child birth, and immune and allergic responses. For example, some types of eicosanoids cause inflammation, whereas other types prevent the inflammation associated with inflammatory diseases and allergic reactions. Other eicosanoids help the blood form clots, whereas other types thin blood and help prevent clots. Still other eicosanoids from omega-6 fats constrict blood vessels and raise blood pressure, yet other omega-6 eicosanoids, along with the omega-3 eicosanoids, lower blood pressure by dilating blood vessels.

Eicosanoids also have other important roles in the body, many of which are only just being discovered. For example, they assist in

- Regulating cell division rates, which may help prevent certain cancers or slow the growth of existing tumors and help prevent cancer from spreading to other parts of the body
- Transporting oxygen from red blood cells to body tissues
- Maintaining normal kidney function and fluid balance
- Directing hormones to their target cells
- Regulating the flow of substances into and out of cells
- Regulating ovulation, body temperature, immune system function, and hormone synthesis

CRITICAL THINKING

Advertisements often claim that fats are bad. Your roommate asks, "If fats are so bad for us, why do we need to have any in our diets?" What would be your answer?

Knowledge Check

1. What are 3 functions of triglycerides?
2. When is fat used as the main fuel in the body?
3. What roles do essential fatty acids play in the body?

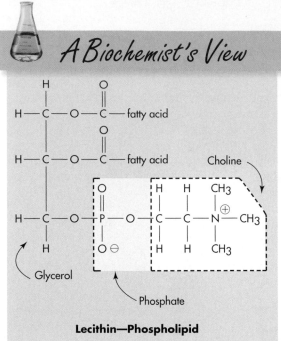

A Biochemist's View

Lecithin—Phospholipid

6.4 Phospholipids

Many types of phospholipids are found in food and the body, especially the brain. The structure of these lipids is very similar to that of triglycerides—with one exception. One fatty acid is replaced with a compound (phosphate) that contains the mineral phosphorus and often has nitrogen attached. Phosphate gives phospholipids an important quality—it lets these fats function in a watery environment (e.g., the blood) without clumping together.

Here's how phospholipids work. The phosphate end (head) of the phospholipid is hydrophilic (water-loving) and is attracted to water. The fatty acid end (tail) of the phospholipid is hydrophobic (water-fearing) and is attracted to fats. When placed in water, phospholipids cluster together, with their hydrophilic phosphate heads facing outward in contact with the water and their hydrophobic tails extending into the cluster away from the water.

Phospholipid Functions

In the body, phospholipids have 2 major roles: cell membrane component and emulsifier. Phospholipids, along with fatty acids and cholesterol, are a primary component of cell membranes (Fig. 6-13). A **cell membrane** is the double-layered outer covering of a cell that corrals the cell's contents and regulates the movement of substances into and out of the cell. Imagine the cell membrane as being like corrugated cardboard. The cardboard has a smooth outside edge and a smooth inside edge, and the corrugated area fills in the space between the 2 edges. The hydrophilic phosphate heads of phospholipids orient themselves to form the cell membrane's outside edge (the part that is exposed to the blood) or inside edge (the part that is exposed to the watery cell components). Regardless of whether the hydrophilic heads are facing toward the inside or outside of the cell, their hydrophobic tails point away from the heads—so they form the "corrugation." Because the heads and tails orient themselves in this way, the cell membrane remains fluid, so that compounds can move into and out of the cell.

Phospholipids also serve as emulsifiers in the body. Bile and lecithins are the body's main emulsifiers. An **emulsifier** is a compound that forms a shell around fat droplets, so that the droplets can be suspended in water and not clump together (Fig. 6-14). The hydrophobic tails of the phospholipids reach toward fat droplets and form the inside of the shell. The outside of the shell is made of the hydrophilic heads that extend away from the fat droplet. With the hydrophilic heads on the outside, fat droplets are attracted to water (stay suspended) and repel other fat droplets (don't clump together). Emulsifiers are essential for fat to be digested and transported through the bloodstream.

The phospholipids in food often are used as an emulsifier in food preparation and manufacturing. Their ability to emulsify fats works the same in foods as it does in the body. For example, eggs are used in many muffin recipes. The lecithins in yolks emulsify fat in muffin batter and keep it suspended in the other ingredients. Mayonnaise is thick because phospholipids in egg yolks and mustard emulsified the oil and vinegar used to make this food. Food manufacturers add emulsifiers to keep the fat and watery compounds in them from separating. Emulsifying fats in foods such as cakes, muffins, and salad dressings gives them body and a smooth texture. Without emulsifiers, these foods would seem oily and have a sandy or rough texture.

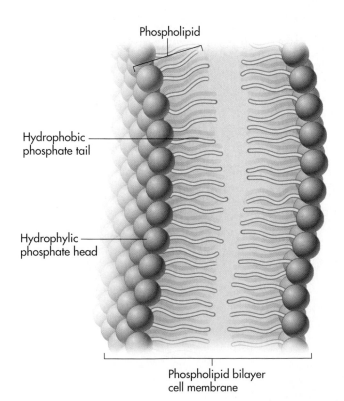

Figure 6-13 Hydrophilic phosphate heads from the outer and inside edges of cell membranes. The hydrophobic tails point away from the heads.

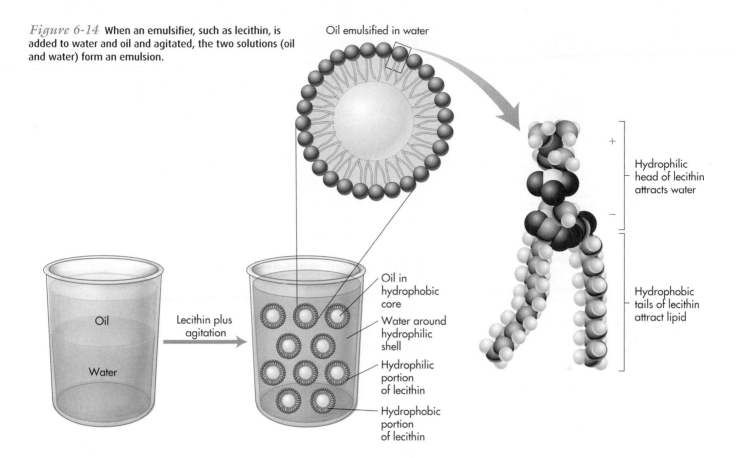

Figure 6-14 When an emulsifier, such as lecithin, is added to water and oil and agitated, the two solutions (oil and water) form an emulsion.

Oil emulsified in water

Hydrophilic head of lecithin attracts water

Hydrophobic tails of lecithin attract lipid

Oil in hydrophobic core

Water around hydrophilic shell

Hydrophilic portion of lecithin

Hydrophobic portion of lecithin

Oil

Water

Lecithin plus agitation

Sources of Phospholipids

Phospholipids can be synthesized by the body or supplied by the diet. For example, lecithins are found in foods such as egg yolks, wheat germ, and peanuts. Although lecithin supplements are available, they are not needed because the liver can produce sufficient amounts of phospholipids. Lecithin supplements have been promoted as a way to lose weight, lower cholesterol, and reduce the risk of Alzheimer's disease. However, studies indicate there is no effect of lecithin on weight loss. Data are conflicting when it comes to lecithin's ability to lower cholesterol or Alzheimer's disease risk.[2, 3] It is important to note that high doses of lecithin can cause gas, diarrhea, and weight gain.

Eggs are the main source of cholesterol in the North American diet. The Food and Nutrition Board suggests limiting intake of high-cholesterol foods.

Knowledge Check

1. What is the main structural difference between phospholipids and triglycerides?
2. What are the main functions of phospholipids?
3. How are phospholipids used in the food industry?

Lecithins are a family of phospholipids synthesized by the body and found in foods such as peanuts, wheat germ, soybeans, egg yolks, and liver.

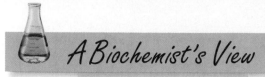

A Biochemist's View

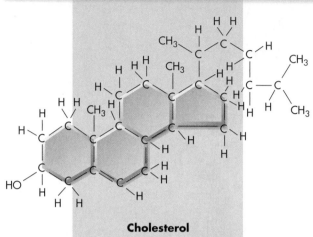

Cholesterol

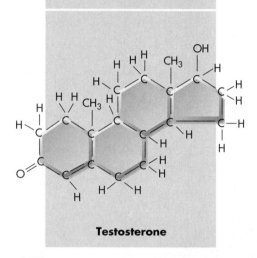

Testosterone

Figure 6-15 The carbons in sterols are arranged in rings. There is a carbon on each corner of this structural drawing of cholesterol and testosterone.

Cholesterol Content of Foods

3 oz beef brains	2635 mg
3 oz beef liver	337 mg
1 large egg yolk*	209 mg
3 oz shrimp	166 mg
3 oz beef*	75 mg
3 oz pork	75 mg
3 oz chicken or turkey (white meat)*	75 mg
1 cup ice cream	63 mg
3 oz trout	60 mg
3 oz tuna	45 mg
3 oz hot dog	38 mg
1 oz cheddar cheese*	30 mg
1 cup whole milk*	24 mg
1 cup 1% milk	12 mg
1 cup fat-free milk	5 mg
1 large egg white	0 mg

*Leading dietary sources of cholesterol in American diets.

 6.5 Sterols

Sterols are the last class of lipids. The structure of sterols is very different from that of the long carbon chains seen in fatty acids and phospholipids. Instead, the carbons are mostly arranged in many rings (Fig. 6-15).

Sterol Functions

From a nutrition perspective, cholesterol is the most well-known sterol. This waxy substance is required to synthesize many compounds. For instance, our bodies use cholesterol to make steroid hormones, such as testosterone, estrogens, the active form of vitamin D hormone, and corticosteroids (cortisone). Cholesterol also is used to make bile, which is required to emulsify fats, so that they can be digested normally.

In addition, cholesterol works with phospholipids to form cell membranes and allow fat-soluble substances to move into and out of the cell. Cholesterol, along with phospholipids and proteins, also forms the shell covering chylomicrons (droplets that transport lipids). This shell is what allows fat droplets to float through the water-based bloodstream (see Section 6.8).

Sources of Sterols

Cholesterol is found in foods of animal origin, such as meat, fish, poultry, eggs, and dairy products. (Foods of plant origin do not contain cholesterol.) Most people get about one-third of their cholesterol from the foods they eat and the rest is manufactured by their bodies. Of the approximately 875 mg of cholesterol produced daily by our bodies, about 400 mg is used to replenish bile stores and about 50 mg is used to make steroid hormones. On average, American diets supply about 180 to 325 mg of cholesterol per day.[4] Of that, we absorb about 40 to 60%. Cholesterol does not need to be supplied by the diet because the body can synthesize all the cholesterol it needs.

Although plants do not contain or produce cholesterol, they do make other sterols, such as ergosterol (a form of vitamin D) and sitostanol (added to some margarines, such as Take Control®). Eating margarine that contains sitostanol can reduce the body's absorption of cholesterol and bile, which is made from cholesterol, thereby reducing blood cholesterol levels, which decreases the risk of heart disease.

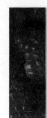

Knowledge Check

1. What is the main structural difference between sterols and triglycerides?
2. What are the main functions of sterols?
3. What are 2 dietary sources of cholesterol?

 6.6 Recommended Fat Intakes

Fats are an essential part of a healthful diet but, for optimal health, the total amount and type of fat consumed need careful attention. There is no RDA for fat, but there is an Adequate Intake for infants. As you can see in Table 6-2, the Institute of Medi-

Table 6-2 Institute of Medicine (IOM) Recommended Daily Fat Intakes[4]

Fat Component	IOM Recommendations
Total Dietary Fat	20 to 35% of calories
Saturated Fat	As low as possible
Trans Fat	As low as possible
Unsaturated Fat	Most of fat intake
Omega 6: linoleic acid	5% of calories
Omega 3: alpha-linolenic acid	0.6 to 1.2% of calories
Cholesterol*	**As low as possible**

*National Cholesterol Education Program daily recommendation for cholesterol is 200 mg or less.

▶ The American Dietetic Association and Dietitians of Canada suggest that adults eat 20 to 35% of their calories as fat, consume diets low in saturated and *trans* fatty acids, and eat more omega-3 fatty acids.[24]

▶ Infants and children younger than 2 years need to get about half of their total calories from fat to meet calorie needs and to obtain sufficient fat for normal brain development. For children 2 to 3 years of age, keep total fat intake between 30 and 35% of calories. Between the ages of 4 and 18 years, keep fat intake between 25 and 35% of calories.

cine's Adequate Macronutrient Distribution Range for total fat is 20 to 35% of calories for most age groups. A total fat intake that exceeds 35% of calories often means saturated fat intake is too high. A low intake of total fat (less than 20% of calories) increases the chances of getting too little vitamin E and essential fatty acids and may adversely affect blood levels of triglycerides and a type of cholesterol called high-density lipoprotein (HDL) cholesterol, which is sometimes called "good" cholesterol (see Section 6.7).

The Institute of Medicine also recommends that saturated fat intake, including *trans* fats, and cholesterol levels be kept as low as possible while still consuming a nutritionally adequate diet. A *Healthy People 2010* goal is to reduce the proportion of people over age 2 years who get more than 10% of their calories from saturated fat. Other expert groups, such as the American Heart Association and the Dietary Guidelines for Americans committee, suggest that healthy people limit saturated fats as well as polyunsaturated fats to no more than 10% of total calories each and minimize *trans* fat intake. Most experts recommend that, when fat calories exceed 30% of total calories, monounsaturated fats supply the extra calories. In addition, cholesterol intake should be limited to about 300 mg daily. The intake levels recommended by these expert groups meet or exceed the body's daily needs while minimizing risk of chronic disease.

Fat intake recommendations are lower for those at risk of heart disease, such as people with high blood levels of low-density lipoprotein (LDL) cholesterol, the so-called bad cholesterol. For example, the American Heart Association recommends that these individuals restrict dietary fat to 20% of total calories, saturated fat to 7% of total calories, and cholesterol to 200 mg or less daily. Even more stringent is Dr. Dean Ornish's recommendation that dietary fat be limited to 10% of total calories.[5] Low-fat diets can help lower the risk of heart disease and, in some cases, partly reverse damage already done to arteries. However, many low-fat diets are high in carbohydrates, which may increase blood triglyceride levels and raise the risk of heart disease. As a result, it's best for those getting less than 20% of total calories from fat to be monitored by a physician. Elevated blood triglycerides often decline over several months, especially if carbohydrate choices are high in fiber, weight is kept at a healthy level, and regular exercise is included.

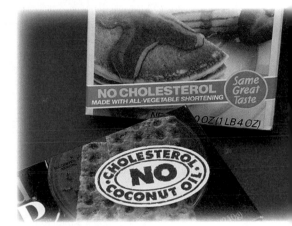

Products with reduced or no cholesterol can help keep cholesterol intake under control.

Mediterranean Diet

There is some evidence that up to 40% of calories from fat can be healthy if monounsaturated fats account for most of the fat. The first evidence that a diet high in monounsaturated fats can be heart healthy was reported over 60 years ago in the 7 countries study conducted by Ancel Keyes and colleagues[6]—this

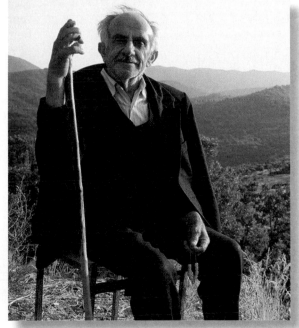

Followers of the traditional Mediterranean Diet, rich in olive oil, have low rates of chronic diseases.

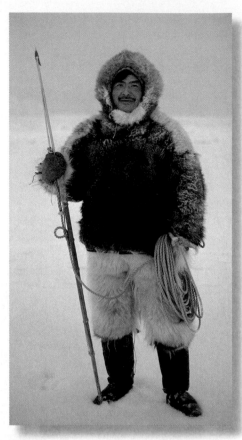

The importance of consuming eicosanoids was discovered many years ago in studies of Greenland Eskimos. Their diet is very high in EPA-rich fish oils, and they exhibit diminished blood clotting and lower risks of heart disease.

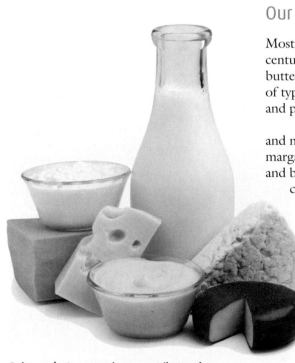

Dairy products are a primary contributor of saturated fat to our diets.

study led to today's popular Mediterranean Diet. Those who follow the traditional Mediterranean Diet enjoy some of the lowest recorded rates of chronic disease in the world. In years gone by, Greek farmers in Crete drank a glass of monounsaturated fat–rich olive oil for breakfast! Even today, the average consumption of olive oil in Greece is 20 liters per person per year.

The traditional Mediterranean Diet features the following:

- Olive oil as the main fat
- Abundant daily intake of fruits, vegetables (especially leafy greens), whole grains, beans, nuts, and seeds
- An emphasis on minimally processed and, wherever possible, seasonally fresh and locally grown foods
- Daily intake of small amounts of cheese and yogurt
- Weekly intake of low to moderate amounts of fish
- Limited use of eggs and red meat
- Regular exercise
- Moderate drinking of wine at mealtime

Essential Fatty Acid Needs

The Institute of Medicine has set Adequate Intakes for essential fatty acids. These recommendations add up to less than 120 calories daily for women and 170 calories for men—that's about 2 to 4 tablespoons daily of oils rich in these fatty acids. An essential fatty acids deficiency is very unlikely to occur, but insufficient intake for many weeks can lead to diarrhea, slowed growth, delayed healing of wounds and infections, and flaky, itchy skin. Although the Institute of Medicine has not yet set an Upper Level for safe intake of omega-3 fats, Greenland Eskimos safely consume about 6.5 g/day, which is 3 to 5 times higher than the Adequate Intake.

Our Fat Intake

Most North Americans get more than enough total dietary fat. In fact, during the last century, our fat intake has doubled. Added fats are those that we add to food, such as butter on bread and shortenings used to make cookies, pastries, and fried foods. In terms of types of fat, many people get too much saturated fat and too little monounsaturated and polyunsaturated fat.

Dairy products (whole milk, cheese, ice cream, butter), beef, chicken, mayonnaise, and margarine are the main contributors of saturated fat. The major *trans* fat sources are margarine and baked goods made with shortening, such as cakes, cookies, crackers, pies, and breads. Vegetable oils are the prime contributors of polyunsaturated fat. Figure 6-16 compares the fat content of a high-fat meal with one lower in fat. What changes can you make to bring your fat intake under control?

Omega-6 fatty acid intakes are usually plentiful, but omega-3 intakes often are lower than optimal. Omega-3 fat needs can be met by eating at least 2 portions of cold-water fish each week. For individuals who do not eat fish regularly, walnuts, flaxseeds, and canola, soybean, and flaxseed oils also supply omega-3 fatty acids. Supplements also are an option. The National Institutes of Health recommends choosing a fish oil supplement that has 650 mg of EPA and 650 mg of DHA. Those who have bleeding disorders, are scheduling surgery, or are taking anticoagulants (e.g., aspirin, warfarin [Coumadin®], or the herb ginkgo biloba) should check with their physician to minimize the risk of harmful side effects from an omega-3 supplement, which can prolong bleeding time.

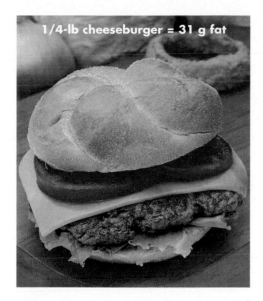

1/4-lb cheeseburger = 31 g fat

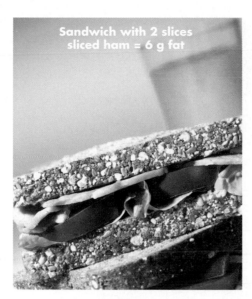

Sandwich with 2 slices sliced ham = 6 g fat

Figure 6-16 Knowing the fat content of foods can help you plan a healthy diet.

Two servings of cold-water fish, such as salmon, each week can meet omega-3 fatty acid needs.

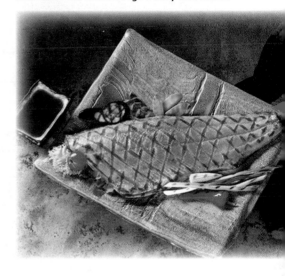

Knowledge Check

1. What are the recommendations regarding total fat intake?
2. What are the main characteristics of the traditional Mediterranean Diet?
3. How does our fat intake compare with recommendations?
4. What are some steps you can take to ensure sufficient intake of omega-3 fatty acids?

CASE STUDY

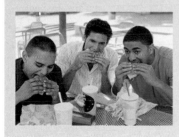

Another typical day at college—Brad, a senior business major, pulls on his favorite pair of jeans and notices they feel tighter than usual. He skips another breakfast to make it to his 8 A.M. class. He is hungry but knows that after the lab class he will stop at the campus union and eat his usual lunch with friends: a double cheeseburger, french fries, and a milkshake. He knows that after that meal he will feel full and not be hungry until later in the afternoon, when his classes end. Then, he'll either call out for a double-cheese pizza or grab another double cheeseburger for dinner. Then, it's off to the library for a long night of studying. What type of fat is he mostly eating? What concerns should Brad have about his diet? What risks does he have for a heart attack, despite the fact that he is only 22 years old? What changes would you recommend?

6.7 Fat Digestion and Absorption

The body is very efficient at digesting and absorbing dietary fat (Fig. 6-17). (For a complete review of the digestive process, see Chapter 4.)

Digestion

Fat digestion begins in the mouth, where lingual lipase is secreted. This enzyme helps break down triglycerides with short and medium chain fatty acids that are found in milk fat. Although this enzyme is active during infancy, it plays only a minor role in fat digestion in adulthood.

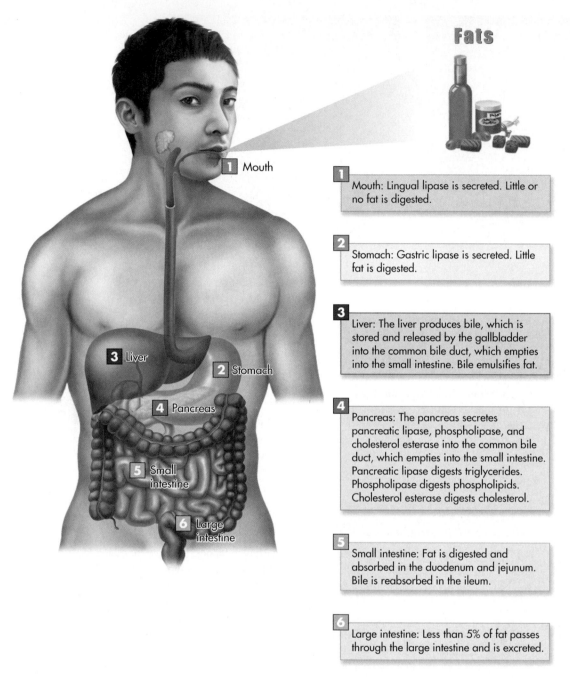

Fats

1 **Mouth:** Lingual lipase is secreted. Little or no fat is digested.

2 **Stomach:** Gastric lipase is secreted. Little fat is digested.

3 **Liver:** The liver produces bile, which is stored and released by the gallbladder into the common bile duct, which empties into the small intestine. Bile emulsifies fat.

4 **Pancreas:** The pancreas secretes pancreatic lipase, phospholipase, and cholesterol esterase into the common bile duct, which empties into the small intestine. Pancreatic lipase digests triglycerides. Phospholipase digests phospholipids. Cholesterol esterase digests cholesterol.

5 **Small intestine:** Fat is digested and absorbed in the duodenum and jejunum. Bile is reabsorbed in the ileum.

6 **Large intestine:** Less than 5% of fat passes through the large intestine and is excreted.

1 Mouth

3 Liver

2 Stomach

4 Pancreas

5 Small intestine

6 Large intestine

Figure 6-17 Lipid digestion and absorption. Enzymes made by the mouth, stomach, pancreas, and small intestine, as well as bile from the liver, participate in the process of digestion. Lipid digestion and absorption mostly take place in the small intestine (see Chapter 4 for details).

In the stomach, gastric lipase helps break triglycerides into monoglycerides, diglycerides, and free fatty acids. Fat floats on top of the watery contents of the stomach, which limits the extent of lipid digestion in the stomach.

Fat digestion occurs mostly in the small intestine. Recall that the presence of fat in the small intestine triggers the release of the hormone cholecystokinin (CCK) from intestinal cells. CCK stimulates the release of bile from the gallbladder and lipase and colipase from the pancreas, all of which are delivered to the small intestine by the common bile duct. Bile emulsifies fats. That is, it breaks fat into many tiny droplets, called **micelles,** and forms a shell around the micelles that keeps the fat droplets suspended in the water-based intestinal contents. Emulsification increases the surface area of lipids and allows pancreatic lipase to efficiently break triglycerides into monoglycerides and free fatty acids. Fat digestion is very rapid and thorough because the amount of pancreatic lipase released usually is much greater than the amount needed. In addition, **colipase** helps lipase latch onto micelles.

Phospholipids and cholesterol also are digested mostly in the small intestine. Phospholipase enzymes from the pancreas and enzymes from the small intestine mucosa break phospholipids into their basic parts: glycerol, fatty acids, phosphoric acid, and other components (e.g., choline). Cholesterol esters (cholesterol with a fatty acid attached) are broken down to cholesterol and free fatty acids by a pancreatic enzyme called cholesterol esterase.

Absorption

The lipid portion of the micelles is absorbed by the brush border of the absorptive cells lining the duodenum and jejunum sections of the small intestine (Fig. 6-18). About 95% of dietary fat is absorbed. The carbon chain length of a fatty acid or

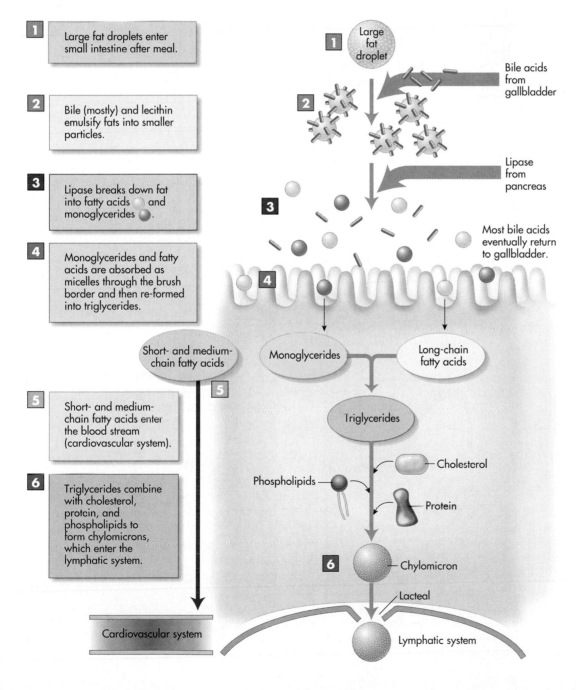

1 Large fat droplets enter small intestine after meal.

2 Bile (mostly) and lecithin emulsify fats into smaller particles.

3 Lipase breaks down fat into fatty acids ○ and monoglycerides ●.

4 Monoglycerides and fatty acids are absorbed as micelles through the brush border and then re-formed into triglycerides.

5 Short- and medium-chain fatty acids enter the blood stream (cardiovascular system).

6 Triglycerides combine with cholesterol, protein, and phospholipids to form chylomicrons, which enter the lymphatic system.

Large fat droplet

Bile acids from gallbladder

Lipase from pancreas

Most bile acids eventually return to gallbladder.

Short- and medium-chain fatty acids

Monoglycerides

Long-chain fatty acids

Triglycerides

Phospholipids

Cholesterol

Protein

Chylomicron

Lacteal

Cardiovascular system

Lymphatic system

Figure 6-18 A simplified look at absorption of triglycerides.

monoglyceride determines whether it is absorbed by the cardiovascular or the lymphatic system. After absorption, short- and medium-chain fatty acids (< 12 carbons) mostly enter the cardiovascular system via the portal vein, which leads directly to the liver. Long-chain fatty acids (≥ 12 carbons) are re-esterified into triglycerides in the absorptive cell. After further packaging (described in Section 6.8), they enter the lymphatic circulation, along with fat-soluble vitamins and dietary cholesterol.

Recall that bile, and the cholesterol it contains, is recycled by enterohepatic circulation. That is, bile is reabsorbed in the ileum and returned to the liver (via the portal vein) to be used again in fat digestion. About 98% of bile is recycled and the rest is eliminated in the feces. Increasing the amount of bile that passes out of the body can help lower blood cholesterol levels because, when less is recycled, the liver takes more cholesterol out of the blood to restore the bile supply. Certain medications and diets rich in soluble fiber, which binds bile and carries it out with the feces, reduce the amount of recycled bile.

Knowledge Check

1. What is the role of cholecystokinin in the digestion of lipids?
2. What is the role of bile in fat digestion?
3. How does the chain length of a fatty acid affect absorption?

6.8 Transporting Fat in the Blood

Transporting fats through the water-based blood and lymphatic system presents a challenge because water and fat do not mix. Fats are transported in the blood as lipoproteins called chylomicrons, very-low-density lipoproteins, intermediate-density lipoproteins, low-density lipoproteins, and high-density lipoproteins. **Lipoproteins** have a core, made of lipids, that is covered with a shell composed of protein, phospholipid, and cholesterol. The shell lets the lipoprotein circulate in the blood. Figure 6-19 and Table 6-3 show the composition role of these lipoproteins.

Transporting Dietary Fats Utilizes Chylomicrons

Triglycerides that are re-formed in the absorptive cells of the intestine are packaged with other lipids, such as cholesterol and phospholipids, into lipoproteins called **chylomicrons**. These large lipid droplets are surrounded by a thin shell of phospholipid, choles-

Table 6-3 Composition and Roles of the Major Lipoproteins in the Blood

Lipoprotein	Primary Component	Key Role
Chylomicron	Triglyceride	Carries dietary fat from the small intestine to cells
VLDL	Triglyceride	Carries lipids both taken up and made by the liver to cells
LDL	Cholesterol	Carries cholesterol made by the liver and from other sources to cells
HDL	Protein	Helps remove cholesterol from cells and, in turn, excretion of cholesterol from the body.

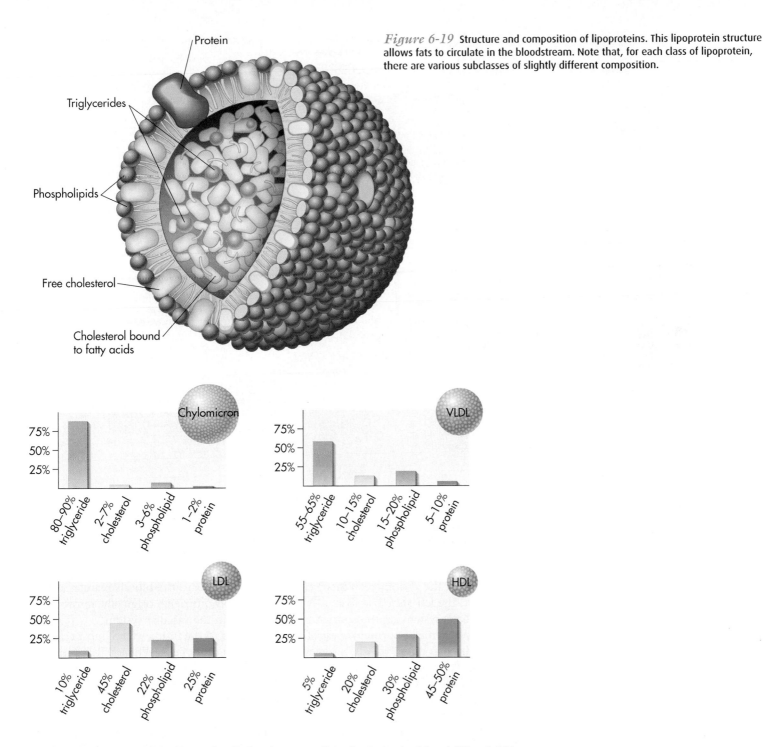

Figure 6-19 Structure and composition of lipoproteins. This lipoprotein structure allows fats to circulate in the bloodstream. Note that, for each class of lipoprotein, there are various subclasses of slightly different composition.

terol, and protein, which allows the chylomicrons to float freely in the blood (Fig. 6-20). The protein portion of the shell lipoproteins contains **apolipoproteins.** A series of letters (A through E) with subclasses are used to identify apolipoproteins. For convenience, they are abbreviated "apo," followed by an identifying letter—that is, apo A, apo B-48, apo C-II, and so on. Apolipoproteins can turn on a lipid transfer enzyme (e.g., apo C-II turns on lipoprotein lipase), assist in binding a lipoprotein to a receptor on cell surfaces (e.g., apo B-48 binds chylomicrons to the liver), or assist enzymes (e.g., apo A-I activates lecithin:cholesterol acyltransferase).

Chylomicrons are secreted from the intestinal cells into the lymphatic system via the lacteals (special lymphatic vessels) in the intestinal villi. Recall that lacteals connect to larger lymphatic vessels, which then connect to the thoracic duct. The thoracic duct

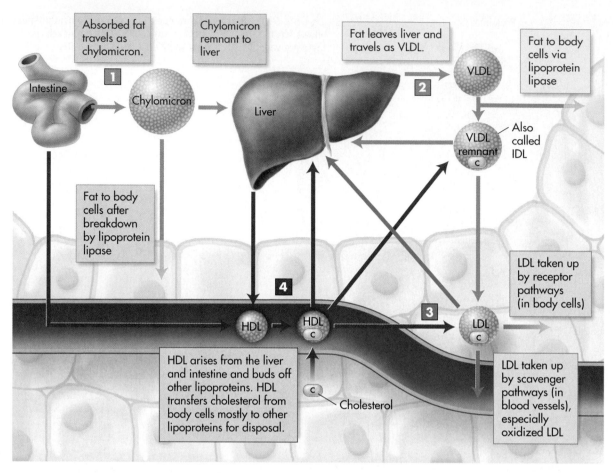

Figure 6-20 Lipoprotein interactions. (1) Chylomicrons carry absorbed fat to body cells. (2) VLDL carries fat taken up from the bloodstream by the liver, as well as any fat made by the liver, to body cells. (3) LDL arises from VLDL and carries mostly cholesterol to cells. (4) HDL arises from body cells, mostly in the liver and intestine, as well as from particles that bud off other lipoproteins. HDL carries cholesterol from cells to other lipoproteins and to the liver for excretion.

extends from the abdomen to the neck, where it connects to the bloodstream at a large vein called the left subclavian vein. Once in the blood, nutrients originally absorbed by the lymphatic system are transported to body tissues in the vascular system.

The enzyme lipoprotein lipase (LPL) is attached to the inside wall of most cells, including those in blood vessels, muscles, fat tissue, and other cells. When LPL is activated by apo C-II, it transfers triglycerides from the chylomicrons to the cells where LPL is attached. Cells can immediately use transferred triglycerides for energy or store them for later use. Certain cells, such as muscles, tend to use the triglycerides as energy, whereas adipose cells tend to store them.

After a meal, the whole process of removing chylomicrons from the blood via LPL activity takes from 2 to 10 hours, depending partly on how much fat was in the meal. After 12 to 14 hours of fasting, no chylomicrons should be in the blood. It is a good idea for people to fast 12 to 14 hours before having blood lipid profiles because the presence of chylomicrons can affect the results.

Transporting Lipids Mostly Made by the Body Utilizes Very-Low-Density Lipoproteins

The liver makes some fat and cholesterol using carbon, hydrogen, and energy from the carbohydrate, protein, and free fatty acids it takes from the blood. Free fatty acids

Expert Perspective *from the Field*

Nuts for Your Heart

Not too long ago, health professionals warned consumers to limit their intake of nuts, including tree nuts (e.g., almonds, walnuts, pistachios) and peanuts (a legume), because they are high in fat and calories. However, according to Dr. Wahida Karmally,* many leading health organizations, such as the American Heart Association, now encourage consumers to substitute healthy (i.e., unsaturated) fats found in nuts, avocados, canola oil, and olive oil for saturated fats found in meat, dairy products, and some processed foods.

Dr. Penny Kris-Etherton** indicated that this shift in thinking about the role of nuts in a healthy diet came about as a result of the substantive and growing body of scientific evidence demonstrating the health benefits of eating nuts frequently (i.e., 1 oz of nuts eaten 5 times/week). The story began with benefits being shown for nut consumption and coronary heart disease and expanded to benefits for other diseases. Large epidemiological studies convincingly demonstrated that frequent intake of nuts decreased risk of coronary heart disease by 30 to 50%. For women, frequent nut consumption also lowered risk of type 2 diabetes and gallstones by 25%. In addition, nuts may help regulate body weight—frequent nut eaters have lower body weights than those who eat nuts infrequently.

Experimental research supported epidemiological findings. Study participants eating diets containing nuts reduced total cholesterol and LDL cholesterol concentrations. In addition, these nut-containing diets did not reduce HDL cholesterol or increase blood triglyceride levels. Dr. Kris-Etherton pointed out that a key research question is "which compounds in nuts caused these effects?" Nuts are a powerhouse of nutrients that promote heart health, including unsaturated fats (both monounsaturated and polyunsaturated), protein, fiber, vitamin E, folic acid, vitamin B-6, niacin, magnesium, copper, zinc, and potassium. In

addition, nuts contain a wide range of phytochemicals, such as ellagic acid, flavonoids, phenolic compounds (including resveratrol), and isoflavones that might play a role in heart health. The plant sterols and omega-3 fatty acid (alpha-linolenic acid) in nuts also may be cardio-protective.

Even though the compounds in nuts that promote heart health are not yet known, the FDA felt that the data supporting the relationship between nuts and reduced cardiovascular disease risk were substantial enough to grant this qualified health claim: "Scientific evidence suggests but does not prove that eating 1.5 ounces of nuts per day as a part of a diet low in saturated fat and cholesterol may reduce the risk for heart disease." Thus, with a new appreciation for the *nut* in *nutrition*, enjoy nuts in moderation for good nutrition and heart health!

Wahida Karmally, DrPH, RD, CDE is Director of Nutrition for the Irving Institute for Clinical and Translational Research and Associate Research Scientist at Columbia University. She chaired the Nutrition Committee for the American Heart Association, New York City Chapter, and the American Dietetic Association committee that developed evidence-based recommendations and practice guidelines for the nutritional management of lipid metabolism disorders.

**Penny Kris-Etherton, PhD, RD is Distinguished Professor of Nutrition in the Department of Nutritional Sciences at Pennsylvania State University and a Fellow of the American Heart Association. She is the recipient of the Lederle Award for Human Nutrition Research from the American Society for Nutritional Sciences and the Foundation Award for Excellence in Research and the Marjorie Hulsizer Copher Award from the American Dietetic Association. She has served on the National Academy of Sciences Panel on Macronutrients, American Heart Association Nutrition Committee, National Cholesterol Education Program Second Adult Treatment Panel, and Dietary Guidelines for Americans 2005 Committee.*

---

are the major source of "ingredients" for tri-glyceride synthesis. The liver coats the cholesterol and triglycerides that collect in that organ with a shell of protein and lipids and produces what are called **very-low-density lipoproteins (VLDLs).**

When VLDLs from the liver enter the circulatory system, the enzyme LPL in the lining of blood vessels transfers the triglycerides in VLDLs to body cells, including adipose tissue for fat storage and muscle tissue for energy. As triglycerides are released, VLDLs get more and more dense and become **intermediate-density lipoproteins (IDLs).** IDLs lose additional triglycerides by activating an enzyme called hepatic trig-lyceride lipase (HTGL) found on the endothelial surface of the liver. HTGL and LPL remove triglycerides from IDLs, causing the proportions of triglyceride to decrease and cholesterol to increase. As more triglycerides are removed, the IDLs become **low-density lipoproteins (LDLs).** LDLs are composed primarily of cholesterol.

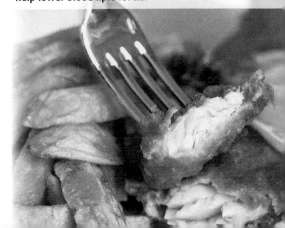

Fried foods are a rich source of fat and *trans* fats. Reducing the intake of these foods can help lower blood lipid levels.

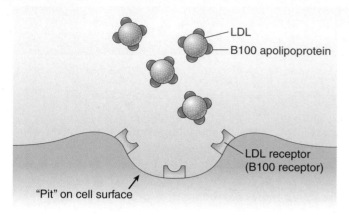

Cells have pits on the surface, which contain LDL receptors.

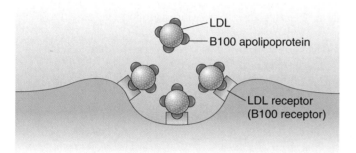

LDL binds to the LDL receptors in the pits.

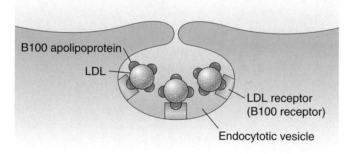

The LDL, bound to LDL receptors, is taken into the cell by endocytosis.

Figure 6-21 **Transport of LDL into cells.** LDL receptors capture circulating LDL and release it inside the cell to be metabolized. Once free of their load, LDL receptors return to the cell surface to await new LDL.

antioxidant Compound that protects other compounds, such as unsaturated fats, and body tissues from the damaging effects of oxygen (*anti* means against; *oxidant* means oxygen).

atherosclerosis Buildup of fatty material (plaque) in the arteries, including those surrounding the heart.

Pathways for Cholesterol Uptake

In the **receptor pathway for cholesterol uptake,** LDL is removed from the blood by cells with the LDL receptor called B-100. The liver, as well as other cells, has this receptor (Fig. 6-21). Once inside a cell, LDL is broken down to protein and free cholesterol. These LDL components are used for maintaining the cell membrane or synthesizing specialized compounds, such as estrogen, testosterone, and vitamin D. When the free cholesterol concentration inside the cell increases to the point at which the cell can no longer take up any more LDL, the B-100 receptor stops taking LDL from the blood. When this occurs, the concentration of LDL increases in the blood. LDL that remains in the blood becomes damaged (oxidized) by free radicals, although a diet rich in **antioxidants** can help reduce LDL oxidation. Recall that oxidized LDL increases the risk for cardiovascular disease and Metabolic Syndrome.[7]

The oxidized LDL is removed from circulation by the **scavenger pathway for cholesterol uptake.** In this pathway, certain "scavenger" white blood cells leave the bloodstream and embed themselves in blood vessels. The scavenger cells detect oxidized LDL, then engulf and digest it. Once engulfed, oxidized LDL generally is prevented from re-entering the bloodstream. Scavenger cells are able to pick up enormous amounts of oxidized LDL.

Over time, cholesterol builds up in the scavenger cells; it does so more quickly when the amount of LDL in the blood is excessive. When scavenger cells have collected and deposited cholesterol for many years at a heavy pace, cholesterol builds up on the inner blood vessel walls—especially in the arteries—and plaque develops. Diets rich in saturated fat, *trans* fat, and cholesterol encourage this process. The plaque eventually mixes with connective tissue (collagen) and is covered with a cap of smooth fibrous muscle cells and calcium. **Atherosclerosis,** also referred to as hardening of the arteries, develops as plaque thickens in the vessel (Fig. 6-22). This thickening eventually chokes off the blood supply to organs, setting the stage for a heart attack and other problems, or it breaks apart and causes a clot to form in an artery.

A final critical participant in this extensive process of fat transport is **high-density lipoprotein (HDL).** Its high proportion of protein makes it the heaviest (most dense) lipoprotein. The liver and intestine produce most of the HDL found in the blood. HDL roams the bloodstream, picking up cholesterol from dying cells and other sources. HDL donates the cholesterol to other lipoproteins for transport back to the liver to be excreted. Some HDL travels directly back to the liver. Another beneficial function of HDL is that it blocks the oxidation of LDL.

Many studies demonstrate that the amount of HDL in the blood can closely predict the risk of cardiovascular disease. Risk increases with low HDL levels because little blood cholesterol is transported back to the liver and excreted. Women tend to have high amounts of HDL, especially before menopause, whereas low amounts are more common in men.

Because high amounts of HDL slow the development of cardiovascular disease, any cholesterol carried by HDL is considered "good" cholesterol. In contrast, cholesterol carried by LDL is termed "bad" cholesterol because high amounts of LDL speed the development of cardiovascular disease. Still, some LDL is needed for normal body functions; LDL is only a problem when there is too much in the blood.

6.9 Health Concerns Related to Fat Intake

Dietary fat is essential for good health. However, high intakes can adversely affect health status.

High Polyunsaturated Fat Intake

Intakes of polyunsaturated fats greater than 10% of total calorie intake seem to increase the amount of cholesterol deposited in arteries, which raises the chances of developing cardiovascular disease. High intakes also may impair the immune system's ability to fight disease.

Excessive Omega-3 Fatty Acid Intake

Diets that include fish rich in omega-3 fatty acids twice a week (8 ounces/week) can reduce blood clotting abilities and may favorably affect heart rhythm in some people—both of these effects help lower the chances of having a heart attack. Larger intakes of fish (4 to 8 ounces/day) further reduce the risk of heart disease by lowering blood triglyceride levels in those whose levels are high. However, an excessive intake of omega-3 fatty acids may impair the function of the immune system, allow uncontrolled bleeding, and cause **hemorrhagic stroke** (bleeding in the brain that damages it). Excessive levels of omega-3s are usually the result of supplement use.

Imbalances in Omega-3 and Omega-6 Fatty Acids

On average, Americans consume 20 times more omega-6 fatty acids than omega-3s. Both fatty acids use the same metabolic pathways; as a result, they compete with one another. Thus, the body may not have enough of some compounds and too much of others. For example, as you saw in Figure 6-10, omega-6 fatty acids can be converted to arachidonic acid, which then can be used to make inflammation-causing eicosanoids called **prostaglandins**. In contrast, the omega-3 fatty acids EPA and DHA can be made into substances that help decrease inflammation, pain, and blood triglycerides.[8] Low intakes of omega-3s can worsen inflammatory diseases, such as arthritis. Although it is not known what causes or cures arthritis, an imbalance in the intakes of omega-3 and omega-6 fatty acids may play a role.[8-10]

Many manufacturers offer products that are lower in fat than traditional products. Even though these products are lower in fat, portion size and total calories provided still must be considered.

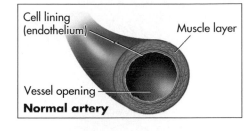
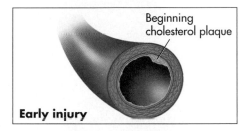
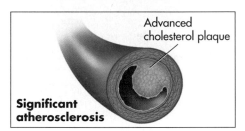
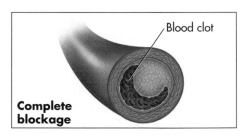

Figure 6-22 **Progression of atherosclerosis.**

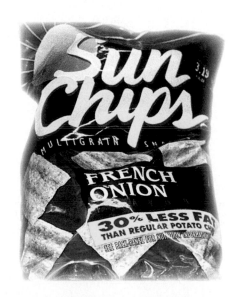

Medical Perspective

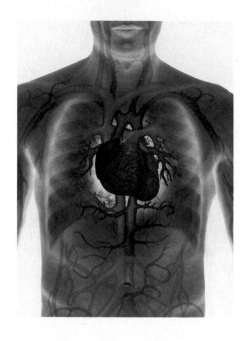

► A *Healthy People 2010* goal is to reduce death from coronary heart disease by 30%, compared with today's incidence.

► CVD typically involves the coronary arteries and thus is frequently termed *coronary heart disease (CHD)* or *coronary artery disease (CAD)*.

homocysteine Amino acid not used in protein synthesis but, instead, produced during metabolism of the amino acid methionine. Homocysteine is likely toxic to many cells, such as those lining the blood vessels.

Cardiovascular Disease (CVD)

Cardiovascular disease (CVD) is the major killer of North Americans. Each year, about 500,000 people die of CVD in the United States, about 60% more than die of cancer. The figure rises to almost 1 million if strokes and other circulatory diseases are included. About 1.5 million people in the United States each year have a heart attack. The overall male-to-female ratio for heart disease is about 2:1. Women generally lag about 10 years behind men in developing the disease. Still, it eventually kills more women than any other disease—twice as many as cancer. And, for each person in North America who dies of CVD, 20 more (over 13 million people) have symptoms of the disease.

High-fat diets, especially those rich in saturated and *trans* fats, increase the risk of CVD. (Recall that the vascular system includes the blood, heart, arteries, and veins.) The symptoms develop over many years and often do not become obvious until old age. Nonetheless, autopsies of those under 20 years of age have shown that many already had atherosclerotic plaque in their arteries.

Development of CVD

Atherosclerotic plaque is probably first deposited to repair injuries in the lining in any artery. The damage that starts plaque formation can be caused by smoking, diabetes, hypertension, **homocysteine** (likely, but not a major factor), and LDL.[14-16] Viral and bacterial infections and ongoing blood vessel inflammation also may promote plaque formation.[17]

As atherosclerosis progresses, plaque thickens over time, causing arteries to harden, narrow, and become less elastic. This makes them unable to expand to accommodate the normal ups and downs of blood pressure. Affected arteries are further damaged as blood pumps through them and pressure increases. In the final phase, a clot or spasm in a plaque-clogged artery blocks the flow of blood and leads to a heart attack (myocardial infarction) or stroke (cerebrovascular accident).

Recall that blood supplies the heart muscle and brain—and other body organs—with oxygen and nutrients. When blood flow via the coronary arteries surrounding the heart is interrupted, a heart attack may occur, which damages the heart muscle. If blood flow to parts of the brain is interrupted long enough, part of the brain dies, causing a stroke. Factors that typically bring on a heart attack in a person at risk include dehydration, severe emotional stress, strenuous physical activity when not otherwise physically fit, sudden awakening during the night or just getting up in the morning (linked to an abrupt increase in blood pressure and stress), and high-fat meals, which increase blood clotting.

Risk Factors for CVD

In addition to a high-fat diet, the American Heart Association has identified several other factors that affect the risk of heart disease. The more risk factors a person has, the greater the risk of CVD. Some of the risk factors cannot be changed, but others can. The risk factors that cannot be changed are age, gender, genetics, and race.

- *Age.* The risk of CVD increases with age. Over 83% of people who die of CVD are at least 65 years old.
- *Gender.* Men have a greater chance of having a heart attack than women do, and they have attacks earlier in life. Even after menopause, when women's death rate from heart disease increases,[18] it's not as great as the risk men face.
- *Genetics.* Having a close relative who died prematurely from CVD, especially before age 50, may increase the risk. Those with the highest risk of premature CVD have genetic

defects that block the removal of chylomicrons and triglycerides from the blood, reduce the liver's ability to remove LDL cholesterol from the blood, limit the synthesis of HDL cholesterol, or increase blood clotting.

- *Race.* Race may affect CVD risk. For example, those of African heritage have more severe high blood pressure levels, compared with Caucasians, which puts them at higher risk of CVD. Heart disease risk also is higher among those of Hispanic/Latino, Native American, and native Hawaiian descent, as well as some Asian groups, which is partly due to higher rates of obesity and diabetes in these groups.

The risk factors that can be modified are blood cholesterol levels, blood triglyceride levels, hypertension, smoking, physical inactivity, obesity, diabetes, liver and kidney disease, and low thyroid hormone levels.

- *Blood cholesterol levels.* A total blood cholesterol level over 200 mg/dl (especially when greater than 240 mg/dl), along with an LDL cholesterol level of 160 mg/dl or higher, increases the risk of CVD. When high blood cholesterol levels accompany other risk factors (e.g., high blood pressure and smoking), CVD risk increases even more. Reducing dietary intakes of cholesterol, saturated fat, and total fat; keeping weight under control; and exercising can help lower blood cholesterol levels, as can prescription medications.
- *Blood triglyceride levels.* Fasting blood triglyceride levels should be below 150 mg/dl. Excess triglycerides in the blood is called **hypertriglyceridemia**. Blood triglycerides are derived from fats in the foods we eat. In some individuals, simple carbohydrates and alcohol raise plasma triglyceride levels. A high triglyceride level in combination with a low HDL and high LDL may speed up atherosclerosis. Individuals with a high triglyceride level should lower their saturated fat intake and increase monounsaturated fat and omega-3 fatty acids.
- *Hypertension.* Hypertension (high blood pressure) damages the heart muscle by making it thicker and stiffer. This damage causes the heart to work harder than normal. It also increases the risk of stroke, heart attack, kidney failure, and congestive heart failure. Hypertension accompanied by high blood cholesterol levels, smoking, obesity, or diabetes raises the risk of heart attack or stroke by several times. Reducing sodium intake, losing weight, and taking medication can help bring hypertension under control. Exercise also may help.
- *Smoking.* Smokers have a 2 to 4 times greater risk of CVD than non-smokers. Even exposure to secondhand smoke can increase the risk of CVD. Smoking boosts a person's genetically linked risk of CVD, increases risk even when blood lipids are low, and makes blood more likely to clot. Smoking also tends to negate the lower CVD risk that females have, compared with males. In fact, smoking is the main cause of about 20% of the CVD cases in women. In addition, women who smoke and take oral contraceptives are at even a greater risk of CVD.
- *Physical inactivity.* Lack of exercise increases the risk of CVD. Regular moderate to vigorous physical activity lowers CVD risk, helps control blood cholesterol levels, reduces the risk of diabetes and obesity, and may even reduce blood pressure.
- *Obesity.* Many adults gain weight as they grow older. This weight gain, especially if it is around the waist, is a chief contributor to the increases in LDL blood cholesterol levels common in older adults. Obesity increases inflammation in the body and reduces the adipose cells' production of the hormone adiponectin. The reduced level of this hormone in the blood elevates the risk of having a heart attack. Obesity also leads to insulin resistance in many people, creating a risk of diabetes.
- *Diabetes.* Diabetes greatly increases the risk of developing CVD. Even when blood glucose (sugar) levels are well controlled, diabetes increases the risk of heart attack and stroke, but the risks are even greater when blood glucose levels are not well controlled. About 75% of those with diabetes die of some form of CVD. Diabetes also negates the female advantage of reduced CVD risk.
- *Liver and kidney disease and low thyroid hormone levels.* Certain forms of liver and kidney disease and low concentrations of thyroid hormone can increase blood LDL cholesterol and thus increase the risk of CVD. Medical treatment can help control these conditions and lower CVD risk.

Assessing CVD Risk

The National Cholesterol Education Program (NCEP) suggests that all adults age 20 years or older have a blood lipoprotein profile done every 5 years. This profile is most useful when the person fasts for 12 to 14 hours before the test. (Only total cholesterol and HDL values are accurate if the person has not fasted.) Table 6-4 shows how blood lipoprotein levels are interpreted.

The NCEP also has developed tables to help you calculate your risk of developing heart disease in the next 10 years. The risk is based on age, total and HDL blood cholesterol levels, blood pressure, and whether you smoke. Knowing your score can help you and your health-care provider determine if you need to make lifestyle changes, go on medication, or both.

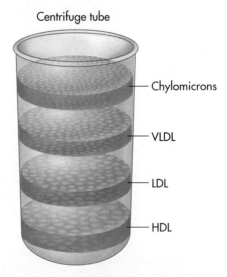

Centrifuge tube

Chylomicrons

VLDL

LDL

HDL

One way to measure the amount of chylomicrons, VLDL, LDL, and HDL particles in the bloodstream is to centrifuge the serum portion of the blood at high speed for about 24 hours in a sucrose-rich solution. The lipoproteins settle out in the centrifuge tube based on their density, with chylomicrons at the top and HDL at the bottom.

(continued)

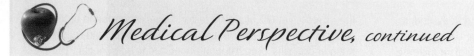

Medical Perspective, continued

▶ **Systolic blood pressure** over 140 mm (millimeters of mercury) and **diastolic blood pressure** over 90 mm indicate hypertension. Healthier blood pressure values are 120 mm and 80 mm, respectively. (**Systolic blood pressure** is the maximum pressure in the arteries when the heart beats. **Diastolic blood pressure** is the pressure in the arteries when the heart is between beats.)

▶ The values in Table 6-4 are for adults. Age-specific values for adolescents, which take their growth and maturation differences into account, have been published.[23]

Table 6-4 Ratings of Blood Lipoprotein Levels (mg/dl)

Lipoprotein (mg/dl)	Rating
Total Cholesterol	
<200	Desirable
200–239	Borderline high
≥240	High
LDL Cholesterol	
<100	Optimal
100–129	Near optimal
130–159	Borderline high
160–189	High
≥190	Very high
HDL Cholesterol	
<30	Low
≥50	High
Triglycerides	
<100	Optimal
100–149	Near optimal
150–199	Borderline high
200–499	High
≥500	Very high

CRITICAL THINKING

As part of his annual health checkup, Juan has a blood sample drawn for the measurement of cholesterol values. The results of the test indicate that his total cholesterol is 210 mg/dl, his HDL cholesterol is 65 mg/dl, and his triglycerides are 100 mg/dl. Juan has read that total cholesterol should be less than 200 mg/dl to minimize cardiovascular problems. However, he is happy with the result of the blood test. How would Juan explain his satisfaction to his parents?

▶ Benecol® and Take Control® margarines contain plant stanols/sterols.

▶ The soluble fiber in 1½ cups of oatmeal a day will reduce blood cholesterol levels by about 15%.

Preventing CVD

The following are lifestyle changes that can lower LDL blood cholesterol levels and reduce health risks.

- Keep total fat intake between 20 and 35% of total calories.
- Keep saturated fat intake to less than 7% of total calories.
- Keep *trans* fat intake low.
- Keep polyunsaturated fat under 10% of total calories.
- Keep monounsaturated fat under 20% of total calories.
- Lower cholesterol intake to less than 200 mg per day.
- Include 2 grams of plant stanols/sterols daily to help reduce cholesterol absorption in the small intestine and lower its return to the liver.
- Increase soluble fiber intake to 20 to 30 grams per day.
- Keep body weight at a healthy level.
- Increase physical activity.

Frequently eating fruits, vegetables, nuts, and plant oils also can help reduce cholesterol buildup in arteries and slow the progression of cardiovascular disease.[19] That's because these foods are rich in antioxidants, which likely reduce LDL oxidation and slow the need for scavenger cells to pick up oxidized LDL. Supplements of antioxidant nutrients, such as vitamins C and E, may help. However, large studies of people with CVD have shown no benefit from megadoses of vitamin E (200–400 mg/day, equaling about 400–800 IU/day).[20, 21] Still, some experts suggest that vitamin E supplements (up to 200 mg [400 IU] per day) may be helpful for *preventing* CVD; these should be taken under a physician's guidance. Note that antioxidant supplements can be harmful to some, especially those taking certain medications that reduce blood clotting (anticoagulants) because vitamin E also reduces blood clotting. High intakes of iron probably speed LDL oxidation, making it unwise to take an iron supplement unless a physician prescribes it. To learn more, visit www.nhlbi.nih.gov/guidelines/cholesterol/atp_iii.htm.

Heart Attack Symptoms

A heart attack can strike with the sudden force of a sledgehammer, with pain radiating up the neck or down the arm. It can sneak up at night, masquerading as indigestion, with slight pain or pressure in the chest. Many times, the symptoms are so subtle in women that it often is too late once she or health professionals realize that a heart attack is taking (or has recently taken) place. If there is any suspicion at all that a heart attack is occurring, the person should first chew an aspirin (325 mg) thoroughly and then call 911. Aspirin helps reduce the blood clotting that precipitates a heart attack. The typical warning signs are

- Intense, prolonged chest pain or pressure, sometimes radiating to other parts of the upper body (men and women)
- Shortness of breath (men and women)
- Sweating (men and women)
- Weakness (men and women)
- Nausea and vomiting (especially women)
- Dizziness (especially women)

- Jaw, neck, and shoulder pain (especially women)
- Irregular heartbeat (men and women)

Symptoms of Stroke

Each year, 700,000 North Americans suffer strokes and almost 25% of them die. Over 90% of strokes (i.e., ischemic strokes) occur when a blood clot blocks blood flow to the brain—think of a stroke as a "brain attack," similar to a heart attack. The other 10% are hemorrhagic strokes, occurring when a blood vessel bursts. The major risk factor for stroke is high blood pressure. Individuals experiencing any of the following symptoms of stroke should seek immediate treatment because physicians can administer drugs that can limit the further death of brain cells and reduce the extent of the damage caused by most strokes (i.e., ischemic strokes). The stroke warning signs are

- Sudden numbness or weakness of the face, arm, or leg, especially on one side of the body
- Sudden confusion and/or trouble speaking or understanding
- Sudden trouble seeing in one or both eyes
- Sudden trouble walking, dizziness, and/or loss of balance or coordination
- Sudden, severe headache with no known cause

Intake of Rancid Fats

Rancid (spoiled) fats smell and taste bad. They also contain compounds (peroxides and aldehydes) that can damage cells. Polyunsaturated fats go rancid fairly easily because their double bonds are easily damaged (broken) by oxygen, heat, metals, or light (sunlight or artificial light). The broken double bonds cause the polyunsaturated fats to decompose. (Saturated and *trans* fats are less susceptible to rancidity because they have no or few double bonds in their carbon chains.)

The foods most likely to become rancid are those high in polyunsaturated fats (e.g., fish and vegetable oils), packaged fried foods (e.g., potato chips), and fatty foods with a large surface area (e.g., powdered egg yolks). To prevent rancidity, food manufacturers can break the double bonds and add hydrogen (hydrogenate them). Or they can protect the double bonds in fats by sealing foods in airtight packages or adding antioxidants, such as certain nutrients (vitamin E, vitamin C), or additives, such as butylated hydroxyanisol (BHA) and butylated hydroxytolune (BHT). (See Chapter 13 to learn more about the antioxidant functions of vitamins and Chapter 3 to learn about additives.)

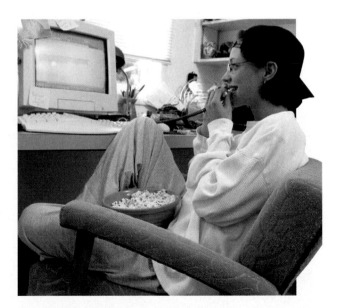

Choosing air-popped popcorn over oil-popped popcorn can help keep fat intake under control.

Diets High in *Trans* Fat

Trans fatty acids from hydrogenated fats have harmful health effects. Hydrogenated fats were popular for many years because they helped food manufacturers produce high-quality baked and fried products. For example, some foods are more pleasing when made with solid fats. Pastries and pies made with oil tend to be oily and mealy, whereas those made with solid fats are flaky and crispy. Although solid fat from animals, such as butter or lard, could be used instead of hydrogenated fat, hydrogenated fat is cholesterol-free. Another advantage of hydrogenation is that it delays fat decomposition and spoilage (rancidity) in packaged foods.

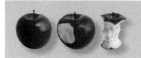

Take Action

What Is Your 10-Year Risk of Cardiovascular Disease?

During the past 2 decades, researchers have identified a number of factors that can contribute to an increased risk of cardiovascular disease. You can estimate your risk of developing cardiovascular disease if you know your blood pressure and blood lipid levels.

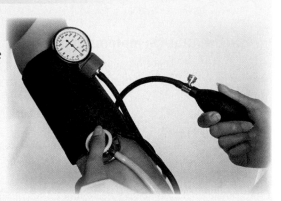

1. Select the chart for your gender.

2. Find your age group and circle your age, smoker, and total cholesterol scores.

3. Circle your systolic blood pressure score.

4. Circle your HDL cholesterol score.

5. Add all your scores and compare them with the risk chart.

    For example, a 21-year-old male smoker with a total cholesterol of 245, untreated systolic blood pressure of 145, and HDL cholesterol less than 40 has a score of 11. He has an 8% risk of cardiovascular disease in the next 10 years. A 35-year-old female non-smoker with a total cholesterol of 180, untreated systolic blood pressure of 125, and HDL cholesterol of 55 has a score of 2. She has a less than 1% risk of cardiovascular disease in the next 10 years.

10-Year Cardiovascular Disease Risk for Women

Age Group	20-34	35-39	40-44	45-49	50-54	55-59	60-64	65-69	70-74	75-79
Age Score	–7	–3	0	3	6	8	10	12	14	16
Smoker Score	9	9	7	7	4	4	2	2	1	1
Total Cholesterol Score										
<160	0	0	0	0	0	0	0	0	0	0
160-199	4	4	3	3	2	2	1	1	1	1
200-239	8	8	6	6	4	4	2	2	1	1
240-279	11	11	8	8	5	5	3	3	2	2
≥280	13	13	10	10	7	7	4	4	2	2

Systolic Blood Pressure Score	≤ 120	120-129	130-139	140-159	≥ 160
Untreated	0	1	2	3	4
Treated	0	3	4	5	6

HDL Cholesterol Score	
< 40	2
40-49	1
50-59	0
≥ 60	–1

Total Cardiovascular Disease Risk Score _____

	Women
Score	10-Year Risk (%)
< 9	< 1
9-12	1
13-14	2
15	3
16	4
17	5
18	6
19	8
20	11
21	14
22	17
23	22
24	27
≥ 25	≥ 30

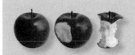

Take Action, *continued*

10-Year Cardiovascular Disease Risk for Men

Age Group	20-34	35-39	40-44	45-49	50-54	55-59	60-64	65-69	70-74	75-79
Age Score	–9	–4	0	3	6	8	10	11	12	13
Smoker Score	8	8	5	5	3	3	1	1	1	1
Total Cholesterol Score										
<160	0	0	0	0	0	0	0	0	0	0
160-199	4	4	3	3	2	2	1	1	1	1
200-239	7	7	5	5	3	3	1	1	0	0
240-279	9	9	6	6	4	4	2	2	1	1
≥280	11	11	8	8	5	5	3	3	1	1

Systolic Blood Pressure Score	≤ 120	120-129	130-139	140-159	≥ 160
Untreated	0	0	1	1	2
Treated	0	1	2	2	3

HDL Cholesterol Score	
< 40	2
40-49	1
50-59	0
≥ 60	–1

	Men
Score	10-Year Risk (%)
< 0	< 1
0-4	1
5-6	2
7	3
8	4
9	5
10	6
11	8
12	10
13	12
14	16
15	20
16	25
≥ 17	≥ 30

Total Cardiovascular Disease Risk Score

CASE STUDY FOLLOW-UP

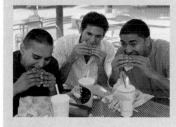

Brad's diet is high in saturated fat and he is consuming more calories than he is expending. Brad's increasing weight and his high-fat diet increase his risk of a heart attack, especially if he keeps eating this way and not getting any exercise. Brad could make improvements by eating a breakfast rich in fiber and nutrients, such as whole-grain cereal, fat-free milk, and fruit juice. Instead of fatty burgers and pizzas, he should choose lean meat, chicken, and fish. To round out meals, he needs to add several servings of fruits and vegetables. To improve his intake of monounsaturated fats, Brad could eat a small handful of peanuts each day as a snack. He could either choose cold-water fish for dinner more often or take an omega-3 fatty acid supplement. Brad also should think about starting an exercise plan to help get his weight under control.

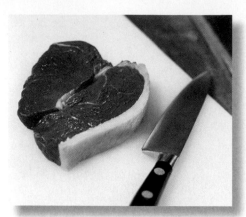

Trimming the fat off meats can help reduce saturated fat intake. Limiting intake of meat that is highly marbled with fat (streaks of fat running through the lean) helps, too.

Despite any advantages of hydrogenation, in recent years scientists have learned that consuming *trans* fatty acids raises blood cholesterol levels, which increases the risk of heart disease. In addition, *trans* fats lower HDL (good) cholesterol and increase inflammation in the body. Recent studies with monkeys indicated that diets rich in *trans* fats raised body weight and the amount of body fat stored in the abdomen, even when calories were at levels that should only maintain weight. Much of the stored abdominal fat was visceral fat, which increases the risk of type 2 diabetes.[11]

To help people control *trans* fat intake, the FDA now requires *trans* fats to be on Nutrition Facts labels (food labels in Canada also must list *trans* fats in foods, as well as their negative health effects). To lower the *trans* fat levels in foods, food manufacturers have reformulated many products to make them *trans* fat free (less than 0.5 g/serving is defined by the FDA as *trans* fat free). *Trans* fat intake can be kept to a minimum when eating out by limiting fried (especially deep fat–fried) foods, pastries, flaky bread products (e.g., pie crusts, crackers, croissants, and biscuits), and cookies. At home, keep *trans* fat intake under control by using little or no stick margarine or shortening. Instead, substitute vegetable oils and softer tub or squeeze margarine. Applesauce and fruit purees can be substituted for shortening in many baked goods. Also, to avoid deep-fat frying in shortening, try baking, pan-frying, broiling, steaming, grilling, or stir frying. Most nondairy creamers are rich in hydrogenated vegetable oils, so replace them with reduced-fat milk or non-fat dry milk.

Diets High in Total Fat

Diets high in total fat increase the risk of obesity (see Chapter 10), certain types of cancer (see Chapter 15), and cardiovascular disease.

Diets high in fat, especially saturated fat, may increase the risk of colon, prostate, and breast cancer.[12, 13] Although it isn't known how high-fat diets increase risk, one theory related to colon cancer is that bile, which is secreted into the intestine to emulsify dietary fat, may irritate colon cells. As fat intake rises, more bile is secreted, which then irritates the cells more intensely and frequently, perhaps damaging them and causing them to become cancerous. In the case of breast and prostate cancer, the risk of both climbs as blood levels of estrogen hormones rise. High-fat diets elevate blood lipid levels, which in turn raise blood estrogen levels. In contrast, low-fat diets seem to lower blood estrogen levels. Another possible explanation of the relationship between high-fat diets and cancer is that high-fat diets usually are low in fiber and other phytonutrients—thus, high-fat diets may lack the protective plant compounds that help prevent certain cancers.

Lowering the intake of dietary fat is one way to help control calorie intake and avoid being overfat. Obesity is linked with a greater risk of cancer of the colon, breast, and uterus. (The risks associated with obesity are discussed in Chapter 10.)

Knowledge Check

1. What is the risk of eating a diet that is low or high in omega-3 fatty acids?
2. What risk factors for cardiovascular disease can be modified by lifestyle changes?
3. What are the risks and benefits of *trans* fatty acids?
4. What health conditions are associated with diets high in total fat?

Summary

6.1 Triglycerides are the most common type of lipid found in foods and in the body. Each triglyceride molecule consists of 3 fatty acids attached to a glycerol. A triglyceride that loses a fatty acid is a diglyceride. A monoglyceride results when 2 fatty acids are lost. The carbon chains of fatty acids can vary in 3 ways: the number of carbons in the chain, the extent to which the chain is saturated with hydrogen, and the shape of the chain (straight or bent). Hydrogenation adds hydrogen to the carbon chain of unsaturated fats. The systems commonly used to name fatty acids, omega and delta, are based on the numbers of carbon atoms and the location of double bonds in a fatty acid's carbon chain. Essential fatty acids (alpha-linolenic acid and linoleic acid) must be obtained from the diet because humans cannot synthesize them.

6.2 Triglycerides are the main fuel source for all body cells, except the nervous system and red blood cells. Triglycerides are the body's main storage form of energy. The insulating layer of fat just beneath the skin is made mostly of triglycerides. Fats in food carry fat-soluble vitamins (vitamins A, D, E, and K) to the small intestine. Essential fatty acids, along with phospholipids and cholesterol, are important structural components of cell walls. They also keep the cell wall fluid and flexible, so that substances can flow into and out of the cell. Eicosanoids, which are made from essential fatty acids, have over 100 different actions, such as regulating blood pressure, blood clotting, sleep/wake cycles, and body temperature.

6.3 Almost all foods provide at least some triglycerides. Most triglyceride-rich foods contain a mixture of fatty acids. The fat in some foods is visible; however, fat is hidden in many foods. Fat replacements help consumers trim fat intake and still enjoy the mouthfeel sensations fat provides.

6.4 The structure of phospholipids is very similar to that of triglycerides, except a fatty acid is replaced with a compound that contains the mineral phosphorus and often has nitrogen attached. Phospholipids function in a watery environment without clumping together. The hydrophilic head of phosphate is attracted to water, and the fatty acid tail of phospholipids is attracted to fats. When placed in water, phospholipids cluster together, with their hydrophilic phosphate heads facing outward in contact with water and their hydrophobic tails extending into the cluster away from the water. In the body, phospholipids have 2 major roles: cell membrane component and emulsifier. Phospholipids can be synthesized by the body or supplied by the diet.

6.5 The carbons in the structure of sterols are mostly arranged in many rings. Cholesterol, the most well-known sterol, is used in the body to make bile and steroid hormones, such as testosterone, estrogens, the active form of vitamin D hormone, and corticosteroids. Cholesterol is found in foods of animal origin, such as meat, fish, poultry, eggs, and dairy products. Foods of plant origin do not contain cholesterol.

6.6 The Adequate Macronutrient Distribution Range for total fat is 20 to 35% of calories for most age groups. Saturated fat intake, including *trans* fats, and cholesterol should be kept as low as possible while still consuming a nutritionally adequate diet. Cholesterol intake should be limited to about 300 mg daily. Fat intake recommendations are lower for those at risk of heart disease. Adequate Intakes for essential fatty acids equal less than 120 calories daily for women and 170 calories for men—that's about 2 to 4 tablespoons daily of oils rich in these fatty acids. Most North Americans get too much saturated and too little monounsaturated and polyunsaturated fat. Omega-6 fatty acid intake is usually plentiful, but omega-3 intakes often are lower than optimal.

6.7 Fat digestion occurs mostly in the small intestine. The presence of fat in the small intestine triggers the release of cholecystokinin from intestinal cells. Cholecystokinin stimulates the release of bile and pancreatic enzymes. Bile emulsifies fats and allows enzymes to efficiently break triglycerides into monoglycerides and free fatty acids. Phospholipids and cholesterol are digested mostly in the small intestine. After absorption, short and medium chain fatty acids mostly enter the circulatory system. Long chain fatty acids enter the lymphatic circulation.

6.8 Fats are transported in the blood as lipoproteins called chylomicrons, very-low-density lipoproteins (VLDLs), intermediate-density lipoproteins (IDLs), low-density lipoproteins (LDLs), and high-density lipoproteins (HDLs). Lipoproteins have a core, made of lipids, that is covered with a shell composed of protein, phospholipid, and cholesterol. The shell lets the lipoprotein circulate in the blood. The receptor pathway for cholesterol uptake removes LDL from the blood, breaks it down, and uses the component parts for maintaining the cell membrane or synthesizing compounds. Oxidized LDL is removed from the blood by the scavenger pathway for cholesterol uptake. Over time, cholesterol builds up in the scavenger cells. When scavenger cells have collected and deposited cholesterol for many years at a heavy pace, cholesterol builds up on the inner blood vessel walls and plaque develops. HDL roams the bloodstream, picking up cholesterol from dying cells and other sources, and donates the cholesterol to other lipoproteins for transport back to the liver to be excreted.

6.9 Intakes of polyunsaturated fats greater than 10% of total calorie intake seem to increase the amount of cholesterol deposited in arteries. Diets that include fish rich in omega-3 twice a week can reduce blood clotting abilities and may favorably affect heart rhythm. Omega-6 and omega-3 fatty acids use the same metabolic pathways; as a result, imbalances in intake of these fatty acids may cause health problems. Rancid fats contain compounds that can damage cells. *Trans* fatty acids raise blood cholesterol levels, lower HDL cholesterol levels, and increase inflammation in the body. Diets high in total fat increase the risk of obesity; colon, prostate, and breast cancer; and cardiovascular disease (CVD). Atherosclerotic plaque is probably first deposited to repair injuries in the lining in any artery. As atherosclerosis progresses, plaque thickens over time, causing arteries to harden, narrow, and become less elastic. CVD risk factors are age, gender, genetics, race, blood cholesterol levels, blood triglyceride levels, hypertension, smoking, physical inactivity, obesity, and diabetes. All adults age 20 years or older should have a blood lipoprotein profile done every 5 years. Lifestyle changes can lower blood LDL cholesterol levels and reduce health risks.

Study Questions

1. All of the following are ways in which fatty acids can differ from one another *except* _____.

   a. number of double bonds
   b. degree of saturation
   c. carbon chain length
   d. number of calories provided

2. Triglycerides consist of _____.

   a. glycerol
   b. cholesterol
   c. 3 fatty acids
   d. a and b
   e. a and c

Match the fat-related terms on the right to their definitions on the left.

3. _____ lipid that is solid at room temperature

4. _____ chief form of fat in food

5. _____ sterol manufactured in the body

6. _____ similar to triglycerides, except a fatty acid has been replaced by a phosphorus

7. _____ lipid that is liquid at room temperature

   a. fat
   b. cholesterol
   c. oil
   d. phospholipid
   e. triglyceride

8. *Trans* fatty acids tend to _____ blood cholesterol.

   a. raise
   b. lower
   c. have no effect on

9. The functions of fat include all of the following *except* _____.

   a. building and repairing tissue
   b. cushioning and protecting vital organs
   c. insulating the body
   d. providing essential fatty acids and fat-soluble vitamins

10. Which of the following lipoproteins is responsible for transporting cholesterol from the liver to tissues?

    a. chylomicrons
    b. low-density lipoprotein (LDL)
    c. high-density lipoprotein (HDL)
    d. very-low-density lipoprotein (VLDL)

11. Which essential fatty acid can help lower the risks of coronary heart disease?

    a. omega-3   c. omega-9
    b. omega-6   d. none of the above

12. Mike has been told to reduce his fat intake to less than 25% of his total calories (2500 per day). How many grams of fat should he consume?

    a. 69 grams or less   c. 89 grams or less
    b. 76 grams or less   d. 93 grams or less

13. Monounsaturated fatty acids _____.

    a. are liquid at room temperature
    b. have 1 double bond in the fatty acid chain
    c. are provided by plants
    d. lower blood cholesterol levels
    e. all of the above

14. Fats liquid at room temperature can be made more solid by the process of _____.

    a. esterification   c. emulsification
    b. hydrogenation   d. calcification

15. The Dietary Guidelines recommend that no more than _____ of total calories be consumed as polyunsaturated fat and that no more than _____ of total calories be consumed in the form of saturated fat.

    a. 20%; 5%   c. 45%; 25%
    b. 10%; 10%   d. 50%; 10%

Answer Key: 1-d; 2-e; 3-a; 4-e; 5-b; 6-d; 7-c; 8-a; 9-a; 10-b; 11-a; 12-a; 13-e; 14-b; 15-b

Websites

To learn more about the topics covered in this chapter, visit these websites.

www.nhlbi.nih.gov/guidelines/cholesterol/atp_iii.htm

www.americanheart.org

www.webmd.com/cholesterol-management

www.medscape.com

www.fda.gov/oc/initiatives/transfat

www.fns.usda.gov/fdd/facts/nutrition/TransFatFactSheet.pdf

www.eatright.org

www.oldwayspt.org

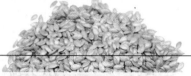

References

1. American Dietetic Association. Position of the American Dietetic Association: Fat replacers. *J Am Diet Assoc.* 2005;105:266.

2. Higgins JP, Flicker L. Lecithin for dementia and cognitive treatment. *Cochrane Database Syst Rev.* 2000:CD 001015.

3. Oosthuizen W and others. Lecithin has no effect on serum lipoprotein, plasma fibrinogen and macro molecular protein complex levels in hyperlipidaemic men in a double-blind controlled study. *Eur J Clin Nutr.* 1998;52:419.

4. Food and Nutrition Board. *Dietary Reference Intakes for energy, carbohydrate, fiber, fat, fatty acids, cholesterol, protein, and amino acids.* Washington, DC: National Academy Press; 2002.

5. Ornish DL and others. Intensive lifestyle changes for reversal of coronary heart disease. *JAMA.* 2007;280:2001.

6. Vanitallie TB. Ancel Keys: A tribute. *Nutr Metab.* 2005;14:4.

7. Holvoet P and others. Association between circulating oxidized low-density lipoprotein and incidence of the Metabolic Syndrome. *JAMA.* 2008; 299:2287.

8. Skulas-Ray AC and others. Omega-3 fatty concentrates in the treatment of moderate hypertriglyceridemia. *Expert Opin Pharmacotner,* 2008; 9:1237.

9. Simopoulos AP. Omega-3 fatty acids in inflammation and autoimmune diseases. *J Am Coll Nutr.* 2002;21:495.

10. Sundrarjun T and others. Effects of n-3 fatty acids on serum interleukin-6, tumour necrosis factor-alpha and soluble tumour necrosis factor receptor p55 in active rheumatoid arthritis. *J Int Med Res.* 2004;32:443.

11. Kavanagh K and others. Trans fat diet induces abdominal obesity and changes in insulin sensitivity in monkeys. *Obesity.* 2007;15:1675.

12. Cho E and others. Premenopausal fat intake and risk of breast cancer. *J Natl Cancer Inst.* 2003;95:1079.

13. Willett WC, Giovannucci E. Epidemiology of diet and cancer risk. In: Shils ME and others, eds. *Modern nutrition in health and disease.* Baltimore: Lippincott Williams & Wilkins; 2005.

14. Coulston AM, Peragallo-Ditto KV. Insulin resistance syndrome: A potent culprit in cardiovascular disease. *J Am Diet Assoc.* 2004;104:176.

15. Greenland P and others. Major risk factors as antecedents of fatal and nonfatal coronary heart disease events. *JAMA.* 2003;290:891.

16. Millen BE and others. Dietary patterns, smoking, and subclinical heart disease in women. *J Am Diet Assoc.* 2004;104:208.

17. Hansson GK. Inflammation, atherosclerosis and coronary artery disease. *N Engl J Med.* 2005;352:1685.

18. Karim R and others. Relationship between serum levels of sex hormones and progression of subclinical atherosclerosis in postmenopausal women. *J Clin Endocrin Metab.* 2008;93:131.

19. Djousse L and others. Fruit and vegetable consumption and LDL cholesterol. *Am J Clin Nutr.* 2004;79:213.

20. Kris-Etherton PM and others. Antioxidant vitamin supplements and cardiovascular disease. *Circulation.* 2004;110:637.

21. Lonn E and others. Effects of long-term vitamin E supplementation on cardiovascular events and cancer: A randomized trial. *JAMA.* 2005;293:1338.

22. Raben A and others. Meals with similar energy densities but rich in protein, fat, carbohydrate, or alcohol have different effects on energy expenditure and substrate metabolism but not on appetite and energy intake. *Am J Clin Nutr.* 2003;77:91.

23. Jolliffe C, Janssen I. Age-specific lipid and lipoprotein thresholds for adolescents. *J Cardio Nurs.* 2008;23:56.

24. American Dietetic Association. Position of the American Dietetic Association and Dietitians of Canada. *J Am Diet Assoc.* 2007; 107:1599.

7 Proteins

Many cultures around the world enjoy the flavors of insects and benefit from the protein they provide—3 ounces of the locusts in this stir-fry provide about 11 grams of protein! Learn more about entomophagy at www.food-insects.com.

STUDENT LEARNING OUTCOMES

After studying this chapter, you will be able to

1. Describe how amino acids form proteins.

2. Define essential and nonessential amino acids and explain why adequate amounts of each of the essential amino acids are required for protein synthesis.

3. Distinguish between high-quality and low-quality proteins and list sources of each.

4. Describe how 2 low-quality proteins can be complementary to each other to provide the required amounts of essential amino acids.

5. Explain the methods used to measure the protein quality of foods, including assessment of biological value.

6. List the factors that influence protein needs. Calculate the RDA for protein for a healthy adult with a given body weight.

7. Explain positive nitrogen balance, negative nitrogen balance, and nitrogen equilibrium and list the conditions under which they occur.

8. Describe how protein is digested and absorbed in the body.

9. List the primary functions of protein in the body.

10. Describe how protein-energy malnutrition can eventually lead to disease in the body.

11. Describe the symptoms and treatment of food allergies.

12. Develop a vegetarian diet plan that meets the body's protein needs.

The term protein comes from the Greek word *protos,* which means "to come first." This is an appropriate name, given that proteins are a primary component of all cells throughout the body. In fact, aside from water, proteins form the major part of lean body tissue, totaling about 17% of body weight.[1] Many of our body proteins are found in muscle, connective tissue, organs, DNA, hemoglobin, antibodies, hormones, enzymes, and other vital compounds.

Proteins are crucial to the regulation and maintenance of essential body functions. For example, maintenance of fluid balance, hormone and enzyme production, vision, and cell synthesis and repair each requires specific proteins. The body synthesizes proteins in many configurations and sizes, so that they can serve these greatly varied functions.[1]

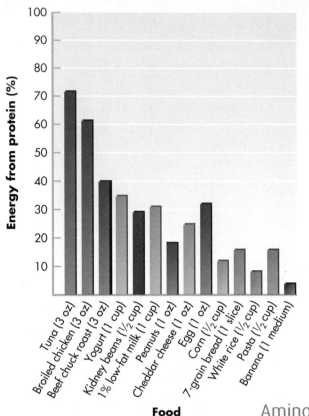

Figure 7-1 **Protein content of foods.**

In countries such as the United States and Canada, most people consume diets rich in protein. In contrast, diets in developing countries often contain insufficient amounts of protein. As you'll see, consuming inadequate amounts of protein can impair many metabolic processes because the body is unable to build the proteins it needs. For example, the immune system no longer functions efficiently when it lacks key proteins, which leads to an increased risk of infection, disease, and if severe, even death. This chapter will examine the functions of protein, its metabolism, the sources of protein, and the consequences of eating diets that are too low or too high in protein.

7.1 Structure of Proteins

Like carbohydrates and lipids, proteins are made of the elements carbon, hydrogen, and oxygen. However, all proteins also contain the element nitrogen and several contain the mineral sulfur. The nitrogen in proteins is in a special form that can be readily used by our bodies for vital functions. Together, these elements form various amino acids, which serve as the building blocks for protein synthesis.

Amino Acids

The amino acids needed to make body proteins are supplied by the protein-containing foods we eat and from cell synthesis (Fig. 7-1). Each amino acid is composed of a central carbon bonded to 4 groups of elements (Fig. 7-2). Three of the groups are a nitrogen group, called an amino (or amine) group; an acid (carboxyl) group; and a hydrogen molecule. The fourth group, called a side chain, is often signified by the letter *R*. The basic, or "generic," model of an amino acid and the structures of 2 amino acids, glycine and alanine, are shown in Figure 7-2. (The chemical structures of the rest of the amino acids are shown in Appendix B.)

The side chain, or R portion, of the amino acid determines the name of the amino acid. For example, if R is a hydrogen, the amino acid is glycine; if R is a methyl group ($-CH_3$), the amino acid is alanine. Some amino acids have chemically similar R portions. These related amino acids form special classes, such as acidic amino acids, basic amino acids, and branched-chain amino acids. For instance, the acidic amino acids lose a hydrogen in reactions and become negatively charged, whereas the basic amino acids gain a hydrogen and become positively charged. This allows them to participate in different enzymatic reactions in the body.

The body needs 20 different amino acids to function. Although they are all important, 11 of these amino acids do not need to be obtained from the diet. They are classified as **non-essential** (or *dispensable*) **amino acids** because our bodies make them,

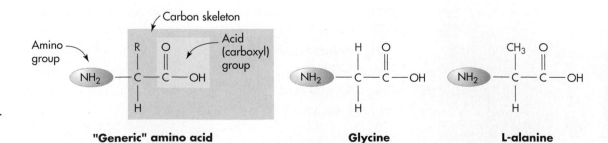

Figure 7-2 **Amino acid structure. The side chain (R) differentiates glycine from alanine.**

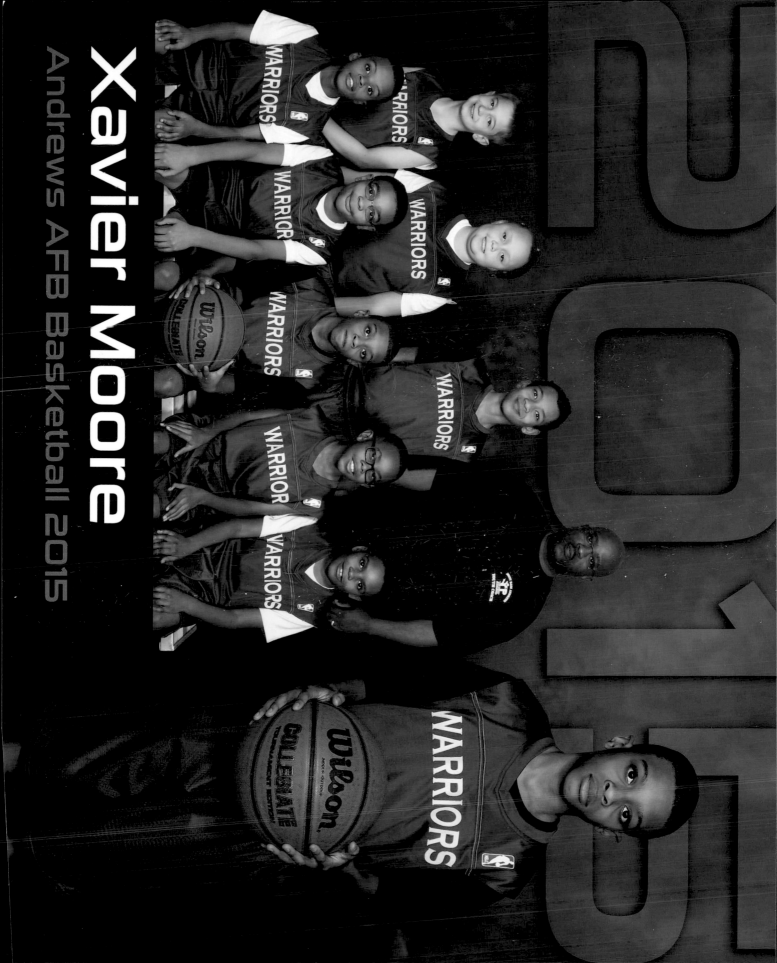

Xavier Moore

Andrews AFB Basketball 2015

using other amino acids we consume (Table 7-1). The 9 amino acids the body cannot make are known as **essential** (or *indispensable*) **amino acids** because they must be obtained from foods. Essential amino acids cannot be synthesized in the body because body cells cannot make the **carbon skeleton** of the amino acid, cannot attach an amino group to the carbon skeleton, or simply cannot do the whole process fast enough to meet the body's needs.

Several nonessential amino acids may be classified as "conditionally essential" amino acids during infancy, disease, or trauma.[1] For example, a person with the genetic disease phenylketonuria (PKU) has a limited ability to metabolize the essential amino acid phenylalanine due to a deficiency of the enzyme phenylalanine hydroxylase. This enzyme is needed to convert phenylalanine to the nonessential amino acid tyrosine. As a result, individuals with PKU cannot produce sufficient tyrosine, thereby making tyrosine a "conditionally" essential amino acid because it must be obtained from the diet. Following trauma and infection, the amino acids glutamine and arginine may be considered conditionally essential because supplemental amounts have been shown to promote recovery.[1]

Table 7-1 Classification of Amino Acids	
Essential Amino Acids	**Non-essential Amino Acids**
Histidine	Alanine
Isoleucine*	Arginine
Leucine*	Asparagine
Lysine	Aspartic acid
Methionine	Cysteine
Phenylalanine	Glutamic acid
Threonine	Glutamine
Tryptophan	Glycine
Valine*	Proline
	Serine
	Tyrosine

*Branched-chain amino acids.

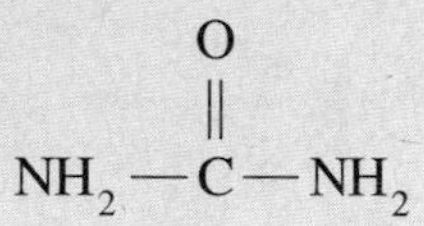

Synthesis of Nonessential Amino Acids

Nonessential amino acids can be synthesized through a process called transamination. **Transamination** involves the transfer of an amino group from 1 amino acid to a carbon skeleton to form a new amino acid. As illustrated in Figure 7-3, glutamic acid donates its amino group to the carbon skeleton of pyruvic acid to become the nonessential amino acid alanine.

Glutamic acid (and several other amino acids) also can lose its amino group without transferring it to another carbon skeleton. This process is called **deamination.** The amino group (in the form of ammonia) is incorporated into **urea** in the liver, transported via the bloodstream to the kidneys, and excreted in the urine. Once an amino acid breaks down to its amino-free carbon skeleton, the carbon skeleton can be used for fuel or synthesized into other compounds, such as glucose (see Chapter 9).

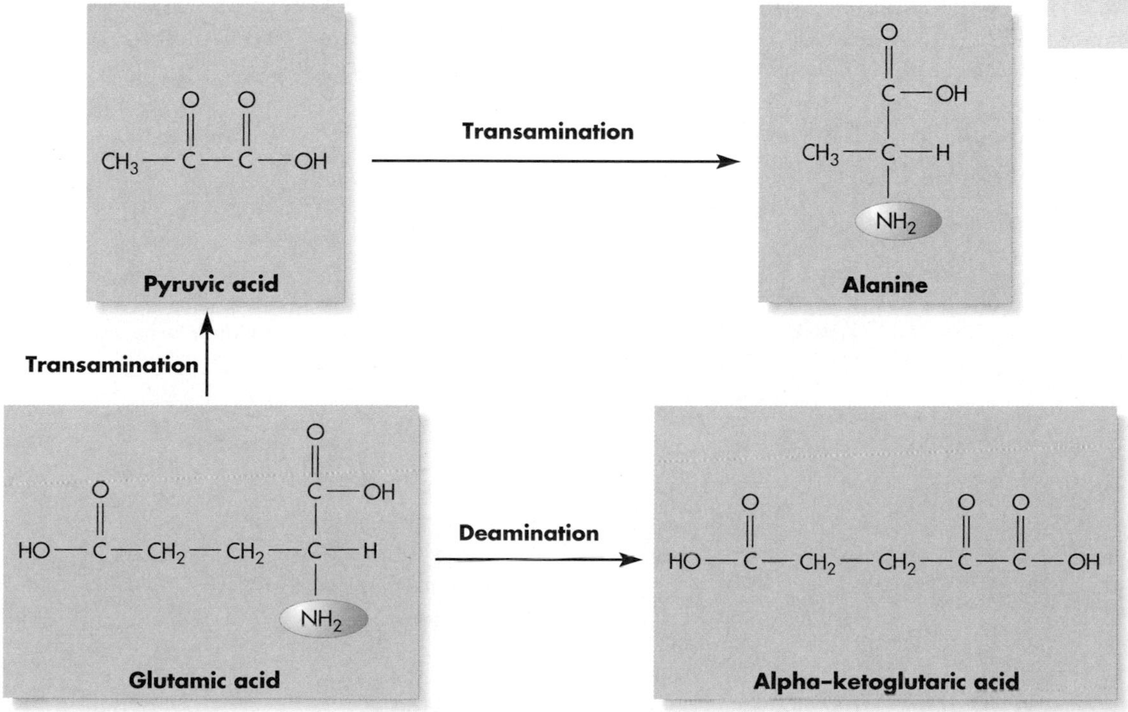

essential amino acids Amino acids that the human body cannot synthesize in sufficient amounts or at all and therefore must be included in the diet.

carbon skeleton Amino acid without the amino group

urea Nitrogenous waste product of protein metabolism and the major source of nitrogen in the urine; chemically depicted as this:

$$NH_2 - \overset{\overset{\displaystyle O}{\|}}{C} - NH_2$$

Figure 7-3 In **transamination**, the pathway allows cells to synthesize non-essential amino acids. In this example, pyruvic acid gains an amino group from glutamic acid to form the amino acid alanine. In deamination, the pathway allows for loss of an amino group without transferring it to another carbon skeleton. In this example, glutamic acid loses its amino group to form alpha-ketoglutaric acid.

Amino Acid Composition: Complete and Incomplete Proteins

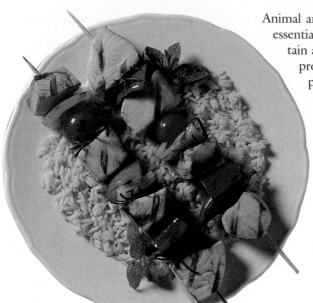

High-protein foods, such as meat can provide all the essential amino acids needed by our bodies.

pool Amount of a nutrient found within the body that can be easily mobilized when needed.

Animal and plant proteins can differ greatly in their proportions of essential and non-essential amino acids. Animal proteins, such as meat, poultry, fish, eggs, and milk, contain ample amounts of all 9 essential amino acids. (Gelatin—made from the animal protein collagen—is an exception because it loses an essential amino acid during processing and is low in other essential amino acids.) In contrast, plant proteins do not contain the needed amounts of essential amino acids. With the exception of soy protein, they are low in at least 1 of the 9 essential amino acids.

Scientists classify dietary proteins according to their amino acid composition. Because they contain sufficient amounts of all the essential amino acids, animal proteins (except gelatin) are classified as complete, or **high-quality,** proteins. Plant proteins (except soybeans) are classified as **incomplete,** or low-quality, proteins because they contain limited amounts of 1 or more of the essential amino acids.

Cells require a **pool** of essential amino acids for the synthesis of body proteins. Thus, a single plant protein, such as wheat (which is low in the amino acid lysine), cannot support the synthesis of body protein if it is the sole source of dietary protein. Even a variety of low-quality proteins may not provide sufficient amounts of essential amino acids for protein synthesis if food choices are not carefully planned. When this occurs, proteins cannot be made and the remaining amino acids may be used for energy or converted to carbohydrate or fat.

The essential amino acid in smallest supply in a food or diet in relation to body needs is called the **limiting amino acid** because it limits the amount of protein the body can synthesize.[1] For example, assume the letters of the alphabet represent the 20 or so different amino acids we consume. If *A* represents an essential amino acid, we need 4 of these letters to spell the hypothetical protein *ALABAMA*. If the body had an *L,* a *B,* and an *M,* but only 3 *A*s, the "synthesis" of *ALABAMA* would not be possible. *A* would be the limiting amino acid, preventing the synthesis of the protein *ALABAMA*.

When 2 or more plant proteins are combined to compensate for deficiencies in essential amino acid content in each protein, the proteins are called **complementary proteins** (Table 7-2). When food protein sources are combined, the amino acids in

Table 7-2 Limiting Amino Acids in Plant Sources of Protein

Food	Primary Limiting Amino Acid	Create a Complete Protein By Combining It With	Complementary Food Protein Combinations
Legumes (peanuts, dry beans, such as navy, black, and kidney beans)	Methionine Tryptophan	Grains, nuts, or seeds	Hummus and pita bread Bean burrito
Nuts and seeds (cashews, walnuts, almonds, sunflower seeds)	Lysine	Legumes	Vegetarian chili with kidney beans and cashews
Grains (wheat, rice, oats, corn)	Lysine	Legumes	Red beans and rice Lentil soup and cornbread

1 source can make up for the limiting amino acid in the other sources to yield a high-quality (complete) protein for the diet. Mixed diets generally provide high-quality protein because these diets often contain complementary proteins. Complementary proteins need not be consumed at the same meal but can be balanced over the course of a day to provide a sufficient supply of amino acids for body cells. For non-vegetarians, adding a small amount of animal protein to a plant-based dish (e.g., pizza with cheese or spaghetti with meatballs) is a way of providing adequate essential amino acids.

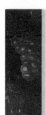

Knowledge Check

1. Why are some amino acids classified as essential and others as non-essential?
2. What are complementary proteins?
3. What does the term *limiting amino acid* mean?

7.2 Synthesis of Proteins

Within body cells, amino acids can be linked together by a chemical bond, called a **peptide bond,** to form needed proteins (Fig. 7-4). Peptide bonds form between the amino group of 1 amino acid and the acid (carboxyl) group of another. Through peptide bonding of amino acids, cells can synthesize dipeptides (joining of 2 amino acids), tripeptides (joining of 3 amino acids), oligopeptides (joining of 4 to 9 amino acids), and **polypeptides** (joining of 10 or more amino acids). Most proteins are polypeptides, ranging from approximately 50 to 2000 amino acids. The body can synthesize many different proteins by joining the 20 amino acids with peptide bonds.

Transcription and Translation of Genetic Information

The synthesis of body proteins is determined through a process called gene expression. **Gene expression** occurs when deoxyribonucleic acid (DNA) replicates, making an exact copy of the gene. Thus, each gene serves as a template to guide the duplication of genetic information carried by the DNA.

As you know, DNA is a double-stranded molecule in a helical form. Each strand of DNA is composed of 4 nucleotides (building blocks of DNA): adenine (A), guanine (G), cytosine (C), and thymine (T). Each of the nucleotides is complementary to (binds to) another nucleotide; A and T are complementary, as are C and G.

DNA-coded instructions for protein synthesis consist of a sequence of 3 nucleotides per unit of instruction (e.g., CTC), which dictate where each amino acid is to be placed in a protein and in which order. These nucleotide units are called **codons,** and each represents a specific amino acid. For example, the codon CTC represents the amino acid glutamic acid. Some amino acids have only 1 possible codon, whereas others have as many as 6. For instance, the amino acid glutamic acid actually has 2 codons: CTC and CTT. Having the correct codons in the right sequence is critical for producing a normal protein. DNA with mistakes in the order or types of amino acids can result in profound health consequences (see the discussion of sickle-cell disease later in this section).

Protein synthesis takes place in the ribosomes located in the cytosol of the cell, not in the nucleus. Thus, the DNA code used for the synthesis of a specific protein must be transferred from the nucleus (where the DNA is) to the cytosol to allow for such synthesis. This transfer is the job of messenger RNA (mRNA). To produce mRNA, the DNA in the nucleus unwinds from its super-coiled state. Enzymes read the code on the DNA

CRITICAL THINKING

Trevor has heard that he should be certain to include complementary proteins in his vegetarian diet. What food combinations would you suggest to him?

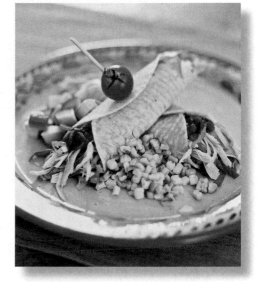

Small amounts of animal protein in a meal quickly add up to meet daily protein needs.

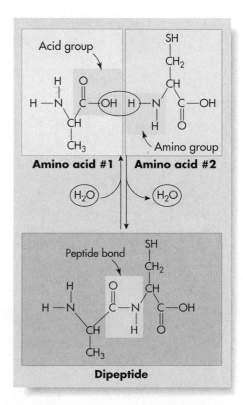

Figure 7-4 Peptide bonds link amino acids.

DNA transcription Process of forming messenger RNA (mRNA) from a portion of DNA.

(i.e., the genes) and transcribe that code into a complementary single-stranded mRNA molecule, called the primary transcript (Fig. 7-5). This is the **DNA transcription** phase of protein synthesis. The nucleotides of mRNA are A, G, C, and U (uracil, which replaces the thymine of DNA) and are organized in complement to the DNA (Table 7-3). Thus, a DNA code of ACTGAT yields an mRNA of UGACUA.

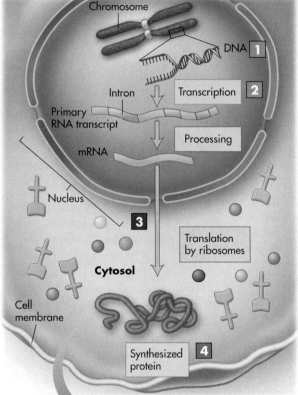

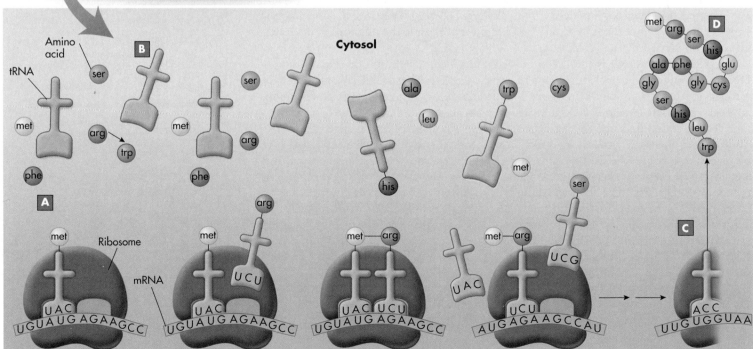

Figure 7-5 **Summary of protein synthesis.** DNA present in the nucleus of the cell is composed of 4 nucleotides: adenine (A), guanine (G), cytosine (C), and thymine (T). The DNA code is read 3 nucleotides at a time, with each specific unit being called a codon. Each DNA codon represents a specific amino acid.

1 The DNA unwinds from its supercoiled state to allow the code for the amino acid sequence to be

2 transcribed into a complementary messenger RNA (mRNA) (labeled as primary RNA transcript).

3 The DNA stays in the nucleus and the mRNA travels to the cytosol.

4 Here the ribosomes read the codons on the mRNA and translate the instructions to produce a specific protein. The lower drawing shows step 4 in more detail.

   A Protein synthesis begins at a specific starting point, indicated by AUG. The initiation complex forms when the ribosomal subunits and the first tRNA molecule locks into a strand of mRNA.

   B Transfer RNA (tRNA) units bring amino acids to the ribosomes as needed during protein synthesis. The tRNA carriers have a complementary code to the mRNA—such that, if the amino acid arginine is needed during synthesis, the AGA on the mRNA would correspond to UCU on the tRNA. Numerous tRNA carriers are present during protein synthesis to continually supply the ribosomes with needed amino acids. ATP is used to supply the energy needed to activate tRNA in order to form each new peptide bond.

   C Protein synthesis continues by adding 1 amino acid at a time to the growing polypeptide chain until a specific ending (stop) codon is reached or when a needed amino acid is not available.

   D The polypeptide is then released from the ribosome when it encounters the ending (stop) codon.

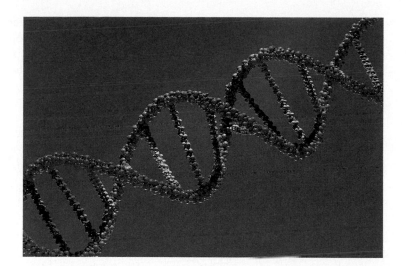

The double stranded, helical shaped DNA, located in the cell nucleus contains the genetic codes for the synthesis of proteins.

Table 7-3 DNA, mRNA, and tRNA Complementary Nucleotides

DNA Nucleotides	Complementary mRNA Nucleotides	Complementary tRNA Nucleotides
Adenine	Uracil	Adenine
Cytosine	Guanine	Cytosine
Thymine	Adenine	Uracil
Guanine	Cytosine	Guanine

mRNA translation Synthesis of polypeptide chains by the ribosome according to information contained in strands of messenger RNA (mRNA).

The primary transcript mRNA undergoes processing in the cell nucleus to remove any parts of the DNA code that do not code for protein synthesis, called introns (these actually make up much of the DNA). The mRNA then travels to the ribosomes. The ribosomes read the codons on the mRNA and translate those instructions to produce a specific protein. This is the **mRNA translation** phase of protein synthesis. Amino acids are added 1 at a time to the polypeptide chain as directed by the instructions on the mRNA. Protein synthesis begins at a specific starting point on the mRNA (indicated by AUG) and continues until a specific ending (stop) codon is reached, such as UAA, UAG, or UGA. Energy input from ATP is needed to add each amino acid to the growing polypeptide chain, making protein synthesis very "costly" to the body in terms of energy use.

One key participant in protein synthesis in the cytosol is transfer RNA (tRNA). The tRNA units take amino acids to the ribosomes as needed during protein synthesis. The tRNA carriers have a complementary code to the mRNA. For example, if the amino acid arginine were needed during synthesis, the AGA on the mRNA would correspond to UCU on the tRNA. Numerous tRNA carriers are present during protein synthesis to continually supply the ribosomes with needed amino acids.

Once synthesis of the polypeptide is completed, indicated by the ending codon, it is released from the ribosome, as is the mRNA. The polypeptide now twists and folds into a very complex 3-dimensional structure (see section on Protein Organization). The DNA code determines not only the shape but also, ultimately, the function of the protein. Thus, if the DNA contains errors, an incorrect mRNA will be produced. The ribosomes, in turn, will read this incorrect message and produce an abnormal polypeptide.

The genetic disorder **sickle-cell anemia** illustrates what can happen when amino acid sequencing errors occur.[2] In this disease, the amino acid valine replaces glutamic acid in the DNA sequence of half of the 4 polypeptide chains of hemoglobin. This error produces a profound change in hemoglobin structure (Fig. 7-6). Instead of forming normal, doughnut-shaped discs, the red blood cells collapse into crescent, or sickle, shapes.

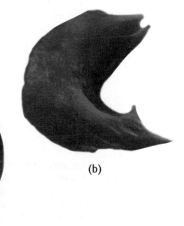

(a)

(b)

Figure 7-6 An example of the consequences of errors in DNA coding of proteins. (*a*) Normal red blood cell; (*b*) red blood cell from a person with sickle-cell anemia—note its abnormal crescent (sicklelike) shape.

Synopsis of the Steps in Protein Synthesis

Part of DNA code (gene) is transcribed to mRNA in the nucleus.

↓

mRNA leaves the nucleus and travels to cytosol.

↓

Ribosomes in the cytosol read the mRNA code and translate it into directions for a specific sequence of amino acids in a polypeptide chain.

↓

To produce the polypeptide, tRNA takes the appropriate amino acid to the ribosome as dictated by the mRNA code. The amino acid is added to the existing amino acid chain, which begins with the amino acid methionine.

↓

When synthesis of the polypeptide is complete, it is released from the ribosome.

↓

The polypeptide folds into its active 3-dimensional form.

 Sulfur-containing amino acids stabilize many compounds, such as the hormone insulin. Sulfur atoms can bond together (—S—S—), creating a bridge between 2 protein strands or 2 parts of the same strand. This stabilizes the structure of the molecule and helps create the *secondary structure.*

This limits their ability to carry oxygen to tissues effectively, resulting in many serious health concerns. The disease can lead to severe bone and joint pain, abdominal pain, headache, convulsions, paralysis, and even death when the sickled cells clump in the capillary beds and impede blood flow. Treatment usually consists of blood transfusions, medications to increase red blood cell synthesis, and bone marrow transplants.

Protein Organization

The sequential order of the amino acids in the polypeptide chain, called *primary structure,* determines a protein's shape. Amino acids must be accurately positioned in order for the amino acids to interact and fold correctly into the intended shape for the protein. This, in turn, allows chemical bonds to form between amino acids near each other and stabilizes the structure. This creates a spiral-like shape called *secondary structure.* The unique 3-dimensional conformation of a protein, called *tertiary structure,* determines its physiological function. Thus, if a protein fails to form the appropriate configuration, it cannot function. In some cases, 2 or more separate polypeptides interact to form a large, new protein, with *quaternary structure* (Fig. 7-7). In this way, a protein may be active when the units are joined but inactive when the units are separate.

Denaturation of Proteins

Exposure to acid or alkaline solutions, enzymes, heat, or agitation can alter a protein's structure, leaving it in a denatured state (Fig. 7-8). **Denaturation** is the alteration of a protein's 3-dimensional structure. Although denaturation does not affect the protein's primary structure, unraveling a protein's shape often destroys its normal biological function.

In some instances, the denaturation of proteins is beneficial. For example, the secretion of hydrochloric acid in the stomach during digestion denatures food proteins, which helps increase their exposure to digestive enzymes and aids in the breakdown of polypeptide chains. The heat produced during cooking also can denature proteins, making them safer to eat (e.g., when pathogenic bacterial protein is denatured) and more pleasing to eat (e.g., when eggs solidify in cooking). However, denaturation also can be harmful to physiological function and overall health. During illness, changes in gastrointestinal acidity, body temperature, or body pH can cause essential proteins to denature and lose their function.

Adaptation of Protein Synthesis to Changing Conditions

Most vital body proteins are in a constant state of breakdown, rebuilding, and repair. This process, called **protein turnover,** allows cells to adapt to changing circumstances. For

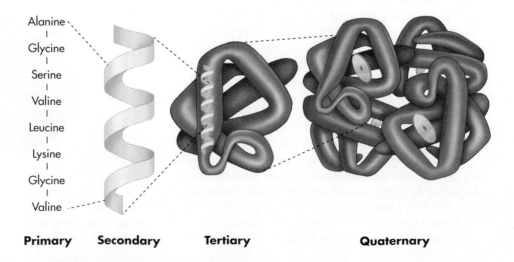

Figure 7-7 **Protein organization. Four** different levels of structure are found in proteins. The primary structure of a protein is the linear sequence of amino acids in the polypeptide chain. Secondary structure consists of areas in the polypeptide chain that have a specific shape stabilized by hydrogen and sulfur bonds. The 3-dimensional shape of proteins is called tertiary structure. It determines the function of the protein. Some proteins also show quaternary structure where 2 or more protein units join together to form a larger protein, such as hemoglobin, depicted in the figure.

Alanine
|
Glycine
|
Serine
|
Valine
|
Leucine
|
Lysine
|
Glycine
|
Valine

Primary   **Secondary**   **Tertiary**   **Quaternary**

example, when we eat more protein than necessary for health, the liver makes more enzymes to process the waste product from the resulting amino acid metabolism—namely, ammonia—into urea. Overall, protein turnover is a process by which a cell can respond to its changing environment and produce needed proteins while reducing the production of proteins not currently needed.[1]

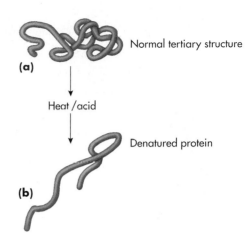

Figure 7-8 **Denaturation.** (*a*) Protein in a typical coiled state. (*b*) Protein is now partly uncoiled, exhibiting a denatured state. This uncoiling typically reduces or eliminates biological activity.

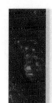

Knowledge Check

1. How are the amino acids in a protein linked together?
2. Why is the structure of a protein important?
3. What effects does denaturation have on a protein?

 ## 7.3 Sources of Protein

Protein is supplied by the diet, as well as by the recycling of body protein. For example, the intestinal tract lining is constantly sloughed off. The digestive tract treats sloughed cells just like food particles and absorbs their amino acids released during digestion. In fact, most protein breakdown products—amino acids—released throughout the body can be recycled and added to the pool of amino acids available for future protein synthesis. By comparing the 250 to 300 g of protein an adult makes and degrades each day with the 65 to 100 g of protein typically consumed by adults, you can see how important recycled amino acids are as a protein source for the body.[3] Nonetheless, dietary protein is needed to replenish and maintain an adequate amino acid pool for protein synthesis and repair.

In typical North American diets, about 70% of dietary protein is supplied by meat, poultry, fish, milk and some milk products, legumes, and nuts (Fig. 7-9).[4] Worldwide, only 35% of protein comes from animal sources. Plants are the major source of protein in many areas of the world.

As shown in Table 7-4, plants can provide ample amounts of dietary protein in addition to providing fiber and a variety of vitamins, minerals, and phytochemicals. Plant proteins also contain no cholesterol and little saturated fat, unless added during processing. North Americans might benefit from adding soy and other plant proteins to their diets because higher intakes of these proteins have been associated with decreased risks of cardiovascular disease, certain cancers, obesity, and diabetes.[5-8] In fact, the FDA has approved a health claim regarding the benefits of soy protein in lowering blood cholesterol levels.

As a way to add more plant proteins to your diet, consider these suggestions:

- At your next cookout, try a veggie burger instead of a hamburger. These are available in the frozen foods section of the grocery store and come in a variety of flavors. Many restaurants have added veggie burgers to their menus.

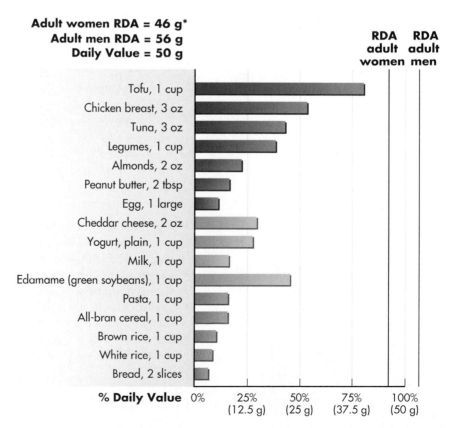

Figure 7-9 **Food sources of protein.**

Table 7-4 Protein Content of Sample Menus Containing 1600 kcal and 2000 kcal

Menu		1600 kcal		2000 kcal	
		Serving Size	Protein (g)	Serving Size	Protein (g)
Breakfast	Low-fat granola	⅔ cup	5	⅔ cup	5
	Blueberries	1 cup	1	1 cup	1
	Fat-free (skim) milk	1 cup	8.5	1 cup	8.5
	Coffee	1 cup	0	1 cup	0
Lunch	Broiled chicken breast	3 oz	25	4 oz	33
	Salad greens	3 cups	5	3 cups	5
	Baked taco shell strips	½ cup	2	½ cup	2
	Low-fat salad dressing	2 tbsp	0	2 tbsp	0
	Fat-free (skim) milk	1 cup	8.5	1 cup	8.5
Dinner	Yellow rice	1¼ cups	5	2½ cups	10
	Shrimp	4 large	5	6 large	7
	Mussels	4 medium	8	6 medium	12
	Clams	5 small	12	10 small	24
	Peas	¼ cup	4	½ cup	4
	Sweet red pepper	¼ cup	0	½ cup	0
Snack	Muffin	1 small	4	1 small	4
	Swiss cheese	1 oz	7.5	1 oz	7.5
	Banana	½ small	0.5	½ small	0.5
	Total		101		132

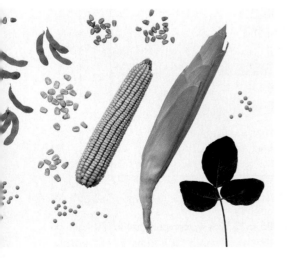

- Sprinkle sunflower seeds or chopped almonds on top of salad to add taste and texture.
- Mix chopped walnuts into the batter of banana bread, muffins, or pancakes to boost your intake of monounsaturated fats and protein.
- Eat edamame (green soybeans) or roasted soy nuts as a snack.
- Spread peanut butter, instead of butter or cream cheese, on bagels.
- Consider using soy milk, especially if you have lactose intolerance. Look for varieties that are fortified with calcium.
- Substitute black beans or vegetarian refried beans for the meat or fish in your tacos.
- Make a stir-fry with tofu, cashew nuts, and a variety of vegetables.

Evaluation of Food Protein Quality

Scientists use various measures to evaluate the protein quality of a food. These measures indicate a food protein's ability to support body growth and maintenance. Protein quality is determined primarily by the food's digestibility (amount of amino acids absorbed) and amino acid composition, compared with a reference protein (e.g., egg white protein) known to provide the essential amino acids in amounts needed to support growth. The digestibility of animal proteins is relatively high (90–100%), in contrast to that of plant proteins (70%).

It is important to note that the concept of protein quality applies only under conditions in which protein intakes are equal to or less than the amount of protein needed to meet the requirement for essential amino acids. When protein intake exceeds this amount, the efficiency of protein use is decreased, even with the highest-quality proteins. This occurs because, once essential amino acid needs have been met, the remaining amino acids (both essential and non-essential) cannot be readily stored and are primarily degraded for use as energy.

Biological Value (BV)

The **biological value (BV)** of a protein is a measure of how efficiently the absorbed food protein is converted into body tissue protein. If a food possesses adequate amounts of all 9 essential amino acids, it should allow a person to efficiently incorporate amino acids from food protein into body protein.

To determine the BV, nitrogen retention in the body is compared with the nitrogen content of the food protein. More nitrogen is retained when a food's amino acid pattern closely matches the amino acid pattern of body protein. The better the match, the higher the BV. In contrast, if the amino acid pattern in a food is quite unlike body tissue amino acid patterns, more nitrogen is excreted because many of the amino acids in the food will not be incorporated into body protein. The BV of such a food protein is low, as little of the nitrogen is retained in body tissues.

Egg white protein has a BV of 100, the highest BV of any single food protein. This means that essentially all nitrogen absorbed from egg protein is retained and incorporated into body tissue protein. Most animal proteins have a high BV, reflecting a tissue amino acid composition similar to that of human tissues. Plants have amino acid patterns that differ greatly from those of humans. Therefore, the BV of plant proteins is usually much lower than that of animal proteins.

Protein Efficiency Ratio (PER)

Protein efficiency ratio (PER) is another method for assessing a food's protein quality. The PER compares the amount of weight gain by a growing laboratory animal consuming a standardized amount of the protein being studied with the weight gain in an animal consuming a standardized amount of a reference protein, such as casein (milk protein). The PER of a food reflects its biological value because the weight gain and growth measured in the PER are dependent on the incorporation of food protein into body tissue. Thus, animal proteins with a high BV also yield a high PER, whereas plant proteins generally yield a lower BV and PER because they are incomplete proteins. The FDA uses this method to set standards for the labeling of foods intended for infants.

Chemical Score

The protein quality of a food also can be evaluated by its chemical score. To calculate a **chemical score**, the amount of each essential amino acid in a gram of the food protein being tested is divided by the "ideal" amount for that amino acid in a gram of the reference protein (usually egg protein). The lowest (or limiting) amino acid ratio that is calculated for the essential amino acids of the test protein is the chemical score of that protein. Chemical scores range from 0 to 1.0.

Protein Digestibility Corrected Amino Acid Score (PDCAAS)

The most widely used measure of protein quality is called the **Protein Digestibility Corrected Amino Acid Score (PDCAAS).** This score is derived by multiplying a food's chemical score by its digestibility. For example, to determine the PDCAAS of wheat, multiply its chemical score (0.47) by its digestibility (0.90). This gives a PDCAAS of approximately

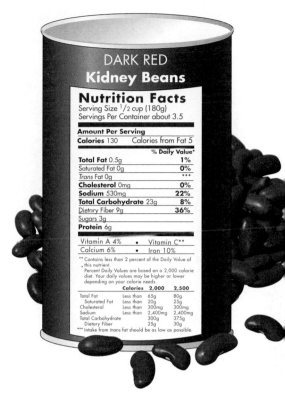

Legumes are rich sources of protein. One-half cup meets about 10% of protein needs but contributes only about 5% of energy needs.

$$BV = \frac{\text{Nitrogen retained (g)}}{\text{Nitrogen absorbed (g)}} \times 100$$

$$PER = \frac{\text{Weight gain (g)}}{\text{Protein consumed}}$$

$$\text{Chemical score} = \frac{\begin{array}{c}\text{mg of limiting amino}\\\text{acid per g of protein}\end{array}}{\begin{array}{c}\text{mg of limiting amino acid}\\\text{per g of an "ideal" protein}\end{array}}$$

$$PDCAAS = \text{Chemical score} \times \text{Digestibility}$$

▶ The concept of biological value has clinical importance whenever protein intake must be limited. This is because it is important that the small amount of protein consumed be used efficiently by the body. For example, protein intake during liver disease and kidney disease may need to be controlled to lessen the effects of the disease. In these cases, most of the protein consumed should be of high biological value, such as eggs, milk, and meat.

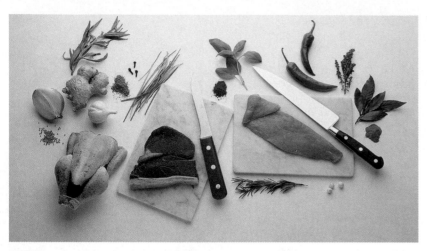

Meat, fish, and poultry are primary sources of high biological value protein.

0.40. The highest PDCAAS is 1.0, which is the score for soy protein and most animal proteins. A protein missing any of the 9 essential amino acids (e.g., gelatin) has a PDCAAS of 0 because its chemical score is 0.

For nutrition labeling purposes, protein content (when listed as % Daily Value) is reduced if the PDCAAS is less than 1. For example, if the protein content of ½ cup of spaghetti noodles is 3 g, only 1.2 g is counted when calculating % Daily Value, since the PDCAAS of wheat is 0.40 (3 g × 0.40 = 1.2). Other PDCAAS values are egg white, 1.0; soy protein, 0.92 to 0.99; beef, 0.92; and black beans, 0.53. Currently, the Nutrition Facts panel rarely contains the % Daily Value for protein because manufacturers do not want to spend the money needed to determine the PDCAAS.

Knowledge Check

1. What are 3 good sources of protein?
2. What are 3 ways of assessing protein quality?
3. What are 2 examples of proteins with high biological value (BV)?
4. What factors affect the protein quality of a food?

CASE STUDY

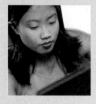

Lily is a college freshman. She lives in a campus residence hall and teaches aerobics in the afternoon. She eats 2 or 3 meals a day at the residence hall cafeteria and snacks between meals. Lily decided to become a vegetarian after reading an article describing the health benefits of a vegetarian diet. Yesterday, her diet consisted of a café latte and Danish pastry for breakfast; a vegetarian tomato-rice dish, pretzels, and a diet soft drink for lunch; 2 cookies in the afternoon after aerobics class; and a vegetarian sub sandwich with 2 glasses of fruit punch for dinner. In the evening, she had a bowl of popcorn. What is missing from Lily's current diet? How can she improve her new diet to meet her nutrient needs? What foods would Lily need to include in her diet to increase her protein intake?

 ## 7.4 Recommended Intakes of Protein

Healthy individuals who are not in periods of growth or recovering from illness or injury need to consume protein in an amount that replaces the protein lost in urine (primarily as urea), feces, sweat, skin cells, hair, and nails. When protein intake equals the amount in losses, protein balance (or equilibrium) is maintained as long as energy intake is adequate to prevent the use of protein for energy.

When protein intake is less than losses, an individual is in negative protein (or nitrogen) balance. Negative protein balance often develops in individuals eating inadequate protein accompanied by a serious, untreated illness or injury (see Section 7.7) and in those with diseases (e.g., **Cushing's disease**) that elevate the production of the hormone cortisol, which increases protein breakdown. For example, individuals with untreated acquired immune deficiency syndrome (AIDS) synthesize protein at rates similar to those of healthy people, but many break down body protein at much higher rates. Over time, the increased rates of protein breakdown result in wasting of lean body mass. Negative protein balance eventually causes blood proteins, skeletal muscles, the heart, the liver, and other organs to decrease in size or volume. Only the brain resists protein breakdown.

Cushing's disease Endocrine disorder characterized by elevated blood levels of the hormone cortisol. High cortisol levels can lead to the breakdown of body proteins, such as those in the skin and muscle.

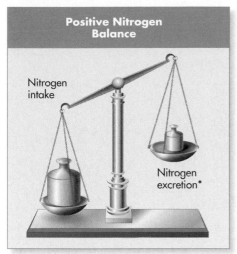

Positive Nitrogen Balance

Nitrogen intake

Nitrogen excretion*

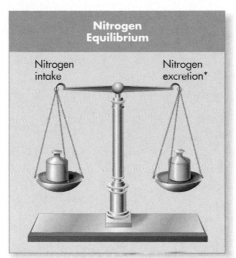

Nitrogen Equilibrium

Nitrogen intake

Nitrogen excretion*

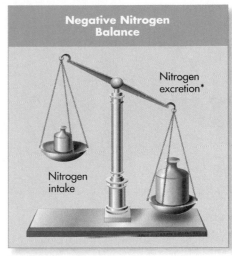

Negative Nitrogen Balance

Nitrogen excretion*

Nitrogen intake

Situations when positive nitrogen balance occurs:

Growth
Pregnancy
Recovery stage after illness/injury
Athletic training resulting in increased lean body mass
Increased secretion of certain hormones, such as insulin, growth hormone, and testosterone

Situations when nitrogen equilibrium occurs:

Healthy adult meeting protein and energy needs

Situations when negative nitrogen balance occurs:

Inadequate intake of protein
Inadequate energy intake
Conditions such as fevers, burns, and infections
Bed rest (for several days)
Deficiency of essential amino acids (e.g., poor-quality protein consumed)
Increased protein loss (as in some forms of disease)
Increased secretion of certain hormones, such as thyroid hormone and cortisol

*Based on losses of urea and other nitrogen-containing compounds in the urine as well as protein losses in feces, skin, hair, nails, and other minor routes.

Figure 7-10 Determining nitrogen balance requires measuring nitrogen intake and loss.

When intake is greater than losses, a state of positive protein balance is attained. During periods of growth and recovery from injury, trauma, or illness, positive protein balance is required to supply sufficient materials for building and repairing tissues. In addition, the hormones insulin, growth hormone, and testosterone all stimulate protein synthesis for the building of new tissue. Merely eating more protein does not build additional body protein, however—protein needs must be increased above normal needs for this to occur.

Researchers and clinicians can measure dietary protein intake and body losses of protein to determine protein balance. Because nitrogen is a component of protein and can be more easily quantified, nitrogen, rather than protein, is measured. Figure 7-10 provides examples of the states of nitrogen (protein) balance. Nitrogen makes up approximately 16% of the weight of an amino acid (16/100 = 6.25). Therefore, nitrogen intake multiplied by 6.25 provides an estimate of protein intake:

$$\text{Nitrogen (g)} \times 6.25 = \text{Protein (g)}$$

Nitrogen balance studies are difficult to conduct because an accurate measure of all sources of nitrogen intake and loss is needed over a 24-hour period. Outside of hospital and research environments, this is not usually feasible. Thus, it is easier to calculate protein needs based on the RDA.

Legumes, such as chickpeas and kidney beans, boost the protein content of meals.

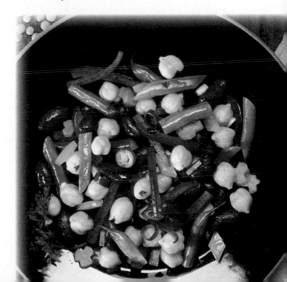

Dietary Reference Intake for Protein

The RDAs for protein are listed in the inside cover of this textbook. These guidelines provide recommendations for healthy individuals during periods of growth and development (infancy, childhood, pregnancy, lactation), as well as during normal adulthood. For most

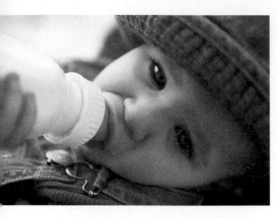

The amount of protein fed to infants should closely follow RDA guidelines. At intakes in excess of the Adequate Intake, their kidneys may have difficulty excreting the large amounts of urea formed in metabolizing the protein. The quantity of protein in breast milk and formula is well matched to infant needs.

adults, the RDA for protein is 0.8 g/kg body weight. Healthy weight is used as a baseline for the RDA because excess fat storage doesn't contribute much to protein needs. As noted in the following equations, the RDAs for adults are 56 g/day for a 154-lb (70-kg) man and 46 g/day for a 125-lb (57-kg) woman.

Convert weight from pounds to kg:

$$\frac{154 \text{ pounds}}{2.2 \text{ pounds/kg}} = 70 \text{ kg} \quad (\text{man})$$

$$\frac{125 \text{ pounds}}{2.2 \text{ pounds/kg}} = 57 \text{ kg} \quad (\text{woman})$$

Calculate RDA:

$$70 \text{ kg} \times \frac{0.8 \text{ g protein}}{\text{kg body weight}} = 56 \text{ g} \quad (\text{man})$$

$$57 \text{ kg} \times \frac{0.8 \text{ g protein}}{\text{kg body weight}} = 46 \text{ g} \quad (\text{woman})$$

The RDA for protein does not address the additional protein amounts needed during recovery from illness or injury or that might be needed to support the needs of highly trained athletes.[3] Protein needs range from approximately 0.8 to 2.0 g/kg body weight in recovery states and 0.8 to 1.7 g/kg body weight in endurance or strength athletes (see Chapter 11). Mental stress, physical labor, and routine weekend sports activities do not require an increase in the protein RDA.[3]

For many North Americans, protein needs are easily met through our typical diets. In fact, North Americans typically consume protein in amounts exceeding the RDA, equaling about 100 g of protein daily for men and 65 g daily for women.[3] Excess protein—whether from dietary sources of protein or amino acid supplements—cannot be stored as such, so the carbon skeletons are put to use for other purposes or metabolized for energy needs.

Knowledge Check

1. When is it important to be in positive nitrogen balance?
2. What situations increase the risk of being in negative nitrogen balance?
3. During what stage of the life cycle are people generally in nitrogen equilibrium?

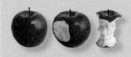 *Take Action*

Meeting Protein Needs When Dieting to Lose Weight

Your father has been gaining weight for the last 5 years. His physician has suggested that he lose 20 pounds to decrease his risk of heart disease and type 2 diabetes. You know that it will be important for your father to meet protein needs as he tries to lose weight. Design a 1-day diet for him that contains about 1500 kcal with 15% of energy intake as protein. A nutrient database, a nutrient analysis computer program, or a website (www.nal. usda.gov/fnic/foodcomp/search/) will provide some help. Does your diet plan meet the RDA for protein and follow MyPyramid guidelines?

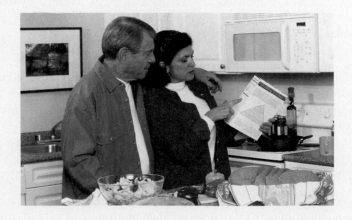

7.5 Protein Digestion and Absorption

For some foods, the first step in protein breakdown takes place during cooking. Cooking unfolds (denatures) proteins and softens the tough connective tissues in meat. This can make many protein-rich foods easier to chew and aids in breakdown during digestion and absorption in the GI tract.

The enzymatic digestion of protein begins in the stomach with the secretion of hydrochloric acid. Once proteins are denatured by stomach acid, **pepsin,** a major enzyme produced by the stomach for digesting proteins, begins to break the long polypeptide chains into shorter chains of amino acids through hydrolysis reactions (Fig. 7-11). Pepsin does not completely separate proteins into amino acids because it can break only a few of the many peptide bonds found in these large molecules.

The release of pepsin is controlled by the hormone **gastrin**. Thinking about food or chewing food stimulates gastrin-producing cells in the terminus of the stomach to release the hormone. Gastrin also strongly stimulates the stomach's parietal cells to produce acid, which aids in digestion and the activation of pepsin. Pepsin is actually stored as an inactive enzyme (called pepsinogen) to prevent it from digesting the stomach lining. Once pepsinogen enters the stomach's acidic environment (pH between 1 and 2), part of the molecule is split off, forming the active enzyme pepsin.

From the stomach, the partially digested proteins move with the rest of the nutrients and other substances in a meal (called chyme) into the duodenum. Once in the

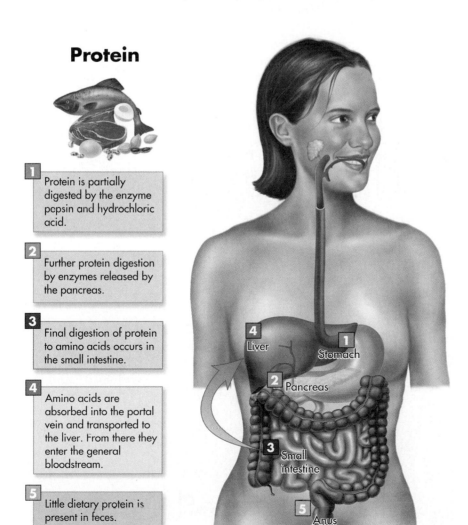

Protein

1. Protein is partially digested by the enzyme pepsin and hydrochloric acid.

2. Further protein digestion by enzymes released by the pancreas.

3. Final digestion of protein to amino acids occurs in the small intestine.

4. Amino acids are absorbed into the portal vein and transported to the liver. From there they enter the general bloodstream.

5. Little dietary protein is present in feces.

Liver

4

1 Stomach

2 Pancreas

3 Small intestine

5 Anus

Figure 7-11 A summary of protein digestion and absorption. Enzymatic protein digestion begins in the stomach and ends in the absorptive cells of the small intestine, where the last peptides are broken down into single amino acids.

small intestine, the polypeptide units, and any fats accompanying them, trigger the release of the hormone cholecystokinin (CCK) from the walls of the small intestine. CCK, in turn, stimulates the pancreas to release the protease or protein-splitting enzymes trypsin, chymotrypsin, and carboxypeptidase into the small intestine. Together, these enzymes digest the polypeptides into short peptides and amino acids.

The short peptides and amino acids in the lumen of the small intestine are actively absorbed into the cells of the small intestine (Fig. 7-12). Approximately 11 different transport mechanisms for amino acids have been identified within the absorptive cells of the small intestine.[1] The remaining short peptides are broken down to individual amino acids by peptidase enzymes. Amino acids then travel via the portal vein to the liver for use in protein synthesis, energy needs, conversion to carbohydrate or fat, or release into the bloodstream for transport to other cells.

Except during infancy, it is uncommon for intact proteins to be absorbed from the digestive tract. However, in early infancy (up to 4 to 5 months of age), the gastrointestinal tract is somewhat permeable to small proteins, so some whole proteins can be absorbed. Because proteins from foods such as cow's milk and egg white may predispose an infant to food allergies, pediatricians and registered dietitians recommend waiting until an infant is 12 months of age or older before introducing common allergenic foods (see Section 7.8).[9]

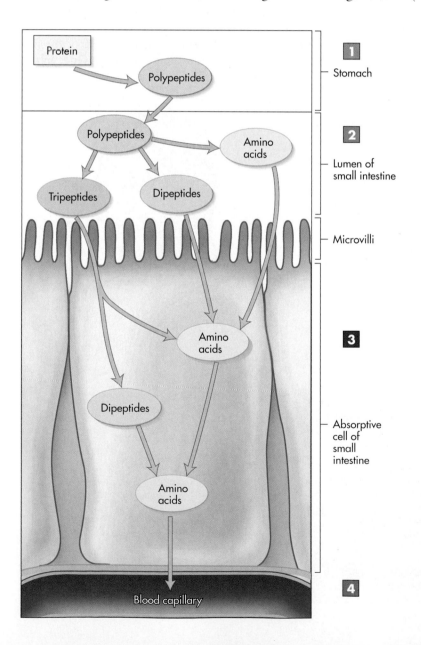

Figure 7-12 Protein digestion takes place in the stomach **1**, the lumen of the small intestine **2**, and the absorptive cells of the small intestine **3**. Then, in a sodium-dependent, energy-requiring process (active absorption), all the end products of protein digestion are absorbed at the microvilli surface. Any remaining peptides are broken down to amino acids within the absorptive cell. These free amino acids are released into the bloodstream **4**. The enzymes used come from the stomach, pancreas, and absorptive and glandular cells that line the small intestine.

Knowledge Check

1. What are 4 enzymes that are involved in protein digestion and absorption?
2. What are the end products of polypeptide digestion?
3. How does the absorption of proteins differ during infancy?

 ## 7.6 Functions of Proteins

Proteins function in many crucial ways in metabolism and in the formation of body structures (Fig. 7-13). Recall that the amino acids needed for the synthesis of proteins are supplied by the diet as well as by the recycling of body protein. However, only when we eat enough carbohydrate and fat can dietary proteins be used efficiently for these functions. If we don't consume enough calories to meet our energy needs, some amino acids will be used to produce energy, rendering them unavailable to build body proteins for other essential functions.

CRITICAL THINKING

Hans eats twice as much protein as his body needs. What happens to this extra protein?

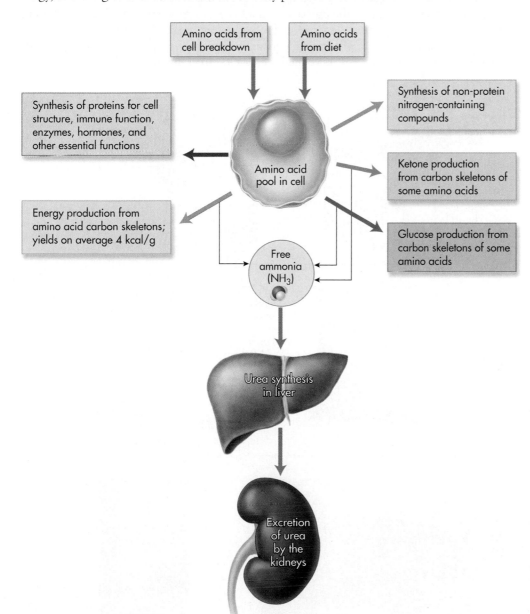

Figure 7-13 Amino acid metabolism. The amino acid pool in a cell can be used to supply amino acids to form body proteins and other compounds from amino acid carbon skeletons. The urea that results is a waste product made from the nitrogen-containing ammonia (NH_3) released during amino acid breakdown. It is excreted in the urine.

Producing Vital Body Structures

One of the primary functions of protein is to provide structural support to body cells and tissues. The key structural proteins (collagen, actin, and myosin) constitute more than a third of body protein and provide a matrix for muscle, connective tissue, and bone. During periods of growth, new proteins are synthesized to support the development of vital body tissues and structures. In periods of malnutrition or disease, protein synthesis drops below normal rates and eventually results in protein wasting and the development of a condition known as kwashiorkor (see Section 7.7).

Maintaining Fluid Balance

capillary beds   Minute blood vessels, 1 cell thick, that create a junction between arterial and venous circulation. Gas and nutrient exchange occurs here between body cells and the blood. Figure A-6 in Appendix A provides a detailed view of a capillary bed.

The blood proteins albumin and globulin are important in maintaining fluid balance between the blood and the surrounding tissue space. Normal blood pressure in the arteries forces blood into **capillary beds**. The blood fluid then moves from the capillary beds into the spaces between nearby cells (**interstitial spaces**) to provide nutrients to those cells (Fig. 7-14). Proteins such as albumin are too large, however, to move out of the capillary beds into the tissues. The presence of these proteins in the capillary beds attracts the right amount of fluid back to the blood, partially counteracting the force of blood pressure to maintain fluid balance.

When protein consumption is inadequate, the concentration of proteins eventually decreases in the bloodstream. Excessive fluid then builds up in the surrounding tissues because

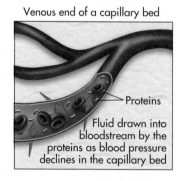

Arterial end of a capillary bed

Venous end of a capillary bed

(a) Fluid forced into interstitial spaces by blood pressure generated by pumping action of heart

Blood cells

Proteins

Fluid drawn into bloodstream by the proteins as blood pressure declines in the capillary bed

(b) Blood pressure is balanced by counteracting force of protein.

Blood pressure exceeds counteracting force of protein, so fluid remains in the tissues.

Normal tissue

Swollen tissue (edema)

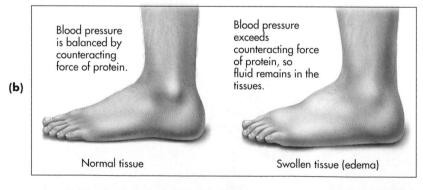
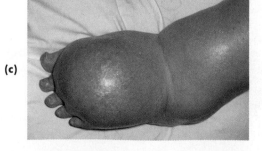
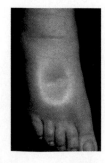

Figure 7-14 Role of protein in maintaining fluid balance. (*a*) Blood proteins help draw fluid back into the capillary bed. (*b*) Without sufficient protein in the bloodstream, edema develops because the counteracting force to blood pressure provided by blood proteins declines. Fluid then remains in the interstitial spaces between cells. (*c*) Examples of feet with edema. In some cases, applying pressure to the swollen area, such as in the photo on the right, causes an indentation that persists after the release of the pressure.

the counteracting force produced by the smaller amount of blood proteins is too weak to pull enough of the fluid back from the tissues into the bloodstream. As fluid builds up in the interstitial spaces, the tissues swell, resulting in **edema.** This can be a sign of a serious medical condition, so it is important for physicians to determine the underlying cause of edema.

Contributing to Acid-Base Balance

The acid-base balance in the body is expressed in terms of pH, which reflects the concentration of hydrogen ions [H]. A solution with a high hydrogen ion concentration has a low pH and is therefore more acidic, whereas a solution with a low hydrogen ion concentration has a high pH and is more alkaline (see Appendix B for additional information). Proteins play an important role in regulating acid-base balance and body pH. For example, proteins located in cell membranes pump chemical ions into and out of cells. The ion concentrations that result from the pumping action help keep the blood slightly alkaline (pH = 7.35–7.45). In this way, proteins act as **buffers**—compounds that help maintain acid-base balance within a narrow range. Proteins are especially good buffers for the body because they have negative charges, which attract positively charged hydrogen ions. This allows them to accept and release hydrogen ions as needed to prevent detrimental changes in pH.

buffers Compounds that help maintain acid-base balance within a narrow range.

Forming Hormones, Enzymes, and Neurotransmitters

Amino acids are required for the synthesis of most hormones in the body. Some hormones, such as the thyroid hormones, are made from only 1 amino acid, whereas others, such as insulin, are composed of many amino acids. Hormones act as messengers in the body and aid in regulatory functions, such as controlling the metabolic rate and the amount of glucose taken up from the bloodstream. Amino acids also are required for the synthesis of enzymes. Cells contain thousands of enzymes that facilitate chemical reactions fundamental to metabolism. Many neurotransmitters, released by nerve endings, also are derivatives of amino acids. This is true for dopamine (synthesized from the amino acid tyrosine), norepinephrine (synthesized from the amino acid tyrosine), and serotonin (synthesized from the amino acid tryptophan).

Contributing to Immune Function

Antibody proteins are a key component of the immune system. Antibodies can bind to foreign proteins (called **antigens**) that invade the body and can prevent their attack on target cells. In a normal, healthy individual, antibodies are very efficient in combating these antigens to prevent infection and disease. However, without sufficient dietary protein, the immune system lacks the material needed to build this defense. Thus, immune incompetence (called **anergy**) develops and reduces the body's ability to fight infection. Anergy can turn measles into a fatal disease for a malnourished child. It also can allow unusual infections to develop in protein-deficient adults.

anergy Lack of an immune response to foreign compounds entering the body.

Transporting Nutrients

Many proteins function as transporters for other nutrients, carrying them through the bloodstream to cells and across cell membranes to sites of action. For instance, the protein hemoglobin carries oxygen from the lungs to cells. Lipoproteins transport large lipid molecules from the small intestine, through the lymph and blood to body cells. Some vitamins and minerals also have specific protein carriers that aid in their transport into and out of tissues and storage proteins. Examples include retinol-binding protein (a carrier protein for vitamin A), transferrin and ferritin (carrier and storage proteins, respectively, for iron), and ceruloplasmin (a carrier protein for copper).

Expert Perspective *from the Field*

Nutrition and Immunity

The immune system is a complex network of organs, tissues, cells, and secretions that protects the body from foreign organisms (pathogens), such as bacteria, viruses, parasites, fungi, and toxins. When the body detects the presence of these "non-self" cells or antigens, innate and acquired immune responses attempt to destroy the antigens.

Innate (non-specific) immunity is present at birth and provides the first barrier of protection against invading antigens. Innate immunity includes *physical barriers,* provided by the skin and mucous membranes, that prevent access to the inside of the body; *chemical secretions,* such as the hydrochloric acid secreted by the stomach, that destroy antigens; *physiological barriers,* such as fever, that prevent the growth of antigens; and *phagocytic cells* that engulf and destroy antigens. Innate immunity provides a general, non-specific response, as it has a limited ability to recognize antigens that have previously attacked the body.

Acquired (specific) immunity provides an immune response that is initiated by the recognition of a specific antigen. Acquired immunity develops over a person's lifetime. Acquired immunity also is referred to as *adaptive immunity* because after exposure to an antigen the immune system can recognize the antigen and adapt its response to it. When the acquired immune system is triggered, the bone marrow and thymus are stimulated to produce *antibodies* (or *immunoglobulins*) and other specialized immune cells that destroy the specific antigens.

Because infants have limited acquired immunity at birth, nutrition experts recommend breastfeeding. Dr. Stephanie Atkinson* is one of many scientists whose research has shown that human milk has high concentrations of many protective immune components, such immunoglobulins and lactoferrin (see Chapter 17). These immune components from the mother can be absorbed by infants and help protect them while their own immune systems are maturing. The immune components in human milk benefit all infants. However, for infants born in underdeveloped countries where exposure to pathogens is much greater than in North America, this immune protection can be life saving.

Nutrition is an important part of maintaining both innate and acquired immunity. According to Dr. Atkinson, nutritional deficiencies can suppress the immune system's ability to prevent infection and disease. Malnutrition results in a loss of antigen-producing tissue, a decreased production of immune cells, the decreased number and effectiveness of antibodies, and a breakdown of physical barriers to antigens. This causes increased risk of infection, disease, and death.

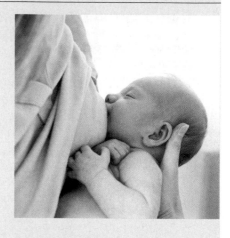

Severe protein-energy malnutrition (PEM) has profound effects on immune function. Dr. Atkinson indicated that this is of particular concern in infants and children with PEM, as they have increased nutritional needs to support growth and often have simultaneous micronutrient deficiencies (e.g., zinc deficiency), infections, and diarrhea, which result in even greater impairment to immune responses. The severity of the nutrient deficiencies and the child's overall health determine whether the impairment can be reversed by supplementing the diet with the deficient nutrients.

Specific nutrients can increase immune protection during critical illness and trauma. For example, the amino acids arginine and glutamine are considered "immunomodulators" because they promote protein synthesis and immune responses. Glutamine also is important in maintaining the integrity of the intestinal mucosa, thereby preventing bacteria in the GI tract from entering the bloodstream. Studies of omega-3 and omega-6 polyunsaturated fatty acids suggest that these essential fatty acids also may be immunomodulators. Specialized nutritional formulas can provide these key nutrients during times of increased nutritional need, such as during disease or injury.

The study of nutrition and immune function is a relatively new field. Thus, scientists' understanding of how nutritional deficiencies and interventions affect immune responses is far from complete. However, it is clear that maintaining optimal nutritional status is an important way to support immune function and reduce the risk of infection and disease.

* Stephanie Atkinson, Ph.D., is Professor, Department of Pediatrics; Associate Chair of Pediatrics (Research); Associate Member, Department of Biochemistry and Biomedical Sciences; and Faculty in the McMaster Medical Sciences Graduate Program and Health Sciences at McMaster University in Hamilton, Ontario, Canada. She directs an internationally recognized research program focused on pediatric nutrition. Among the many honors she has received are a Career Scientist Award from the Ministry of Health in Ontario, the McHenry Award from the Canadian Society for Nutritional Sciences, and a distinguished service award from the Dietitians of Canada.

Forming Glucose

The body must maintain a fairly constant concentration of blood glucose to supply energy, especially for red blood cells, brain cells, and other nervous tissue cells that rely almost exclusively on glucose for energy. If carbohydrate intake is inadequate to maintain blood glucose levels, the liver (and kidneys, to a lesser extent) is forced to make glucose from the amino acids present in body tissues (see Fig. 7-13). This process is called gluconeogenesis (see Chapter 9).

Making glucose from amino acids is normal. For example, when you skip breakfast and haven't eaten since 7 P.M. the preceding evening, glucose must be synthesized from amino acids. However, when this occurs chronically, such as in starvation, the conversion of amino acids into glucose results in the development of widespread muscle wasting in the body (called **cachexia**).

Providing Energy

Proteins supply very little energy for healthy individuals. Under most conditions, body cells use primarily fats and carbohydrates for energy. Although proteins and carbohydrates contain the same amount of usable energy—on average, 4 kcal/g—proteins are a very costly source of energy, considering the amount of metabolism and processing the liver and kidneys must perform to use this energy source (see Fig. 7-13).

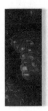

Knowledge Check

1. What are 3 functions of proteins?
2. How do proteins help maintain fluid balance?
3. How do proteins contribute to immune function?

 ## 7.7 Health Concerns Related to Protein Intake

Many people living in developing countries suffer ill health because dietary protein supplies are limited.[10] In contrast, the residents of developed countries tend to eat more protein than they need and may boost their intake even higher by consuming protein or amino acid supplements.[3] As you know, getting sufficient amounts of protein is required for good health, but getting too little or too much can have serious health consequences.[10, 11]

Protein-Energy Malnutrition

Protein deficiency rarely develops as an isolated condition. It most often occurs in combination with a deficiency of energy (and other nutrients) and results in a condition known as **protein-energy malnutrition (PEM),** or protein-calorie malnutrition (PCM). In many developing areas of the world where diets are low in protein and energy, PEM is a very serious public health concern. Although PEM can affect people of all ages, its most devastating consequences are seen in children. Without adequate protein and energy, children fail to grow normally, and many develop diarrhea, infections, and diseases and die early in life. Of the 55,000 people who die of hunger each day, nearly two-thirds are children.[10]

PEM often occurs as either marasmus or kwashiorkor. These conditions differ in the severity of the overall energy and protein deficit and the related clinical characteristics (Fig. 7-15). **Marasmus** develops slowly from a severe deficiency of energy (and, in turn, protein and micronutrients). Over time, this leads to extreme weight loss, muscle and fat loss, and growth impairment. **Kwashiorkor** occurs more rapidly in response to a severe protein deficit, typically accompanied by underlying infections or disease. Kwashiorkor

protein-energy malnutrition (PEM) Condition resulting from insufficient amounts of energy and protein, which eventually result in body wasting and an increased susceptibility to infections.

marasmus Condition that results from a severe deficit of energy and protein, which causes extreme loss of fat stores, muscle mass, and strength. Death from infections is common.

kwashiorkor Condition occurring primarily in young children who have an existing disease and consume a marginal amount of energy and severely insufficient protein. It results in edema, poor growth, weakness, and an increased susceptibility to further infection and disease.

Figure 7-15 Classification of undernutrition in children.

Protein Energy Malnutrition

Severe protein (with moderate energy) deficit; often accompanied by infections or other diseases

Severe energy and protein deficit

Characteristics of Kwashiorkor

Edema
Mild to moderate weight loss
Maintenance of some muscle and
  subcutaneous fat
Growth impairment (60–80% of normal weight
  for age)
Rapid onset
Fatty liver

Characteristics of Marasmus

Severe weight loss
Wasting of muscle and body fat (skin and
  bones appearance)
Severe growth impairment (less than 60% of
  normal weight for age)
Develops gradually

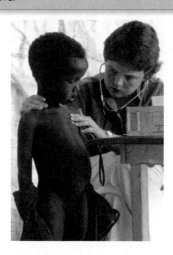
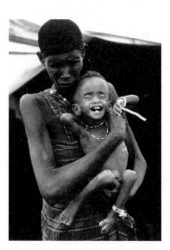

is characterized by edema, mild to moderate weight loss, growth impairment, and the development of a fatty liver (excess accumulation of fat in the liver).

PEM is most prevalent in parts of Africa, Southeast Asia, Central America, and South America.[1] However, it also is seen in some population groups in industrialized countries. Those at greatest risk are individuals living in poverty and/or isolation and those with substance abuse problems, anorexia nervosa, or debilitating diseases (e.g., AIDS or cancer). Some hospitalized patients also are at increased risk of PEM because of poor prior health, low dietary intakes, and increased protein needs for recovery from surgery, trauma, and/or disease. Malnourished patients face a much greater risk of complications and even death. Consequently, hospitals have developed nutrition support teams to ensure appropriate nutritional care for at-risk patients.

Kwashiorkor

Kwashiorkor is a word from Ghana that means "the disease that the first child gets when the new child comes." From birth, an infant in developing areas of the world is usually breastfed. Often by the time the child is 12 to 18 months old, the mother is pregnant or has already given birth again. The mother's diet is usually so marginal that she cannot produce sufficient milk to continue breastfeeding the older child. This child's diet then abruptly changes from nutritious human milk to starchy roots and gruels. These foods have low protein densities, compared with their energy content. Additionally, the foods are usually high in plant fibers and bulk, making it difficult for the child to consume enough to meet energy needs and nearly impossible to meet protein needs. Many children in these areas also have infections and parasites that elevate protein and energy needs and often precipitate the development of kwashiorkor.

The presence of edema in a child who has some subcutaneous fat still present is the hallmark of kwashiorkor (see Fig. 7-15). Other major symptoms of kwashiorkor are apathy, diarrhea, listlessness, failure to grow and gain weight, infections, and withdrawal from the environment. These symptoms also complicate other diseases that may be present. For example, measles, a disease that normally makes a healthy child ill for only a week or so, can become severely debilitating and even fatal in a child with kwashiorkor.

Many symptoms of kwashiorkor can be explained based on what is known about proteins. Proteins play important roles in fluid balance, growth, immune function, and the transport of other nutrients. Thus, protein deficiency can severely compromise these functions.

If children with kwashiorkor are helped in time—infections are treated and a diet ample in protein, energy, and other essential nutrients is provided—the disease process often reverses and they begin to grow again. Unfortunately, by the time many of these children reach a hospital or care center, they already have severe infections. Thus, despite good medical care, many still die. Those who survive often continue to battle chronic infections and diseases.[10]

Marasmus

Marasmus is the result of chronic PEM. It is caused by diets containing minimal amounts of energy, protein, and other nutrients. The word *marasmus* means "to waste away." Over time, the severe lack of energy and protein results in a "skin and bones" appearance, with little or no subcutaneous fat (see Fig. 7-15).

Marasmus usually develops in infants who either are not breastfed or have stopped breastfeeding in the early months. Often, the weaning formula used is incorrectly prepared because of unsafe water and because the parents cannot afford sufficient infant formula for the child's needs. The latter problem may lead the parents to dilute the formula to provide more feedings, not realizing that this deprives the infant of essential calories, protein, and other nutrients.

Marasmus in infants commonly occurs in the large cities of poverty-stricken countries. In the cities, bottle-feeding is often necessary because the infant must be cared for by others when the mother is working or away from home.

An infant with marasmus requires large amounts of energy and protein; unless the child receives them, full recovery from the disease may never occur. Most brain growth occurs between conception and the child's first birthday. If the diet does not support brain growth during the first months of life, the brain may not fully develop, resulting in poor cognitive and intellectual growth.

High-Protein Diets

In addition to recommending adequate protein consumption, the Food and Nutrition Board also suggests that protein intake not exceed 35% of energy intake.[3] Diets containing an excessive or disproportionate amount of protein do not provide additional health benefits. Instead, high protein intakes may increase health and disease risks. One area of concern is the effect of excess protein on the kidneys.[12, 13] Recall that the kidneys are responsible for excreting excess nitrogen as urea. Thus, high-protein diets may overburden the kidney's capacity to excrete nitrogen wastes. Additionally, because water is needed to dilute and excrete urea, inadequate fluid intake can increase the risk of dehydration as the kidneys use body water to dispose of the urea. These concerns are greatest for people who already have impaired kidney function. A lower-protein diet with adequate fluid intake is recommended for these individuals to help preserve kidney health.[13]

When excess protein is primarily from a high intake of animal proteins, the overall diet is likely to be low in plant-based foods and consequently low in fiber, some vitamins (vitamins C and E and folate), minerals (magnesium and potassium), and beneficial phytochemicals. Animal proteins are often rich in saturated fat and cholesterol. As a result, these diets can increase the risk of cardiovascular disease.[5, 6, 8] Diets that also contain high amounts of red meat (especially in cured forms, such as hot dogs, ham, salami, and luncheon meats) have been associated with an increased risk of certain cancers.[14]

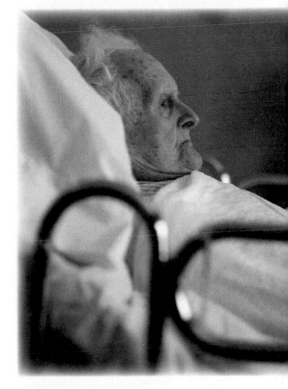

Some hospitalized patients are at risk of protein-energy malnutrition (PEM) because of poor dietary intakes and increased needs for recovery from surgery, trauma, or disease.

High-protein diets also may increase urinary calcium loss and eventually lead to a loss of bone mass and an increased risk of osteoporosis.[5] These findings are somewhat controversial, however, and are less of a concern for individuals with adequate calcium intakes.

Another concern, particularly with athletes, is the health risks associated with excess protein and amino acid supplementation. As described earlier, our bodies are designed to obtain amino acids from dietary sources of whole proteins. This assures a supply of amino acids in proportions needed for body functions and prevents amino acid toxicity, especially for methionine, cysteine, and histidine—the most toxic amino acids.[11] When individual amino acid supplements are taken, chemically similar amino acids can compete for absorption, resulting in amino acid imbalances and toxicity risk.

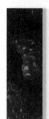

Knowledge Check

1. How does kwashiorkor differ from marasmus?
2. Which individuals might be at greatest risk of PEM in the United States?
3. What areas of the world have the highest incidence of PEM?
4. Why might an excessive protein intake be harmful?

7.8 Food Protein Allergies

Allergies, including food allergies, involve responses of the immune system designed to eliminate foreign proteins (antigens). These responses occur when the body mistakenly reacts to a food as though it were a harmful invader.[15] In some people, certain food proteins (called **allergens**) cause hypersensitivity reactions and trigger this response. These allergens stimulate white blood cells to produce antibodies (specifically, the **immunoglobulin IgE**) that bind to antigens and cause the symptoms associated with an allergic reaction.

Fortunately, most allergic reactions are mild, such as a runny nose, sneezing, itching skin, hives, or digestive upset (indigestion, nausea, vomiting, diarrhea). For those who are severely allergic, exposure to the allergenic food may cause a generalized life-threatening reaction involving all body systems (known as **anaphylaxis,** or anaphylactic shock). Anaphylaxis causes decreased blood pressure and respiratory distress so severe that the person cannot breathe—death will occur without immediate medical help. Unfortunately, in the U.S., allergic reactions result in 30,000 emergency room visits and 150 to 200 deaths per year.

The protein in any food can trigger an allergic reaction. However, 8 foods account for 90% of all food allergies: peanuts, tree nuts (e.g., walnuts and cashews), milk, eggs, fish, shellfish, soy, and wheat (Fig. 7-16). Other foods frequently identified as causing allergic reactions are meat and meat products, fruits, and cheese.

The only way to prevent allergic reactions is to avoid foods known to trigger reactions. Carefully reading food labels and asking questions when eating out are essential, perhaps life-saving steps for those with food allergies.[15] In addition, individuals preparing foods at home or in restaurants need to know their menu ingredients and take steps to ensure that foods that cause an allergic reaction in a person do not come in contact with the food to be served to that individual. Even trace amounts of an allergen can cause a reaction. To prevent cross-contact, anything that will be used to prepare an allergen-free meal (i.e., hands, workspace, pans, utensils, plates) should be washed thoroughly before preparing the allergen-free meal. Unlike foodborne illness pathogens, such as bacteria and viruses, cooking an allergenic food often does not render its allergens harmless.[16]

Food allergies are a common, but sometimes fatal, problem. In fact, almost 11 million Americans have food allergies. The number of children developing food allergies has risen sharply in recent years. For instance, from 1997 to 2002, the number of children with peanut allergies doubled.[1] Experts are not certain what has caused this dramatic increase.

It is unclear why some people develop allergies. Although some studies have shown that pregnant women can help prevent or delay the onset of food allergies in their child by avoiding peanuts and tree nuts during their last 3 months of pregnancy, currently it

allergen Protein (e.g., those in food) that induces a hypersensitive response, with excess production of certain immune system antibodies. Subsequent exposure to the same protein leads to allergic symptoms.

immunoglobulins Proteins (also called antibodies) in the blood that are responsible for identifying and neutralizing antigens as well as pathogens that bind specifically to antigens.

CRITICAL THINKING

Jocelyn developed hives and swelling of her lips, tongue, and throat after eating her friend's homemade chili. She learned that her friend used peanut butter as a special ingredient in her chili. How could this have caused Jocelyn's symptoms?

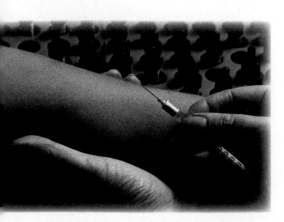

People with hypersensitivity to certain foods can be tested to determine which food allergens cause their symptoms.

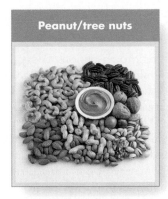

Peanut/tree nuts

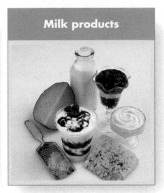

Milk products

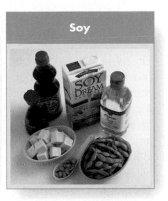

Soy

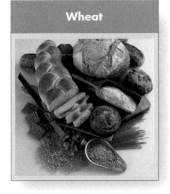

Wheat

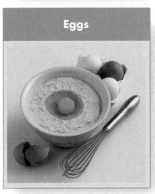

Eggs

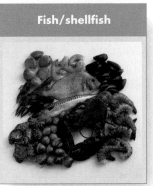

Fish/shellfish

Figure 7-16 These foods account for the vast majority of all food allergies.

appears that maternal dietary restrictions do not play a significant role in preventing food allergies in their children.[17] After the child is born, the American Academy of Pediatrics advises the following steps to help prevent food allergies.[9] These guidelines are especially important for families with a history of any type of allergy.

- Avoid eating highly allergenic foods, such as peanuts, while breastfeeding.
- Feed babies only breast milk or infant formula until they are at least 6 months old.
- Delay feeding infants cow's milk and milk products until infants are at least 1 year of age.
- Serve egg whites only after children reach age 2 years.
- Keep diets free of peanuts, tree nuts, fish, and shellfish until children are at least 3 years old.

The outlook for children with food allergies that first appear before 3 years of age is good. About 80% of young children with food allergies outgrow them before 3 years.[18] Thus, parents should not assume that the allergy will be long-lasting. Food allergies diagnosed after 3 years of age, however, are often more long-lived. In these cases, about 33% of children outgrow their food allergies within 3 years. For others, food allergies can last a lifetime, especially allergies to peanuts, tree nuts, and shellfish. Offending foods that have not previously caused anaphylaxis can be tested every 6 to 12 months or so to see whether the allergic reaction has decreased. If so, the food(s) can be gradually reintroduced into the diet and eaten safely.

▶ Food allergies and food intolerances are not the same. Food allergies cause an immune response as a result of exposure to certain food proteins (allergens). In contrast, food intolerances (see Chapter 4) are caused by an individual's inability to digest certain food components, usually due to low amounts of specific enzymes. Generally, larger amounts of an offending food are required to produce the symptoms of food intolerance than to trigger allergic symptoms. Food allergies tend to be far more life-threatening than food intolerances.

▶ The American Academy of Allergy and Immunology has a 24-hour toll-free hot line (800-822-2762) to answer questions about food allergies and help direct people to specialists who treat allergy problems. Free information on food allergies is available by contacting The Food Allergy & Anaphylaxis Network at www.foodallergy.org.

Knowledge Check

1. What are the symptoms of food allergies?
2. Which foods cause most food allergies?
3. What steps can parents take to help prevent food allergies in their children?

7.9 Vegetarian Diets

Vegetarianism has evolved over the centuries from a necessity into an option. Today, approximately 2.5% of adults in the United States and 4% of adults in Canada follow a vegetarian diet. Additionally, 20 to 25% of Americans report that they eat at least 4 meatless meals a week.[5] Most people choose vegetarian diets for religious, philosophical, ecological, or health-related reasons. For example, Hindus, Seventh Day Adventists, and Trappist monks follow vegetarian diets as a part of their religious practices. Others adopt vegetarian practices because they are concerned with the economic and ecological impact of eating meat-based diets. They recognize that meat is not an efficient way of obtaining protein because it requires the use of approximately 40% of the world's grain production to raise meat-producing animals. Diets rich in fruits, vegetables, legumes, and grains frequently result in increased intakes of antioxidant nutrients, such as vitamins C and E and carotenoids; dietary fiber; and healthful phytochemicals and decreased intakes of saturated fat and cholesterol. Thus, the American Cancer Society, the World Cancer Research Fund, the American Heart Association, and the Heart and Stroke Foundation of Canada all promote plant-based diets to promote health and reduce risk of chronic disease.[5, 19-23]

The eating patterns of vegetarians can vary considerably, depending on the extent to which animal products are excluded. Vegans follow the most restrictive diet, as they eat only plant foods. Because they do not eat any animal foods, their diets may be low in high biological value protein, riboflavin, vitamin D, vitamin B-12, calcium, and zinc unless carefully planned.[5] Lacto-vegetarians are similar to vegans, because their diets exclude meat, poultry, eggs, and fish but differ in that they include dairy products in their diets. Lacto-ovo-vegetarians include eggs in their diets but avoid meat, poultry, and fish. These last 2 groups eat some animal foods, so their diets often contain ample amounts of nutrients that may be low or missing in strictly plant-based diets. However, to reduce the risk of nutrient deficiencies, all vegetarians need to follow nutritional recommendations (Table 7-5) when making daily food choices.[24, 25]

Vegetarian diets require knowledge and creative planning to yield high-quality protein and other key nutrients without animal products. Earlier in this chapter, you learned about complementary proteins, whereby the essential amino acids deficient in 1 protein source are supplied by those of another consumed at the same meal or the next. Recall that many legumes are deficient in the essential amino acid methionine, whereas cereals are

The amino acids in legumes are best used when combined with nuts, seeds, or grains.

Table 7-5 Food Plan for Vegetarians Based on MyPyramid

| Food Group | MyPyramid Servings | | Key Nutrients Supplied[c] |
	Lactovegetarian[a]	Vegan[b]	
Grains	6–11	8–11	Protein, thiamin, niacin, folate, vitamin E, zinc, magnesium, iron, and fiber
Beans and other legumes	2–3	3	Protein, vitamin B-6, zinc, magnesium, and fiber
Nuts, seeds	2–3	3	Protein, vitamin E, and magnesium
Vegetables	3–5 (include 1 dark green or leafy variety daily)	4–6 (include 1 dark green or leafy variety daily)	Vitamin A, vitamin C, folate, vitamin K, potassium, and magnesium
Fruits	2–4	4	Vitamin A, vitamin C, and folate
Milk	3	———	Protein, riboflavin, vitamin D, vitamin B-12, and calcium
Fortified soy milk	———	3	Protein, riboflavin, vitamin D, vitamin B-12, and calcium

[a]This plan contains about 75 grams of protein in 1650 kcal.
[b]This plan contains about 79 grams of protein in 1800 kcal.
[c]One serving of vitamin- and mineral-enriched ready-to-eat breakfast cereal is recommended to meet possible nutrient gaps. Alternatively, a balanced multivitamin and mineral supplement can be used. Vegans also may benefit from the use of fortified soy milk to provide calcium, vitamin D, and vitamin B-12.

limited in lysine. Thus, eating a combination of legumes and cereals, such as beans and rice, will supply the body with adequate amounts of all essential amino acids. Variety is an especially important characteristic of a nutritious vegan diet.[25]

At the forefront of nutritional concerns for vegetarians are riboflavin, vitamins D and B-12, calcium, iron, and zinc.[5, 26, 27] A major source of riboflavin, vitamin D, and calcium in the typical North American diet is milk, which is omitted from the vegan diet. However, riboflavin can be obtained from green leafy vegetables, whole-grain breads and cereals, yeast, and legumes—components of most vegan diets. Alternate sources of vitamin D include fortified foods (e.g., soy milk) and dietary supplements, as well as regular sun exposure (see Chapter 12).

Calcium-fortified foods are the vegan's best option for obtaining calcium. These include fortified soy milk, fortified orange juice, calcium-rich tofu (check the label), and certain ready-to-eat breakfast cereals, breads, and snacks. Green leafy vegetables and nuts also contain calcium, but the mineral is either not well absorbed or not very plentiful from these sources.[28] Dietary supplements provide another option for meeting calcium needs (see Chapter 14). It is important to read supplement labels and to plan supplement use carefully because even a typical multivitamin and mineral supplement will not supply enough calcium to meet the body's needs.[29]

Vitamin B-12 occurs naturally only in animal foods. Plants can contain soil or microbial contaminants that provide trace amounts of vitamin B-12, but these are negligible sources of the vitamin. Therefore, vegans need to eat food fortified with vitamin B-12 or take supplements to protect against deficiency.[26]

To obtain iron, vegans can consume whole-grain breads and cereals, dried fruits and nuts, and legumes.[5, 25] The iron in these foods is not absorbed as well as the iron in animal foods, but eating a good source of vitamin C with these foods enhances iron absorption (see Chapter 15).

Vegans can find zinc in whole-grain breads and cereals, nuts, and legumes, but phytic acid and other substances in these foods limit zinc absorption. Grains are most nutritious when consumed as breads, because the leavening (rising of the bread dough) reduces the influence of phytic acid.[5]

Special Concerns for Infants and Children

Infants and children are at highest risk of nutrient deficiencies as a result of poorly planned vegetarian diets.[5] However, with the use of complementary proteins and good sources of problem nutrients discussed earlier, the energy, protein, vitamin, and mineral needs of vegetarian and vegan infants and children can be met. The most common nutritional concerns for infants and children following vegetarian and vegan diets are deficiencies of iron, vitamin B-12, vitamin D, zinc, and calcium.[5, 27]

Vegetarian and vegan diets tend to be high in bulky, high-fiber, low-calorie foods that cause fullness. Although this side effect can be a welcome advantage for adults, children have a small stomach volume and relatively high nutrient needs for their size and may feel full before their energy needs are met. For this reason, the fiber content of a child's diet may need to be decreased by replacing high-fiber sources with some refined grain products, fruit juices, and peeled fruit. Including concentrated sources of energy, such as fortified soy milk, nuts, dried fruits, and avocados, can help meet calorie and nutrient needs.

Overall, vegetarian and vegan diets can be appropriate during infancy and childhood. However, to achieve normal growth and ensure adequate intake of all nutrients, these diets must be implemented with knowledge and, ideally, professional guidance.[5, 25]

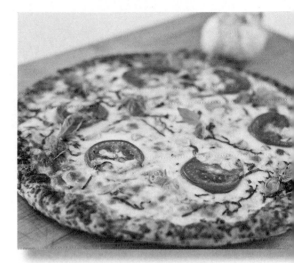

Vegetarian versions of common foods are becoming more readily available in groceries and restaurants.

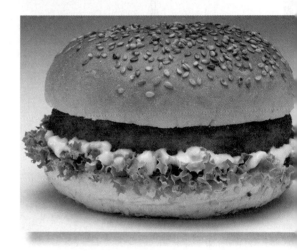

Vegetarianism Websites

www.ivu.org

www.vrg.org

www.vegetariannutrition.net

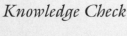

Knowledge Check

1. How does a vegan diet differ from a lacto-vegetarian diet?
2. Which nutrients are likely to be low in a vegan diet?
3. What are 2 nutritional risks for children on vegetarian diets?

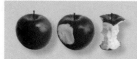

Take Action

Protein and the Vegan

Alana is excited about the possible health benefits of her new vegan diet. However, she is concerned that her diet may not contain enough protein, vitamins, and minerals. Use a nutrient database, a nutrient analysis computer program, or a website (www.nal.usda.gov/fnic/foodcomp/search) to calculate her protein intake and see if her concerns are valid.

Breakfast	**Protein (g)**
Calcium-fortified orange juice, 1 cup	
Soy milk, 1 cup	
Fortified bran flakes, 1 cup	
Banana, medium	
Snack	
Calcium-enriched granola bar	
Lunch	
Garden Veggie Burger, 4 oz	
Whole-wheat bun	
Mustard, 1 tbsp	
Soy cheese, 1 oz	
Apple, medium	
Green leaf lettuce, 1½ cups	
Peanuts, 1 oz	
Sunflower seeds, ¼ cup	
Tomato slices, 2	
Mushrooms, 3	
Vinaigrette salad dressing, 2 tbsp	
Iced tea	
Dinner	
Kidney beans, ½ cup	
Brown rice, ¾ cup	
Fortified margarine, 2 tbsp	
Mixed vegetables, ¼ cup	
Hot tea	
Snack	
Strawberries, ½ cup	
Angel food cake, 1 small slice	
Soy milk, ½ cup	

Total Protein: _____

Alana's diet contained 2150 kcal, with _____ g (you fill in) of protein (is this adequate for her?), 57 g of total dietary fat (only 9 g of which came from saturated fat), and 50 g of fiber. Her vitamin and mineral intake with respect to those of concern to vegetarians—vitamin B-12, vitamin D, calcium, iron, and zinc—met her needs.

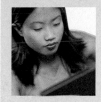

Lily's dietary intake for this day is not as healthy as it could be because it does not come close to following recommendations. Many of the components of a healthy vegetarian diet—whole grains, nuts, soy products, beans, 2 to 4 servings of fruit, and 3 to 5 servings of vegetables per day—are missing. With so few fruits and vegetables, her diet also is low in the many phytochemicals that may provide numerous health benefits. It is apparent that Lily has not yet learned to implement the concept of complementary proteins, so the quality of the protein in her diet is low. Unless she makes a more informed effort at diet planning, Lily will not reap the health benefits she had hoped for when she chose to follow a vegetarian diet.

Summary

7.1 Amino acids, the building blocks of proteins, contain a usable form of nitrogen for humans. Of the 20 amino acids needed by the body, 9 must be provided in the diet (essential). The other 11 can be synthesized by the body (nonessential) from amino acids in the body's amino acid pool. High-quality, also called complete, proteins contain ample amounts of all 9 essential amino acids. Foods derived from animal sources provide high-quality, or complete, protein. Lower-quality, or incomplete, proteins lack sufficient amounts of 1 or more essential amino acids. This is typical of plant foods. Different types of plant foods eaten together often complement each other's amino acid deficits, thereby providing high-quality protein in the diet.

7.2 Individual amino acids are linked together to form proteins. The sequential order of amino acids determines the protein's ultimate shape and function. This order is directed by DNA in the cell nucleus. Diseases, such as sickle-cell anemia, can occur if the amino acids are incorrect in a polypeptide chain. When the 3-dimensional shape of the protein is unfolded—denatured—by treatment with heat, acid, or alkaline solutions, or other processes, the protein also loses its biological activity.

7.3 Almost all animal products are rich sources of protein. The high quality of these proteins means that they can be easily converted into body proteins. Legumes, nuts, seeds, and grains are good sources of plant protein. Protein quality can be measured by determining the extent to which the body can retain the nitrogen contained in the amino acids absorbed. This is called biological value. In addition, the balance of essential amino acids in a food can be compared with an ideal pattern to determine chemical score. When multiplied by the degree of digestibility, the chemical score yields the Protein Digestibility Corrected Amino Acid Score (PDCAAS).

7.4 The adult RDA for protein is 0.8 g per kg of healthy body weight. For a typical 154-lb (70-kg) person, this corresponds to 56 g of protein daily; for a 125-lb (57-kg) person, this corresponds to 46 g/day. The North American diet generally supplies plenty of protein: men typically consume about 100 g of protein daily, and women consume about 65 g. These intakes are also of sufficient quality to support body functions.

7.5 Protein digestion begins in the stomach, where proteins are broken down into shorter polypeptide chains of amino acids. In the small intestine, these polypeptide chains are digested into dipeptides and amino acids, which are absorbed by the small intestine, where any remaining peptides are broken down into amino acids. Absorbed amino acids then travel via the portal vein to the liver.

7.6 Important body components—such as muscles, connective tissue, transport proteins, enzymes, hormones, and antibodies—are made of proteins. Proteins also provide carbon skeletons, which can be used to synthesize glucose when necessary.

7.7 Undernutrition can lead to protein-energy malnutrition in the form of kwashiorkor or marasmus. Kwashiorkor results primarily from an inadequate energy intake with a severe protein deficit, often accompanied by disease and infection. Kwashiorkor frequently occurs when a child is weaned from human milk and fed mostly starchy gruels. Marasmus results from extreme starvation—a negligible intake of both protein and energy. Marasmus commonly occurs during famine, especially in infants. These conditions have been noted in some North Americans with cancer, AIDS, malabsorption disease, anorexia nervosa, alcoholism, or limited income and resources to obtain food. High-protein diets (above 35% of energy intake) do not provide additional health benefit. They are associated with dehydration, overburdening of the kidneys' capacity to excrete nitrogen wastes, increased risk of cardiovascular disease and certain cancers, increased urinary calcium loss, and risk of amino acid imbalance and toxicity.

7.8 Food allergies involve immune system responses designed to eliminate allergens that the body mistakenly reacts to as though they were harmful invaders. Symptoms range from mild to life-threatening. The only way to prevent reactions is to avoid foods known to trigger allergic reactions.

7.9 Vegetarian diets are becoming more popular as individuals recognize the possible health benefits of plant-based diets. Low intakes of riboflavin, vitamins D and B-12, calcium, iron, and zinc are of greatest concern in vegetarian diets. Vegetarian diets require knowledge and creative planning to obtain high-quality protein and other key nutrients but can be nutritionally adequate when guidelines are followed.

253

Study Questions

1. Essential amino acids must be supplied by the diet because the body cannot synthesize them in adequate amounts.

    a. true   **b.** false

2. A process involved in the synthesis of nonessential amino acids is called _____.

    a. ketogenesis   **c.** transamination
    b. gluconeogenesis   **d.** supplementation

3. The carbon skeleton of an amino acid is the portion remaining after an amino group has been removed.

    a. true   **b.** false

4. Which of the following is classified as a complete protein?

    a. kidney beans   **c.** whole-grain bread
    b. fat-free milk   **d.** corn tortillas

5. The sequential order of amino acids in a polypeptide chain is called the _____.

    a. primary structure   **c.** tertiary structure
    b. secondary structure   **d.** quaternary structure

6. Which of the following is a rich source of protein?

    a. citrus fruits   **c.** enriched grains
    b. dark leafy greens   **d.** barbequed chicken

7. Which of the following is *not* a means of determining the protein quality of a food?

    a. biological value
    b. chemical score
    c. protein efficiency ratio
    d. complementary score

8. Hospitalized patients recovering from illness or trauma usually need additional protein to attain positive nitrogen balance.

    a. true   **b.** false

9. Proteins are involved in all of the following functions *except* _____.

    a. providing energy   **c.** promoting bowel health
    b. aiding in immune function   **d.** providing cell structure

10. Which of the following population groups is at increased risk of PEM?

    a. college athletes   **c.** the elderly
    b. obese individuals   **d.** adolescents

11. Many children with kwashiorkor maintain some muscle and subcutaneous fat.

    a. true   **b.** false

12. Which of the following is *not* a usual characteristic of marasmus?

    a. edema   **c.** impaired growth
    b. severe weight loss   **d.** muscle wasting

13. Which of the following is associated with excessive protein intakes?

    a. dehydration   **c.** diarrhea
    b. anemia   **d.** diabetes

14. Which of the following foods is a common cause of food allergies?

    a. peanuts   **c.** eggs
    b. shellfish   **d.** all of the above

15. Which of the following nutrients would most likely be low in a vegan diet?

    a. vitamin C   **c.** vitamin B-12
    b. thiamin   **d.** dietary fiber

Answer Key: 1-a; 2-c; 3-a; 4-b; 5-a; 6-d; 7-d; 8-a; 9-c; 10-c; 11-a; 12-a; 13-a; 14-d; 15-c

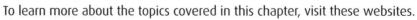

Websites

To learn more about the topics covered in this chapter, visit these websites.

Food Allergies

www.foodallergy.org

www.foodallergy.rutgers.edu

Vegetarianism

www.ivu.org

www.vrg.org

www.vegetariannutrition.net

vegrd.vegan.com

fnic.nal.usda.gov

www.vegdining.com

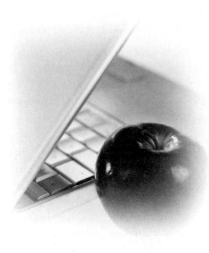

References

1. Matthews E. Proteins and amino acids. 10th ed. In: Shils M and others, eds. *Modern nutrition in health and disease.* Philadelphia: Lippincott Williams & Wilkins; 2006.

2. Bonds D. Three decades of innovation in the management of sickle cell disease: The road to understanding the sickle cell disease clinical phenotype. *Blood Rev.* 2005;19:99.

3. Institute of Medicine, Food and Nutrition Board. *Dietary Reference Intakes for energy, carbohydrate, fiber, fat, fatty acids, cholesterol, protein, and amino acids.* Washington, DC: National Academy Press; 2002.

4. U.S. Department of Agriculture. *Nutrient content of the US food supply.* Research Report 57. Washington, DC: U.S. Department of Agriculture; 2007.

5. Dawson-Hughes B. Interaction of dietary calcium and protein in bone health in humans. *J Nutr.* 2003;133:852S.

6. Kelemen L and others. Associations of dietary protein with disease and mortality in a prospective study of postmenopausal women. *Am J Epidemiol.* 2005;161 239.

7. Leitzman C. Vegetarian diets: What are the advantages? *Forum Nutr.* 2005;57:147.

8. McVeigh B and others. Effect of soy protein varying in isoflavone content on serum lipids in healthy young men. *Am J Clin Nutr.* 2006;83:244.

9. Zeiger R. Food allergen avoidance in the prevention of food allergy in infants and children. *Pediatrics.* 2003;111:1662.

10. Muller O, Krawinkel M. Malnutrition and health in developing countries. *Can Med Assoc J.* 2005;173:279.

11. Garlick P. The nature of human hazards associated with excessive intakes of amino acids. *J Nutr.* 2004;134:1633S.

12. Eating a high protein diet may accelerate kidney problems. *Today's Dietitian.* 2004; April:26.

13. Knight E and others. The impact of protein intake on renal function decline in women with normal renal function or mild renal insufficiency. *Ann Intern Med.* 2003;138:460.

14. Chao A and others. Meat consumption and colorectal cancer. *JAMA.* 2005;293:172.

15. Kline D. Food allergy symptoms and causes. *Today's Dietitian.* 2005; August:10.

16. Mondoulct L and others. Influence of thermal processing on the allergenicity of peanut proteins. *J Agric Food Chem.* 2005;53:4547.

17. Greer FR and others. American Academy of Pediatrics Committee on Nutrition, American Academy of Pediatrics Section on Allergy and Immunology. Effects of early nutritional interventions on the development of atopic disease in infants and children: The role of maternal dietary restriction, breastfeeding, timing of introduction of complementary foods, and hydrolyzed formulas. *Pediatrics.* 2008;121:183.

18. Kleinman R, ed. *Pediatric nutrition handbook.* Chicago: American Academy of Pediatrics; 2004.

19. Berkow S, Barnard N. Blood pressure regulation and vegetarian diets. *Nutr Rev.* 2005;63:1.

20. Gardner C and others. The effect of a plant-based diet on plasma lipids in hyper-cholesterolemic adults. *Ann Intern Med.* 2005;142:725.

21. Hu F. Plant-based foods and prevention of cardiovascular disease: An overview. *Am J Clin Nutr.* 2003;78:544S.

22. Newby P. Risk of overweight and obesity among semivegetarian, lactovegetarian, and vegan women. *Am J Clin Nutr.* 2005;81:1267.

23. Sabate J. The contribution of vegetarian diets to human health. *Forums of Nutrition.* 2005;56:218.

24. Davis B, Kris-Etherton P. Achieving optimal essential fatty acid status in vegetarians: Current knowledge and practical implications. *Am J Clin Nutr.* 2003;78:640S.

25. Messina V and others. A new food guide for North American vegetarians. *Can J Diet Pract Res.* 2003;64:82.

26. Antony A. Vegetarianism and vitamin B-12 (cobalamin) deficiency. *Am J Clin Nutr.* 2003;78:3.

27. Weiss R and others. Severe vitamin B-12 deficiency in an infant associated with a maternal deficiency and a strict vegetarian diet. *J Pediatr Hematol Oncol.* 2004;26:270.

28. Titchenal AC, Dobbs J. A system to assess the quality of food sources of calcium. *J Food Comp Analysis.* 2007;20:717.

29. Aronson D. Vegetarian nutrition. *Today's Dietitian.* 2005; March:3.

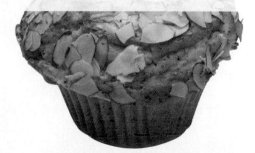

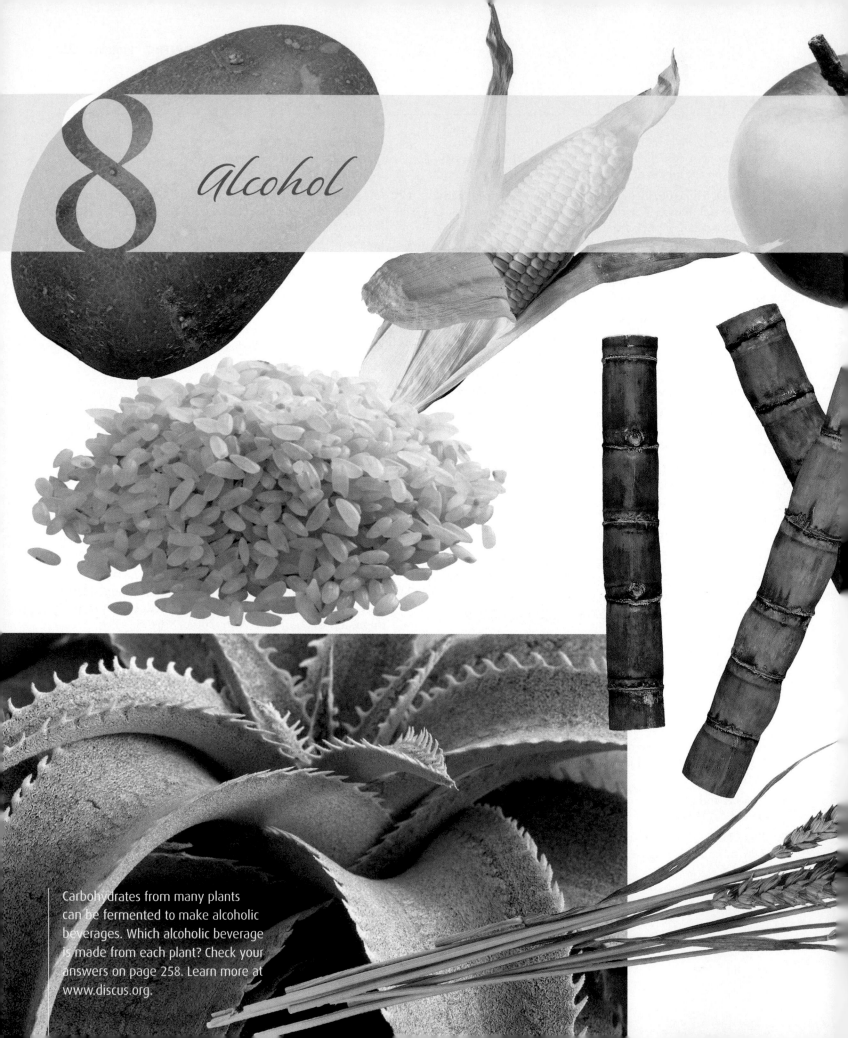

8 Alcohol

Carbohydrates from many plants can be fermented to make alcoholic beverages. Which alcoholic beverage is made from each plant? Check your answers on page 258. Learn more at www.discus.org.

STUDENT LEARNING OUTCOMES

After studying this chapter, you will be able to:

1. Describe the sources of alcohol and the calories it provides.

2. Define standard sizes of alcoholic beverages and the term *moderate drinking*.

3. Summarize how alcoholic beverages are produced.

4. Outline the process of alcohol absorption, transport, and metabolism.

5. Define binge drinking and explain how it increases the risk of alcohol poisoning.

6. Explain how alcohol consumption affects blood alcohol concentration.

7. Describe guidelines for using alcohol safely.

8. Discuss potential benefits of using alcohol.

9. Summarize the risks of alcohol consumption.

10. Describe the effects of chronic alcohol use on the body and nutritional status.

11. List the signs of alcohol dependency and abuse.

12. Outline the methods used to diagnose alcohol abuse.

13. List the strategies and resources available for the treatment of alcoholism.

Beer, wine, and hard liquor, or spirits, are consumed by about 60% of the adult population in North America.[1] The alcohol in these beverages, when averaged across the population, provides about 3% of the total energy intake. Although not an essential nutrient, alcohol also contributes about 7 kcal/g of energy to the diet.

For some individuals, alcohol adds to the enjoyment of a meal or social times shared with friends and family. For others, moderate alcohol use may relieve tensions and enhance relaxation. In middle-aged and older adults, moderate alcohol consumption may even reduce the risk of cardiovascular disease. Unfortunately, moderate use of alcohol can escalate to alcohol dependence and abuse in susceptible individuals.

Alcohol is a **narcotic,** an agent that reduces sensations and consciousness, and a central nervous system depressant. It is the most commonly abused drug in North America. The harmful effects of alcohol are well known. Alcoholism and alcohol abuse can cause motor vehicle accidents, destroy families and friendships, and spur deadly behaviors, such as suicide, rape, and other types of violence. Too much alcohol damages almost every organ in the body—the liver and brain are especially vulnerable to its

Sugar cane—rum

Grapes—wine

Wheat—beer

Potato—vodka

Apple—cider, brandy

Barley—ale, porter, stout, Scotch

Rice—sake

Agave—tequila

Corn—bourbon

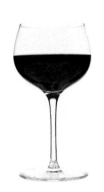

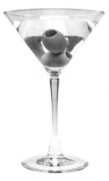

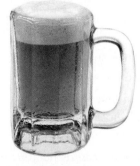

The following servings of each type of alcoholic beverage provide the same amount of alcohol (about 15 g): wine—5 oz, hard liquor—1.5 oz, beer or wine cooler—12 oz. In determining a safe level of intake, it is important to observe these serving sizes.

toxic effects. Nutrient deficiencies are widespread in alcoholics. Alcohol abuse, behind smoking and obesity, is the third leading cause of preventable death in adults. Because alcohol is so widely consumed and its abuse touches many lives, this chapter will examine this substance in detail. It will explore the sources of alcohol, the production of alcohol, the metabolism of alcohol, and the health concerns related to intakes of alcohol.

 8.1 Sources of Alcohol

The form of alcohol we consume, chemically known as ethanol, is supplied mostly by beverages such as beer, wine, distilled spirits (or hard liquor, such as vodka and rum), liqueurs, cordials, and hard cider. It also is sometimes used as an ingredient in foods, such as chicken cooked in wine (coq au vin), flaming desserts, and chocolate candy filling.

As shown in Table 8-1, beverages vary in alcohol and calorie content. Most beers are about 5% alcohol or less, although some beers exceed 11% alcohol. Wines generally range in alcohol content from approximately 5 to 14%. Fortified wines (wines that have spirits added to increase their alcohol content) typically contain 15 to 22% alcohol. Distilled wine spirits, such as brandy, contain more than 22% alcohol. For hard liquor (distilled spirits), alcohol content is listed by "proof" rather than by percentage. The "proof" is actually twice the percentage of alcohol content. Thus, an 80-proof vodka or gin is 40% alcohol.

A standard drink is usually defined as the size that provides approximately 15 g of alcohol. In general, this equates to a 12-ounce beer, 10-ounce wine cooler, 5-ounce glass of wine, or 1.5-ounce pour of hard liquor. These serving sizes are used as the basis for recommendations of moderate and excessive drinking. Many individuals are not

Table 8-1 Alcohol and Energy Content of Alcoholic Beverages

Beverage		Amount (Fluid oz)	Alcohol (g)	Energy (kcal)
Beer				
Regular		12	12	150
Light		12	10	75–100
Distilled Spirits				
Gin, rum, vodka, bourbon, tequila, whiskey (80 proof)		1.5	14	95
Liqueurs		1.5	14	160
Wine				
Red		5	14	100
White		5	14	100
Dessert, sweet		5	23	225
Rose		5	14	100
Mixed Drinks				
Martini		3.5	32	220
Manhattan		3.5	30	225
Whiskey sour		3.5	17	135
Margarita (frozen)		8	20	175
Rum and cola		8	15	170

aware of these definitions of serving sizes—some may consider a 20-ounce glass of beer or an 8-ounce glass of wine to be a "drink," when, in fact, these servings are both closer to 2 drinks.

Most guidelines for "moderate alcohol intake" suggest no more than 1 standard-size drink per day for women and no more than 2 per day for men. This does not mean that one can abstain from drinking during the week and then safely consume 7 or more drinks on a single day. As discussed in a later section, this is defined as binge drinking, and it can have serious consequences.

Production of Alcoholic Beverages

The alcohol we consume is produced by fermentation. The process of fermenting foods to produce mead (fermented honey), beer, wine, and other alcoholic products dates back to prehistoric times. Grains, cereals, fruits, honey, milk, potatoes, and other carbohydrate-rich foods can be used to make alcoholic beverages.

Fermentation occurs when yeast, a microorganism, consumes carbohydrates and converts them to alcohol and carbon dioxide. The carbohydrate must be in the form of simple sugars, such as maltose or glucose, for yeast to use it as food. If the carbohydrate is a starch, such as that found in cereal grain seeds (e.g., barley), it must be broken down to simpler forms, or "malted," before fermentation can occur. During malting, the grain seeds are allowed to sprout; the sprouting process produces enzymes in the seed that break starches into simple sugars. Each molecule of glucose that is fermented produces 2 molecules of ethanol, 2 molecules of carbon dioxide, and 2 molecules of water. Additionally, the reaction yields energy that the yeast can use.

Fermentation begins when a food rich in simple sugars, yeast, and water are combined and left at room temperature. During the first stage, the yeast cells multiply, using the sugars for energy, and produce small amounts of alcohol. When the oxygen in the container holding the mixture of water, yeast, and sugars is depleted, the second stage begins, during which the yeast ferments the remaining sugar to produce alcohol and carbon dioxide under anaerobic (without oxygen) conditions. After fermentation has ceased (when the sugar is used up or the alcohol content is high enough to inactivate the yeast), the product can be finished in a variety of ways, or the alcohol itself can be recovered from the product by **distilling** it into spirits, such as gin or whiskey.

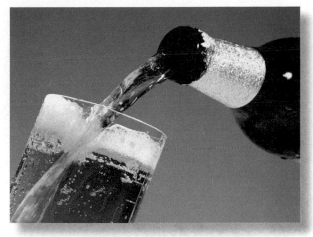
Beer is a source of alcohol and carbohydrates.

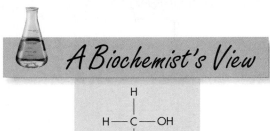
A Biochemist's View

Ethanol

distill To separate 2 or more liquids that have 2 different boiling points. Alcohol is boiled off and the vapors are collected and condensed. Distillation produces a high alcohol content in hard liquor.

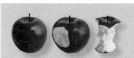 *Take Action*

Investigate the Energy Cost of Alcohol Use

On an upcoming weekend (Friday night through Sunday night), have a few friends keep a careful log of their alcoholic beverage intake. Include males and females. Then use Table 8-1 or nutrient analysis software to calculate the amount of energy provided by alcoholic beverages over that time period. Assuming that many college-age men need about 2500 kcal/day and women need about 2000 kcal/day, is the amount of energy provided by alcoholic beverages large (e.g., 25% or more of needs) or small (e.g., 10% or less of needs) in comparison?

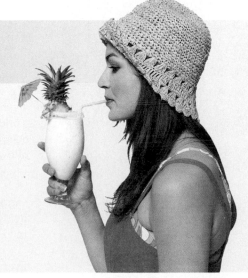

Knowledge Check

1. What amounts of beer, wine, and hard liquor each contain 15 g alcohol?
2. What ingredients are required for fermentation?
3. What process is used to increase the alcohol of fermented beverages?

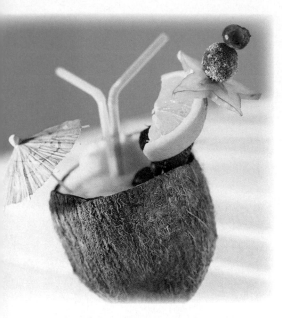

Distilled spirits, used to make many popular drinks, have the highest alcohol content of the alcohol-containing beverages.

Women are smaller, have less body water, and have less alcohol dehydrogenase in their stomachs. This makes them more susceptible than men to the effects of alcohol.

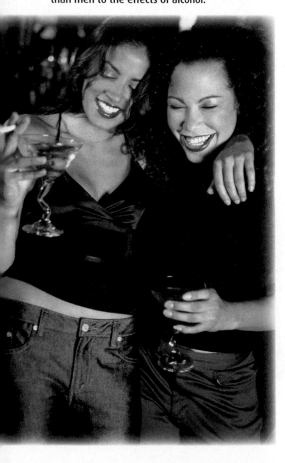

8.2 Alcohol Absorption and Metabolism

Alcohol, unlike carbohydrates, protein, and fat, requires no digestion. It also does not need specific transport mechanisms or receptors to enter cells. Therefore, it is absorbed rapidly throughout the digestive tract, including the stomach, by simple diffusion.

In general, the upper parts of the small intestine, the duodenum and jejunum, absorb alcohol more quickly than other parts of the digestive tract, although this depends on how quickly food leaves the stomach.[2] As you know from Chapter 4, the rate at which food leaves the stomach depends on the types and amount of food consumed. Larger meals containing foods high in fat leave the stomach most slowly, thereby slowing the absorption of any alcohol consumed. In contrast, alcohol consumed on an empty stomach is absorbed quickly from the stomach and small intestine into the bloodstream.

Alcohol is readily dispersed throughout the body because alcohol is found wherever water is distributed in the body. Alcohol moves easily through the cell membranes; however, as it does, it damages proteins in the membranes.[3]

Alcohol Metabolism

Because alcohol cannot be stored in the body, it has absolute priority in metabolism as a fuel source, taking precedence over other energy sources, such as carbohydrate. At low to moderate intakes, alcohol is metabolized through a series of reactions called the alcohol dehydrogenase (ADH) pathway. This pathway requires 2 enzymes (alcohol dehydrogenase and aldehyde dehydrogenase) to convert ethanol to the toxic intermediate compound acetaldehyde and then to acetyl-CoA. Acetyl-CoA can be readily metabolized to yield energy or can be used for fatty acid synthesis (see Chapter 9). Although the cells lining the stomach metabolize 10 to 30% of alcohol via the ADH pathway, the liver is the chief site for alcohol metabolism.

$$\text{Ethanol} \xrightarrow{\textit{alcohol dehydrogenase}} \text{Acetaldehyde} \xrightarrow{\textit{aldehyde dehydrogenase}} \text{Acetyl-CoA}$$

When a person drinks moderate to excessive amounts of alcohol, the ADH pathway cannot keep up with the demand to metabolize all the alcohol. Under these circumstances, the liver treats the alcohol as a foreign substance and activates the microsomal ethanol oxidizing system (MEOS) to help metabolize alcohol. The MEOS pathway produces the same compounds as the ADH pathway, but it requires energy to function (see Chapter 9). As a person's alcohol intake increases over time, the MEOS becomes increasingly active, allowing for more efficient metabolism of alcohol and a greater tolerance to alcohol, meaning that increasing amounts of alcohol are necessary to produce the same effect.[3]

The MEOS also metabolizes drugs and other substances foreign to the body. Activation of the MEOS by excessive alcohol intake reduces the liver's capacity for metabolizing drugs because the metabolism of alcohol takes priority.[3] Thus, MEOS activation increases the potential for drug toxicities.

A third metabolic pathway for metabolizing alcohol—the catalase pathway—in the liver and other cells makes a minor contribution to alcohol metabolism in comparison

Table 8-2 Alcohol Metabolism Summary

Alcohol Metabolic Pathway	Main Location of Pathway Activity	Alcohol Intake Level That Activates Pathway	Extent of Participation in Alcohol Metabolism
Alcohol dehydrogenase pathway (ADH)	Stomach Liver (mostly)	Low to moderate intake	Major role (metabolizes about 90% of alcohol)
Microsomal ethanol oxydizing system (MEOS)	Liver	Moderate to excessive intake	Role increases in importance with increasing alcohol intake levels
Catalase pathway	Liver Other cells	Moderate to excessive intake	Minor

with the alcohol dehydrogenase pathway and the MEOS. Table 8-2 summarizes alcohol metabolism.

The 3 metabolic pathways (ADH, MEOS, and catalase) metabolize nearly all the alcohol consumed. Only a small percentage of alcohol intake is excreted unmetabolized through the lungs, urine, and sweat.[3]

Factors Affecting Alcohol Metabolism

The key to alcohol metabolism lies in one's ability to produce the enzymes used in the alcohol dehydrogenase pathway because this pathway metabolizes about 90% of the alcohol consumed.[3] Ethnicity, gender, and age affect the production and activity of enzymes in the alcohol dehydrogenase pathway. For instance, many individuals of Asian descent have normal to high alcohol dehydrogenase enzyme activity, allowing a very rapid conversion of alcohol by the first enzyme (alcohol dehydrogenase), but they have very low activity of the second enzyme (aldehyde dehydrogenase) needed to complete alcohol breakdown. The resulting buildup of acetaldehyde commonly causes flushing, dizziness, nausea, headaches, rapid heartbeat (tachycardia), and rapid breathing (hyperventilation). These reactions can be so severe that it's uncomfortable to drink more or even at all.[4]

Compared with men, women produce less of the alcohol dehydrogenase enzyme in the cells that line their stomachs—as a result, women absorb about 30 to 35% more unaltered alcohol from the stomach directly into the bloodstream. Another gender-related factor is that, in comparison with men, women are generally smaller in body size, have more body fat, and have less muscle tissue and total body water (as do older men and older women). As a result, alcohol becomes more concentrated in the blood and body tissues of a woman than in a similar-size man because alcohol can be diluted by water-holding muscle tissue, but not by adipose. For these reasons, a woman becomes intoxicated on less alcohol than a similar-size man.

Other factors that can affect alcohol metabolism include the alcohol content of the beverage, the amount of alcohol consumed, and the individual's usual alcohol intake.[5] Compared with an occasional drinker, the MEOS is more active in individuals who drink large amounts of alcohol regularly, which increases the chronic drinker's alcohol metabolism as well as tolerance.

Rate of Alcohol Metabolism

Although the body is fairly well equipped to metabolize alcohol, this process is not instantaneous. A social drinker who weighs 150 pounds (about 70 kg) and has normal liver function metabolizes about 5 to 7 g of alcohol per hour. This is the amount in about half of a 12-ounce beer, 5-ounce glass of wine, or 1.5 ounce shot of distilled spirits.

▶ The mind-altering effects of alcohol begin soon after it enters the bloodstream. Within minutes, alcohol inhibits nerve cells in the brain. As a drug, alcohol eventually produces a narcotic effect on the body. The heart muscle strains to cope with alcohol's depressive action. If drinking continues, rising blood alcohol impairs speech, vision, balance, and judgment. Extremely high blood alcohol content can lead to respiratory failure.

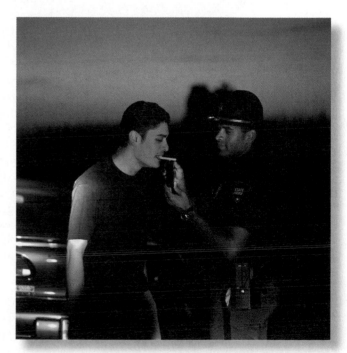

One is legally intoxicated at a blood alcohol concentration of 0.08 in the United States and Canada. However, for many individuals driving is often noticeably impaired at a blood alcohol concentrations of 0.02 to 0.05.

Table 8-3 Blood Alcohol Concentration (BAC) and Symptoms

BAC	Behavior	Impairment
.01–.06	• Relaxation • Sense of well-being • Loss of inhibition • Lowered alertness • Joy	• Thought • Judgment • Coordination • Concentration
.06–.10	• Blunted feelings • Disinhibition • Extroversion • Diminished sexual pleasure	• Reflexes • Reasoning • Depth perception • Distance acuity • Peripheral vision • Glare recovery
.11–.20	• Overexpression of emotions • Emotional swings • Angry or sad • Boisterous	• Reaction time • Gross motor control • Walking (staggering) • Speech (slurred)
.21–.29	• Stupor • Loss of understanding • Loss of sensations	• Gross motor control • Consciousness loss • Memory (blackouts)
.30–.39	• Severe depression • Unconsciousness • Possible death	• Bladder function • Breathing • Heart rate
> .40	• Unconsciousness • Death	• Breathing • Heart rate

CRITICAL THINKING

Kevin went out with his friends to celebrate the end of the semester. Over an hour's time, he had 4 beers. Kevin weighs approximately 160 lb. According to Figure 8-1, what would Kevin's blood alcohol level be? Is this within a legally safe limit to drive?

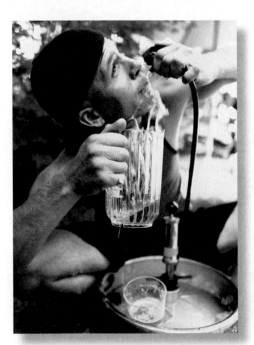

Although many young adults do not recognize the true impact of binge-drinking habits, it poses a risk to their nutritional health, overall health, and safety.

When the rate of alcohol consumption exceeds the liver's metabolic capacity, blood alcohol levels rise and the symptoms of intoxication appear as the brain and central nervous system are exposed to alcohol (Table 8-3).[6]

Blood alcohol levels can be determined by measuring the amount of alcohol excreted through the lungs because the alcohol content of exhaled air and blood are directly related (Fig. 8-1). The constant relationship between the alcohol content of blood and exhaled air makes it possible to use breathalyzer tests as a legal basis for defining alcohol impairment and intoxication.

If blood alcohol levels rise high enough, the person experiences acute alcohol toxicity, also known as alcohol poisoning (Table 8-4). This dangerous condition requires immediate medical treatment—left untreated, alcohol poisoning can cause respiratory failure and death. Inhalation of vomit also can result in death and has occurred at levels lower than those that cause alcohol poisoning. The risk of consuming toxic levels of alcohol is greater when drinking distilled spirits because their higher alcohol content makes it is easier to ingest more alcohol in less volume and less time than with beer or wine. **Binge drinking,** defined as having 4 or more drinks for females and 5 or more drinks for males on a single occasion, also increases the risk of alcohol poisoning.

Knowledge Check

1. How does the body metabolize low to moderate amounts and large amounts of alcohol?
2. What factors affect alcohol metabolism?
3. How quickly can most people metabolize 1 alcoholic beverage?
4. Why does binge drinking increase the risk of alcohol poisoning?

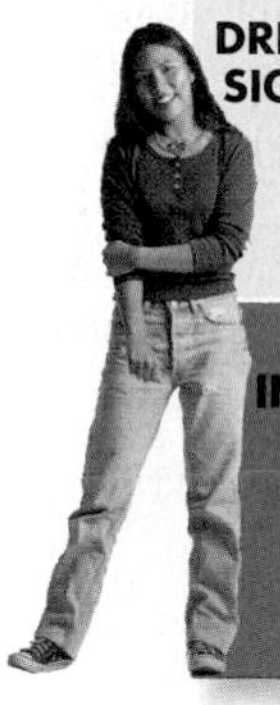

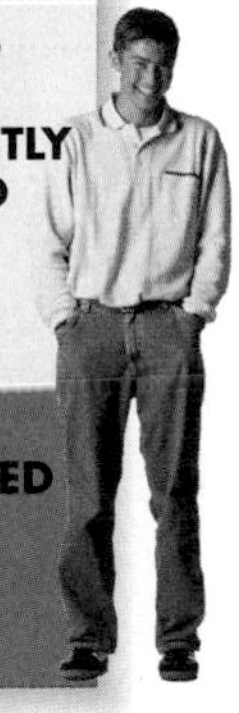

	Effect on Women									Drinks	Effect on Men								
Body weight in pounds	90	100	120	140	160	180	200	220	240		100	120	140	160	180	200	220	240	**Body weight in pounds**
ONLY SAFE DRIVING LIMIT	.00	.00	.00	.00	.00	.00	.00	.00	.00	0	.00	.00	.00	.00	.00	.00	.00	.00	**ONLY SAFE DRIVING LIMIT**
IMPAIRMENT BEGINS	.05	.05	.04	.03	.03	.03	.02	.02	.02	1	.04	.03	.03	.02	.02	.02	.02	.02	**IMPAIRMENT BEGINS**
DRIVING SKILLS SIGNIFICANTLY AFFECTED	.10	.09	.08	.07	.06	.05	.05	.04	.04	2	.08	.06	.05	.05	.04	.04	.03	.03	**DRIVING SKILLS SIGNIFICANTLY AFFECTED**
	.15	.14	.11	.11	.09	.08	.07	.06	.06	3	.11	.09	.08	.07	.06	.06	.05	.05	
	.20	.18	.15	.13	.11	.10	.09	.08	.08	4	.15	.12	.11	.09	.08	.08	.07	.06	
	.25	.23	.19	.16	.14	.13	.11	.10	.09	5	.19	.16	.13	.12	.11	.09	.09	.08	
LEGALLY INTOXICATED	.30	.27	.23	.19	.17	.15	.14	.12	.11	6	.23	.19	.16	.14	.13	.11	.10	.09	**LEGALLY INTOXICATED**
	.35	.32	.27	.23	.20	.18	.16	.14	.13	7	.26	.22	.19	.16	.15	.13	.12	.11	
	.40	.36	.30	.26	.23	.20	.18	.17	.15	8	.30	.25	.21	.19	.17	.15	.14	.13	
	.45	.41	.34	.29	.26	.23	.20	.19	.17	9	.34	.28	.24	.21	.19	.17	.15	.14	
	.51	.45	.38	.32	.28	.25	.23	.21	.19	10	.38	.31	.27	.23	.21	.19	.17	.16	

Approximate blood alcohol percent (Women)   **Approximate blood alcohol percent** (Men)

Figure 8-1 Approximate relationship between alcohol consumption and blood alcohol concentration (units are % or mg of alcohol per 100 ml of blood). Note that effects can vary among people and whether food also is consumed. A blood alcohol concentration of 0.02 begins to impair driving. One is legally intoxicated at a blood alcohol concentration of 0.08 in the United States and Canada.

Table 8-4 Signs and Symptoms of Alcohol Poisoning

- Confusion, stupor
- Vomiting
- Low blood sugar (hypoglycemia)
- Severe dehydration
- Seizures
- Slow or irregular breathing and heartbeats
- Blue-tinged or pale skin
- Low body temperature (hypothermia)
- Unconsciousness

Call 911 or your local emergency number if you suspect alcohol poisoning and the person cannot be roused or is unconscious. If the person is conscious, you can call 1-800-222-1222 to be routed to your local poison control center for further instructions.

8.3 Alcohol Consumption

Currently, about 62% of North American adults consume alcohol. Approximately 42% are light drinkers (consuming 3 or fewer drinks per week), 14% have moderate alcohol consumption (no more than 7 or 14 drinks per week for women and men, respectively), and 4.8% consume alcohol excessively (more than 7 to 14 drinks weekly). Thirty-eight percent abstain from consuming alcohol.[1]

The largest drinking population in North America consists of young, White college students, many of whom are not yet of legal drinking age. College students are drinking more heavily and more frequently than ever before. In fact, excessive alcohol consumption is a bigger problem than illicit drug use on most college campuses. Many young adults consider drinking alcohol to be a "rite of passage" into adulthood and incorporate drinking competitions into initiations to clubs and social circles. Alcohol producers also target college

CRITICAL THINKING

Imagine that you are president of a sorority or fraternity where there is a tradition of the "fourth-year fifth," a long-standing practice of seniors to consume a fifth of liquor during the semester prior to graduation. Every weekend, between 3 and 10 students arrive in the local emergency room with alcohol poisoning or alcohol-related injuries, and there are several alcohol-related deaths each year. As the president of the organization, what might you recommend to prevent alcohol-related accidents and deaths?

▶ *Healthy People 2010* set important goals regarding alcohol use:
- Reduce by 25% the proportion of adults who exceed the guidelines for appropriate alcohol use.
- Reduce the number of high school and college students engaging in binge drinking by at least 50%.

students with advertising and other marketing efforts. Unfortunately, many young drinkers have little or no knowledge of the potentially harmful acute and chronic effects of alcohol.

Of the 70% of college students who report using alcohol, approximately 45% or more engage in binge drinking. Binge drinking is associated with vandalism, violent crime, traffic accidents and injuries, sexual abuse, suicide, hazing deaths, and serious acute health risks.[7,8] As noted in Table 8-5, binge drinking has serious consequences, which affect virtually all college campuses, college communities, and college students, even those who choose not to drink alcohol. Thus, it is important that binge drinkers be aware that these habits can cause lifelong problems, especially when drinking becomes habitual.[7]

According to the National Institute on Alcohol Abuse and Alcoholism, nearly 4% of the adult U.S. population is dependent on alcohol.[9] In young adults, ages 18 to 29 years, these rates jump to 9%. Underage drinking also is a significant public health and safety issue. By age 14 to 15, approximately half of all adolescents have consumed alcohol and approximately 20% have been drunk at least once.[10] Underage drinkers are particularly vulnerable to alcohol's damaging effects and are at much greater risk of alcoholism in adulthood.[11]

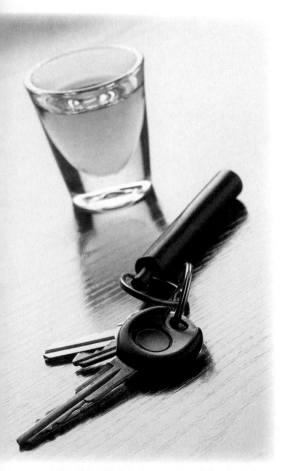

Thirty-nine percent of all motor vehicle fatalities are alcohol-related.

Table 8-5 Impact of Binge Drinking on College Campuses

Death: 1700 college students between the ages of 18 and 24 die each year from alcohol-related unintentional injuries, including motor vehicle crashes.

Injury: 599,000 students between the ages of 18 and 24 are unintentionally injured each year under the influence of alcohol.

Assault: More than 696,000 students between the ages of 18 and 24 are assaulted each year by another student who has been drinking.

Sexual abuse: More than 97,000 students between the ages of 18 and 24 are victims of alcohol-related sexual assault or date rape each year.

Unsafe sex: Each year about 400,000 students between the ages of 18 and 24 have unprotected sex and more than 100,000 students between the ages of 18 and 24 have been too intoxicated to know if they consented to having sex.

Academic problems: About 25% of college students report academic consequences of their drinking, including missing class, falling behind, doing poorly on exams or papers, and receiving lower grades overall.

Health problems/suicide attempts: More than 150,000 students develop an alcohol-related health problem and between 1.2 and 1.5% of students indicate that they tried to commit suicide within the past year because of drinking or drug use.

Drunk driving: 2.1 million students between the ages of 18 and 24 drive under the influence of alcohol each year.

Vandalism: About 11% of college student drinkers report that they have damaged property while under the influence of alcohol.

Property damage: More than 25% of administrators from schools with relatively low drinking levels and more than 50% from schools with high drinking levels say their campuses have a "moderate" or "major" problem with alcohol-related property damage.

Police involvement: About 5% of 4-year college students are involved with the police or campus security as a result of their drinking, and an estimated 110,000 students between the ages of 18 and 24 are arrested for an alcohol-related violation, such as public drunkenness or driving under the influence.

Alcohol abuse and dependence: 31% of college students met the criteria for a diagnosis of alcohol abuse and 6% for a diagnosis of alcohol dependence in the past 12 months, according to questionnaire-based self-reports about their drinking.

The consequences of excessive and underage drinking affect virtually all college campuses, college communities, and college students whether they choose to drink or not.

Source: www.collegedrinkingprevention.gov/facts/snapshot.aspx.

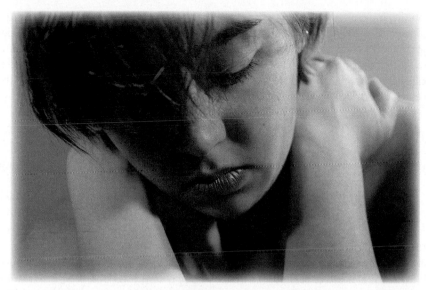

Many colleges require students who break alcohol and drug rules to attend counseling or educational programs to reduce their alcohol intake and binge-drinking episodes. Colleges and communities offer a variety of educational and treatment strategies for individuals with alcohol dependency.

CASE STUDY

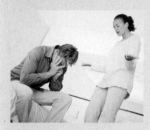

Alyssa and her boyfriend, Todd, are college juniors. Todd was a very serious student in high school and achieved excellent grades, but as a college student he has begun binge drinking. His grades have fallen sharply and he is becoming socially isolated. He was even arrested once for drunk driving.

Last night, Todd had 8 beers and 3 shots of whiskey at an off-campus party he attended with Alyssa. Unfortunately, everyone who knows Todd says he tends to get angry and says things he doesn't mean when he drinks too much. He often becomes cruel and destructive to those he cares for and respects. He also has been involved in several fights. As the party began to die down, Alyssa tried to get Todd to leave. He responded rudely and forcefully grabbed her arm. She became frightened with his aggressive behavior and left without him.

The next morning, Alyssa noticed a large bruise on her arm where Todd had grabbed her. She decided to tell Todd about her anxiety about the events from the night before and his alcohol abuse. She did not want to see everything he had worked so hard for be ruined by alcohol. What should Alyssa say and do?

8.4 Health Effects of Alcohol

Low to moderate use of alcohol has been associated with several social and health-related benefits. However, despite the possible benefits of regular, moderate alcohol use, excessive alcohol intake has serious effects on health and nutritional status.

Guidance for Using Alcohol Safely

The U.S. Surgeon General's office, National Academy of Science, U.S. Department of Agriculture, and U.S. Department of Health and Human Services do not recommend that a non-drinker start consuming alcohol because risks often outweigh possible benefits. However, they do not specifically discourage moderate alcohol use. The Dietary Guidelines for Americans (see Chapter 2) provide the following suggestions for individuals who choose to drink alcohol.

- Drinking alcohol should be done sensibly and in moderation—defined as the consumption of up to 1 drink per day for women and up to 2 drinks per day for men.

- Alcoholic beverages should not be consumed by some individuals, including those who cannot restrict their alcohol intake, women of childbearing age who may become pregnant, pregnant and lactating women, children and adolescents, individuals taking medications that can interact with alcohol, and those with specific medical conditions.
- Alcoholic beverages should be avoided by individuals engaging in activities that require attention, skill, or coordination, such as driving or operating machinery.

Potential Benefits of Alcohol Intake

Many people enjoy meeting a friend for a beer or having a glass of wine in the evening with dinner. Others report a reduced feeling of anxiety and stress after having a drink at the end of their workday. In elderly individuals, moderate alcohol use can stimulate appetite and increase dietary intake. These behaviors are not considered harmful as long as they are practiced by individuals of a legal drinking age, continue in moderation, and cause no obvious harm.[12]

In middle-aged and older adults, moderate alcohol use has been shown to lower the risk of cardiovascular disease and overall mortality in comparison with non-drinkers.[13, 14] Alcohol can lower serum low-density lipoprotein (LDL) levels, increase protective high-density lipoprotein (HDL) levels, and decrease platelet aggregation (blood cell accumulation)—all of which help reduce the risk of heart disease. Some studies suggest that the heart disease prevention benefits are predominantly associated with red wine consumption and may be attributed to a phytochemical in red wine called resveratrol.[15] However, other compounds and types of alcohol may produce similar benefits.

Although the heart health benefits of alcohol have received the most attention, a few studies have shown an association between moderate alcohol use and reduced risk of type 2 diabetes and dementia.[14, 16, 17] These associations are more controversial and require additional research.

Risks of Excessive Alcohol Intake

The excessive consumption of alcohol contributes significantly to 5 of the 10 leading causes of death in North America—heart failure, certain forms of cancer, cirrhosis of the liver, motor vehicle and other accidents, and suicides. Alcohol-related conditions lead to 100,000 deaths in the United States each year.

As shown in Figure 8-2, excessive alcohol intake affects many organs and systems in the body. Heavy drinkers may develop heart damage that causes arrhythmias (abnormal heartbeats) and fluid retention in the lungs. Excess alcohol intake also can contrib-

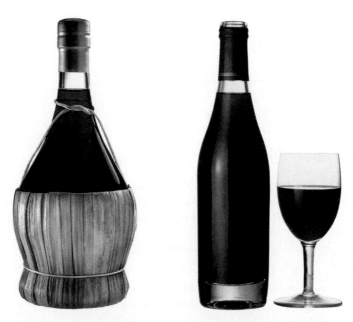

Of all the alcohol sources, red wine is often singled out as the best choice because of the added bonus of the many phytochemicals (e.g., resveratrol) present. These leach out of the grape skins when red wine is made. Dark beer contains some phytochemicals, but in lower amounts.

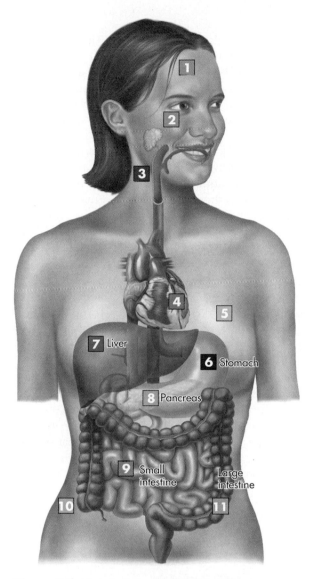

1	Impaired brain function and resulting brain damage
2	Vasodilation and flushing of the skin
3	Cancer of the oral cavity, throat, larynx, and esophagus
4	Heart muscle damage and resulting heart failure
5	Breast cancer
6	Irritation of the stomach lining and stomach cancer
7	Fatty infiltration of the liver, alcoholic hepatitis, cirrhosis, and ultimate liver failure
8	Impaired pancreatic function and related hypoglycemia; pancreatic cancer
9	Malabsorption of nutrients in the small intestine
10	Abdominal fat deposition and fluid accumulation (ascites)
11	Cancer of the colon and rectum

Figure 8-2 **Alcohol affects virtually every organ.**

ute to high blood pressure and the risk of stroke. Limiting alcohol intake to no more than 2 drinks per day (men) and 1 drink per day (women) may help prevent or improve these conditions.[18] Several cancers also are related to alcohol consumption. Cancers of the oral cavity, throat, larynx, and esophagus are the most strongly related to alcohol consumption, with heavy drinking (5 to 6 drinks per day) increasing the risk 50-fold.[19, 20] Tobacco, often used simultaneously with alcohol, interacts with alcohol to further increase the risk of these cancers. Alcohol ingestion also elevates the risk for colorectal and breast cancers, although to a much lesser extent.

Prolonged, excessive alcohol intake can cause significant liver damage and lead to the development of cirrhosis of the liver. Alcohol-related liver damage also can increase the risk of liver cancer. Other adverse effects of excessive alcohol include osteoporosis, brain damage, inflammation of the stomach lining, intestinal bleeding, suppression of the immune system (with an increased risk of infections), sleep disturbances, impotence, hypoglycemia (effect of acute excessive alcohol intake), hyperglycemia (effect of chronic excessive alcohol intake), abdominal obesity, high blood triglyceride levels, and nutrient deficiencies.

Cirrhosis of the Liver

The liver is one of the largest organs in the body. It has many functions, including nutrient storage, protein and enzyme synthesis, and the metabolism of protein, fats, and carbohydrates. It is also vital for removing toxins from the body and for metabolizing drugs. Because the liver is the main organ for alcohol metabolism, long-term excessive alcohol intake can damage the liver.

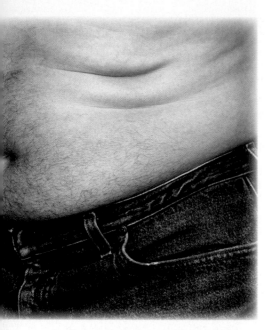

The "beer belly," common in many drinkers, occurs because alcohol promotes the synthesis of fat in the liver and promotes a positive energy balance that contributes to a risk of obesity, especially abdominal obesity.

The first change seen in the liver is fat accumulation, known as fatty liver, or steatosis. Fatty liver occurs in response to the increased synthesis of fat and trapping of fat in the liver. This condition is reversible, but only if alcohol is eliminated from the diet.

If alcohol consumption persists, inflammation of the liver cells, known as alcoholic hepatitis, develops. Alcoholic hepatitis produces symptoms of nausea, poor appetite, vomiting, fever, pain, and **jaundice** (yellow-orange coloration of the skin and whites of the eyes), resulting from the liver's inability to excrete bile pigments, which instead spill from damaged hepatocytes (liver cells) into the blood. Alcoholic hepatitis is a serious condition, which frequently progresses to the chronic, irreversible liver disease known as cirrhosis.

Cirrhosis is characterized by the loss of functioning hepatocytes (Fig. 8-3). As cirrhosis progresses, the synthesis of proteins, such as those required for normal blood clotting, decreases dramatically. Ascites, abnormal fluid retention in the abdomen amounting to as much as 4 gallons (15 liters), is another common complication of cirrhosis. Nutritional status also is often poor.[21]

Whereas the early stages of alcoholic liver injury (fatty liver and alcoholic hepatitis) are reversible, cirrhosis usually is not; thus, liver failure develops. The overt signs of liver failure associated with cirrhosis are jaundice, ascites, and loss of liver functions. Once a person has cirrhosis, there is a 50% chance of death within 4 years. Approximately 28,000 people die from cirrhosis each year in the United States—most of these deaths are of people between the ages of 40 and 65 years. A liver transplant is necessary for long-term survival, and successful liver transplantation requires that patients abstain from consuming any alcohol.

Cirrhosis develops in about 10 to 15% of cases of alcoholism and affects about 2 million people in the U.S. Although cirrhosis can be caused by any substance that poisons liver cells, in North America most cases of cirrhosis are caused by excess alcohol consumption. Cirrhosis is commonly associated with a 10-year or longer consumption of approximately 80 g of alcohol (the equivalent of 7 beers) per day. Some evidence suggests that damage is caused by chronic intakes as low as 40 g/day for men (about 3 beers) and 20 g/day for women. In addition to the amount and duration of alcohol consumption, genetic factors and individual factors, such as obesity, diabetes, exposure to hepatotoxins (e.g., acetaminophen

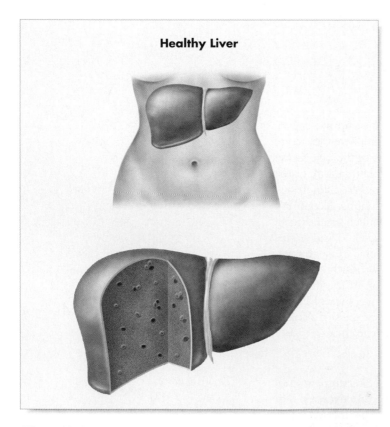

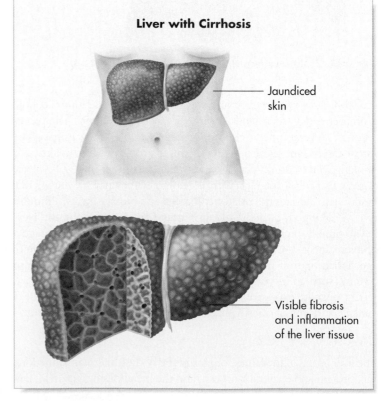

Figure 8-3 Notice the difference in the healthy liver on the left and the liver with cirrhosis on the right.

[Tylenol®]), iron overload disorders, and infections with hepatitis, determine one's risk of the disease. (About 4 million people in the U.S. are infected with the virus that causes hepatitis C.)

A number of possible mechanisms are thought to cause the liver damage that results from alcohol abuse. In chronic alcoholism, the increased concentration of acetaldehyde (a compound formed during alcohol metabolism) in the liver is thought to damage this organ. The accumulation of fat in liver cells causes inflammation and cell damage. Scientists also believe that the production of free radicals from alcohol metabolism contributes to liver damage. The highly reactive free radical molecules destroy cell membranes and DNA and lead to chronic inflammation.[3]

A nutritious diet can help prevent some of the complications associated with alcoholism and alcoholic liver disease. However, alcoholism usually brings about the serious destruction of vital tissues regardless of the quality of the food consumed. Laboratory animal studies clearly show that, even when a nutritious diet is consumed, alcohol abuse leads to cirrhosis. Still, nutrient deficiencies compound the problem of cirrhosis by making the liver more vulnerable to toxic substances produced by alcohol metabolism and by increasing complications caused by malnutrition.[3]

Effects of Alcohol Abuse on Nutritional Status

Many alcohol abusers have poor nutritional status and are at risk of developing many nutrient deficiencies because they tend to replace some or all of the food in their diets with alcohol, a poor source of nutrients.[22] For instance, if a person were to use beer as a nutrient source, he or she would need to consume daily 40 to 55 bottles (12 oz each) to meet protein needs and 65 bottles for thiamin needs.

When an individual relies on alcohol for the majority of his or her energy needs, protein-energy malnutrition can result. The symptoms of protein-energy malnutrition are similar to those seen in individuals with kwashiorkor (see Chapter 7). In addition to potential protein deficiencies, deficiencies of vitamins and minerals also are likely. These deficiencies, which are usually the result of decreased intake, impaired absorption, altered metabolism, and alcohol-related tissue damage, have profound effects on the body.

It is important for medical personnel to be aware of the severe consequences of alcohol abuse on nutritional health. Early intervention, guided by a dietitian and physician, is an essential part of the treatment for alcoholism to correct nutrient deficiencies, minimize tissue damage, and restore overall health.

Water-Soluble Vitamins

Excessive alcohol intake can lead to deficiencies of the water-soluble vitamins thiamin, niacin, vitamin B-6, vitamin B-12, and folate (see Chapter 13). For example, chronic alcohol abuse often leads to a severe form of thiamin deficiency called Wernicke-Korsakoff Syndrome. This causes significant changes in brain and nervous system function, which, if untreated, result in irreversible paralysis of the eye muscles, loss of sensation in lower extremities, loss of balance with abnormal gait, and memory loss.[3]

Alcoholics are at increased risk of developing niacin deficiency because alcohol metabolism requires large quantities of this vitamin. The metabolism of alcohol can increase the excretion of vitamin B-6 in the urine, which, if not offset with increased dietary intake, increases the risk of developing anemia and peripheral neuropathy (weakness or numbness in the arms and legs). Excessive alcohol intake also can impair the absorption of vitamin B-12, which also increases the risk of anemia and neuropathy.

Fat-Soluble Vitamins

Excessive alcohol intake can result in deficiencies of the fat-soluble vitamins A, D, E, and K (see Chapter 12). Chronic alcohol abuse damages the liver and pancreas, which impairs the liver's ability to secrete bile and the pancreas's ability to secrete fat-digesting enzymes. Recall that bile and pancreatic lipases are needed to digest fat—decreased bile and pancreatic lipase secretions lead to poor absorption of fat and fat-soluble vitamins.

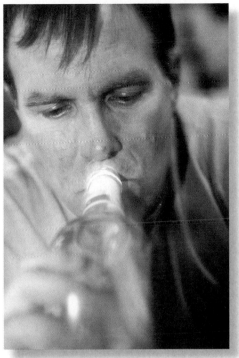

Alcohol abusers are at increased risk for protein, vitamin, and mineral deficiencies.

The risk of vitamin A deficiency is compounded by the liver's increased rate of breakdown and excretion of this vitamin, as well as the liver's inability to produce the protein needed to deliver vitamin A to all parts of the body. Alcohol also can decrease the amount of beta-carotene (a precursor of vitamin A) that the liver converts to vitamin A. Because of these changes in liver function, vitamin A stores in individuals with alcoholism are diminished, regardless of whether dietary vitamin A intake is low, adequate, or high. This alcohol-induced vitamin A deficiency often causes alcoholics to have trouble seeing in the dark (called night blindness).

Individuals with alcoholic liver disease are less able to synthesize vitamin K–containing compounds that are needed to help blood clot, in turn increasing the risk of bleeding. Additionally, damage to the liver can lead to a vitamin D deficiency because the liver plays a key role in converting vitamin D to its biologically active form. Vitamin D is required for calcium absorption and bone health; thus, a deficiency can cause bone loss and increase the risk of osteoporosis.

Minerals

Individuals who abuse alcohol and eat a poor diet are at increased risk of mineral deficiencies as well. Deficiencies of calcium, magnesium, zinc, and iron are most common (see Chapters 14 and 15). Poor absorption of calcium contributes to a deficiency of this mineral. Increased urinary excretion of magnesium contributes to low blood concentrations of magnesium and deficiency symptoms. One of the classic symptoms of magnesium deficiency is tetany, a condition characterized by muscle twitches, cramps, spasms, and seizures. Decreased absorption and increased urinary excretion both contribute to zinc deficiency, which leads to changes in taste and smell, loss of appetite, and impaired wound healing.

Iron deficiency is possible in alcoholics. Excessive alcohol consumption can damage gastrointestinal tissues, causing bleeding, malabsorption, and the eventual development of iron deficiency.

Alcohol Consumption during Pregnancy and Breastfeeding

More than half of all women in the United States of childbearing age drink alcohol. Alcohol slows nutrient and oxygen delivery to the developing offspring, thereby retarding growth and development. Alcohol also may displace nutrient-dense foods in the mother's diet. Although the most severe damage occurs during the first 12 to 16 weeks or so of pregnancy, when organs are undergoing major developmental steps, consuming alcohol at any time during pregnancy can cause lifelong damage.

Of every 1000 babies born in the United States each year, as many as 30 have alcohol-related health consequences. About one-tenth of these babies suffer the greatest damage and are classified as having an irreversible condition called **fetal alcohol syndrome.**[23] The main features of fetal alcohol syndrome are characteristic facial malformations (Fig. 8-4), growth retardation, and central nervous system defects, including profound mental retardation and a small brain size. These children are among the smallest in height, weight, and head circumference for their age.

Prenatal exposure to alcohol also may cause somewhat lesser effects known as **fetal alcohol effects.** These children may experience behavioral, learning, or nervous system abnormalities caused by alcohol exposure. They may have lifelong learning difficulties, short attention spans, and hyperactivity. Some also have physical birth defects similar to those associated with fetal alcohol syndrome.

It is not clear how alcohol causes physical malformations and disabilities. It may be the result of alcohol itself or

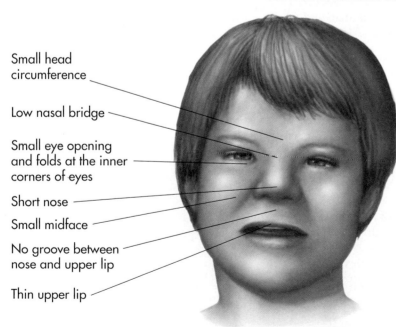

Small head circumference

Low nasal bridge

Small eye opening and folds at the inner corners of eyes

Short nose

Small midface

No groove between nose and upper lip

Thin upper lip

Figure 8-4 **The facial features shown are typical of children with fetal alcohol syndrome. Additional abnormalities in the brain and other internal organs accompany fetal alcohol syndrome but are not immediately apparent from simply looking at the child. Milder forms of alcohol-induced changes from a lower alcohol exposure to the fetus are known as fetal alcohol effects.**

compounds produced during alcohol metabolism. Within minutes after consumption, the alcohol travels through the mother's blood to the developing offspring. The effects of alcohol are intensified by the offspring's small size and are prolonged because the fetus is unable to metabolize the alcohol and must wait for maternal blood to carry it away.

No one is sure how much alcohol it takes to cause developmental problems. However, consuming as little as 1 ounce per day has resulted in mental and physical defects. The more alcohol consumed during pregnancy, the worse the effects are likely to be. Until a safe level of alcohol consumption during pregnancy is known, experts recommend that pregnant women drink no alcohol. Because of the potentially deleterious effect during the early part of pregnancy, experts recommend that women planning a pregnancy avoid alcohol, in case they do become pregnant, and that women who drink alcohol avoid becoming pregnant. For more information about fetal alcohol syndrome, visit the website www.cdc.gov/ncbddd/fas/default.htm.

For centuries, health-care providers advised new mothers to drink wine or beer before breastfeeding to relax and allow babies to suckle longer. However, alcohol actually reduces the mother's ability to produce milk and causes babies to drink less and have disrupted sleep patterns. Infants are not as efficient at breaking down alcohol as adults, so the effects linger longer. The safest route for mothers and babies is to avoid alcohol altogether.[24] However, breastfeeding women who want to drink alcohol are advised to limit their intake and wait 3 to 4 hours before breastfeeding again. The amount of alcohol in breast milk peaks about 30 to 60 minutes after the mother ingests it, then declines.[25]

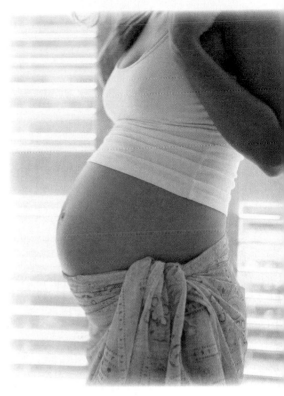

Consuming alcohol during pregnancy poses grave danger for the developing offspring.

Knowledge Check

1. What are the guidelines for using alcohol safely?
2. What are some possible benefits of moderate alcohol intake by middle-aged and older adults?
3. What levels of alcohol intake are associated with the development of cirrhosis?
4. How does alcohol abuse impair nutritional status?
5. What are the dangers of consuming alcohol during pregnancy?

 8.5 Alcohol Use Disorders: Alcohol Abuse and Alcoholism

Alcohol abuse and alcoholism (also known as alcohol dependency) pose serious risks for many individuals. **Alcohol abuse** is characterized by a pattern of drinking accompanied by at least 1 of these problems:

- Failing to fulfill major responsibilities at work, school, or home because of drinking
- Drinking when it is physically dangerous, such as while driving a car
- Having recurring alcohol-related legal problems, such as physically hurting someone while drunk
- Having social or relationship problems that are worsened by alcohol intake[26]

Alcohol dependency, or alcoholism, is a chronic disease that includes the following symptoms:

- Craving—a strong need to drink
- Loss of control—not being able to stop drinking once started
- Withdrawal symptoms—such as nausea, sweating, anxiety, or shakiness after stopping drinking
- Tolerance—the need to drink larger amounts of alcohol in order to feel its effects
- Unsuccessful attempts to cut down on use[26]

Nearly 1 in 3 Americans abuses or becomes dependent on alcohol over a lifetime.[27] At any given time, about 8.5% (or 1 in 12 persons) of people in the United States meet the criteria for either alcohol abuse or alcohol dependence.[9] About 30% of people in the United States can be considered at high risk of alcohol-related problems because of excessive intakes.[28] The factors linked to developing alcohol-related problems include genetics, gender, age of drinking onset, and ethnicity. Parental and peer attitudes favoring excessive drinking and the presence of mental health disorders, such as depression and anxiety disorder, are other significant risk factors.[9]

Genetic Influences

Genetic factors account for approximately 40 to 50% of a person's risk of alcoholism. Twins and first-degree relatives (parents, siblings, and offspring) share a tendency toward alcohol addiction. Children of alcoholics have a 4 times greater risk of developing alcoholism, even when adopted by a family with no history of alcoholism.

Scientists are actively studying the genetic basis for alcohol dependency. The genes regulating alcohol metabolism enzymes—alcohol dehydrogenase and aldehyde dehydrogenase—have been of particular interest to researchers.[29, 30] These genes have several possible variants (polymorphisms) that can occur. Scientists are trying to understand how polymorphisms alter alcohol metabolism and increase the risk of developing alcohol dependency or alcoholic liver disease. For example, as discussed earlier, the inability to completely metabolize alcohol quickly may cause a person to feel ill, causing him or her to be unlikely to drink large amounts of alcohol.[4] Other genes, such as those that make antioxidant enzymes, neurotransmitters and their receptors, and immune factors, are also under study.

Individuals with a family history of alcoholism need to be especially alert for evidence of the early signs of alcohol dependence. However, it is important to recognize that genetic risk is not destiny—not all children of alcoholic parents go on to develop alcohol use problems. Some alcoholics have no family history of alcohol problems at all, so genetic factors do not fully explain why some individuals develop alcohol-related problems but others do not.

Effect of Gender

Gender plays a key role in alcohol dependency and metabolism. The male:female ratio of alcohol dependency is 4:1. However, women are more susceptible to the adverse effects of alcohol—liver disease, heart muscle damage, cancer, and brain injury. As previously noted, the recommended limit for alcohol use is lower for women than for men because an equivalent amount of alcohol is more concentrated in women because they are smaller, have more fat, and have less muscle tissue and body water. Additionally, women cannot metabolize alcohol as quickly as men, due to lower activity of the alcohol dehydrogenase in the stomach, so blood alcohol concentrations remain elevated for longer periods.

Age of Onset of Drinking

Not only does alcohol consumption in underage youths contribute to approximately 4500 deaths in the United States each year (mainly from homicides, motor vehicle accidents, and suicides),[31] but drinking at a young age also is an important risk factor for later alcohol dependence. Researchers have found that drinking before age 14 is especially problematic. In fact, 45% of these adolescents go on to develop alcohol dependence, compared with 10% of those who wait until age 21 years or later to begin drinking.[11] This is particularly worrisome, considering that about 40% of high school students report that they currently consume alcohol.[10, 11]

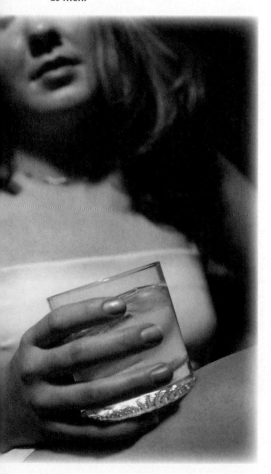

Women cannot metabolize alcohol as efficiently as men.

Ethnicity and Alcohol Abuse

Patterns of alcohol use vary among ethnic groups. In North America, Native American Indians, Alaska Natives, and Native Hawaiians have the highest alcohol use, whereas Asian Americans have the lowest use. The major causes of death among Native Americans are motor vehicle accidents and unintentional injuries related to alcohol use. Native American populations also have a higher rate of alcohol-related suicide, homicide, domestic abuse, and fetal alcohol syndrome than other ethnic groups. Differences in alcohol use may result from social factors such as the availability of alcohol in communities and biological factors that affect vulnerability to alcohol. As discussed previously, many Asian Americans experience uncomfortable effects after drinking alcohol, which likely accounts for low alcohol use in this population.

Drinking alcohol at a young age increases the risk for alcohol addiction.

Mental Health and Alcohol Abuse

Mental health disorders, such as depression and generalized anxiety disorder, often go hand in hand with alcohol use disorders.[32] Alcohol dependence and abuse may aggravate or even cause mental health disorders. Conversely, individuals with depression or other disorders may use alcohol to self-medicate their conditions. It's important that both mental health disorders and alcohol abuse be identified and treated.

The majority of suicides and interfamily homicides are alcohol-related. Alcohol consumption appears to increase the risk of youth suicide—the younger the drinker, the more likely he or she is to commit suicide.

Each year in the United States, the cost of alcohol abuse is about $185 billion in lost productivity, premature deaths, direct treatment expenses, and legal fees. A liver transplant costs about $300,000 and is needed in cases of excessive alcohol use. On the positive side, a typical counseling program to treat a person who is abusing alcohol costs only about $5000.

Knowledge Check

1. What are 3 factors that predispose a person to alcohol dependency?
2. Why is the age at which a person started drinking alcohol of concern?
3. Why might women suffer more ill effects from alcohol consumption than men?
4. Which ethnic groups are at increased risk of alcohol-related problems?

CASE STUDY FOLLOW-UP

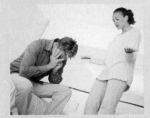

As a close friend, Alyssa has a responsibility to hold Todd accountable for his actions. Sometimes, it is difficult to realize that one has a drinking problem, although it may be obvious to others. Alyssa should talk privately to Todd about the most recent incident when he is sober and calm. It is important to deal with situations such as these very carefully because the problem drinker will probably respond defensively. She can explain how his drinking is causing problems for both of them, she can tell him about the harmful consequences of his drinking, and she can refuse to go with him to any alcohol-related events, but she must be prepared to carry out her refusal. This is especially important for her because she does not want to risk further physical harm from Todd. Alyssa should talk with a counselor, who may help her learn ways to approach Todd effectively. Offering to go with Todd to a treatment program or an AA meeting and get help is one idea. There is strength in numbers, so other members of Todd's family or close friends also should be enlisted to help, under the guidance of a therapist trained in treating alcoholism.

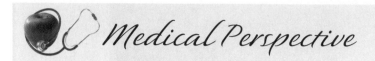

Medical Perspective

Diagnosis and Treatment of Alcoholism

Alcoholism is often considered a 2-phase problem. Initially, it begins as problem drinking. This includes the repetitive use of alcohol, often to alleviate anxiety or solve other emotional problems. Alcohol addiction, the second phase of alcoholism, then follows. In addition to the symptoms listed at the beginning of Section 8.5, other signs of alcoholism include frequent alcohol odor on the breath, flushed face, and nervous system disorders, such as tremors. Unexplained work absences, frequent accidents, and falls or injuries of vague origin may be other signs. Laboratory tests also are helpful. These tests include measures of impaired liver function and high triglyceride and uric acid concentrations in the blood.

Determining Whether a Problem with Alcohol Intake Exists

Asking a person about the quantity and frequency of his or her alcohol consumption is an important means of detecting abuse and dependence. The CAGE questionnaire is commonly used in routine health care:[33]

C: Have you ever felt you ought to *cut* down on drinking?
A: Have people *annoyed* you by criticizing your drinking?
G: Have you ever felt bad or *guilty* about your drinking?
E: Have you ever had a drink first thing in the morning (an *eye-opener*) to steady your nerves or get rid of a hangover?

More than a single positive response in the CAGE questionnaire suggests an alcohol problem. Other questions to ask along with the CAGE questionnaire are the following:

1. Does it take more to make you inebriated than it did in the past? That is, do you have an increased tolerance for alcohol?
2. Have you had memory lapses or blackouts due to drinking?
3. Do you continue to drink, even though you have health problems caused by alcohol?
4. Do you get withdrawal symptoms, such as headaches, chills, shakes, and a strong craving for alcohol and, as a result, drink more to get rid of these symptoms?
5. Do you take part in high-risk behaviors, such as having unsafe sex or driving a car or boat when under the influence of alcohol?
6. Has drinking caused trouble at school, at home, at work, or in relationships with others?
7. Do you have to drink alcohol for any of the following reasons?
   a. To get through the day or unwind at the end of the day
   b. To cope with stressful life events
   c. To escape from ongoing problems

An affirmative answer to any of these questions indicates an individual should seek help from a physician or a certified counselor. Unfortunately, about 75% of people with alcohol problems do not seek treatment.[9]

Recovery from Alcoholism

The treatment of alcoholism or alcohol abuse typically involves behavioral therapy, along with medication.[34] Behavioral therapy is usually facilitated by a psychologist, social worker, or counselor. An important goal of counseling is to identify ways to compensate for the loss of pleasure from drinking. This helps the drinker confront the immediate problem of how to stop drinking. Total abstinence must be the ultimate objective because, for most alcoholics, there is no such thing as controlled drinking. Most problem drinkers cannot return safely to social drinking.[6] Because other mental health disorders, such as depression, bipolar disorder,

▶ Swiss chemist Paracelsus (1493–1541) made the observation that "the dose determines the poison." This is true for alcohol because, the greater the dose of alcohol, the greater the risk of alcohol poisoning and death.

▶ Uric acid is the end product of the metabolism of the purines (double-ringed nitrogen containing bases), adenine, and guanine from DNA and RNA. When uric acid production exceeds the kidneys' ability to excrete it, uric acid crystals form in joints and the very painful condition known as gout results. Gout is well known as a disease of affluence—its risk factors include overweight, excessive alcohol intake, and high purine intake (gravies, organ meats, fish eggs, anchovies, sardines, and many meats are high in purines), along with genetics, male sex, and older age.

▶ Another common screening tool for alcohol abuse is the Michigan Alcohol Screening Test (MAST). Screening tools are available at the following website: www. niaaa.nih.gov/publications/niaaa_guide.

CRITICAL THINKING

José is a well-liked 17-year old. It always seems as if everything is going his way—an A on a test, a scholarship to college, you name it. Lately, however, José has experienced some disappointments. His grandfather has just passed away and he and his girlfriend have broken up. When he arrived home late with the smell of alcohol on his breath, his parents started to worry. What signs and symptoms should they be aware of that indicate a problem with alcohol?

and mood and anxiety disorders, often go hand in hand with alcoholism or alcohol abuse, these conditions must be treated as well for successful outcomes.

Three medications are approved in the U.S. to treat alcoholism:[35]

- Naltrexone (ReVia®) blocks the craving for alcohol and the pleasure of intoxication (Fig. 8-5).
- Acamprosate (Campral®) is thought to act on neurotransmitter pathways in the brain to decrease the desire to drink.
- Disulfiram (Antabuse®) causes physical reactions, such as vomiting, when drinking alcohol. It does so by blocking the complete breakdown of alcohol in the liver in a way similar to that experienced naturally by some individuals of Asian decent (as described earlier in the chapter).

Self-help programs also facilitate the recovery from alcohol dependency. Alcoholics Anonymous® (AA),[36] a 12-step program, is one of the most well-known programs that helps many individuals with alcoholism. At AA meetings, men and women share their experiences, strengths, challenges, and hopes with each other as they try to solve their common problems and help each another recover from alcoholism. As an informal society chartered in 1935, AA includes more than 2 million recovered alcoholics. The only requirement for membership is the desire to stop drinking. There are no rules, regulations, dues, or fees. In addition, the group is not a political or formal organization. Further information about AA is available at www.alcoholics-anonymous.org. Another organization, Al-Anon, helps family members and friends recover from the effects of living with an alcohol-dependent person; visit www.al-anon.alateen.org for more information.

Current research does not support the generally negative public opinion about the prognosis for recovery from alcoholism. In most job-related alcoholism treatment programs, where workers are socially stable and well motivated (because of the risk of job and pension loss), recovery rates reach 60% or more.[6] This remarkably high cure rate is probably accounted for by early detection. Once a person moves from problem drinking to an advanced stage of alcoholism, treatment success seldom exceeds 50%. Early identification and intervention remain the most important steps in the treatment of alcoholism.

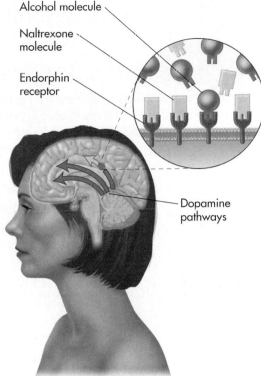

Figure 8-5 **The euphoria that arises from alcohol use involves alcohol binding to endorphin receptors in the brain. Endorphins are chemical compounds produced in the brain that act as natural painkillers and elicit feelings of well-being. It is likely that this binding, in turn, causes a release of the neurotransmitter dopamine, which is thought to cause the characteristic high associated with alcohol use. Naltrexone (ReVia®) works by blocking alcohol's ability to bind to brain receptors. This, then, reduces dopamine release and blocks the pleasant feelings elicited by alcohol use.**

▶ Alcoholics who stop drinking may substitute caffeine, nicotine, and/or sweets for alcohol. Because alcoholics usually have poor nutritional status, these substitutions often have a significant negative impact on their overall nutritional status. However, these substitutions are not as harmful as alcohol abuse.

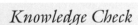

Knowledge Check

1. Why is tolerance to alcohol considered a risk factor for alcohol dependence?
2. How might the CAGE questionnaire be used to identify those with alcohol problems?
3. How do medications currently approved to treat alcoholism limit alcohol intake?
4. In addition to medications, what programs are available to help individuals with alcohol use problems?

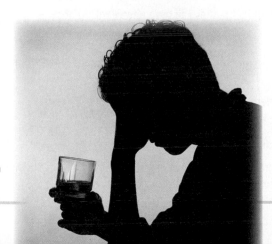

Alcohol abuse and dependency often begin during young adulthood.

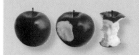

Take Action

Might You or Someone You Know Have a Problem with Alcoholism?

Problem drinking often has its seeds in the teen years. Significant health consequences of this practice typically occur in adulthood. Alcohol abuse is a prominent contributor to 5 of the 10 leading causes of death in North America. The social consequences of alcohol dependency include divorce, unemployment, and poverty. The following questionnaire was developed by the National Council on Alcoholism. With this assessment, you can determine whether you or someone you know might need help.

Yes	No	1.	Do you occasionally drink heavily after disappointment, after a quarrel, or when someone gives you a hard time?
Yes	No	2.	When you have trouble or feel under pressure, do you drink more heavily than usual?
Yes	No	3.	Have you ever noticed that you're able to handle liquor better than you did when you first started drinking?
Yes	No	4.	Do you ever wake up the morning after you've been drinking and discover that you can't remember part of the evening before, even though your friends tell you that you didn't pass out?
Yes	No	5.	When drinking with other people, do you try to have a few extra drinks when others won't know it?
Yes	No	6.	Are there certain occasions when you feel uncomfortable if alcohol isn't available?
Yes	No	7.	Have you recently noticed that, when you begin drinking, you're in more of a hurry to get the first drink than you used to be?
Yes	No	8.	Do you sometimes feel a little guilty about your drinking?
Yes	No	9.	Are you secretly irritated when your family or friends discuss your drinking?
Yes	No	10.	Have you recently noticed an increase in the frequency of memory blackouts?
Yes	No	11.	Do you often find that you wish to continue drinking after your friends say they've had enough?
Yes	No	12.	Do you usually have a reason for the occasions when you drink heavily?
Yes	No	13.	When you're sober, do you often regret things you have done or said while drinking?
Yes	No	14.	Have you tried switching brands or following different plans to control your drinking?
Yes	No	15.	Have you often failed to keep promises you've made to yourself about controlling or stopping your drinking?
Yes	No	16.	Have you ever tried to control your drinking by changing jobs or moving to a new location?
Yes	No	17.	Do you try to avoid family or close friends while you're drinking?
Yes	No	18.	Are you having an increasing number of financial and work problems?
Yes	No	19.	Do more people seem to be treating you unfairly without good reason?
Yes	No	20.	Do you eat very little or irregularly when you're drinking?
Yes	No	21.	Do you sometimes have the "shakes" in the morning and find that it helps to have a little drink?
Yes	No	22.	Have you recently noticed that you can drink more than you once did?
Yes	No	23.	Do you sometimes stay drunk for several days at a time?
Yes	No	24.	Do you sometimes feel very depressed and wonder whether life is worth living?
Yes	No	25.	Sometimes after periods of drinking do you see or hear things that aren't there?
Yes	No	26.	Do you get terribly frightened after you have been drinking heavily?

Interpretation

These are all symptoms that may indicate alcoholism. "Yes" answers to several of the questions indicate the following stages of alcoholism.

> Questions 1 to 8: Potential drinking problem
>
> Questions 9 to 21: Drinking problem likely
>
> Questions 22 to 26: Definite drinking problem

It is vital to assess yourself honestly. If you or someone you know demonstrates some of these symptoms, it is important to seek help. If there is even a question in your mind, talk to a professional about it.

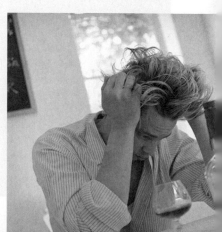

Summary

8.1 Alcohol, chemically known as ethanol, is found in beer, wine, distilled spirits (or hard liquor, such as vodka and rum), liqueurs, cordials, and hard cider. These beverages range from 5% alcohol to more than 40% alcohol. A standard drink is defined as 15 g of alcohol, and that equates to 12 oz of beer, 5 oz of wine, and 1.5 oz of distilled spirits. Ethanol is produced by the chemical process known as fermentation. Grains, cereals, fruits, honey, milk, potatoes, and other carbohydrate-rich foods are used to make alcoholic beverages.

8.2 Alcohol is readily absorbed in the GI tract because it does not require digestion. The rate of absorption is affected by gender, ethnicity, body size and composition, and alcohol and food intake. Alcohol is primarily metabolized in the liver, although small amounts also are metabolized in the stomach. The body uses the alcohol dehydrogenase (ADH) pathway to metabolize small amounts of alcohol and the microsomal ethanol oxidizing system (MEOS) to metabolize moderate to large amounts of alcohol. Blood alcohol levels can be determined by measuring the amount of alcohol excreted through the lungs with a breathalyzer test. A blood alcohol content of 0.08% is the legal definition of intoxication and is associated with impaired judgment and coordination. Alcohol poisoning, a very dangerous condition, occurs when blood alcohol content continues to rise, causing vomiting, irregular breathing and heartbeats, low blood sugar, severe dehydration, seizures, confusion, coma, and death.

8.3 About 62% of North American adults consume alcohol; most are light or moderate drinkers, but 5% consume excessive amounts. College students are frequent drinkers and many engage in binge drinking. Binge drinking is a dangerous practice associated with a variety of accidents, crimes, health risks, and even death.

8.4 If alcohol is consumed, it should be consumed in moderation with meals. Women are advised to drink no more than 1 drink per day; men, no more than 2 drinks a day. The benefits of alcohol use are associated with low to moderate alcohol consumption. These benefits include the pleasurable and social aspects of alcohol use and possibly a reduced risk of cardiovascular disease. Excessive consumption of alcohol contributes significantly to 5 of the 10 leading causes of death in North America. Alcohol increases the risk of developing heart damage, inflammation of the pancreas, GI tract damage, certain forms of cancer, and hypertension. The liver is particularly vulnerable to the toxic effects of alcohol. Liver damage occurs as fatty liver, alcoholic hepatitis, and cirrhosis. Fatty liver can be relieved by abstention from alcohol, but cirrhosis cannot. Cirrhosis results in the impaired synthesis of vital proteins and abnormal fluid retention. Most people with cirrhosis are malnourished. Liver failure is the typical outcome of cirrhosis. Nutritional problems are common among alcoholics. Alcohol abuse can impair nutrient intake and absorption, alter nutrient metabolism, and increase nutrient excretion. Deficiencies of protein, fat- and water-soluble vitamins, and the minerals calcium, magnesium, iron, and zinc are most common.

8.5 Alcoholism and alcohol abuse affect 8.5% of the adult population in the U.S. Many personal, social, and employment problems result from excessive alcohol use. Genetic factors account for 40 to 50% of a person's risk of alcoholism. Differences in the alcohol-metabolizing genes may account for some of these genetic risks. Males have higher rates of alcoholism, but women are at higher risk of alcohol-related damage throughout the body. Drinking at a young age puts one at risk of alcohol problems later in life. Some ethnic groups, particularly Native American Indians, have higher rates of alcohol use and abuse. Mental health and alcohol use disorders often occur together. The CAGE questionnaire is one of several that can help a person determine whether he or she has an alcohol problem. The treatment of alcoholism or alcohol abuse includes behavioral and pharmacologic therapy. Three medications are approved to treat alcoholism. Alcoholics Anonymous® is another avenue for help. Recovery rates from alcoholism and alcohol abuse can be high, especially with early detection.

Study Questions

1. An 80-proof alcohol is approximately 80% alcohol.

   a. true   b. false

2. A standard drink is defined as the amount that provides approximately 15 g of alcohol. Which of the following is considered a standard-size drink?

   a. 16-ounce beer
   b. 20-ounce wine cooler
   c. 5-ounce glass of wine
   d. 4-ounce pour of hard liquor

3. Alcohol requires no digestion and can enter cells without specific transport mechanisms.

   a. true   b. false

4. Which of the following is the primary pathway used in the metabolism of small amounts of alcohol?

   a. alcohol dehydrogenase pathway
   b. microsomal ethanol oxidizing system
   c. catalase pathway
   d. none of the above

5. Which of the following affects the metabolism of alcohol?

   a. gender   c. ethnicity
   b. diet composition   d. all of the above

6. What blood alcohol concentration denotes legal intoxication in the U.S. and Canada?

   a. 1.0%   c. 0.05%
   b. 0.08%   d. 0.10%

7. Compared with individuals who begin drinking alcohol at a legal age, those who begin drinking as teenagers have higher rates of alcohol dependency and alcohol abuse in adulthood.

   a. true   b. false

8. Which of the following would be considered moderate drinking?

   a. 1 drink per day for women and 2 drinks per day for men
   b. 2 drinks per day for both men and women
   c. 2 drinks per day for women and 3 drinks per day for men
   d. 4 drinks on any single occasion for men and women

9. In moderation, alcohol may help raise HDL cholesterol.

   a. true   b. false

10. Risk of cancer of the _____ increases greatly with high alcohol consumption.

    a. esophagus   c. bone
    b. lung   d. all of the above

11. The first stage of alcoholic liver disease is _____.

    a. cirrhosis   c. steatosis
    b. alcoholic hepatitis   d. inflammation of the liver

12. The symptoms of cirrhosis include _____.

    a. abnormal fluid retention   c. poor nutritional status
    b. jaundice of the liver   d. all of the above

13. Alcohol intake should be avoided during pregnancy.

    a. true   b. false

14. Which of the following is *not* a common nutritional concern in alcoholics?

    a. vitamin B-12 deficiency   c. vitamin A toxicity
    b. protein-energy malnutrition   d. iron deficiency

15. Medications used to treat alcohol dependence act on _____.

    a. the brain to reduce alcohol cravings
    b. the liver to block complete metabolism of alcohol
    c. the stomach to prevent alcohol absorption
    d. both a and b

Answer Key: 1-b; 2-c; 3-a; 4-a; 5-d; 6-b; 7-a; 8-a; 9-a; 10-a; 11-c; 12-d; 13-a; 14-c; 15-d

Websites

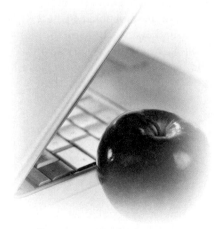

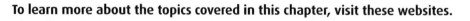

To learn more about the topics covered in this chapter, visit these websites.

www.niaaa.nih.gov

www.asam.org

www.mentalhelp.net/selfhelp

www.nlm.nih.gov/medlineplus

alcoholconsumption.html

www.findtreatment.samhsa.gov

www.nacoa.org

www.alcoholics-anonymous.org

www.al-anon.alateen.org

www.cdc.gov/ncbddd/fas/default.htm

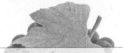

References

1. National Institute on Alcohol Abuse and Alcoholism. Database resources/statistical tables. 2007; www.niaaa.nih.gov.

2. Clairmont M. Alcohol dependence and abuse. *Today's Dietitian*. 2005;7:44.

3. Lieber C. Nutrition in liver disorders and the role of alcohol. In: Shils ME and others, eds. *Modern nutrition in health and disease*. Philadelphia: Lippincott Williams & Wilkins; 2006.

4. Crabb D and others. Overview of the role of alcohol dehydrogenase and aldehyde dehydrogenase and their variants in the genesis of alcohol-related pathology. *Proceedings of the Nutrition Society*. 2004;63:49.

5. Parlesak A and others. Gastric alcohol dehydrogenase in man: Influence of gender, age, alcohol consumption and smoking in a Caucasian population. *Alcohol Alcohol*. 2002;37:338.

6. Schuckit M. Alcohol and alcoholism. In: Kasper D and others, eds. *Harrison's principles of internal medicine*. New York: McGraw-Hill; 2004.

7. Brewer R, Swahn M. Binge drinking and violence. *JAMA*. 2005;294:6165.

8. National Highway Traffic Safety Administration. Fatality analysis reporting system. 2004; www.nhtsa.gov.

9. National Institute on Alcohol Abuse and Alcoholism. Alcohol alert 70. National Epidemiologic Survey on Alcohol and Related Conditions. 2006; pubs.niaaa.nih.gov/publications/AA70/AA70.htm.

10. Moritsugu K. Underage drinking: A call to action. *J Am Diet Assoc*. 2007;107:1464.

11. Hingson RW and others. Age at drinking onset and alcohol dependence: Age at onset, duration, and severity. *Arch Pediatr Adolesc Med*. 2006;160:739.

12. Klasky A. Drink to your health? *Sci Am*. 2003; September:75.

13. Mukamal K and others. Alcohol and risk of ischemic stroke in men: The role of drinking pattern and usual beverages. *Ann Int Med*. 2005;142:11.

14. Renaud S and others. Moderate wine drinkers have lower hypertension-related mortality: A prospective cohort study in French men. *Am J Clin Nutr*. 2004;80:621.

15. Tolstrup J and others. Prospective study of alcohol drinking patterns and coronary heart disease in women and men. *BMJ*. 2006; 332:1224.

16. Wannamethee S and others. Alcohol drinking patterns and risk of type 2 diabetes mellitus among younger women. *Arch Int Med*. 2003;163:1329.

17. Mehlig, K and others. Alcoholic beverages and the incidence of dementia: 34-year follow-up of the prospective population study of women in Goteborg. *Am J Epidemiol*. 2008; 167:684.

18. National Heart Lung and Blood Institute. The seventh report of the Joint National Committee on Prevention, Detection, Evaluation and Treatment of High Blood Pressure. Accessed June 28, 2007; www.nhlbi.nih.gov/guidelines/hypertension/jnc7full.htm.

19. Warnakulasuriya S and others. Demonstration of ethanol-induced protein adducts in oral leukoplakia (pre-cancer) and cancer. *J Oral Pathol Med*. 2008;37:157.

20. World Cancer Research Fund/American Institute for Cancer Research. Food, nutrition, physical activity and the prevention of cancer: a global perspective. Washington, DC: AICR, 2007.

21. Everitt H and others. Nutrition and alcoholic liver disease. *Br Nutr Foundation*. 2007;32:138.

22. Leevy M, Moroianu S. Nutritional aspects of liver disease. *Clin Liver Dis*. 2005;9:67.

23. Eustace L and others. Fetal alcohol syndrome: A growing concern for health care professionals. *J Ob Gyn Neonat Nurs*. 2003;32:215.

24. American Academy of Pediatrics. Breastfeeding and the use of human milk. *Pediatrics*. 2005;115:496.

25. Mennella J, Gerrish C. Effects of exposure to alcohol in mother's milk on infant sleep. *Pediatrics*. 1998;101:e2.

26. Midanik LT and others. Alcohol-attributable deaths and years of potential life lost. *MMWR*. 2004;53:866.

27. Hasin DS and others. Prevalence, correlates, disability, and comorbidity of DSM-IV alcohol abuse and dependence in the United States: Results from the National Epidemiologic Survey on Alcohol and Related Conditions. *Arch Gen Psychiatry*. 2007;64:830.

28. U.S. Department of Health and Human Services. *Healthy People 2010. With understanding and improving health and objectives for improving health*. 2000; www.healthypeople.gov.

29. Edenberg HJ and others. Association of alcohol dehydrogenase genes with alcohol dependence: A comprehensive analysis. *Hum Mol Genet*. 2006;15:1539.

30. National Institute on Alcohol Abuse and Alcoholism. Alcohol alert 60. The genetics of alcoholism. 2003; pubs.niaaa.nih.gov/publications/aa60.htm.

31. Centers for Disease Control and Prevention. Alcohol-related disease impact. 2004; apps.nccd.cdc.gov/ardi/homepage.aspx.

32. Grant B and others. Prevalence and co-occurrence of substance use disorders and independent mood and anxiety disorders. Results from the National Epidemiologic Survey on Alcohol and Related Conditions. *Arch Gen Psychiatry*. 2004;61:807.

33. U.S. Preventive Services Task Force. Screening and behavioral counseling interventions in primary care to reduce alcohol misuse: Recommendation statement. *Am Fam Physician*. 2004;70:353.

34. Anton RF and others. Combined pharmacotherapies and behavioral interventions for alcohol dependence: The COMBINE Study: A randomized controlled trial. *JAMA*. 2006;295:2003.

35. Laaksonen E and others. A randomized, multicentre, open-label, comparative trial of disulfiram, naltrexone and acamprosate in the treatment of alcohol dependence. *Alcohol Alcohol*. 2008;43:53.

36. Gossop M and others. Attendance at Narcotics Anonymous and Alcoholics Anonymous meetings, frequency of attendance and substance use outcomes after residential treatment for drug dependence: A 5-year follow-up study. *Addiction*. 2008;103:119.

9

Energy Metabolism

Life depends on energy from the sun. During photosynthesis, plants transform solar energy into chemical energy in the form of carbohydrates. During energy metabolism, we transform this chemical energy into ATP. Learn more at health.nih.gov.

STUDENT LEARNING OUTCOMES

After studying this chapter, you will be able to

1. Explain the differences among metabolism, catabolism, and anabolism.

2. Describe aerobic and anaerobic metabolism of glucose.

3. Illustrate how energy is extracted from glucose, fatty acids, amino acids, and alcohol using metabolic pathways, such as glycolysis, beta-oxidation, the citric acid cycle, and the electron transport system.

4. Describe the role that acetyl-CoA plays in cell metabolism.

5. Identify the conditions that lead to ketogenesis and its importance in survival during fasting.

6. Describe the process of gluconeogenesis.

7. Discuss how the body metabolizes alcohol.

8. Compare the fate of energy from macronutrients during the fed and fasted states.

9. Describe common inborn errors of metabolism.

The macronutrients and alcohol are rich sources of energy; however, the energy they provide is neither in the form that cells can use nor in the amount needed to carry out the thousands of chemical reactions that occur every day in the human body. Thus, the body must have a process for breaking down energy-yielding compounds to release and convert their chemical energy to a form the body can use.[1] That process is energy metabolism—an elaborate, multistep series of energy-transforming chemical reactions. Energy metabolism occurs in all cells every moment of every day for your entire lifetime; it is slowest when we are resting and fastest when we are physically active.

Understanding energy metabolism clarifies how carbohydrates, proteins, fats, and alcohol are interrelated and how they serve as fuel for body cells. In this chapter, you will see how the macronutrients and alcohol are metabolized and discover why proteins can be converted to glucose but most fatty acids cannot. Studying energy metabolism pathways in the cell also sets the stage for examining the roles of vitamins and minerals. As you'll see in this and subsequent chapters, many micronutrients contribute to the enzyme activity that supports metabolic reactions in the cell.[2] Thus, both macronutrients and micronutrients are required for basic metabolic processes.

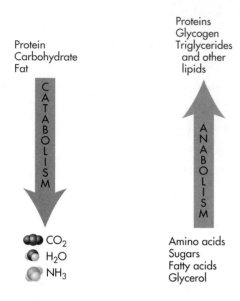

Protein
Carbohydrate
Fat

C A T A B O L I S M

CO_2
H_2O
NH_3

Proteins
Glycogen
Triglycerides
and other
lipids

A N A B O L I S M

Amino acids
Sugars
Fatty acids
Glycerol

Figure 9-1 Anabolism relies on catabolism to provide the energy (ATP) required to build compounds.

9.1 Metabolism: Chemical Reactions in the Body

Metabolism refers to the entire network of chemical processes involved in maintaining life. It encompasses all the sequences of chemical reactions that occur in the body. Some of these biochemical reactions enable us to release and use energy from carbohydrate, fat, protein, and alcohol. They also permit us to synthesize 1 substance from another and prepare waste products for excretion.[1] A group of biochemical reactions that occur in a progression from beginning to end is called a **metabolic pathway**. Compounds formed in 1 of the many steps in a metabolic pathway are called **intermediates**.

All of the pathways that take place within the body can be categorized as either anabolic or catabolic. **Anabolic** pathways use small, simpler compounds to build larger, more complex compounds (Fig. 9-1). The human body uses compounds, such as glucose, fatty acids, cholesterol, and amino acids, as building blocks to synthesize new compounds, such as glycogen, hormones, enzymes, and other proteins, to keep the body functioning and to support normal growth and development. For example, to make glycogen (a storage form of carbohydrate), we link many units of the simple sugar glucose. Energy must be expended for anabolic pathways to take place.

Conversely, **catabolic** pathways break down compounds into small units. The glycogen molecule discussed in the anabolism example is broken down into many glucose molecules when blood levels of glucose drop. Later, the complete catabolism of this glucose results in the release of carbon dioxide (CO_2) and water (H_2O). Energy is released during catabolism: some is trapped for cell use and the rest is lost as heat.

The body strives for a balance between anabolic and catabolic processes. However, there are times when one is more prominent than the other. For example, during growth there is a net anabolic state because more tissue is being synthesized than broken down. However, during weight loss or a wasting disease, such as cancer, more tissue is being broken down than synthesized.

Energy for the Cell

Cells use energy for the following purposes: building compounds, contracting muscles, conducting nerve impulses, and pumping ions (e.g., across cell membranes).[1] This energy comes from catabolic reactions that break the chemical bonds between the atoms in carbohydrate, fat, protein, and alcohol. This energy is originally produced during photosynthesis, when plants use solar energy to make glucose and other organic (carbon-containing) compounds (see Chapter 5). The chemical reactions in photosynthesis form compounds that contain more energy than the building blocks used—carbon dioxide and water. Virtually all organisms use the sun—either indirectly, as we do, or directly—as their source of energy.[1]

As shown in Figure 9-2, the series of catabolic reactions that produce energy for body cells begins with digestion and continues when monosaccharides, amino acids, fatty acids, glycerol, and alcohol are sent through a series of metabolic pathways, which finally trap a portion of the energy they contain into a compound called **adenosine triphosphate (ATP)**—the main form of energy the body uses. Heat, carbon dioxide, and water also result from these catabolic pathways. The heat produced helps maintain body temperature. Plants can use the carbon dioxide and water to produce glucose and oxygen via photosynthesis.

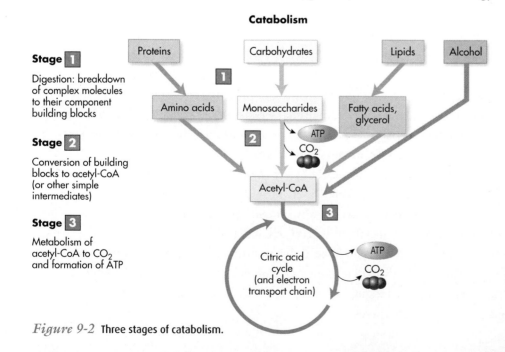

Catabolism

Stage 1

Digestion: breakdown of complex molecules to their component building blocks

Stage 2

Conversion of building blocks to acetyl-CoA (or other simple intermediates)

Stage 3

Metabolism of acetyl-CoA to CO_2 and formation of ATP

Proteins → Amino acids

Carbohydrates → Monosaccharides → ATP → CO_2

Lipids → Fatty acids, glycerol

Alcohol

Acetyl-CoA

Citric acid cycle (and electron transport chain) → ATP → CO_2

Figure 9-2 Three stages of catabolism.

Adenosine Triphosphate (ATP)

Only the energy in ATP and related compounds can be used directly by the cell.[3] A molecule of ATP consists of the organic compound adenosine (comprised of the nucleotide adenine and the sugar ribose) bound to 3 phosphate groups (Fig. 9-3). The bonds between the phosphate groups contain energy and are called high-energy phosphate bonds. Hydrolysis of the high-energy bonds releases this energy. To release the energy in ATP, cells break a high-energy phosphate bond, which creates **adenosine diphosphate (ADP)** plus P_i, a free (inorganic) phosphate group (Fig. 9-4). Hydrolysis of ADP results in the compound **adenosine monophosphate (AMP)** in a reaction muscles are capable of performing during intense exercise when ATP is in short supply (ADP + ADP → ATP + AMP). ATP can be regenerated by adding the phosphates back to AMP and ADP.

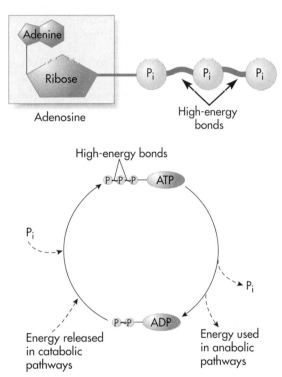

Figure 9-3 ATP is a storage form of energy for cell use because it contains high-energy bonds. P_i is the abbreviation for an inorqanic phosphate group.

Figure 9-4 ATP stores and yields energy. ATP is the high-energy state; ADP is the lower-energy state. When ATP is broken down to ADP plus P_i, energy is released for cell use. When energy is trapped by ADP plus P_i, ATP can be formed.

Every cell requires energy from ATP to synthesize new compounds (anabolic pathways), to contract muscles, to conduct nerve impulses, and to pump ions across membranes. Catabolic pathways in cells release energy, which allows ADP to combine with P_i and form ATP. Every cell has pathways to break down and resynthesize ATP. A cell is constantly breaking down ATP in one site while rebuilding it in another. This recycling of ATP is an important strategy because the body contains only about 0.22 lb (100 g) of ATP at any given time, but a sedentary adult uses about 88 lb (40 kg) of ATP each day. The requirement increases even more during exercise—during 1 hour of strenuous exercise, an additional 66 lb (30 kg) of ATP are used. In fact, the runner who currently holds the American record for the men's marathon was estimated to use 132 lb (65 kg) to run the race.[24]

Oxidation-Reduction Reactions: Key Processes in Energy Metabolism

The synthesis of ATP from ADP and P_i involves the transfer of energy from energy-yielding compounds (carbohydrate, fat, protein, and alcohol). This process uses oxidation-reduction reactions, in which electrons (along with hydrogen ions) are transferred in a series of reactions from energy-yielding compounds eventually to oxygen. These reactions form water and release much energy, which can be used to produce ATP.

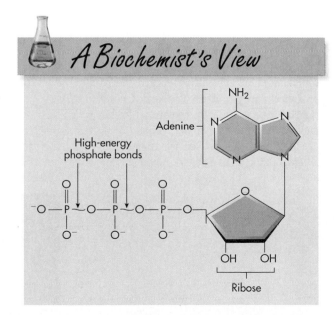

A Biochemist's View

▶ The mnemonic "**LEO** [loss of electrons is oxidation] the lion says **GER** [gain of electrons is reduction]" can help you differentiate between oxidation and reduction.

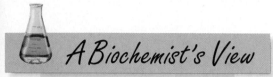

A Biochemist's View

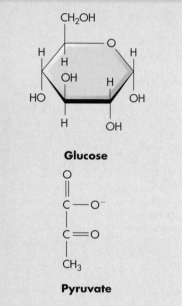

Glucose

Pyruvate

coenzyme Compound that combines with an inactive protein, called an apoenzyme, to form a catalytically active protein, called a holoenzyme. In this manner, coenzymes aid in enzyme function.

▶ The term *antioxidant* is typically used to describe a compound that can donate electrons to oxidized compounds, putting them into a more reduced (stable) state. Oxidized compounds tend to be highly reactive; they seek electrons from other compounds to stabilize their chemical configuration. Dietary antioxidants, such as vitamin E, donate electrons to these highly reactive compounds, in turn, putting these oxidized compounds into a less reactive state (see Chapter 12).

A substance is *oxidized* when it loses 1 or more electrons. For example, copper is oxidized when it loses an electron:

$$Cu^+ \rightleftharpoons Cu^{2+} + e^-$$

A substance is *reduced* when it gains 1 or more electrons. For example, iron is reduced when it gains an electron:

$$Fe^{3+} + e^- \rightleftharpoons Fe^{2+}$$

The movement of electrons governs oxidation-reduction processes. If 1 substance loses electrons (is oxidized), another substance must gain electrons (is reduced). These processes go together; one cannot occur without the other.[2] In the previous examples, the electron lost by copper can be gained by the iron, resulting in this overall reaction;:

$$Cu^+ + Fe^{3+} \rightarrow Cu^{2+} + Fe^{2+}$$

Oxidation-reduction reactions involving organic (carbon-containing) compounds are somewhat more difficult to visualize. Two simple rules help identify whether these compounds are oxidized or reduced:

If the compound gains oxygen or loses hydrogen, it has been *oxidized*.

If it loses oxygen or gains hydrogen, the compound has been *reduced*.

Enzymes control oxidation-reduction reactions in the body. Dehydrogenases, one class of these enzymes, remove hydrogens from energy-yielding compounds or their breakdown products. These hydrogens are eventually donated to oxygen to form water. In the process, large amounts of energy are converted to ATP.[1]

Two B-vitamins, niacin and riboflavin, assist dehydrogenase enzymes and, in turn, play a role in transferring the hydrogens from energy-yielding compounds to oxygen in the metabolic pathways of the cell.[2] In the following reaction, niacin functions as the **coenzyme** nicotinamide adenine dinucleotide (NAD). NAD is found in cells in both its oxidized form (NAD) and reduced form (NADH). During intense (anaerobic) exercise, the enzyme lactate dehydrogenase helps reduce pyruvate (made from glucose) to form lactate. During reduction, 2 hydrogens, derived from NADH + H⁺, are gained. Lactate is oxidized back to pyruvate by losing 2 hydrogens. NAD⁺ is the hydrogen acceptor. That is, the oxidized form of niacin (NAD⁺) can accept 1 hydrogen ion and 2 electrons to become the reduced form NADH + H⁺. (The plus [+] on NAD⁺ indicates it has 1 less electron than in its reduced form. The extra hydrogen ion [H⁺] remains free in the cell.) By accepting 2 electrons and 1 hydrogen ion, NAD⁺ becomes NADH + H⁺, with no net charge on the coenzyme.

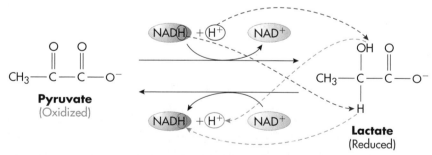

Pyruvate
(Oxidized)

Lactate
(Reduced)

Riboflavin plays a similar role. In its oxidized form, the coenzyme form is known as flavin adenine dinucleotide (FAD). When it is reduced (gains 2 hydrogens, equivalent to 2 hydrogen ions and 2 electrons), it is known as $FADH_2$.

The reduction of oxygen (O) to form water (H_2O) is the ultimate driving force for life because it is vital to the way cells synthesize ATP. Thus, oxidation-reduction reactions are a key to life.

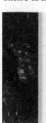

Knowledge Check

1. What is the main form of energy used by the body?
2. What are catabolic and anabolic reactions?
3. What is the difference between oxidation and reduction reactions?
4. How do niacin and riboflavin play a role in metabolism?

9.2 ATP Production from Carbohydrates

Cells release energy stored in food fuels and then trap as much of this energy as possible in the form of ATP. The body cannot afford to lose all energy immediately as heat, even though some heat is necessary for the maintenance of body temperature. This section examines how ATP is produced from carbohydrates. Subsequent sections will explore how ATP is produced using the energy stored in fats, proteins, and alcohol. Along the way, you will see how these energy-yielding processes are interconnected.

ATP is generated through cellular respiration. The process of **cellular respiration** oxidizes (removes electrons) food molecules to obtain energy (ATP). Oxygen is the final electron acceptor. As you know, humans inhale oxygen and exhale carbon dioxide. When oxygen is readily available, cellular respiration may be **aerobic**. When oxygen is not present, **anaerobic** pathways are used. Aerobic respiration is far more efficient than anaerobic metabolism at producing ATP. As an example, the aerobic respiration of a single molecule of glucose will result in a net gain of 30 to 32 ATP. In contrast, the anaerobic metabolism of a single molecule of glucose is limited to a net gain of 2 ATP.

The 4 overall stages of aerobic cellular respiration of glucose are as follows (Fig. 9-5).[1,4]

Stage 1: Glycolysis. In this pathway, glucose (a 6-carbon compound) is oxidized and forms 2 molecules of the 3-carbon compound pyruvate, produces NADH + H[+], and generates a net of 2 molecules of ATP. Glycolysis occurs in the **cytosol** of cells.

▶ A new tool for understanding how individuals differ in the metabolic response to nutrients may lie in the ability to track the actual metabolic intermediates made during metabolism, such as how we respond to exposure to different fatty acids. This approach, called *metabolomics*, should be more accurate than looking for differences in DNA between individuals to predict dietary responses.

aerobic Requiring oxygen.

anaerobic Not requiring oxygen.

cytosol Water-based phase of a cell's cytoplasm; excludes organelles, such as mitochondria.

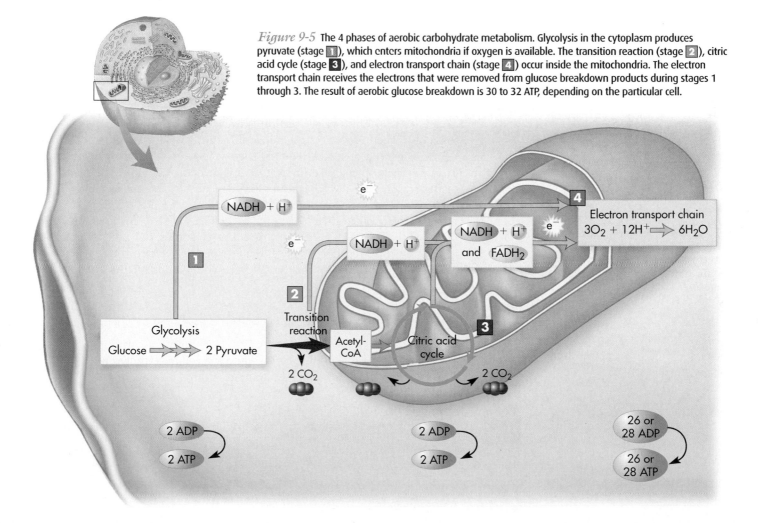

Figure 9-5 The 4 phases of aerobic carbohydrate metabolism. Glycolysis in the cytoplasm produces pyruvate (stage **1**), which enters mitochondria if oxygen is available. The transition reaction (stage **2**), citric acid cycle (stage **3**), and electron transport chain (stage **4**) occur inside the mitochondria. The electron transport chain receives the electrons that were removed from glucose breakdown products during stages 1 through 3. The result of aerobic glucose breakdown is 30 to 32 ATP, depending on the particular cell.

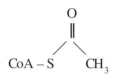

mitochondria Main sites of energy production in a cell. They also contain the pathway for oxidizing fat for fuel, among other metabolic pathways.

▶ A number of defects are related to the metabolic processes that take place in mitochondria. A variety of medical interventions, some of which use specific nutrients and related metabolic intermediates, can be used to treat the muscle weakness and muscle destruction typically arising from these disorders.

acetyl-CoA

$$\text{CoA} - \text{S} \underset{}{\overset{\displaystyle \overset{\text{O}}{\|}}{\diagup \diagdown}} \text{CH}_3$$

▶ *CoA* is short for *coenzyme A*. The *A* stands for *acetylation* because CoA provides the 2-carbon acetyl group to start the citric acid cycle.

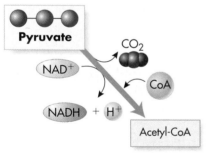

Figure 9-6 **Pyruvate dehydrogenase assists in the transition reaction where pyruvate is metabolized to acetyl-CoA. It is acetyl-CoA that actually enters the citric acid cycle. In the process, NADH + H$^+$ is produced and CO$_2$ is lost.**

Stage 2: Synthesis of acetyl-CoA. In this stage, pyruvate is further oxidized and joined with coenzyme A (CoA) to form acetyl-CoA. The transition reaction also produces NADH + H$^+$ and releases carbon dioxide (CO$_2$) as a waste product. The transition reaction takes place in the **mitochondria** of cells.

Stage 3: Citric acid cycle. In this pathway, acetyl-CoA enters the citric acid cycle, resulting in the production of NADH + H$^+$, FADH$_2$, and ATP. Carbon dioxide is released as a waste product. Like the transition reaction, the citric acid cycle takes place within the mitochondria of cells.

Stage 4: Electron transport chain. The NADH + H$^+$ produced by stages 1 through 3 of cellular respiration and FADH$_2$ produced in stage 3 enter the electron transport chain, where NADH + H$^+$ is oxidized to NAD$^+$, and FADH$_2$ is oxidized to FAD. At the end of the electron transport chain, oxygen is combined with hydrogen ions (H$^+$) and electrons to form water. The electron transport chain takes place within the mitochondria of cells. Most ATP is produced in the electron transport chain; thus, the mitochondria are the cell's major energy-producing organelles.

Glycolysis

Because glucose is the main carbohydrate involved in cell metabolism, we will track its step-by-step metabolism as an example of carbohydrate metabolism. Glucose metabolism begins with **glycolysis**, which means "breaking down glucose." Glycolysis has 2 roles: to break down carbohydrates to generate energy and to provide building blocks for synthesizing other needed compounds. During glycolysis, glucose passes through several steps, which convert it to 2 units of a 3-carbon compound called pyruvate. The details of glycolysis can be found in Figure 9-6.

Synthesis of Acetyl-CoA

Pyruvate passes from the cytosol into the mitochondria, where the enzyme pyruvate dehydrogenase converts pyruvate into the compound acetyl-CoA in a process called a transition reaction[5] (Fig. 9-7). This overall reaction is irreversible, which has important metabolic consequences. Whereas glycolysis requires only the B-vitamin niacin as NAD, the conversion of pyruvate to acetyl-CoA requires coenzymes from 4 B-vitamins—thiamin, riboflavin, niacin, and pantothenic acid. In fact, CoA is made from the B-vitamin pantothenic acid. For this reason, carbohydrate metabolism depends on an ample supply of these vitamins (see Chapter 13).[2]

The transition reaction oxidizes pyruvate and reduces NAD$^+$. Each glucose yields 2 acetyl-CoA. As with the NADH + H$^+$ produced by glycolysis, the 2 NADH + 2 H$^+$ produced by the transition reaction will eventually enter the electron transport chain. Carbon dioxide is a waste product of the transition reaction and is eventually eliminated by way of the lungs.

Knowledge Check

1. What is the first step to bring glucose into the cell to start glycolysis?
2. How many 3-carbon compounds are made from a 6-carbon glucose molecule?
3. What is the end product of glycolysis?
4. What nutrients are involved in the transition reaction?

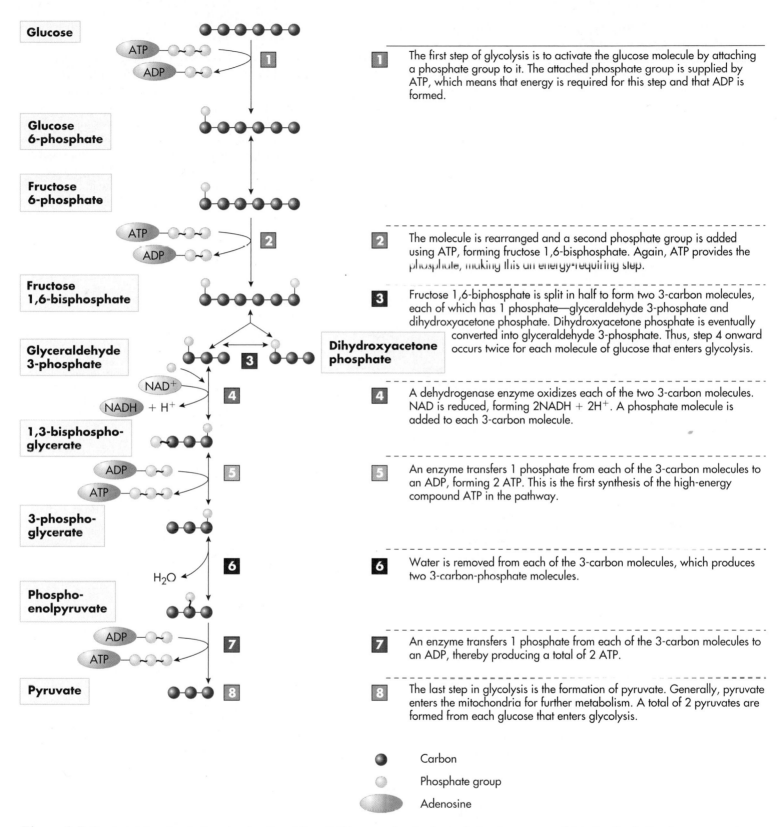

Glucose

The first step of glycolysis is to activate the glucose molecule by attaching a phosphate group to it. The attached phosphate group is supplied by ATP, which means that energy is required for this step and that ADP is formed.

Glucose 6-phosphate

Fructose 6-phosphate

The molecule is rearranged and a second phosphate group is added using ATP, forming fructose 1,6-bisphosphate. Again, ATP provides the phosphate, making this an energy-requiring step.

Fructose 1,6-bisphosphate

Fructose 1,6-biphosphate is split in half to form two 3-carbon molecules, each of which has 1 phosphate—glyceraldehyde 3-phosphate and dihydroxyacetone phosphate. Dihydroxyacetone phosphate is eventually converted into glyceraldehyde 3-phosphate. Thus, step 4 onward occurs twice for each molecule of glucose that enters glycolysis.

Glyceraldehyde 3-phosphate

Dihydroxyacetone phosphate

A dehydrogenase enzyme oxidizes each of the two 3-carbon molecules. NAD is reduced, forming 2NADH + 2H$^+$. A phosphate molecule is added to each 3-carbon molecule.

1,3-bisphospho-glycerate

An enzyme transfers 1 phosphate from each of the 3-carbon molecules to an ADP, forming 2 ATP. This is the first synthesis of the high-energy compound ATP in the pathway.

3-phospho-glycerate

Water is removed from each of the 3-carbon molecules, which produces two 3-carbon-phosphate molecules.

Phospho-enolpyruvate

An enzyme transfers 1 phosphate from each of the 3-carbon molecules to an ADP, thereby producing a total of 2 ATP.

Pyruvate

The last step in glycolysis is the formation of pyruvate. Generally, pyruvate enters the mitochondria for further metabolism. A total of 2 pyruvates are formed from each glucose that enters glycolysis.

- Carbon
- Phosphate group
- Adenosine

Figure 9-7 Glycolysis takes place in the cytosol portion of the cell. This process breaks glucose (a 6-carbon compound) into 2 units of a 3-carbon compound called pyruvate. More details can be found in Appendix A.

Citric Acid Cycle

The acetyl-CoA molecules produced by the transition reaction enter the citric acid cycle, which also is known as the tricarboxylic acid cycle (TCA cycle) and the Krebs cycle. The citric acid cycle is a series of chemical reactions that cells use to convert the carbons of an acetyl group to carbon dioxide while harvesting energy to produce ATP.[3]

It takes 2 turns of the citric acid cycle to process 1 glucose molecule because glycolysis and the transition reaction yield 2 acetyl-CoA. Each complete turn of the citric acid cycle produces 2 molecules of CO_2 and 1 potential ATP in the form of 1 molecule of guanosine triphosphate (GTP), as well as 3 molecules of NADH + H^+ and 1 molecule of $FADH_2$. Oxygen does not participate in any of the steps in the citric acid cycle; however, it does participate in the electron transport chain. The details of the citric acid cycle can be found in Figure 9-8; further details are in Appendix A.

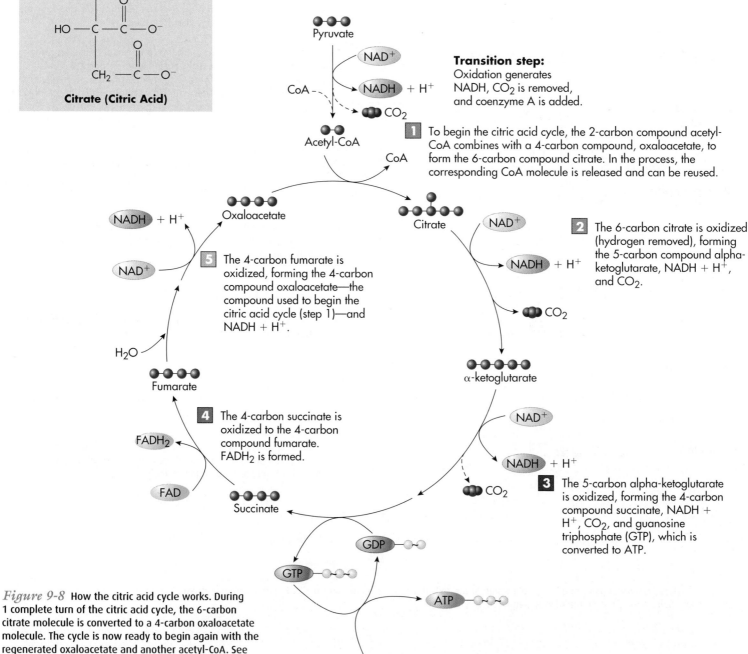

Figure 9-8 How the citric acid cycle works. During 1 complete turn of the citric acid cycle, the 6-carbon citrate molecule is converted to a 4-carbon oxaloacetate molecule. The cycle is now ready to begin again with the regenerated oxaloacetate and another acetyl-CoA. See Figure A-2 in Appendix A for a more detailed view of the citric acid cycle.

A Biochemist's View

Oxaloacetate

Citrate (Citric Acid)

Transition step:
Oxidation generates NADH, CO_2 is removed, and coenzyme A is added.

1 To begin the citric acid cycle, the 2-carbon compound acetyl-CoA combines with a 4-carbon compound, oxaloacetate, to form the 6-carbon compound citrate. In the process, the corresponding CoA molecule is released and can be reused.

2 The 6-carbon citrate is oxidized (hydrogen removed), forming the 5-carbon compound alpha-ketoglutarate, NADH + H^+, and CO_2.

3 The 5-carbon alpha-ketoglutarate is oxidized, forming the 4-carbon compound succinate, NADH + H^+, CO_2, and guanosine triphosphate (GTP), which is converted to ATP.

4 The 4-carbon succinate is oxidized to the 4-carbon compound fumarate. $FADH_2$ is formed.

5 The 4-carbon fumarate is oxidized, forming the 4-carbon compound oxaloacetate—the compound used to begin the citric acid cycle (step 1)—and NADH + H^+.

Electron Transport Chain

The final pathway of aerobic respiration is the electron transport chain located in the mitochondria. The electron transport chain functions in most cells in the body. Cells that need a lot of ATP, such as muscle cells, have thousands of mitochondria, whereas cells that need very little ATP, such as adipose cells, have fewer mitochondria. Almost 90% of the ATP produced from the catabolism of glucose is produced by the electron transport chain.

The electron transport chain involves the passage of electrons along a series of electron carriers. As electrons are passed from one carrier to the next, small amounts of energy are released. NADH + H$^+$ and FADH$_2$, produced by glycolysis, the transition reaction, and the citric acid cycle, supply both hydrogen ions and electrons to the electron transport chain. The metabolic process, called **oxidative phosphorylation**, is the way in which energy derived from the NADH + H$^+$ and FADH$_2$ is transferred to ADP + P$_i$ to form ATP (Fig. 9-9). Oxidative phosphorylation requires the minerals copper and iron. Copper is a component of an enzyme, whereas iron is a component of **cytochromes** (electron-transfer compound) in the electron transport chain. In addition to ATP production, hydrogen ions, electrons, and oxygen combine to form water. The details of the electron transport chain are presented in Figure 9-10.

▶ Intermediates of the citric acid cycle, such as oxaloacetate, can leave the cycle and go on to form other compounds, such as glucose. Thus, the citric acid cycle should be viewed as a traffic circle, rather than as a closed circle.

▶ How many ATP are produced by 1 molecule of glucose? The metabolism of 1 glucose molecule yields

Glycolysis	2 NADH and 2 ATP
Transition reaction	2 NADH
Citric acid cycle	6 NADH, 2 FADH$_2$, and 2 GTP
Total	**10 NADH, 2 FADH$_2$, 2 GTP, and 2 ATP**

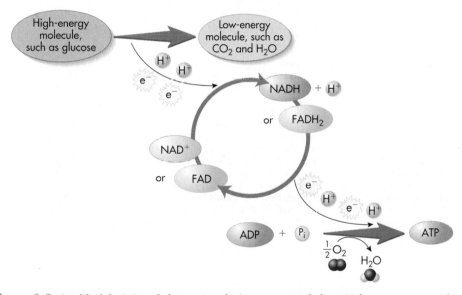

Figure 9-9 Simplified depiction of electron transfer in energy metabolism. High-energy compounds, such as glucose, give up electrons and hydrogen ions to NAD$^+$ and FAD. The NADH + H$^+$ and FADH$_2$ that are formed transfer these electrons and hydrogen ions, using specialized electron carriers, to oxygen to form water (H$_2$O). The energy yielded by the entire process is used to generate ATP from ADP and P$_i$.

The NADH and FADH$_2$ generated undergo oxidative phosphorylation in the electron transport chain to yield

2.5 ATP molecules per NADH

1.5 ATP molecules per FADH$_2$

Thus, 28 ATP molecules are synthesized in the electron transport chain.

Total ATP Produced from Each Glucose Molecule

Glycolysis ATP	2 ATP
Citric acid cycle GTP	2 ATP
Citric acid cycle ATP	28 ATP
Total	**32 ATP**

The Importance of Oxygen

NADH + H$^+$ and FADH$_2$ produced during the citric acid cycle can be regenerated into NAD$^+$ and FAD only by the eventual transfer of their electrons and hydrogen ions to oxygen, as occurs in the electron transport chain. The citric acid cycle has no ability to oxidize NADH + H$^+$ and FADH$_2$ back to NAD$^+$ and FAD. This is ultimately why oxygen is essential to many life forms—it is a final acceptor of the electrons and hydrogen ions generated from the breakdown of energy-yielding nutrients. Without oxygen, most of our cells are unable to extract enough energy from energy-yielding nutrients to sustain life.[1]

▶ Coenzyme Q-10 is sold as a nutrient supplement in health food stores (*10* signifies that it is the form found in humans). However, when the mitochondria need coenzyme Q, they make it. Thus, to maintain overall health, coenzyme Q is not needed in the diet or as a supplement. (Such use may be helpful, however, in people with heart failure.)

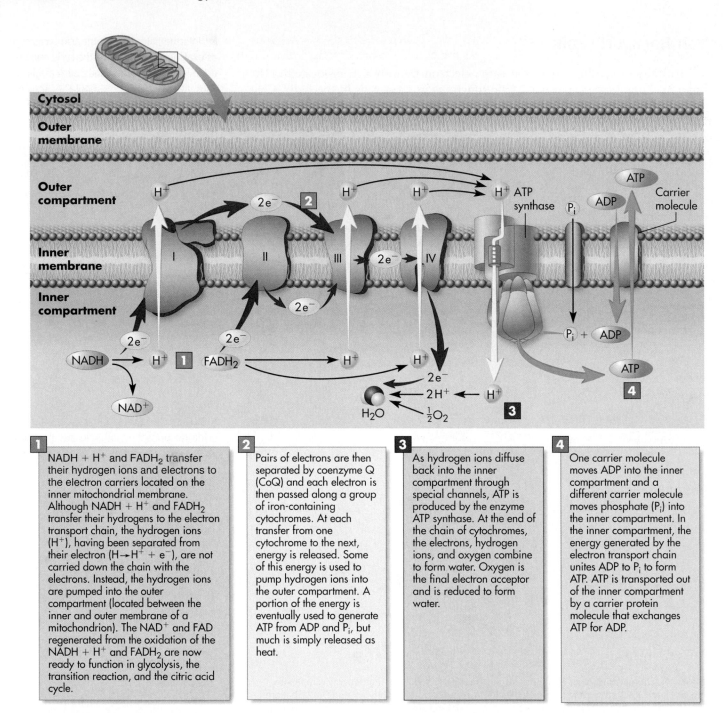

Cytosol

Outer membrane

Outer compartment

Inner membrane

Inner compartment

H⁺

2e⁻   **2**

H⁺   H⁺   H⁺   ATP synthase

Pᵢ   ADP   Carrier molecule

ATP

I   II   III   2e⁻   IV

2e⁻

2e⁻   H⁺   **1**   FADH₂   H⁺   H⁺

Pᵢ + ADP

ATP

NADH

H⁺

2e⁻
2H⁺ ← H⁺
H₂O   ½O₂   **3**

NAD⁺

4

1 NADH + H⁺ and FADH₂ transfer their hydrogen ions and electrons to the electron carriers located on the inner mitochondrial membrane. Although NADH + H⁺ and FADH₂ transfer their hydrogens to the electron transport chain, the hydrogen ions (H⁺), having been separated from their electron (H→H⁺ + e⁻), are not carried down the chain with the electrons. Instead, the hydrogen ions are pumped into the outer compartment (located between the inner and outer membrane of a mitochondrion). The NAD⁺ and FAD regenerated from the oxidation of the NADH + H⁺ and FADH₂ are now ready to function in glycolysis, the transition reaction, and the citric acid cycle.

2 Pairs of electrons are then separated by coenzyme Q (CoQ) and each electron is then passed along a group of iron-containing cytochromes. At each transfer from one cytochrome to the next, energy is released. Some of this energy is used to pump hydrogen ions into the outer compartment. A portion of the energy is eventually used to generate ATP from ADP and Pᵢ, but much is simply released as heat.

3 As hydrogen ions diffuse back into the inner compartment through special channels, ATP is produced by the enzyme ATP synthase. At the end of the chain of cytochromes, the electrons, hydrogen ions, and oxygen combine to form water. Oxygen is the final electron acceptor and is reduced to form water.

4 One carrier molecule moves ADP into the inner compartment and a different carrier molecule moves phosphate (Pᵢ) into the inner compartment. In the inner compartment, the energy generated by the electron transport chain unites ADP to Pᵢ to form ATP. ATP is transported out of the inner compartment by a carrier protein molecule that exchanges ATP for ADP.

Figure 9-10 **The electron transport chain.**

▶ In Figure 9-10, step 1, NADH + H⁺ donates its chemical energy to an FAD-related compound called flavin mononucleotide (FMN). In contrast, FADH₂ donates its chemical energy at a later point in the electron transport chain. This different placement of FAD and NAD⁺ in the electron transport chain results in a difference in ATP production. Each NADH + H⁺ in a mitochondrion releases enough energy to form the equivalent of 2.5 ATP, whereas each FADH₂ releases enough energy to form the equivalent of 1.5 ATP.[1]

Anaerobic Metabolism

Some cells lack mitochondria and, so, are not capable of aerobic respiration. Other cells are capable of turning to anaerobic metabolism when oxygen is lacking. When oxygen is absent, pyruvate that is produced through glycolysis is converted into lactate, or lactic acid. Anaerobic metabolism is not nearly as efficient as aerobic respiration because it converts only about 5% of the energy in a molecule of glucose to energy stored in the high-energy phosphate bonds of ATP.[1]

The anaerobic glycolysis pathway encompasses glycolysis and the conversion of pyruvate to lactate (Fig. 9-11). The 1-step reaction, catalyzed by the enzyme pyruvate dehydrogenase, involves a simple transfer of a hydrogen from NADH + H⁺ to pyruvate

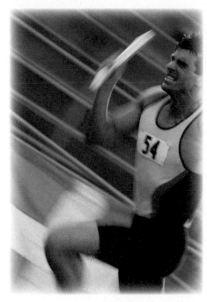

Quick bursts of activity rely on the production of lactate to help meet the ATP energy demand.

to form lactate and NAD⁺. The synthesis of lactate regenerates the NAD⁺ required for the continued function of glycolysis. The reaction can be summarized as

$$\text{Pyruvate} + \text{NADH} + \text{H}^+ \rightarrow \text{Lactate} + \text{NAD}^+$$

For cells that lack mitochondria, such as red blood cells, anaerobic glycolysis is the only method for making ATP because they lack the electron transport chain and oxidative phosphorylation. Therefore, when red blood cells convert glucose to pyruvate, NADH + H⁺ builds up in the cell. Eventually, the NAD⁺ concentration falls too low to permit glycolysis to continue.[5] The anaerobic glycolysis pathway produces lactate to regenerate NAD⁺. The lactate produced by the red blood cell is then released into the bloodstream, picked up primarily by the liver, and used to synthesize pyruvate, glucose, or some other intermediate in aerobic respiration.

Even though muscles cells contain mitochondria, during intensive exercise they also produce lactate when NAD⁺ is depleted. By regenerating NAD⁺, the production of lactate allows anaerobic glycolysis to continue. Muscle cells can then make the ATP required for muscle contraction even if little oxygen is present. However, as you will find out in Chapter 11, it becomes more difficult to contract those muscles as the lactate concentration builds up.

▶ In anaerobic environments, some microorganisms, such as yeast, produce ethanol, a type of alcohol, instead of lactate from glucose. Other microorganisms produce various forms of short-chain fatty acids. All this anaerobic metabolism is referred to as fermentation.

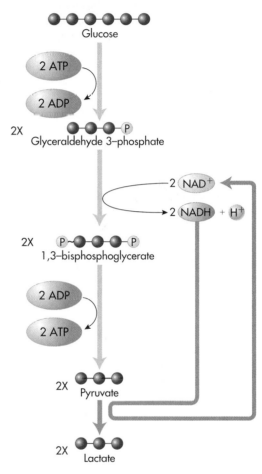

Figure 9-11 Anaerobic glycolysis "frees" NAD⁺ and it returns to the glycolysis pathway to pick up more hydrogen ions and electrons.

Knowledge Check

1. How is citric acid in the citric acid cycle formed?
2. How many NADH + H⁺ are formed in the citric acid cycle?
3. Why is the citric acid cycle called a cycle?
4. What is the purpose of the electron transport chain?
5. What are the end products of the electron transport chain?

CASE STUDY

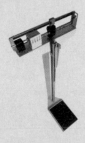

Melissa is a 45-year-old woman who is obese. At her last physical, her doctor told her that she needs to lose weight. Melissa purchased a low-carbohydrate, high-protein diet book and has read it and is now ready to try the diet. She knows it will be difficult to follow because many of the foods Melissa likes are rich in carbohydrates, and the first 2 weeks of the diet eliminates almost all carbohydrates from her diet. Although she is ready to try the diet, she is confused about certain phases of the program, especially the part where the author talks about ketones. In the book, the author states that anyone going on this diet should purchase ketone strips to dip in his or her urine for the detection of ketones. The author strongly suggests these tests, especially during the extremely low-carbohydrate part of the diet. Melissa wonders if she should be considering this diet if the author is telling her to check something and she wonders what ketones are.

What are ketones and why does a very-low-carbohydrate diet produce an increase in ketones in both the blood and the urine? Can you speculate at this time why low carbohydrates cause ketones? Why do some fad diets produce ketones?

9.3 ATP Production from Fats

▶ Carnitine is a popular nutritional supplement. In healthy people, cells produce the carnitine needed, and carnitine supplements provide no benefit. In patients hospitalized with acute illnesses, however, carnitine synthesis may be inadequate. These patients may need to have carnitine added to their intravenous feeding (total parenteral nutrition) solutions.

Just as cells release the energy in carbohydrates and trap it as ATP, they also release and trap energy in triglyceride molecules. This process begins with **lipolysis,** the breaking down of triglycerides into free fatty acids and glycerol. The further breakdown of fatty acids for energy production is called **fatty acid oxidation** because the donation of electrons from fatty acids to oxygen is the net reaction in the ATP-yielding process. This process takes place in the mitochondria.

Fatty acids for oxidation can come from either dietary fat or fat stored in the body as adipose tissue. Following high-fat meals, the body stores excess fat in adipose tissue. However, during periods of low calorie intake or fasting, triglycerides from fat cells are broken down into fatty acids by an enzyme called hormone-sensitive lipase and released in the blood. The activity of this enzyme is increased by hormones such as glucagon, growth hormone, and epinephrine and is decreased by the hormone insulin. The fatty acids are taken up from the bloodstream by cells throughout the body and are shuttled from the cell cytosol into the mitochondria using a carrier called **carnitine** (Fig. 9-12).[6]

Figure 9-12 Lipolysis. Because of the action of hormone-sensitive lipase, fatty acids are released from triglycerides in adipose cells and enter the bloodstream. The fatty acids are taken up from the bloodstream by various cells and shuttled by carnitine into the inner portion of the cell mitochondria. The fatty acid then undergoes beta-oxidation, which yields acetate molecules equal in number to half of the carbons in the fatty acid.

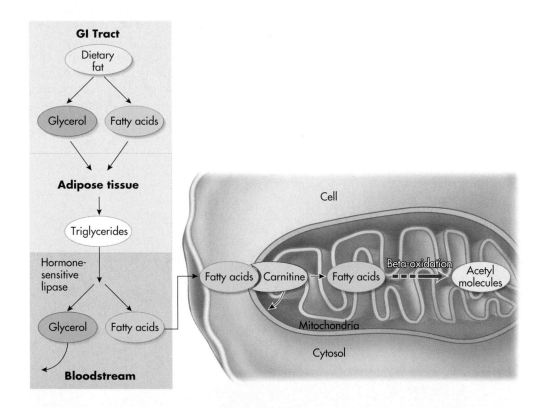

ATP Production from Fatty Acids

Almost all fatty acids in nature are composed of an even number of carbons, ranging from 2 to 26. The first step in transferring the energy in such a fatty acid to ATP is to cleave the carbons, 2 at a time, and convert the 2-carbon fragments to acetyl-CoA. The process of converting a free fatty acid to multiple acetyl-CoA molecules is called **beta-oxidation** because it begins with the beta carbon, the second carbon on a fatty acid (counting after the carboxyl [acid] end).[1] (See Chapter 6.) During beta-oxidation, NADH + H$^+$ and FADH$_2$ are produced (Fig. 9-13). Thus, as with glucose, a fatty acid is eventually degraded into a number of the 2-carbon compound acetyl-CoA (the exact number produced depends on the number of carbons in the fatty acid). Some of the chemical energy contained in the fatty acid is transferred to NADH + H$^+$ and FADH$_2$.

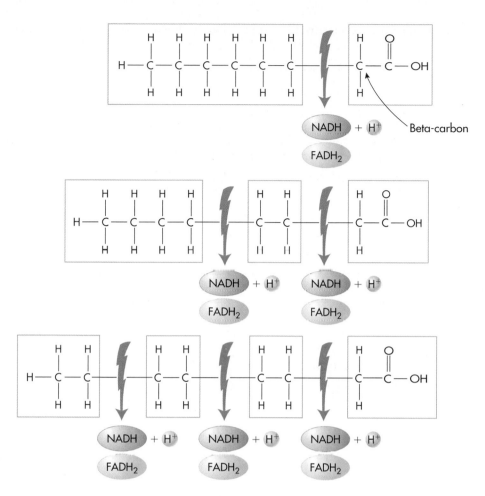

Figure 9-13 In beta-oxidation, each 2-carbon fragment cleaved from a fatty acid (acetyl group) yields electrons and hydrogen ions to form NADH + H⁺ and FADH₂ as the fragments are split off the parent fatty acid. The 2-carbon acetyl molecule then typically enters the citric acid cycle (as acetyl-CoA).

The acetyl-CoA enters the citric acid cycle, and 2 carbon dioxides are released, just as with the acetyl-CoA produced from glucose. Thus, the breakdown product of both glucose and fatty acids—acetyl-CoA—enter the citric acid cycle. One big difference, however, is that a 16-carbon fatty acid yields 104 ATP, whereas the 6-carbon glucose yields only 30 to 32 ATP. The difference in ATP production occurs because each 2-carbon segment in the fatty acid goes around the citric acid cycle; thus, a 16-carbon fatty acid goes around the citric acid cycle 8 times. Additionally, each fatty acid carbon results in about 7 ATP, whereas about 5 ATP per carbon result from glucose oxidation. This is because fatty acids have more carbon-hydrogen bonds and fewer carbon-oxygen atoms than glucose. The carbons of glucose exist in a more oxidized state than fat; as a result, fats yield more energy than carbohydrates (9 kcal/g versus 4 kcal/g).[1]

Occasionally, a fatty acid has an odd number of carbons, so the cell forms a 3-carbon compound (propionyl-CoA) in addition to the acetyl-CoA. The propionyl-CoA enters the citric acid cycle directly, bypassing acetyl-CoA. It can then go on to yield NADH + H⁺ and FADH₂, CO_2, and even other products, such as glucose (see Section 9.4).

Carbohydrate Aids Fat Metabolism

In addition to its role in energy production, the citric acid cycle provides compounds that leave the cycle and enter biosynthetic pathways. This results in a slowing of the cycle, as eventually not enough oxaloacetate is formed to combine with the acetyl-CoA entering the cycle. Cells are able to compensate for this by synthesizing additional oxaloacetate. One potential source of this additional oxaloacetate is pyruvate (Fig. 9-14). Thus, as fatty acids create acetyl-CoA, carbohydrates (e.g., glucose) are

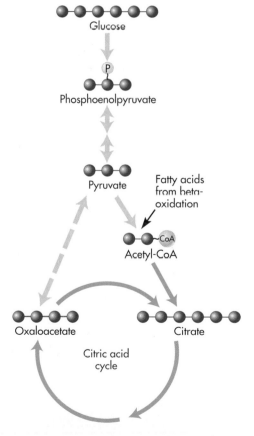

Figure 9-14 As acetyl-CoA concentrations increase due to beta-oxidation, oxaloacetate levels are maintained by pyruvate from carbohydrate metabolism. In this way, carbohydrates help oxidize fatty acids.

A Biochemist's View

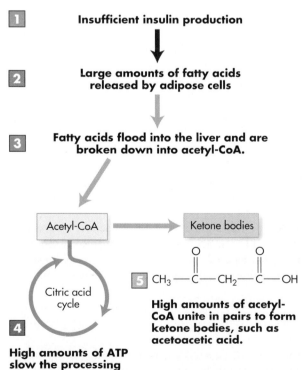

Pyruvate

CH_3 — C — C — O⁻

CO_2

Oxaloacetate

---

ketone bodies Incomplete breakdown products of fat, containing 3 or 4 carbons. Most contain a chemical group called a ketone. An example is acetoacetic acid.

ketosis Condition of having a high concentration of ketone bodies and related breakdown products in the bloodstream and tissues.

---

needed to keep the concentration of pyruvate high enough to resupply oxaloacetate to the citric acid cycle. Overall, the entire pathway for fatty acid oxidation works better when carbohydrate is available.

Ketogenesis

Ketone bodies are products of incomplete fatty acid oxidation.[7] This occurs mainly with hormonal imbalances—chiefly, inadequate insulin production to balance glucagon action in the body. These imbalances lead to a significant production of ketone bodies and a condition called **ketosis.** The key steps in the development of ketosis are shown in Figure 9-15.

Most ketone bodies are subsequently converted back into acetyl-CoA in other body cells, where they then enter the citric acid cycle and can be used for fuel. One of the ketone bodies formed (acetone) leaves the body via the lungs, giving the breath of a person in ketosis a characteristic, fruity smell.

Ketosis in Diabetes

In type 1 diabetes, little to no insulin is produced. This lack of insulin does not allow for normal carbohydrate and fat metabolism. Without sufficient insulin, cells cannot readily utilize glucose, resulting in rapid lipolysis and the excess production of ketone bodies.[8] If the concentration of ketone bodies rises too high in the blood, the excess spills into the urine, pulling the electrolytes sodium and potassium with it. Eventually, severe ion imbalances occur in the body. The blood also becomes more acidic because 2 of the 3

---

1 **Insufficient insulin production**

2 **Large amounts of fatty acids released by adipose cells**

3 **Fatty acids flood into the liver and are broken down into acetyl-CoA.**

Acetyl-CoA → Ketone bodies

Citric acid cycle

4 **High amounts of ATP slow the processing of acetyl-CoA to ATP.**

5 CH_3 — C — CH_2 — C — OH

High amounts of acetyl-CoA unite in pairs to form ketone bodies, such as acetoacetic acid.

Stage 1
Blood insulin drops, usually as a result of type 1 diabetes or low carbohydrate intake.

Stage 2
A fall in blood insulin promotes lipolysis, which causes fatty acids stored in adipose cells to be released rapidly into the bloodstream.

Stage 3
Most of the fatty acids in the blood are taken up by the liver.

Stage 4
As the liver oxidizes the fatty acids to acetyl-CoA, the capacity of the citric acid cycle to process the acetyl-CoA molecules decreases. This is mostly because the metabolism of fatty acids to acetyl-CoA yields many ATP. When the cells have plenty of ATP, there is no need to use the citric acid cycle to produce more.

Stage 5
These metabolic changes encourage liver cells to combine a 2 acetyl-CoA molecules to form a 4-carbon compound. This compound is further metabolized and eventually secreted into the bloodstream as ketone bodies (acetoacetic acid and the related compounds, beta-hydroxybutyric acid and acetone).

Figure 9-15 Key steps in ketosis. Any condition that limits insulin availability to cells results in some ketone body production.

forms of ketone bodies contain acid groups. The resulting condition, known as **diabetic ketoacidosis**, can induce coma or death if not treated immediately, such as with insulin, electrolytes, and fluids (see Chapter 5). Ketoacidosis usually occurs only in ketosis caused by uncontrolled type 1 diabetes; in fasting, blood concentrations of ketone bodies typically do not rise high enough to cause the problem.

Ketosis in Semistarvation or Fasting

When a person is in a state of semistarvation or fasting, the amount of glucose in the body falls, so insulin production falls. This fall in blood insulin then causes fatty acids to flood into the bloodstream and eventually form ketone bodies in the liver. The heart, muscles, and some parts of the kidneys then use ketone bodies for fuel. After a few days of ketosis, the brain also begins to metabolize ketone bodies for energy.

This adaptive response is important to semistarvation or fasting. As more body cells begin to use ketone bodies for fuel, the need for glucose as a body fuel diminishes. This then reduces the need for the liver and kidneys to produce glucose from amino acids (and from the glycerol released from lipolysis), sparing much body protein from being used as a fuel source (see Section 9.4). The maintenance of body protein mass is a key to survival in semistarvation or fasting—death occurs when about half of the body protein is depleted, usually after about 50 to 70 days of total fasting.[9]

Knowledge Check

1. What is anaerobic glycolysis?
2. What cells use anaerobic glycolysis?
3. How do fatty acids enter the citric acid cycle?
4. What conditions must exist in the body to promote the formation of ketones?

 ## 9.4 Protein Metabolism

The metabolism of protein (i.e., amino acids) takes place primarily in the liver. Only branched-chain amino acids—leucine, isoleucine, and valine—are metabolized mostly at other sites—in this case, the muscles.[2]

Protein metabolism begins after proteins are degraded into amino acids. To use an amino acid for fuel, cells must first deaminate them (remove the amino group) (see Chapter 7). These pathways often require vitamin B-6 to function. Removal of the amino group produces carbon skeletons, most of which enter the citric acid cycle. Some carbon skeletons also yield acetyl-CoA or pyruvate.[5]

Some carbon skeletons enter the citric acid cycle as acetyl-CoA, whereas others form intermediates of the citric acid cycle or glycolysis (Fig. 9-16). Any part of the carbon skeleton that can form pyruvate (i.e., alanine, glycine, cysteine, serine, and threonine) or bypass acetyl-CoA and enter the citric acid cycle directly (such amino acids include asparagine, arginine, aspartic acid, histidine, glutamic acid, glutamine, isoleucine, methionine, proline, valine, and phenylalanine) are called **glucogenic** amino acids because these carbons can become the carbons of glucose. Any parts of carbon skeletons that become acetyl-CoA (leucine and lysine, as well as parts of isoleucine, phenylalanine, tryptophan, and tyrosine) are called **ketogenic** amino acids because these carbons cannot become parts of glucose molecules. The factor that determines whether an amino acid is glucogenic or ketogenic is whether part or all of the carbon skeleton of the amino acid can yield a "new" oxaloacetate molecule during metabolism, 2 of which are needed to form glucose.

CRITICAL THINKING

The use of a very low carbohydrate diet to induce ketosis for weight loss is covered in Chapter 10. Why is careful physician monitoring needed if this type of diet is followed?

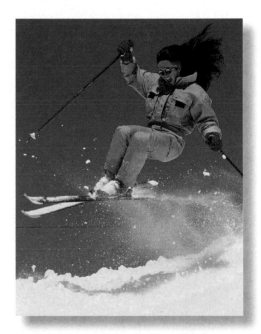

Metabolism is part of everyday life; metabolic activity increases when we increase physical activity and slows during fasting and semi-starvation.

▶ Branched-chain amino acids are added to some liquid meal replacement supplements given to hospitalized patients. Some fluid replacement formulas marketed to athletes also contain branched-chain amino acids (see Chapter 11).

Figure 9-16 Gluconeogenesis. Amino acids that can yield glucose can be converted to pyruvate **1**, directly enter the citric acid cycle **3**, or be converted directly to oxaloacetate **4**. Amino acids that cannot yield glucose are converted to acetyl Co-A and are metabolized in the citric acid cycle **2**. The glycerol portion of triglycerides **5** can be converted to glucose. All amino acids except ketogenic amino acids can be used to make glucose. Fatty acids with an even number of carbons and ketogenic amino acids cannot become glucose **2**.

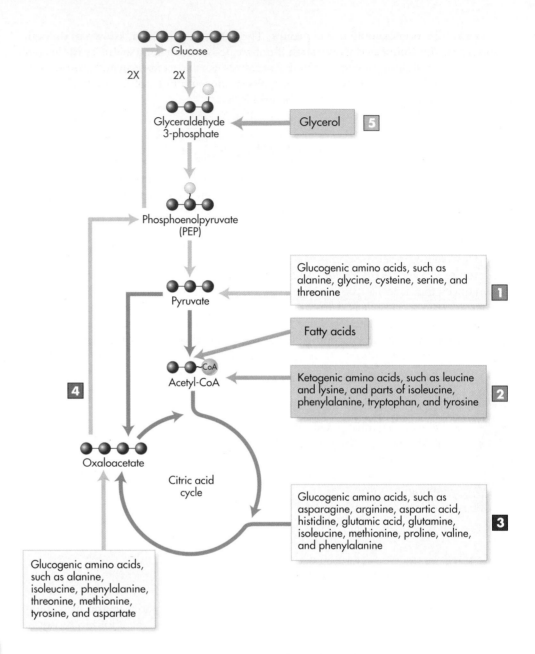

gluconeogenesis Generation (*genesis*) of new (*neo*) glucose from certain (glucogenic) amino acids.

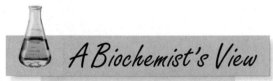

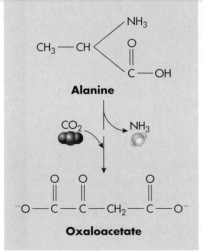

Gluconeogenesis: Producing Glucose from Glucogenic Amino Acids and Other Compounds

The pathway to produce glucose from certain amino acids—**gluconeogenesis**—is present only in liver cells and certain kidney cells. The liver is the primary gluconeogenic organ. A typical starting material for this process is oxaloacetate, which is derived primarily from the carbon skeletons of some amino acids, usually the amino acid alanine. Pyruvate also can be converted to oxaloacetate (see Fig. 9-14).

   Gluconeogenesis begins in the mitochondria with the production of oxaloacetate. The 4-carbon oxaloacetate eventually returns to the cytosol, where it loses 1 carbon dioxide, forming the 3-carbon compound phosphoenolpyruvate, which then reverses the path back through glycolysis to glucose. It takes 2 of this 3-carbon compound to produce the 6-carbon glucose. This entire process requires ATP, as well as coenzyme forms of the B-vitamins biotin, riboflavin, niacin, and B-6.[5]

To learn more about gluconeogenesis, examine Figure 9-16 and trace the pathway that converts the amino acid glutamine to glucose. Glutamine first loses its amino group to form its carbon skeleton, which enters the citric acid cycle directly and is converted by stages to oxaloacetate. Oxaloacetate loses 1 carbon as carbon dioxide, and the 3-carbon phosphoenolpyruvate produced then moves through the gluconeogenic pathway to form glucose. Eventually, 2 glutamine molecules are needed to form 1 glucose molecule.

Gluconeogenesis from Typical Fatty Acids Is Not Possible

Typical fatty acids cannot be turned into glucose because those with an even number of carbons—the typical form in the body—break down into acetyl-CoA molecules. Acetyl-CoA can never re-form into pyruvate; the step between pyruvate and acetyl-CoA is irreversible. The options for acetyl-CoA are forming ketones and/or combining with oxaloacetate in the citric acid cycle. However, 2 carbons of acetyl-CoA are added to oxaloacetate at the beginning of the citric acid cycle, and 2 carbons are subsequently lost as carbon dioxide when citrate converts back to the starting material, oxaloacetate. Thus, at the end of 1 cycle, no carbons from acetyl-CoA are left to turn into glucose; it is impossible to convert typical fatty acids into glucose.[5]

The glycerol portion of a triglyceride is the part that can become glucose. Glycerol enters the glycolysis pathway and can follow the gluconeogenesis pathway from glyceraldehyde 3-phosphate to glucose. Glucose yield from glycerol is insignificant.[1]

Disposal of Excess Amino Groups from Amino Acid Metabolism

The catabolism of amino acids yields amino groups ($-NH_2$), which then are converted to ammonia (NH_3). The ammonia must be excreted because its buildup is toxic to cells. The liver prepares the amino groups for excretion in the urine with the urea cycle. Some stages of the urea cycle occur in the cytosol and some in the mitochondria. During the urea cycle, 2 nitrogen groups—1 ammonia group and 1 amino group—react through a series of steps with carbon dioxide molecules to form urea and water. Eventually, urea is excreted in the urine (Fig. 9-17).[5] In liver disease, ammonia can build up to toxic concentrations in the blood, whereas in kidney disease the toxic agent is urea. The form of nitrogen in the blood—ammonia or urea—is a diagnostic tool for detecting liver or kidney disease.

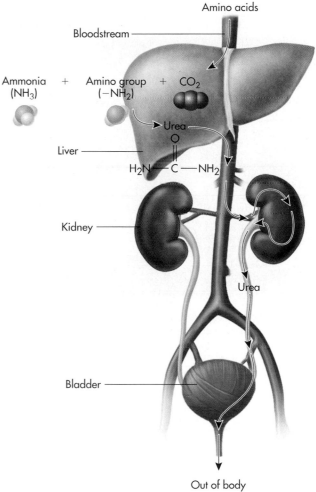

Figure 9-17 **Disposal of excess amino groups.** The nitrogen groups, one as ammonia and the other as an amino group, form part of urea, which is excreted in urine. The nitrogen groups originally came from amino acids that went through transamination reactions and ultimately deamination to yield the free nitrogen groups.

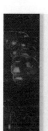

Knowledge Check

1. In order to use amino acids as a fuel, what must happen to the nitrogen attached to the amino acid?
2. Where does the nitrogen attached to an amino acid used as fuel end up?
3. What part of the amino acid is used in the metabolic pathways?
4. What is the name of the pathway that converts amino acids to glucose?
5. Can fat be used to synthesize glucose? Why or why not?

9.5 Alcohol Metabolism

The alcohol dehydrogenase (ADH) pathway is the main pathway for alcohol metabolism. In the first step of this pathway, alcohol is converted in the cytosol to acetaldehyde by the action of the enzyme alcohol dehydrogenase and the coenzyme NAD^+. NAD^+ picks up 2 hydrogen ions and 2 electrons from the alcohol to form $NADH + H^+$ and produces the intermediate acetaldehyde (Fig. 9-18). In the next step of the ADH pathway, the acetaldehyde formed is converted to acetyl-CoA, again yielding $NADH + H^+$ with the aid of the enzyme aldehyde dehydrogenase and coenzyme A.

The metabolism of alcohol occurs predominantly in the liver, although approximately 10 to 30% of alcohol is metabolized in the stomach. Different forms (known as polymorphisms) of alcohol dehydrogenase and aldehyde dehydrogenase are found in the stomach and the liver.

The acetyl-CoA formed through the ADH pathway has several metabolic fates. Small amounts can enter the citric acid cycle to produce energy. However, the breakdown of alcohol in the ADH pathway utilizes NAD^+ and converts it to NADH. As NAD^+ supplies become limited and NADH levels build, the citric acid cycle slows and blocks the entry of acetyl-CoA. Because of the toxic effects of alcohol and acetaldehyde, the metabolism of alcohol takes priority over continuation of the citric acid cycle. Thus, most of the acetyl-CoA is directed toward fatty acid and triglyceride synthesis, resulting in the accumulation of fat in the liver (called steatosis). Clinicians are often alerted to this condition by high levels of triglycerides in the blood.

When a person drinks moderate to excessive amounts of alcohol, the ADH pathway cannot keep up with the demand to metabolize all the alcohol and acetaldehyde. To prevent the toxic effects of alcohol and acetaldehyde, the body utilizes a second pathway, called the microsomal ethanol oxidizing system (MEOS), to metabolize the excess alco-

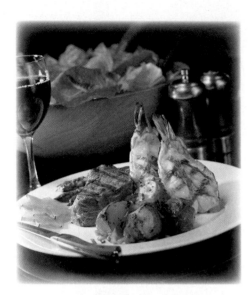

Alcohol, carbohydrate, protein, and fat all contribute chemical energy to the body.

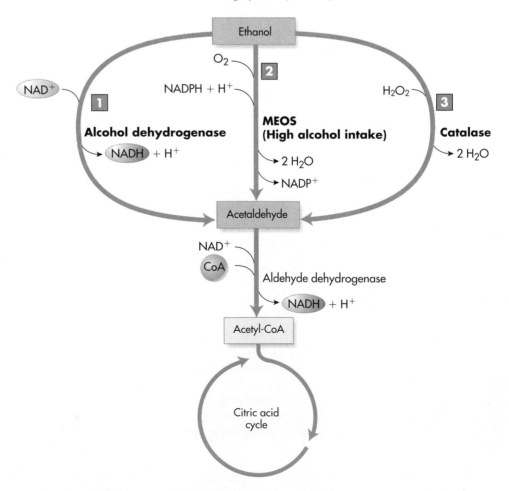

Figure 9-18 **1** At low levels of alcohol intake, the alcohol dehydrogenase pathway in the cytoplasm is used. **2** At high alcohol intake, the microsomal ethanol oxidizing system (MEOS) in the cytoplasm is used. The MEOS uses rather than yields energy and accounts in general for about 10% of alcohol metabolism. **3** Catalase occurs in the peroxisomes of cells and is a minor pathway.

hol. As shown in Figure 9-18, this system uses oxygen and a different niacin-containing coenzyme (NADP) and produces water and acetaldehyde. When excessive amounts of alcohol are consumed at one time, the ability of these enzyme systems to metabolize alcohol completely is exceeded, and the result is alcohol poisoning (see Chapter 8).

The MEOS differs in several ways from the ADH pathway. First, the MEOS uses potential energy (in the form of NADPH + H$^+$, another niacin coenzyme), rather than yielding potential energy (as NADH + H$^+$ in the ADH pathway) in the conversion of ethanol to acetaldehyde. This use of energy may, in part, explain why individuals who consume large amounts of alcohol do not gain as much weight as might be expected from the amount of alcohol-derived energy they consume.

The body has an additional pathway, called the catalase pathway, for metabolizing alcohol. However, this is a relatively minor pathway in comparison with the ADH and MEOS pathways.

Knowledge Check

1. Where does the alcohol dehydrogenase pathway function?
2. Which intermediate in the alcohol dehydrogenase pathway is toxic?
3. In addition to the ADH pathway, what other pathways allow the metabolism of alcohol?

9.6 Regulation of Energy Metabolism

As shown in Figure 9-19, energy metabolism can take many forms in the body. Carbohydrates can be used for fat synthesis—the acetyl-CoA from the breakdown of carbohydrate is the building block for fatty acid synthesis. By stringing together glycolysis and the citric acid cycle, cells can convert carbohydrates into carbon skeletons for the synthesis of certain amino acids and can use the energy in carbohydrates to form ATP. These pathways also can turn the carbon skeletons of some amino acids into the carbon skeletons of others. They also can convert carbon skeletons from some amino acids to glucose or have them drive ATP synthesis by serving as substrates (precursors) for intermediates in the citric acid cycle. Finally, fatty acids can provide energy for ATP synthesis or produce ketone bodies; however, they cannot become glucose. The glycerol part of the triglyceride either can be converted into glucose and be used for fuel or can contribute to ATP synthesis via participation in glycolysis, the citric acid cycle, and electron transport chain metabolism (Table 9-1).

When it comes to regulating these metabolic pathways, the liver plays the major role—it responds to hormones and makes use of vitamins. Additional means of regulating metabolism involve ATP concentrations, enzymes, hormones, vitamins, and minerals.[1]

The Liver

The liver is the location of many nutrient interconversions (Fig. 9-20). Most nutrients must pass first through the liver after absorption into the body. What leaves the liver is often different from what entered. The key metabolic functions of the liver include conversions between various forms of simple sugars, fat synthesis, the production of ketone bodies, amino acid metabolism, urea production, and alcohol metabolism. Nutrient storage is an additional liver function.[2]

Table 9-1 What Happens Where: A Review	
Pathway	**Location**
Glycolysis (glucose → pyruvate)	Cytosol
Transition reaction (pyruvate → acetyl-CoA)	Mitochondria
Fatty acid oxidation (fatty acid → acetyl-CoA)	Mitochondria
Glucogenic amino acid oxidation (amino acids → pyruvate)	Cytosol
Non-glucogenic amino acid oxidation (amino acids → acetyl-CoA)	Mitochondria
Alcohol oxidation (ethanol → acetaldehyde) (acetaldehyde → acetyl-CoA)	Cytosol Mitochondria
Citric acid cycle (acetyl-CoA → CO2)	Mitochondria
Gluconeogenesis	Begins in mitochondria, then moves to cytosol

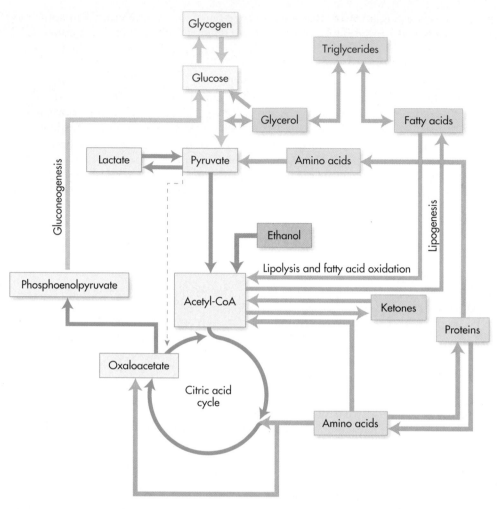

Figure 9-19 Overview of cell metabolism. Note that acetyl-CoA forms a crossroads for many pathways and that the citric acid cycle also can be used to help build compounds. Anabolic and catabolic processes may appear to share the same pathways, but generally this is true for only a few steps. Because a specific set of enzymes must be activated to promote anabolism and a different set to activate catabolism, the cell has significant control over metabolism.

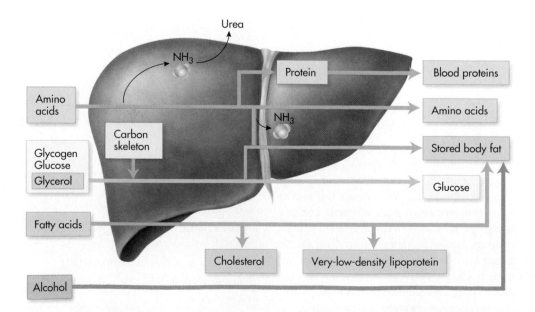

Figure 9-20 Most nutrients must pass first through the liver after absorption into the body. What leaves the liver is often different from what entered.

ATP Concentrations

ATP concentration in a cell helps regulate metabolism. High ATP concentrations decrease energy-yielding reactions, such as glycolysis, and promote anabolic reactions, such as protein synthesis, that use ATP. High ADP concentrations, on the other hand, stimulate energy-yielding pathways.[10]

Enzymes, Hormones, Vitamins, and Minerals

Enzymes are key regulators of metabolic pathways; both their presence and their rate of activity are critical to chemical reactions in the body. Enzyme synthesis and rates of activity are controlled by cells and by the products of the reactions in which the enzymes participate. For example, a high-protein diet leads to increased synthesis of enzymes associated with amino acid catabolism and gluconeogenesis. Within hours of a shift to a low-protein diet, the synthesis of enzymes associated with amino acid metabolism slows.[5]

Hormones, including insulin, regulate metabolic processes. Low levels of insulin in the blood promote gluconeogenesis, protein breakdown, and lipolysis. Increased blood insulin levels promote the synthesis of glycogen, fat, and protein.

Many vitamins and minerals are needed for metabolic pathways to operate (Fig. 9-21). Most notable are the B-vitamins thiamin, riboflavin, niacin, pantothenic acid, biotin, vitamin B-6, folate, and vitamin B-12, as well as the minerals iron and copper. Because so many metabolic pathways depend on nutrient input, health problems can develop from nutrient deficiencies.[2] (The roles that vitamins and minerals play in metabolism are discussed in greater detail in Chapters 12 through 15.)

Knowledge Check

1. Where does glycolysis take place in a cell?
2. What factors determine the regulation of glycolysis and citric acid cycle pathways?
3. What factors regulate energy metabolism?

> ### CRITICAL THINKING
>
> If you had unlimited resources to design a drug that inhibits fat synthesis, which type of metabolism (aerobic or anaerobic) would you look to affect? What unintended metabolic consequences might result from using such a drug? Reviewing Figure 9-21 might help you answer this question.

Figure 9-21 **Many vitamins and minerals participate in the metabolic pathways.**

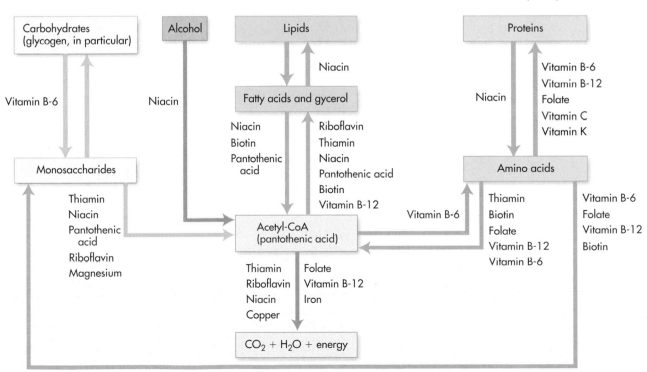

Postprandial fasting (0 to 6 hours after eating)

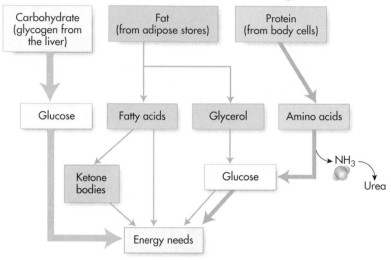

Short-term fasting (3 to 5 days)

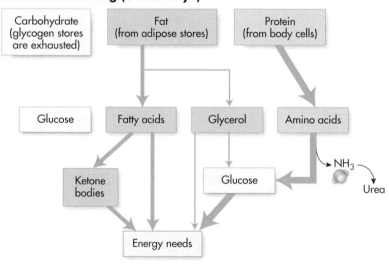

Long-term fasting (5 to 7 days and beyond)

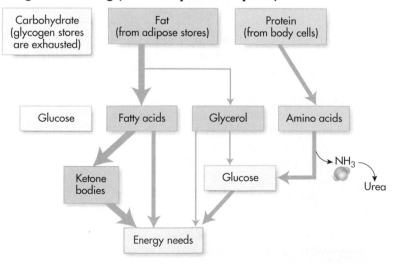

 # 9.7 Fasting and Feasting

Both fasting and feasting affect metabolism. The form of each macronutrient and the rate at which it is used vary when the calorie supplies are insufficient or exceed needs.

Fasting

In the first few hours of a fast, the body fuels itself with stored liver glycogen and fatty acids from adipose tissue. As the fast progresses, body fat continues to be broken down and liver glycogen becomes exhausted. Although most cells can use fatty acids for energy, the nervous system and red blood cells use only glucose for energy. To provide the needed glucose, the body begins breaking down lean body tissue and converts glucogenic amino acids, via gluconeogenesis, to glucose (Fig. 9-22).[6, 7] During the first few days of a fast, body protein is broken down rapidly—in fact, it supplies about 90% of needed glucose, with the remaining 10% coming from glycerol. At this rate of breakdown, body protein would be quickly depleted and death would occur within 2 to 3 weeks. (Death would occur regardless of the amount of body fat a person has because fatty acids cannot be used for gluconeogenesis.) Sodium and potassium depletion also can result during fasting because these elements are drawn into the urine along with ketone bodies. Finally, blood urea levels increase because of the breakdown of protein.

Fortunately, the body undergoes a series of adaptations that prolong survival. One of these adaptations is the slowing of metabolic rate and a reduction in energy requirements. This helps slow the breakdown of lean tissue to supply amino acids for gluconeogenesis. Another adaptation allows the nervous system to use less glucose (and, hence, less body protein) and more ketone bodies. After several weeks of fasting, half or more of the nervous system's energy needs are met by ketone bodies; nonetheless, some glucose must still be supplied via the catabolism of lean body mass. When lean body mass declines by about 50% (usually within 7 to 10 weeks of total fasting), death occurs.

Feasting

The most obvious result of feasting is the accumulation of body fat. In addition, feasting increases insulin production by the pancreas, which in turn encourages the burning of glu-

Figure 9-22 Postprandial fasting encourages the use of mostly glucose, as well as some fatty acids and amino acids for energy needs. As the fast progresses, glycogen stores are depleted, which causes the rapid use of carbon skeletons of certain amino acids from body protein to produce glucose. This supplies glucose to glucose-dependent cells, such as red blood cells. Long-term fasting leads to reduced breakdown of body protein and increased use of adipose stores, which are used to produce ketones. Ketones can provide a significant proportion of the fuel required by glucose-dependent cells, thereby sparing body protein and prolonging life. Note that the thickness of the arrows in the figures conveys the relative use of each energy source during the stages of fasting.

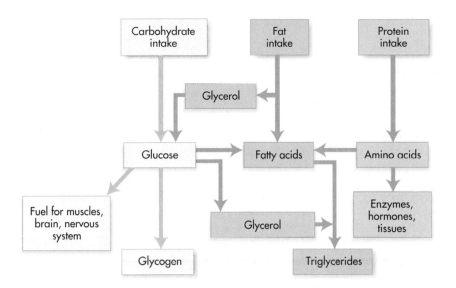

Figure 9-23 Feasting encourages glycogen and triglyceride synthesis and storage and allows amino acids to participate in the synthesis of body proteins. Minimal synthesis of fatty acids using glucose or carbon skeletons of amino acids occurs unless intake is quite excessive in comparison with overall energy needs.

cose for energy, as well as the synthesis of glycogen and, to a lesser extent, protein and fat (Fig. 9-23).[6, 11]

Fat consumed in excess of need goes immediately into storage in adipose cells.[2] Compared with the conversion of carbohydrate and protein, relatively little energy is required to convert dietary fat into body fat. Therefore, high-fat, high-energy diets promote the accumulation of body fat.

Protein consumed in excess of need—contrary to popular belief—does not promote muscle development. Some of the excess protein can reside in amino acid pools in the body, but the amount is not significant. Amino acids left over in the body after a large meal can be used to synthesize fatty acids, but this is typically of minor importance in humans.[11] The process of storing amino acids as fat requires ATP and the B-vitamins biotin, niacin, and pantothenic acid.[2] The energy cost of converting dietary protein to body fat is higher than it is for the conversion of dietary fat to body fat.

Carbohydrate consumed in excess of need is used first to maximize glycogen stores. Once glycogen stores are filled, carbohydrate consumption stimulates the use of carbohydrate as fuel and the storage of excess amounts as body fat. This then lessens the need for any fat catabolism. However, the pathway for storing carbohydrate as body fat is not very active in humans.[11] In addition, it requires the B-vitamins biotin, niacin, and pantothenic acid, and it is energetically expensive to convert carbohydrate to body fat (Table 9-2). Anyone who consumes more calories from any of the energy-yielding nutrients than what the body can expend will gain weight.

▶ Fasting encourages the following:

Glycogen breakdown

Fat breakdown

Gluconeogenesis

Synthesis of ketone bodies

▶ Feasting encourages the following:

Glycogen synthesis

Protein synthesis

Fat synthesis

Urea synthesis

Feasting especially encourages the synthesis of glycogen and the storage of fat.

Table 9-2 Metabolism of ATP-Yielding Compounds

Nutrient	Yields Glucose?	Yields Amino Acids for Body Proteins?	Yields Fat for Adipose Tissue Stores?	Energy Cost of Conversion to Adipose Tissue Stores
Carbohydrate (glucose)	Yes	No	Yes, but is inefficient	High
Triglycerides				
Fatty acids	No	No	Yes	Minimal
Glycerol	Yes, but not a major pathway	No	Yes	High
Protein (amino acids)	Yes	Yes	Yes, but is inefficient	High
Alcohol	No	No	Yes	High

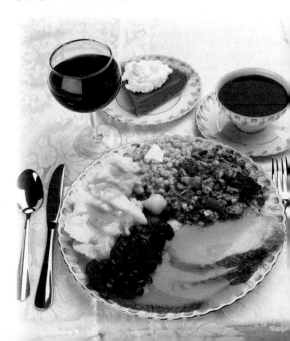

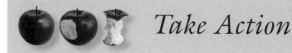

Take Action

Weight Loss and Metabolism

A friend is very overweight and describes to you his method of weight loss. He fasted completely for 1 week and is now on a strict diet of 400 to 600 kcal/day under a physician's supervision. The food energy comes from a liquid formula, which he drinks for breakfast. He skips lunch and eats a small dinner of 3 ounces of protein, ½ cup of vegetables, 1 cup of fruit, and 2 starch items (a small potato, a piece of bread, etc.). He has lost approximately 25 lb in 12 weeks.

Based on your knowledge of energy metabolism, answer the following questions he poses.

1. During the fasting stage, what were the likely sources of energy for the body's cells? What metabolic adaptations occurred to provide glucose for the nervous system?

2. When he began eating 400 to 600 kcal/day, how did the metabolic processes in the body most likely change from the fasting state?

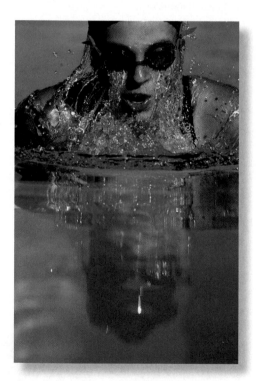

The energy used to perform physical activity is in the form of ATP, which can be supplied by carbohydrate, fat, or protein. The proportion supplied by each macronutrient depends on length of time after eating and type and intensity of exercise.

The pathways for the synthesis of fat from excess carbohydrate or protein intake, called lipogenesis, are found primarily in the cytosol of liver cells. Synthesis involves a series of steps that link the acetyl-CoA formed from either glucose or amino acids into a 16-carbon saturated fatty acid, palmitic acid. Insulin increases the activity of a key enzyme—fatty acid synthase—used in the pathway. Palmitic acid can later be lengthened to an 18- or 20-carbon chain either in the cytosol or in the mitochondria.[1] Ultimately, the fatty acids and glycerol (produced during glycolysis from glyceraldehyde 3-phosphate) are used to synthesize triglycerides, which are subsequently delivered by very-low-density lipoproteins (see Chapter 6) via the bloodstream to adipose tissues for storage.

Knowledge Check

1. In the first few hours of a fast, what is the primary fuel for the body?
2. What adaptations occur that help slow the breakdown of lean body mass during prolonged fasting?
3. What happens to excess amounts of ingested fat, protein, and carbohydrate?

CASE STUDY FOLLOW-UP

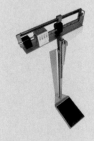

A very low carbohydrate diet that produces ketones is not the best way to lose body fat. Although body weight may decline, the large production of ketones means that the body is not capable of oxidizing fatty acids and therefore excretes them in the urine. The body is using protein (amino acids) as a fuel source for the brain and nervous system. This loss of amino acids, especially from muscle, is part of the loss of body mass. A better weight-loss program would be to reduce total calories to create a calorie deficit and maintain an exercise or fitness program.

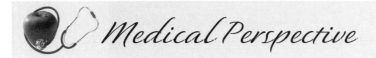

Medical Perspective

Inborn Errors of Metabolism

Some people lack a specific enzyme to perform normal metabolic functions—they are said to have an inborn error of metabolism. The metabolic pathway in which the enzyme is supposed to participate does not function normally. Typically, this causes alternative metabolic products to be formed, some of which are toxic to the body.

Inborn errors of metabolism occur when a person inherits a defective gene coding for a specific enzyme from both parents. Both parents are likely to be carriers of the defective gene—that is, they have 1 healthy gene and 1 defective gene for the enzyme in their chromosomes. When each parent donates the defective form of the gene to the offspring, the offspring has 2 defective copies of the gene and therefore little or no activity of the enzyme that the gene normally would produce. If a person has a defective gene, he or she produces a defective protein based on the instructions contained in that defective gene. It also is possible that 1 or both parents have the disease and are not simply carriers. Generally, however, individuals who have an inborn error of metabolism are advised to see a genetic counselor to assess the risk of passing on the inborn error of metabolism to their offspring (see chapter 1).

The following are some characteristics of inborn errors of metabolism.[12]

- They appear soon after birth. Such a disorder is suspected when otherwise physically well children develop a loss of appetite, vomiting, dehydration, physical weakness, or developmental delays soon after birth. For some of these conditions, infants are screened for the potential to have a specific inborn error of metabolism.

- They are very specific, involving only 1 or a few enzymes. These enzymes usually participate in catabolic pathways (in which compounds are degraded).

- No cure is possible, but typically the disorders can be controlled. The type of control depends on the inborn error—control might include reducing intake of the substance they are unable to metabolize normally, taking pharmacological doses of vitamins, and replacing a compound that cannot be synthesized.[13]

Some of the most common inborn errors of metabolism are phenylketonuria (PKU), galactosemia, and glycogen storage disease. A number of other, very rare inborn errors of metabolism involve various amino acids, fatty acids, and the sugars fructose and sucrose. Typically, in large hospitals and in state health departments, physicians, nurses, and registered dietitians can help affected persons and their families cope with these and other inborn errors of metabolism.[12]

Newborn Screening

Newborn screening is the process of testing newborn babies for treatable genetic errors of metabolism.[14] Newborn screening

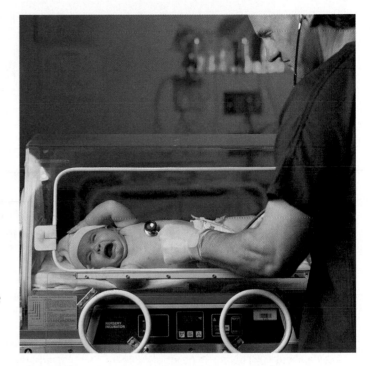

An infant who does not develop normally may have an inborn error of metabolism. A physician should investigate this possibility.

is a public health program that provides early identification and follow-up for the treatment of infants with genetic and metabolic disorders. There are no national mandates to test newborns. Currently, each state determines which newborn screening tests are required—as a result, required tests vary widely among states. In 2004, the American College of Medical Genetics recommended that all states test for 29 conditions—only 15 states and the District of Columbia require all of these tests. To learn more, visit www.marchofdimes.com/298_834.asp.

Phenylketonuria (PKU)

PKU is estimated to occur in about 1 per 13,500 to 1 in 19,000 births.[14] Most carriers can be detected with a simple blood test. People of Irish descent are especially affected.[15] Today, most infants in the United States are diagnosed within a few days of life because all states require them to be tested for this inborn error of metabolism.[16]

The majority of PKU cases occur because the enzyme phenylalanine hydroxylase does not function efficiently in the liver. Normally, phenylalanine hydroxylase converts the amino acid phenylalanine into the amino acid tyrosine. If this reaction does not take place, phenylalanine accumulates in the blood and tyrosine is deficient. If not corrected within 30 days of birth, this phenylalanine buildup leads to the production of toxic

Medical Perspective continued

phenylalanine by-products, such as phenylpyruvic acid, which then can lead to severe, irreversible mental retardation.[17]

Normal: Phenylalanine $\xrightarrow{\text{Sufficient phenylalanine hydroxylase activity}}$ Tyrosine

PKU: Phenylalanine $\xrightarrow{\text{Reduced phenylalanine hydroxylase activity}}$ Phenylpyruvic acid
Phenyllactic acid
Other related products

As soon as they are diagnosed, infants are started on a phenylalanine-restricted diet.[18] Recall that phenylalanine is an essential amino acid, which means that even someone with PKU has to obtain phenylalanine from his or her diet; however, the amount of phenylalanine consumed needs to be controlled carefully to prevent toxic amounts from building up.[17, 19] During infancy, nutritional needs can change frequently, so these infants are monitored continually through blood phenylalanine testing.

Starting in infancy, special formulas are used to provide nutrients for individuals with PKU. Because infants have high protein needs, satisfying protein requirements—without also having high intakes of phenylalanine—is impossible without these specially prepared formulas. For infants, formulas are designed to provide about 90% of protein needs and 80% of energy needs. Human milk or regular infant formula then can be used to make up the difference and supply small amounts of phenylalanine.[12]

Later in life, foods can be used to make up the difference, especially foods low in phenylalanine. Fruits and vegetables are naturally low in phenylalanine, and breads and cereals have a moderate amount. Dairy products, eggs, meats, nuts, and cheeses are very high in amino acids, including phenylalanine, and, so, are not allowed in the diet. Foods and beverages that contain the alternative sweetener aspartame also are not allowed because aspartame contains phenylalanine (see Chapter 5). Older children and adults can use a formula (such as Phenyl-Free®) that is very low in phenylalanine, which allows the person to consume more foods but limits phenylalanine intake. Overall, the majority of the person's nutrient intake throughout life will come from a special formula.

Ideally, the low-phenylalanine diet is followed for life.[20] At one time, health-care professionals thought it was appropriate to end the diet after age 6 years because brain development was complete. However, it is now known that discontinuing this diet leads to decreased intelligence and behavior problems, such as aggressiveness, hyperactivity, and decreased attention span.[12]

If a woman with PKU has abandoned the diet, she needs to return to it at least 6 months before becoming pregnant.[21] Otherwise, the fetus—even though it does not have PKU—will be exposed to a high blood phenylalanine level and related toxic products from the mother. This can result in miscarriage or birth defects. All pregnancies for women with PKU are high-risk and require close medical supervision.

Children with PKU must restrict their intake of high-protein foods, such as milk and meat.

▶ A new drug, sapropterin dihydrochloride, 6-R-L-erythro-5,6,7,8-tetrahydrobiopterin (BH4), which has been used in Europe to treat mild forms of PKU, has been approved for use in the U.S. Although the drug cannot cure PKU, it appears to lower blood levels of phenylalanine.[25, 26]

Galactosemia

Galactosemia is a rare genetic disease—the most common form occurs in 1 in 47,000 births.[14, 22] It is more common in those of Italian and Irish descent.[23] In galactosemia, 2 specific enzyme defects lead to a reduction in the metabolism of the monosaccharide galactose to glucose (a third form is very rare). Galactose then builds up in the bloodstream, which can lead to very serious bacterial infections, mental retardation, and cataracts in the eyes.

An infant with galactosemia typically develops vomiting after a few days of consuming infant formula or breast milk. Both contain much galactose as part of the milk sugar lactose. This child is then switched to a soy formula. In addition, all dairy products and other lactose-containing products (butter, milk solids), organ meats, and some fruits and vegetables must be avoided. Strict label reading also is important for controlling the disease because lactose can be found in a variety of products. Even in well-controlled cases, slight mental retardation (e.g., speech delays) and cataracts occur.

Glycogen Storage Disease

Glycogen storage disease is a group of diseases that occurs in 1 in 60,000 births. In glycogen storage disease, the liver is unable to convert glycogen to glucose. There are a number of possible enzyme defects along the pathway from glycogen to glucose. The most common forms cause poor physical growth, low blood glucose, and liver enlargement. Low blood glucose results because liver glycogen breakdown is typically used to maintain blood glucose between meals (see Chapter 5). People with glycogen storage disease typically have to consume frequent meals in order to regulate blood glucose. They also consume raw cornstarch between meals because it is slowly digested and helps maintain steady blood glucose. Careful monitoring of blood glucose is very important for these people, so that low blood glucose levels can be detected and treated quickly.[12]

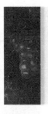

Knowledge Check

1. What are the characteristics of inborn errors of metabolism?
2. What is the cause of PKU?
3. What dietary restrictions must those with galactosemia observe?

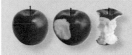

Take Action

Newborn Screening in Your State

There are no mandatory national newborn screening standards in the U.S., even though dozens of metabolic diseases are detectable by newborn screening tests. Each state has developed its own newborn screening program for infants born there. To learn which metabolism disorder tests are required for newborns in your state, visit this website: genes-r-us.uthscsa.edu. Why don't all states require the same tests? Once a newborn has tested positive, what resources and professionals can help the family manage the disorder?

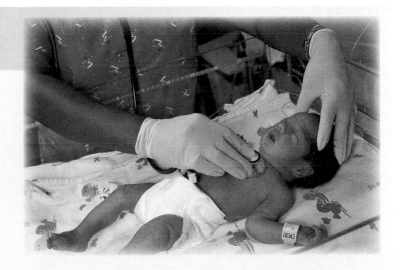

Summary

9.1 *Metabolism* refers to the entire network of chemical processes involved in maintaining life. It encompasses all the sequences of chemical reactions that occur in the body. Some of these biochemical reactions enable us to release and use energy from carbohydrate, fat, protein, and alcohol. Metabolism is the sum total of all anabolic and catabolic reactions. A molecule of ATP consists of the organic compound adenosine (comprised of the nucleotide adenine and the sugar ribose) bound to 3 phosphate groups. ATP is the energy currency for the body. As ATP is broken down to ADP plus P_i, energy is released from the broken bond. Every cell contains catabolic pathways, which release energy to allow ADP to combine with P_i to form ATP. The synthesis of ATP from ADP and P_i involves the transfer of energy from energy-yielding compounds (carbohydrate, fat, protein, and alcohol). This process uses oxidation-reduction reactions, in which electrons (along with hydrogen ions) are transferred in a series of reactions from energy-yielding compounds eventually to oxygen. The process of cellular respiration oxidizes (removes electrons) to obtain energy

(ATP). Oxygen is the final electron acceptor. When oxygen is readily available, cellular respiration may be aerobic. When oxygen is not present, anaerobic pathways are used.

9.2 Glucose metabolism begins with glycolysis, which literally means "breaking down glucose." Glycolysis has 2 roles: to break down carbohydrates to generate energy and to provide building blocks for synthesizing other needed compounds. During glycolysis, glucose passes through several steps, which convert it to 2 units of a 3-carbon compound called pyruvate. Glycolysis nets 2 ATP. Pyruvate passes from the cytosol into the mitochondria, where the enzyme pyruvate dehydrogenase converts pyruvate into the compound acetyl-CoA in a process called a transition reaction. Acetyl-CoA molecules enter the citric acid cycle, which is a series of chemical reactions that convert carbons in the acetyl group to carbon dioxide while harvesting energy to produce ATP. In the citric acid cycle, acetyl-CoA undergoes many metabolic conversions, which result in the production of GTP, ATP, NADH, and FADH$_2$. NADH and FADH$_2$ enter the electron transport chain, which passes electrons along a series of electron carriers. As electrons pass from one carrier to the next, small amounts of energy are released. This metabolic process is called oxidative phosphorylation, and it is the pathway in which energy derived from glycolysis, the transition reaction, and the citric acid cycle is transferred to ADP + P$_i$ to form ATP and water.

9.3 The first step in generating energy from a fatty acid is to cleave the carbons, 2 at a time, and convert the 2-carbon fragments to acetyl-CoA. The process of converting a free fatty acid to multiple acetyl-CoA molecules is called beta-oxidation, because it begins with the beta carbon, which is the second carbon on a fatty acid chain. Fatty acids can be oxidized for energy but cannot be converted into glucose. During low carbohydrate intakes and uncontrolled diabetes, more acetyl-CoA is produced in the liver than can be metabolized. This excess acetyl-CoA is synthesized into ketone bodies, which can be used as an energy source by other tissues or excreted in the urine and breath.

9.4 Protein metabolism begins after proteins are degraded into amino acids. To use an amino acid for fuel, cells must first deaminate them (remove the amino group, NH$_2$). Resulting carbon skeletons mostly enter the citric acid cycle. Some carbon skeletons also yield acetyl-CoA or pyruvate. The process of generating glucose from amino acids is called gluconeogenesis. Acetyl-CoA molecules cannot participate in gluconeogenesis; thus, ketogenic amino acids cannot participate in gluconeogenesis.

9.5 The alcohol dehydrogenase (ADH) pathway is the main pathway for alcohol metabolism. Alcohol is converted in the cytosol to acetaldehyde by the action of the enzyme alcohol dehydrogenase and the coenzyme NAD$^+$. NAD$^+$ picks up 2 hydrogen ions and 2 electrons from the alcohol to form NADH + H$^+$ and produces the intermediate acetaldehyde. Acetaldehyde is converted to acetyl-CoA, again yielding NADH + H$^+$ with the aid of the enzyme aldehyde dehydrogenase and coenzyme A. Most of the acetyl-CoA is used to synthesize fatty acids and triglycerides, resulting in the accumulation of fat in the liver. When an individual consumes too much alcohol, a second pathway—called the microsomal ethanol oxidizing system (MEOS)—is activated to help metabolize the excess alcohol.

9.6 The liver plays the major role in regulating metabolism. Additional means of regulating metabolism involve enzymes, ATP concentrations, and minerals. Many micronutrients (thiamin, niacin, riboflavin, biotin, pantothenic acid, vitamin B-6, magnesium, iron, and copper) play important roles in the metabolic pathway.

9.7 During fasting, the body breaks down both amino acids and fats for energy. The body undergoes a series of adaptations that prolong survival. One of these adaptations is the slowing of metabolic rate and the reduction in energy requirements. This helps slow the breakdown of lean tissue to supply amino acids for gluconeogenesis. Another adaptation allows the nervous system to use less glucose and more ketone bodies. Fat consumed in excess of need goes into storage in adipose cells. Compared with the conversion of carbohydrate and protein, relatively little energy is required to convert dietary fat into body fat. Therefore, high-fat diets promote the accumulation of body fat. Inborn errors of metabolism occur when a person inherits a defective gene coding for a specific enzyme from one or both parents. Some of the most common inborn errors of metabolism are phenylketonuria (PKU), galactosemia, and glycogen storage disease. Strict diets can help those with these inborn errors of metabolism minimize many of the serious effects of these diseases.

Study Questions

1. The energy currency in the body is _____.

   a. NAD
   b. FAD
   c. TCA
   d. ATP

2. Glycolysis is a biochemical pathway that _____.

   a. breaks down glucose
   b. generates energy
   c. takes place in the cytosol
   d. all of the above

3. Glycolysis begins with_____ and ends with_____.

   a. pyruvate; water
   b. pyruvate; glucose
   c. glucose; pyruvate
   d. pyruvate; acetyl-CoA

4. When muscle tissue is exercising under anaerobic conditions, the production of _____ is important because it assures a continuous supply of NAD.

   a. glucose-6-phosphate
   b. pyruvate
   c. lactic acid
   d. glycogen

5. The net energy production of ATP via glycolysis is _____.

   a. 1 ADP
   b. 2 ATP
   c. 4 FADH
   d. 2 GTP
   e. none of the above

6. The common pathway for the oxidation of glucose and fatty acid is _____ .

   a. glycolysis
   b. the urea cycle
   c. the citric acid cycle
   d. ketosis

7. The oxidation of fatty acids occurs in the _____.

   a. cell membrane
   b. mitochondria
   c. nucleus
   d. cytosol

Match the definitions on the right with the terms on the left.

8. beta-oxidation
9. ketosis
10. electron transport chain
11. gluconeogenesis
12. glycolysis

   a. breakdown of glucose to pyruvate
   b. breakdown of fat to 2-carbon units called acetyl-CoA
   c. synthesis of glucose from non-carbohydrate sources
   d. formation of excess ketone bodies
   e. electrons transferred back and forth to make ATP

13. Metabolism is regulated by _____.

   a. hormones
   b. enzymes
   c. the energy status of the body
   d. all of the above

14. During periods of starvation, the body uses protein as a fuel source for the brain and central nervous system in a pathway called gluconeogenesis.

   a. true
   b. false

15. Insulin is _____.

   a. a coenzyme in the glycolytic pathway
   b. a cofactor needed for gluconeogenesis
   c. an anabolic hormone
   d. a catabolic hormone

Answer Key: 1-d; 2-d; 3-c; 4-c; 5-b; 6-c; 7-b; 8-b; 9-d; 10-e; 11-c; 12-a; 13-d; 14-a; 15-c

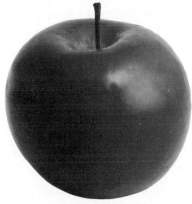

Websites

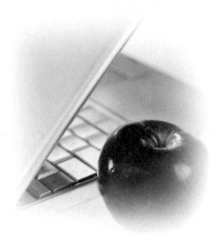

To learn more about the topics covered in this chapter, visit these websites.

Metabolic Pathways

www.johnkyrk.com/glycolysis.html

metacyc.org/

Inborn Errors of Metabolism

www.marchofdimes.com

genes-r-us.uthscsa.edu

www.nlm.nih.gov/medlineplus

www.aafp.org

References

1. Berg J and others. *Biochemistry.* 5th ed. New York: WH Freeman; 2002.

2. Gropper S and others. *Advanced nutrition and human metabolism.* 4th ed. Belmont, CA: Thomson/Wadsworth; 2005.

3. Mayes P, Bender D. The citric acid cycle: The catabolism of acetyl-CoA. In: Murray R and others, eds. *Harper's biochemistry.* 26th ed. New York: Appleton & Lange Medical Books/McGraw-Hill; 2003.

4. Mayes P, Bender D. Overview of metabolism. In: Murray R and others, eds. *Harper's biochemistry.* 26th ed. New York: Appleton & Lange Medical Books/McGraw-Hill; 2003.

5. Champe P and others. *Biochemistry.* 3rd ed. Philadelphia: Lippincott Williams & Wilkins; 2005.

6. Foster D. The role of the carnitine system in human metabolism. *Ann NY Acad Sci.* 2004;1033:1.

7. Mayes P, Botham K. Oxidation of fatty acids: Ketogenesis. In: Murray R and others, eds. *Harper's biochemistry.* 26th ed. New York: Appleton & Lange Medical Books/McGraw-Hill; 2003.

8. Trachtenbarg D. Diabetic ketoacidosis. *Am Family Phys.* 2005;71:659.

9. VanItallie T, Nufert T. Ketones: Metabolism's ugly duckling. *Nutrition Reviews.* 2003;61:327.

10. Mayes P and others. Bioenergetics. In: Murray R and others, eds. *Harper's biochemistry.* 26th ed. New York: Appleton & Lange Medical Books/McGraw-Hill: 2003.

11. Timlin M, Parks E. Temporal pattern of denovo lipogenesis in the postprandial state in healthy men. *Am J Clin Nutr.* 2005;81:35.

12. Trahms C. Medical nutrition therapy for metabolic disorders. In: Mahan L, Escott-Stump S, eds. *Krause's food, nutrition and diet therapy.* 11th ed. Philadelphia: WB Saunders; 2004.

13. Marriage B and others. Nutritional cofactor treatment in mitochondrial disorders. *J Am Diet Assoc.* 2003;103:1029.

14. Kaye C, Committee on Genetics. Newborn screening fact sheets. *Pediatrics.* 2006;118:934.

15. Woolf L. A study of the cause of the high incidence of phenylketonuria in Ireland and west Scotland. *J Irish Med Assoc.* 1976;69:398.

16. March of Dimes. Newborn screening. 2007; www.marchofdimes.com.

17. Gassio R and others. Cognitive functions in classic phenylketonuria and mild hyperphenylalanemia: Experience in paediatric population. *Dev Med Child Neurol.* 2005;47:443.

18. National Institutes of Health. Consensus Development Conference statement: Phenylketonuria: Screening and management. *Pediatrics.* 2001;108:972.

19. Acosta P and others. Nutrient intakes and physical growth of children with phenylketonuria undergoing nutrition therapy. *J Am Diet Assoc.* 2003;103:1167.

20. Ney DM and others. Dietary glycomacropeptide supports growth and reduces the concentrations of phenylalanine in plasma and brain in a murine model of phenylketonuria. *J Nutr.* 2008;138:316.

21. American Academy of Pediatrics, Genetics Committee. Maternal phenylketonuria. *Pediatrics.* 2001;107:427.

22. Ridel K and others. An updated review of the long-term neurological effects of galactosemia. *Pediatr Neurol.* 2005;33:153.

23. Murphy M and others. Genetic basis of transferase-deficient galactosemia in Ireland and the population history of the Irish Travellers. *Eur J Hum Genet.* 1999;7:549.

24. Buono MJ, Kolkhorst FW. Estimating ATP synthesis during a marathon run: A method to introduce metabolism. *Adv Physiol Educ.* 2001;25:70.

25. Thompson CA. First drug approved for treatment of phenylketonuria. *Am J Health-Sys Pharm.* 2008;65:100.

26. Michals-Matalon K. Sapropterin dihydrochloride, 6-R-L-erythro-5,6,7,8-tetrahydrobiopterin, in the treatment of phenylketonuria. *Expert Opin Invest Drugs.* 2008;17:245.

10

Energy Balance, Weight Control, and Eating Disorders

How much popcorn do you eat? Research shows that, the more you are served (even if it is stale!), the more you will eat. Learn more at mindlesseating.org.

STUDENT LEARNING OUTCOMES

After studying this chapter, you will be able to

1. Describe energy balance and uses of energy by the body.

2. Compare methods used to measure energy expenditure by the body.

3. Explain internal and external regulation of hunger, appetite, and satiety.

4. Discuss methods for assessing body composition and determining whether body weight and composition are healthy.

5. Describe the impact of genetics and environment on body weight and composition.

6. Outline the key components of programs designed to treat overweight and obesity.

7. Discuss the characteristics of fad diets.

8. Evaluate weight-loss programs to determine whether they are safe and likely to result in long-term weight loss.

9. Describe treatments for severe obesity.

10. Outline recommendations for treating underweight.

11. Describe the causes of, effects of, typical persons affected by, and treatment for anorexia nervosa, bulimia nervosa, and binge-eating disorder.

12. Explain methods for reducing the development of eating disorders, including the use of warning signs to identify early cases.

This chapter begins with some good news and some bad news. The good news is that, if you stay at a healthy body weight, you increase your chances of living a long and healthy life. The bad news is that, in the last 20 years, there has been a dramatic increase in the percentage of individuals who are obese. This problem is occurring not only in the U.S. but also in many other countries—including developing countries where Westernized dietary patterns (high-fat, high-calorie) are increasing in popularity. In 1990, no state in the U.S. had an obesity prevalence rate exceeding 14%. By 2006, obesity prevalence rates exceeded 14% in every state—and, in almost half of the states, the prevalence rate exceeded 30%.[1] Currently in North America, 2 out of 3 adults weigh more than is healthy. The current trend is not likely to be reversed without a national commitment to weight maintenance and approaches that make our social environment more favorable to maintaining a healthy weight.[2] There is a good chance that many of us will become part of those statistics if we do not pay attention to preventing significant weight gain in adulthood.[3] Despite the many health risks associated with obesity and all our efforts to lose weight, obesity rates continue to climb.[4] There is no quick cure for overweight, despite what advertisements claim. Any success comes from hard work and commitment. Unfortunately, for most people, weight-reduction efforts fizzle before they achieve a healthy weight range (Fig. 10-1).

Popular ("fad") diets are generally monotonous, ineffective, and confusing; they may even be dangerous for some population groups and individuals with health disorders. The relentless pursuit of thinness may drive some individuals to develop eating disorders, which involve severe distortions of the eating process. The safest and most logical approach to maintaining a healthy weight is to watch calorie intake, exercise regularly, and get problem eating behaviors under control.[5] Preventing excess weight gain in the first place is the most successful approach of all.[4]

Figure 10-1 Obesity trends among U.S. adults: 1990, 1998, 2006 (BMI ≥ 30, or about 30 lb overweight for 5'4" person).

Source: CDC Behavioral Risk Factor Surveillance System.

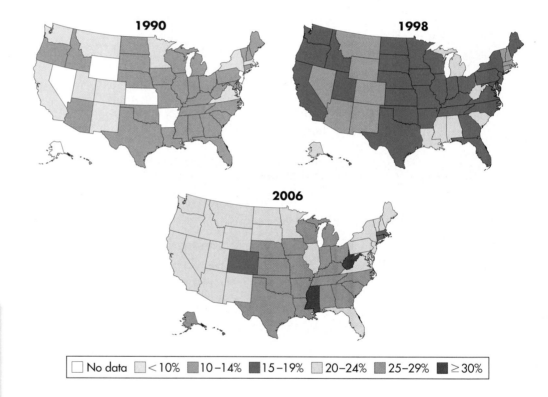

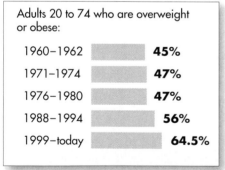

Adults 20 to 74 who are overweight or obese:

1960–1962		**45%**
1971–1974		**47%**
1976–1980		**47%**
1988–1994		**56%**
1999–today		**64.5%**

CRITICAL THINKING

A 20-year-old classmate of yours has been watching her parents and grandparents gain weight over the years. How should she explain energy balance to them?

10.1 Energy Balance

Energy balance is the relationship between energy intake and energy expenditure. When the calories consumed from food and beverages (energy intake) match the amount of energy expended, **energy equilibrium** occurs. If energy intake exceeds energy expended, the result is a **positive energy balance**. The excess energy consumed is stored, resulting in weight gain (Fig. 10-2). There are some situations in which positive energy balance is desired, such as during the growth stages of the life cycle (pregnancy, infancy, childhood, adolescence) and to restore body weight to healthy levels after losses caused by starvation, disease, or injury. However, during other times, such as adulthood, positive energy balance over time can cause body weight to climb to unhealthy levels. The process of aging itself does not cause weight gain; rather, weight

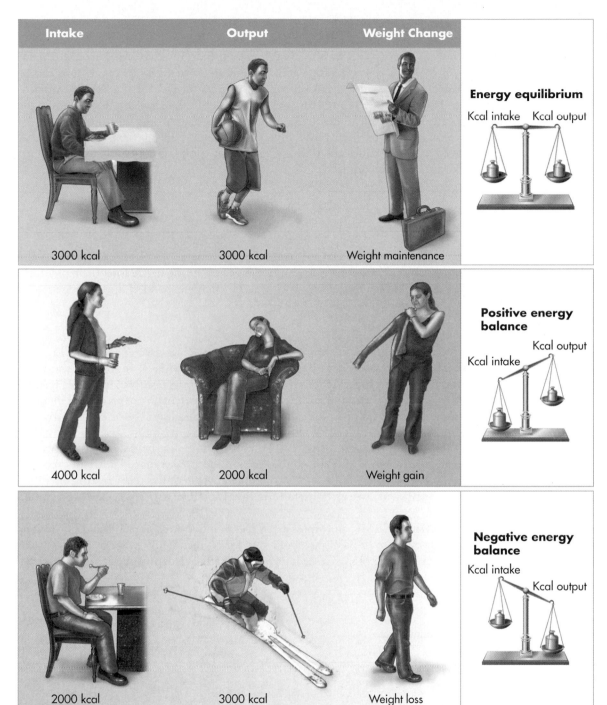

Figure 10-2 States of energy balance.

gain stems from a pattern of excess food intake coupled with limited physical activity and slower metabolism.[4]

Negative energy balance results when energy intake is less than energy expenditure. Weight loss occurs because energy stored in the body—fat and muscle—is used to make up for the shortfall in energy intake. Negative energy balance is desired in adults when body fatness exceeds healthy levels. Negative energy balance during growth stages of the life cycle generally is not recommended because it can impair normal growth.

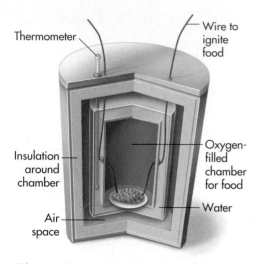

Figure 10-3 Bomb calorimeters measure calorie content by igniting and burning a dried portion of food. The burning food raises the temperature of the water surrounding the chamber holding the food. The increase in water temperature indicates the number of kilocalories in the food because 1 kilocalorie equals the amount of heat needed to raise the temperature of 1 kg of water by 1°C.

▶ When a person is resting, the following are the approximate percentages of total energy used by the body's organs.

Liver	27%	380 kcal/day
Brain	19%	265 kcal/day
Skeletal muscle	18%	250 kcal/day
Kidney	10%	140 kcal/day
Heart	7%	100 kcal/day
Other	19%	265 kcal/day

Energy Intake

The amount of energy in a food or beverage can be estimated using nutrient databases or nutrient analysis software. Calorie values in these tables and programs can be derived by directly measuring calorie content using a device called a **bomb calorimeter** (Fig. 10-3). Calorie content is most commonly calculated by determining the grams of carbohydrate, protein, and fat (and possibly alcohol) in a food and multiplying these compounds by their physiological fuel values. (Recall from Chapter 1 that the physiological fuel values are 4 kcal/g for carbohydrates and proteins, 9 kcal/g for fat, and 7 kcal/g for alcohol.)

Energy Expenditure

The body uses energy for 3 general purposes: basal metabolism; physical activity; and the digestion, absorption, and processing of ingested nutrients. A fourth, minor form of energy output, known as thermogenesis, is the energy expended during fidgeting or shivering in response to cold (Fig.10-4).[4]

Basal Metabolism

Basal metabolism (expressed as **basal metabolic rate [BMR]**) represents the minimum amount of energy expended in a fasting state (12 hours or more) to keep a resting, awake body alive in a warm, quiet environment. For a sedentary person, basal metabolism accounts for about 60 to 70% of total energy expenditure. Some of the processes involved include the beating of the heart, respiration by the lungs, and the activity of other organs, such as the liver, brain, and kidney.[4] It does not include energy expended for physical activity or the digestion, absorption, and processing of nutrients recently consumed. If the person is not fasting or completely rested, the term **resting metabolism** is used (expressed as **resting metabolic rate [RMR]**). RMR is typically 6% higher than BMR.

Both BMR and RMR are expressed as the number of calories burned per unit of time. A rough estimate of basal metabolic rate for women is 0.9 kcal/kg per hour and 1.0 kcal/kg per hour for men. To see how basal metabolism contributes to energy needs,

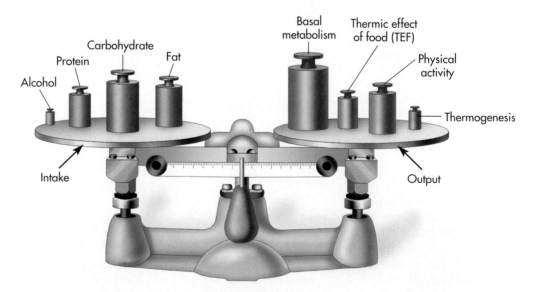

Figure 10-4 Major components of energy intake and expenditure. The size of each component shows the relative contribution of that component to energy balance. Alcohol is an additional source of energy only for those who consume it.

consider a 130-lb woman. First, knowing that there are 2.2 lb for every kg, convert her weight into metric units:

$$130 / 2.2 = 59 \text{ kg}$$

Then, using a rough estimate of the basal metabolic rate of 0.9 kcal/kg per hour for an average female, calculate her basal metabolic rate:

$$59 \times 0.9 = 53 \text{ kcal/hour}$$

Finally, use this hourly basal metabolic rate to find her basal metabolic rate for an entire day:

$$53 \times 24 = 1272 \text{ kcal/day}$$

These calculations are only an estimate of actual basal metabolism—it can vary 25 to 30% among individuals. The following factors increase basal metabolism.

- Greater muscle mass
- Larger body surface area
- Male gender (males typically have more lean body mass than females)
- Body temperature (fever or cold environmental conditions)
- Thyroid hormones (a key regulator of basal metabolism; high levels increase BMR)
- Aspects of nervous system activity (e.g., the release of stress hormones)
- Growth stages of the life cycle
- Caffeine and tobacco use (using tobacco to control body weight is not recommended because too many health risks are increased)

Of these factors, the amount of lean body mass a person has is the most important.

The factors that decrease basal metabolism include lower than normal secretions of thyroid hormones (hypothyroidism), restricted calorie intake, and loss of lean body mass. Basal metabolism decreases by about 10 to 20% (about 150 to 300 kcal/day) when calorie intake declines and the body shifts into a conservation mode. This shift helps us survive during periods of famine and starvation, but it also is a barrier to sustained weight loss during dieting that involves extremely low calorie intake.[5] Basal metabolism drops 1 to 2% for each decade past the age of 30 years as a result of the lean body mass loss that typically occurs with advancing age. However, physical activity helps maintain lean body mass and helps preserve BMR throughout adulthood.[6]

Energy for Physical Activity

Physical activity increases energy expenditure above and beyond basal energy needs by as much as 25 to 40%. In choosing to be active or inactive, we determine much of our total energy expenditure for a day. Climbing stairs rather than riding the elevator, walking rather than driving to the store, and standing in a bus rather than sitting increase physical activity and, hence, energy expenditure. The increased rate of obesity in North America is caused, in part, by our inactivity.[6]

Thermic Effect of Food

The **thermic effect of food (TEF)** is the energy the body uses to digest, absorb, transport, store, and metabolize the nutrients consumed in the diet. The TEF accounts for about 5 to 10% of the energy consumed each day. If daily energy intake were 3000 kcal, TEF would account for 150 to 300 kcal. As with other components of energy output, the total amount varies somewhat among individuals.[4] In addition, food composition influences TEF. For example, the TEF value for a protein-rich meal (20 to 30% of the energy consumed) is higher than that of a carbohydrate-rich (5 to 10%) or fat-rich (0 to 3%) meal because it takes more energy to metabolize amino acids into fat than to convert glucose into glycogen or transfer absorbed fat into adipose stores. In addition, large meals result in higher TEF values than the same amount of food eaten over many hours.[4]

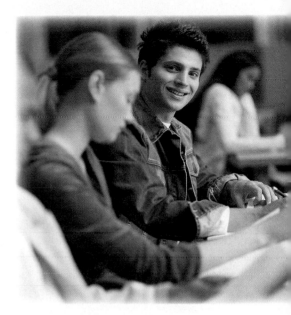

Classwork leads to mental activity, but little physical activity. Hence, energy is burned at a rate of only about 1.5 kcal per minute.

▶ The TEF of alcohol is 20%. About 90% of the energy in food can be used by the body as an energy source, whereas only 80% of the energy in alcohol can be used by the body to make energy.[48]

Adaptive Thermogenesis

Thermogenesis, the process of heat production by humans and other organisms, makes a fairly small contribution to overall energy expenditure. Thermogenesis goes by other names, such as thermoregulation and non-exercise activity thermogenesis (NEAT). Adaptive thermogenesis heat is produced when the body expends energy for non-voluntary physical activity triggered by cold conditions or overeating. Examples of non-voluntary activities include fidgeting, shivering when cold, maintaining muscle tone, and holding the body up when not lying down. Some studies show that certain people are able to resist weight gain from overeating by inducing thermogenesis, whereas others experience little thermogenesis.

Brown adipose tissue is a specialized form of fat tissue that participates in thermogenesis. The brown appearance results from the large number of capillaries it contains. It is found in small amounts in infants and hibernating animals. Brown fat contributes to thermogenesis because it releases much of the energy from energy-yielding nutrients as heat. Brown fat has a protein (uncoupling protein) that uses the food we consume to generate heat for the body instead of creating energy in the form of ATP. Adults have very little brown fat and its role in adulthood is not known. It is thought to be important mostly for thermoregulation during infancy, when brown fat accounts for as much as 5% of body weight. Hibernating animals use brown fat to generate heat during cold winter months.

Expert Perspective *from the Field*

High-Fructose Corn Syrup and Your Waistline

High-fructose corn syrup (HFCS) is a common sweetener in the U.S. food supply. Although it is called fructose, HFCS really is a combination of glucose and fructose. One of the main types is HFCS-42, which is 42% fructose, 53% glucose, and 5% other saccharides. It is used to sweeten baked goods, canned fruit, condiments, jams, jellies, and some dairy products, such as yogurt. HFCS-55, used to sweeten beverages, ice cream, and frozen desserts, is 55% fructose, 42% glucose, and 3% other saccharides. The very sweet HFCS-90 contains 90% fructose and is used in tiny amounts to sweeten some low-sugar foods.[7]

HFCS is made by milling corn to produce cornstarch. Then, in a series of steps, enzymes are used to break the long chains of glucose in the cornstarch into glucose. Finally, other enzymes are used to convert some of the glucose into fructose.

Food manufacturers use HFCS instead of table sugar (sucrose) because it costs less to produce—corn is more abundant in the U.S., and this crop is subsidized by the U.S. government. Another reason manufacturers favor HFCS is that it is easier to use because it is a liquid and dissolves easily. HFCS first entered the U.S. food supply in 1966 and, by 2005, the per capita availability of the sweetener was about 59 lb per year.[8] During the same time period, the per capita availability of table sugar (made from sugar cane and sugar beets) dropped to 63 lb, down from a peak of 102 lb per capita in 1972.[8]

In 2004, some respected nutrition scientists noted that the rate of HFCS use paralleled the rising rates of obesity.[9] They hypothesized that the high intakes of HFCS may be linked to excess weight gain. According to Maureen Storey, Ph.D.,* several theories have been proposed to explain how HFCS might be related to weight gain. One theory suggests that HFCS triggers a desire to eat sweet foods and beverages, which leads to excessive energy consumption. However, as Storey explains, HFCS-42 is less sweet than sucrose, and HFCS-55 has the same sweetness as sucrose. Another theory speculates that, as intake of HFCS increases and that of sucrose decreases, this change in the fructose:glucose ratio in our diets leads to adverse metabolic consequences, such as greater fat synthesis in the liver and diminished release of satiety hormones. However, the fructose:glucose ratio in the food supply has not changed.[7] Storey also notes that there is no scientific evidence that the body metabolizes HFCS and sucrose differently. A recent study found that the impacts of HFCS and sucrose on fasting plasma glucose, insulin, and the appetite-regulating hormones ghrelin and leptin were the same.[10]

Currently, scientific evidence does not support the theory that HFCS promotes weight gain to a greater extent than sucrose or any other caloric sweetener. However, since 1970 the consumption of all caloric sweeteners has increased nearly 20%, likely contributing to excessive energy intake and weight gain in many individuals.

Maureen Storey is Senior Vice President, Science Policy, American Beverage Association, and Affiliate Research Professor, Department of Nutrition and Food Science, University of Maryland.

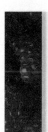

Knowledge Check

1. What percentage of total energy expenditure is spent on basal metabolism?
2. What factors increase basal metabolism?
3. How much energy is expended via the thermic effect of food?
4. What is adaptive thermogenesis?
5. What is brown fat and what function does it play in an infant?

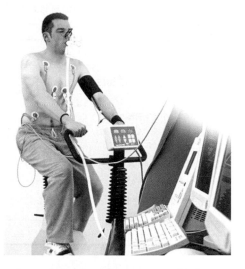

Indirect calorimetry measures oxygen intake and carbon dioxide output to determine energy expended during daily activities.

 ## 10.2 Measuring Energy Expenditure

The amount of energy a body uses can be measured by both direct and indirect calorimetry or can be estimated based on height, weight, degree of physical activity, and age.

Direct calorimetry estimates energy expenditure by measuring the amount of body heat released by a person. Direct calorimetry works because almost all the energy the body uses eventually leaves as heat. Heat release is measured by placing a person in an insulated chamber, often the size of a small bedroom, that is surrounded by a layer of water. The change in water temperature before and after the body releases heat is used to determine the amount of energy the person has expended. Recall that a calorie is related to the amount of heat required to raise the temperature of water. Few studies use direct calorimetry, mostly because it is expensive and complex to use.

Indirect calorimetry, the most commonly used method to determine energy use by the body, involves collecting expired air from an individual during a specified amount of time. This method works because a predictable relationship exists between the body's use of energy and the amount of oxygen consumed and carbon dioxide produced. The procedure to collect the air can be done in a laboratory or with a handheld device that allows the individual to be mobile and not restricted to the lab. Data tables showing energy costs of different exercises are based on information from indirect calorimetry studies.

Another approach to indirect calorimetry uses **stable isotopes** of oxygen and hydrogen. In this method, a person drinks doubly labeled water (^2H_2O and $H_2{}^{18}O$); then, his or her urine and blood samples are analyzed to examine ^2H and ^{18}O excretion. The labeled oxygen is eliminated from the body as water and carbon dioxide, whereas the labeled hydrogen is eliminated only as water. Subtracting hydrogen losses from oxygen losses provides a measure of carbon dioxide output. This stable isotope method is quite accurate but also very expensive. It is the basis for determining Estimated Energy Requirements for humans.

Estimated Energy Requirements (EERs) are measurements based on formulas, developed by the Food and Nutrition Board, that can estimate energy needs using a person's weight, height, gender, age, and physical activity level. The following are the formulas for adults (remember to do the multiplication and division before the addition and subtraction).

Men 19 Years and Older

$$EER = 662 - (9.53 \times AGE) + PA \times (15.91 \times WT + 539.6 \times HT)$$

Women 19 Years and Older

$$EER = 354 - (6.91 \times AGE) + PA \times (9.36 \times WT + 726 \times HT)$$

The variables in the formulas correspond to the following:

EER = Estimated Energy Requirement
AGE = Age in years
 PA = Physical Activity Estimate (see the accompanying table)
WT = Weight in kg (lb ÷ 2.2)
HT = Height in meters (inches ÷ 39.4)

stable isotope Specific, non-radioactive form of a chemical element. It differs from atoms of other forms (isotopes) of the same element in the number of neutrons in its nucleus. *Stable* means that the isotope is not radioactive.

Children	Sedentary ⟶	Active
2–3 years	1000 ⟶	1400

Females	Sedentary ⟶	Active
4–8 years	1200 ⟶	1800
9–13	1600 ⟶	2200
14–18	1800 ⟶	2400
19–30	2000 ⟶	2400
31–50	1800 ⟶	2200
51+	1600 ⟶	2200

Males	Sedentary ⟶	Active
4–8 years	1200 ⟶	2000
9–13	1800 ⟶	2600
14–18	2200 ⟶	3200
19–30	2400 ⟶	3000
31–50	2200 ⟶	3000
51+	2000 ⟶	2800

Energy expenditure estimates from MyPyramid.

▶ Resting Energy Expenditure (REE) is the amount of calories needed during a non-active period. It is used to estimate calorie needs in clinical situations. The Harris-Benedict Equation can be used to estimate resting energy expenditure:

Men
REE = 66.5 + (13.8 × WT) + (5 × HT) −(6.8 × AGE)

Women
REE = 655.1 + (9.6 × WT) + (1.9 × HT) − (4.7 × AGE)

The variables in the formulas correspond to the following:

REE = Resting energy expenditure
WT = Weight in kg (lb ÷ 2.2)
 HT = Height in cm (inches × 2.54)
AGE = Age in years

Physical Activity (PA) Estimates

Activity Level	PA (Men)	PA (Women)
Sedentary (e.g., no exercise)	1.00	1.00
Low activity (e.g., walks the equivalent of 2 miles per day at 3 to 4 mph)	1.11	1.12
Active (e.g., walks the equivalent of 7 miles per day at 3 to 4 mph)	1.25	1.27
Very active (e.g., walks the equivalent of 17 miles per day at 3 to 4 mph)	1.48	1.45

Consider a man who is 25 years old, is 5 feet 9 inches (1.75 meters) tall and 154 lb (70 kg), and has an active lifestyle. His EER is

$$\text{EER} = 662 - (9.53 \times 25) + 1.25 \times (15.91 \times 70 + 539.6 \times 1.75) = 2997$$

Remember, EERs are only estimates—many other factors, such as genetics and hormones, can affect actual energy needs.

A simple method of tracking energy expenditure, and thus energy needs, is to use the forms in Appendix M. Begin listing all the activities performed (including sleep) in a 24-hour period and recording the number of minutes spent in each activity; the total should be 1440 minutes (24 hours). Next, record the energy cost for each activity in kcal per minute, following the directions in Appendix M. Multiply the energy cost by the minutes to determine the energy expended for each activity. Finally, total all the kcal values to calculate your estimated energy expenditure for the day.

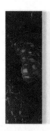

Knowledge Check

1. How do direct and indirect calorimetry differ?
2. Why is it possible to use direct calorimetry and indirect calorimetry to measure energy expenditure?
3. What is your Estimated Energy Requirement?

CASE STUDY

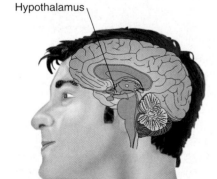

Christy is a college freshman. She is excited about college and has good support from her family and friends to help her succeed. Her greatest concerns this first semester are to establish good study habits and time management, to get along with her new roommate, and to avoid the "Freshman 15." For the last 3 months, all she has heard about is the amount of weight that she will gain in her freshman year. She has never had a weight problem, but in high school she was on the track team and played basketball. She is not quite sure what she should be eating, so for now she has a salad for lunch and dinner and skips breakfast because she has an 8 A.M. class. She gets very hungry at around 10 P.M. and her roommate has been having pizza delivered to the dorm—she cannot resist having several slices. What advice would you give Christy? With these eating habits, is the Freshman 15 likely to happen to Christy? Why can't she resist eating pizza?

Hypothalamus

The hypothalamus is the site in the brain that does most of the processing of signals regarding food intake.

 10.3 Eating Behavior Regulation

Two drives influence our desire to eat and thus take in food: hunger and appetite (Fig. 10-5). **Hunger**, the physiological drive to find and eat food, is controlled primarily by internal body mechanisms, such as organs, hormones, hormonelike factors, and the nervous system.[11] **Appetite**, the psychological drive to eat, is affected mostly by external factors that encourage us to eat, such as social custom, time of day, mood (e.g., feeling sad or happy), memories of pleasant tastes, and the sight of a tempting dessert.

Internal and external signals that drive hunger and appetite generally operate simultaneously and lead us to decide whether to reject or eat a food. For example, external signals can cause cephalic phase responses by the body—that is, saliva flows and digestive hormones and insulin are released in response to seeing, smelling, and initially tasting food. These physiological responses encourage eating and prepare the body for the meal.[11]

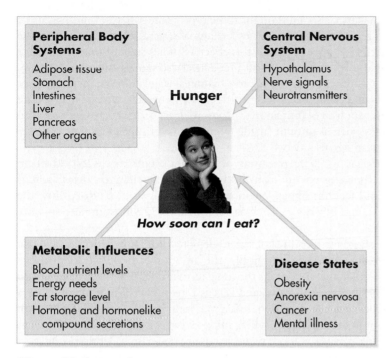

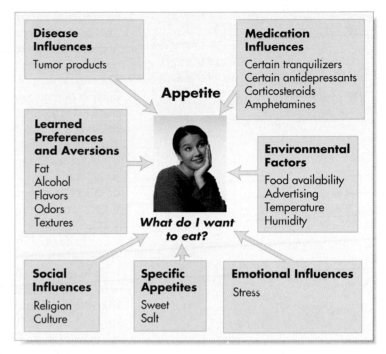

Figure 10-5 Although some factors have an impact on both hunger and appetite, internal factors are mainly responsible for hunger, whereas external factors primarily influence appetite. These factors combine to play a role in the complex and interrelated processes that help determine when, what, and how much we eat.

Although hunger and appetite are closely intertwined, they don't always coincide. Almost everyone has encountered a mouthwatering dessert and devoured it, even on a full stomach. Alternately, there are times when we are hungry but have no appetite for the food being served. Where food is ample, appetite—not hunger—mostly triggers eating.

Fulfilling either or both drives by eating sufficient food normally brings a state of **satiety**, in which we feel satisfaction and no longer have the drive to eat. The hypothalamus, a portion of the brain, is the key integration site for the regulation of satiety. The hypothalamus communicates with the endocrine and nervous systems and integrates many internal cues, including blood glucose levels, hormone secretions, and **sympathetic nervous system** activity, that both inhibit and encourage food intake.[11] If these internal signals stimulate the satiety centers of the hypothalamus, we stop eating. If they stimulate the feeding centers in the hypothalamus, we eat more.[11] Surgery and some cancers and chemicals can harm the hypothalamus. Damage to the satiety center causes humans to become obese, whereas damage to the feeding center inhibits eating and eventually leads to weight loss.[11]

Feelings of satiety are elicited first by the sensory aspects of food (e.g., food flavor and smell, the size and shape of the portion served, and dietary variety) and the knowledge that a meal has been eaten (Fig. 10-6). Chewing also seems to contribute to satiety, in part linked to the release of the neurotransmitter histamine, which affects the satiety center in the brain. Next, the stomach and intestines expand (called **gastrointestinal distension**) as they fill with digesting food and drink, which further contributes to satiety. Low-energy-dense foods (those high in water and/or fiber) promote satiety because they expand the stomach and intestines to a greater extent than lighter-weight foods (e.g., oils and snack foods).

Finally, the effects of digestion, absorption, and metabolism promote satiety. For example, the secretion of hormones, such as cholecystokinin, glucagon-like peptide-1 (GLP-1), and peptide YY_{3-36}, during digestion helps shut off hunger. **Nutrient**

We have an innate taste for sweet and acquire a taste for fat.

sympathetic nervous system Part of the nervous system that regulates involuntary vital functions, including the activity of the heart muscle, smooth muscle, and adrenal glands.

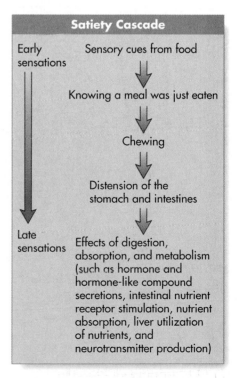

Figure 10-6 Factors affecting satiety.

receptors in the small intestines also are thought to help promote satiety. (Infusing fats or carbohydrates directly in the small intestine causes feelings of satiety, whereas infusing these nutrients directly into the blood does not cause this effect.) Studies suggest that an apolipoprotein on chylomicrons absorbed into the blood after a meal also signals satiety to the brain. The metabolism of certain nutrients, especially carbohydrates, is linked to an increased production of serotonin (a brain neurotransmitter), which causes us to feel calm and may reduce our food intake.[11] The metabolism of protein may promote short-term satiety by decreasing the secretion of hormones, such as **ghrelin** (made by the stomach), that stimulate eating.[12] Nutrient use in the liver also signals satiety.

Several hours after eating, concentrations of macronutrients in the blood begin to fall and the body starts using energy from body stores. This change causes feelings of satiety to diminish, and feeding signals begin to dominate again.[11] **Endorphins**, the body's natural painkillers, and hormones, such as cortisol and ghrelin, stimulate appetite and increase food intake.

In addition to the short-term control of satiety depicted in Figure 10-6, food intake also is affected by body composition—specifically, the amount of body fat. **Leptin** is a protein made by adipose tissue that influences the long-term regulation of fat mass. Leptin was isolated from the obesity gene (ob gene) and acts as a hormone. When the ob gene is functioning normally, leptin is made. When there is a mutation in the ob gene, leptin is not made in sufficient quantities. Theoretically, when adipose tissue stores are increasing, leptin signals satiety. Conversely, when adipose tissue stores are decreasing, leptin production drops and the desire to eat is enhanced. Because treating people with leptin doesn't cause significant weight loss, experts suggest that, instead of protecting against obesity, leptin may be more important for signaling low body fat stores and setting in motion adaptations that promote energy conservation, delaying the effects of starvation.[11]

As you can see, the regulation of food intake and satiety is complex and involves body cells (brain, adipose tissue, stomach, intestine, liver, and other organs), hormones (e.g., cholecystokinin and ghrelin), neurotransmitters (e.g., serotonin), dietary components, and social customs. This system is not perfect, however; your body weight can increase (or decrease) over time if you are not careful to balance your energy intake with your energy output.

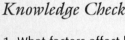

Knowledge Check

1. What factors affect hunger?
2. What factors affect appetite?
3. What factors affect satiety?
4. How do body fat stores affect food intake?

10.4 Estimating Body Weight and Composition

Over the last 50 years, the use of the weight-for-height tables issued by the Metropolitan Life Insurance Company has been the typical method for determining if a person's weight was healthy. These tables considered gender and frame size, predicting the weight range at a specific height that was associated with the greatest longevity. The latest table (issued in 1983) and methods for determining frame size can be found in Appendix G.

Most of the weight-for-height tables came from studies of large populations. When applied to the population, they provide a good estimate of weights associated with health and longevity (Fig. 10-7). However, these tables did not necessarily refer directly to an individual's health status. As a result, in recent years the focus has shifted from using weight-for-height tables to considering the components of body weight (e.g., body fat and lean) and their relative proportions because of the increased health risks associated

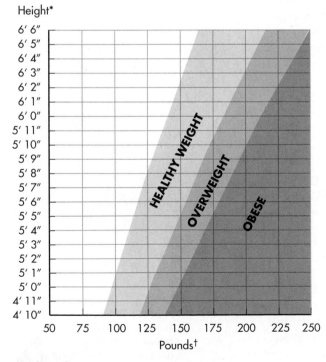

*Without shoes.
†Without clothes. The higher weights apply to people with more muscle and bone, such as many men.

Figure 10-7 Height-weight table based on BMI.

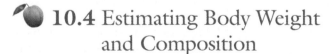

with excess body fatness. Instead of just assessing body weight, experts now recommend evaluating total amount of body fat, the location of body fat, and the presence or absence of weight-related medical problems.[5]

Body Mass Index

Currently, body mass index (BMI) is the preferred weight-for-height standard because it is most closely related to body fat content (Fig. 10-8).[4] BMI is convenient to use because it is easier to measure height and weight than body fat and because BMI values apply to both men and women. Table 10-1 lists the BMI for

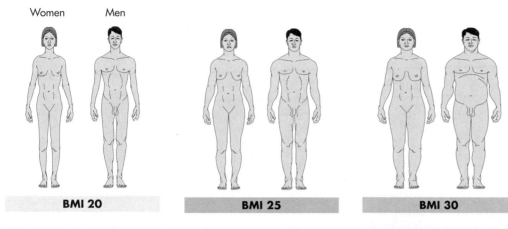

Women   Men

BMI 20   BMI 25   BMI 30

Figure 10-8 Examples of body shapes associated with different BMI values.

Table 10-1 Body Weight in Pounds According to Height and Body Mass Index (BMI)

Height (Inches)	Healthy BMI						Overweight BMI					Obese BMI		
	19	20	21	22	23	24	25	26	27	28	29	30	35	40
	Body Weight (Pounds)													
58	91	96	100	105	110	115	119	124	129	134	138	143	167	191
59	94	99	104	109	114	119	124	128	133	138	143	148	173	198
60	97	102	107	112	118	123	128	133	138	143	148	153	179	204
61	100	106	111	116	122	127	132	137	143	148	153	158	185	211
62	104	109	115	120	126	131	136	142	147	153	158	164	191	218
63	107	113	118	124	130	135	141	146	152	158	163	169	197	225
64	110	116	122	128	134	140	145	151	157	163	169	174	204	232
65	114	120	126	132	138	144	150	156	162	168	174	180	210	240
66	118	124	130	136	142	148	155	161	167	173	179	186	216	247
67	121	127	134	140	146	153	159	166	172	178	185	191	223	255
68	125	131	138	144	151	158	164	171	177	184	190	197	230	262
69	128	135	142	149	155	162	169	176	182	189	196	203	236	270
70	132	139	146	153	160	167	174	181	188	195	202	207	243	278
71	136	143	150	157	165	172	179	186	193	200	208	215	250	286
72	140	147	154	162	169	177	184	191	199	206	213	221	258	294
73	144	151	159	166	174	182	189	197	204	212	219	227	265	302
74	148	155	163	171	179	186	194	202	210	218	225	233	272	311
75	152	160	168	176	184	192	200	208	216	224	232	240	279	319
76	156	164	172	180	189	197	205	213	221	230	238	246	287	328

Each entry gives the body weight in pounds for a person of a given height and BMI (kg/m²). Pounds have been rounded off. To use the table, find the appropriate height in the far left column. Move across the row to a weight. The number at the top of the column is the BMI for the height and weight.

► One BMI unit equals about 6 to 7 lb.

► *Healthy weight* is currently the preferred term to use for weight recommendations. Older terms, such as *ideal weight* and *desirable weight,* are no longer used in medical literature, although you still may hear them used in clinical practice.

Pounds per Inch Shortcut for Estimating Healthy Body Weight

Women: Start with 100 lb; then add 5 lb for each inch of height above 5 feet.

Men: Start with 106 lb; then add 6 lb for each inch of height above 5 feet.

The weight estimate is given a ±10% range.

Example: A 6-foot-tall man's healthy weight is 178 lb (106 + [12 × 6 = 178]).

The 10% range is about 18 lb (178 × 10%).

His healthy weight range = 160 to 196 (178 ± 18).

various heights and weights. Either of the following equations can be used to calculate BMI.

$$\frac{\text{Body weight (in kg)}}{\text{Height}^2 \text{ (in meters)}} \quad \text{or} \quad \frac{\text{Body weight (in lb)} \times 703}{\text{Height}^2 \text{ (in inches)}}$$

A healthy weight-for-height is a BMI ranging from 18.5 to 24.9. Health risks from excess weight may begin when the BMI is 25 or more. When interpreting BMI, it is important to remember that any weight-for-height standard is a crude measure of body fat—a BMI of 25 to 29.9 is a marker of overweight, not necessarily a marker of overfat. Even agreed-upon standards for BMI are not appropriate for everyone; they do not apply to children, teens, frail older adults, and pregnant and lactating women. Many men (especially athletes) have a BMI greater than 25 because of extra muscle tissue. Adults less than 5 feet tall may have high BMIs but are not overweight or overfat. For this reason, BMI alone should not be used to diagnose overweight or obesity. Still, overfat and overweight conditions generally appear together.

Measuring Body Fat Content

Body fat can range from 2 to 70% of body weight. Desirable amounts of body fat are about 8 to 24% of body weight for men and 21 to 35% for women. Men with over 24% body fat and women with over about 35% body fat are considered obese. Women need more body fat because some "sex-specific" fat is associated with reproductive functions. This fat is normal and factored into calculations. The farther body fatness rises above desirable levels, the greater the health risks are likely to be (Table 10-2).

To measure body fat content accurately using typical methods, both body weight and body volume must be measured. Body weight is easy to measure. Of the typical methods used to estimate body volume, **underwater weighing** is one of the most accurate (2 to 3% error margin).[13] This technique determines body volume by measuring body weight when under

Table 10-2 Obesity-Related Health Conditions
Surgical risk
Pulmonary disease and sleep disorders
Type 2 diabetes
Hypertension
Cardiovascular disease (e.g., coronary heart disease and stroke)
Bone and joint disorders (including gout)
Gallstones
Skin disorders
Various cancers, such as kidney, gallbladder, colon and rectum, and uterus (women) and prostate gland (men)
Shorter stature (in some cases of obesity)
Pregnancy risks
Reduced physical agility and increased risk of accidents and falls
Menstrual irregularities and infertility
Vision problems
Premature death
Infections
Liver damage and eventual failure
Erectile dysfunction in men

The greater the degree of obesity, the more likely and the more serious these health problems generally become. They are much more likely to appear among people who have excess upper-body fat distribution and/or are greater than twice healthy body weight.

water and body weight in air and entering these values into a mathematical formula that accounts for the differences in the relative densities of fat tissue and lean tissue (Fig. 10-9). **Air displacement**, another method for determining body volume, measures the space a person takes up inside a small chamber, such as the BodPod® (Fig. 10-10). This method also has a 2 to 3% error margin and is an accurate alternative to underwater weighing.[14]

Once body weight and body volume are known, body density and body fat can be calculated:

$$\text{Body density} = \frac{\text{Body weight}}{\text{Body volume}} \qquad \text{\% body fat} = (495 \,/\, \text{Body density}) - 450$$

For example, if the person in the underwater weighing tank in Figure 10-9 has a body density of 1.06 g/cm³, he has 17% body fat ([495 / 1.06] − 450 = 17).

▶ Another method to assess body fat is to measure total-body electrical conductance (TOBEC) when placed in an electromagnetic field. Still another method exposes the bicep muscle to a beam of near-infrared light and assesses interactions of the light beam with fat and lean tissues. This inexpensive, flashlight-size device can quickly estimate body composition; however, this method is not very accurate.

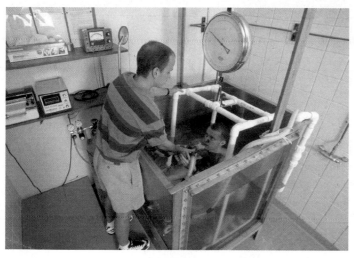

Figure 10-9 During underwater weighing, the person exhales as much air as possible and then holds his or her breath and bends over at the waist. When the person is totally submerged, underwater weight is recorded. Body volume is calculated by entering this value and weight in air into a formula.

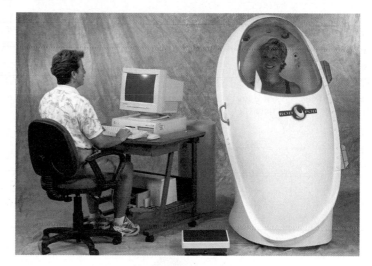

Figure 10-10 A BodPod® determines body volume by measuring the volume of air displaced when a person sits in a sealed chamber for a few minutes.

Skinfold thickness is a common anthropometric method to estimate total body fat content. Technicians use calipers to measure the fat layer directly under the skin at multiple sites and then enter those values into a mathematical formula (Fig. 10-11). The accuracy of this method is good (3 to 4% error margin) when performed by a trained technician.[13]

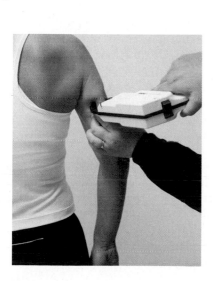

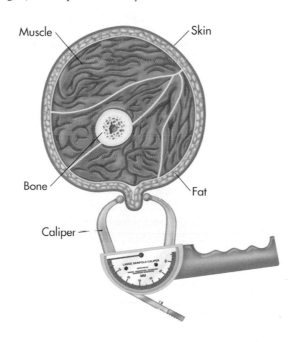

Muscle Skin

Bone Fat

Caliper

Figure 10-11 In about 10 minutes, a skilled technician can take skinfold measurements around the body, such as the arm, back, and abdomen, and use them to predict body fat content.

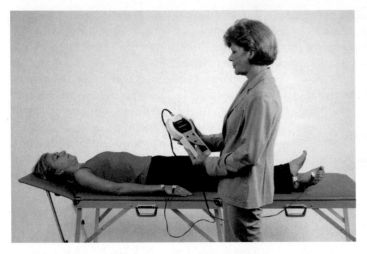

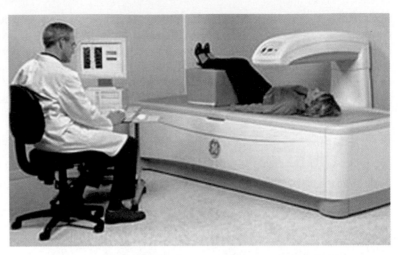

Figure 10-12 Bioelectrical impedance estimates total body fat in less than 5 minutes and is based on the principle that body fat resists the flow of electricity, since it is low in water and electrolytes. The degree of resistance to electrical flow is used to estimate body fatness.

Figure 10-13 Dual energy X-ray absorptiometry (DEXA) measures body fat by releasing small doses of radiation through the body to assess body fat and bone density. DEXA is considered the most accurate method for determining body fat.

Bioelectrical impedance estimates body fat content by sending a painless, low-energy electrical current through the body. Researchers surmise that adipose tissue resists electrical flow more than lean tissue does because adipose tissue contains less electrolytes and water than lean tissue. Thus, greater electrical resistance is associated with more adipose tissue. Electrical resistance measurements can be used to estimate total body fat (3 to 4% error margin) if the individual has prepared by having normal body hydration, resting for 12 hours, fasting for 4 hours, and not drinking alcohol for 48 hours before the test (Fig. 10-12).

Dual energy X-ray absorptiometry (DEXA) is considered the most accurate way to determine body fat (1 to 4% error margin), but the equipment is very expensive and not widely available. The usual whole-body scan requires about 5 to 20 minutes and the dose of radiation is less than a chest X-ray. This method can estimate body fat, fat-free soft tissue, and bone minerals. Thus, obesity, osteoporosis, and other health conditions can be investigated using DEXA (Fig. 10-13).

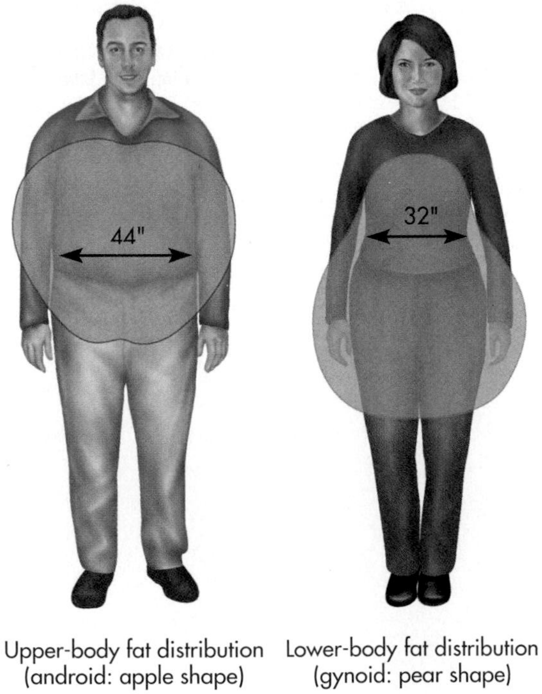

Assessing Body Fat Distribution

Some people store fat in upper-body areas. Others accumulate fat lower on the body. Excess fat in either place generally presents health risks, but each storage space also has its unique risks. Upper-body (android) obesity is more often related to cardiovascular disease, hypertension, and type 2 diabetes.[15] Instead of emptying fat directly into general circulation like other adipose cells, abdominal adipose cells release fat directly to the liver by way of the portal vein. This direct delivery to the liver likely interferes with the liver's ability to clear insulin and alters the liver's lipoprotein metabolism. Abdominal adipose cells also make substances that increase inflammation, insulin resistance, blood clotting, and blood vessel constriction. All these changes can lead to long-term health problems.

High blood testosterone (primarily a male hormone) levels apparently encourage upper-body fat storage, as does a diet with a high glycemic load, alcohol intake, and smoking. This characteristic male pattern of fat storage appears in an apple shape (large abdomen [potbelly] and thinner buttocks and thighs). Upper-body obesity is assessed by simply measuring the waist at the narrowest point just above the navel when relaxed. A waist circumference more than 40 inches (102 cm) in men and more than 35 inches (88 cm) in women indicates upper-body obesity (Fig. 10-14).[4]

Upper-body fat distribution
(android: apple shape)

Lower-body fat distribution
(gynoid: pear shape)

Figure 10-14 Body fat stored primarily in the upper-body (android) form brings higher risks of ill health associated with obesity than does lower-body (gynoid) fat. The woman's waist circumference of 32 inches and the man's waist circumference of 44 inches indicate that the man has upper-body fat distribution but the woman does not, based on a cutoff of 35 inches for women and 40 inches for men.

Estrogen and progesterone (primarily female hormones) encourage the storage of fat in the lower body. The small abdomen and much larger buttocks and thighs give a pearlike appearance. After menopause, blood estrogen levels fall, encouraging upper-body fat distribution in women.

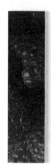

Knowledge Check

1. What is body mass index and how is it calculated?
2. When determining if a person's weight is healthy, what factors should be considered?
3. What are 3 techniques used to assess body fat?
4. How is body fat distribution used to assess health risks?
5. Which body shape is at the greatest risk of health problems?

▶ To determine if body weight is healthy, consider these factors:

- Weight
- Body composition
- Body fat distribution
- Age and physical development
- Health status
- Family history of obesity and weight-related diseases
- Personal feelings about one's body weight

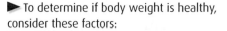

10.5 Factors Affecting Body Weight and Composition

Observations indicate that a child with no obese parent has only a 10% chance of becoming obese. When a child has 1 obese parent, that risk rises to 40%; when both parents are obese, it soars to 80%. This section explores whether this increasing risk is due to nature or nurture.

Role of Genetics

Studies of **identical twins** provide some insight into the contribution of nature (or genetics) to body weight. Even when identical twins are raised apart, they tend to show similar weight-gain patterns, both in overall weight and in body fat distribution. Nurture—eating habits and nutrition, which vary between twins who are raised apart— seems to have less to do with weight-gain patterns than nature does.[4]

Research suggests that genes account for up to 40 to 70% of weight differences between people. The genes may be those that determine body type, metabolic rate, and the factors that affect hunger and satiety. For example, basal metabolism increases as body surface increases, and therefore those who inherited genes that cause them to grow tall use more energy than shorter people, even at rest. As a result, tall people appear to have an inherently easier time maintaining healthy body weight. Some individuals are thought to have a genetic predisposition to obesity because they inherit a "thrifty metabolism"— one that uses energy frugally. This metabolism enables them to store fat readily and use less energy to perform tasks than a typical individual. In earlier times when food supplies were scarce, a thrifty metabolism would have been a safeguard against starvation. Now, with the abundant food supply available in Westernized countries, people with a thrifty metabolism need to engage in physical activity and make wise food choices to prevent storing excess amounts of fat. If you think you are prone to weight gain, you may have inherited a thrifty metabolism.

The **set-point theory** proposes that humans have a genetically predetermined body weight or body fat content, which the body closely regulates. It is not known what cells control this set point or how it actually functions in weight regulation. There is evidence, however, that mechanisms exist that help regulate weight. For example, some research suggests that the hypothalamus monitors the amount of body fat and tries to keep that amount constant over time. Recall from earlier in the chapter that the hormone leptin forms a communication link between adipose cells and the brain, which allows for some weight regulation.[11]

identical twins Two offspring that develop from a single ovum and sperm and, consequently, have the same genetic makeup.

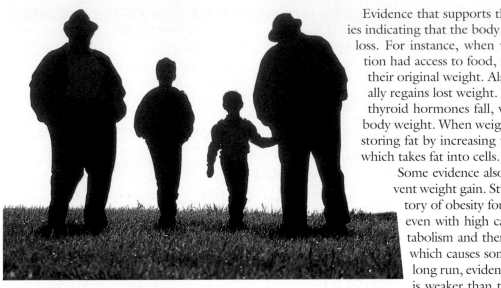

Does the difference in body fat between the grandfathers and the grandsons arise from nature, from nurture, or both?

Evidence that supports the set-point theory includes numerous studies indicating that the body tries to maintain its weight and resist weight loss. For instance, when volunteers who lost weight through starvation had access to food, they tended to eat in such a way as to regain their original weight. Also, after an illness is resolved, a person generally regains lost weight. When energy intake is reduced, secretions of thyroid hormones fall, which slows basal metabolism and conserves body weight. When weight is lost, the body becomes more efficient at storing fat by increasing the activity of the enzyme lipoprotein lipase, which takes fat into cells.

Some evidence also supports the idea that a set point helps prevent weight gain. Studies in the 1960s using prisoners with no history of obesity found it was hard for some men to gain weight, even with high calorie intakes. If a person overeats, basal metabolism and thermogenesis tend to increase in the short run, which causes some resistance to weight gain. However, in the long run, evidence that the set point helps us resist weight gain is weaker than the evidence that the set point helps us resist weight loss. When a person gains weight and stays at that weight for a while, the body tends to establish a new set point.

Opponents of the set-point theory argue that weight does not remain constant throughout adulthood—the average person gains weight slowly, at least until old age. In addition, if an individual is placed in a different social, emotional, or physical environment, weight can be altered and maintained at markedly higher or lower levels. These arguments suggest that humans, rather than having a set point determined by genetics or number of adipose cells, actually settle into a particular stable weight based on their circumstances, often referred to as a "settling point."

Role of Environment

Some researchers argue that body weight similarities among family members stem more from learned behaviors than from genetic similarities. Even couples and friends (who generally have no genetic link) may behave similarly toward food and eventually assume similar degrees of leanness or fatness.[16] The effects of environment are supported by the fact that our gene pool has not changed much in the last 50 years, but the ranks of obese people recently have grown in what the U.S. Centers for Disease Control and Prevention describes as epidemic proportions.

Environmental factors have important effects on what we eat. These factors may define when eating is appropriate, what is preferable to eat, and how much food should be eaten. As you recall from Chapter 1 (Fig. 1-5), our food choices are affected by numerous environmental factors, including food availability and preferences, food marketing, social networks, culture, education, lifestyle, health concerns, and income—all of which can affect calorie intake and weight gain. For example, those with limited incomes tend to have a greater risk of obesity. People who experience significant emotional stress, are members of a cultural or ethnic group that prefers higher body weight, have a social network of overweight friends, or get insufficient sleep are more likely to carry excess body fat. These patterns suggest the important role of nurture in determining body weight and composition.

Genetic and Environmental Synergy

Even though our genetic backgrounds have a strong influence on body weight and composition, genes are not destiny—both nature and nurture are involved (Table 10-3). Hereditary factors interact with environmental factors to determine actual body weight and composition. Even with a genetic potential for leanness, it is possible for a person who over-

Student life is often full of physical activity. This is not necessarily true for a person's later working life; hence, weight gain is a strong possibility.

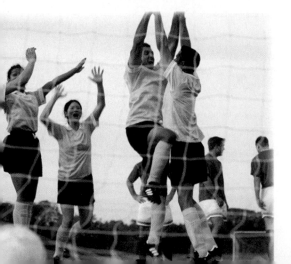

Table 10-3 Factors That Encourage Excess Body Fat Storage and Obesity

Factors	How They Promote Fat Storage
Aging	Adults tend to gain weight as they age due to the slowing of basal metabolism and increasingly sedentary lifestyles.
Female gender	Women naturally have greater fat stores than men. Women may not lose all weight gained in pregnancy. At menopause, abdominal fat deposition is favored.
High-calorie diet	Excess energy intake, binge eating, and preference for high energy density foods favor weight gain.
Sedentary lifestyle	A low or decreasing amount of physical activity ("couch potato") favors weight gain.
Weight history	Overweight children and teens have an increased risk of being overweight in adulthood.
Social and behavioral factors	Lower socioeconomic status, overweight friends and family, a cultural/ethnic group that prefers higher body weight, a lifestyle that discourages healthy meals and adequate exercise, easy availability of inexpensive high-calorie food, excessive television viewing, smoking cessation, lack of adequate sleep, emotional stress, and frequently eaten meals away from home are linked with increased fat storage.
Certain medications	Certain medications stimulate appetite, causing food intake to increase.
Geographic location	Regional differences, such as high-fat diets and sedentary lifestyles in the Midwest and areas of the South, lead to different rates of obesity in different places.
Genetic characteristics	These affect basal metabolic rate, the thermic effect of food, adaptive thermogenesis, the efficiency of storing body fat, the relative proportion of fat and carbohydrate used by the body, and possibly increased hunger sensations linked to the activity of various brain chemicals.

eats to gain excess fat. Conversely, an individual genetically predisposed to obesity can avoid excess fat storage with a healthy diet and sufficient amounts of regular physical activity.

Diseases and Disorders

Body weight and fatness can be affected by certain diseases, hormonal abnormalities, rare genetic disorders, and psychological disturbances. For instance, cancer, AIDS, hyperthyroidism, **Marfan syndrome,** and anorexia nervosa tend to cause a person to have limited fat stores. A very small percentage of obesity cases are caused by brain tumors, ovarian cysts, hypothyroidism, and congenital syndromes, such as **Prader-Willi syndrome**.

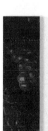

Knowledge Check

1. What evidence supports the role of genetics in determining body weight?
2. What evidence supports the role of the environment in determining body weight?
3. Why is it likely that both genetics and the environment determine body weight?

Marfan syndrome Genetic disorder affecting muscles and skeleton, characterized by tallness, long arms, and little subcutaneous fat. Some medical historians speculate that Abraham Lincoln suffered from Marfan syndrome.

Prader-Willi syndrome Genetic disorder characterized by shortness, mental retardation, and uncontrolled appetite, caused by a dysfunction of the nervous system, leading to extreme obesity.

Weight-Control Objectives from *Healthy People 2010*

· Increase by 40% the proportion of adults who are at a healthy weight (BMI between 18.5 and 25).
· Reduce by 50% the proportion of adults who are obese (BMI of 30 or more).
· Reduce by 50% the proportion of children and adolescents who are overweight or obese.

 ## 10.6 Treatment of Overweight and Obesity

The treatment of overweight and obesity should be considered similar to the treatment of any chronic disease: it requires long-term lifestyle changes.[5] Too often, however, people view a "diet" as something they go on temporarily and, once the weight is lost, they revert to their old dietary habits and physical activity routines. It is mostly for this reason that so many people regain lost weight (called weight cycling). Instead, overweight and

Figure 10-15 Characteristics of a sound weight-loss diet. The body makes numerous physiological adjustments during times of underfeeding or overfeeding that resist weight change. This compensation is most pronounced during times of underfeeding and is why slow, steady weight loss is advocated.

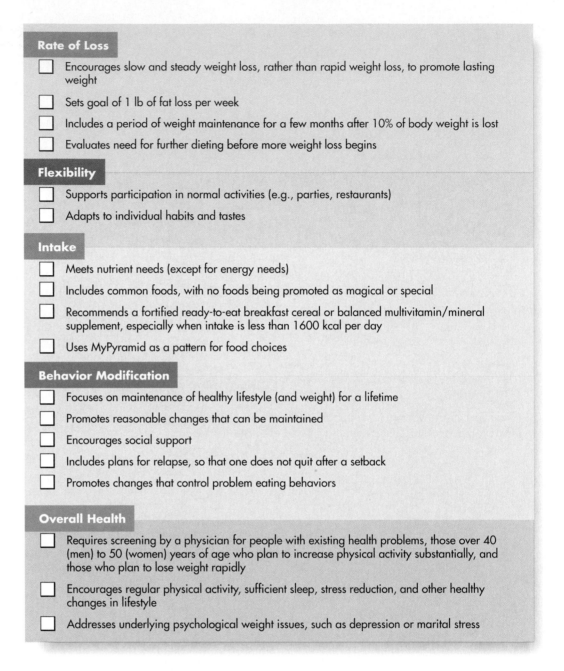

Rate of Loss

☐ Encourages slow and steady weight loss, rather than rapid weight loss, to promote lasting weight

☐ Sets goal of 1 lb of fat loss per week

☐ Includes a period of weight maintenance for a few months after 10% of body weight is lost

☐ Evaluates need for further dieting before more weight loss begins

Flexibility

☐ Supports participation in normal activities (e.g., parties, restaurants)

☐ Adapts to individual habits and tastes

Intake

☐ Meets nutrient needs (except for energy needs)

☐ Includes common foods, with no foods being promoted as magical or special

☐ Recommends a fortified ready-to-eat breakfast cereal or balanced multivitamin/mineral supplement, especially when intake is less than 1600 kcal per day

☐ Uses MyPyramid as a pattern for food choices

Behavior Modification

☐ Focuses on maintenance of healthy lifestyle (and weight) for a lifetime

☐ Promotes reasonable changes that can be maintained

☐ Encourages social support

☐ Includes plans for relapse, so that one does not quit after a setback

☐ Promotes changes that control problem eating behaviors

Overall Health

☐ Requires screening by a physician for people with existing health problems, those over 40 (men) to 50 (women) years of age who plan to increase physical activity substantially, and those who plan to lose weight rapidly

☐ Encourages regular physical activity, sufficient sleep, stress reduction, and other healthy changes in lifestyle

☐ Addresses underlying psychological weight issues, such as depression or marital stress

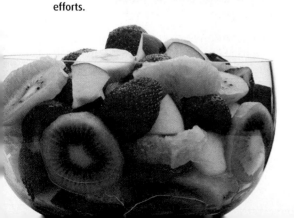

Foods, such as fruit, that are nutrient dense and have low energy density help weight-control efforts.

obese (as well as underweight) people should emphasize healthy, active lifestyles with lifelong dietary modifications (Fig. 10-15)—if started early, these modifications also can help prevent obesity.[17]

A sound weight-loss program should include 3 key components:[6, 18, 19]

1. Control of energy intake
2. Regular physical activity
3. Control of problem behaviors

A 1-sided approach that focuses only on restricting energy intake is a difficult plan of action. Instead, adding physical activity and the control of problem behaviors will contribute to success in weight loss. Accepting that these changes must be maintained for a lifetime improves the likelihood that lost weight will not be regained (Fig. 10-16).

A weight-loss program should be considered successful only when the subjects involved in the process remain at or close to their lower weights. Only about 5% of people who follow commercial diet programs actually lose weight and then remain close to that weight. Typically, one-third of the weight lost during dieting is regained within a year

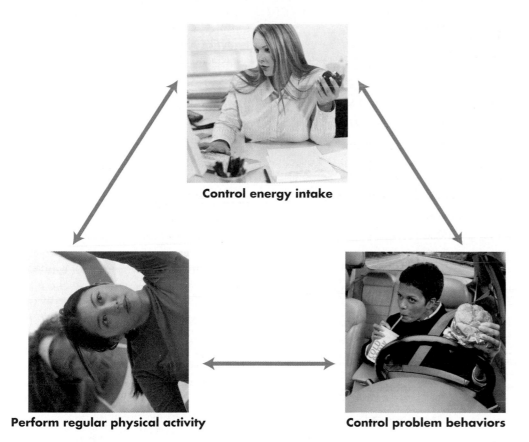

Control energy intake

Perform regular physical activity

Control problem behaviors

Figure 10-16 The key to weight loss and maintenance can be thought of as a triangle, in which the 3 corners consist of controlling energy intake, performing regular physical activity, and controlling problem behaviors. The 3 corners of the triangle support each other—without 1 corner, the triangle becomes incomplete.

▶ As you read brochures, articles, or research reports about specific diet plans, look beyond the weight loss promoted by the diet's advocate to see if the reported weight loss was maintained. If the weight maintenance aspect is missing, then the program is not successful.

after the diet ends, and almost all weight lost is regained within 3 to 5 years. Some programs have success rates higher than 5%, as do some people who simply lose weight on their own without enrolling in a supervised plan. Overall, however, the statistics are grim. Currently, only the surgical approaches to obesity treatment routinely show success in maintaining the weight loss in most people.

Because lost weight is frequently regained, many dieters try a variety of weight-loss diets. The negative health consequences associated with this weight cycling are an increased risk of upper-body fat deposition, discouragement, diminished self-esteem, and possibly a decline in high-density lipoprotein (HDL) cholesterol and immune system function. Nevertheless, experts still encourage obese people to attempt weight loss, with a strong focus on maintaining that lower weight.

Control of Energy Intake

Adipose tissue, which is mostly fat, contains about 3500 kcal/lb. Therefore, to lose 1 pound of adipose tissue per week, energy intake must be decreased by approximately 500 kcal/day or physical activity must be increased by 500 kcal per day. Alternately, a combination of both strategies can be used.[4] A goal of losing 1 lb or so of stored fat per week may require limiting energy intake to 1200 kcal/day for women and 1500 kcal/day for men. The energy allowance could be higher for very active people. Keep in mind that, in our very sedentary society, decreasing energy intake is a vital component of weight loss.

To reduce energy intake, some experts suggest consuming less fat (especially saturated fat and *trans* fat), whereas others suggest consuming less carbohydrate, especially from refined (high glycemic load) carbohydrate sources. Protein intakes in excess of what is typically needed by adults are also sometimes used as a weight-loss strategy (especially plant protein sources).[20] All these approaches can be used simultaneously. It currently appears that low energy density (low-fat, high-fiber) approaches are the most successful in

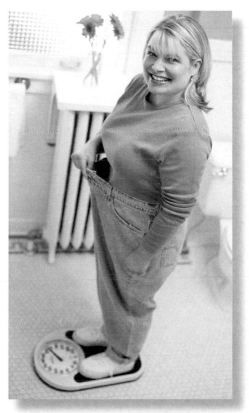

Slow, steady weight loss is one of the characteristics of a sound weight-loss program.

Table 10-4 Saving Calories: Ideas for Getting Started

Save	140 kcal	by choosing	3 oz lean beef	instead of	3 oz well-marbled beef
Save	175 kcal	by choosing	½ broiled chicken	instead of	½ batter-fried chicken
Save	210 kcal	by choosing	3 oz lean roast beef	instead of	½ cup beef stroganoff
Save	65 kcal	by choosing	½ cup boiled potatoes	instead of	½ cup fried potatoes
Save	140 kcal	by choosing	1 cup raw vegetables	instead of	½ cup potato salad
Save	150 kcal	by choosing	2 tbsp low-kcal salad dressing	instead of	2 tbsp regular salad dressing
Save	310 kcal	by choosing	1 apple	instead of	1 slice apple pie
Save	150 kcal	by choosing	1 English muffin	instead of	1 Danish pastry
Save	60 kcal	by choosing	1 cup cornflakes	instead of	1 cup sugar-coated cornflakes
Save	45 kcal	by choosing	1 cup 1% milk	instead of	1 cup whole milk
Save	150 kcal	by choosing	6 oz wine cooler made with sparkling water	instead of	6 oz gin and tonic
Save	150 kcal	by choosing	1 cup plain popcorn	instead of	1 oz potato chips
Save	185 kcal	by choosing	1 slice angel food cake	instead of	1 slice white iced cake
Save	150 kcal	by choosing	12 oz sugar-free soft drink	instead of	12 oz regular soft drink
Save	140 kcal	by choosing	12 oz light beer	instead of	12 oz regular beer

long-term studies. There is no long-term evidence for the effectiveness of the other approaches.[21]

The success of low-energy-density diets may be because foods low in energy density provide bigger portions for a given number of calories. Water is the dietary component that has the biggest impact on the energy density of foods; water adds weight but no calories and therefore decreases energy density. Increasing the water content of recipes (e.g., by adding vegetables) helps reduce energy intake and enhance satiety. A surprising finding in recent years is that people tend to eat a consistent weight or volume of food over a day or two. Thus, when foods contain fewer calories per gram, people consume less energy but still report feeling just as full and satisfied. Using energy density as a guide to food selection helps individuals consume foods that health professionals recommend—fruits, vegetables, legumes, low-fat dairy products, and whole grains.[22]

Overall, it is best to consider healthy eating a lifestyle change, rather than simply a weight-loss plan. Healthy eating choices that bring calories under control start with eating smaller portions and using MyPyramid as a pattern for daily intake. Many people often underestimate portion size, so measuring cups and a food weighing scale can help them learn appropriate portion sizes. Reading Nutrition Facts panels also can help individuals find low-energy-density foods. Learning to identify lower-calorie versions of favorites also is helpful (Table 10-4). Note that liquids do not stimulate satiety mechanisms as strongly as solid foods; thus, experts advise choosing beverages that have few or no calories. Another method is to become aware of calorie and nutrient intake by writing down food intake for 24 hours, calculating energy intake by using nutrient analysis software, and then adjusting future food choices as needed.

▶ Meal replacement formulas to replace a meal or snack are appropriate to use once or twice a day, if one desires. These are not a magic bullet for weight loss, but they have been shown to help some people control calorie intake.

Regular Physical Activity

Regular physical activity is very important for everyone, especially people who are trying to lose weight or maintain a lower body weight.[6] Obviously, more energy is burned during physical activity than at rest. Even expending only 100 to 300 extra kcal/day above and beyond normal daily activity, while controlling energy intake, can lead to a steady weight loss. Physical activity also has so many other benefits, including a boost for overall self-esteem and maintenance of bone mass.

Physical activity complements any diet plan.

Table 10-5 Approximate Energy Costs of Various Activities

Activity	Kcal/kg per Hour	Activity	Kcal/kg per Hour	Activity	Kcal/kg per Hour
Aerobics—heavy	8.0	Dressing/showering	1.6	Running or jogging (10 mph)	13.2
Aerobics—medium	5.0	Driving	1.7	Downhill skiing (10 mph)	8.8
Aerobics—light	3.0	Eating (sitting)	1.4	Sleeping	1.2
Backpacking	9.0	Food shopping	3.6	Swimming (.25 mph)	4.4
Basketball—vigorous	10.0	Football—touch	7.0	Tennis	6.1
Cycling (5.5 mph)	3.0	Golf	3.6	Volleyball	5.1
Bowling	3.9	Horseback riding	5.1	Walking (2.5 mph)	3.0
Calisthenics—heavy	8.0	Jogging—medium	9.0	Walking (3.75 mph)	4.4
Calisthenics—light	4.0	Ice skating (10 mph)	5.8	Water skiing	7.0
Canoeing (2.5 mph)	3.3	Jogging—slow	7.0	Weight lifting—heavy	9.0
Cleaning (female)	3.7	Lying—at ease	1.3	Weight lifting—light	4.0
Cleaning (male)	3.5	Racquetball—social	8.0	Window cleaning	3.5
Cooking	2.8	Roller skating	5.1	Writing (sitting)	1.7
Cycling (13 mph)	9.7				

The values refer to total energy expenditure, including that needed to perform the physical activity plus that needed for basal metabolism, the thermic effect of food, and thermogenesis.
Example: For a 150-lb person who played tennis for 1.5 hours,
150 lb/2.2 = 68 kg
68 kg × 6.1 kcal/hr × 1.5 hr = 622 kcal expenditure

Adding any of the activities in Table 10-5 to one's lifestyle can increase energy expenditure. Duration and regular performance, rather than intensity, are the keys to success with this weight-loss approach. Another key is finding activities that are enjoyable and can be continued throughout life. There is no one activity that is better than another—for example, walking vigorously 3 miles daily can be as helpful as aerobic dancing or jogging. Activities of lighter intensity are less likely to lead to injuries, as well. Some resistance exercises, such as weight training, also should be added to increase lean body mass and, in turn, fat use (see Chapter 11). As lean muscle mass increases, so does overall metabolic rate.

Unfortunately, opportunities to expend energy in our daily lives continue to diminish as technology eliminates almost every reason to move our muscles.[2] The easiest way to increase physical activity is to make it an enjoyable part of a daily routine. To start, one might wear walking shoes and walk between classes and to and from the parking lot. Some people find wearing a pedometer helps motivate them to walk. There are also plenty of other simple ways to increase the activity of daily living, such as parking the car farther away from the shopping mall entrance or getting up to change the channels on the television.

▶ Spot-reducing by using diet and physical activity is not possible. "Problem" local fat deposits can be reduced in size, however, using lipectomy (surgical removal of fat). This procedure carries some risks and is designed to help a person lose about 4 to 8 lb per treatment.

▶ A pedometer is a low-cost device that monitors the number of steps taken. An often-stated goal for activity is to take 10,000 steps/day—typically, we take half that many or less.

Control of Problem Behaviors

Controlling energy intake and increasing physical activity also means modifying problem behaviors.[6, 18] Only the dieter can decide which behaviors derail weight-loss efforts. What events start (or stop) the action of eating or exercising? Becoming aware of these events can help dieters change their behaviors and improve habits. The following key behavior modification techniques help organize intervention strategies into manageable steps and bring problem behaviors under control.

- **Chain-breaking** breaks the link between behaviors that tend to occur together—for example, snacking on chips while watching television (Fig. 10-17).
- **Stimulus control** alters the environment to minimize the stimuli for eating—for example, storing foods out of sight and avoiding the path by the vending machines.

Positive stimulus control includes keeping low-fat snacks on hand to satisfy hunger/appetite or placing walking shoes in a convenient, visible location.

- **Cognitive restructuring** changes one's frame of mind regarding eating—for example, instead of using a difficult day as an excuse to overeat, substitute another pleasure or reward, such as a relaxing walk with a friend.
- **Contingency management** prepares one for situations that may trigger overeating (e.g., when snacks are within arm's reach at a party) or hinder physical activity (e.g., rain).
- **Self-monitoring** tracks which foods are eaten, when, why, how one feels (usually using a diary), which physical activities are completed, and body weight. Self-monitoring helps people understand more about their habits and reveals patterns—such as unconscious overeating—that may explain problem behaviors that lead to weight gain.

Controlling energy intake and boosting energy expenditure are critical for losing and maintaining lost weight. Many times, we know what we should do, but some eating and exercise behaviors keep us from reaching our goals. Table 10-6 lists steps for modifying behaviors that promote weight loss and maintenance.

Figure 10-17 Examining behavior chains helps you learn more about habits and how to control them. The earlier in the chain that you can substitute a nonfood link, the easier it is to stop the chain reaction. You could substitute a fun activity (take a walk, call a friend), a necessary activity (type a paper, clean a room, take a shower), or an urge-delaying activity (set a timer and wait 30 minutes before eating).

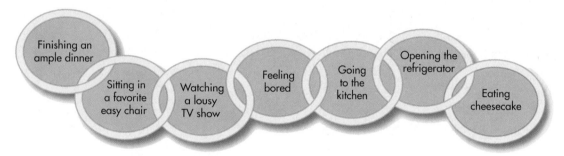

Finishing an ample dinner · Sitting in a favorite easy chair · Watching a lousy TV show · Feeling bored · Going to the kitchen · Opening the refrigerator · Eating cheesecake

Weight-Loss Maintenance

Losing excess weight might be easier than keeping it off. Several studies from the National Weight Registry have identified 4 behaviors for successful maintainers.[6, 23]

1. Eat a low-fat, high-carbohydrate diet. Individuals who have been successful at losing weight and keeping it off appear to eat about 25% of their total intake as fat and eat about 56% of their calories as carbohydrates, mainly in the form of fruits, vegetables, and whole grains.
2. Eat breakfast. About 90% of the participants in the National Weight Registry eat breakfast at least 4 days a week. By eating breakfast, the body burns more fat throughout the day and there is less tendency to overeat due to hunger.[24, 25] Most of the participants in the study eat whole-grain cereal, skim milk, and fruit for breakfast.
3. Self-monitor by regularly weighing oneself and keeping a food journal. Self-monitoring helps individuals know when weight is creeping up and signals them to pay more attention to their diets and exercise.
4. Have a physical activity plan. Participants in the National Weight Registry program exercise about 1 hour a day. A regular exercise program helps individuals maintain lost weight and feel better.

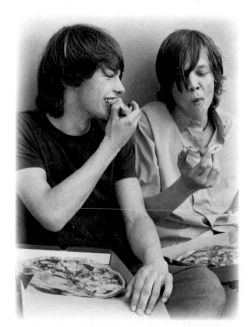

We are faced with many opportunities to overeat. It takes much perseverance to control dietary intake.

Knowledge Check

1. What are the 3 components of a sound weight-loss program?
2. What are key behavior modification techniques that can help bring problem behaviors under control?
3. What are 4 behaviors that help keep weight off?

Table 10-6 Behavior Modification Principles for Weight Loss and Control

Shopping

1. Shop for food after eating—buy nutrient-dense foods.
2. Shop from a list; limit purchases of irresistible "problem" foods. It helps to shop first for fresh foods around the perimeter of the store. Shopping online also can help control purchases of problem foods.
3. Avoid ready-to-eat foods.

Plans

1. Plan to limit food intake as needed.
2. Plan meals, snacks, and physical activity.
3. Eat meals and snacks at scheduled times; don't skip meals.
4. Exercise with a partner and schedule a time together.
5. Plan to take an exercise class at the YMCA or local recreation center.

Activities

1. Store food out of sight, preferably in the freezer, to discourage impulsive eating.
2. Eat food only in a "dining" area.
3. Keep serving dishes off the table, especially dishes of sauces and gravies.
4. Use smaller dishes, glasses, and utensils.
5. Keep exercise equipment handy and visible.

Holidays and Parties

1. Drink fewer alcoholic beverages.
2. Plan eating behavior before parties.
3. Eat a low-calorie snack before parties.
4. Practice polite ways to decline food.
5. Take opportunities to dance, swim, or engage in other physical activities at parties.

Eating Behavior

1. Put your fork down between mouthfuls and chew thoroughly before taking the next bite.
2. Leave some food on the plate.
3. Concentrate on eating; do nothing else while eating (e.g., do not watch TV).
4. Don't label certain foods "off limits;" this sets up an internal struggle that can keep you feeling deprived and defeated. Control problem foods by buying small amounts and eating a little at a time, such as 1 snack-size candy bar.
5. Limit eating out to once or twice a week.

Portion Control

1. Make substitutions, such as a regular hamburger instead of a "quarter pounder" or cucumbers instead of croutons in salads.
2. Think small. Share an entrée with another person. Order a cup of soup instead of a bowl or an appetizer in place of an entrée.
3. Use a to-go container (doggie bag). Ask your server to put half the entrée in a to-go container before bringing it to the table.
4. Become aware of portion sizes and use guides (see Chapter 2, Fig. 2-7) to judge portions.
5. Learn to recognize feelings of satiety and stop eating.

Reward

1. Plan specific non-food rewards for specific behavior (behavioral contracts).
2. Solicit help from family and friends and suggest how they can help you. Encourage family and friends to provide this help in the form of praise and non-food rewards.
3. Use self-monitoring records as basis for rewards.

Self-Monitoring

1. Keep a diet diary (note the time and place of eating, the type and amount of food eaten, who is present, and how you feel) and use it to identify problem areas.
2. Keep a physical activity diary (note which exercise is done, when, and how long) and use it to identify when more physical activity can be included.
3. Check body weight regularly.

Cognitive Restructuring

1. Avoid setting unreasonable goals.
2. Think about progress, not shortcomings.
3. Avoid imperatives, such as *always* and *never*.
4. Counter negative thoughts with positive restatements.
5. Don't get discouraged by an occasional setback. Take charge immediately—think about how progress got disrupted and make a plan for avoiding it next time.
6. Eating a particular food doesn't make a person "bad" and shouldn't lead to feelings of guilt. Change responses such as "I ate a cookie, so I'm a failure" to "I ate a cookie and enjoyed it. Next time, I'll have a piece of fruit."
7. Seek professional help before weight, dietary intake, and/or sedentary behavior get out of control.

10.7 Fad Diets

Fad diets claim miraculous weight loss or improved health—often by unhealthy or unrealistic eating plans and, perhaps, touting "miracle" foods, specific rituals (e.g., eating only fruit for breakfast or cabbage soup every day), or certain foods that people would not normally eat in large amounts. Some are so monotonous that they are hard to follow for more than a short time. Fad diets may lead to some immediate weight loss simply because daily energy intake is monitored and food choices are monotonous. Fad diets rarely lead to lasting weight loss or help retrain eating and exercise habits. Plus, some can actually cause harm (Table 10-7).

Instead of adding to the $33 billion a year Americans already spend on fad diets,[26] a better choice for losing weight and keeping it off is to follow an eating and exercise plan that you can live with every day for the rest of your life. The goal should be lifelong weight control, not immediate weight loss. How can you tell if a program or diet plan is a fad diet? The American Dietetic Association published 10 red flags to help consumers determine if the diet or nutrition information they are receiving is credible.[26]

1. Recommendations that promise a quick fix

2. Dire warnings of danger from a single product or regimen

3. Claims that sound too good to be true

4. Simplistic conclusions drawn from a complex study

5. Recommendations based on a single study

6. Dramatic statements that are refuted by reputable scientific organizations

7. Lists of "good" and "bad" foods

8. Recommendations made to help sell a product; often, testimonials are used

9. Recommendations based on studies published without peer review

10. Recommendations from studies that ignore differences among individuals or groups

Fad diets often promise rapid weight loss. Unfortunately, quick weight loss cannot consist primarily of fat because a high energy deficit is needed to lose a large amount of adipose tissue. Diets that promise a weekly weight loss of 10 to 15 lb cannot ensure that the weight loss is from adipose tissue stores alone. Subtracting enough energy from one's daily intake to lose that amount of adipose tissue simply is not possible. Lean tissue and water, rather than adipose tissue, account for the major part of the weight lost when weight loss exceeds a few pounds weekly.

Probably the cruelest characteristic of these diets is that they essentially guarantee failure for the dieter. The diets are not designed for permanent weight loss. Habits are not changed, and the food selection is so limited that the person cannot follow the diet for long. Although dieters assume they have lost fat, they have actually lost mostly muscle and other lean tissue mass. As soon as they begin eating normally again, much of the lost weight returns in a matter of weeks. The dieter appears to have failed, when actually the diet has failed. The gain and loss cycle (or "yo-yo" dieting) can cause blame, guilt, and negative health effects.

Health professionals can help dieters design and follow a healthy weight-loss plan—unfortunately, current trends suggest that people are spending more time and money on fad diets and quick fixes than on professional help.[3, 5]

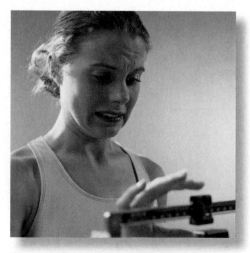

People on diets often have healthy BMIs—rather than worrying about weight loss, these individuals should focus on a healthy lifestyle that promotes weight maintenance and acceptance of one's body characteristics. For those at a healthy weight, the desire to lose weight may stem from unrealistic weight expectations (especially for women) and lack of appreciation for the natural variety in body shape and weight. Not everyone can look like a movie star, but all of us can strive for good health and a healthy lifestyle.

Table 10-7 A Summary of Popular Diet Approaches to Weight Control

Approach	Examples		Characteristics	Outcomes

Moderate energy restriction	Set-Point Diet
	Slim Chance in a Fat World
	Weight Watcher's Diet
	Mary Ellen's Help Yourself
	  Diet Plan
	Beyond Diet
	Staying Thin
	Callaway Diet
	Living without Dieting
	Volumetrics
		Lose the Last 10 Pounds
		Dieting with the Duchess
		Dieting for Dummies
		Wedding Dress Diet
		Dr. Shapiro's Picture Perfect
		  Diet
		French Women Don't Get Fat
		No Fad Diet: A Personal Plan
		  for Healthy Weight
		Sonoma Diet
			Generally, 1200 to 1800
			  kcal/day, with moderate
			  fat intake
			Reasonable balance of
			  macronutrients
			Encourage exercise
			May use behavioral approach
				Acceptable if a balanced
				multivitamin and mineral
				supplement is used and if
				physician approval is
				obtained

Restricted carbohydrate	Dr. Atkins' New Diet
	  Revolution
	Calories Don't Count
	Miracle Diet for Fast
	  Weight Loss
	Woman Doctor's Diet for
	  Women
	Doctor's Quick Weight
	  Loss Diet
	Complete Scarsdale
	  Medical Diet
		Four Day Wonder Diet
		Endocrine Control Diet
		Enter the Zone
		Protein Power
		Five-Day Miracle Diet
		Healthy for Life
		Carbohydrate Addicts Diet
		Sugar Busters
		South Beach Diet (especially
		  initial phases)
			Generally, less than 100 g of
			  carbohydrate per day
				Ketosis; reduced exercise
				capacity due to poor
				glycogen stores in the
				muscles; excessive animal
				fat and cholesterol intake;
				constipation, headaches,
				halitosis (bad breath), and
				muscle cramps

Low-fat	Rice Diet Report
	Macrobiotic Diet (some
	  versions)
	Pritikin Diet
	Eat More, Weigh Less
	35+ Diet
	20/30 Fat and Fiber
	Fat to Muscle Diet
	T-Factor Diet
	Fit or Fat
	Two-Day Diet
		Maximum Metabolism Diet
		Pasta Diet
		McDougall Plan
		Ultrafit Diet
		Stop the Insanity
		G-Index Diet
		Outsmarting the Female
		  Fat Cell
		Foods That Cause You to
		  Lose Weight
		Lean Bodies
		Turn Off the Fat Genes
			Generally, less than 20% of
			  energy intake from fat
			Limited (or elimination of)
			  animal protein sources; also
			  limited fats, nuts, and seeds
				Flatulence; possibly poor
				mineral absorption from
				excess fiber; limited food
				choices sometimes lead
				to deprivation
				Not necessarily to be
				avoided, but certain
				aspects of many of the
				plans possibly
				unacceptable

Novelty diets	Dr. Abravenel's Body Type
	  and Lifetime Nutrition Plan
	  (or his other books)
	Dr. Berger's Immune Power
	  Diet
	Fit for Life
	New Hilton Head
	  Metabolism Diet
	Beverly Hills Diet
	Dr. Debetz Champagne Diet
	Sun Sign Diet
	F-Plan Diet
	Fat Attack Plan
	Autohypnosis Diet
	Princeton Diet
	Diet Bible
		Eat to Succeed
		Underburner's Diet
		Eat to Win
		Paris Diet
		Cabbage-Soup Diet
		Eat Great, Lose Weight
		Eat Smart Think Smart
		*Scents*ational Weight Loss
		Eat Right 4 Your Type
		Greenwich Diet
		3 Season Diet
		Metabolize
		God's Diet
		Weigh Down Diet
		Paleo Diet
			Promote certain nutrients,
			  foods, or combinations of
			  foods as having unique,
			  magical, or previously
			  undiscovered qualities
				Malnutrition, no change in
				habits, which leads to
				relapse; unrealistic food
				choices lead to possible
				bingeing

Low-carbohydrate diets lead to reduced glycogen synthesis and therefore reduced amounts of water in the body (about 3 g of water are stored per gram of glycogen). As discussed in Chapter 9, a very low carbohydrate intake forces the liver to produce glucose via gluconeogenesis. The source of carbons for this glucose is mostly body proteins. (Recall also from Chapter 9 that typical fatty acids cannot form glucose.) Thus,

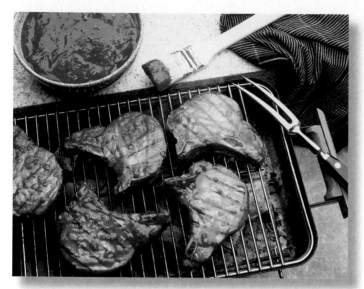

In time, very-low-carbohydrate, high-protein diets typically leave a person wanting more variety in meals, so the diets are abandoned. Dropout rates are very high on these diets.

a low-carbohydrate diet results in the loss of lean body tissue, which is about 72% water, as well as the loss of ions, such as potassium, in the urine. Because lean tissue is mostly water, dieters lose weight very rapidly, but, when a normal diet is resumed, protein tissue is rebuilt and the weight is regained.

Low-carbohydrate diets work primarily in the short run because they limit total food intake. In long-term studies, these diets have not shown an advantage over diets that simply limit energy intake in general.[27]

When you see a new diet advertisement, look first to see how much carbohydrate it contains. If breads, cereals, fruits, and vegetables are extremely limited, you are probably looking at a low-carbohydrate diet (see Table 10-7). Diet plans that use a low-carbohydrate approach are the Dr. Atkins' New Diet Revolution, the Scarsdale Diet, and the Four-Day Wonder Diet. More moderate approaches are found in the South Beach (especially initial phases), Zone, and Sugar Busters diets.

Low-fat diets, especially those that are very low in fat, turn out to be very-high-carbohydrate diets. These diets contain approximately 5 to 10% of energy intake as fat. The most notable are the Pritikin Diet and Dr. Dean Ornish's Eat More, Weigh Less plans. Low-fat diets are not harmful for healthy adults, but they are difficult to follow. These diets contain mostly grains, fruits, and vegetables. Eventually, many people get bored with this type of diet because they cannot eat favorite foods—they want some foods higher in fat or protein. Low-fat diets are very different from the typical North American diet, which makes it hard for many adults to follow them consistently.

Novelty diets are built on gimmicks. Some emphasize 1 food or food group and exclude almost all others. They might include only grapefruit, rice, or eggs. The rationale behind these diets is that you can eat only these foods for just so long before becoming bored and, in theory, reduce your energy intake. However, chances are that you will abandon the diet entirely before losing much weight.

The most questionable of the novelty diets propose that "food gets stuck in your body." Examples are Fit for Life, Beverly Hills Diet, and Eat Great, Lose Weight. The supposition is that food gets stuck in the intestine, putrefies, and creates toxins that cause disease. In response, these diets recommend not consuming certain foods or eating them only at certain times of the day. These recommendations make no physiological sense, however—as you know from Chapter 4, the digestive tract is efficient at digesting foods and eliminating waste.

Quack fad diets usually involve a costly product or service that doesn't lead to weight loss. Often, those offering the gimmick don't realize that they are promoting quackery because they have been victims themselves. For example, they tried the product and by pure coincidence lost weight, and they erroneously believe it worked for them, so they wish to sell it to others. Numerous weight-loss gimmicks have come and gone and are likely to resurface again.[28] If you hear that an important aid for weight loss is discovered, you can feel confident that, if it is legitimate, major peer-reviewed journals and authorities, such as the Surgeon General's Office or the National Institutes of Health, will make North Americans aware of it. Information in diet books, websites, infomercials, and advertisements needs to be viewed with a scientist's skeptical, questioning eye.

▶ Operation Waistline is a program designed by the U.S. Federal Trade Commission to stop fraudulent claims made by weight-loss charlatans. The program hopes to put an end to the billions of dollars spent annually in the United States on counterfeit products.

Knowledge Check

1. What are the 10 red flags that can help you determine if nutrition information is credible?
2. Why can't rapid weight loss consist mainly of fat?
3. What are the characteristics of each of the main types of fad diets?

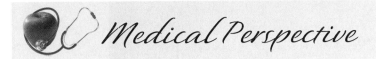

Medical Perspective

Professional Help for Weight Control

The first professional to see for weight control advice is one's family physician. Doctors are best equipped to assess overall health and the appropriateness of weight loss and weight gain. The physician may then recommend a registered dietitian for a specific eating plan and answers to diet-related questions. Registered dietitians are uniquely qualified to help design eating plans for weight control because they understand both food composition and the psychological importance of food. Exercise physiologists also can provide advice about physical activity. The expense for professional interventions is tax deductible in the U.S. in some cases (see a tax advisor) and often covered by health insurance if prescribed by a physician.

Drug Treatment for Weight Loss

In skilled hands, prescription medications can aid weight loss in some instances. However, drug therapy alone has not been found to be successful. Success with medications has been shown only in those who also modify their behavior, decrease their energy intake, and increase their physical activity.[5, 29]

People who are candidates for medications for obesity include those with a BMI of 30 or more or a BMI of 27 to 29.9 with weight-related (i.e., comorbid) conditions, such as type 2 diabetes, cardiovascular disease, hypertension, or excess waist circumference; those with no contraindications to the use of the medication; and those ready to undertake lifestyle changes that support weight loss. The following are the general classes of medications used.[30]

- Medications that enhance norepinephrine and serotonin activity in the brain by reducing the re-uptake of these neurotransmitters by nerve cells (sibutramine [Meridia®]). This effect causes the neurotransmitters to remain active in the brain longer, which prolongs a sense of reduced hunger. These medications appear to be effective in helping some people who eat healthy diets but who simply eat too much.[5]
- Amphetamine-like medication (phenteramine [Fastin® or Ionamin®]), which prolongs epinephrine and norepinephrine activity in the brain. This therapy is effective for some people in the short run but has not yet been proven effective in the long run.
- Medications that inhibit lipase enzyme action in the small intestine, thereby reducing fat digestion by about 30% (orlistat [Xenical®, Alli®]). Malabsorbed fat is deposited in the feces. Fat intake has to be controlled, however, because large amounts of fat in the feces can cause gas, bloating, and oily discharge. The malabsorbed fat also carries fat-soluble vitamins into the feces, so a multivitamin and mineral supplement is recommended.
- Medications that are not approved for weight loss, per se, can have weight loss as a side effect. For example, certain antidepressants (e.g., bupropion [Wellbutrin®]) have this effect.[29] Using a medication in this way is termed off-label because the product label does not include weight loss as an FDA-approved use.

Treatment of Severe Obesity

Severe (morbid) obesity—weighing at least 100 lb over healthy body weight (or twice one's healthy body weight)—requires professional treatment. Because of the serious health implications of severe obesity, drastic measures may be necessary. Such treatments are recommended only when traditional diets fail because they have serious physical and psychological side effects that require careful monitoring by a physician. These practices include very-low-calorie diets and gastroplasty.

Very-low-calorie diets (VLCDs), or modified fasts, are used to treat severe obesity if more traditional dietary changes have failed. Optifast® is one such commercial program. VLCDs provide 400 to 800 calories daily, often in liquid form, and tend to be used if a person has obesity-related diseases that are not well controlled (e.g., hypertension, type 2 diabetes).[5] About half the calories in these diets are carbohydrate, and the rest is high-quality protein. This low-carbohydrate intake often causes ketosis, which may help decrease hunger. However, the main reasons for weight loss are minimal calorie intake and absence of food choice. About 3 to 4 lb can be lost per week; men tend to lose at a faster rate than women. Careful monitoring by a physician is crucial throughout this very restrictive form of weight loss. Major health risks include heart problems and gallstones. If behavioral therapy and physical activity supplement a long-term support program, maintenance of the weight loss is more likely but still difficult. Medications for obesity also may be included in the maintenance phase of a VLCD.

Gastroplasty (gastric bypass surgery, also called stomach stapling) may be recommended for those who are morbidly obese, have been obese for at least 5 years with several non-surgical attempts to lose weight, and have no history of alcoholism or major psychiatric disorders. Gastroplasty works by reducing the stomach capacity to about 30 ml (the volume of 1 egg or shot glass) and bypassing a short segment of the upper small intestine (Fig. 10-18). Another surgical approach is banded gastroplasty. In vertical-banded gastroplasty, a vertical staple line is made down the length of the stomach to create a small stomach pouch. At the pouch outlet, a band is placed to keep the opening from stretching. With gastric banding, a band is placed around the upper portion of the stomach to create a small stomach pouch. A salt solution can be injected into the band through a port to adjust the size of the pouch over time.

(continued)

Medical Perspective, continued

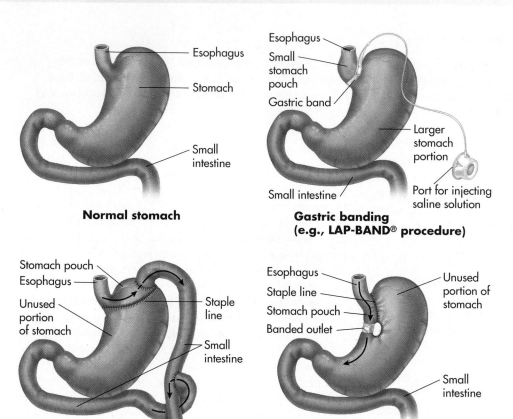

Normal stomach

Gastric banding (e.g., LAP-BAND® procedure)

Gastric bypass

Vertical-banded gastroplasty

Figure 10-18 The most common forms of gastroplasty for treating severe obesity. The gastric bypass is the most effective method. In banded gastroplasty, the band prevents expansion of the outlet for the stomach pouch.

With gastroplasty, weight loss is achieved because most of the food bypasses the stomach and small intestine, which results in less digestion and absorption of nutrients. Gastroplasty requires major lifestyle changes, such as the need for frequent, small meals and the elimination of sugars from the diet, to avoid **dumping syndrome** (severe diarrhea that begins almost immediately after eating concentrated sugar, such as regular soft drinks, candy, and cookies).

The surgery is costly and may not be covered by health insurance. In addition, the patient faces months of difficult adjustments. However, with gastroplasty, about 75% of people with severe obesity eventually lose half or more of their excess body weight. In addition, the surgery's success at long-term maintenance often leads to dramatic health improvements, such as reduced blood pressure and the elimination of type 2 diabetes. The risks of this very serious surgery include bleeding, blood clots, hernias, and severe infections. About 2% die from the surgery itself. In the long run, nutrient deficiencies can develop if the person is not adequately treated in the years following the surgery (chewable multivitamin and mineral supplements are often used). Follow-up surgery often is needed after weight loss to remove excess skin that was previously padded with fat.

Treatment of Underweight

Being underweight (BMI below 18.5) also carries health risks, including loss of menstrual function, low bone mass, complications with pregnancy and surgery, and slow recovery after illness. In growing children and teens, underweight can interfere with normal growth and development. Significant underweight also is associated with increased death rates, especially when combined with cigarette smoking.

Underweight can be caused by excess physical activity, severely restricted calorie intake, and health conditions such as cancer, infectious disease (e.g., tuberculosis), digestive tract disorders (e.g., chronic inflammatory bowel disease), and mental stress or depression. Active children and teens who do not take the time to consume enough energy to support their needs may become underweight. Genetic background may confer characteristics that promote low body weight, such as a higher metabolic rate, a lean or petite body frame, or both.

treating underweight individuals is to replace less-energy-dense foods with higher-energy-dense foods. For example, a cup of granola instead of bran flakes can add an extra 300 to 500 calories. Choosing bean soup over vegetable soup adds 50 calories or more. Portion sizes may need to be increased gradually. Having a regular meal and snack schedule also aids in weight gain and maintenance. Making time to eat regular meals can help underweight individuals attain an appropriate weight and help with digestive disorders, such as constipation, that are sometimes associated with irregular eating schedules. Excessively physically active people can reduce their activity. If their weight remains low, they can add muscle mass through resistance training (weight lifting), but to gain weight they must increase energy intake to support that physical activity. If these changes do not lead to weight gain within a few weeks, the underweight person should seek medical intervention to identify the cause of this condition and get appropriate treatment.

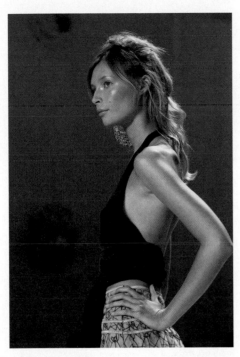

Although the media and the fashion world promote a very thin physique, being underweight carries severe risks.

Gaining weight can be a formidable task for an underweight person. An extra 500 calories per day may be required to gain weight, even at a slow pace, in part because of the increased expenditure of energy from thermogenesis. One approach for

Knowledge Check

1. Which weight-loss medications may be used to treat obesity?
2. Who should use a modified fast for weight loss?
3. What is gastroplasty?
4. What health risks are associated with being underweight?

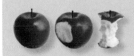

Take Action

Changing for the Better

Even if you are satisfied with your current weight, many people see their weight climb as they get older, so it is a good idea to be aware of how to keep weight under control. This behavioral change method can help you do just that. It also can be applied to changing exercise habits, self-esteem, and many other behaviors (Fig. 10-19).

1. **Become aware of the problem.** Calculate your current weight status to determine if you have a weight problem. First, measure your height and weight. Then, using Table 10-1, record your BMI: _____. When BMI exceeds 25, health risks from overweight may start. It is especially advisable to consider weight loss if your BMI exceeds 30.

   Now, use a tape measure to measure the circumference of your waist (at the narrowest point just above the navel with stomach muscles relaxed). Record the circumference: _____ inches.

When BMI exceeds 25 and a waist circumference is more than 40 inches (102 cm) in men or 35 inches (88 cm) in women, health risks rise. Does your waist circumference exceed the standard for your gender? _____

Whether you feel the need to pursue a program of weight loss now or in future, it is important to find out more about how to make changes.

2. **Gather baseline data.** Look back at the food diary you completed in Chapter 1. What factors most influence your eating habits? Do you eat out of stress, boredom, or depression? Is eating too much food your problem or do you mainly eat a poor diet? Next, think about whether it is worth changing these practices—a cost:benefit analysis can help you decide (Fig. 10-20).

(continued)

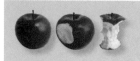

Take Action, *continued*

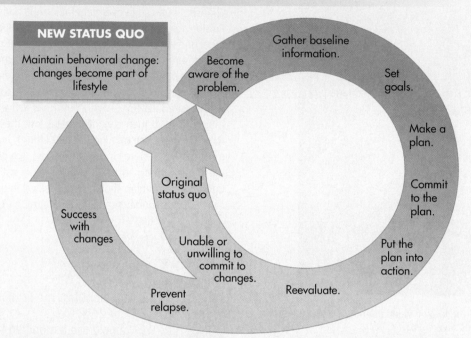

NEW STATUS QUO

Maintain behavioral change: changes become part of lifestyle

Gather baseline information.

Become aware of the problem.

Set goals.

Make a plan.

Commit to the plan.

Original status quo

Put the plan into action.

Success with changes

Unable or unwilling to commit to changes.

Reevaluate.

Prevent relapse.

Figure 10-19 **A model for behavioral change. It starts with awareness of the problem and ends with the incorporation of new behaviors intended to address the problem.**

3. **Set goals.** Setting realistic, achievable goals and allowing a reasonable amount of time to pursue them increase the likelihood of success. What final goal would you like to achieve? Why do you want to pursue this goal (e.g., improve health, lose weight, boost self-esteem)?

4. **Make a plan.** List several steps that will be necessary to achieve your goal. Changing only a few behaviors at a time increases the chances of success. You might choose to walk 60 minutes daily, eat less fat, eat more whole grains, or not eat after 8 P.M. What steps will you take to achieve the goal? If you are having trouble

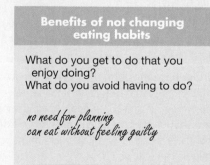

Benefits of changing eating habits

What do you expect to get, now or later, that you want?
What may you avoid that would be unpleasant?

feel better physically and psychologically
look better

Benefits of not changing eating habits

What do you get to do that you enjoy doing?
What do you avoid having to do?

no need for planning
can eat without feeling guilty

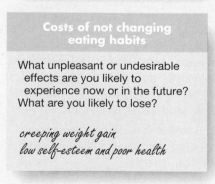

Costs involved in changing eating habits

What do you have to do that you don't want to do?
What do you have to stop doing that you would rather continue doing?

take time to plan meals and shop
must give up some food volume

Costs of not changing eating habits

What unpleasant or undesirable effects are you likely to experience now or in the future?
What are you likely to lose?

creeping weight gain
low self-esteem and poor health

Figure 10-20 **Benefits and costs analysis applied to changing eating habits. This process helps put behavior change into the context of total lifestyle.**

Name _Alan Young_

Goal
I agree to _ride my exercise bike_
_____
(specify behavior)
under the following circumstances _for 30 minutes, 4 times per week_
in the evening.
(specify where, when, how much, etc.)

Substitute behavior and/or reinforcement schedule _I will reinforce myself_
if I've acheived my goal after a month with a weekend off campus.

Charting progress
To keep track of my progress, _I will mark the days I exercise on a calendar._

Environmental planning
To help me do this, I am going to (1) arrange my physical and social environment
by _buying a new portable DVD player_

and (2) control my internal environment (thoughts, images) by _coordinating riding_
the bike with the first T.V. watching I do in the evening.

Reinforcements
Reinforcements provided by me daily or weekly (if contract is kept):
I will buy myself a new piece of clothing for off-campus trip.

Reinforcements provided by others daily or weekly (if contract is kept):
at the end of a month if I've completed my goal my parents will buy me
a fitness club membership for winter.

Social support
Behavioral change is more likely to take place when other people support you.
During the quarter/semester, please meet with the other person at least 3 times
to discuss your progress.
The name of my "significant helper" is _Mr. and Mrs. Young_

Figure 10-21 Completing such a contract can help generate commitment to behavior change. What would your contract look like?

listing the steps, you may want to consult a health professional for assistance.

5. **Commit to the plan.** Next, ask yourself, "Can I do this?" Be honest with yourself. Commitment is an essential component in the success of behavioral change. Permanent change is not quick or easy. Drawing up a behavioral contract often adds incentive to follow through with a plan (Fig. 10-21). The contract can list goal behaviors and objectives, milestones for measuring progress, and regular rewards for meeting the terms of the contract. After finishing a contract, you should sign it in the presence of some friends. This formality encourages commitment.

6. **Put the plan into action.** Thinking of a lifetime commitment can be overwhelming, so start with a trial of 6 or 8 weeks. Aim for a total duration of 6 months of new activities before giving up. To keep your plan on track:

   • Focus on reducing, but not necessarily extinguishing, undesirable behaviors. For example, it's usually unrealistic to say, "I'll never eat a certain food again." It's better to say, "I won't eat that problem food as often as before."

   • Monitor progress. Note your progress in a diary and reward positive behaviors. While conquering some habits and seeing improvement, you may find yourself quite encouraged about your plan of action— that can motivate you to move ahead with the plan.

   • Control environments. In the early phases of behavioral change, try to avoid problem situations, such as parties, favorite restaurants, and people who try to derail your plans. Once new habits are firmly established, you can probably more successfully resist the temptations of these environments.

7. **Reevaluate and prevent relapse.** After practicing a program for several weeks to months, take a close and critical look at your original plan. Does it actually lead to the goals you set? Are there any new steps toward your goal that you want to add? Do you need new reinforcements? Have you have experienced relapses? What triggered these relapses? How can you avoid future relapses? You may have noticed a behavior chain in some of your relapses (see Fig. 10-17)—how can you break the chain?

8. **Maintain behavioral change.** If you have used the activities in this section, you are well on your way to permanent behavioral change. Change isn't easy, but the results can be worth the effort.

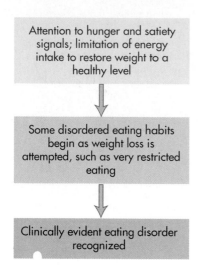

Figure 10-22 **Progression from ordered to disordered eating.**

 ## 10.8 Eating Disorders

Disordered eating can be defined as mild and short-term changes in eating patterns that occur in response to a stressful event, an illness, or a desire to modify the diet for health and/or personal appearance reasons. The problem may be no more than a bad habit, a style of eating adapted from friends or family members, or an aspect of preparing for athletic competition. Although disordered eating can lead to changes in body weight and certain nutritional problems, it rarely requires in-depth professional attention. However, in today's world, given the common practice of dieting, skipping meals, eating at odd times, and having hectic jobs and schedules, it may not be obvious when disordered eating stops and an eating disorder begins (Fig. 10-22).

Although obesity is the most common eating disorder in our society, the eating disorders explored in this section involve much more severe distortions of the eating process that can develop into life-threatening conditions if left untreated.[31] What is most alarming about these disorders is the increasing number of cases reported each year.[32] Some people are more susceptible to these disorders than others for genetic, psychological, and physical reasons. Until recently, most researchers reported that eating disorders primarily affect middle- and upper-class white women. Although some non-white cultures may be more accepting of larger body shapes, studies show greater similarities in the rates of body dissatisfaction and disordered eating behaviors across ethnic and cultural groups. Eating disorders are not restricted to any socioeconomic class, ethnicity, age group, or gender.

Many eating disorders start with a simple diet. Stress and a lack of appropriate coping mechanisms, dysfunctional family relationships, and drug abuse may cause dieting to get out of control.[33] Stress may be caused by physical changes associated with entering puberty, having to maintain a certain weight to look attractive or competent on a job, leaving home for college, or losing a friend. Disordered eating can escalate into physiological changes associated with sustained food restriction, binge eating, purging, and fluctuations in weight that interfere with everyday activities. They also involve emotional and cognitive changes that affect how people perceive and experience their bodies, such as feelings of distress or extreme concern about body shape or weight.[31]

Eating disorders are not due to a failure of will power or behavior; rather, they are real, treatable medical illnesses that require complex professional intervention that must go beyond nutritional therapy.[34] Without treatment, eating disorders can cause serious physical health complications, including heart conditions and kidney failure, which may even lead to death. Self-help groups for those with eating disorders, as well as their families and friends, represent non-threatening first steps into treatment. People also can attend self-help group meetings to get a sense of whether they really do have an eating disorder.

The main types of eating disorders are anorexia nervosa and bulimia nervosa. A third type, binge-eating disorder, has been recognized by the psychiatric community

Even well-intentioned parents may place expectations on their children that compound the anxiety felt during turbulent periods of childhood and adolescence. As a result, children and teens may find comfort in exerting control over their environment through the restrictive behaviors associated with eating disorders.

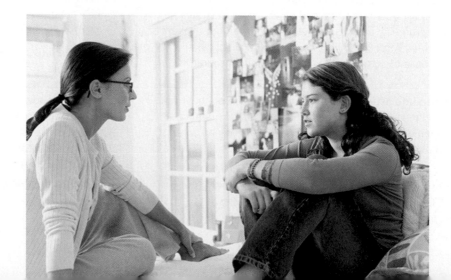

since 1994. Currently, health professions are determining whether binge-eating disorder should be included as a diagnosable disease.[35] More than 5 million people in North America have 1 of these disorders; females outnumber males 5 to 1. Eating disorders develop 85% of the time during adolescence or early adulthood, but some reports indicate that their onset can occur during childhood or later in adulthood. Currently, up to 5% of women in North America will develop some form of anorexia nervosa or bulimia nervosa in their lifetimes.[35] Eating disorders frequently co-occur with other psychological disorders, such as depression, substance abuse, and anxiety disorders.[31]

Anorexia Nervosa

The term **anorexia** implies a loss of appetite; however, a denial of appetite more accurately describes the behavior of people with anorexia nervosa. The term **nervosa** refers to disgust with one's body. Anorexia nervosa is characterized by extreme weight loss, a distorted body image, and an irrational, almost morbid fear of obesity and weight gain. These individuals believe they are fat, even though they are not and others tell them so. Some realize they are thin but continue to be haunted by certain areas of their bodies that they believe to be fat (e.g., thighs, buttocks, and stomach). The discrepancy between actual and perceived body shape is an important gauge of the severity of the disease.

Estimating the prevalence of this eating disorder is difficult because of underreporting, but approximately 1 in 200 (0.5%)[31] adolescent girls in North America eventually develops anorexia nervosa. This relatively high number may be due to girls' tendency to blame themselves for weight gain associated with puberty. It happens less commonly among adult women and African-American women. Men account for approximately 10% of cases of anorexia nervosa, partly because the ideal image conveyed for men is big and muscular. Among men, athletes are most prone to develop anorexia nervosa, especially those who participate in sports that require weight classes, such as boxers, wrestlers, and jockeys. Other activities that may foster eating disorders in men include swimming, dancing, and modeling.[35]

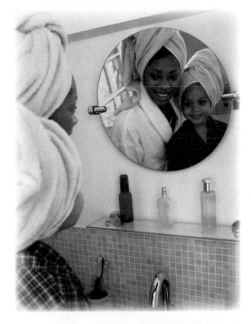

Concern over self-image begins early in life—we develop images of "acceptable" and "unacceptable" body types. Of all the attributes that constitute attractiveness, many people view body weight as the most important. Fatness is the most dreaded deviation from our cultural ideals of body image, the one most derided and shunned, even among schoolchildren.

disordered eating Mild and short-term changes in eating patterns that occur in relation to a stressful event, an illness, or a desire to modify one's diet for a variety of health and personal appearance reasons.

eating disorder Severe alterations in eating patterns linked to physiological changes; the alterations include food restricting, binge eating, purging, weight fluctuations, and emotional and cognitive changes in perceptions of one's body.

anorexia nervosa Eating disorder involving a psychological loss or denial of appetite followed by self-starvation; it is related, in part, to a distorted body image and to social pressures.

bulimia nervosa Eating disorder in which large quantities of food are eaten at one time (binge eating) and counteracted by purging food from the body, fasting, and/or excessive exercise.

binge-eating disorder Eating disorder characterized by recurrent binge eating and feelings of loss of control over eating.

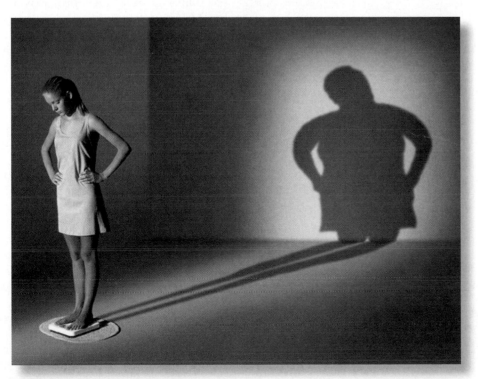

For people with eating disorders, the difference among real, perceived, and desired body images may be too difficult to accept.

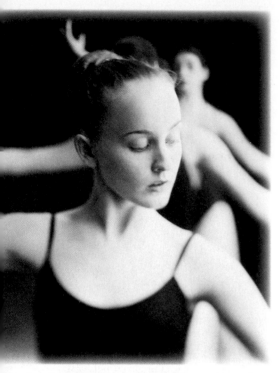

Eating disorders are commonly seen in people who must maintain low body weight, such as ballet dancers.

The *Diagnostic and Statistical Manual of Mental Disorders* lists these criteria for diagnosing anorexia nervosa:[35]

- Refusal to maintain body weight at or above a minimally normal weight for age and height
- Intense fear of gaining weight or becoming fat, even though underweight
- Disturbance in the way in which one's body weight or shape is experienced, undue influence of body weight or shape on self-evaluation, or denial of the seriousness of the current low body weight
- Amenorrhea (absence of at least 3 consecutive menstrual cycles) in females who have passed puberty

Although food is entwined in this disease, it stems more from psychological conflict. A common thread underlying many—but not all—cases of anorexia nervosa is conflict within the family structure, typically manifested by an overbearing mother and an emotionally absent father. When family expectations are too high, including those regarding body weight, frustration leads to fighting. Overinvolvement, rigidity, overprotection, and denial are typical daily transactions of such families.

Issues of control are central to the development of anorexia nervosa. The eating disorder can allow an anorexic person to exercise control over an otherwise powerless existence.[34] Losing weight may be the first independent success the person has had. People with anorexia evaluate their self-worth almost entirely in terms of self-control. Some sexually abused children develop anorexia nervosa, believing that, if they control their appetite for food, they can control and thereby eliminate their shameful feelings. Moreover, food restriction, which arrests development and shuts down sexual impulses, may be a strategy to prevent future victimization and guilt feelings. Often, anorexic persons feel hopeless about human relationships and socially isolated because of their dysfunctional families. They focus on food, eating, and weight instead of human relationships.

Some characteristics of those with anorexia nervosa are listed in Table 10-8. Keep in mind that only a health professional can correctly evaluate the diagnostic criteria required to make a diagnosis of eating disorders and exclude other possible diseases. If you think you know someone who is at risk for this or other eating disorders, suggest that the person seek professional evaluation because, the sooner treatment begins, the better the chances are for recovery.[36]

Physical Effects of Anorexia Nervosa

Rooted in the emotional state of the victim, anorexia nervosa produces profound physical effects.[37] The anorexic person often appears to be skin and bones. Body weight less than 85% of that expected is 1 clinical indicator of anorexia nervosa.[38] BMI is a more reliable indicator of the degree of malnourishment; generally, a BMI of 17.5 or less indicates a severe case. For children under age 18, growth charts should be used to assess weight status (see Chapter 17).

This state of semi-starvation forces the body to conserve as much energy as possible and results in most of the physical effects of anorexia nervosa (Fig. 10-23). Thus, many complications can be ended by returning to a healthy weight, provided the

Table 10-8 Typical Characteristics of Those with Eating Disorders

Anorexia Nervosa	Bulimia Nervosa
• Rigid dieting causing dramatic weight loss, generally to less than 85% of what would be expected for one's age (or BMI of 17.5 or less)	• Secretive binge eating; generally not overeating in front of others
• False body perception—thinking "I'm too fat," even when extremely underweight; relentless pursuit of control	• Eating when depressed or under stress
• Rituals involving food, excessive exercise, and other aspects of life	• Bingeing on a large amount of food, followed by fasting, laxative or diuretic abuse, self-induced vomiting, or excessive exercise (at least twice a week for 3 months)
• Maintenance of rigid control in lifestyle; security found in control and order	• Shame, embarrassment, deceit, and depression; low self-esteem and guilt (especially after a binge)
• Feeling of panic after a small weight gain; intense fear of gaining weight	• Fluctuating weight (±10 lb or 5 kg) resulting from alternate bingeing and fasting
• Feelings of purity, power, and superiority through maintenance of strict discipline and self-denial	• Loss of control; fear of not being able to stop eating
• Preoccupation with food, its preparation, and observing another person eat	• Perfectionism, "people pleaser;" food as the only comfort/escape in an otherwise carefully controlled and regulated life
• Helplessness in the presence of food	• Erosion of teeth, swollen glands
• Lack of menstrual periods after what should be the age of puberty for at least 3 months	• Purchase of syrup of ipecac, a compound sold in pharmacies that induces vomiting
• Possible presence of bingeing and purging practices	

People who exhibit only 1 or a few of these characteristics may be at risk but probably do not have either disorder. They should, however, reflect on their eating habits and related concerns and take appropriate action, such as seeking a careful evaluation by a physician.

duration of anorexia nervosa has not been too long. These are predictable effects caused by hormonal responses to and nutrient deficiencies from semistarvation.[31, 34, 35, 39]

- Low body weight (15% or more below what is expected for age, height, and activity level)
- Lowered body temperature and cold intolerance caused by loss of an insulating fat layer
- Slower metabolic rate caused by decreased synthesis of thyroid hormones
- Decreased heart rate as metabolism slows, leading to easy fatigue, fainting, and an overwhelming need for sleep. Other changes in heart function also may occur, including loss of heart tissue and poor heart rhythm.
- Iron deficiency anemia, which leads to further weakness
- Rough, dry, scaly, and cold skin from a deficient nutrient intake, which may show multiple bruises because of the loss of protection from the fat layer normally present under the skin
- Low white blood cell count, which increases the risk of infection and potentially death
- Abnormal feeling of fullness or bloating, which can last for several hours after eating
- Loss of hair
- Appearance of **lanugo**—downy hairs that appear on the body after a person has lost much body fat through semistarvation—that help trap air, reducing heat loss that occurs with the loss of fat tissue
- Constipation from semistarvation and laxative abuse
- Low blood potassium caused by a deficient nutrient intake, a loss of potassium from vomiting, and the use of some types of diuretics. Low blood potassium increases the risk of heart rhythm disturbances, another leading cause of death in anorexic people.

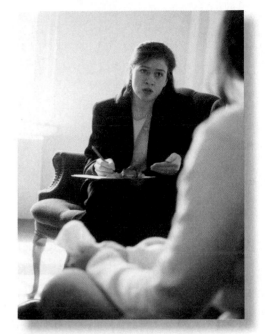

Early treatment of eating disorders improves chances of success. Note that such help is commonly available at student health centers and student guidance/counseling facilities on college campuses.

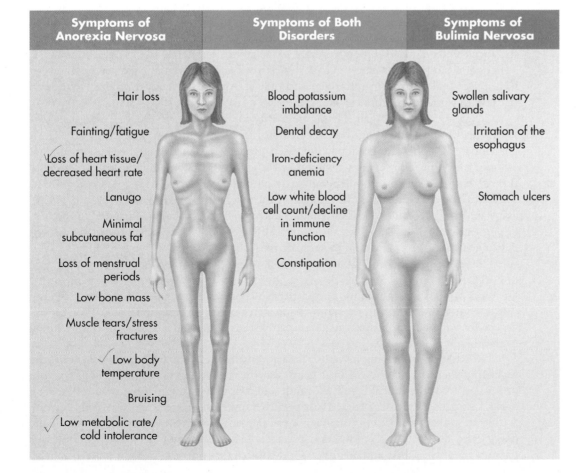

Symptoms of Anorexia Nervosa	Symptoms of Both Disorders	Symptoms of Bulimia Nervosa
Hair loss	Blood potassium imbalance	Swollen salivary glands
Fainting/fatigue	Dental decay	Irritation of the esophagus
Loss of heart tissue/ decreased heart rate	Iron-deficiency anemia	
Lanugo	Low white blood cell count/decline in immune function	Stomach ulcers
Minimal subcutaneous fat		
Loss of menstrual periods	Constipation	
Low bone mass		
Muscle tears/stress fractures		
Low body temperature		
Bruising		
Low metabolic rate/ cold intolerance		

Figure 10-23 This figure contains many potential consequences associated with anorexia nervosa and bulimia nervosa, but it is not an exhaustive list. These physical effects also can serve as warning signs that a problem exists and professional evaluation is needed.

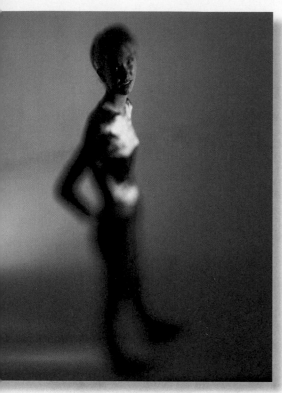

A young woman in a self-help group for those with anorexia nervosa explained her feelings to the other group members: "I have lost a specialness that I thought it gave me. I was different from everyone else. Now I know that I'm somebody who's overcome it, which not everybody does."

- Loss of menstrual periods because of low body weight, low body fat content, and the stress of the disease. Accompanying hormonal changes cause a loss of bone mass and increase the risk of osteoporosis later in life.
- Changes in neurotransmitter function in the brain, leading to depression
- Eventual loss of teeth caused by acid erosion if frequent vomiting occurs. Loss of teeth (along with low bone mass) can be lasting signs of the disease, even if the other physical and mental problems are resolved.
- Muscle tears and stress fractures in athletes caused by decreased bone and muscle mass

Treatment of Anorexia Nervosa

The longer someone suffers from this eating disorder, the poorer the chances are for complete recovery. However, with prompt, vigorous, and professional help, many people with anorexia nervosa can lead normal lives. Treatment requires a multidisciplinary team of experienced physicians, registered dietitians, psychologists, and other health professionals.[31] An ideal setting is an eating disorders clinic in a medical center. Outpatient therapy, day hospitalization (6–12 hours), or total hospitalization may be used. Hospitalization is necessary once a person falls below 75% of expected weight, experiences acute medical problems, and/or exhibits severe psychological problems or suicidal risk.[31] Still, even in the most skilled hands at the finest facilities, efforts may fail. Thus, the prevention of anorexia nervosa is of utmost importance.

Experienced professional help is the key. An anorexic patient may be on the verge of suicide and near starvation. In addition, many anorexic people are very clever and resistant. They may try to hide weight loss by wearing many layers of clothes, putting coins in their pockets or underwear, and drinking numerous glasses of water before stepping on a scale. Currently, the average time for recovery from anorexia nervosa is 7 years; many insurance companies cover only a fraction of the cost of treatment.

Nutrition Therapy   The first goal of nutrition therapy is to gain the patient's cooperation and trust in order to increase oral food intake. Ideally, weight gain must be enough to raise the metabolic rate to normal and reverse as many physical signs of the disease as possible. Food intake is designed first to minimize or stop any further weight loss. Then, the focus shifts to restoring appropriate food habits. After this, the expectation can be switched to slow weight gain—2 to 3 lb per week is appropriate. Tube feeding and/or total parenteral nutrition support is used only if immediate renourishment is required because this drastic measure can cause the patient to distrust medical staff.

During the weight-gain phase, an energy intake goal of 1000 to 1600 kcal/day, with a distribution of 50 to 55% carbohydrate, 15 to 20% protein, and 25 to 30% fat, is appropriate. Calories are gradually increased until the patient is gaining an appropriate amount of weight. For females, an appropriate weight is one in which normal menstruation is restored. This nutrition therapy may ultimately require a daily intake of 3000 to 4000 kcal to attain a goal weight because of the increase in body metabolism and anxiety associated with feeding.[40] A multivitamin and mineral supplement is added, as well as enough calcium to raise intake to about 1500 mg/day. As noted previously, nutrient deficiencies are commonly seen in anorexic persons.[31]

Patients need considerable reassurance during the refeeding process because of uncomfortable effects, such as bloating, increase in body heat, and increase in body fat. This process is frightening because these changes can lead to the patient feeling out of control. Monitoring for rapid changes in electrolytes and minerals in the blood, especially potassium, phosphorus, and magnesium, is critical as more food is included in the diet.[34]

In addition to helping patients reach and maintain adequate nutritional status, the registered dietitian on the medical team also provides accurate nutrition information, promotes a healthy attitude toward food, and helps the patient learn to eat based on natural hunger and satiety cues. Nutrition therapy with anorexic persons can be frustrating for a dietitian because many anorexic persons are very knowledgeable about the energy and fat content of most food products. The focus should be on helping these patients identify healthy and adequate food choices that promote weight gain to achieve and maintain a clinically estimated goal weight (e.g., BMI of 20 or more).[32] The medical team also should assure patients that they will not be abandoned after gaining weight.

Psychological and Related Therapy   Once the physical problems of anorexic patients are addressed, the treatment focus shifts to the underlying emotional problems of the disorder. To heal, these patients must reject the sense of accomplishment they associate with an emaciated body and begin to accept themselves at a healthy body weight. Establishing a strong relationship with either a therapist or another supportive person is an especially important key to recovery. If therapists can discover reasons for the disorder, they can develop psychological strategies for restoring normal weight and eating habits. A key aspect of psychological treatment is showing affected individuals how to regain control of other facets of their lives and cope with tough situations. As eating evolves into a normal routine, they can return to previously neglected activities.

Family therapy often is important, especially for younger patients who still live at home. Family therapy focuses on the role of the illness among family members, the reactions of individual family members, and the ways in which their subconscious behavior might contribute to the abnormal eating patterns.[31] Frequently, a therapist finds family struggles at the heart of the problem. As the disorder resolves, patients must relate to family members in new ways to gain the attention that was needed and previously tied to the disease. For example, the family may need to help the young person ease into adulthood and accept its responsibilities as well as its advantages.

Medications are sometimes part of the therapy for anorexic patients. However, their use is aimed primarily at preventing relapse in patients who have been treated but have an existing psychiatric disorder, such as depression, anxiety, or obsessive-compulsive disorder.

Bulimia Nervosa

Bulimia nervosa (*bulimia* means "great [ox] hunger") is characterized by episodes of binge eating followed by attempts to purge the excess energy consumed by vomiting or misusing laxatives, diuretics, or enemas. Some people exercise excessively to try to burn off a binge's high energy intake. Those with bulimia nervosa may think of food constantly. Unlike an anorexic person, who turns away from food when faced with problems, a bulimic person turns toward food in critical situations.[41] Also, unlike those with anorexia nervosa, people with bulimia nervosa recognize their behavior as abnormal.[38] These individuals often have very low self-esteem and are depressed—about half have major depression. The lingering effects of child abuse or sexual abuse may be one reason for these feelings. The world sees their competence, but inside they feel out of control, ashamed, and frustrated.

Up to 4% of adolescent and college-age women suffer from bulimia nervosa. About 10% of the cases occur in men.[35] However, many people with bulimic behavior are probably never diagnosed, perhaps because their symptoms are not obvious and many with bulimia nervosa lead secret lives, hiding their abnormal eating habits. Most diagnoses of bulimia nervosa are based on self-reports; consequently, current estimates of the number of cases are probably low. This disorder, especially in its milder forms, may be much more widespread than commonly thought.

Many susceptible people have genetic factors and lifestyle patterns that predispose them to becoming overweight, and many frequently try weight-reduction diets as teenagers. Like people with anorexia nervosa, those with bulimia nervosa are usually female and successful. Unlike anorexics, however, they are usually at or slightly above a normal weight.[42] Females with bulimia nervosa also are more likely to be sexually active than are those with anorexia nervosa.

The *Diagnostic and Statistical Manual of Mental Disorders* gives these criteria for diagnosing bulimia nervosa:[35]

- Recurrent **binge eating episodes** (eating during a discrete period of time, such as 2 hours, an amount of food that is larger than most people would eat during a similar

CRITICAL THINKING

Jennifer is an attractive 13-year-old. However, she's very compulsive. Everything has to be perfect—her hair, her clothes, even her room. Since her body started to mature, she's become quite obsessed with having perfect physical features as well. Her parents are worried about her behavior. The school counselor told them to look for certain signs that could indicate an eating disorder. What might those signs be?

time period and under similar circumstances, coupled with feeling a lack of control over what or how much one is eating)

- Recurrent inappropriate compensatory behavior to prevent weight gain, such as self-induced vomiting; misuse of laxatives, diuretics, enemas, or other medications; fasting; or excessive exercise
- Binge eating episodes and inappropriate compensatory behaviors both occurring, on average, at least twice a week for 3 months
- Undue influence of body weight or shape on self-evaluation
- Disturbance does not occur exclusively during episodes of anorexia nervosa.

▶ Bulimia nervosa is rare in developing countries, which suggests that our culture is an important causal factor.

Over a third of individuals initially diagnosed with anorexia nervosa may cross over to bulimia nervosa, although the crossover from bulimia nervosa to anorexia nervosa is much less likely. Typically, the crossover between eating disorders occurs within the first 5 years of the illness. Anorexic persons who perceive their parents as being highly critical are most likely to cross over to bulimia nervosa. In contrast, bulimic individuals who struggle with alcohol abuse are most likely to cross over to anorexia nervosa.

The typical characteristics of those with bulimia nervosa are described in Table 10-8. In addition to binging and purging, those with bulimia nervosa often have elaborate food rules, such as avoiding all sweets. Thus, eating just 1 cookie or doughnut may cause bulimic persons to feel guilty that they have broken a rule and proceed to binge. Usually, this action leads to significant overeating. A binge can be triggered by a combination of hunger from recent dieting, stress, boredom, loneliness, and depression. Bingeing often follows a period of strict dieting and thus can be linked to intense hunger. The binge is not at all like normal eating; once begun, it seems to propel itself. The person not only loses control but generally doesn't even taste or enjoy the food that is eaten during a binge. This separates the practice from simple overeating. Binge-purge cycles may be practiced daily, weekly, or at longer intervals. Often, a special time is set aside. Most binge eating occurs at night, when others are less likely to interrupt them, and usually lasts from 30 minutes to 2 hours.

Most commonly, bulimic people consume cakes, cookies, ice cream, and similar high-carbohydrate convenience foods during binges because these foods can be purged relatively easily and comfortably by vomiting. In a single binge, foods supplying 3000 kcal or more may be eaten.[34] Purging follows, in hopes that no weight will be gained. However, even when vomiting follows the binge, 33 to 75% of the food energy taken in is still absorbed, which causes some weight gain. When laxatives or enemas are used, about 90% of the energy is absorbed because these products act in the large intestine, beyond the point of most nutrient absorption. Clearly, the belief of bulimic persons that purging soon after bingeing will prevent excessive energy absorption and weight gain is a misconception.

Early in the onset of bulimia nervosa, sufferers often induce vomiting by placing their fingers (or other objects) deep into the throat. They may inadvertently bite down on fingers, such that the resulting bite marks around the knuckles are a characteristic sign of this disorder. Once the disease is established, however, a person can often vomit simply by contracting the abdominal muscles. Vomiting also may occur spontaneously.

Another way bulimic people attempt to compensate for a binge is by engaging in excessive exercise to expend a large amount of energy. Exercise is considered excessive when it is done at inappropriate times or settings or when a person continues to exercise despite injury or medical complications. Some bulimic people try to estimate the amount of energy eaten in a binge and then exercise to counteract this energy intake. This practice, referred to as "debting," represents an effort to control their weight.[42]

After binging and purging, those with bulimia nervosa usually feel guilty and depressed.[38] Over time, they experience

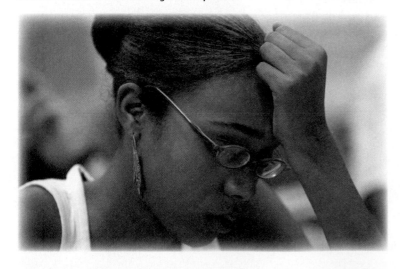

Bulimia nervosa can lead to tragic consequences.

low self-esteem and feel hopeless about their situation (Fig. 10-24). Sufferers gradually distance themselves from others, spending more and more time preoccupied by and engaging in bingeing and purging.

Physical Effects of Bulimia Nervosa

Most of the health problems associated with bulimia nervosa arise from vomiting.[35, 42, 43]

- Repeated exposure of teeth to the acid in vomit causes demineralization, making the teeth painful and sensitive to heat, cold, and acids. Eventually, the teeth may decay severely, erode away from fillings, and finally fall out.
- Blood potassium can drop significantly because of regular vomiting or the use of certain diuretics. This drop can disturb the heart's rhythm and even cause sudden death.
- Salivary glands may swell as a result of infection and irritation from persistent vomiting.
- Stomach ulcers and tears in the esophagus develop, in some cases.
- Constipation may result from frequent laxative use.
- Ipecac syrup, sometimes used to induce vomiting, is toxic to the heart, liver, and kidneys and can cause accidental poisoning when taken repeatedly.
- Overall, bulimia nervosa is a potentially debilitating disorder that can lead to death, usually from suicide, low blood potassium, or overwhelming infections.

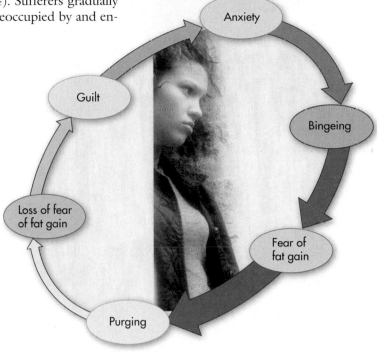

Figure 10-24 Bulimia nervosa's vicious cycle of obsession.

Treatment of Bulimia Nervosa

Therapy for bulimia nervosa, as for anorexia nervosa, requires a team of experienced psychotherapists and nutritionists.[42] Bulimic patients are less likely than those with anorexia to enter treatment in a state of semistarvation. However, if a bulimic patient has lost significant weight, this weight loss must be treated before psychological treatment and nutrition counseling begin. Although clinicians have yet to agree on the best therapy for bulimia nervosa, they generally agree that treatment should last at least 16 weeks. Hospitalization may be necessary in cases of extreme laxative abuse, regular vomiting, substance abuse, and depression, especially if physical harm is evident.

The first goal of treatment for bulimia nervosa is to decrease the amount of food consumed in a binge session in order to reduce the risk of esophageal tears from related purging by vomiting. Patients also are given information about bulimia nervosa and its consequences. They must recognize that they are dealing with a serious disorder that can have grave medical complications if not treated. Next follows nutrition counseling and psychotherapy.

Excessive tooth decay is common in bulimic patients. Dental professionals are sometimes the first health professionals to notice signs of bulimia nervosa.

Nutrition Therapy In general, the focus of nutrition therapy is not on stopping bingeing and purging but, rather, on developing regular eating habits and correcting misconceptions about food. To establish regular eating patterns, some specialists encourage patients to self-monitor by keeping a food diary, in which they record food intake, internal sensations of hunger, environmental factors that trigger binges, and thoughts and feelings that accompany binge-purge cycles. Avoiding binge foods and not constantly stepping on a scale may be recommended early in treatment. Patients also are discouraged from following strict rules about healthy food choices because such rules simply mimic the typical obsessive attitudes associated with bulimia nervosa. Rather, they should be encouraged to adopt a mature perspective on food intake—that is, regularly consume moderate amounts from a variety of foods from each food group.[32] Once the goals of developing regular eating habits and correcting misconceptions about food are achieved, the binge-purge cycle should start to break down.

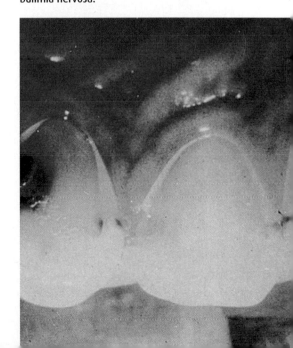

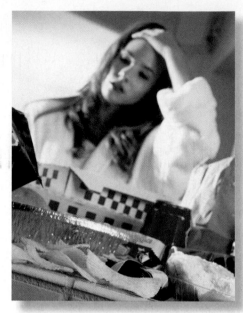

Purging episodes add to the despair felt by people with bulimia nervosa.

Binge eaters usually consume foods that carry the social stigma of so-called junk foods—ice cream, cookies, sweets, potato chips, and similar snack foods.

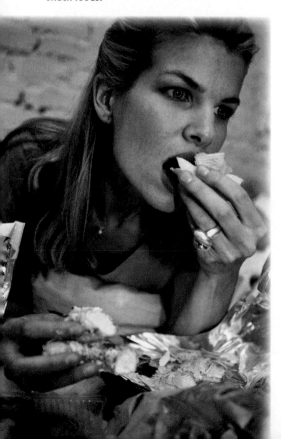

Psychological and Related Therapy People with bulimia nervosa need psychological help because they can be very depressed and are at a high risk of suicide. The primary aims of psychotherapy are to improve patients' self-acceptance and to help them to be less concerned about body weight. Psychotherapy helps correct the all-or-none thinking typical of bulimic persons: "If I eat 1 cookie, I'm a failure and might as well binge." In addition, the therapist guides the person in using methods other than bingeing and purging to cope with stressful situations. Group therapy often is useful in fostering strong social support. One goal of therapy is to help bulimic persons accept some depression and self-doubt as normal. Certain antidepressants may be used to treat the bulimic patient; however, they should be used in conjunction with other therapies.

Because relapse is likely, therapy should be long-term. About 50% of people with bulimia nervosa recover completely from the disorder. Others continue to struggle with it, to varying degrees, for the rest of their lives. This fact underscores the need for prevention because treatment is difficult.

Eating Disorders Not Otherwise Specified (EDNOS)

EDNOS is a broad category of eating disorders in which individuals have partial syndromes that do not meet the strict criteria for anorexia nervosa or bulimia nervosa.[35] About 50% of people with eating disorders fall into this EDNOS category, especially adolescents. Examples of disordered eating in this category include (1) a woman who meets all the criteria for anorexia nervosa but continues to menstruate; (2) an individual who meets all the criteria for anorexia nervosa but, despite a significant weight loss, has a current weight in the normal range (perhaps a person who was once obese); (3) a person who meets all the criteria for bulimia nervosa but who binges less than twice a week; (4) a person who meets all the criteria for bulimia nervosa but does not binge (this person might eat normal amounts of food but purges regularly out of fear of weight or fat gain); and (5) a person who repeatedly chews and spits out food but does not swallow it.

EDNOS also includes binge-eating disorder. The *Diagnostic and Statistical Manual of Mental Disorders* gives these criteria for binge-eating disorder:

- Recurrent binge-eating episodes
- During most binge episodes, at least 3 of these occur: eating much more rapidly than usual, eating until feeling uncomfortably full, eating large amounts of food when not feeling physically hungry, eating alone because of being embarrassed by how much one is eating, and/or feeling disgusted with oneself, depressed, or very guilty after overeating.
- Marked feelings of distress regarding binge eating
- Binge-eating episodes occur, on average, at least 2 days a week for 6 months.
- Binge eating does not occur only during the course of bulimia nervosa or anorexia nervosa.

Although people with anorexia nervosa and bulimia nervosa exhibit a persistent preoccupation with body shape, weight, and thinness, binge eaters do not necessarily share these concerns. Thus, neither purging nor prolonged food restriction is characteristic of binge-eating disorder. Some physicians classify binge-eating disorder as an addiction to food involving psychological dependence. The person becomes attached to the behavior itself and has a drive to continue it, senses only limited control over it, and needs to continue, despite negative consequences.

Note that obesity and binge eating are not necessarily linked. Not all obese people are binge eaters, and, although obesity may result, it is not necessarily an outcome of binge eating. Nonetheless, binge-eating disorder is most common among the severely obese and those with a long history of frequent restrictive dieting, although obesity is not a criterion for having binge-eating disorder. Approximately 30 to 50% of subjects in organized weight-control programs have binge-eating disorder, whereas about 1 to 2% of North Americans in general have this disorder. Many more people in the general population have less severe forms of the disease but do not meet the formal criteria for diagnosis. The number of cases of binge-eating disorder is far greater than that of either anorexia nervosa or bulimia nervosa.

For some people, frequent dieting beginning in childhood or adolescence is a precursor to binge-eating disorder. During periods when little food is eaten, they get very hungry and feel driven to eat in a compulsive, uncontrolled way. Many individuals with binge-eating disorder (about 40% of whom are males) perceive themselves as hungry more often than normal. They usually started dieting at a young age, began bingeing during adolescence or in their early twenties, and did not succeed in commercial weight-control programs. Almost half of those with severe binge-eating disorder exhibit clinical depression symptoms and isolate themselves from others.

Stressful events and feelings of depression or anxiety can trigger this binge eating. Giving themselves "permission" to eat a "forbidden" food also can precipitate a binge. Other triggers include loneliness, anxiety, self-pity, depression, anger, rage, alienation, and frustration.[44] In general, people engage in binge eating to induce a sense of well-being and perhaps even emotional numbness, usually in an attempt to avoid feeling and dealing with emotional pain and anxiety.

Binge eaters consume food without regard to biological need and often in a recurrent, ritualized fashion. Some people with this disorder eat food continually over an extended period; others cycle episodes of bingeing with normal eating.[44] For example, someone with a stressful or frustrating job might come home every night and eat until bedtime. Another person might eat normally most of the time but find comfort in consuming large quantities of food when an emotional setback occurs.

People with binge-eating disorder may come from families with alcoholism or may have suffered sexual abuse. Members of such dysfunctional families often do not know how to deal effectively with emotions. They cope by turning to substances. Family members learn to cover up dysfunctional patterns and learn to nurture the behavior of others at the expense of their own needs.

Overall, people who have binge-eating disorder are usually unsuccessful in controlling it without professional help.[44] Depending on the specific symptoms, these individuals may need treatment as outlined earlier for anorexia nervosa or bulimia nervosa.

The focus of nutrition therapy for people with binge-eating disorder mirrors that of controlling the bingeing associated with bulimia nervosa. Psychological therapy involves helping those with binge-eating disorder identify personal emotional needs and express emotions. Because this problem is a common predisposing factor in binge eating, communication issues should be addressed during treatment. Binge eaters often must be helped to recognize their own buried emotions in anxiety-producing situations, and learning simple but appropriate phrases to say to oneself can help stop bingeing when the desire is strong. Self-help groups, such as Overeaters Anonymous, aim to help recovery from binge-eating disorder. The treatment philosophy attempts to create an environment of encouragement and accountability to overcome this eating disorder. Antidepressants, as well as other medications, may be prescribed to help reduce binge eating in these individuals by decreasing depression.

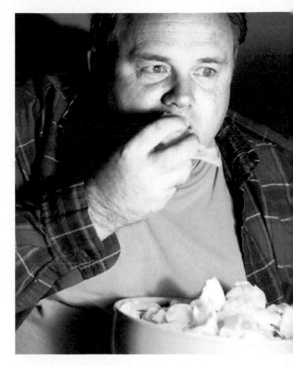

Night eating syndrome is an eating disorder under study. In this disorder, people eat a lot in the late evening or eat food in order to fall asleep again once awakened in the night. This night eating can contribute to weight gain, so affected persons are urged to seek treatment.

Prevention of Eating Disorders

A key to developing and maintaining healthful eating behavior is to realize that some concern about diet, health, and weight is normal, as are variations in what we eat, how we feel, and even how much we weigh. For example, most people experience some minimal weight change (up to 2 to 3 lb) throughout the day and even more over the course of a week. A large weight fluctuation or an ongoing weight gain or weight loss is more likely to indicate that a problem is present. If you notice a large change in your eating habits, how you feel, or your body weight, it is a good idea to consult your physician. Treating physical and emotional problems early helps prevent eating disorders and promotes good health.

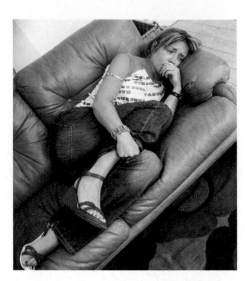

Eating disorders affect many college students. Counselors are aware of this and are available to help.

Not only is the treatment of eating disorders far more difficult than prevention, but these disorders also have devastating effects on the entire family. For this reason, parents, friends, and professionals working with children and teens must emphasize the importance of an overall healthful diet that focuses on moderation, as opposed to restriction and perfection. These caregivers also can help children and teens form positive habits and appropriate expectations, especially regarding body image.[45] The following is some advice that these caregivers and health professionals can extend to growing children and adolescents to help them avoid eating disorders:

- Discourage restrictive dieting, meal skipping, and fasting (except for religious reasons).
- Encourage children to eat only when hungry.
- Promote good nutrition and regular physical activity in school and at home.
- Promote regularly eating meals as a family unit.[46]
- Provide information about normal changes that occur during puberty.
- Correct misconceptions about nutrition, healthy body weight, and approaches to weight loss.
- Carefully phrase any weight-related recommendations and comments.
- Don't overemphasize numbers on a scale. Instead, primarily promote healthful eating irrespective of body weight.
- Increase self-acceptance and appreciation of the power and pleasure emerging from one's body.
- Encourage coaches to be sensitive to weight and body-image issues among athletes.
- Emphasize that thinness is not necessarily associated with better athletic performance.
- Enhance tolerance for diversity in body weight and shape.
- Encourage normal expression of emotions.
- Build respectful environments and supportive relationships.
- Provide adolescents with an appropriate, but not unlimited, degree of independence, choice, responsibility, and self-accountability for their actions.

Knowledge Check

1. What is the difference between eating disorders and disordered eating?
2. What are the characteristics of anorexia nervosa, bulimia nervosa, and binge-eating disorder?
3. What kinds of therapy are appropriate for anorexia nervosa?
4. What kinds of therapy are appropriate for bulimia nervosa?

CASE STUDY FOLLOW-UP

There is a good chance that, if Christy keeps eating as she is, she will gain weight in her freshman year of college. Christy skips breakfast, eats a light lunch and dinner, and then becomes hungry late at night and cannot resist the high-calorie, high-fat pizza that is delivered to the dorm. Recent data show that women who skip breakfast are more likely to weigh more than those who eat breakfast.[24] This pattern of eating will lead to weight gain. Christy needs to wake up and eat a simple breakfast, such as a bowl of cereal with fat-free milk and a banana. In addition, she needs to eat a balanced lunch and dinner and find ways to add exercise to her daily routine to avoid the Freshman 15.

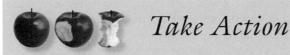

Take Action

Assessing Risk of Developing an Eating Disorder

British investigators have developed a 5-question screening tool, called the **SCOFF** Questionnaire, for recognizing eating disorders.[47]

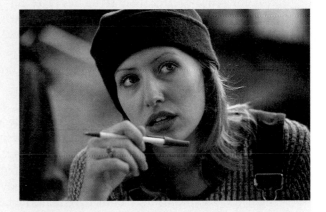

1. Do you make yourself **S**ick because you feel full?

2. Do you lose **C**ontrol over how much you eat?

3. Have you lost more than **O**ne stone (about 13 lb) recently?

4. Do you believe yourself to be **F**at when others say you are thin?

5. Does **F**ood dominate your life?

Two or more positive responses suggest an eating disorder.

1. After completing this questionnaire, do you feel that you might have an eating disorder or the potential to develop one?

2. Do you think any of your friends might have an eating disorder?

3. What counseling and education resources exist in your area or on your campus to help with a potential eating disorder?

4. If a friend has an eating disorder, what do you think is the best way to assist him or her in getting help?

Summary

10.1 Energy balance considers energy intake and energy output. Negative energy balance occurs when energy output surpasses energy intake, resulting in weight loss. Positive energy balance occurs when energy intake is greater than output, resulting in weight gain. Basal metabolism, the thermic effect of food, physical activity, and thermogenesis account for total energy use by the body. Basal metabolism, which represents the minimum amount of energy used to keep the resting, awake body alive, is primarily affected by lean body mass, body surface area, and thyroid hormone concentrations. Physical activity is energy use above the amount expended when at rest. The thermic effect of food describes the increase in metabolism that facilitates digestion, absorption, and processing of nutrients recently consumed. Thermogenesis is heat production caused by shivering when cold, fidgeting, and other stimuli. In a sedentary person, about 70 to 80% of energy use is accounted for by basal metabolism and the thermic effect of food.

10.2 Direct calorimetry estimates energy expenditure by measuring the amount of body heat released by a person. Indirect calorimetry, the most commonly used method to determine energy use by the body, involves collecting expired air from an individual during a specified amount of time. This method works because a predictable relationship exists between the body's use of energy and the amount of oxygen consumed and carbon dioxide produced. Estimated Energy Requirements (EERs) are based on formulas developed by the Food and Nutrition Board that can be used to estimate energy needs.

10.3 Groups of cells in the hypothalamus and other regions in the brain affect hunger, the primarily internal desire to find and eat food. These cells monitor macronutrients and other substances in the blood and read low amounts as a signal to promote feeding. A variety of external (appetite-related) forces, such as food availability, affect satiety. Hunger cues combine with appetite cues to promote feeding. Numerous factors elicit satiety, such as flavor, smell, chewing, and the effects of digestion, absorption, and metabolism.

10.4 A person of healthy weight generally shows good health and performs daily activities without weight-related problems. A body mass index (weight in kilograms/height² in meters) of 18.5 to 25 is one measure of healthy weight, although weight in excess of this value may not lead to ill health. A healthy weight is best determined in conjunction with a thorough health evaluation by a health-care provider. A body mass index of 25 to 29.9 represents overweight. Obesity is defined as a total body fat percentage over 25% (men) or 35% (women), or a body mass index of 30 or more. Fat distribution greatly determines health risks from obesity. Upper-body fat storage, as measured by a waist circumference greater than 40 inches (102 cm) (men) or 35 inches (88 cm) (women), increases the risks of hypertension, cardiovascular disease, and type 2 diabetes more than does lower-body fat storage.

10.5 Research suggests that genes account for up to 40 to 70% of weight differences between people. The genes may be those that determine body type, metabolic rate, and the factors that affect hunger and satiety. Some individuals are thought to have a genetic predisposition to obesity because they inherit a thrifty metabolism. The set-point theory proposes that humans have a genetically predetermined body weight or body fat content, which the body closely regulates. Environmental factors have important effects on what we eat. These factors may define when eating is appropriate, what is preferable to eat, and how much food should be eaten. Even though our genetic backgrounds have a strong influence on body weight and composition, genes are not destiny—both nature and nurture are involved.

10.6 A sound weight-loss program emphasizes a wide variety of low-energy-density foods; adapts to the dieter's habits; consists of readily obtainable foods; strives to change poor eating habits; stresses regular physical activity; and stipulates the participation of a physician if weight is to be lost rapidly or if the person is over the age of 40 (men) or 50 (women) years and plans to perform substantially greater physical activity than usual. A pound of adipose tissue contains about 3500 kcal. Thus, if energy output exceeds intake by about 500 kcal per day, a pound of adipose tissue can be lost per week. Physical activity as part of a weight-loss program should be focused on duration, rather than intensity. Behavior modification is a vital part of a weight-loss program because the dieter may have many habits that discourage weight maintenance.

10.7 Many fad diets promise rapid weight loss; however, these diets are not designed for permanent weight loss. Low-carbohydrate diets work in the short run because they limit total food intake; however, long-term studies have shown that the weight generally returns in about a year. Weight-loss drugs are reserved for those who are obese or have weight-related problems, and they should be administered under close physician supervision. The treatments for severe obesity include surgery to reduce stomach volume to approximately 1 oz (30 ml) and very-low-calorie diets containing 400 to 800 kcal/day. Both of these measures should be reserved for people who have failed at more conservative approaches to weight loss. They also require close medical supervision. Underweight can be caused by a variety of factors, such as excessive physical activity and genetic background. Sometimes being underweight requires medical attention. A physician should be consulted first to rule out underlying disease. The underweight person may need to increase portion sizes and include energy-dense foods in the diet.

10.8 Anorexia nervosa usually starts with dieting in early puberty and proceeds to the near-total refusal to eat. Early warning signs include intense concern about weight gain and dieting, as well as abnormal food habits. Eventually, anorexia nervosa can lead to numerous negative physical effects. The treatment of anorexia nervosa includes increasing food intake to support gradual weight gain. Psychological counseling attempts to help patients establish regular food habits and to find means of coping with the life stresses that led to the disorder. Bulimia nervosa is characterized by secretive bingeing on large amounts of food within a short time span and then purging by vomiting or misusing laxatives, diuretics, or enemas. Alternately, fasting and excessive exercise may be used to offset calorie intake. Both men and women are at risk. Vomiting as a means of purging is especially destructive to the body. The treatment of bulimia nervosa includes psychological as well as nutritional counseling. During treatment, bulimic persons learn to accept themselves and to cope with problems in ways that do not involve food. Binge-eating disorder is most common among people with a history of frequent, unsuccessful dieting. Binge eaters binge without purging. Thus, this condition falls under the category Eating Disorders Not Otherwise Specified (EDNOS). Emotional disturbances are often at the root of this disordered form of eating. Treatment addresses deeper emotional issues, discourages food deprivation and restrictive diets, and helps restore normal eating behaviors. The treatment of eating disorders may include certain medications.

Study Questions

1. Positive energy balance occurs when energy output surpasses energy intake.

   a. true
   b. false

2. What is the approximate basal metabolism of a 175-pound man?

   a. 3840 kcal/day
   b. 1227 kcal/day
   c. 1909 kcal/day
   d. 1745 kcal /day

3. All the following raise basal metabolism rate *except* _____.

   a. growing
   b. muscle mass
   c. fever
   d. starvation

4. Direct calorimetry estimates energy expenditure by collecting expired air from an individual during a specified amount of time.

   a. true
   b. false

5. Which protein produced in fat tissue regulates body weight by signaling the brain that the body has low body fat stores?

   a. ghrelin
   b. leptin
   c. thyroid hormone
   d. cholecystokinin

6. The most accurate method for diagnosing obesity is _____.

   a. underwater weighing
   b. dual energy X-ray absorptiometry (DEXA)
   c. skinfold thickness
   d. body mass index

7. Jane's waist measurement is 35 inches. Which of the following statements about Jane's body fat distribution is correct?

   a. Jane is at an increased risk of developing diabetes, hypertension, and heart disease.
   b. Jane's waist circumference indicates central body fat distribution.
   c. Jane has a "pear" shape.
   d. Both a and c are correct.
   e. Both a and b are correct.

8. The set-point theory proposes that humans have a genetically predetermined body weight or body fat content, which the body closely regulates.

   a. true
   b. false

9. A sound weight-loss program _____.

   a. includes a wide variety of low-energy-density foods
   b. stresses regular physical activity
   c. includes behavior modification to change problem behaviors
   d. all of the above

10. The danger of low-carbohydrate diets is that they cause fast weight loss in the form of _____.

    a. fat tissue
    b. water
    c. muscles
    d. a and b
    e. b and c

11. Surgery to reduce stomach volume should be reserved for people who have failed at more conservative approaches to weight loss.

    a. true
    b. false

12. Which eating disorder starts with dieting and proceeds to near total refusal to eat?

    a. bulimia nervosa
    b. binge eating
    c. anorexia nervosa
    d. none of the above

13. What is lanugo?

    a. downy, soft hair that develops on people with anorexia nervosa
    b. a sudden drop in blood pressure from excessive dieting
    c. a popular fad diet
    d. a code word for an eating disorder

14. Bulimia nervosa is characterized by all of the following *except* _____.

    a. refusal to eat
    b. secretive bingeing
    c. purging
    d. misuse of laxatives

15. Binge-eating disorder is more widespread than anorexia or bulimia.

    a. true
    b. false

Answer Key: 1-a; 2-c; 3-d; 4-b; 5-b; 6-b; 7-e; 8-a; 9-d; 10-e; 11-a; 12-c; 13-a; 14-a; 15-a

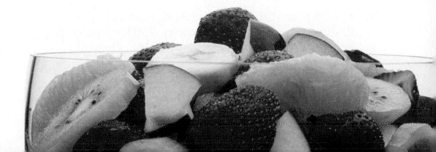

Websites

To learn more about the topics covered in this chapter, visit these websites.

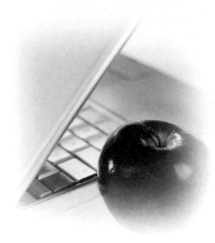

Weight Control, Obesity, and Nutrition

www.niddk.nih.gov/health/nutrit/win.htm (or call 800-WIN-8098)

www.nhlbi.nih.gov/guidelines/index.htm

www.caloriecontrol.org

www.weight.com

www.obesity.org

www.cyberdiet.com

Eating Disorders

www.acadeatdis.org

www.aabainc.org/home.html

www.nationaleatingdisorders.org

www.hedc.org

www.nimh.nih.gov/publicat/eatingdisordersmenu.cfm

www.4women.gov/bodyimage

References

1. Centers for Disease Control and Prevention. *U.S. obesity 1985–2006.* Atlanta: CDC; 2007.

2. Booth K and others. Obesity and the built environment. *J Am Diet Assoc.* 2005;105:s110.

3. Davidson K, Birch L. Lean and weight stable: Behavioral predictors and psychological correlates. *Obes Res.* 2004;12:1085.

4. Hill J and others. Obesity: Etiology. In: Shils M and others, eds. *Modern nutrition in health and disease.* 10th ed. Philadelphia: Lippincott Williams & Wilkins; 2006.

5. Wadden T and others. Obesity: Management. In: Shils M and others, eds. *Modern Nutrition in health and disease.* 10th ed. Philadelphia: Lippincott Williams & Wilkins; 2006.

6. Jakicic J, Otto A. Physical activity considerations for the treatment and prevention of obesity. *Am J Clin Nutr.* 2005;82:226s.

7. Forshee R and others. A critical examination of the evidence relating high fructose corn syrup and weight gain. *Crit Rev Food Sci Nutr.* 2007;47:561.

8. United States Department of Agriculture, Economic Research Service. Food availability. 2007; www.ers.usda.gov/Data/FoodConsumption/FoodAvailIndex.htm.

9. Bray G and others. Consumption of high-fructose corn syrup in beverages may play a role in the epidemic of obesity. *Am J Clin Nutr.* 2004;79: 537.

10. Melanson K and others. Effects of high-fructose corn syrup and sucrose consumption on circulating glucose, insulin, leptin, and ghrelin and on appetite in normal-weight women. *Nutrition.* 2007;23:103.

11. Smith G. Control of food intake. In: Shils M and others, eds. *Modern nutrition in health and disease.* 10th ed. Philadelphia: Lippincott Williams & Wilkins; 2006.

12. Bowen J and others. Appetite hormones and energy intake in obese men after consumption of fructose, glucose and whey protein beverages. *Int J Obes.* 2007;31:1696.

13. Heyward V, Wagner D. *Applied body composition assessment.* 2nd ed. Champaign, IL: Human Kinetics; 2004.

14. McCrory M and others. Body composition by air-displacement plethysmography by using predicted and measured thoracic gas volumes. *J Appl Physio.* 1998;84:1475.

15. Lofgren I and others. Waist circumference is a better predictor than body mass index of coronary heart disease risk in overweight premenopausal women. *J Nutr.* 2004;134:1071.

16. Christakis N, Fowler J. The spread of obesity in a large social network over 32 years. *New Eng J Med.* 2007;357:370.

17. Wing R, Phelan S. Long-term weight loss maintenance. *Am J Clin Nutr.* 2005;82:222s.

18. Foster G and others. Behavioral treatment of obesity. *Am J Clin Nutr.* 2005;82:230s.

19. Hill J and others. Obesity and the environment: Where do we go from here? *Science*. 2003;299:853.

20. Hu F. Protein, body weight, and cardiovascular health. *Am J Clin Nutr*. 2005;82:242s.

21. Ornish D. Was Dr. Atkins right? *J Am Diet Assoc*. 2004;104:537.

22. Ello-Martin J and others. Dietary energy density in the treatment of obesity: A year-long trial comparing 2 weight-loss diets. *Am J Clin Nutr*. 2007;85:1465.

23. Shick S and others. Persons successful at long term weight loss and maintenance continue to consume a low energy, low fat diet. *J Am Diet Assoc*. 1998;98:1273.

24. Wyatt H and others. Long term weight loss and breakfast in subjects in the National Weight Control Registry. *Obes Res*. 2002;10:78.

25. Barton B and others. The relationship of breakfast and cereal consumption to nutrient intake and body mass index: The National Heart, Lung, and Blood Institute Growth and Health Study. *J Am Diet Assoc*. 2005;105:1383.

26. ADA. Position of the American Dietetic Association: Food and nutrition misinformation. *J Am Diet Assoc*. 2006;106:601.

27. Dansinger M and others. Comparison of the Atkins, Ornish, Weight Watchers and Zone diets for weight loss and heart disease risk reduction: A randomized trial. *JAMA*. 2005;293:173.

28. Pittler M, Ernst E. Dietary supplements for body-weight reduction: A systematic review. *Am J Clin Nutr*. 2004;79:529.

29. Moyers S. Medications as adjunct therapy for weight loss: Approved and off-label agents in use. *J Am Diet Assoc*. 2005;105:948.

30. Li Z and others. Meta-analysis: Pharmacologic treatment of obesity. *Ann Intern Med*. 2005:142:532.

31. Yager J, Andersen A. Anorexia nervosa. *New Eng J Med*. 2005;353:1441.

32. ADA. Position of the American Dietetic Association: Nutrition intervention in the treatment of anorexia nervosa, bulimia nervosa and eating disorders not otherwise specified (EDNOS). *J Am Diet Assoc*. 2001;101:810.

33. Courbasson C and others. Substance use disorders, anorexia, bulimia, and concurrent disorders. *Can J Public Health*. 2005;96:102.

34. Coughlin J, Guarda A. Behavioral disorders affecting food intake: Eating disorders and other psychiatric conditions. In: Shils M and others, eds. *Modern nutrition in health and disease*. 10th ed. Philadelphia: Lippincott Williams & Wilkins; 2006.

35. American Psychiatric Association. *Diagnostic and statistical manual of mental disorders (DSM-IV-TR)*. 4th ed. Washington, DC: American Psychiatric Association; 2000.

36. Woods S. Untreated recovery from eating disorders. *Adolescence*. 2004;39:361.

37. Holtkamp K and others. Depression, anxiety and obsessionality in long-term recovered patients with adolescent onset anorexia nervosa. *Eur Child Adol Psychiatry*. 2005;14:106.

38. Walsh B. Eating disorders. In: Kaser D and others, eds. *Harrison's principles of internal medicine*. New York: McGraw-Hill; 2004.

39. Miller K and others. Medical findings in outpatients with anorexia nervosa. *Arch Intern Med*. 2005;165:561.

40. Van Wymelbeke V and others. Factors associated with the increase in resting energy expenditure during refeeding in malnourished anorexia nervosa patients. *Am J Clin Nutr*. 2004;80:1469.

41. Broussard B. Women's experiences of bulimia nervosa. *J Adv Nurs*. 2005;49:43.

42. Mehler P. Bulimia nervosa. *New Eng J Med*. 2003;349:875.

43. Frydrych A and others. Eating disorders and oral health. *Aust Dent J*. 2005;50:6.

44. Shanta-Retelny V. Binge eating into obesity. *Today's Dietitian*. 2004;May:34.

45. Jackson K. Eating disorders revealed. *Today's Dietitian*. 2004;March:37.

46. Neumark-Sztainer D and others. Family meals and disordered eating in adolescents: Longitudinal findings from Project EAT. *Arch Pediatr Adol Med*. 2008;162:17.

47. Morgan J and others. The SCOFF Questionnaire. *Br Med J*. 1999;319:1467.

48. Suter P and others. Effect of ethanol on energy expenditure. *Am J Physiol Regul Integr Comp Physiol*. 1994;266:4.

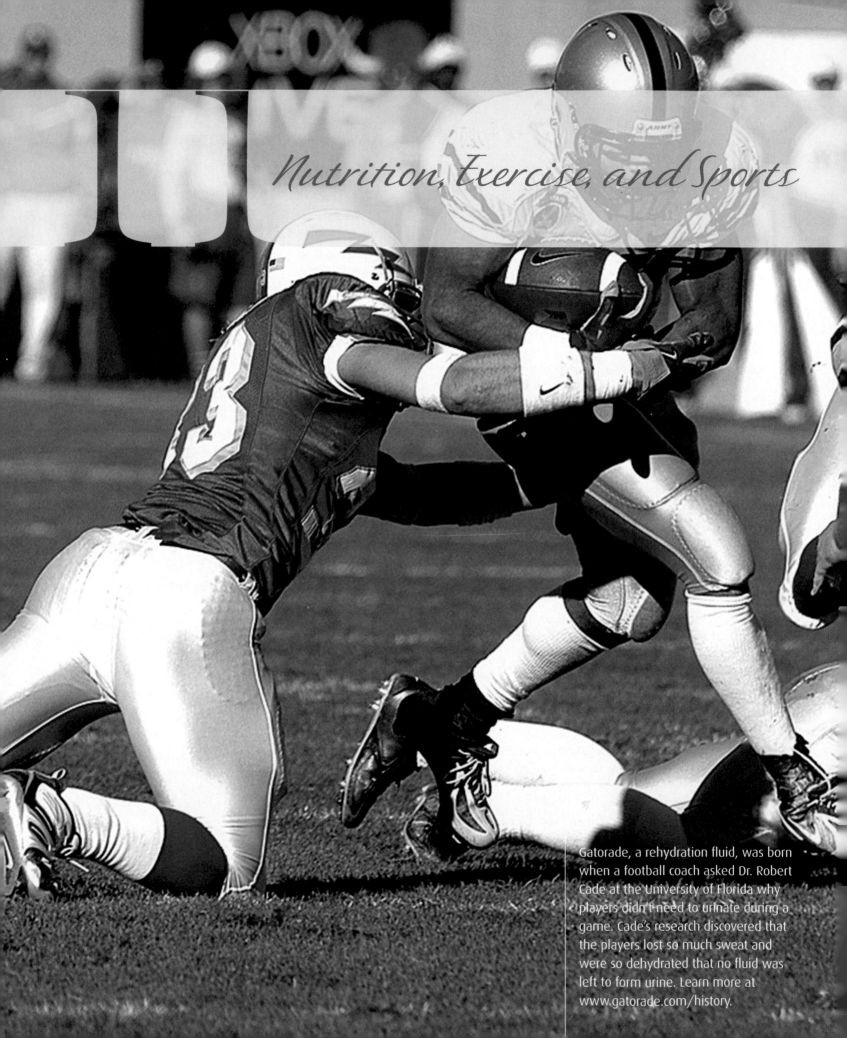

Nutrition, Exercise, and Sports

Gatorade, a rehydration fluid, was born when a football coach asked Dr. Robert Cade at the University of Florida why players didn't need to urinate during a game. Cade's research discovered that the players lost so much sweat and were so dehydrated that no fluid was left to form urine. Learn more at www.gatorade.com/history.

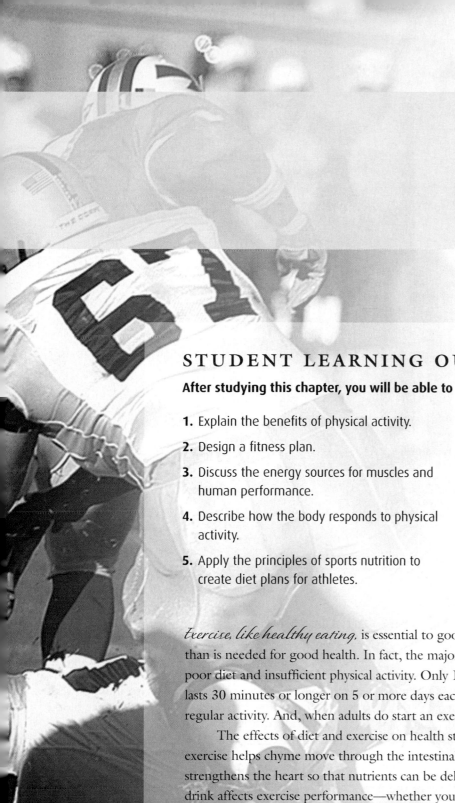

STUDENT LEARNING OUTCOMES

After studying this chapter, you will be able to

1. Explain the benefits of physical activity.

2. Design a fitness plan.

3. Discuss the energy sources for muscles and human performance.

4. Describe how the body responds to physical activity.

5. Apply the principles of sports nutrition to create diet plans for athletes.

6. Describe the fluid needs of athletes and how to avoid dehydration and hyponatremia.

7. Describe how the composition of food eaten before, during, and after exercise training sessions can affect performance.

8. Explain the role of ergogenic aids and describe their effect on athletic performance.

Exercise, like healthy eating, is essential to good health. However, many people get far less exercise than is needed for good health. In fact, the majority of health problems in North America are related to poor diet and insufficient physical activity. Only 15% of adults report engaging in physical activity that lasts 30 minutes or longer on 5 or more days each week. Approximately 40% do not participant in any regular activity. And, when adults do start an exercise program, about half quit within 3 months.

The effects of diet and exercise on health status are closely related to each other. Recall that regular exercise helps chyme move through the intestinal tract, promotes calcium deposition in the bones, and strengthens the heart so that nutrients can be delivered to cells efficiently. Similarly, what you eat and drink affects exercise performance—whether you are a recreational athlete or an elite athlete or you just want to maintain your health.

Athletes invest a lot of time and effort in training; their quest to find a competitive edge has spurred research studies designed to determine how diet affects exercise performance. Good eating habits can't substitute for physical training and genetic endowment, but healthy food and beverage choices are crucial for top-notch performance, contributing to endurance and helping speed the repair of injured tissues.[1] Unfortunately, there is much misinformation regarding the effect of diet and nutrients on exercise performance. A good working knowledge and understanding of sports nutrition can help individuals choose diets that help them perform as close to their potential as possible. In this chapter, you will discover how exercise benefits the entire body and how nutrition relates to fitness and sports performance.

Figure 11-1 The benefits of regular, moderate physical activity and exercise.

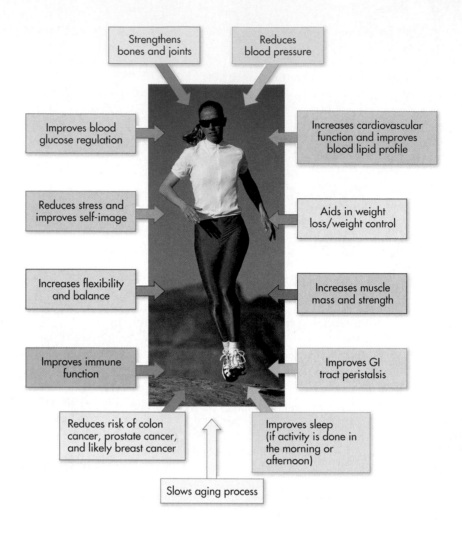

Strengthens bones and joints

Reduces blood pressure

Improves blood glucose regulation

Increases cardiovascular function and improves blood lipid profile

Reduces stress and improves self-image

Aids in weight loss/weight control

Increases flexibility and balance

Increases muscle mass and strength

Improves immune function

Improves GI tract peristalsis

Reduces risk of colon cancer, prostate cancer, and likely breast cancer

Improves sleep (if activity is done in the morning or afternoon)

Slows aging process

🍑 11.1 Benefits of Fitness

The benefits of regular physical activity (and exercise) include enhanced heart function, improved balance, a reduced risk of falling, better sleep habits, healthier body composition (less body fat, more muscle mass), and reduced injury to muscles, tendons, and joints. Physical activity also can reduce stress and positively affect blood pressure, blood cholesterol levels, blood glucose regulation, and immune function. In addition, physical activity aids in weight control, both by raising resting energy expenditure for a short period of time after exercise and by increasing overall energy expenditure (Fig. 11-1).[2-7]

Almost everyone can benefit from regular exercise. *Healthy People 2010* has set the following objectives for U.S. adults.

- Reduce by 50% the proportion of adults engaging in no leisure-time physical activity (currently 27% of adults).
- Double the proportion of adults engaging regularly, preferably daily, in moderate exercise for at least 30 minutes per day (currently 45% of adults).
- Increase by 50% the proportion of adults who perform exercises that enhance and maintain muscular strength and endurance (currently 19% of adults).

The 2005 Dietary Guidelines for Americans recommend 3 daily time goals for physical activity.

- Thirty minutes per day of moderate-intensity physical activity, in addition to usual activity, for individuals trying to reduce their risk of chronic disease in adulthood.

▶ Recall how the terms *physical activity* and *exercise* are related. Exercise is physical activity done with the intent to gain health and fitness benefits, whereas physical activity is simply part of day-to-day activities.

Doing more than 30 minutes or increasing the intensity of the workout can lead to even greater benefits.

• Sixty minutes per day of moderate- to vigorous-intensity physical activity to help adults manage body weight and prevent gradual weight gain.

• Ninety minutes per day of moderate-intensity physical activity may be needed for some adults to sustain weight loss; at the same time, these individuals also need to monitor their energy intakes.

Knowledge Check

1. What are 3 benefits of physical activity?
2. What are the specific physical activity objectives set by *Healthy People 2010*?
3. What amount of time should be devoted to physical activity to reduce the risk of chronic diseases?

 ## 11.2 Characteristics of a Good Fitness Program

A good fitness program is one that meets a person's needs—the ideal program for one individual may not be right for another. The first step in designing a fitness program is to define goals. Some may want a program that trains them for athletic competition; others may want to lose weight or just increase their stamina or improve their balance. Different goals mean different fitness programs. To reach goals, fitness program planning should consider the mode, duration, frequency, intensity, and progression of exercise, as well as consistency and variety. Also, a good fitness program must help individuals achieve and maintain fitness.

Mode

Mode refers to the type of exercise performed. The American College of Sports Medicine (ACSM) defines **aerobic exercise** as "any activity that uses large muscle groups, can be maintained continuously, and is rhythmic in nature." It is a type of exercise that causes the heart and lungs to work harder than at rest. Aerobic exercise usually involves using large muscle groups, for activities such as brisk walking, running, lap swimming, or cycling. **Resistance exercise,** or strength training, is defined as activities that use muscular strength to move a weight or work against a resistant load. **Flexibility exercise** is the ability of a joint to move through its entire range of motion.

Duration

Duration is the amount of time spent in an exercise or physical activity session. Generally, exercise should last at least 30 minutes, not counting time for warm-up and cool-down. Ideally, exercise should be continuous (without stopping), but research has shown that 10-minute bouts of exercise done 3 times throughout the day can lower the risk of cardiovascular disease, cancer, and diabetes.[8]

Frequency

Frequency is the number of times the activity is performed weekly. For the best fitness level, daily aerobic activity is recommended. However, aerobic exercise performed 3 to 5 days a week appears to achieve cardiovascular fitness. To meet desired weight-loss goals,

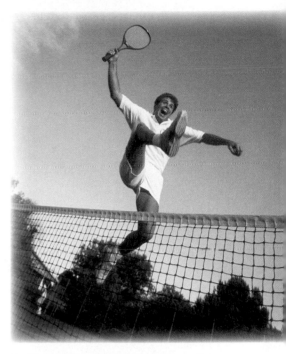

The best exercise is one you want to continue to do.

▶ To stick with an exercise program, experts recommend the following:

• Start slowly.
• Vary activities; make exercise fun.
• Include friends and others.
• Set specific attainable goals and monitor progress.
• Set aside a specific time each day for exercise; build it into daily routines, but make it convenient.
• Reward yourself for being successful in keeping up with your goals.
• Don't worry about occasional setbacks; focus on long-term benefits to your health.

Figure 11-2 Heart rate training chart. This chart shows the number of heart beats per minute that corresponds to various exercise intensities.

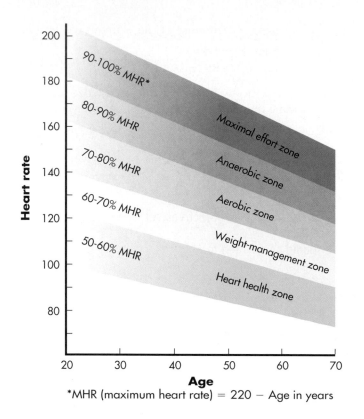

*MHR (maximum heart rate) = 220 − Age in years

▶ The maximum heart rate for a 20-year-old person is 200 beats per minute:

220 − Age in years = Maximum heart rate
220 − 20 = 200

The target zone for a 20-year-old person is 120 to 180 heartbeats per minute:

Maximum heart rate × 0.6 = Low end of maximum heart rate target zone
200 × 0.6 = 120

Maximum heart rate × 0.9 = High end of maximum heart rate target zone
200 × 0.9 = 180

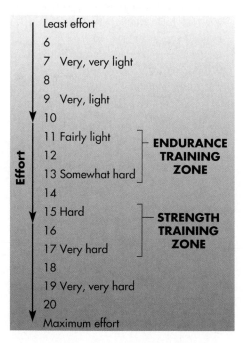

Figure 11-3 Rating of Perceived Exertion (RPE) scale. This scale is used to estimate exercise intensity. A rating between 12 and 15 is recommended to achieve a high physical fitness level.

the frequency of exercise may need to be 5 to 6 times per week. To achieve muscular fitness, 2 to 3 days of resistance training are needed weekly. Similarly, 2 to 3 days per week of flexibility exercises are recommended.

Intensity

Intensity is the level of effort required, or how hard the exercise is to perform. Intensity can be described as low-intensity (very mild increased heart rate exercise), moderate-intensity (exercise that increases breathing, sweating, and beat but permits one to carry on a conversation), or vigorous-intensity (exercise that significantly increases breathing, sweating, and heart rate, which makes it difficult to carry on a conversation).

Traditionally, heart rate has been used to define intensity (Fig. 11-2). This popular and simple method uses a percentage of age-predicted maximum heart rate. To estimate maximum heart rate in beats per minute, subtract a person's age from 220. The range of heart rates between 60 and 90% of maximum is sometimes called the target zone. The lower end of this range is calculated by multiplying maximum heart rate by 0.6; the upper end is computed by multiplying maximum heart rate by 0.9. Medications, such as those for high blood pressure, may affect maximum heart rate. A physician can help those with health conditions personalize their target zone.

Another way to determine exercise intensity is the Borg Scale of Perceived Exertion, which often is called the **Rating of Perceived Exertion (RPE)** scale. The scale ranges from 6 to 20, with numbers corresponding to a subjective feeling of exertion (Fig. 11-3). For example, the number 9 is rated as "very light" exertion and the number 19 is considered close to maximal effort, or "very, very hard," such as would occur in an all-out sprint. To achieve fitness, aim for an intensity of 12 to 15. At this level, you are working at a moderate intensity but can still talk to an exercise partner.

Individuals need to monitor how their bodies feel during exercise. A jogger who wants to engage in moderate-intensity exercise should aim for a Borg Scale rating of "somewhat hard" (12 to 14), which is of moderate intensity. If the jogger felt muscle fatigue and breathing was "very light" (9), then he or she could increase the intensity.

On the other hand, if the jogger felt the exertion was "extremely hard" (19), he or she should slow down to achieve the moderate-intensity range.

Because this rating is what the exerciser perceives, the actual exertion differs among those with different levels of fitness. That is, a very fit person will have a lower Borg scale rating when jogging than a less fit person engaging in the same activity. Similarly, as a less fit person becomes more fit, his or her RPE will drop over time as the same exercise becomes easier. To continue to increase fitness levels, the exerciser would always aim to exercise at a moderate intensity.

Energy needs dictate the amount of oxygen used by the body's cells (1.5 or 2.5 ATP molecules are produced from each molecule of oxygen). Thus, another way to determine exercise intensity is to measure oxygen consumption during exercise. A treadmill test is commonly used to determine the maximum amount of oxygen a person can consume in a unit of time (ml/min). In this test, oxygen consumption is measured as the treadmill speed and/or grade is gradually increased until the subject can no longer increase oxygen use as workload increases. The oxygen consumption measured at this point is VO_{2max}. Because of individual differences in VO_{2max}, it is generally best to express exercise intensity as a percentage of VO_{2max}.

Exercise intensity also is sometimes expressed in units called metabolic equivalents (METs). One MET is the expenditure of 1 kcal/kg/hour, or on average 3.5 ml O_2/kg/minute. This approximates resting energy expenditure. A brisk walk represents about 4.5 METs of energy expenditure. Exercise prescriptions given to people recovering from a heart attack often are in MET units.[1]

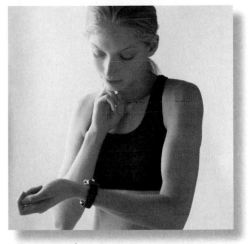

Taking your pulse determines if your exercise output is in the target zone. To measure heart rate (pulse), count the number of heartbeats for 6 seconds and then multiply that number by 10 to determine heart rate per minute. There also are watches that contain heart rate monitors.

Progression

Progression describes how the duration, frequency, and intensity of exercise increase over time. The first 3 to 6 weeks of an exercise program make up the initiation phase. This phase corresponds to the time it takes for the body to adapt to the exercise program. The next 5 to 6 months of training are the improvement stage, during which intensity and duration increase to a point that no further physical gains are achieved. This plateau marks the beginning of the maintenance stage. At this stage, exercisers may want to evaluate their fitness goals. If their goals have been achieved, the fitness program can continue in the same way to maintain the level of fitness achieved. If the goals have not been reached, exercise duration, frequency, intensity, and/or mode can be adjusted.

Consistency

The easiest way to have consistency in physical activity is to make it part of a daily routine, similar to other regular activities, such as eating. The best time to exercise is whenever it fits best into one's lifestyle—first thing in the morning, at lunchtime, before dinner, or later. Many people find that the best time to exercise is when they need an energy pick-me-up or a break from work or studying. When schedules are tight, exercise can occur in short segments, such as breaks between classes.

Variety

Although some people enjoy doing the same activities day after day, boredom is one reason many people abandon fitness programs. Just as a variety of foods helps ensure a nutritious diet, a varied fitness routine helps exercise different muscles for overall fitness, keeps exercising interesting and fun, and helps individuals stick with their fitness programs. Variety can be achieved in a number of ways, such as exercising indoors or outdoors or alternating aerobic exercise with resistance exercise. The Physical Activity Pyramid (Fig. 11-4) shows how to add variety to fitness programs and to increase fitness levels.

> ### CRITICAL THINKING
>
> Pedro started going to the gym about 8 weeks ago. At first, he noticed that he began huffing and puffing about 7 minutes into his aerobic workout. Now, however, he can work out for about 25 minutes without tiring. What is a possible explanation for his ability to work out longer?

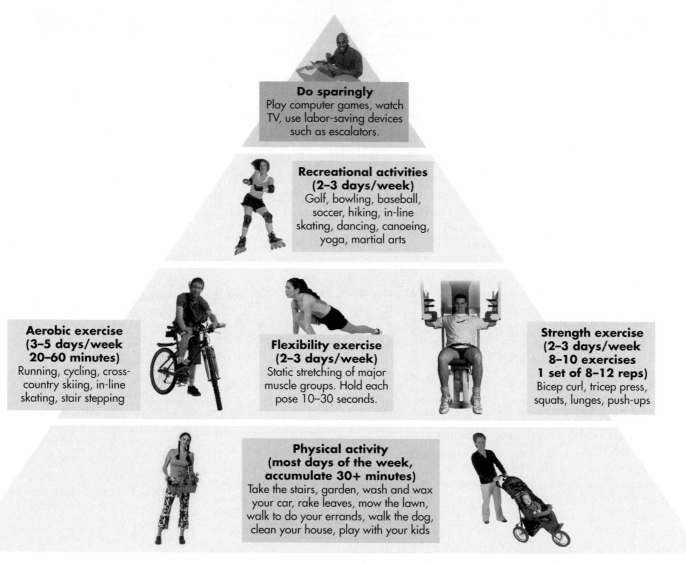

Figure 11-4 Each week, try to balance your physical activity using this guide.

Achievement and Maintenance of Fitness

Starting a new fitness program has 2 main activities. The first is to discuss the fitness program goals with a health-care provider. This is especially important for men over 40 and women over 50 years of age who have been inactive for many years or have existing health problems. The second is to assess and record baseline fitness scores—these provide benchmarks against which to measure progress. Benchmarks should be based on fitness program goals. A benchmark for a person wanting to increase muscle strength might be the amount of weight that can be lifted with the arms or the number of push-ups that can be done without stopping. The amount of time it takes to walk a mile and the heart rate after the walk may be appropriate benchmarks for individuals wanting to build stamina. Determining how far a person can bend or stretch can be a benchmark for those wanting to improve flexibility.

Most new exercise programs should start with short intervals of exercise at the lower end of the maximum heart rate target zone and work up to a total of 30 minutes of activity incorporated into each day. If necessary, exercise can be broken into 3 sessions lasting 10 minutes each. When individuals are able to perform physical activity for 30 minutes daily, they can begin concentrating on the goals of their physical activity program. As fitness progresses, exercisers can work up to a higher level of their maximum heart rate target zone.

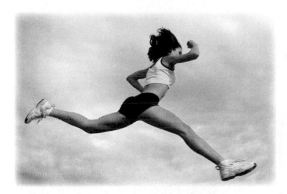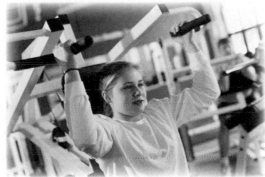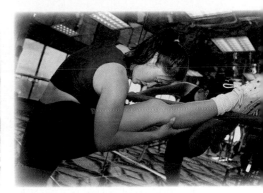

A total fitness plan includes aerobic training, strength training, and flexibility exercise.

To prepare and recover safely from an exercise session, warm-up and cool-down periods should be included. Warm-up includes 5 to 10 minutes of low-intensity exercises, such as walking, slow jogging, or stretching, and calisthenics that warm muscles and prepare them for exercise. The warm-up should be gradual and sufficient to increase muscle and body temperature, but it should not cause fatigue or deplete energy stores. Cool-down activities help prevent injury and soreness. These activities are like those performed during the warm-up and should be done gradually and allow the body to recover slowly.

Knowledge Check

1. How do aerobic and resistance exercise differ?
2. What are the components of a good fitness program?
3. What is perceived exertion and how is it measured?

 ## 11.3 Energy Sources for Muscle Use

Recall that cells cannot directly use the energy released from breaking down macronutrients. Rather, to utilize the chemical energy in foods, body cells must first convert the energy in foods to adenosine triphosphate (ATP).

ATP: Immediately Usable Energy

When the body uses energy, 1 of the phosphates in ATP is cleaved off, releasing usable energy for cell functions, including muscle contractions. The product remaining is ADP and inorganic phosphate (P_i). A resting muscle cell contains a small amount of ATP—just enough to keep the muscle working maximally for about 2 to 4 seconds. To produce more ATP for muscle contraction over extended periods, the body uses phosphocreatine. In addition, dietary carbohydrates, fats, and proteins are used as energy sources (Fig. 11-5). The breakdown of all these compounds releases energy to make more ATP (Table 11-1).

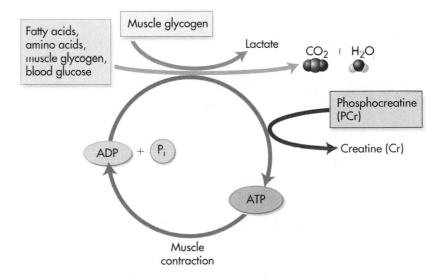

Figure 11-5 Energy sources for muscular activity. Different fuels are used for ATP synthesis. As shown, ATP also can be synthesized rapidly using phosphocreatine.

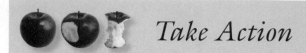

Take Action

How Physically Fit Are You?

The fitness assessments presented here are easy to do and require little equipment. Also included are charts to compare your results with those typical of your peers.

Cardiovascular Fitness: 1-Mile Walk

Measure a mile on a running track or on a little-trafficked neighborhood street. With a stopwatch or watch with a second hand, walk the mile as fast as you can. Note the time it took.

Strength: Push-Ups

Lie face down on the floor. Get up on your toes and hands. Women can use the same position or can use knees if necessary instead of toes. Keep your back straight, with hands flat on the floor directly below your shoulders. Lower your body, bending your elbows, until your chin grazes the floor. Push back up until your arms are straight. Count the number of push-ups you can do (you can rest when in the up position).

Strength: Curl-Ups

Lie on the floor on your back with your knees bent, feet flat. Rest your hands on your thighs. Now, squeeze your stomach muscles, push your back flat, and raise your upper body high enough for your hands to touch the tops of your knees. Don't pull with your neck or head, and keep your lower back on the floor. Count how many curl-ups you can do in 1 minute.

Flexibility: Sit-and-Reach

Place a yardstick on the floor and apply a 2-foot piece of tape on the floor perpendicular to the yardstick, crossing at the 15-inch mark.

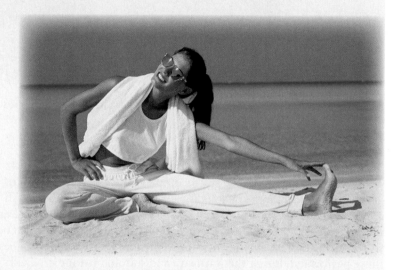

Sit on the floor with your legs extended and the soles of your feet touching the tape at the 15-inch mark, the 0-inch facing you. Your feet should be about 12 inches apart. Put 1 hand on the other, exhale, and very slowly reach forward as far as you can along the yardstick, lowering your head between your arms. Don't bounce! Note the farthest inch mark you reach. Don't hurt yourself by reaching farther than your body wants to. Relax, and then repeat 2 more times.

Now, check your results. If you want to improve:

- Do aerobic exercise that makes you breathe hard for at least half an hour on almost or all days of the week.
- Lift weights that challenge you 2 or 3 times per week.
- Stretch after activity at least a couple of times per week.
- Walk more.

Cardiovascular: 1-Mile Walk (Time, in Minutes)				
	Under 40 Years		**Over 40 Years**	
	Men	**Women**	**Men**	**Women**
Excellent	13:00 or less	13:30 or less	14:00 or less	14:30 or less
Good	13:01–15:30	13:31–16:00	14:01–16:30	14:31–17:00
Average	15:31–18:00	16:01–18:30	16:31–19:00	17:01–19:30
Below average	18:01–19:30	18:31–20:00	19:01–21:30	19:31–22:00
Poor	19:31 or more	20:01 or more	21:31 or more	22:01 or more

Source: Cooper Institute.

(continued)

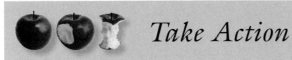

Take Action

Strength: Push-Ups (Number Completed without Rest)

	Ages 17–19		Ages 20–29		Ages 30–39		Ages 40–49		Ages 50–59		Ages 60–65	
	Men	Women	Men	Women	Men	Women	Men	Women	Men	Women	Men	Women
Excellent	> 56	> 35	> 47	> 36	> 41	> 37	> 34	> 31	> 31	> 25	> 30	> 23
Good	47–56	27–35	39–47	30–36	34–41	30–37	28–34	25–31	25–31	21–25	24–30	19–23
Above average	35–46	21–27	30–39	23–29	25–33	22–30	21–28	18–24	18–24	15–20	17–23	13–18
Average	19–34	11–20	17–29	12–22	13–24	10–21	11–20	8–17	9–17	7–14	6–16	5–12
Below average	11–18	6–10	10–16	7–11	8–12	5–9	6–10	4–7	5–8	3–6	3–5	2–4
Poor	4–10	2–5	4–9	2–6	2–7	1–4	1–5	1–3	1–4	1–2	1–2	1
Very poor	< 4	0–1	< 4	0–1	< 2	0	0	0	0	0	0	0

Source: topendsports.com.

Strength: Curl-Ups (Number Completed in 60 Seconds)

	Ages 18–25		Ages 26–35		Ages 36–45		Ages 46–55		Ages 56–65		Ages 65+	
	Men	Women	Men	Women	Men	Women	Men	Women	Men	Women	Men	Women
Excellent	> 49	> 43	> 45	> 39	> 41	> 33	> 35	> 27	> 31	> 24	> 28	> 23
Good	44–49	37–43	40–45	33–39	35–41	27–33	29–35	22–27	25–31	18–24	22–28	17–23
Above average	39–43	33–36	35–39	29–32	30–34	23–26	25–28	18–21	21–24	13–17	19–21	14–16
Average	35–38	29–32	31–34	25–28	27–29	19–22	22–24	14–17	17–20	10–12	15–18	11–13
Below average	31–34	25–28	29–30	21–24	23–26	15–18	18–21	10–13	13–16	7–9	11–14	5–10
Poor	25–30	18–24	22–28	13–20	17–22	7–14	13–17	5–9	9–12	3–6	7–10	2–4
Very poor	< 25	< 18	< 22	< 20	< 17	< 7	< 9	< 5	< 9	< 3	< 7	< 2

Source: topendsports.com.

Flexibility: Sit-and-Reach (in Inches)

	Men	Women
Super	> +27	> +30
Excellent	+17 – +27	+21 – +30
Good	+6 – +16	+11 – +20
Average	0 – +5	+1 – +10
Fair	–8 – –1	–7 – 0
Poor	–19 – –9	–14 – –8
Very poor	< – 20	< – 15

Source: topendsports.com.

These charts are typical of those used by health and fitness experts. For a more thorough assessment of fitness or for development of an exercise plan appropriate for your fitness level, consult a certified personal trainer or another fitness professional.

Table 11-1 Energy Stored in the Human Body as ATP, Phosphocreatine PCr, and Various Forms of Carbohydrate and Fat Site

Energy Source	Major Storage	When Used	Activity
ATP	All Tissues	All the time	Sprinting (0–3 sec)
Phosphocreatine (PCr)	All Tissues	Short bursts	Shot put, high jump, bench press
Carbohydrate (anaerobic)	Muscles and liver	High intensity lasting 30 seconds to 2 minutes	200-meter sprint
Carbohydrate (aerobic)	Muscles and liver	Exercise lasting 2 minutes to 3 hours or more	Jogging, soccer, basketball, swimming, gardening, car washing
Fat (aerobic)	Muscles and fat cells	Exercise lasting more than a few minutes; greater amounts are used at lower exercise intensities	Long-distance running, marathons, ultra endurance events, cycling, day-long hikes

The total amount of energy is approximate and may vary considerably between individuals.

phosphocreatine (PCr) High-energy compound that can be used to re-form ATP from ADP.

creatine Organic molecule in muscle cells that is a part of the high-energy compound creatine phosphate, or phosphocreatine.

Phosphocreatine: Initial Resupply of Muscle ATP

Phosphocreatine (PCr) is a high-energy compound created from ATP and **creatine (Cr)** and is stored in small amounts in muscle cells. Creatine is an organic molecule in muscle cells that is synthesized from 3 amino acids: glycine, arginine, and methionine.[9] As soon as ADP from the breakdown of ATP begins to accumulate in a contracting muscle, an enzyme is activated, transferring a high-energy P_i from PCr to ADP—this transfer reforms ATP (Fig. 11-6).

Figure 11-6 Quick energy for muscle use includes a supply of phosphocreatine (PCr). Phosphocreatine can rapidly replenish ATP stores as activity begins, but in less than 60 seconds it can become nearly depleted in maximally contracting human forearm muscles. It takes 4 minutes of rest to replenish half the PCr and 7 minutes to replenish 95% of the PCr. Similarly, it takes about 7 minutes of rest to replenish 95% of the PCr depleted with repeated knee extensions against resistance.

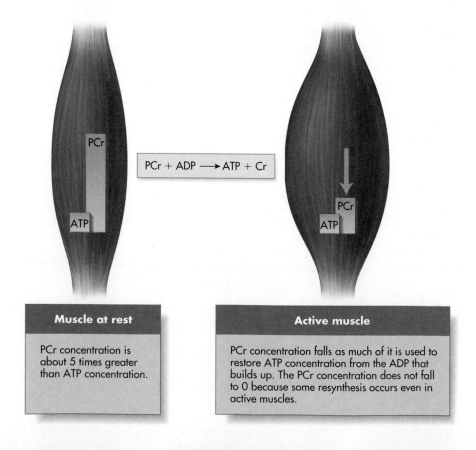

PCr + ADP ⟶ ATP + Cr

Muscle at rest

PCr concentration is about 5 times greater than ATP concentration.

Active muscle

PCr concentration falls as much of it is used to restore ATP concentration from the ADP that builds up. The PCr concentration does not fall to 0 because some resynthesis occurs even in active muscles.

If no other system for resupplying ATP were available, PCr could probably maintain maximal muscle contractions for about 10 seconds.[1] However, because the energy released from the metabolism of glucose and fatty acids also begins to contribute ATP and thus spares some PCr use, PCr can function as the major source of energy for events lasting up to about 1 minute.

The main advantage of PCr is that it can be activated instantly and can replenish ATP quickly enough to meet the energy demands of the fastest and most powerful sports events, such as jumping, lifting, throwing, and sprinting. The disadvantage of PCr is that too little is made and stored in muscles to sustain a high rate of ATP resupply for more than a few minutes.

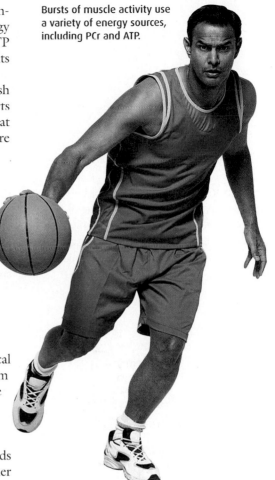

Bursts of muscle activity use a variety of energy sources, including PCr and ATP.

Carbohydrate: Major Fuel for Short-Term, High-Intensity, and Medium-Term Exercise

As you know, glucose breaks down during glycolysis, producing a 3-carbon compound called pyruvate. Glycolysis does not require oxygen, but it yields only a small amount of ATP. If oxygen is present, pyruvate is metabolized further, yielding much more ATP.

Anaerobic Pathway

When the oxygen supply in muscle is limited (anaerobic state) or when the physical activity is intense (e.g., running 400 meters or swimming 100 meters), pyruvate from glycolysis accumulates in the muscle and is converted to lactate (Fig. 11-7). Because the breakdown of 1 glucose molecule to 2 pyruvates yields 2 ATP, glycolysis can resupply some ATP depleted in muscle activity.[9] Carbohydrate is the only fuel that can be used for this process.

Glycolysis provides most of the energy for physical activity from about 30 seconds to 2 minutes after it has started. The advantage of the anaerobic pathway is that, other than PCr breakdown, it is the fastest way to resupply ATP in muscle.[1] The anaerobic pathway has 3 major disadvantages.

- It cannot sustain ATP production for long.
- Only about 5% of the energy available from glucose is released during glycolysis.
- The rapid accumulation of lactate from anaerobic glycolysis greatly increases the acidity of muscle cells. Because high acidity inhibits the activity of key enzymes in glycolysis, anaerobic ATP production soon slows and fatigue sets in. The acidity also leads to a net potassium loss from muscle cells, providing another cause of fatigue.[9] By trial and error, we learn an exercise pace that controls muscle lactate concentrations from anaerobic glycolysis.

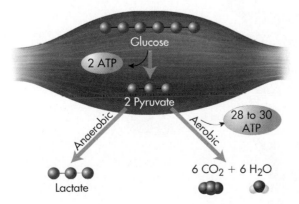

Figure 11-7 Both anaerobic and aerobic pathways can supply ATP. However, the aerobic pathway can supply more ATP but does it at a slower rate, whereas the anaerobic pathway supplies less ATP at a more rapid rate.

Most of the lactate that accumulates in active muscle cells is eventually released into the bloodstream. The heart can use lactate directly for its energy needs, as can less active muscle cells situated near active ones. The liver (and to some extent the kidneys) takes up some of the lactate from the blood and resynthesizes it into glucose, using an energy-requiring process. This glucose then can reenter the bloodstream and be used by cells for energy.

Aerobic Pathway

If plenty of oxygen is available in muscle tissue (aerobic state) and physical activity is moderate- to low-intensity (e.g., jogging or distance swimming), most of the pyruvate produced by glycolysis in the cell cytoplasm is shuttled to the mitochondria and metabolized into carbon dioxide and water by a series of oxygen-requiring reactions (see Chapter 9). About 95% of the ATP produced from the complete metabolism of glucose is formed aerobically in the mitochondria (Fig. 11-8).

The aerobic pathway supplies ATP more slowly than the anaerobic pathway, but it releases much more energy. Also, ATP production via the aerobic pathway can be sustained for hours. As a result, this pathway of glucose metabolism makes an important

▶ When acids lose a hydrogen ion, as typically happens at the pH level of the body, they are given the ending -*ate*. Thus, pyruvic acid is called pyruvate and lactic acid is called lactate when in the context of body metabolism.

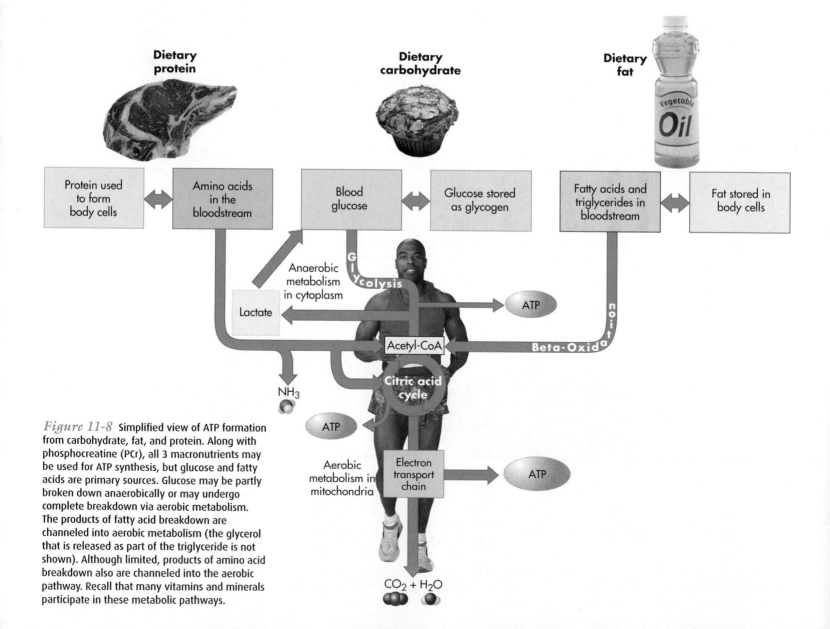

Figure 11-8 Simplified view of ATP formation from carbohydrate, fat, and protein. Along with phosphocreatine (PCr), all 3 macronutrients may be used for ATP synthesis, but glucose and fatty acids are primary sources. Glucose may be partly broken down anaerobically or may undergo complete breakdown via aerobic metabolism. The products of fatty acid breakdown are channeled into aerobic metabolism (the glycerol that is released as part of the triglyceride is not shown). Although limited, products of amino acid breakdown also are channeled into the aerobic pathway. Recall that many vitamins and minerals participate in these metabolic pathways.

energy contribution to physical activity lasting from about 2 minutes through 3 hours or more (Fig. 11-9).[1]

Muscle Glycogen versus Blood Glucose as Muscle Fuel

Recall that glycogen is the temporary storage form of glucose in the liver (about 100 g) and muscles (about 350 g in sedentary people). Glycogen is broken down to glucose, which can be metabolized by both the anaerobic and aerobic pathways. Liver glycogen is used to maintain blood glucose levels, whereas muscle glycogen supplies the glucose to the working muscle. Glycogen is, in fact, the primary source of glucose for ATP production in muscle cells during fairly intense activities that last for less than about 2 hours.

In short events (e.g., less than 30 minutes or so), muscles rely primarily on muscle glycogen stores for carbohydrate fuel. Muscles do not take up much blood glucose during short-term exercise because the action of insulin, which increases glucose uptake by muscles, is blunted by other hormones, such as epinephrine and glucagon, that increase initially during exercise.[1] As exercise time increases, muscle glycogen stores decline and the muscles begin to take up blood glucose to use as an energy source. The depletion of glycogen in the muscles contributes to fatigue, whereas the depletion of glycogen in the liver leads to a fall in blood glucose.[9]

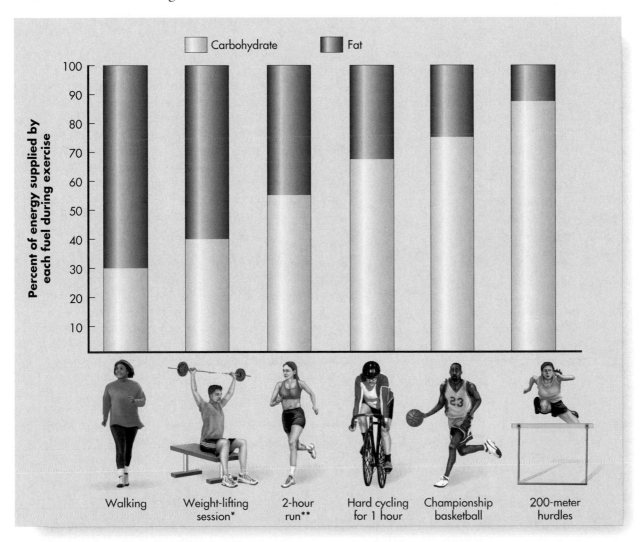

Figure 11-9
Rough estimates of carbohydrate and fat use during various forms of exercise.

*With regard to weight lifting, carbohydrate use can be somewhat greater and fat use somewhat less if the session is intense and fast-paced (e.g., circuit training). Fat use generally is higher because much of the time spent weight lifting is for rest periods.

**With regard to endurance running, the balance of fat and carbohydrate used will vary somewhat depending on whether the athlete is consuming carbohydrate during the run. The values shown are for a runner consuming carbohydrate during the run; more fat and less carbohydrate would be used if carbohydrates were not consumed.

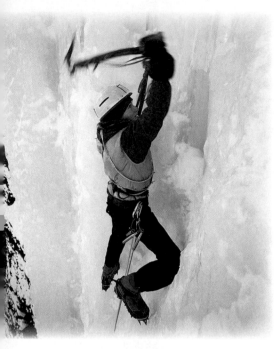

The energy to perform comes from carbohydrate, fat, and protein. The relative mix of fuels depends on the pace of exercise.

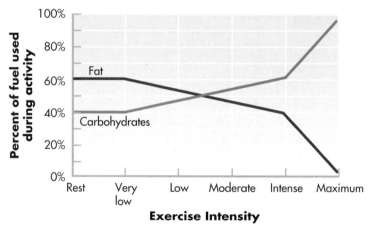

Figure 11-10 As the intensity of exercise increases, the exercising muscles tend to rely more on carbohydrates and less on fat. At lower intensities of exercise, fat is the predominant fuel.

Once glycogen stores are exhausted, a person can continue working at only about 50% of maximal capacity. Athletes call this point of glycogen depletion "hitting the wall," because further exertion is hampered. Thus, for exercise that requires 70% or more of maximal effort for more than an hour or so, athletes (e.g., long-distance runners or cyclists) should consider increasing the amount of carbohydrate stored in their muscles. Diets high in carbohydrate can be used to increase muscle glycogen stores—up to double the typical amounts—in advance of competition, thereby delaying the onset of fatigue and improving endurance (see Section 11.5).

The maintenance of blood glucose becomes an increasingly important consideration as exercise duration increases beyond about 20 to 30 minutes. By maintaining blood glucose levels, muscle glycogen is saved for muscle use during sudden bursts of effort, such as a sprint to the finish in a marathon race. Without the maintenance of blood glucose, irritability, sweating, anxiety, weakness, headache, and confusion may occur (cyclists call this "bonking"). A carbohydrate intake of 0.7 g/kg/hour (about 30–60 g/hour) during strenuous endurance exercise, such as cycling, that lasts about 1 hour or more, can help maintain adequate blood glucose concentrations, which in turn results in delay of fatigue (see Section 11.5).[10]

Fat: Main Fuel for Prolonged, Low-Intensity Exercise

Fat is the predominant fuel source during prolonged exercise, especially when exercise remains at a low or moderate (aerobic) rate (Fig. 11-10). In fact, during very lengthy activities, such as a triathlon, an ultra-marathon, occupations requiring manual labor, or even work at a desk for 8 hours a day, fat supplies about 50 to 90% of the energy required.[1]

The rate at which muscles use fatty acids is affected by training level. The more trained a muscle, the greater its ability to use fat as a fuel. Training increases the size and number of mitochondria and the levels of enzymes involved with the aerobic synthesis of ATP. Training also increases muscle myoglobin, which enhances oxygen availability in muscles needed to metabolize fat (Table 11-2). Overall, training allows an athlete to use fat for fuel more readily, thereby conserving glycogen for when it is really needed—such as for a burst of speed at the end of a race.

As you know, most of the energy stored in the body is in fat, stored as triglycerides. Most of this energy resides in adipose tissue, although some is stored in the muscle itself. That stored in muscles is especially used as activity increases from a low to a moderate pace.

The advantage of fat over other energy sources is that it provides more than twice (9 kcal/g) as much energy and thus can provide more ATP. In addition, there is plenty of fat stored in the body, compared with the very limited carbohydrate stores. How-

Table 11-2 Adaptations to Endurance Exercise Training in Skeletal Muscle	
Changes	**Advantage**
Increased ability of muscle to store glycogen (high-carbohydrate diet increases this even further)	More glycogen fuel available for the final minutes of an event
Increased triglyceride storage in muscle	Conserves glycogen by allowing for increased fat use
Increased mitochondrial size and number	Conserves glycogen by allowing for increased fat use (even at high exercise outputs)
Increased myoglobin content	Increased oxygen delivery to muscles and increased ability to use fat for fuel

ever, carbohydrate metabolism is more efficient than fat because it produces more ATP per unit of oxygen and it is the only fuel source that can support intense (anaerobic) activity. Fat utilization simply cannot occur fast enough to meet the ATP demands of short-duration, high-intensity physical activity—if fat were the only available fuel, we would be unable to carry out physical activity more intense than a fast walk or jog.[1]

Protein: A Minor Fuel Source during Exercise

Most of the energy supplied from protein comes from metabolism of the branched-chain amino acids—leucine, isoleucine, and valine. These amino acids can be used to make glucose, or they can enter the citric acid cycle as precursors to glucose and provide energy during exercise.

Although amino acids derived from protein can fuel muscles, their contribution is relatively small, compared with that of carbohydrate and fat. As a rough guide, only about 5% of the body's general energy needs, as well as the typical energy needs of exercising muscles, is supplied by amino acid metabolism.[9] However, proteins can contribute to energy needs in endurance exercise, perhaps as much as 15%, especially as glycogen stores in the muscle are exhausted.[9] Endurance exercise is when protein is most likely to make its most significant contribution as a fuel source—but, even then, it provides limited energy, with estimates ranging from 3 to 15%.[9,11] In contrast, protein is used least in resistance exercise (e.g., weight lifting).

Despite the fact that the primary muscle fuels for weight lifting are phosphocreatine (PCr) and carbohydrate, high-protein supplements are marketed to weight lifters and bodybuilders and sold in nearly every health food and fitness store. Consuming more protein than the body needs or can use will not lead to greater muscle mass. Eating high-carbohydrate, moderate-protein foods immediately after a weight-training workout can enhance the anabolic effect of the activity. This most likely increases blood concentrations of insulin and growth hormone and contributes to protein synthesis.[1] Remember, it is impossible to increase muscle mass simply by eating protein; putting physical strain on muscle through strength training or other physical activity is needed, as is adequate protein intake to support growth and recovery.

Fuel Use and VO_{2max}

As you can see in Table 11-3, fuel sources for muscle cells can be estimated based on percent of VO_{2max}. For example, fat use drops as exercise intensity increases. Carbohydrate use then becomes more important for meeting energy needs. In very-high-intensity activities, the ATP equivalent to the "extra" 50% above 100% of VO_{2max} is produced anaerobically from PCr and glycolysis.

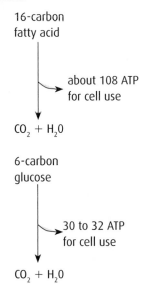

ATP Yield from Aerobic Fatty Acid Metabolism and Aerobic Glucose Metabolism

16-carbon fatty acid

about 108 ATP for cell use

$CO_2 + H_2O$

6-carbon glucose

30 to 32 ATP for cell use

$CO_2 + H_2O$

CASE STUDY

Jake, a college junior, is currently 6 feet tall and weighs 175 pounds. He has been lifting weights since he was a college freshman. Although he has gotten significantly stronger over the last 2 years, he decided he wants to have more muscle definition. He read (mainly on the Internet) a lot about nutrition and resistance training, especially about the role of protein and muscle growth and decided to take a protein supplement to get bigger muscles and more definition. He has been taking the supplement for about 3 weeks. It consists of a whey protein powder, which he mixes with either water or milk. It contains about 60 grams of protein per serving and he has 2 protein drinks per day.

His breakfasts consist of a protein shake and for lunch he has a sandwich with extra meat and a small salad with fat-free dressing. He consumes another shake around 4 P.M. and isn't hungry again until about 7 P.M. Yesterday for dinner, he ate 2 chicken breasts with ½ cup of rice, a small salad with fat-free dressing, and an iced tea.

Unfortunately, this past week he noticed that during his lifting he was tired and could not lift as much weight as the week before. Today while lifting, he started to feel fatigued 20 minutes into the training session. He is not sure why he can't finish his workout and thinks maybe he should eat more protein.

What role does protein have in resistance exercise? What is causing him to be so fatigued that he cannot finish his workout? Should he consume more protein?

Table 11-3 Fuel Use Estimate Based on Percent VO_{2max}

VO_{2max}	Muscle Glycogen	Muscle Triglyceride	Blood Glucose	Free Fatty Acids in the Bloodstream
Low-intensity (e.g., fast walk)—30 to 50% of VO_{2max}	5%	20%	5%	70%
Moderate-intensity (e.g., fast jog)—50 to 65% of VO_{2max}	30%	30%	10%	30%
High-intensity (e.g., 3-hour marathon pace)—70 to 80% of VO_{2max}	55 %	15%	15%	15%
Very-high-intensity (e.g., sprints)—85 to 150% of VO_{2max}	70%	10%	10%	10%

Knowledge Check

1. What is the main form of energy that cells use?
2. What fuels anaerobic exercise?
3. What fuels aerobic exercise?
4. Why is creatine so important for fueling high-intensity, short-duration exercise?
5. How does fitness level affect the fuels burned for exercise?
6. When is protein used as a fuel source during exercise?

muscle fiber Essentially a single muscle cell; an elongated cell, with contractile properties, that forms the muscles of the body.

Relative Distribution of Muscle Fiber Types

Activity Level	Type 1	Type IIA + Type IIX
Non-athlete	45–50%	50–55%
Sprinter	20–35%	65–85%
Marathoner	80%	20%

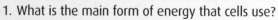

11.4 The Body's Response to Physical Activity

Physical activity has many effects on the body. The most pronounced effects are typically seen in the muscular, circulatory, and skeletal systems.

Specialized Functions of Skeletal Muscle Fiber Types

The body contains 3 major types of muscle tissue: skeletal muscle (the type involved in locomotion); smooth muscle (the type found in internal organs, except the heart); and cardiac (heart) muscle. Skeletal muscle is composed of 3 main types of **muscle fibers**, which have distinct characteristics (Table 11-4).[9]

Table 11-4 Muscle Fiber Summary

Muscle Fiber	Description	Structure	Primary Fuel Source	Activities When Used
Type I	Slow-twitch; high oxidative metabolism capacity	High density of capillaries, mitochondria, myoglobin	Aerobic metabolism of fat	Aerobic activity, such as endurance exercise
Type IIA	Fast-twitch; moderate oxidative metabolism capacity	Rich in capillaries and mitochondria	Anaerobic glycolysis; aerobic metabolism of fat and glucose	Aerobic/anaerobic activities, such as middle-distance running, swimming
Type IIX	Fast-twitch; lower oxidative metabolism capacity	Less dense in mitochondria and myoglobin	Anaerobic glycolysis	Anaerobic activity, such as sprinting

- *Type I (slow-twitch—oxidative).* These muscle fibers contract slowly and have a high capacity for oxidative metabolism. They also are called red fibers because of their high myoglobin content. Type I fibers are fueled by the aerobic metabolism of fat.
- *Type IIA (fast-twitch—oxidative, glycolytic).* These muscle fibers have moderate oxidative capacity and are fueled by glycolysis using glucose (anaerobic) plus the aerobic metabolism of both fat and glucose.
- *Type IIX (fast-twitch—glycolytic).* These muscle fibers have less oxidative capacity than other muscle fibers. They also are called white fibers (in rodents, type IIX fibers are called type IIB) because they have less mitochondria and myoglobin than other fibers. Type IIX fibers are fueled by glycolysis using glucose (anaerobic).

Prolonged, low-intensity exercise, such as a slow jog, mainly uses type I muscle fibers, so the predominant fuel is fat. As exercise intensity increases, type IIA and type IIX fibers are gradually recruited; in turn, the contribution of glucose as a fuel increases. Type IIA and type IIX fibers also are important for rapid movements, such as a jump shot in basketball.

The relative proportions of the 3 fiber types throughout the muscles of the body vary from person to person and are constant throughout each person's life. The individual differences in fiber-type distribution are partially responsible for producing elite marathon runners who could never compete at the same level as sprinters, or elite gymnasts who could never be competitive as long-distance swimmers. Although the proportion of muscle fiber types is largely determined by genetics, appropriate training can develop muscles within limits. For example, aerobic training enhances the capacity of type IIA muscle fibers to produce ATP and may bring about a relative change in size. Overall, great athletes are born, but their genetic potential must be nurtured by training.[9]

Adaptation of Muscles and Body Physiology to Exercise

With training, muscle strength becomes matched to the muscles' work demands. Muscles enlarge after being made to work repeatedly, a response called **hypertrophy**. Certain cells in the muscles gain bulk and improve their ability to work. Conversely, after several days without activity, muscles diminish in size and lose strength, a response called **atrophy**. Both hypertrophy and atrophy are forms of adaptation to the workload applied. Thus, many marathon runners have well-developed leg muscles but little arm or chest muscle development.

Repeated aerobic exercise produces beneficial changes in the circulatory system. Because the body needs more oxygen during exercise, it responds to training by producing more red blood cells and expanding total blood volume. Training also leads to an increase in the number of capillaries in muscle tissue; as a result, oxygen can be delivered more easily to muscle cells. Finally, training causes the heart, a muscle itself, to strengthen. Then, each contraction empties the heart's chamber more efficiently, so more blood is pumped with each beat. As exercise increases the heart's efficiency, its rate of beating at rest and during submaximal exercise decreases.[1]

The more physically fit a person is, the more work the muscles and body can do and the more oxygen the person can consume. Typical VO_{2max} values range from 20–65 ml O_2/kg/min depending on age, gender and fitness level. Most people can improve their VO_{2max} by 15 to 20% or more with training.[9]

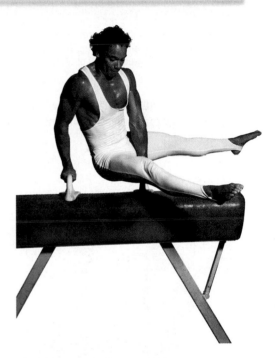

The quick, powerful movements of the gymnast rely primarily on type IIA and type IIX muscle fibers. What sort of physiological changes would you expect to occur in a gymnast who has trained diligently for many years?

	Typical VO_{2max} ml O_2/kg/min
Sedentary elderly person	15
Typical middle-aged adult	35–45
Elite athlete	65–75

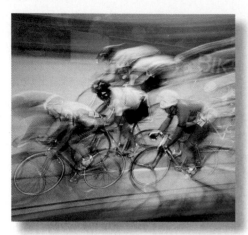

Athletes often expend much energy. An increase in food and beverage intake can easily provide ample carbohydrate, protein, and other nutrients to support activity.

▶ Review Table 10-5 in Chapter 10, which lists the energy costs of typical forms of physical activity.

Another adaptation that occurs with exercise is increased bone density. By placing a mechanical stress on bone, exercise stimulates bone development by promoting the deposition of calcium in bones. Weight-bearing exercise, such as running, gymnastics, basketball, soccer, walking, and volleyball, is essential for the normal development and maintenance of a healthy skeleton.

Knowledge Check

1. How do the functions of the muscle fiber types differ?
2. What is the predominant fuel used by each muscle fiber type?
3. How does repeated exercise affect the circulatory system?

 11.5 Power Food: Dietary Advice for Athletes

Athletic training and genetic makeup are very important determinants of athletic performance. A good diet won't substitute for either factor, but making wise food choices will allow an athlete to maximize his or her athletic potential. On the other hand, poor food choices can seriously reduce performance.

Energy Needs

Athletes need varying amounts of food energy, depending on their body size, their body composition, and the type of training or competition. A petite gymnast may need only 1800 kcal/day to sustain normal daily activities without losing body weight; a tall, muscular swimmer may need 4000 kcal/day. If an athlete experiences daily fatigue and/or weight loss, the first consideration should be whether that person is consuming enough food. Up to 6 meals per day may be needed, including 1 before each workout.

Monitoring body weight is an easy way to assess the adequacy of calorie intake. Athletes should strive to maintain weight during competition and training. Generally, if athletes are losing weight, then energy intake is inadequate; however, if athletes are gaining weight, then energy intake is too high. If an athlete needs to lose weight, his or her food intake should be lowered by 200 to 500 kcal per day. This slight reduction will allow the athlete to continue to train and compete yet will create a calorie deficit, so that weight loss can be achieved. Reducing fat intake is the best way to cut calories and not affect performance. On the other hand, if an athlete needs to gain weight, increasing food intake by 500 to 700 kcal/day will eventually achieve that goal. The extra calories should come from a healthy balance of carbohydrate, protein, and fat; exercise needs to be maintained to make sure this gain is mostly in the form of lean muscle mass.

Some athletes compete in sports that require them to maintain a lean profile, whereas others must maintain a certain weight. Gymnasts, swimmers, figure skaters, and dancers are required to maintain a lean profile, whereas wrestlers, boxers, jockeys, judoists, and rowers are often weighed before matches to verify they meet weight restrictions. Athletes in sports such as these tend to eat and drink less than needed to support training and competition needs—this puts them at risk of eating disorders and the effects of poor nutritional status, including osteoporosis, menstrual dysfunction, kidney failure, heat-related illness, dehydration, and even death (Fig. 11-11).

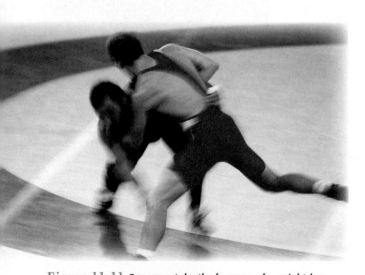

Figure 11-11 To prevent deaths from unsafe weight-loss practices in wrestlers, the National Collegiate Athletic Association and many states now establish a weight class at the beginning of the season to eliminate the severe weight-loss practices that often happen at the end of the season. Each school must have a physician or an athletic trainer conduct an initial weight assessment during the first week of October using body weight, body composition (body fat), and specific gravity of urine (to determine level of hydration at time of weighing). Minimum wrestling weight is set at the student-athlete's lean body weight plus 5% body fat. Each wrestler has the option of modifying his weight over an 8-week period under the following guidelines: no more than 1.5% of body weight can be lost per week, and the final weight cannot fall below the calculated minimum wrestling weight. A national certification period is held the first week of December. At that time, the process is repeated and a weight class is set that remains in place for the rest of the wrestling season.

Carbohydrate Needs

Carbohydrates are the primary energy source for exercising muscles. Anyone who exercises vigorously, especially for more than an hour per day on a regular basis, needs to consume moderate to high amounts of carbohydrates. Numerous servings of grains, starchy vegetables, and fruits provide enough carbohydrate to maintain adequate liver and muscle glycogen stores, especially for replacing glycogen losses from workouts on the previous day. Table 11-5 shows some nutritious, carbohydrate-rich foods.

Carbohydrate intake should be at least 5 to 7 g/kg of body weight. Athletes engaged in aerobic training and endurance activities (duration 60 minutes or more per day) may need as much as 7 to 9 g/kg of body weight. When exercise duration approaches several hours per day, the carbohydrate recommendation increases up to

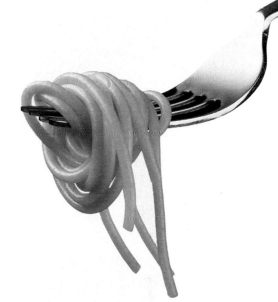

High-carbohydrate foods should form the basis of an athlete's diet.

Table 11-5 Grams of Carbohydrate Based on Serving Size of Typical Carbohydrate-Rich Foods

Starches—15g Carbohydrate per Serving (80 kcal)

One Serving

Dry breakfast cereal,* ½–¾ cup	Baked potato, ¼ 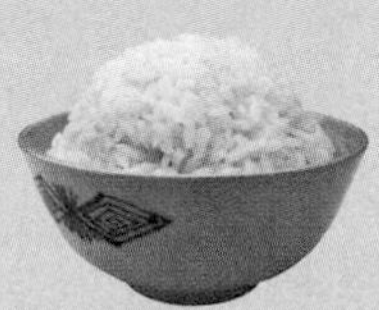
Cooked breakfast cereal, ½ cup	Bagel, ¼ (4 oz)
Cooked grits, ½ cup	English muffin, ½
Cooked rice, ⅓ cup	Bread, 1 slice
Cooked pasta, ⅓ cup	Pretzels, ¾ oz
Cooked beans, ⅓ cup	Saltine crackers, 6
Cooked corn, ½ cup	Pancake, 4 inches in diameter, 1
Cooked/dry beans, ½ cup	Taco shells, 2 (add 45 kcal)

Vegetables—5 g Carbohydrate per Serving (25 kcal)

One Serving

Cooked or canned vegetables, ½ cup
Raw vegetables, 1 cup
Vegetable juice, ½ cup

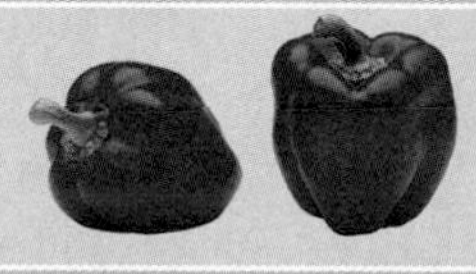

Fruits—15 g Carbohydrate per Serving (60 kcal)

One Serving

Canned fruit, ½ cup	Grapes, 17 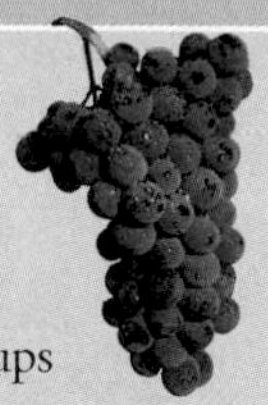
Fruit juice, ½ cup	Grapefruit, ½
Figs (dried), 1½	Dates, 3
Apple or orange, 1 small	Peach, 1
Apricots (dried), 8	Watermelon cubes, 1¼ cups
Banana, 1 small	

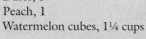

Milk—12 g Carbohydrate per Serving

One Serving

Milk, 1 cup	Soy milk, 1 cup
Plain low-fat yogurt, ⅔ cup	

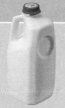

Sweets—15 g Carbohydrate per Serving (variable kcal)

One Serving

Cake, 2-inch square	Ice cream, ½ cup 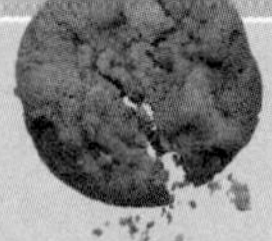
Cookies, 2 small	Sherbet, ½ cup

*The carbohydrate content of dry cereal varies widely. Check the labels of those you choose and adjust the serving size accordingly.
Modified from *Exchange Lists for Meal Planning* by the American Diabetes Association and American Dietetic Association, 2003, Chicago, American Dietetic Association.

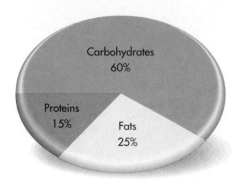

Figure 11-12 Recommended nutrient intakes for athletes.

10 g/kg of body weight.[12] In other words, triathletes and marathon runners should consider eating close to 500 to 600 grams of carbohydrates daily. Even more may be necessary to prevent chronic fatigue and to load the muscles and liver with glycogen. Attention to carbohydrate intake is especially important when performing multiple training bouts in a day, such as swim practices or track and field events, as well as tournament play, such as volleyball, basketball, or soccer. The depletion of carbohydrate ranks just behind the depletion of fluid and electrolytes as a major cause of fatigue.

Athletes should obtain at least 60% of total energy needs from carbohydrates, rather than the 50% typical of most North American diets, especially if exercise duration is expected to exceed 2 hours and total energy intake is about 3000 kcal per day or less (Fig. 11-12). Diets providing 4000 to 5000 kcal/day can have as little as 50% of energy content coming from carbohydrate and still provide sufficient carbohydrate (e.g., 500 to 600 g or so per day).[12] Table 11-6 shows sample menus for diets providing food energy ranging from 1800 to 5000 kcal/day. In addition, the Exchange System

Table 11-6 Sample Daily Menus, Based on MyPyramid, That Provide Various Total Energy Intakes

1800 kcal	3000 kcal	4000 kcal	5000 kcal
Breakfast	**Breakfast**	**Breakfast**	**Breakfast**
1 cup fat-free milk	1 cup fat-free milk	3 slices French toast	4 slices whole-wheat toast
1 cup Cheerios®	2 cups Cheerios®	2 tbsp syrup	2 tsp margarine
½ whole-wheat bagel	1 whole-wheat bagel	1 tsp margarine	2 poached eggs
1 tsp margarine	1 tsp margarine	1 banana	1 cup low-fat yogurt
	½ cup grapes	1 cup low-fat yogurt	½ cup granola
	1 large muffin		
Lunch	**Lunch**	**Lunch**	**Lunch**
2 oz sliced turkey breast	3 oz sliced turkey breast	4 medium beef and bean	3 chicken enchiladas
2 slices whole-wheat bread	2 slices whole-wheat bread	tacos topped with lettuce	1 oz shredded cheese
1 tsp mayonnaise	1 oz cheese	and shredded cheese	1 cup romaine lettuce with 1 cup
½ cup carrots	1 tsp mayonnaise	1 cup Spanish rice	carrots, celery, and green peppers
1 medium banana	1 banana	1 cup romaine lettuce	2 tbsp salad dressing
1 cup apple juice	½ cup carrots	2 tbsp salad dressing	1 banana
	1 cup yogurt	1½ cups orange juice	1 cup apple juice
	1 cup apple juice		1 fresh orange
			2 oz peanuts
Snack	**Snack**	**Snack**	**Snack**
1 granola bar	1 granola bar	2 slices whole-wheat bread	2 whole-grain bagels
1 cup low-fat yogurt	1 cup applesauce	4 tbsp peanut butter	3 tbsp almond butter
			1 cup grapes
Dinner	**Dinner**	**Dinner**	**Dinner**
3 oz roast beef	1 cup spaghetti with meat sauce	4 oz turkey breast	5 oz grilled salmon (or other fish)
1 medium baked potato	1½ cups pasta	2 cups mashed potatoes	2 cups rice pilaf
1 tsp margarine	1 tbsp Parmesan cheese	½ cup corn	1 cup asparagus
1 cup romaine lettuce	1 cup romaine lettuce	1 roll	1 cup green beans
2 tsp salad dressing	2 tsp salad dressing	1 tsp margarine	2 tsp margarine
1 cup green beans	1 cup green beans	1 cup vanilla pudding	1 cup low-fat yogurt topped with
1 cup fat-free milk	½ cup fat-free milk	½ cup sliced fruit	½ cup melon and ½ cup granola
		1 cup fat-free milk	1½ cups fat-free milk
Nutrient Contribution	**Nutrient Contribution**	**Nutrient Contribution**	**Nutrient Contribution**
57% carbohydrate	64% carbohydrate	50% carbohydrate	48% carbohydrate
20% protein	16% protein	17% protein	18% protein
25% fat	21% fat	33% fat	34% fat

(Appendix E) is a useful tool for planning all types of diets, including high-carbohydrate diets for athletes.

Boosting Glycogen Stores

The first source of glucose for the exercising muscle is its own glycogen store. During endurance exercise that exceeds 90 minutes, such as marathon running, muscle glycogen stores progressively decline. When they drop to critically low levels, high-intensity exercise cannot be maintained. In practical terms, the athlete is exhausted and must either stop exercising or drastically reduce the pace.

Glycogen depletion also may be a gradual process, occurring over repeated days of heavy training in which muscle glycogen breakdown exceeds its replacement, as well as during high-intensity exercise that is repeated several times during competition or training. For example, a distance runner who averages 10 miles per day, but does not take the time to consume enough carbohydrates, or a swimmer who completes several interval sets at above maximal oxygen consumption can deplete his or her glycogen stores rapidly.

Because carbohydrates are such an important fuel for exercise and the body has limited capacity to store them, researchers have investigated ways to maximize the body's ability to store carbohydrates. The regimen of getting the body to store more glycogen than typical is called **carbohydrate loading,** or **glycogen loading.** It involves altering both exercise and diet. The classic method of carbohydrate loading depleted muscle glycogen stores with 3 days of heavy training and a very-low-carbohydrate diet. This was followed by 3 days of high carbohydrate intake and rest to promote muscle glycogen synthesis. This classic method often left athletes exhausted and prone to injuries during the first 3 days. A modified method tapers off training intensity and duration on consecutive days after a bout of glycogen-depleting exercise 6 days before competition. During the first 3 days of tapering, the athlete consumes a normal mixed diet, followed by a high-carbohydrate diet 3 days before competition.

Carbohydrate-Loading Regimen						
Days before Competition	6	5	4	3	2	1
Exercise Time (Minutes)	60	40	40	20	20	Rest
Carbohydrate (g/kg Body Weight)	5	5	5	10	10	10

Carbohydrate-loading regimens usually increase muscle glycogen stores 50 to 85% over typical conditions, when dietary carbohydrate intake is only about 50% of total intake. However, the process is relatively slow. It takes from 2 to 6 days to fully load the muscles with glycogen. These regimens pose problems for athletes who compete on back-to-back days or who do not want to alter their training before a competition. Some preliminary research[13] indicates that 1 day of a high-carbohydrate diet (10.3 g/kg body weight) after a short bout of high-intensity exercise can increase muscle glycogen levels above typical levels. Although more studies need to confirm these results, this "new" carbohydrate-loading technique might result in better compliance and less disruption to training than the older carbohydrate-loading regimens.

Carbohydrate loading is for athletes who compete in continuous, intense aerobic events lasting more than 60 to 90 minutes or in shorter events taking place more than once within a 24-hour period. Above normal glycogen stores do not allow an athlete to work harder during shorter exercise periods, such as 5- and 10-km races, and may harm performance because of muscle stiffness and heaviness. With each gram of glycogen stored in the muscle, 3 to 4 grams of water also are stored. Although this water aids in maintaining hydration, this additional water weight may make the muscles feel stiff and therefore make carbohydrate loading inappropriate. Athletes who want to try carbohydrate loading should do so during training, and long before an important competition, to experience its effects on performance.

Appropriate Activities for Carbohydrate Loading

Marathons

Long-distance swimming

Cross-country skiing

30-kilometer runs

Triathlons

Tournament-play basketball

Soccer

Cycling time trials

Long-distance canoe racing

Inappropriate Activities for Carbohydrate Loading

American football games

10-kilometer or shorter runs

Walking and hiking

Most swimming events

Single basketball games

Weight lifting

Most track and field events

Table 11-7   Current Recommendations for Protein Intake Based on Body Weight (kg)*

Group	g/kg	Amount for a 70-kg Person (g)
RDA for adults	0.8	56
Strength-trained athletes, muscle mass maintenance phase	1.0–1.2	70–84
Strength-trained athletes, muscle mass gain phase	1.5–1.7	105–119
Moderate-intensity endurance activity athletes	1.2	84
High-intensity endurance athletes	1.7	112

*Calculate kilograms by dividing pounds by 2.2.
Adapted from Burke L, Deakin V. .*Clinical sports nutrition.* Roseville NSW2069, Australia: McGraw-Hill; 2000.

Fat Needs

A fat intake of 15 to 25% of energy is generally recommended for athletes. Rich sources of monounsaturated fat, such as canola and olive oil, should be emphasized, and saturated fat and *trans* fat intake should be limited.[12]

Protein Needs

Typical recommendations for protein intake for most athletes range from 1.0 to 1.7 g of protein/kg of body weight, which is considerably higher than the RDA of 0.8 g/kg of body weight for adults. As you can see in Table 11-7, recommended protein intake is at the lower end of the range for strength-training maintenance and moderate-intensity endurance activities. The highest recommendations are for high-intensity endurance training and during the muscle mass gain phase of strength training.

Energy needs are not the reason for the higher protein recommendations for athletes (recall that protein is not a major fuel for exercise). The extra protein is needed for the repair of tissue and the synthesis of the new muscle that results from training. The high level set for muscle mass gain during strength training, theoretically, is required for the synthesis of new muscle tissue brought on by the loading effect of this training. Once the desired muscle mass is achieved, protein intake need not exceed 1.2 g/kg of body weight.

Although it has long been a popular belief among athletes that additional protein increases strength and enhances performance, sports nutritionists and exercise physiologists generally agree that consuming protein at levels above recommendations does not build bigger or stronger muscles. Protein intakes above recommendations result in an increased use of amino acids for energy needs and has disadvantages, such as insufficient carbohydrate intake and increased urine production, which may interfere with body hydration. No advantages, such as an increase in muscle protein synthesis, are seen. Despite marketing claims, protein supplements are an expensive and unnecessary part of a fitness plan.

Any athlete not specifically on a low-calorie regimen can easily meet protein recommendations simply by eating a variety of foods (see Table 11-6). To illustrate, a 116-lb (53-kg) woman performing endurance activity can meet daily protein needs of 64 g (53 × 1.2) by eating a 3-oz chicken breast, a small hamburger (3 oz), and 2 glasses of milk. Similarly, a 170-lb (77-kg) man wanting to gain muscle mass through strength training needs to consume just 6 oz of chicken, ½ cup of cooked beans, 6 oz of canned tuna, and 3 glasses of milk to achieve an intake of 130 g of protein (77 × 1.7) in a day. Plus, for both athletes, these calculations do not include the protein they will get from

Weight-restricted athletes who feel they must significantly limit their energy intake and athletes who are vegetarians should be sure to consume at least 1.2 g of protein per kg of body weight each day, the upper recommendation for most athletes.

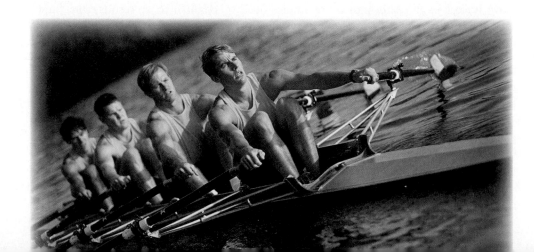

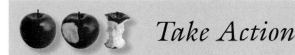

Take Action

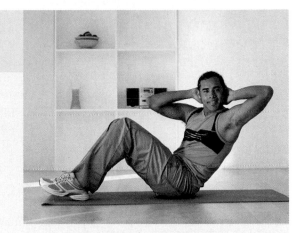

Meeting the Protein Needs of an Athlete—a Case Study

Mark is a college student who has been lifting weights at the student recreation center. Mark's weight has been stable at 154 lb (70 kg). An analysis of the total energy and protein content of Mark's current diet is 3470 kcal, 125 g of protein (14% of total energy intake supplied by protein). This diet is representative of the food choices and amounts of food that Mark chooses on a regular basis. The trainer at the center recommended a protein drink to help Mark build muscle mass. Answer the following questions and determine whether a protein drink is needed to supplement Mark's diet.

1. Determine Mark's protein needs based on the RDA (0.8 g/kg).

   a. Mark's estimated protein RDA: _____

   b. What are the maximum recommendations for protein intake for athletes?

   _____

   c. Calculate the maximum protein recommendation for Mark.

   _____

2. Compare Mark's protein intake with the recommended intake amounts.

   a. What is the difference between Mark's estimated protein needs as an athlete (from question 1) and the amount of protein that his current diet provides? _____

   b. Is his current protein intake inadequate, adequate, or excessive? _____

3. Mark takes his trainer's advice and goes to the supermarket to purchase a protein drink to add to his diet. Four products are available; they contain the following label information.

	Amino Fuel	Sugar-Free 90% Plus Protein	Dynamic Muscle Builder	Super Mega Mass 2000
Serving size	3 tbsp	3 tbsp	3 tbsp	1/4 scoop
Kcal	104	110	103	104
Protein (g)	15	24	10	5

The trainer recommends that Mark add the supplement to his diet 2 times a day. Mark chooses Dynamic Muscle Builder.

   a. How much protein would be added to Mark's diet daily from 2 servings of the supplement alone?

   b. How much total protein would Mark now consume in 1 day?

   c. What is the difference between Mark's estimated protein needs as an athlete and his total protein intake with the supplement?

4. What is your conclusion—does Mark need the protein supplement?

Answers to Calculations

1a. Mark's estimated protein RDA: 70 kg × 0.8 g/kg = 56 g

1b. Maximum recommendation for protein intake for athletes = 1.7 g/kg

1c. Applied to Mark: 1.7 × 70 = 119 g

2a. Difference between Mark's diet and the maximum amount recommended for athletes: 125 − 119 = 6 g

2b. Mark's current diet is adequate.

3a. Two servings of protein supplement alone = 20 g of protein

3b. Mark's total protein consumption: 125 g + 20 g = 145 g protein

3c. Difference between Mark's estimated maximum protein needs as an athlete and total protein consumption: 145 g − 119 g = 26 g of protein

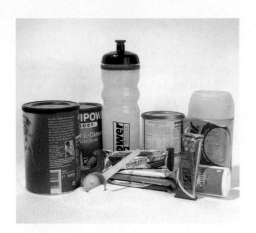

High-protein drinks, bars, and other products, which are often marketed to athletes, are unnecessary in most cases.

▶ At one time in his career, long-distance runner Alberto Salazar experienced problems sleeping and performed poorly because of low iron intake and related iron deficiency anemia.

the grains they eat. As you can see, simply by meeting their energy needs, many athletes consume much more protein than is required.

As you know, consuming carbohydrates immediately after exercise helps reload the muscles with glycogen for the next day's exercise. Including protein in these recovery meals or in a beverage consumed during exercise does not help muscle resynthesize glycogen;[14] however, it may help repair and synthesize muscle proteins. A small amount of protein (0.1–0.2 g/kg/hour) combined with sufficient amounts of carbohydrates (1.2 g/kg/hour) can enhance the muscles' ability to make new proteins during recovery from both endurance and resistance exercise.[11]

Vitamin and Mineral Needs

Vitamin and mineral needs are the same or slightly higher for athletes, compared with those of sedentary adults. Still, because athletes usually have such high energy intakes, they tend to consume plenty of vitamins and minerals. An exception is athletes consuming low-calorie diets (about 1200 kcal or less), such as some female athletes participating in events in which maintaining a low body weight is crucial. These diets may not meet B-vitamin and other micronutrient needs.[15] To meet vitamin and mineral needs, athletes consuming low-calorie diets and vegetarian athletes should consume fortified foods, such as ready-to-eat breakfast cereals, or a balanced multivitamin and mineral supplement.

Iron Deficiency and Impaired Performance

Because iron is involved in red blood cell production, oxygen transport, and energy production, a deficiency of this mineral can noticeably detract from optimal athletic performance.[16] The potential causes for iron deficiency in athletes vary. As in the general population, female athletes are most susceptible to low iron status due to monthly menstrual losses. Special diets followed by athletes, such as low-energy and vegetarian (especially vegan) diets, are likely to be low in iron. Distance runners should pay special attention to iron intake because their intense workouts may lead to gastrointestinal bleeding.

Another concern is sports anemia, which occurs because exercise causes blood plasma volume to expand, particularly at the start of a training regimen before the synthesis of red blood cells increases. This expansion results in dilution of the blood. In sports anemia, even if iron stores are adequate, blood iron tests may appear low. Sports anemia is not detrimental to performance, but it is hard to differentiate between sports anemia and true anemia.

True anemia, noted as a reduced blood hemoglobin level, may affect up to about 15% of males and 30% of females athletes. It is a good idea, especially for women athletes, to have their iron status checked at the beginning of a training season and at least once during midseason, as well as to monitor their dietary iron intake. Once depleted, iron stores can take months to replenish. For this reason, athletes must be especially careful to meet their iron needs.

Any blood test indicating low iron status—sports anemia or not—is cause for follow-up. For some athletes, the use of iron supplements may be advisable. However, the indiscriminate use of iron supplements is not advised because toxic effects are possible. It is important that physicians investigate the cause of the deficiency because iron deficiency can be caused by blood loss. If caught early, serious medical conditions often can be treated or prevented.

Calcium Intake and the Female Athlete Triad

Athletes, especially women trying to maintain a lean profile, can have marginal or low intakes of dietary calcium if they restrict their intake of milk and other dairy products. This practice compromises optimal bone health. Of still greater concern are women athletes who suffer from the female athlete triad, consisting of 3 conditions: menstrual disorders, low energy availability, and low bone mineral density.[17]

Research has clearly documented the importance of regular menstruation to maintain bone mineral density. Disturbing reports show that female athletes who do not menstruate regularly have far less dense spinal bones than both non-athletes and female athletes who menstruate regularly. These female athletes are at increased risk of bone fractures during training and competition. If irregular menstrual cycles persist, severe bone loss, much of which is not reversible, and osteoporosis can result.[18] This combination of risks outweighs the benefits of weight-bearing exercise for bone density.

Women with symptoms of the female athlete triad are best treated by a team that includes a physician, a registered dietitian, a psychologist, and an athletic trainer. The primary goals of treatment are to control and manage the athlete's diet, to restore normal hormone levels and menstruation, and to monitor and treat any injuries or other medical complications. Treatment strategies to reach these goals may include a slight reduction (10 to 20%) in the amount of training and a higher energy intake for a 2 to 5% increase in weight. Some amenorrheic athletes who gain weight either by cutting back on training or by consuming more energy have a better chance of resuming normal menstrual activity. Most amenorrheic athletes fear weight gain and must be counseled that an increase in muscle weight can improve their stamina and performance. Extra calcium in the diet does not necessarily compensate for the effects of menstrual irregularities, but inadequate dietary calcium can make matters worse. Calcium supplementation should be implemented in all athletes presenting with amenorrhea.

Knowledge Check

1. What is the easiest way for athletes to assess calorie intake?
2. What is the primary source of energy for an exercising muscle?
3. What is glycogen loading?
4. How does iron deficiency anemia affect athletic performance?
5. What is the female athlete triad?

11.6 Fluid Needs for Active Individuals

Active individuals need more fluids than those who are sedentary to replace fluid lost in sweat and, thereby, allow the body to regulate internal temperature normally.[10] Exercise can raise muscle temperature 15 to 20 times above resting muscle temperature—this heat can be dissipated through the evaporation of sweat from the skin. During prolonged exercise, sweat loss ranges from 3 to 8 cups (750–2000 ml) per hour. Sweat losses tend to be greatest during hot weather and in endurance sports or those that require athletes to wear heavy equipment (e.g., football). When humidity rises, especially above 75%, evaporation slows and sweating becomes an inefficient way to cool the body. The result is rapid fatigue, increased work for the heart, and difficulty with prolonged exertion.

To maintain the body's ability to regulate internal temperature, athletes must consume sufficient fluids because dehydration leads to a decline in endurance, strength, and overall performance and sets the stage for heat exhaustion, heat cramps, and potentially fatal heatstroke (Fig. 11-13).[19] Increased body temperature associated with dehydration is evident when the amount of water loss exceeds just 2% of body weight, especially in hot weather. From 1995 to 2001, 25 young football players died from heatstroke caused by dehydration; these types of tragic deaths continue.[20]

Insufficient fluid intake is dangerous at any age, but it is particularly dangerous for young children participating in activities such as youth soccer, T-ball, and basketball. That's because, for any given level of dehydration, children's core body temperatures rise faster than those of adults, putting them at far greater risk of heat stress. Children who participate in sports activities must be taught to prevent dehydration by drinking above and beyond thirst and drinking at frequent intervals—for example, every 20 minutes.[21]

CRITICAL THINKING

Joe is a wrestler who qualified for the 125-lb weight classification in the annual state high school competition. After a few matches, he began to feel dizzy and faint. He was disqualified because he was unable to continue the match. Later, the coach found out that Joe had spent 2 hours in the sauna before weighing in, which had made him dehydrated. What are the consequences of dehydration? What can you suggest as a safer alternative for weight loss?

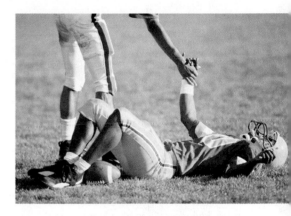

Wearing football equipment in hot weather can lead to a loss of 2% of body weight in 30 minutes.

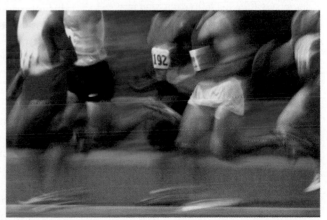

Marathon runners can lose 6 to 10% of their body weight during a race.

Relative humidity (%)	70°	75°	80°	85°	90°	95°	100°	105°	110°
100	72°	80°	91°	108°					
90	71°	79°	88°	102°	122°				
80	71°	78°	86°	97°	113°	136°			
70	70°	77°	85°	93°	106°	124°	144°		
60	69°	76°	82°	90°	100°	114°	132°	149°	
50	70°	75°	81°	88°	96°	107°	120°	135°	150°
40	68°	74°	79°	86°	93°	101°	110°	123°	137°
30	67°	73°	78°	84°	90°	96°	104°	113°	123°
20	66°	72°	77°	82°	87°	93°	99°	105°	112°
10	65°	70°	75°	80°	85°	90°	95°	100°	105°
0	64°	69°	73°	78°	83°	87°	91°	95°	99°

Air temperature (°F)

Heat index	Heat disorders possible with prolonged exposure and/or physical activity
80°–89°	Fatigue
90°–104°	Sunstroke, heat cramps, and heat exhaustion
105°–129°	Sunstroke, heat cramps, or heat exhaustion likely and heatstroke possible
130° or higher	Heatstroke/sunstroke highly likely

NOTE: Direct sunshine increases the heat index by up to 15°F.

Figure 11-13 Heat index chart showing associated heat disorders.

heat exhaustion First stage of heat-related illness that occurs because of depletion of blood volume from fluid loss by the body. This depletion increases body temperature and can lead to headache, dizziness, muscle weakness, visual disturbances, and other effects.

heat cramps Frequent complication of heat exhaustion. Cramps usually occur in individuals who have experienced large sweat losses from exercising for several hours in a hot climate and have consumed a large volume of water. The cramps occur in skeletal muscles and consist of contractions for 1 to 3 minutes at a time.

heatstroke Condition in which the internal body temperature reaches 104°F. Blood circulation is greatly reduced. Nervous system damage may ensue, and death is likely. Sweating generally ceases, which causes the skin of individuals who suffer heatstroke to feel hot and dry.

Heat exhaustion and heatstroke are on a continuum. Common symptoms of **heat exhaustion** include profuse sweating, headache, dizziness, nausea, vomiting, muscle weakness, visual disturbances, and flushing of the skin. A person with heat exhaustion should be taken to a cool environment immediately, and excess clothing should be removed. The body should be sponged with cool water. Fluid replacement, as tolerated, should be provided.[19] It is critical that the individual get immediate medical attention to prevent tissue damage and possible death.

Heat cramps are a frequent complication of heat exhaustion, but they may appear without other symptoms of dehydration. Cramps usually occur in individuals who have experienced significant sweating from exercising for several hours in a hot climate and who have consumed a large volume of water without replacing sodium losses. It is important not to confuse heat cramps with other forms of muscle cramps, such as those caused by intestinal tract upset. Heat cramps occur in skeletal muscles, including those of the abdomen and extremities. They consist of contractions lasting 1 to 3 minutes at a time. The cramp moves down the muscle and causes excruciating pain. The best way to prevent heat cramps is to exercise moderately at first, have adequate salt intake before engaging in long and strenuous activity in hot conditions, and avoid becoming dehydrated.[19]

Left unchecked, heat exhaustion can rapidly lead to **heatstroke.** Heatstroke can occur when the internal body temperature reaches 104°F or more. Related symptoms include nausea, confusion, irritability, poor coordination, seizures, hot and dry skin, rapid heart rate, vomiting, diarrhea, and coma. Exertional heatstroke results from high blood flow to exercising muscles, which overloads the body's cooling capacity. Sweating generally ceases, and the body temperature may become dangerously high. If heatstroke is left untreated, circulatory collapse, nervous system damage, and death are likely. The death rate from heatstroke is approximately 10%.[19]

For heatstroke victims, cooling the skin with ice packs or cold water is the usually recommended immediate treatment until medical help can be summoned. To decrease the risk of developing heatstroke, athletes should watch for rapid changes in body weight (2% or more), replace lost fluids and sodium, and avoid exercising in extremely hot, humid conditions.

Fluid Intake and Replacement Strategies

Paying attention to fluid intake before exercising can help ensure that athletes begin with optimal fluid levels. During exercise, the recommended fluid status goal is a loss of no more than 2% of body weight, especially in hot weather. Athletes should first calculate 2% of their body weight and then by trial and error determine how much fluid they must drink to avoid losing more than this amount of weight during exercise. This determination is most accurate if an athlete is weighed before and after a typical workout. For every pound (½ kg) lost, 3 cups (about ¾ liter) of fluid should be consumed during or immediately after exercise. If weight change can't be monitored, urine color is another measure of hydration status—it should be no darker than the color of lemonade (Fig. 11-14).[1]

Thirst is a late sign of dehydration and, so is not a reliable indicator of an athlete's need to replace fluid during exercise. An athlete who drinks only when thirsty is likely to take 48 hours to replenish fluid loss. After several days of training, an athlete relying on thirst as an indicator can build up a fluid debt that will impair performance.

Fluid intake during exercise, when possible, can help minimize fluid loss and a drop in body weight. Drinking fluids during practice is a good idea, even when sweating can go unnoticed, such as when swimming or during the winter.[10] However, fluid replacement mostly has to take place after exercise because it is difficult to consume enough fluid during exercise to prevent weight loss.

The following guidelines can meet most athletes' fluid needs.[12]

Before Exercise
- Freely drink beverages (e.g., sports drinks, water, diluted fruit juice) during the 24-hour period before an event, even if not thirsty.
- Drink 2 to 3 cups of fluid (500 to 750 ml) 2 to 3 hours before exercise. This allows time for both adequate hydration and the excretion of excess fluid.
- Drink 1 to 1.5 cups (250 to 375 ml) of fluid 10 to 15 minutes prior to the exercise or competition, especially if it is a long event.

During Exercise
- Drink 1 to 1.5 cups (250 to 375 ml) of fluid every 10 to 15 minutes.
- Fluids that are flavored and cooler than the environmental temperature promote fluid replacement.
- Drink enough fluids to maintain weight during the exercise bout.
- If exercise lasts more than 1 hour, fluid replacement beverages should contain 4 to 8% carbohydrates to maintain blood glucose levels. Sodium also should be included in the beverage in amounts of 0.5 to 0.7 gram of sodium per liter of water to replace sodium lost in sweat.

After Exercise
- Drink 3 cups of fluid for each pound lost during exercise.
- Restore weight before the next exercise period.

Hyponatremia

In athletes, hyponatremia (water intoxication) is most often caused by overdrinking before, during, or after exercise. To prevent hyponatremia, athletes should drink beverages containing sodium and should consume enough fluid during exercise to minimize loss of body weight (i.e., to avoid significant dehydration), but they should avoid overdrinking. Sports drinks containing at least 100 mg of sodium per 8-ounce serving have been shown to help maintain blood sodium level better than plain water.[22]

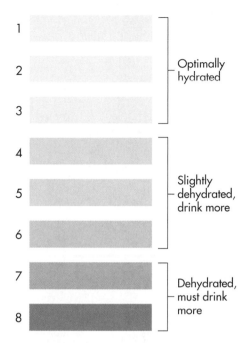

1
2 — Optimally hydrated
3
4
5 — Slightly dehydrated, drink more
6
7 — Dehydrated, must drink more
8

Figure 11-14 Urine color chart.

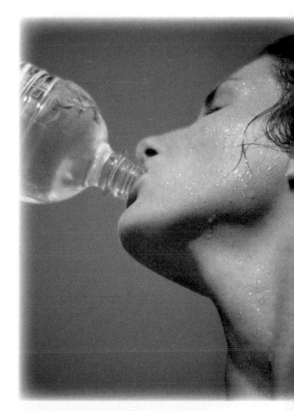

Adequate fluid intake is important before, during, and after exercise. Skipping fluids before or during events will almost certainly impair performance. For peak performance, it is important that weight be restored before the next exercise period.

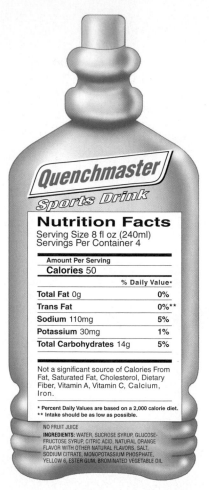

Figure 11-15 Sports drinks for fluid and electrolyte replacement typically contain simple carbohydrates plus sodium and potassium. The various sugars in this product total 14 g per 1-cup (240-ml) serving. In percentage terms based on weight, the sugar content is about 6% ([14 g sugar per serving / 240 g per serving] × 100 = 5.8%). (*Note:* 1 ml of water weighs 1 g.) Sports drinks typically contain about 6 to 8% sugar. This provides ample glucose and other monosaccharides to aid in fueling working muscles, and it is well tolerated.

Sports Drinks

It was once thought that, if physical activity lasted less than an hour, water was the best choice for fluid replacement. However, researchers[23] are finding that using a sports drink during high-intensity stop-and-go sports, such as basketball, volleyball, and sprint cycling, can delay fatigue and maintain hydration. Athletes of all ages who consume only water as a fluid replacement, even for short-term exercise, risk diluting the blood (plasma sodium, in specific) and increasing their urine output, thus shutting off the drive to drink and becoming dehydrated.

When exercise extends beyond 60 minutes, a sports drink becomes even more important. The use of sports drinks during these longer bouts of exercise—even more so in hot weather—can offer several advantages over water alone (Fig. 11-15).

- The carbohydrates in sports drinks supply glucose to muscles as they become depleted of glycogen, thus enhancing performance.
- The electrolytes in sports drinks help maintain blood volume, enhance the absorption of water and carbohydrates from the intestines, and stimulate thirst.

Beverages containing alcohol should be avoided because they increase urine output and reduce fluid retention. In addition, high intakes of caffeine (greater than 500 mg per day, or the amount in 4 to 5 cups of brewed coffee) can increase urine output. Carbonated beverages also should be avoided, as they reduce the desire to consume fluids because the carbonation leads to feelings of stomach fullness. Drinks with a sugar content above 10%, such as soft drinks or fruit juices, take longer to absorb, less efficiently contribute to hydration, and are not recommended.

Overall, most experts prefer sports drinks to water.[24] In fact, the American College of Sports Medicine suggests that the consumption of beverages containing electrolytes and carbohydrates (sports drinks) can provide benefits to athletes over water alone.[24] If athletes have not consumed a sports drink and want to try one, they can experiment with them during practice before using them during competition.

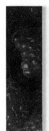

Knowledge Check

1. What are the symptoms of heat exhaustion?
2. What are the symptoms of heatstroke?
3. How much fluid should an athlete drink after exercise?
4. How should athletes determine if they are dehydrated?
5. What are the advantages of sports drinks, compared with water?

11.7 Food Intake before, during, and after Exercise

The composition of food eaten before, during, and after athletic events or exercise training sessions can affect performance and the speed with which the athlete recovers from the exercise bout. Careful planning is needed to ensure food intake meets the athlete's needs.

Pre-Exercise Meal

The pre-event or pre-exercise training meal keeps the athlete from feeling hungry before and during the exercise bout and it maintains optimal levels of blood glucose for the exercising muscles. A pre-exercise meal has been shown to improve performance, compared with exercising in a fasted state. Athletes who train early in the morning before eating or drinking risk developing low liver glycogen stores, which can impair performance, particularly if the exercise regimen involves endurance training.

Allowing for personal preferences and psychological factors, the pre-exercise meal should be high in carbohydrate, non-greasy, and readily digested. Recall that eating carbohydrate before exercise can help restore suboptimal liver glycogen stores, which may be called on during prolonged training and high-intensity competition. Fat in pre-exercise meals should be limited because it delays stomach-emptying time and takes longer to digest.

A meal eaten 3.5 to 4 hours before exercising can have as much as 4 g of carbohydrate per kg of body weight and 26% of the calories from fat. To avoid indigestion, nausea, vomiting, and gastrointestinal distress, the carbohydrate and fat content of the meal should be reduced the closer the meal is to the exercise time (Table 11-8). For example, 1 hour before exercising, the athlete should consume only 1 g carbohydrate/kg body weight.[25] Likewise, fat in meals eaten closer to exercise start time should provide less than 26% of calories. Allowing time for partial digestion and absorption provides for a final addition to muscle glycogen, additional blood sugar, and relatively complete emptying of the stomach.

Commercial liquid formulas providing a high-carbohydrate meal are popular with athletes because they leave the stomach rapidly. Other appropriate pregame meals are toast with jelly, a baked potato, spaghetti with tomato sauce, cereal with skim milk, and low-fat yogurt with fruit-sugar flavorings (Table 11-9).

In addition to food, recall that, within 10 to 15 minutes of a long event, athletes should drink 8 to 12 oz of water or other fluid. This prehydration allows for maximal absorption of fluid without urination. After exercise begins, the kidney slows down urine production to compensate for water loss.

Table 11-8 Rule of Thumb for Approximate Pre-event Carbohydrate Intake

Hours Before	Grams per Kilogram Body Weight	For a 70-kg Person
1	1	70
2	2	140
3	3	210
4	4	280

Table 11-9 Convenient Pre-Event Meals

Breakfast Options

Cornflakes, ¾ cup Reduced-fat milk, 1 cup Blueberry muffin, 1 Orange juice, 4 oz	450 kcal 82% carbohydrate (92 g)
Low-fat fruit yogurt, 1 cup Plain bagel, ½ Apple juice, 4 oz Peanut butter (for bagel), 1 tbsp	482 kcal 68% carbohydrate (84 g)
Whole-wheat toast, 1 slice Jam, 1 tsp Apple, 1 large Reduced-fat milk, 1 cup Oatmeal, ½ cup (with reduced-fat milk, ½ cup)	507 kcal 73% carbohydrate (98 g)

Lunch or Dinner Options

Chili with beans, 8 oz Baked potato with sour cream and chives Chocolate milk shake	900 kcal 65% carbohydrate (150 g)
Spaghetti noodles, 2 cups Spaghetti sauce, 1 cup Reduced-fat milk, 1½ cups Green beans, 1 cup	761 kcal 66% carbohydrate (129 g)
Orange, 1 large Reduced-fat milk, 1½ cups Chicken noodle soup, 1 cup Saltine crackers, 12 Buttered beans, 1 cup Corn, 1 cup Angelfood cake, 1 slice	829 kcal 70% carbohydrate (160 g)

The rule of thumb when timing preactivity meals is to allow 4 hours for a big meal (about 1200 kcal), 3 hours for a moderate meal (about 800 to 900 kcal), 2 hours for a light meal (about 400 to 600 kcal), and an hour or less for a snack (about 300 kcal).

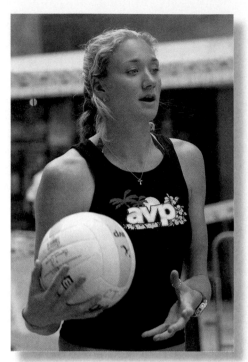

Elite athletes, such as Olympic beach volleyball gold medal winner Kerri Walsh, know that modifying their diet and training regimens to match up the specific needs of their sports is key to optimum performance. Replenishing carbohydrates and fluids is especially important when training.

Fueling during Exercise

For sporting events that are longer than 60 minutes, consuming carbohydrate during activity can improve athletic performance because prolonged exercise depletes muscle glycogen stores, and low levels of blood glucose lead to both physical and mental fatigue.[10] Recall that, when the supply of energy from carbohydrates runs low, athletes often complain of "hitting the wall," the point at which maintaining a competitive pace seems impossible. To avoid this situation, a general guideline for endurance events is to consume 30 to 60 g of carbohydrate per hour; however, an athlete should experiment during training sessions to establish the level that leads to optimal performance.[10]

As you know, sports drinks are a good source of carbohydrates for endurance events. They supply the necessary fluid, electrolytes, and carbohydrate to keep athletes performing at their best. An alternative to sports drinks are carbohydrate gels (e.g., PowerGel™ and Clif Shot®) and energy bars (e.g., PowerBar®). Gels contain about 25 g of carbohydrate per serving and popular energy bars range from 2 to 45 g of carbohydrate per serving. Sports drinks, by comparison, contain about 14 g of carbohydrate per 8-oz serving. Overall, choose a bar with about 40 g of carbohydrate and no more than 10 g of protein, 4 g of fat, and 5 g of fiber. The bars also are typically fortified with vitamins and minerals, often to 100% of the Daily Values. As such, these bars can be seen as a convenient, although somewhat expensive, source of nutrients. If the athlete prefers solid sources of carbohydrate, fig cookies, gummy bears, and jellybeans yield a quick source of glucose at a much lower cost. However, any carbohydrate-containing food, including energy bars and gels, must be accompanied by fluid to ensure adequate hydration.[1]

Recovery Meals

Carbohydrate-rich foods providing 1 to 2 g of carbohydrate per kg of body weight should be consumed 30 minutes after exercise and again at 2 hours after exercise (Table 11-10). Immediately after exercise is when glycogen synthesis is greatest because the muscles are very insulin-sensitive at this point.[1] Athletes who are training hard can consume a simple sugar candy, a sugared soft drink, fruit or fruit juice, or a sports or recovery drink right after training as they attempt to reload their muscles with glycogen. Later, bread, mashed potatoes, and rice can contribute to additional carbohydrate consumption during a meal. All these high glycemic load carbohydrates especially contribute to glycogen synthesis (Table 5-7 in

Table 11-10 Sample Postexercise Meals for Rapid Muscle Glycogen Replacement

Option 1

Bagel, 1 regular
Peanut butter, smooth, 2 tbsp
Fat-free milk, 8 oz
Banana, 1 medium
Chocolate beverage powder, 1 tbsp
600 kcal, 87 g carbohydrate, 23 g protein, 18 g fat

Option 2

Carnation® Instant Breakfast, 1 packet
Fat-free milk, 8 oz
Banana, 1 medium
Peanut butter, 1 tbsp
Blend until smooth.
438 kcal, 70 g carbohydrate, 17 g protein, 10 g fat

Option 3

Gatorade® Nutrition Shake, 1.5 cans (1.1 fl oz per can)
555 kcal, 81 g carbohydrate, 30 g protein, 12 g fat

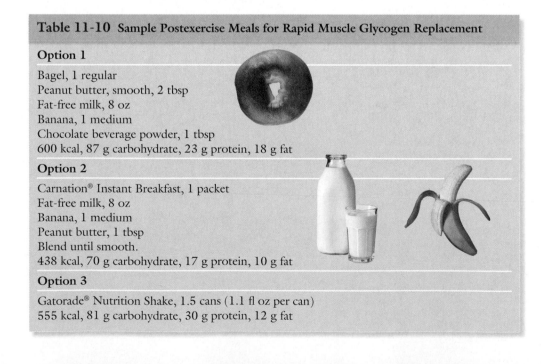

Chapter 5 shows the glycemic load of various foods). Remember, adding a small amount of protein immediately after exercise helps with muscle synthesis. For a 154-lb (70-kg) athlete, the amount of carbohydrate needed for recovery corresponds to about 70 g of carbohydrate while the amount of protein needed is 7–8 g of protein in each 2-hour interval.

In summary, the following are key factors for achieving the most rapid replenishment of muscle glycogen after exercise:

- The availability of adequate carbohydrate
- The ingestion of carbohydrate as soon as possible after the completion of exercise
- The selection of high glycemic load carbohydrates

Fluid and electrolyte intake is also an essential component of an athlete's recovery diet.[24] Recall that replenishing body fluids as quickly as possible is especially important if more than 1 workout a day is performed or if the environment is hot and humid. If food and fluid intake is sufficient to restore weight loss, it generally also will supply enough electrolytes to meet needs during recovery from endurance activities.

Knowledge Check

1. What is the purpose of the pre-exercise meal?
2. What is the primary nutrient that should be consumed in the pre-exercise meal?
3. How important is timing in pre-exercise and recovery meals?
4. What effect does glycemic index have on the recovery meal?

11.8 Ergogenic Aids to Enhance Athletic Performance

Today's athletes are as likely as their predecessors to seek ways to improve performance. Most don't want to miss out on any advantage, whether real or perceived, that might give them the winning edge. As a result, many experiment with diet composition, supplements, and other aids in hopes of gaining an ergogenic (work-producing) benefit. An **ergogenic aid** is a nutritional, psychological, pharmacological, mechanical, or physiological substance or treatment intended to improve exercise performance. Most of these aids, such as artichoke hearts, bee pollen, dried adrenal glands from cattle, seaweed, freeze-dried liver flakes, gelatin, and ginseng, are ineffective. In fact, scientific support for ergogenic effectiveness exists for only a few dietary substances: sufficient water and electrolytes, abundant carbohydrates, a healthy, varied diet, and caffeine.[1, 26] Protein and amino acid supplements are not among those aids because athletes can easily meet protein needs from foods, as Table 11-6 demonstrates. Nutrient supplements should be used only to meet specific dietary shortcomings, such as inadequate iron intake.

As summarized in Table 11-11, no scientific evidence supports the effectiveness of many substances touted as performance-enhancing aids. Many are useless; some are dangerous. The risk-benefit ratio of any ergogenic aid merits careful evaluation before use.[1] Athletes should be skeptical of any substance until its ergogenic effect is scientifically verified. The FDA has a limited ability to regulate dietary supplements (see Chapter 1), and the manufacturing processes for dietary supplements are not as tightly regulated as they are for medications. As a result, some supplements do not contain the substance and/or the amount listed on the label and may contain substances that will cause athletes to test positive for various banned substances. Even substances that have been supported by systematic scientific studies should be used with caution because the conditions under which they were tested may not match those of the intended use. Finally, rather than waiting for a magic bullet to enhance performance, athletes should concentrate their efforts on improving their training routines and sport techniques while consuming healthy diets.

▶ Why hasn't fat been mentioned as a way to improve athletic performance during an endurance event? Although it is true that fat is used along with carbohydrate as fuel during prolonged aerobic activity, the processes of digestion, absorption, and metabolism of fat are relatively slow. Therefore, the consumption of fat during activity is not likely to translate into better athletic performance.

▶ For more information on sports nutrition, visit the Gatorade Sport Science Institute web page (www.gssiweb.com). For more information on sports medicine, visit www.physsportsmed.com. This home page of The *Physician and Sports Medicine* journal details current issues in sports medicine, including injury prevention, nutrition, and exercise. Also helpful are the web pages of the American College of Sports Medicine (www.acsm.org), Centers for Disease Control and Prevention (www.cdc.gov/nccdphp/dnpa), and American Council on Exercise (www.acefitness.org).

CRITICAL THINKING

How would you advise someone who was planning to buy a purported "muscle-building" protein supplement? What risks are important to point out?

Table 11-11 Evaluation of Popular Ergogenic Aids

Substance/Practice	Rationale for Use	Reality
Useful in Some Circumstances		
Creatine	Increase phosphocreatine (PCr) in muscles to keep ATP concentration high	Use of 20 g per day for 5 to 6 days and then a maintenance dose of 2 g per day may improve performance in athletes who undertake repeated bursts of activity, such as in sprinting and weight lifting. Vegetarian athletes may especially show benefits because creatine is low or nonexistent in their diets. Some of the muscle weight gain noted with use results from water contained in muscles. Endurance athletes do not benefit from use. Little is known about the safety of long-term creatine use. Continual use of high doses has led to kidney damage in a few cases. Cost: $25 to $65 per month.
Sodium bicarbonate (baking soda)	Counter lactic acid buildup	Partially effective in some circumstances in which lactate is rapidly produced, such as wrestling, but induces nausea and diarrhea. The dose used is 300 mg/kg, given 1 to 3 hours before exercise. Cost: nil.
Caffeine	Stimulate nervous system, heighten sense of awareness and may enhance nerve conduction	Drinking 2 to 3 5-ounce cups of coffee (3-9 milligrams of caffeine per kg of body weight) about 1 hour before events lasting about 5 minutes or longer is useful for some athletes; benefits are less apparent in those who habitually consume caffeine. Intakes of more than about 600 milligrams (6 to 8 cups of coffee) elicits a urine concentration illegal under NCAA rules (greater than 15 mg per ml). Possible side effects are increased blood pressure, increased heart rate, intestinal distress, and insomnia. Cost: $0.08 per 300 mg.
Possibly Useful, Still under Study		
Beta-hydroxy-beta methylbutyric acid (HMB)	Decrease protein catabolism, causing a net growth-promoting effect	Research in livestock and humans suggests that supplementation with this substance may increase muscle mass. Still, safety and effectiveness of long-term HMB use in humans are unknown. Cost: $100 per month.
Glutamine (an amino acid)	Enhance immune function, preserve lean body mass	Study results are mixed and difficult to draw a conclusion at this time. Long-term studies are lacking. Protein foods are a rich source of glutamine. Cost: $10 to $20 per month for 1 to 2 g per day.
Branched-chain amino acids (BCAA) (leucine, isoleucine, valine)	Important energy source, especially when carbohydrate stores are depleted	Supplementation of BCAA (10 to 30 g/day) during exercise can increase BCAA in the blood when levels are low due to exercise. However, supplemental BCAA have not been shown to delay fatigue or improve endurance performance. Carbohydrate feeding, by delaying use of BCAA as fuel, may negate the need for BCAA supplementation. Protein-rich foods (especially dairy proteins) are rich in BCAA. Cost: $20 per month.
Glucosamine	Aid in repair of joint damage	Most of the positive evidence is for repair of knee damage in older people, but a large study showed no clear benefit for such use. May be of use to athletes experiencing knee damage, but reliable evidence is lacking. Cost: $30 per month.
Dangerous or Illegal Substances/Practices		
Anabolic steroids (and related substances, such as androstenedione and tetrahydrogestrinone [THG])	Increase muscle mass and strength	Although effective for increasing protein synthesis, anabolic steroids are illegal in the U.S. unless prescribed by a physician. They have numerous potential side effects, such as premature closure of growth plates in bones (possibly limiting potential height of a teenage athlete), bloody cysts in the liver, increased risk of cardiovascular disease, increased blood pressure, and reproductive dysfunction. Possible psychological consequences include increased aggressiveness, drug dependence (addiction), withdrawal symptoms (e.g., depression), sleep disturbances, and mood swings (known as "roid rage"). Use of needles for injectable forms adds further health risk. They are banned by the International Olympic Committee, National Football League, Major League Baseball, and other sports organizations.
Growth hormone	Increase muscle mass	It may increase height; at critical ages, it also may cause uncontrolled growth of the heart and other internal organs and even death; it is potentially dangerous and requires careful monitoring by a physician. The use of needles for injections adds further health risk. It is banned by the International Olympic Committee.

Table 11-11 Continued

Substance/Practice	Rationale for Use	Reality
Dangerous or Illegal Substances/Practices, continued		
Blood doping	Enhance aerobic capacity by injecting red blood cells harvested previously from the athlete, or alternately the athlete may use the hormone erythropoietin (Epogen®) to increase red blood cell number	It may offer aerobic benefit, but very serious health consequences are possible, including thickening of the blood, which puts extra strain on the heart. It is an illegal practice under Olympic guidelines.
Gamma hydroxybutyric acid (GHB)	Promoted as a steroid alternative for body building	The FDA has never approved it for sale as a medical product; it is illegal to produce or sell GHB in the U.S. GHB-related symptoms include vomiting, dizziness, tremors, and seizures. Many victims require hospitalization, and some have died. Clandestine laboratories produce virtually all the chemical accounting for GHB abuse. The FDA is working with the U.S. Attorney's office to arrest, indict, and convict individuals responsible for the illegal operations.

Substances that are promoted to athletes but have yet to show any clear ergogenic effects include pyruvic acid (pyruvate), glycerol, ribose, chromium, coenzyme Q-10, medium-chain triglycerides, L-carnitine, conjugated linoleic acid (CLA), bovine colostrum, insulin, and amino acids not already mentioned in this section. Any use of these products is not recommended at this time. Some of these substances are defined in the glossary.

The National Collegiate Athletic Association's Committee on Competitive Safeguards and Medical Aspects of Sports has developed lists of supplements that are permissible and non-permissible for athletic departments to dispense. The following are some key examples.

Permissible	*Non-permissible*
Vitamins and minerals	Amino acids
Energy bars (if no more than 30% protein)	Creatine
	Glycerol
Sports drinks	Beta-hydroxy-beta methylbutyric acid (HMB)
Meal replacement drinks (Ensure Plus®, Boost®)	L-carnitine
	Protein powders

Knowledge Check

1. What is an ergogenic aid?
2. When should supplements be used?
3. Should all athletes take a supplement?

CASE STUDY **FOLLOW-UP**

Jake decided to see the sports dietitian at his college. She asked him to keep a 3-day food record, so that she could analyze his diet. When they met to go over his diet, she told him that he was overconsuming protein and underconsuming carbohydrate. Jake told her he needed more protein due to his lifting, but the dietitian pointed out that he was consuming almost 300 g/day of protein. When the dietitian calculated his protein requirement using the recommended protein requirements for athletes, he actually needed 120 g/day. He was eating so much protein that he was not getting enough carbohydrate to fuel his workouts. To increase carbohydrate intake, they worked out a plan to add more whole-grain cereals for breakfast instead of the protein shake. He added rice, potatoes, or pasta and vegetables with his chicken for the evening meal and cut back his protein shake to once a day. A couple of weeks later, Jake's energy returned, he was lasting longer in the weight room, and he was lifting more weight.

Summary

11.1 The benefits of regular physical activity include enhanced heart function, improved balance, reduced risk of falling, better sleep habits, healthier body composition, and reduced injury to muscles, tendons, and joints. A gradual increase in regular physical activity is recommended for all healthy persons. A minimum plan includes 30 minutes of physical activity on most (or all) days; 60 to 90 minutes per day provides even more benefit, especially if weight control is an issue.

11.2 A good fitness program is one that meets a person's needs. To reach goals, fitness program planning should consider the mode, duration, frequency, intensity, and progression of exercise, as well as consistency and variety. Before starting a new fitness program, discuss program goals with a health-care provider. Also, assess and record baseline fitness scores. Most new exercise programs should start with short intervals of exercise at the lower end of the maximum heart rate target zone and work up to a total of 30 minutes of activity incorporated into each day. To prepare and recover safely from an exercise session, a warm-up and cooldown period should be included.

11.3 At rest, muscle cells mainly use fat for fuel. For intense exercise of short duration, muscles mostly use phosphocreatine (PCr) for energy. During more sustained intense activity, muscle glycogen breaks down to lactic acid, providing a small amount of ATP. For endurance exercise, both fat and carbohydrate are used as fuels; carbohydrate is used increasingly as activity intensifies. Little protein is used to fuel muscles. Fuel sources for muscle cells can be estimated based on percent of VO_{2max}.

11.4 Physical activity has many effects on the body. The most pronounced effects are typically seen in the muscular, circulatory, and skeletal systems. The body contains 3 major types of muscle tissue: skeletal muscle, smooth muscle, and cardiac muscle. Skeletal muscle is composed of 3 main types of muscle fibers, which have distinct characteristics. Prolonged, low-intensity exercise, such as a slow jog, mainly uses type I muscle fibers, so the predominant fuel is fat. As exercise intensity increases, type IIA and type IIX fibers are gradually recruited; in turn, the contribution of glucose as a fuel increases. Type IIA and type IIX fibers are also important for rapid movements, such as a jump shot in basketball. The relative proportions of the 3 fiber types throughout the muscles of the body vary from person to person and are constant throughout each person's life. With training, muscle strength becomes matched to the muscles' work demands. Muscles enlarge after being made to work repeatedly. Repeated aerobic exercise strengthens the heart and increases in the number of capillaries in muscle tissue; as a result, oxygen can be delivered more easily to muscle cells. Another adaptation that occurs with exercise is increased bone density.

11.5 Athletic training and genetic makeup are very important determinants of athletic performance. Monitoring body weight is an easy way to assess the adequacy of calorie intake. Athletes should strive to maintain weight during competition and training. Athletes should obtain at least 60% of total energy needs from carbohydrates. Carbohydrate-loading regimens usually increase muscle glycogen stores 50 to 85% over typical conditions. Carbohydrate loading is for athletes who compete in continuous, intense aerobic events lasting more than 60 to 90 minutes. A fat intake of 15 to 25% of energy is generally recommended for athletes. Typical recommendations for protein intake for most athletes range from 1.0 to 1.7 g of protein/kg of body weight. The extra protein is needed for the repair of tissue and the synthesis of new muscle that results from training. Vitamin and mineral needs are the same or slightly higher for athletes, compared with those of sedentary adults. The female athlete triad consists of 3 conditions: menstrual disorders, low energy availability, and low bone mineral density.

11.6 To maintain the body's ability to regulate internal temperature, athletes must consume sufficient fluids because dehydration leads to a decline in endurance, strength, and overall performance and sets the stage for heat exhaustion, heat cramps, and potentially fatal heatstroke. During exercise, the recommended fluid status goal is a loss of no more than 2% of body weight. To prevent hyponatremia, athletes should drink beverages containing sodium and should consume enough fluid during exercise to minimize the loss of body weight. Most experts recommend drinking sports drinks instead of water.

11.7 The composition of food eaten before, during, and after athletic events or exercise training sessions can affect performance and the speed with which the athlete recovers from the exercise bout. Pre-exercise training meals keep the athlete from feeling hungry before and during the exercise bout and maintain optimal levels of blood glucose for the exercising muscles. The pre-exercise meal should be high in carbohydrate, non-greasy, and readily digested. For sporting events lasting more than 60 minutes, consuming carbohydrate during activity can improve athletic performance. Carbohydrate-rich foods should be consumed 30 minutes after exercise and again 2 hours after exercise.

11.8 An ergogenic aid is a nutritional, psychological, pharmacological, mechanical, or physiological substance or treatment intended to improve exercise performance. Most of these aids are ineffective.

Study Questions

1. The benefits of regular physical activity include _____.
   a. a reduced risk of falling
   b. better sleep habits
   c. healthier body composition
   d. all of the above

2. Which mode of exercise is defined as any activity that uses large muscle groups, can be maintained continuously, and is rhythmic in nature?
   a. aerobic
   b. resistance
   c. flexibility
   d. none of the above

3. The predominant fuels for the 50-meter sprint are _____.
   a. fat and protein
   b. carbohydrate and protein
   c. protein and phosphocreatine
   d. ATP and phosphocreatine

4. The predominant fuel for a 2-hour marathon is _____.
   a. protein
   b. fat
   c. carbohydrate
   d. water

5. The amount of ATP stored in a muscle cell can keep a muscle active for about _____.
   a. 2 to 4 seconds
   b. 10 to 30 seconds
   c. 1 to 3 minutes
   d. 1 to 3 hours

6. There are 4 main types of muscle fibers.
   a. true
   b. false

7. Although genetics largely determines the proportion of muscle fiber type, training can develop muscle fibers within some limits.
   a. true
   b. false

8. Which of the following athletes would *not* benefit from carbohydrate loading?
   a. marathon runner
   b. long-distance cyclist
   c. triathlete
   d. football player

9. Athletes who are involved in endurance activities may need to consume _____ grams of carbohydrates per kilogram of body weight.
   a. 5 to 7
   b. 7 to 8
   c. up to 10
   d. 3 to 4

10. All athletes should consume at least 2.0 grams of protein/kg of body weight.
    a. true
    b. false

11. Iron deficiency can impair athletic performance.
    a. true
    b. false

12. What 3 factors are included in the female athlete triad?
    a. _____
    b. _____
    c. _____

13. Hyponatremia is a condition that can occur when athletes drink too much _____.
    a. alcohol
    b. water
    c. sports drinks
    d. milk

14. Thirst is an accurate indicator of fluid needs.
    a. true
    b. false

15. Most ergogenic aids are effective and enhance athletic performance.
    a. true
    b. false

Answer Key: 1-d; 2-a; 3-d; 4-b; 5-a; 6-b; 7-a; 8-d; 9-c; 10-b; 11-a; 12-menstrual disorders, low energy availability, low bone mass; 13-b; 14-b; 15-b

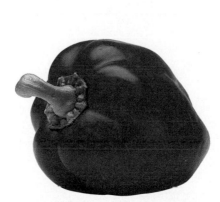
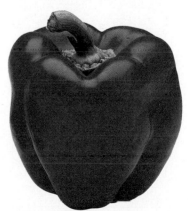

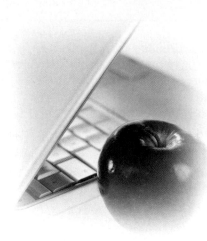

Websites

To learn more about the topics covered in this chapter, visit these websites.

American College of Sports Medicine
www.acsm.org

Sports and Cardiovascular and Wellness Nutritionists, a Practice Group of the American Dietetic Association
www.scandpg.org

NIH Office of Dietary Supplements
dietary-supplements.info.nih.gov

American Alliance for Health, Physical Education, Recreation, and Dance
www.aahperd.org

Gatorade Sport Science Institute
www.gssiweb.com

The Physician and Sports Medicine journal
www.physsportsmed.com.

Centers for Disease Control and Prevention
www.cdc.gov/nccdphp/dnpa

American Council on Exercise
www.acefitness.org

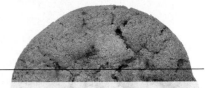

References

1. Williams M. *Nutrition for health, fitness, and sport.* 7th ed. Boston: McGraw-Hill; 2005.

2. Bacon S and others. Effects of exercise, diet and weight loss on high blood pressure. *Sports Med.* 2004;34:307.

3. Laaksonen D and others. Increased physical activity is a cornerstone in the prevention of type 2 diabetes in high risk individuals. *Diabetologia.* 2007;50:1432.

4. Ross R and others. Exercise induced reduction in obesity and insulin resistance in women: A randomized control trial. *Obesity Res.* 2004;12:789.

5. Thompson P and others. Exercise and physical activity in the prevention and treatment of athlerosclerotic cardiovascular disease. *Circulation.* 2003;107:3109.

6. Zanker C, Cook C. Energy balance, bone turnover, and skeletal health in physically active individuals. *Med Sci Sports Exerc.* 2004;36:1372.

7. Chan B and others. Incident fall risk and physical activity and physical performance among older men: The osteoporotic fractures in men study. *Am J Epidemiol.* 2007;165:696.

8. Haskell W and others. Physical activity and public health: Update recommendation for adults from the American College of Sports Medicine and the American Heart Association. *Circulation.* 2007;39:1081.

9. Hunter G. Physical activity, fitness, and health. In: Shils M and others, eds. *Modern nutrition in health and disease.* 10th ed. Philadelphia: Lippincott Williams & Wilkins; 2006.

10. Coyle E. Fluid and fuel intake during exercise. *J Sport Sci.* 2004;22:39.

11. Tarnopolsky M. Protein requirements for endurance athletes. *Nutrition.* 2004;20:7.

12. ACSM. Nutrition and athletic performance. *Med Sci Sports Exerc.* 2000;32.

13. Bassau V and others. Carbohydrate loading in human muscle: An improved 1 day protocol. *Eur J Appl Physiol.* 2002;87:290.

14. Betts J and others. Recovery of endurance running capacity effect of carbohydrate-protein mixtures. *Int J Sport Nutr Exerc Metab.* 2005;15:590.

15. Lukaski H. Vitamin and mineral status: Effects on physical performance. *Nutrition.* 2004;20:632.

16. Sinclair L, Hinton P. Prevalence of iron deficiency with and without anemia in recreationally active men and women. *J Am Diet Assoc.* 2005;105:975.

17. Nattiv A and others. American College of Sports Medicine position stand. The female athlete triad. *Med Sci Sports Exerc.* 2007;39:1867.

18. Harber V. Energy balance and reproductive function in active women. *Can J App Physiol.* 2004;29:48.

19. Glazer J. Management of heat stroke and heat exhaustion. *Am Family Phys.* 2005;71:2133.

20. Bergeron M and others. Youth football: Heat stress and injury risk. *Med Science Sports Exerc.* 2005;37:1421.

21. AAP. Climatic heat stress and the exercising child and adolescent. *Pediatrics.* 2007;120:683.

22. Montain S and others. Exercise associated hyponatremia: Quantitative analysis to understand the aetiology. *Br J Sports Med.* 2006;40:98.

23. Davis J and others. Carbohydrate drinks delay fatigue during intermittent high intensity cycling in active men and women. *Int J Sport Nutr Exerc Metab.* 1997;7(261).

24. Sawka M and others. American College of Sports Medicine position stand. Exercise and fluid replacement. *Med Sci Sports Exerc.* 2007;39:377.

25. Sherman W and others. Carbohydrate feedings 1 hour before exercise improves cycling performance. *Am J Clin Nutr.* 1991;54:866.

26. Foad, AJ and others. Pharmacological and psychological effects of caffeine ingestion in 40-km cycling performance. *Med Sci Sports Exerc.* 2008;40:158.

12

the Fat-Soluble Vitamins

One pound of polar bear liver contains enough vitamin A to keep a human healthy for several years. A team of early Arctic explorers became gravely ill from vitamin A toxicity after eating polar bear liver. Learn more about vitamin toxicity at www.unu.edu.

STUDENT LEARNING OUTCOMES

After studying this chapter, you will be able to:

1. Define the term *vitamin* and list 3 characteristics of vitamins as a group.

2. Classify the vitamins according to whether they are fat soluble or water soluble.

3. List 3 important food sources for each fat-soluble vitamin.

4. List the major functions for each fat-soluble vitamin.

5. Describe the deficiency symptoms for each fat-soluble vitamin and state the conditions in which deficiencies are likely to occur.

6. Describe the toxicity symptoms caused by excess consumption of certain fat-soluble vitamins.

7. Evaluate the use of vitamin and mineral supplements with respect to their potential benefits and risks to health.

When it comes to vitamins, we often hear, "If a little is good, then more must be better." Some people believe that consuming vitamins far in excess of their needs provides them with extra energy, protection from disease, and prolonged youth. Actually, our total vitamin needs to prevent deficiency are quite small. In general, humans require about 1 oz (28 g) of vitamins for every 150 lb (70 kg) of food they consume. Although plants can synthesize all the vitamins they need, animals vary in their ability to synthesize vitamins. For example, guinea pigs and humans are among the few organisms that cannot make their own supply of vitamin C.

Long before any vitamins were identified, certain foods were known to cure conditions brought on by what we now know to be vitamin deficiencies. The ancient Greeks, for example, treated night blindness with beef liver, a rich source of vitamin A. As you'll see, vitamin A plays a critical role in vision. During the 15th and 16th centuries, many British sailors on long sea voyages died from the disease scurvy. After it was discovered that eating lemons and limes prevents scurvy, citrus was included as a routine part of British sailors' rations, and deaths from scurvy declined sharply. We now know that scurvy results from a deficiency of vitamin C.

Today, consumers in developed countries rarely consider vitamin deficiencies when making choices about diet and vitamin supplements. Instead, the focus has switched to the ability of vitamins, and of diets rich in vitamins, to decrease the risk of developing chronic diseases, such as cancer, heart disease, and bone disease. However, some vitamin deficiencies are still a public health concern in specific groups

Fat-Soluble Vitamins

Vitamin A

Vitamin D

Vitamin E

Vitamin K

Water-Soluble Vitamins

B-vitamins

Thiamin

Riboflavin

Niacin

Pantothenic acid

Biotin

Folic acid

Vitamin B-6 (pyridoxine)

Vitamin B-12 (cobalamin)

Vitamin C

▶ The synthetic and natural forms of most vitamins have similar characteristics. One exception, natural vitamin E, is about twice as potent as the synthetic form. In contrast, synthetic folic acid is almost twice as potent as the natural form.

Foods provide a wide array of vitamins.

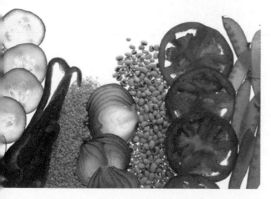

of people in developed countries and in large populations in many developing countries. Vitamin A deficiency, for example, is a primary cause of childhood blindness in many developing countries.

Vitamins are divided into fat-soluble vitamins and water-soluble vitamins. This chapter will provide an overview of vitamins and an in-depth discussion of fat-soluble vitamins.

12.1 Vitamins: Essential Dietary Components

Vitamins are essential, organic (containing carbon bonded to hydrogen) substances needed in small amounts in the diet. They are not a source of energy. Instead, they aid in the growth, development, and maintenance of body tissues.

During the first half of the 20th century, scientists identified each of the 13 vitamins now recognized as essential. For the most part, as the vitamins were discovered, they were named alphabetically: A, B, C, D, and E. Later, some substances originally classified as B-vitamins were dropped from the list because they were shown to be non-essential substances. The B-vitamins originally were thought to have a single chemical form but turned out to exist in many forms. Thus, the label "vitamin B" now comprises 8 B-vitamins. Vitamins A, D, E, and K dissolve in organic solvents, such as ether and benzene, and are referred to as **fat-soluble vitamins**. The B-vitamins and vitamin C, in contrast, dissolve in water and are classified as **water-soluble vitamins**.

Vitamins are indispensable in human diets because they either cannot be synthesized in the body at all or are synthesized in insufficient quantities. However, a substance does not qualify as a vitamin merely because the body can't make it. Evidence must suggest that health declines when the substance is not consumed.[1-3] In fact, when vitamin intake is insufficient to meet needs, a deficiency develops, accompanied by a measurable decline in health. If the deficiency is not in advanced stages, the deficiency and related symptoms can be alleviated by increased intakes of the vitamin.

In addition to correcting deficiency diseases, a few vitamins have been useful as pharmacological agents (drugs) in treating several non-deficiency conditions. These treatments often require the administration of **megadoses,** amounts much higher than typical human needs for the vitamin. For example, megadoses of a form of niacin can be used as part of blood cholesterol–lowering treatment for certain individuals. Nevertheless, any claimed benefits for the use of vitamin supplements, especially intakes above the Upper Level (if set), should be viewed critically because many unproved claims are continually being made.[1-3]

Foods of both plant and animal origin supply vitamins in the diet. Dietary supplements also can provide needed vitamins. Whether vitamins in supplements are isolated from foods or synthesized in a laboratory, these vitamins are usually similar chemical compounds and generally work equally well in the body. Contrary to claims in the health-food literature, "natural" vitamin supplements isolated from foods are, for the most part, no more healthful than those synthesized in a laboratory. However, vitamins consumed in foods as part of a varied diet may be more beneficial than vitamins taken separately as dietary supplements. Because some vitamins exist in several related forms that differ in chemical or physical properties, it is important to consume enough vitamins in the forms the body can use.

Absorption of Vitamins

Fat-soluble vitamins are absorbed along with dietary fat. Thus, adequate absorption of fat-soluble vitamins depends on the efficient use of bile and pancreatic lipase in the small intestine to digest dietary fat and the adequate absorptive capacity of the intestinal mucosa (Fig. 12-1). Under optimal conditions, about 40 to 90% of the fat-soluble vitamins are absorbed when they're consumed in recommended amounts. In contrast, the

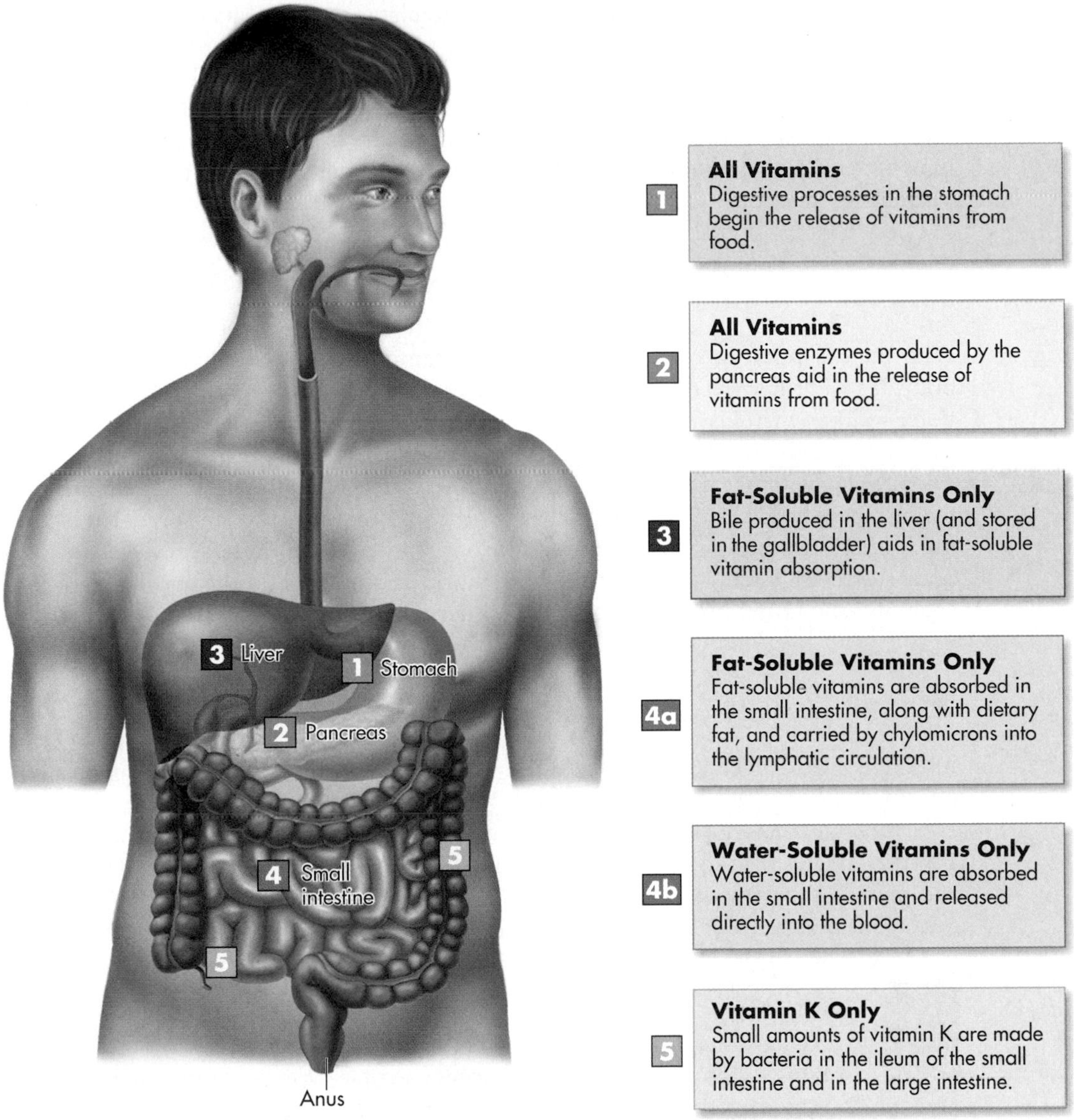

Figure 12-1 An overview of the digestion and absorption of vitamins.

1 All Vitamins
Digestive processes in the stomach begin the release of vitamins from food.

2 All Vitamins
Digestive enzymes produced by the pancreas aid in the release of vitamins from food.

3 Fat-Soluble Vitamins Only
Bile produced in the liver (and stored in the gallbladder) aids in fat-soluble vitamin absorption.

4a Fat-Soluble Vitamins Only
Fat-soluble vitamins are absorbed in the small intestine, along with dietary fat, and carried by chylomicrons into the lymphatic circulation.

4b Water-Soluble Vitamins Only
Water-soluble vitamins are absorbed in the small intestine and released directly into the blood.

5 Vitamin K Only
Small amounts of vitamin K are made by bacteria in the ileum of the small intestine and in the large intestine.

B-vitamins and vitamin C are water soluble and can be absorbed in the small intestine independent of dietary fat. Absorption of water-soluble vitamins typically ranges from 90 to 100%.

Malabsorption of Vitamins

Vitamins consumed in food must be absorbed efficiently from the small intestine to meet body needs. If the absorption of a vitamin is decreased, a person must consume larger amounts of it to avoid deficiency symptoms. For example, fat malabsorption (resulting from GI tract and pancreatic disease) may cause poor absorption of fat-soluble vitamins.[1-3] Alcohol abuse and certain intestinal diseases also can lead to malabsorption of some B-vitamins (see Chapter 13). Individuals with these diseases usually require vitamin supplements to prevent deficiencies.

Transport of Vitamins

Once absorbed, fat-soluble vitamins are packaged for transport through the lymphatic system and delivered by the bloodstream to target cells throughout the body in a manner similar to that for dietary fats—namely, by way of chylomicrons and other blood

▶ People with diseases that result in poor fat absorption, such as cystic fibrosis, celiac disease, and Crohn's disease, are at high risk of fat-soluble vitamin deficiencies. Medications, such as the weight-loss drug orlistat (Xenical®, Alli®), also interfere with fat absorption. Unabsorbed fat carries fat-soluble vitamins to the large intestine, where they are incorporated into the feces and excreted. A multivitamin and mineral supplement usually is prescribed as part of the treatment for preventing nutrient deficiencies associated with fat malabsorption.

lipoproteins.[1-3] Recall that, as a chylomicron circulates, much of its triglyceride content is removed by body cells. What remains—the remnant—is taken up by the liver. This remnant contains the fat-soluble vitamins absorbed from the diet. The liver then "repackages" fat-soluble vitamins with new proteins for transport in the blood, or it stores them in adipose tissue or the liver for future use. In contrast to the fat-soluble vitamins, water-soluble vitamins are delivered directly to the bloodstream and distributed throughout the body.

Storage of Vitamins in the Body

With the exception of vitamin K, fat-soluble vitamins are not readily excreted from the body. Instead, they are often stored in the liver and/or adipose tissue. In contrast, most water-soluble vitamins are excreted from the body quite rapidly, resulting in limited stores. Two exceptions are vitamin B-12 and vitamin B-6, which are stored to a greater extent than the other water-soluble vitamins. Because of the limited storage of many vitamins, they should be consumed daily. However, the signs and symptoms of a deficiency usually do not occur until the vitamin is lacking in the diet for at least several weeks and body stores are essentially depleted. Thus, an occasional lapse in dietary intake of most vitamins is not a serious health concern in otherwise healthy individuals.

Vitamin Toxicity

Although the toxic effects of an excessive intake of any vitamin is theoretically possible, toxicity from the fat-soluble vitamins A and D is the most likely to occur.[2, 3] However, these vitamins are unlikely to cause toxicities unless taken in amounts at least 5 to 10 times greater than the DRI guidelines. Because the daily use of balanced multivitamin and mineral supplements usually supplies less than twice the Daily Value of the components, this practice is unlikely to cause toxic effects in adults.

Knowledge Check

1. Which vitamins are classified as water soluble? Which are fat soluble?
2. How does the absorption of fat-soluble vitamins differ from that of water-soluble vitamins?
3. Why are large doses of certain fat-soluble vitamins more likely to cause toxic effects than large intakes of water-soluble vitamins?

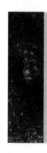

12.2 Vitamin A

Although vitamins per se were not discovered until the 20th century, vitamin A was known for more than 3500 years as a factor needed to prevent night blindness. Ancient Egyptians and the Greek physician Hippocrates recommended the consumption of beef liver, a cure that still works today. *Vitamin A* refers to the preformed retinoids and provitamin A carotenoids that can be converted to vitamin A activity.

Retinoids is a collective term for the biologically active forms of vitamin A. They are called preformed vitamin A because, unlike carotenoids, they do not need to be converted to become biologically active. Retinoids exist in 3 forms: retinol (an alcohol), retinal (an aldehyde), and retinoic acid. The tail segment of the vitamin A structure terminates in 1 of these 3 chemical groups (alcohol, aldehyde, or acid) and determines the name or classification. To some extent, these forms can be interconverted (Fig. 12-2).

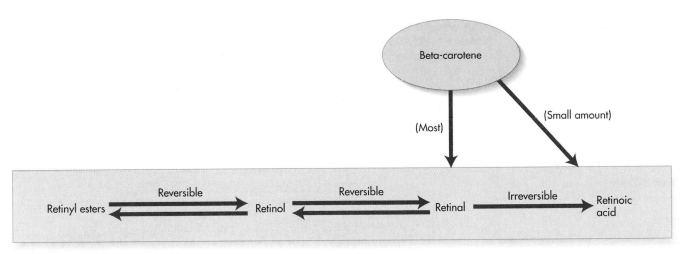

Figure 12-2 Interconversions of beta-carotene and various retinoids. Notice that the synthesis of retinoic acid is a "dead end" in metabolic terms.

However, retinoic acid cannot be converted back to the other forms. The ability to interconvert forms helps maintain adequate amounts of each retinoid form for its unique functions.

Retinol   Retinal   Retinoic acid

The tail of the vitamin A molecule can vary from *cis* to *trans* configuration. This orientation influences the function of the specific retinoid.

Cis   *Trans*

Carotenoids are yellow-orange pigmented materials in fruits and vegetables, some of which are **provitamins**—that is, they can be converted into vitamin A. Of the 600 or more known carotenoids, only alpha-carotene, beta-carotene, and beta-cryptoxanthin can be converted to biologically active forms of vitamin A. Other carotenoids, such as lycopene, do not have vitamin A activity in humans.[4]

Vitamin A in Foods

Retinoids (preformed vitamin A) are found in liver, fish, fish oils, fortified milk, and eggs. Margarine is fortified with vitamin A, as are fat-free, low-fat, and reduced-fat milks. The provitamin A carotenoids are found mainly in dark green and yellow-orange vegetables and fruits, such as carrots, spinach and other greens, winter squash, sweet potatoes, broccoli, mangoes, cantaloupe, peaches, and apricots. About 70% of the vitamin A in the typical North American diet comes from animal (preformed vitamin A) sources, whereas plant-based carotenoids (provitamin A) provide most of the vitamin A in the diet among poor people in other parts of the world. Figure 12-3 displays the vitamin A content of various foods.

A Biochemist's View

Beta-carotene

Retinal

Retinol

Retinoic acid

Vitamin A family

CRITICAL THINKING

Check out the ready-to-eat breakfast cereals at your local supermarket. Which ones have beta-carotene added? Why do you think the manufacturers are using this kind of fortification?

Figure 12-3 Food sources of vitamin A.

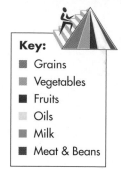

Key:
- Grains
- Vegetables
- Fruits
- Oils
- Milk
- Meat & Beans

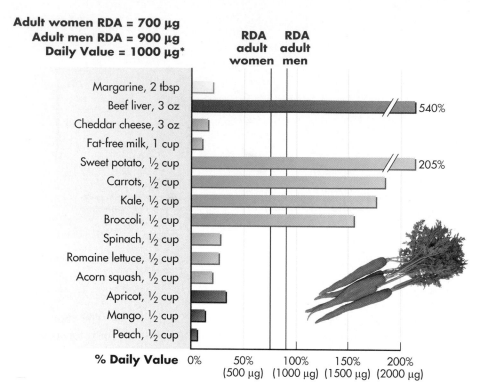

Adult women RDA = 700 μg
Adult men RDA = 900 μg
Daily Value = 1000 μg*

* Calculated from International Units.

Beta-carotene accounts for some of the orange color in carrots and other carotenoid-rich foods. In dark green vegetables, this yellow-orange coloring is masked by the dark green pigment chlorophyll, although these vegetables do contain provitamin A. Therefore, consuming a varied diet rich in both dark green and yellow-orange vegetables can provide vitamin A.

At one time, the amounts of vitamin A (and most other nutrients) were expressed in International Units (IUs). Today, there are more sensitive means for measuring nutrients. Consequently, milligram (1/1000 of a gram) and microgram (1/1,000,000 of a gram) measurements have generally replaced IUs as the units of measure. However, some food and vitamin supplement labels may still display the older IU values.

Dietary vitamin A activity is currently expressed in Retinol Activity Equivalents (RAE). One RAE is equal to 1 μg of retinol, 12 μg of beta-carotene, and 24 μg of the other 2 provitamin A carotenoids (alpha-carotene and beta-cryptoxanthin).[1,2] Table 12-1 is a tool for converting the amounts of vitamin A and carotenes expressed in 1 unit of measure into another unit of measure.

The retinol equivalent (RE) is an older unit of measurement for vitamin A activity. The RE was based on the assumption that carotenoids made a greater contribution to vitamin A needs than is now known to be the case. Nutrient databases may contain this older RE standard because it will take some time to update these resources.

Many vegetables are rich in provitamin A carotenoids.

To compare the older RE or IU standards with current RAE recommendations, assume that, for any preformed vitamin A in a food or added to food, 1 RE (or 3.3 IU) = 1 RAE. There is no easy way to convert RE or IU units to RAE units for foods that naturally contain provitamin A carotenoids, such as carrots, spinach, and apricots. A general rule of thumb is to divide the older values for foods containing carotenoids by 2, and then do the conversion from RE to IU to RAE, as shown in Table 12-1. There also is no easy way to do this calculation for food containing a mixture of pre-

Table 12-1 Conversion Values for Retinol Activity Equivalents

1 Retinol Activity Equivalent (RAE)	1 IU vitamin A activity
= 1 µg retinol	= 0.3 µg retinol
= 12 µg beta-carotene	= 3.6 µg beta-carotene
= 24 µg alpha-carotene and beta-cryptoxanthin	= 7.2 µg alpha-carotene and beta-cryptoxanthin

formed vitamin A and carotenoids. Generally speaking, these foods contain less vitamin A than the RE or IU values suggest.

Vitamin A Needs

The RDA for vitamin A is 900 µg Retinol Activity Equivalents (RAE) per day for adult men and 700 µg RAE per day for adult women.[2] At this intake, adequate body stores of vitamin A are maintained in healthy adults. The Daily Value used on food packages and supplements is 5000 IU, or about 1000 µg. At present, there is no DRI for beta-carotene or any of the other provitamin A carotenoids.[1] The average intakes of adult men and women in North America currently meet DRI guidelines for vitamin A.

Absorption, Transport, Storage, and Excretion of Vitamin A

Preformed vitamin A is found in foods of animal origin as retinol and retinyl ester-compounds (retinol attached to a fatty acid). Retinyl esters don't have vitamin A activity until the retinol and fatty acid are separated in the intestinal tract.[2] This process requires bile and pancreatic lipase enzymes. Up to 90% of retinol is absorbed into the cells of the small intestine. After absorption, a fatty acid is attached to retinol to form a new retinyl ester. These retinyl esters are packaged into chylomicrons before entering the lymphatic circulation.

The provitamin A carotenoids can be enzymatically split within the intestinal cells or liver cells to form retinal or, to a lesser extent, retinoic acid. The carotenoid absorption is much lower than that of retinol. After being absorbed in the small intestine, carotenoids can be cleaved to yield retinal, which is then converted to retinol. Retinol can then have a fatty acid attached to it to become a retinyl ester and enter the lymphatic system as part of a chylomicron. The chylomicrons deliver vitamin A to tissues for storage or cellular use. Carotenoids also can enter the bloodstream directly; however, this occurs to a lesser extent.[4]

Over 90% of the body's vitamin A stores are found in the liver, with small amounts in adipose tissue, kidneys, bone marrow, testicles, and eyes. Normally, the liver stores enough vitamin A to last for several months to protect against vitamin A deficiency.[2]

When vitamin A (as a retinoid) is released from the liver into the bloodstream, it is bound to a retinol-binding protein (RBP) (Fig. 12-4). In the bloodstream, retinol-binding protein is bound to another protein called transthyretin (commonly known as prealbumin). In contrast, when carotenoids are released from the liver, they are carried by the lipoprotein VLDL.[4] Within the body's cells, retinoids are bound to specific RBPs, which direct them to functional sites in the cell. Nearly all cells contain 1 or more of these binding proteins. The distribution of the cellular RBPs differs among tissues, possibly reflecting their different functional needs for vitamin A.[4]

Although vitamin A is not readily excreted by the body, some is lost in the urine. Kidney disease increases the risk of vitamin A toxicity because this urinary route of excretion is compromised.[4]

▶ During protein-energy malnutrition, the synthesis of retinol-binding protein and transthyretin (prealbumin) is reduced by the lack of sufficient amino acids and energy. These proteins often are used as clinical indicators of protein status in a person because decreased concentrations in the blood can suggest inadequate protein intake.

Figure 12-4 The mechanism of the action of vitamin A (as retinoic acid) on the target cell.

1 Vitamin A is carried by retinal-binding protein and transthyretin in the blood.

2 On release, vitamin A enters the target cell.

3 The vitamin A binds to cellular retinoid-binding protein.

4 Once released from this protein, vitamin A then enters the nucleus and binds to its nuclear-retinoid receptors (RAR and RXR). Nearly all cells have a least 1 member of the RAR and RXR families of vitamin A–binding proteins.

5 This complex then binds to DNA, activating gene transcription.

6 The resulting messenger RNA (mRNA) has the code for the protein.

7 The protein ultimately produces the cellular responses.

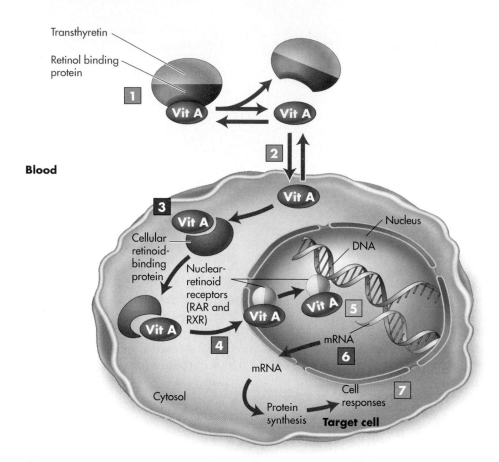

RXR, RAR Abbreviations for *retinoid X receptor* and *retinoid acid receptor.*

stem cells Unspecialized cells that can be transformed into specialized cells.

Functions of Vitamin A (Retinoids)

Vitamin A retinoids perform different functions in the body. Their key functions include growth and development, cell differentiation, vision, and immune function.

Growth and Development

Retinoids play an important role in embryonic development. From studies of animals, scientists learned that vitamin A is involved in the development of eyes, limbs, the cardio-vascular system, and the nervous system. They also noted that a lack of vitamin A during early stages of pregnancy resulted in birth defects and fetal mortality (death). Retinoic acid also is necessary for the production, structure, and normal function of epithelial cells in the lungs, the trachea, the skin, the GI tract, and many other systems. It is important for the formation and maintenance of mucous-forming cells in these organs.

Cell Differentiation

In the cell nucleus, retinoids bind to 2 main families of retinoid receptors (see Fig. 12-4). These receptors (called **RXR** and **RAR**) bind to specific DNA sites that regulate the formation of messenger RNA (needed to copy genetic material from DNA) and the subsequent formation of proteins through gene expression. Gene expression directs **cell differentiation**—the process in which **stem cells** develop into specialized cells with unique functions in the body. Vitamin A is especially important in maintaining normal differentiation of the cells that make up the structural components of the eye, such as the cornea (clear lens) and the retina (rod and cone cells).[4]

Vision

Vitamin A (as retinal) is needed in the **retina** of the eye to turn visual light into nerve signals to the brain. The sensory elements of the retina consist of the rods and cones. **Rods** are responsible for the visual processes that occur in dim light, translating objects

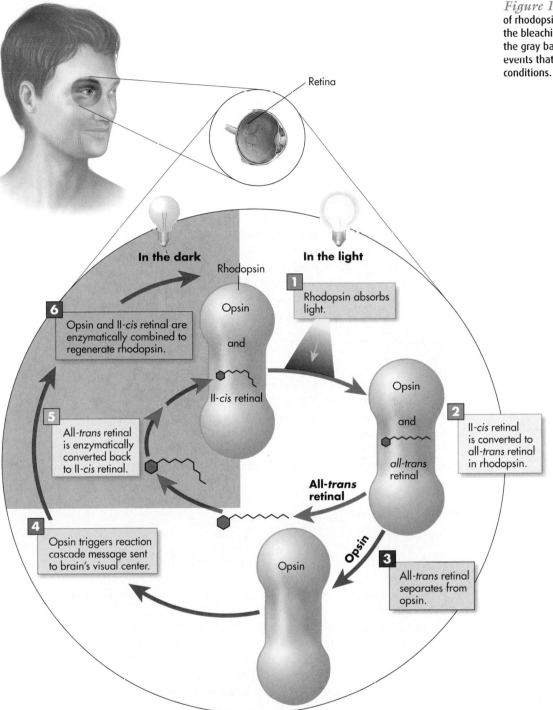

Figure 12-5 The bleaching and regeneration of rhodopsin. The yellow background indicates the bleaching events that occur in the light; the gray background indicates the regenerative events that can occur in either light or dark conditions.

In the dark

In the light

Rhodopsin

1 Rhodopsin absorbs light.

6 Opsin and ll-*cis* retinal are enzymatically combined to regenerate rhodopsin.

Opsin

and

ll-*cis* retinal

Opsin

and

all-trans retinal

2 ll-*cis* retinal is converted to all-*trans* retinal in rhodopsin.

5 All-*trans* retinal is enzymatically converted back to ll-*cis* retinal.

All-*trans* retinal

4 Opsin triggers reaction cascade message sent to brain's visual center.

Opsin

Opsin

Opsin

3 All-*trans* retinal separates from opsin.

into black-and-white images and detecting motion. **Cones** are responsible for the visual processes occurring under bright light, translating objects into color images.

In the rods, ll-*cis*-retinal binds to a protein called **opsin** to form the visual pigment **rhodopsin** (Fig. 12-5). The absorption of light catalyzes a change in the shape of ll-*cis*-retinal to all-*trans*-retinal, causing opsin to separate from all-*trans*-retinal.[4] (The separation is a **bleaching process**.) This leads to a cascade of biochemical events that trigger a change in the ion permeability of the photoreceptor cells and initiate a signal to the nerve cells that communicate with the brain's visual center. Thousands of rod cells containing millions of molecules of rhodopsin are triggered simultaneously to produce this signal. During exposure to bright light, the rod's rhodopsin is completely activated and cannot respond to more light. To keep the visual process functioning, all-*trans*-retinal must

bleaching process Process by which light depletes the rhodopsin concentration in the eye by separating opsin from all-*trans*-retinal. This fall in rhodopsin concentration allows the eye to become adapted to bright light.

dark adaptation Process by which the rhodopsin concentration in the eye increases in dark conditions, allowing improved vision in the dark.

eventually be converted back to ll-*cis*-retinal. This regeneration occurs within several minutes. The ll-*cis*-retinal then moves back to the photoreceptor cells, where it recombines with the opsin, forming rhodopsin, and is ready for another visual cycle.

Not all retinal is used in each cycle. Some is stored in the eye to maintain vitamin A pools. If vitamin A pools become depleted, the process of **dark adaptation** is impaired, making it difficult to adjust to seeing in dim light, known as night blindness. You may have had a brief experience similar to night blindness when you walked into a dark movie theatre or when a bright light was suddenly shined in your eyes. However, this brief difficulty in seeing is not related to vitamin A deficiency because your vision quickly returns once your eyes have adjusted to the change in light.

Immune Function

As early as the 1920s, researchers recognized that vitamin A (mostly as retinoic acid) was important for immune system functions. They observed that increased incidence of infection was one of the first symptoms of vitamin A deficiency. Many studies since have shown that vitamin A deficient individuals have greater susceptibility to illness and infection. This may be, in part, because vitamin A helps maintain the **epithelium,** a barrier that protects the body against the entry of disease pathogens. In many regions of the world where vitamin A deficiency is common, vitamin A supplementation has been shown to reduce the severity of some infections, such as measles and diarrhea, in vitamin A deficient children.

Use of Vitamin A Analogs in Dermatology

Several synthetic compounds with a chemical makeup similar to that of vitamin A (called analogs) have been used in topical and oral medications (e.g., Retin-A® and Accutane®) to treat acne and **psoriasis.** Retinoid-based medications also have been used topically to lessen the damage from excess sun and UV-light exposure. It is important that a physician monitor the use of these medications because high doses of oral, and even topical, retinoids can cause serious toxic effects. A pregnancy test is required before Accutane® is prescribed to women because high doses of vitamin A can cause birth defects.

Carotenoid Functions

Scientists have known for many years that several dietary carotenoids can be converted to vitamin A within the body. More recently, evidence from research studies suggests that carotenoids may have functions other than provitamin A activity. These studies indicate that diets high in carotenoid-rich fruits and vegetables may decrease the risk of certain eye diseases, cancers, and cardiovascular disease.[5-7] This has sparked interest in the potential benefits of supplementing diets with specific carotenoids to lower disease risks.

The most familiar carotenoid is beta-carotene, the carotenoid with the most vitamin A activity. Because of its chemical structure, beta-carotene may act as an antioxidant within tissues, thereby protecting them from free radical damage. Evidence that beta-carotene might protect eye tissues was suggested by epidemiological studies showing a decreased risk of cataracts in people with high blood levels of antioxidant nutrients.[7] However, in follow-up studies, long-term supplementation of beta-carotene (and vitamin E) did not prevent or reduce the incidence of cataracts.

Several other studies have focused on a possible role for beta-carotene in the prevention of lung cancer. Although the consumption of fruits and vegetables rich in beta-carotene has been associated with a reduced risk of lung cancer, large studies examining the effectiveness of beta-carotene supplements in preventing lung cancer in high-risk populations (smokers and asbestos workers) revealed that these supplements actually increased the risk of lung cancer. Thus, beta-carotene supplements are not an effective means of reducing the risk of cancer and may even increase the risk in certain individuals.[8]

Studies of diets that contain high amounts of the carotenoids lutein and zeaxanthin suggest that they may help protect against age-related **macular degeneration** of the eye (Fig. 12-6).[7] To date, however, a direct link between increased intake of lutein and zeaxanthin

---

dark adaptation Process by which the rhodopsin concentration in the eye increases in dark conditions, allowing improved vision in the dark.

epithelium Covering of internal and external surfaces of the body, such as the lungs, GI tract, blood vessel linings, and skin.

psoriasis Immune system disorder that causes a chronic inflammatory skin condition (painful patches of red, scaly skin).

macular degeneration Chronic eye disease that occurs when tissue in the macula (the part of the retina responsible for central vision) deteriorates. It causes a blind spot or blurred vision in the center of the visual field.

▶ Concentrations of lutein and zeaxanthin are 500–1,000 times higher in the macula of the eye than in other tissues. Spinach and kale are 2 notable sources of these carotenoids.

and the prevention of age-related macular degeneration has not been demonstrated. Thus, as with beta-carotene, taking supplements of these carotenoids is not recommended.

Over the last decade, there has been increased interest in a carotenoid pigment found in tomatoes, called lycopene.[9] Much of this interest developed when scientists observed that men with greater intakes of tomato products and higher blood levels of lycopene had a reduced risk of prostate cancer. However, tomatoes may contain many phytochemicals in addition to lycopene, some of which may provide protection against disease. Thus, increased blood lycopene levels may simply reflect increased tomato intake and may not be responsible for reduced cancer risk.

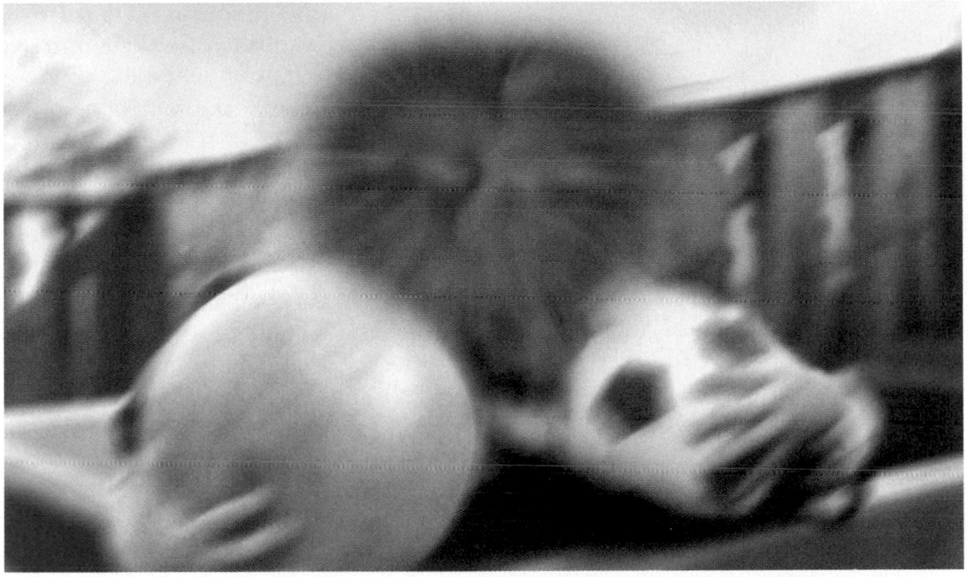

Both beta-carotene and lycopene have been studied for their possible role in reducing the risk of cardiovascular disease (CVD). Because carotenoids are carried in the blood with lipoproteins, scientists have proposed that they may inhibit oxidation of the lipoprotein LDL. Beta-carotene supplementation alone has not been consistently shown to decrease risk of CVD.[10] However, there is evidence that lycopene may reduce the CVD risk by decreasing LDL oxidation and cholesterol synthesis, as well as by increasing LDL receptor activity in cells. Until these complex relationships are more clearly understood, nutritionists do not recommend carotenoid supplements. Instead, they advocate increased intakes of carotenoid-rich fruits and vegetables.

Figure 12-6 Age-related macular degeneration causing a blind spot in the center of the visual field. Increased dietary lutein and zeaxanthin are associated with decreased risk of macular degeneration. Further research is needed to better understand the relationship between macular degeneration and carotenoids.

Vitamin A Deficiency Diseases

North Americans have little risk of developing vitamin A deficiency because this vitamin is abundant in our food supply.[2] Vitamin A deficiency, however, is one of the major public health problems in developing countries. Worldwide, vitamin A deficiency is the leading cause of non-accidental blindness. Children in impoverished nations in Africa, Asia, and South America are especially susceptible because inadequate intakes and low stores of vitamin A fail to meet their needs for growth. In the most destitute nations, approximately 500,000 children become blind each year because of vitamin A deficiency.[11]

Although vitamin A deficiency is not commonly seen in North America, several population groups are considered at risk. Impoverished and older adults, people with alcoholism or liver disease (which limits vitamin A storage), and individuals with severe fat malabsorption, such as gluten-sensitive enteropathy (celiac disease), chronic diarrhea, pancreatic insufficiency, Crohn's disease, cystic fibrosis, and AIDS, may develop vitamin A deficiency. Premature infants also are at risk of deficiency because they are born with low stores of vitamin A.[2, 4]

Vitamin A deficiency results in many changes in the eye. When the retinol in the blood is insufficient to replace the retinal lost during the visual cycle, the rods in the retina regenerate rhodopsin more slowly. The resulting night blindness is a common early symptom of vitamin A deficiency, as discussed earlier. Without enough retinoic acid, mucous-forming cells deteriorate and are no longer able to synthesize mucous. The eye, especially the cornea, is adversely affected by the loss of mucous because mucous helps keep the eye surface moist and washes away dirt particles that settle on the eye. This leads to the development of conjunctival xerosis (abnormal dryness of the **conjunctiva** of the eye). Bitot's spots (foamy gray spots on the eye consisting of hardened epithelial cells) also appear as vitamin A deficiency worsens. These conditions often progress to keratomalacia (softening

conjunctiva Mucous membrane covering the front surface of the eye and the lining of the eyelids.

xerophthalmia Condition marked by dryness of the cornea and eye membranes that results from vitamin A deficiency and can lead to blindness.

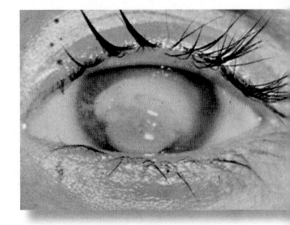

Figure 12-7 Vitamin A deficiency can have severe effects on the eye, eventually leading to blindness.

of the cornea) and scarring (Fig. 12-7). This sequence of changes in the eye—collectively known as **xerophthalmia**—causes irreversible blindness in millions of people worldwide.

Vitamin A deficiency also produces skin changes, referred to as **follicular hyper-keratosis**. Keratin, the normal component in the outer layers of the skin, protects the inner layers and reduces water loss through the skin. During severe vitamin A deficiency, keratinized cells, which are normally present only in the outer layers, replace normal epithelial cells in the underlying skin layers. Hair follicles become plugged with keratin, giving a dry, rough, sandy texture to the skin.

In infants and young children, vitamin A deficiency can impair growth. If adequate vitamin A stores are established before an infant is **weaned**, they can help protect against deficiency. Vitamin A supplementation for infants and young children at risk also may protect them. Finding suitable foods to improve vitamin A intake is essential as a long-term solution to vitamin A deficiency.[12]

wean To accustom an infant to a diet containing foods rather than just milk.

Vitamin A Toxicity

The signs and symptoms of toxicity from excessive vitamin A—called hypervitaminosis A—appear with long-term supplement use at 5 to 10 times the RDA for retinoids[2] (Fig. 12-9). Correspondingly, the Upper Level is set at 3000 μg/day of retinol to prevent harmful effects. No Upper Level is set for carotenoids because vitamin A toxicity results only from excess intakes of retinoids.[1]

Three kinds of vitamin A toxicity occur: acute, chronic, and teratogenic.[13] Acute toxicity is caused by the ingestion of 1 very large dose of vitamin A or several large doses taken over a few days (about 100 times the RDA). The effects of acute toxicity include GI tract upset, headache, blurred vision, and poor muscle coordination. Once the dosing is stopped, the signs disappear. Extraordinarily large doses of 500 mg in children and 10 g in adults can be fatal.

In chronic toxicity, infants and adults show a wide range of signs and symptoms: joint pain, loss of appetite, skin disorders, headache, reduced bone minerals, liver damage, double vision, hemorrhage, and coma. These symptoms occur with repeated intakes of at least 10 times the RDA guidelines. The treatment is simply to discontinue the sup-

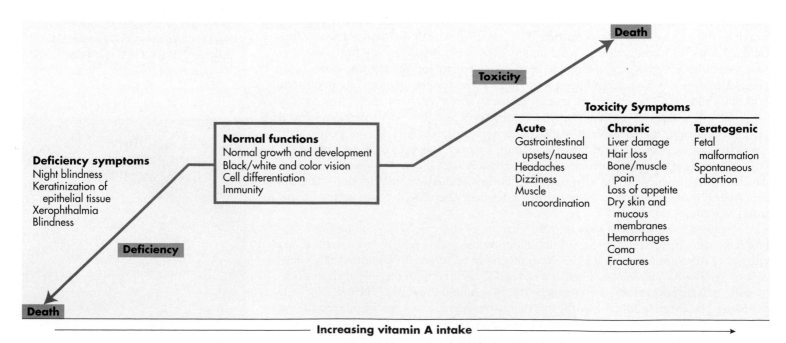

Figure 12-9 Consuming the right amount of vitamin A is critical to overall health. A very low (deficient) or very high (toxic) vitamin A intake (as retinoids) can produce harmful symptoms and can even lead to death.

plement. The symptoms then decrease over the next few weeks as blood concentrations fall within a normal range. Permanent damage to the liver, bones, and eyes, however, can occur with the chronic ingestion of excessive amounts of the vitamin.

The most serious and tragic effects of hypervitaminosis A are **teratogenic** (causing birth defects). Vitamin A and its related analog forms (all-*trans*-retinoic acid [topical tretinoin, or Retin-A®] and 13-*cis*-retinoic acid [oral isotretinoin, or Accutane®]) are used to treat various skin disorders, such as acne and psoriasis. However, these analogs are teratogenic in humans and can cause spontaneous abortion and birth defects in laboratory animals, including congenital malformations of the head (because neural crest cells, which are important in the development of the head and brain, are known to be very sensitive to excess amounts of vitamin A). Women of childbearing age should be cautioned against using these medications or should use reliable methods to prevent pregnancies that might result in fetal malformations.

It is even possible for pregnant women to get too much vitamin A from food if they frequently consume increased amounts of foods rich in vitamin A, such as liver or fortified ready-to-eat breakfast cereals. For this reason, pregnant women should limit their intake of these foods and, if taking supplements, should check that much of the supplemental vitamin A is in the form of beta-carotene. The FDA recommends that women of childbearing age limit their intake of preformed vitamin A to 100% of the Daily Value.[2]

Consuming carotenoids in large amounts from foods does not readily result in toxicity. The carotenoids' rate of conversion to vitamin A is relatively slow. In addition, the efficiency of carotenoid absorption from the small intestine decreases markedly as dietary intake increases.[1] If one consistently consumes large amounts of carrots, carrot juice, or winter squash, the resulting high carotenoid concentrations in the body can turn the skin a yellow-orange color, a condition termed hypercarotenemia, or carotenemia.[1] (*Hyper* means "high" and *emia* means "in the bloodstream.")

CRITICAL THINKING

Julie bought a new juice maker machine and has been making carrot and mango juice, which she drinks 2 or 3 times daily. She has noticed recently that the palms of her hands are turning orange. What is likely causing this? Is she at risk of vitamin A toxicity?

CASE STUDY

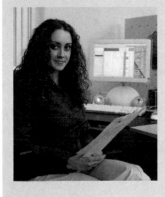

Kristin has been under a lot of stress and is concerned about her overall health. She works nights at a local package distribution center and takes a full course load during the day at the local community college. At lunch one day, her friend Jessi suggested that she take Nutrimega supplements to help prevent colds, flu, and other illnesses and reduce her stress. Jessi said that she had been taking Nutrimega for several months and feels great.

Kristin was a little surprised to learn that a month's supply of Nutrimega costs about $50, but she decided to buy the supplements, anyway. The Nutrimega label recommends taking 2 or 3 tablets daily for health maintenance and 2 or 3 tablets every 3 hours at the first sign of illness. When Kristin read the label on the bottle, she noted that each tablet contained the following nutrients (listed as % Daily Value): 33% vitamin A (75% as preformed vitamin A), 700% vitamin C, 50% zinc, and 10% selenium.

If you were Kristin's dietitian, health clinician, or nutritionist, would you recommend that Kristin use this product? Are there any health risks associated with its use, considering the dosages recommended on the label for maintenance and illness? What alternative suggestions might you give Kristin to help her maintain her overall health?

Knowledge Check

1. What are 3 sources of provitamin A and 3 sources of preformed vitamin A?
2. Why is the carotenoid beta-carotene classified as a provitamin?
3. How does vitamin A affect vision?
4. What are 2 symptoms of vitamin A deficiency?
5. What population groups are at highest risk of vitamin A deficiency?
6. What are the signs and symptoms of vitamin A toxicity?

Global Perspective

Vitamin A Deficiency

In many parts of the developing world, vitamin A deficiency is a major public health concern (Fig. 12-8). Recent estimates indicate that 100 to 140 million children worldwide suffer from vitamin A deficiency. Women of childbearing years also are at increased risk of deficiency, especially in impoverished areas of Africa and Southeast Asia. In many of these areas, where HIV infection also is prevalent, vitamin A deficiency in pregnancy increases the likelihood of the transmission of HIV to the developing fetus and increases the risk of maternal mortality. Approximately 600,000 women die each year from pregnancy- and childbirth-related causes. Many of these deaths result from complications secondary to poor vitamin A and overall nutritional status.[11]

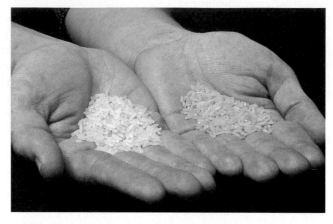

Golden rice was genetically engineered to synthesize beta-carotene. This rice was developed for use as a fortified food in areas of the world that have limited access to vitamin A–rich foods.

As discussed in this chapter, vitamin A deficiency can lead to serious consequences, such as night blindness, total blindness, impaired growth, and an increased incidence of infections. Due to the prevalence of vitamin A deficiency worldwide, it is the leading cause of preventable blindness in children, resulting in 250,000 to 500,000 cases annually. Approximately half of these children die within a year from severe infections, measles, diarrhea, and anemia.[11]

In 1998, a partnership was formed among the World Health Organization (WHO), the United Nations Children's Fund (UNICEF), the Canadian International Development Agency (CIDA), the U.S. Agency for International Development (U.S.AID), and the Micronutrient Initiative (MI) to combat vitamin A deficiency.[11] This coalition of international agencies, called the Vitamin A Global Initiative, has worked to decrease vitamin A deficiency by promoting breastfeeding, the fortification of foods (e.g., sugar fortification in Guatemala), and educational programs to increase home gardening of vitamin A–rich fruits and vegetables in rural areas of Africa and Southeast Asia. WHO, UNICEF, and other international agencies also have provided vitamin A supplements (as a complement to immunization programs) to populations at increased risk of vitamin A deficiency. Vitamin A supplements, which cost pennies, have been shown to decrease vitamin A–related mortality by almost 25% in these areas. Although these organizations have made important strides in the effort to combat worldwide vitamin A deficiency, continued nutritional and medical support is needed to eradicate global vitamin A deficiency. Programs to increase production and access to nutrient-rich foods (e.g., fish) that are native to the diets and livelihoods of the individuals in many at-risk rural areas are food-based strategies that can help prevent nutrient deficiencies.

Countries categorized by degree of public health importance of vitamin A deficiency

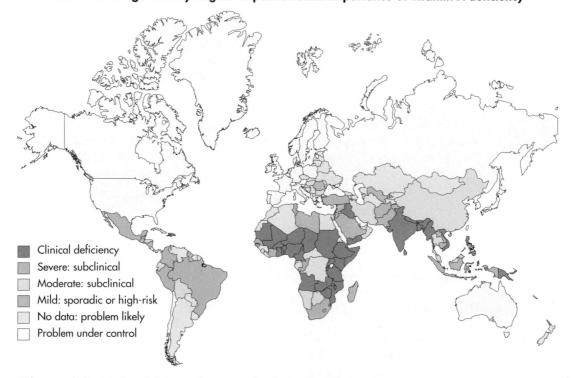

- Clinical deficiency
- Severe: subclinical
- Moderate: subclinical
- Mild: sporadic or high-risk
- No data: problem likely
- Problem under control

Figure 12-8 Vitamin A deficiency affects many developing countries.

12.3 Vitamin D

Bone deformities that were likely caused by the vitamin D deficiency disease, rickets, have been described since ancient times.[14] It wasn't until 1918, when scientists cured rachitic dogs (dogs affected with rickets) by feeding them cod liver oil, that diet was linked with this disease. Soon after, vitamin D was discovered and cod liver oil became a daily supplement for millions of children.

Most scientists classify vitamin D as a vitamin. However, in the presence of sunlight, skin cells can synthesize a sufficient supply of vitamin D from a derivative of cholesterol. Because a dietary source is not required if synthesis is adequate to meet needs, the vitamin is more correctly classified as a "conditional" vitamin, or prohormone (a precursor of an active hormone). In the absence of UV light exposure, an adequate dietary intake of vitamin D is essential to prevent the deficiency diseases rickets and osteomalacia and to provide for cellular needs.

After exposure to the sun, humans produce vitamin D_3 (cholecalciferol) from a derivative of cholesterol. The liver and kidneys each add a hydroxyl group (–OH) to this to yield the active form of vitamin D (1,25 dihydroxy D_3, or calcitriol).

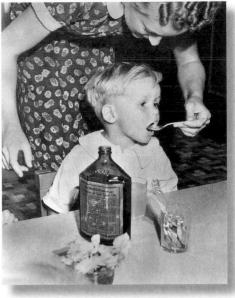

Cod liver oil was a common supplement for children in the United States until 1933, when milk was first fortified with vitamin D.

Vitamin D_2 in Foods

The best food sources of vitamin D are fatty fish (e.g., sardines, mackerel, and salmon), cod liver oil, fortified milk, and some fortified breakfast cereals (Fig. 12-10). In North America, milk is generally fortified with 10 µg (400 IU) of vitamin D per quart. Although eggs, butter, liver, and a few brands of margarine contain some vitamin D, large servings must be eaten to obtain an appreciable amount of the vitamin. Thus, these foods are not considered a significant source. Most fortified foods and supplements containing vitamin D are in the form of ergocalciferol, or vitamin D_2, the same form found naturally in foods. Ergocalciferol has vitamin D activity in humans, but in lesser amounts than provided by cholecalciferol (vitamin D_3).

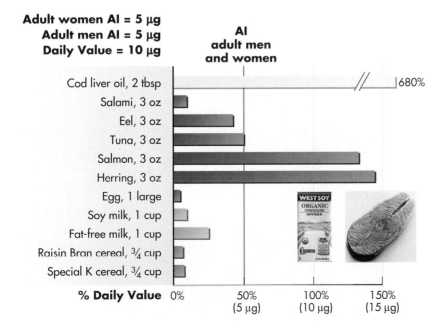

Figure 12-10 Food sources of vitamin D.

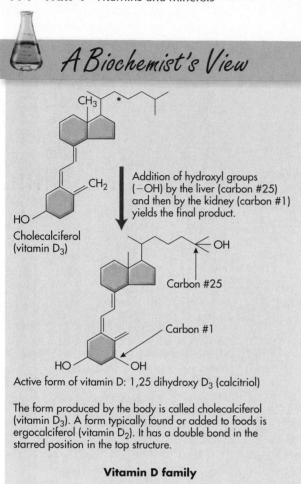

A Biochemist's View

Addition of hydroxyl groups (–OH) by the liver (carbon #25) and then by the kidney (carbon #1) yields the final product.

Cholecalciferol (vitamin D_3)

Carbon #25

Carbon #1

Active form of vitamin D: 1,25 dihydroxy D_3 (calcitriol)

The form produced by the body is called cholecalciferol (vitamin D_3). A form typically found or added to foods is ergocalciferol (vitamin D_2). It has a double bond in the starred position in the top structure.

Vitamin D family

previtamin D_3 Precursor of 1 form of vitamin D, produced as a result of sunlight opening a ring on 7-dehydrocholesterol in the skin.

Vitamin D_3 Formation in the Skin

The synthesis of vitamin D_3 begins with a compound called 7-dehydrocholesterol, a precursor of cholesterol synthesis located in the skin. During exposure to sunlight, 1 ring on the molecule undergoes a chemical transformation, forming the more stable vitamin D_3 (cholecalciferol). This change allows vitamin D_3 to enter the bloodstream for transport to the liver and kidneys, where it undergoes hydroxylation (the addition of –OH) and subsequent conversion to its bioactive form 1,25 dihydroxy D_3 (calcitriol).

For many individuals, sun exposure provides 80 to 100% of the vitamin D_3 required by the body.[3] The amount of sun exposure needed, however, depends on the time of day, the geographic location, the season of the year, one's age, one's skin color, and the use of sunscreen. For example, in Boston, Massachusetts, the production of vitamin D_3 from UV light exposure is adequate to meet needs from March through October. From November through February, however, UV light availability is too low at this latitude (42° N) to produce enough vitamin D_3. In Los Angeles, California (34° N), the production of vitamin D_3 in the skin occurs throughout the year because of greater UV light availability (Fig. 12-11). The production of vitamin D_3 in the skin decreases by about 70% when one reaches the age of 70. Older people are advised to get small amounts of sun exposure, especially during early morning and late afternoon (to minimize skin cancer risk), or to take vitamin D supplements to prevent deficiency.

The large amount of melanin (skin pigment) in dark-skinned individuals may block UV light and prevent adequate vitamin D_3 synthesis. Using sunscreens with an SPF higher than 8, although useful in decreasing the risk of skin cancer, also may prevent adequate vitamin D_3 synthesis. Scientists recommend that people expose their hands, face, and arms to UV light at least 2 or 3 times a week for 10 to 15 minutes. Individuals with dark skin may need sun exposure of 30 minutes or more (or vitamin D supplementation). Prolonged sun exposure is not likely to result in vitamin D synthesis beyond needs or in toxic amounts, as excess amounts of **previtamin D_3** in the skin are rapidly degraded. Overall, those who do not receive enough UV light exposure to synthesize adequate amounts of vitamin D_3 should make certain that they have adequate sources of vitamin D in their diets.

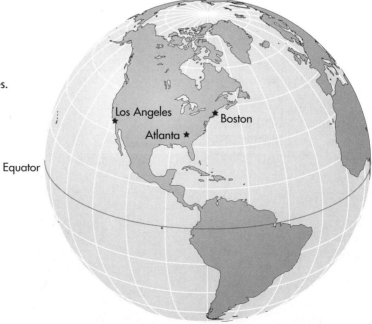

Figure 12-11 As the distance from the equator increases, available UV light decreases.

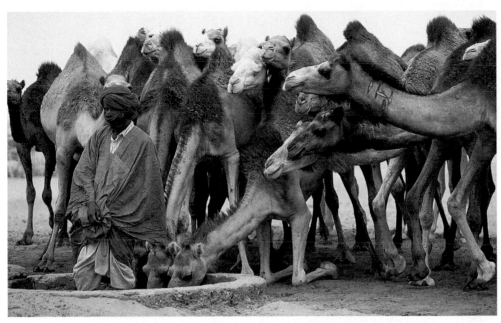

People who remain almost fully covered during the day produce little vitamin D_3.

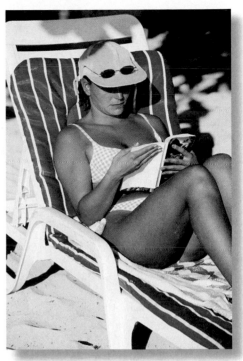

Ultraviolet light on the skin provides about 80 to 100% of the vitamin D humans use. Few foods provide significant amounts of vitamin D; thus, sun exposure often provides the most reliable way of maintaining vitamin D status.

Vitamin D Needs

The Food and Nutrition Board has set an Adequate Intake, rather than an RDA, for vitamin D (see Chapter 2). A more precise RDA level could not be set because the amount of vitamin D produced by sun exposure varies considerably among individuals. The Adequate Intake for vitamin D is 5 µg/day (200 IU/day) for people under age 51, 10 µg/day (400 IU/day) for people between 51 and 70, and 15 µg/day (600 IU/day) for older adults.[3] Older adults as well as others who have limited sun exposure may need 20 to 25 µg (800 to 1000 IU) from a combination of vitamin D–fortified foods and a supplement to decrease the risk of bone loss and other chronic diseases.[15-18] The Daily Value used on food and supplement labels is 10 µg.

Although full-term infants are born with a supply of vitamin D, the American Academy of Pediatrics recommends that breastfed infants be given a vitamin D supplement of 5 µg/day (200 IU) until they are weaned to infant foods fortified with, or rich in, vitamin D.

Absorption, Transport, Storage, and Excretion of Vitamin D

Milk is usually fortified with vitamin D, so even fat-free and low-fat milk contain vitamin D.

Following the consumption of vitamin D_2–containing foods, about 80% of vitamin D_2 is incorporated (along with other dietary fats) into micelles in the small intestine, absorbed, and transported to the liver by chylomicrons through the lymphatic system (Fig. 12-12). Patients with diseases that may result in fat malabsorption syndromes (e.g., cystic fibrosis, Crohn's disease, and celiac disease) are at increased risk of vitamin D_2 malabsorption and deficiency.

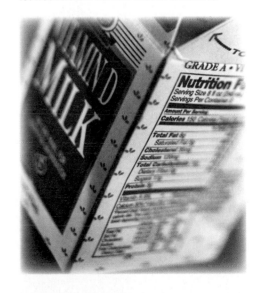

When vitamin D (either D_3 synthesized in the skin or D_2 consumed in food or supplements) enters the general circulation, it is bound to a protein for transport to the adipose cells for storage or to the liver and kidneys. In the liver, vitamin D is hydroxylated on carbon 25, converting it to 25–OH vitamin D_3. This inactive form circulates in the blood for many weeks. The next stop is the kidney, the principal site for the production of $1,25(OH)_2$ vitamin D_3, also known as calcitriol. This is the active form of the vitamin that, as needed, binds to specific receptors in target tissues to induce vitamin D functions.

The synthesis of $1,25(OH)_2$ vitamin D_3 is tightly regulated by the parathyroid gland and the kidneys. When there's a shortage of calcium in the blood, the parathyroid gland increases the production of parathyroid hormone (PTH). PTH then increases the production of $1,25(OH)_2$ vitamin D_3 in the kidneys.

Vitamin D is primarily excreted through the small amount of bile that is lost during digestion. Small amounts of vitamin D also are excreted in the urine.

Figure 12-12 Whether synthesized in the skin or obtained from dietary sources, vitamin D ultimately functions as a hormone: $1,25(OH)_2$ vitamin D_3 (calcitriol).

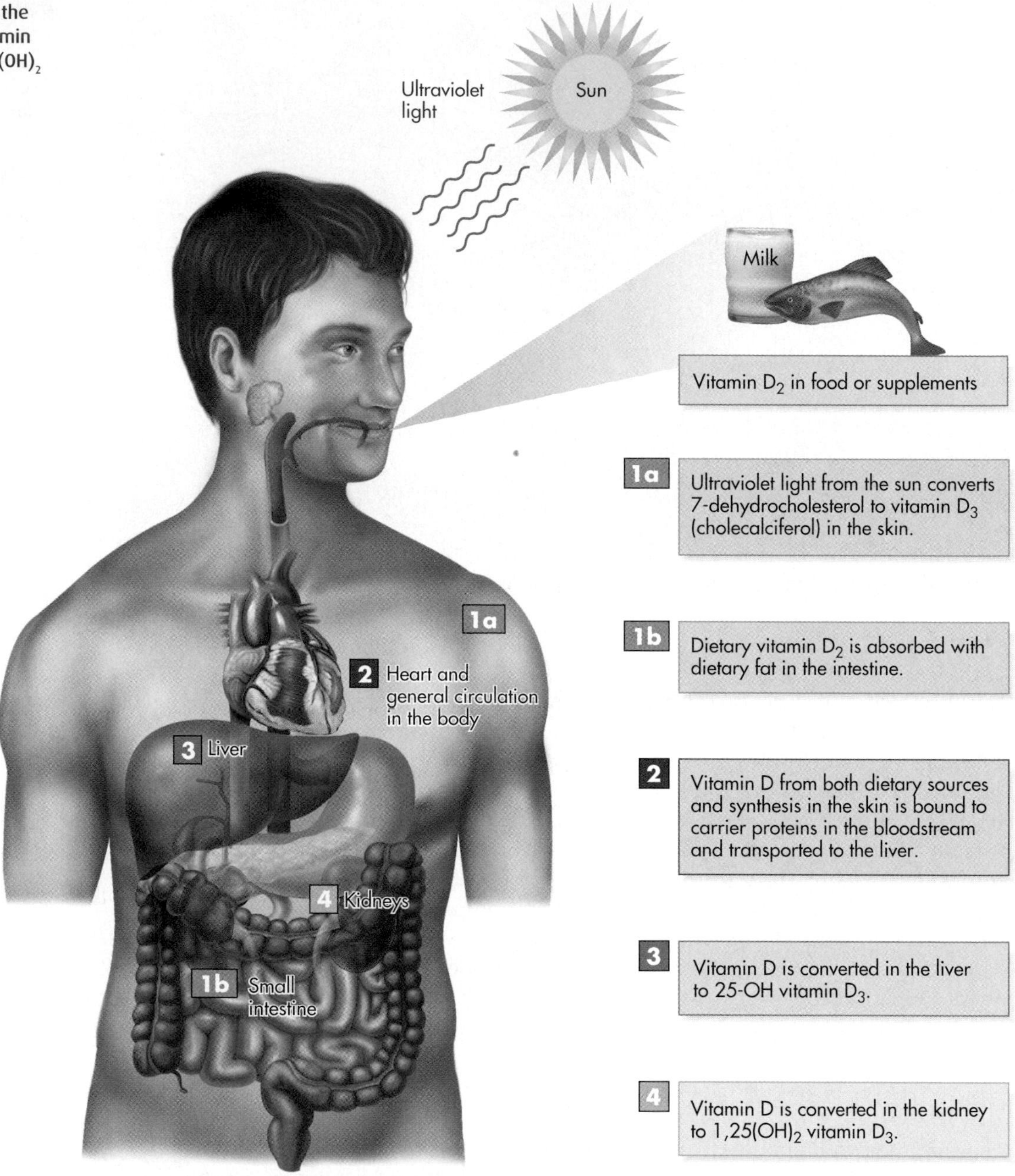

Ultraviolet light

Sun

Milk

Vitamin D_2 in food or supplements

1a Ultraviolet light from the sun converts 7-dehydrocholesterol to vitamin D_3 (cholecalciferol) in the skin.

1b Dietary vitamin D_2 is absorbed with dietary fat in the intestine.

2 Vitamin D from both dietary sources and synthesis in the skin is bound to carrier proteins in the bloodstream and transported to the liver.

3 Vitamin D is converted in the liver to 25-OH vitamin D_3.

4 Vitamin D is converted in the kidney to $1,25(OH)_2$ vitamin D_3.

2 Heart and general circulation in the body

3 Liver

4 Kidneys

1b Small intestine

Functions of Vitamin D

Vitamin D has hormonelike functions, which help regulate the body's concentration of calcium and phosphorus (Fig. 12-13).[16] The effects can have somewhat opposite impacts on bone. On the one hand, vitamin D promotes increased intestinal absorption of calcium and phosphorus from foods to maintain blood levels of these minerals. This makes calcium and phosphorus available for body cells and for incorporation into bones when there is more than needed for basic functions. On the other hand, when blood levels of calcium and phosphorus start to fall, vitamin D (with PTH from the parathyroid gland) can release calcium and phosphorus from bone into the blood to restore blood levels of these minerals. Although this action can eventually weaken the bones if it continues for a prolonged period of time, it helps provide the calcium and phosphorus needed for many basic life functions (see Chapter 14). If the bones did not supply calcium and phosphorus for these functions, a person could quickly have serious, even fatal, health consequences.

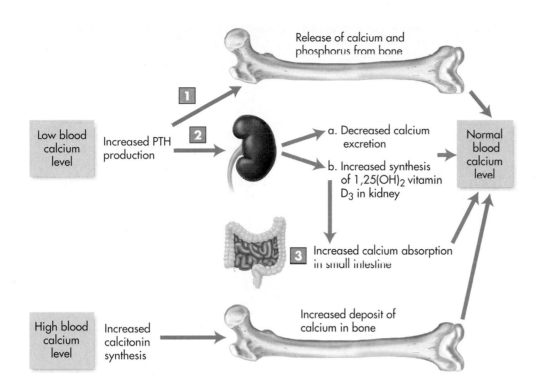

Figure 12-13 The active vitamin D hormone—1,25(OH)$_2$ vitamin D$_3$—and parathyroid hormone interact to control blood calcium concentration. Low blood calcium is a trigger for the following actions, all of which raise blood calcium levels.

1 Parathyroid hormone (PTH) and 1,25(OH)$_2$ vitamin D$_3$ mobilize calcium from the bone.

2 PTH also
   a. Reduces calcium excretion by the kidneys
   b. Stimulates kidney synthesis of 1,25(OH)$_2$ vitamin D$_3$.

3 1,25(OH)$_2$ vitamin D$_3$ stimulates intestinal calcium absorption.

Conversely, when calcium levels in the blood become too high, the hormone calcitonin responds by promoting calcium deposition in the bone (see Chapter 14).

Thus, vitamin D preserves these important functions even if dietary intakes of these minerals are inadequate.[19]

Vitamin D has important functions beyond its role in maintaining calcium and phosphorus homeostasis and bone health.[19] The discovery of vitamin D receptors in immune cells and many other cells throughout the body indicates that vitamin D also is involved in immune function and cellular metabolism. Although the exact role of vitamin D in many tissues is not fully known, studies suggest that it may be involved in cell cycle regulation. Additionally, vitamin D may decrease the risk of certain types of infections and autoimmune diseases, such as multiple sclerosis, through its actions in the immune system and offer protection against diabetes, hypertension, and certain cancers.[20, 21, 22] Much of this evidence has come from observational studies; thus, intervention studies of vitamin D supplementation are needed to determine its role in these diseases.

Vitamin D Deficiency Diseases

Without adequate calcium and phosphorus in the blood available for deposition in the bone, the skeleton fails to mineralize normally. This causes the bones to weaken and bow under pressure. When these effects occur in the growing bones of a child, the disease is called **rickets** (Fig. 12-14). The signs of rickets include enlarged head, joints, and rib cage; a deformed pelvis; and bowed legs. In developed countries, rickets is most commonly associated with fat malabsorption, such as is seen in children with cystic fibrosis. However, an increase in cases has been seen in children who have dark skin, children with low milk intakes, and children with minimal sun exposure due to protective clothing, sunscreens, and/or limited outdoor activity.[20, 23, 24] In fact, many scientists are concerned about an epidemic of vitamin D deficiency and rickets reemerging in industrialized and developing countries.[20, 23, 24]

Vitamin D deficiency in adults is called **osteomalacia**, which means "soft bones." It is characterized by poor calcification of newly synthesized bone, resulting in fractures in the hip, spine, and other bones. (Do not confuse this disease with osteoporosis, which is discussed in Chapter 14.) Osteomalacia is most likely to occur in adults with kidney, liver, gallbladder, or intestinal disease because these diseases affect both vitamin D metabolism and calcium absorption.[3] Other individuals at risk include those with dark skin and with limited UV exposure.[20, 23, 24]

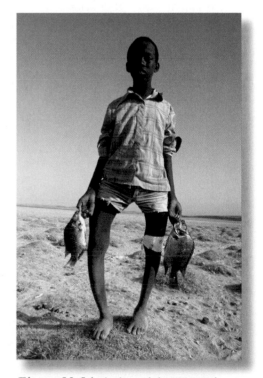

Figure 12-14 The bone deformities and bowed legs of rickets, a vitamin D deficiency disease in children.

Expert Perspective *from the Field*

Vitamin D: "The Iceberg below the Surface"

The fortification of milk with vitamin D and the prophylactic use of cod liver oil almost completely eradicated the epidemic of rickets in the 19th century, convincing many health-care professionals that vitamin D–related health problems had been resolved. However, vitamin D deficiency is reemerging as a global health concern in children and adults. According to Dr. Robert P. Heaney,* low intakes of vitamin D, coupled with behaviors that limit UV light exposure (e.g., time spent indoors, the use of sunscreen, the use of clothing to fully cover the skin), have resulted in widespread reports of inadequate vitamin D status.

The current DRIs for vitamin D were based on intakes shown to promote calcium homeostasis and prevent vitamin D–related bone disorders. However, Dr. Heaney suggests that this is only the "tip of the iceberg" with regard to the role of vitamin D in the body. He notes that, in the last 10 years, scientists have gained vast knowledge about vitamin D functions that have no connection to calcium economy and bone health. The discovery that vitamin D plays an important role in gene control and cell cycle regulation in most tissues of the body has provided new insights into the role of vitamin D in decreasing the risk of many chronic illnesses, including diabetes; colon, prostate, and breast cancer; cardiovascular disease; and autoimmune diseases, such as multiple sclerosis. These insights have led Heaney and other scientists to argue that the current vitamin D intake recommendations (200–600 IU [5–15 µg] daily in adults age 19 years and older) are set too low.

To support the diverse functions of vitamin D, Heaney estimates that the body requires approximately 3000 to 4000 IU (75–100 µg) of vitamin D daily to maintain optimal blood levels of 25(OH)D. However, typical inputs from UV exposure (2000 IU), food sources (150–200 IU), and dietary supplements (200 IU) often provide 2400 IU daily or less for the average individual. Although 90% or more of the body's vitamin D stores are supplied by sunlight exposure, increased skin pigmentation, geographic latitude, seasonal alterations in the angle of the sun, the use of sunscreens, and aging all dramatically affect vitamin D_3 production in the skin and, in turn, increase the risk of vitamin D deficiency. Thus, an oral intake of approximately 1000 to 4000 IU daily might be necessary to maintain optimal vitamin D status in people who have limited sun exposure.

One of the barriers to increasing the dietary recommendations for vitamin D is the Tolerable Upper Intake Level (UL), currently set at 2000 IU daily (50 µg). Heaney and other scientists believe that clinical data published after the vitamin D UL was established in 1997 provide sound evidence that vitamin D is not toxic at much higher intakes than previously considered safe. They urge an increase of the UL to 10,000 IU daily (250 µg) to permit increased intakes of vitamin D for optimal health benefits.

Robert P. Heaney, MD, FACP, FACN, is the John A. Creighton University Professor and Professor of Medicine, Department of Medicine, Creighton University, Omaha, Nebraska. Among his many honors, Dr. Heaney has been awarded the Frederic C. Bartter Award of the American Society for Bone and Mineral Research, the Best Scientific Paper Award of the American College of Nutrition, the Scientific Prize of the Institut Candia (France), the E.V. McCollum Award of the American Society for Clinical Nutrition, the McCollum International Lectureship of the American Society of Nutritional Sciences, and the W.O. Atwater Award of the U.S. Dept. of Agriculture.

Many older adults who live in northern climates or reside in nursing homes also are at increased risk of vitamin D deficiency. Not only do many of these individuals have little sun exposure, they also may have reduced vitamin D levels from low dietary intakes and impaired kidney function, which limit the conversion to $1,25(OH)_2$ vitamin D_3, the active form of the vitamin.[20]

A person with a low circulating concentration of 25-OH vitamin D_3 should take at least 20 to 25 µg (800–1000 IU) of vitamin D each day until the concentration reaches the normal range.[3, 20] After blood concentrations are normal, 10 µg (400 IU/day) from a supplement should be sufficient for most people.[3]

Vitamin D Toxicity

Vitamin D toxicity can occur from excessive vitamin D supplementation. It does not result from excess sun exposure (vitamin D in the skin is readily broken down) or from natural sources in the diet. However, because of the serious consequences of vitamin D toxicity, an Upper Level of intake for vitamin D (50 µg /day [2000 IU/day]) has been set.[3] This UL was established because high intakes of vitamin D can cause an overabsorption of calcium and hypercalcemia (increased calcium in the blood). Excess blood calcium, in turn, leads to deposits of calcium in the kidneys, heart, and lungs; anorexia; nausea; vomiting; bone demineralization; weakness; joint pain; and disorientation. In the early stages of toxicity, the symptoms often are treatable if vitamin D is withdrawn. However, if excess supplementation continues, vitamin D toxicity eventually can be fatal.

Knowledge Check

1. Why is vitamin D often classified as a conditional vitamin, or pro-hormone?
2. What are the rich dietary sources of vitamin D?
3. What are 3 functions of vitamin D?
4. What are the consequences of vitamin D deficiency?
5. Why are those who live in northern latitudes at risk of vitamin D deficiency?
6. Why was an Upper Level of intake established for vitamin D?

 ## 12.4 Vitamin E

The importance of vitamin E was first noted in 1922, when researchers discovered that a substance in vegetable oil was needed for normal reproduction in rats. They later named the substance tocopherol, from the Greek words *toco*, meaning "childbirth" and *pherein*, meaning "to bear." Vitamin E was not fully recognized as an essential nutrient in humans until the mid-1960s, when vitamin E deficiency was observed in children with fat malabsorption diseases. The first RDA for vitamin E was established in 1968. Like RDAs for other nutrients, it has been subsequently revised as knowledge about vitamin E has grown.

Vitamin E is a family of 8 naturally occurring compounds—4 tocopherols (alpha, beta, gamma, delta) and 4 tocotrienols (alpha, beta, gamma, delta)—with widely varying degrees of biological activity. Vitamin E has a long carbon chain tail attached to a ringed structure. This tail exists in many possible isomer forms. The most active form of the vitamin is alpha-tocopherol. This is the form found in some foods and in varying amounts in vitamin supplements. Gamma-tocopherol is a potentially beneficial form of vitamin E found in many vegetable oils. However, it does not have as much biological activity as alpha-tocopherol.[1]

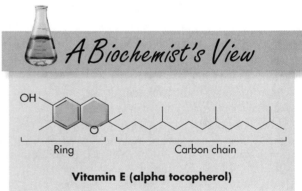

A Biochemist's View

Ring   Carbon chain

Vitamin E (alpha tocopherol)

Vitamin E in Foods

Good food sources of vitamin E include plant oils (e.g., cottonseed, canola, safflower, and sunflower oils), wheat germ, asparagus, almonds, peanuts, and sunflower seeds (Fig. 12-15). Products made from the plant oils—margarine, shortenings, and salad dressings—also are good sources. Animal fats and dairy products contain little vitamin E.

The vitamin E content of a food depends on harvesting, processing, storage, and cooking because vitamin E is highly susceptible to destruction by oxygen, metals, light, and deep-fat frying. Thus, foods that are highly processed and/or deep-fried are usually poor sources of vitamin E.

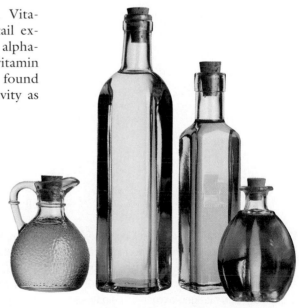

Plant oils are rich sources of vitamin E.

Figure 12-15 Food sources of vitamin E.

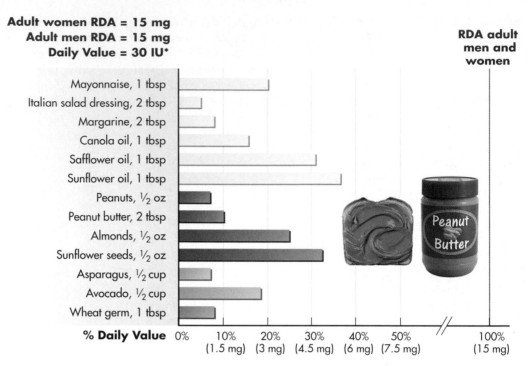

Adult women RDA = 15 mg
Adult men RDA = 15 mg
Daily Value = 30 IU*

RDA adult men and women

% Daily Value scale: 0% | 10% (1.5 mg) | 20% (3 mg) | 30% (4.5 mg) | 40% (6 mg) | 50% (7.5 mg) | 100% (15 mg)

Food sources: Mayonnaise, 1 tbsp; Italian salad dressing, 2 tbsp; Margarine, 2 tbsp; Canola oil, 1 tbsp; Safflower oil, 1 tbsp; Sunflower oil, 1 tbsp; Peanuts, ½ oz; Peanut butter, 2 tbsp; Almonds, ½ oz; Sunflower seeds, ½ oz; Asparagus, ½ cup; Avocado, ½ cup; Wheat germ, 1 tbsp

*Approximately 16.8 mg if half is from synthetic and half is from natural sources.

▶ When you look at food or supplement labels, the type of vitamin E they contain will be labeled as "d" or "l." If you see "d" next to vitamin E on a label, all of that vitamin E will be active in the body. If you see "dl" on a label, only about half of the vitamin E will be active in the body.

Vitamin E Needs

The RDA for vitamin E is 15 mg/day of alpha-tocopherol for both men and women. The recommendation is based on the amount of vitamin E needed to prevent a breakdown of red blood cell membranes, a process called **hemolysis.**[1] The 15-mg allotment is equivalent to 22 IU of a natural source and 33 IU of a synthetic source of vitamin E.

Adults consume, on average, only two-thirds of the RDA for vitamin E each day.[25, 26] In addition to an increased intake of vitamin E–rich foods, the daily consumption of a ready-to-eat breakfast cereal containing vitamin E or the use of a supplement can close this gap between typical vitamin E intakes and needs.

Food and supplement labels often report vitamin E activity in IUs. When converting IUs of vitamin E in synthetic form (as in most supplements) to milligrams, 1 IU equals about 0.45 mg. If the vitamin E is from a natural source, 1 IU equals 0.67 mg because the natural form of vitamin E is more potent than the synthetic form. The Daily Value for vitamin E used on food and supplement labels is 30 IU.

Absorption, Transport, Storage, and Excretion of Vitamin E

The degree of vitamin E absorption depends on the amount consumed and the absorption of dietary fat. Absorption can vary from 20 to 70% of dietary intake. As with other fat-soluble nutrients, vitamin E must be incorporated into micelles in the small intestine, a process dependent on bile and pancreatic enzymes. Once taken up by the intestinal cells, vitamin E is incorporated into chylomicrons for transport by the lymph and eventually the blood.[27]

As chylomicrons are broken down, most of the vitamin E is carried to the liver as chylomicron remnants. A small amount is carried directly to other tissues. The liver repackages the vitamin E from the chylomicron remnants with other lipoproteins (VLDL, LDL, and HDL) for delivery to body tissues.[27] Unlike other fat-soluble vitamins, vitamin E does not have a specific transport protein in the blood, so it's carried by these lipoproteins. Vitamin E also differs from other fat-soluble vitamins in that it does not accumulate in the liver; instead, most of the vitamin E in the body is localized in adipose tissue.

▶ Oxidizing agents that cause cell damage include highly reactive oxygen species, such as the singlet oxygen ($^1O_2$), hydrogen peroxide (H_2O_2), hydroxyl radical ($\cdot OH$), superoxide ($O_2^{\cdot-}$), ozone (O_3), and nitrogen-oxygen combinations that are typical of air pollutants ($NO^{\cdot}$).

Vitamin E can be excreted via the bile, urine, and skin. However, because vitamin E absorption is often low, most vitamin E is excreted via the small amount of bile that exits the body in the feces.

Functions of Vitamin E

Vitamin E is an important part of the body's antioxidant network. It functions as an antioxidant that stops chain reactions caused by free radicals that can potentially damage cells. **Free radicals** are very unstable compounds that have an unpaired electron. Normally, atoms left with an unpaired electron after oxidation reactions immediately pair with one another, creating more stable compounds. However, when this does not occur, free radicals remain and act as strong oxidizing (electron-seeking) agents. These can be very destructive to electron-dense cell components, such as cell membranes and DNA.

Antioxidants function in a variety of ways to prevent the damage caused by free radicals. As a fat-soluble compound, vitamin E acts primarily in lipid-rich areas of the body, where free radicals can initiate a chain of reactions known as peroxidation.[27] Lipid peroxidation reactions break apart fatty acids and create free radicals called lipid **peroxyl radicals** (also called reactive oxygen species because they contain oxygen radicals). The chain of reactions continues to break apart fatty acids until 2 free radicals pair and stabilize each other. However, many lipid peroxyl radicals may be produced through these reactions before stabilization occurs.

Vitamin E is one of the most effective mechanisms for stopping lipid peroxidation chain reactions in the body. By donating a hydrogen to lipid radicals, vitamin E stops the chain of oxidation reactions, which protects the lipids in the body. For example, recall that cell membranes are composed of a phospholipid bilayer (Fig. 12-16). Vitamin E protects cell membrane integrity by neutralizing lipid peroxyl radicals and preventing lipid peroxidation. In this way, vitamin E reduces **oxidative stress** (damage to proteins, lipids, and DNA caused by free radicals) in the body. This reduction in oxidative stress, in turn, may be important in lowering the risk of cardiovascular disease, certain cancers, cognitive decline, and impaired immune function.[28-31]

As damaging as free radicals can be, they play important roles in the body. For example, as part of the immune system's arsenal against invading pathogens, white blood cells (leukocytes) generate free radicals to destroy the agents that cause infections. Although free radicals are a part of life and play essential roles, the body must be able to regulate exposure to free radicals and avoid the undesirable effects, a task assigned to antioxidants.

A vitamin E molecule is "used up" during chain-breaking action. However, there is some evidence that vitamin C may aid in partial regeneration of vitamin E to allow it to function again.

In addition to vitamin E, the body has various other antioxidant compounds, such as glutathione peroxidase, catalase, and superoxide dismutase, to protect against oxidative damage (Fig. 12-17).

Glutathione peroxidase catalyzes the breakdown of hydrogen peroxides and lipid peroxides. These compounds are not radicals, but they can easily become radicals. Glutathione peroxidase eliminates these peroxides before this happens. In this way, glutathione peroxidase helps vitamin E reduce oxidative damage to cells. The activity of glutathione peroxidase depends on the mineral selenium (the functional part of this enzyme). Thus, an adequate dietary intake of selenium reduces the need for vitamin E, whereas an inadequate intake of selenium increases the need. The enzyme **catalase** performs a function similar to that of glutathione peroxidase, but in a different cell location (peroxisomes).

Another vital defense system in cells is provided by a family of enzymes known as superoxide dismutase. These enzymes are important in eliminating superoxide radicals. Two of the superoxide dismutase enzymes contain copper and zinc. One of these enzymes is located inside the cell cytosol and the other is found outside of cells. The third superoxide dismutase enzyme is found in the mitochondria and requires the mineral manganese.

free radical Compound with an unpaired electron, which causes it to seek an electron from another compound. Free radicals are strong oxidizing agents.

peroxyl radical Peroxide compound containing a free radical; designated R-O-O•, where R is a carbon-hydrogen chain broken off of a fatty acid and the dot is an unpaired electron.

Antioxidants versus Redox Agents

Because an antioxidant protects other compounds by becoming oxidized itself, in a chemical sense antioxidants are more correctly termed **redox agents**. In other words, they can undergo both oxidation (loss of an electron) and later reduction (regaining an electron). Nevertheless, *antioxidant* is still the most common term, even in the scientific literature.

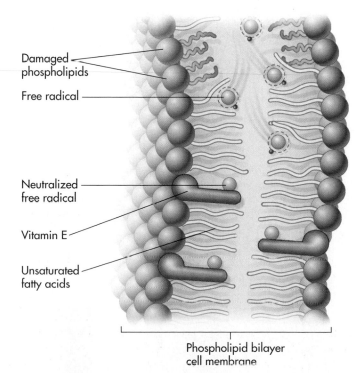

Damaged phospholipids

Free radical

Neutralized free radical

Vitamin E

Unsaturated fatty acids

Phospholipid bilayer cell membrane

Figure 12-16 Fat-soluble vitamin E can donate an electron to stop free radical chain reactions. If not interrupted, these reactions cause extensive oxidative damage to cell membranes.

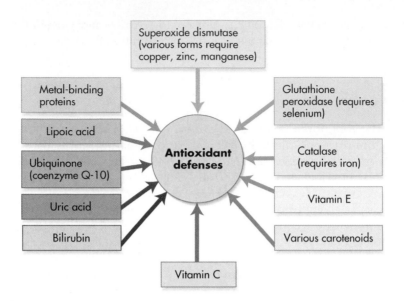

Figure 12-17 The body does not rely solely on vitamin E for antioxidant protection. Such protection is a team effort, utilizing a number of nutrients, metabolites, and enzyme systems.

preterm Born before 37 weeks of gestation (also referred to as premature).

hemolytic anemia Disorder that causes red blood cells to break down faster than they can be replaced.

hemorrhaging Bleeding.

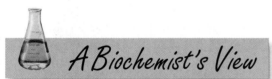

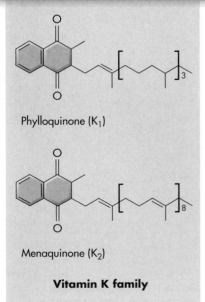

Phylloquinone (K₁)

Menaquinone (K₂)

Vitamin K family

[ ] = Repeated section

Vitamin E Deficiency

Overt vitamin E deficiency is rare in humans. Individuals with fat malabsorption conditions, such as cystic fibrosis and Crohn's disease; smokers; and **preterm** infants are at greatest risk.[1] Preterm infants are particularly susceptible because they are born with limited stores of vitamin E and have insufficient intestinal absorption of this vitamin. Smokers are at increased risk of deficiency because of oxidative stress caused by smoke.[32]

Vitamin E deficiency is characterized by the premature breakdown of red blood cells (hemolysis) and the development of **hemolytic anemia**. Because of the serious risk of this, preterm infants are given supplemental vitamin E and specialized formulas containing vitamin E early in life.

Vitamin E deficiency also can impair immune function and cause neurological changes in the spinal cord and peripheral nervous system. These symptoms have been noted in individuals who developed vitamin E deficiency as a result of a genetic abnormality in lipoprotein synthesis, which decreases vitamin E transport and distribution in the body.[27]

Vitamin E Toxicity

Although vitamin E is relatively non-toxic, excessive amounts can interfere with the role of vitamin K in blood clotting. This causes insufficient clotting and a risk of **hemorrhaging**. These risks are of particular concern in individuals taking daily aspirin or anticoagulation medications, such as warfarin (Coumadin®), to prevent blood clots. Megadoses of vitamin E can result in severe hemorrhaging in these individuals. To prevent toxicity-related problems, the Upper Level for vitamin E is set at 1000 mg (1500 IU) of alpha-tocopherol from natural sources or 1100 IU from synthetic sources.[1]

Taking large amounts of alpha-tocopherol also might decrease gamma-tocopherol activity in the body. To compensate, some experts recommend that vitamin E supplements contain a mixture of natural tocopherols. This form is more expensive, however, than the natural or synthetic alpha-tocopherol alone.

Knowledge Check

1. How does vitamin E function as an antioxidant in the body?
2. What are 3 foods rich in vitamin E?
3. Why is excess supplementation of vitamin E of concern in individuals taking daily aspirin or anticoagulation medications?

12.5 Vitamin K

The discovery of vitamin K centered on its role in blood clotting (Fig. 12-18). A Danish researcher first noted the relationship between vitamin K and blood clotting when he observed that chicks fed a diet with the fat extracted developed hemorrhages. Thus, he named this new lipid-soluble factor "vitamin K" after *koagulation*, the Danish spelling for **coagulation**.

The family of compounds known as vitamin K, or the quinones, include **phylloquinones** (vitamin K_1) from plants and **menaquinones** (vitamin K_2) found in fish oils and meats. Menaquinones also are synthesized by bacteria in the human colon. A synthetic compound, called menadione, can be converted to menaquinone in body tissues. Phylloquinone, the main dietary form of the vitamin, is the most biologically active form.

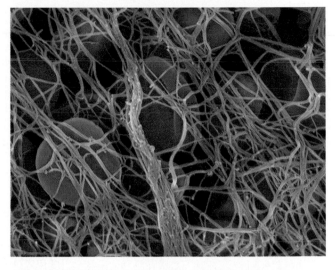

Figure 12-18 Vitamin K is essential for normal blood clotting.

Vitamin K Sources

About 10% of the vitamin K absorbed each day comes from bacterial synthesis in the colon. The remainder comes from dietary sources. Although the vitamin K content of individual foods varies, green leafy vegetables (e.g., kale, turnip greens, parsley, salad greens, cabbage, and spinach), broccoli, peas, and green beans are the best sources (Fig. 12-19). Vegetable oils, such as soy and canola, also are good sources. Vitamin K is relatively stable to heat processing, but it can be destroyed by exposure to light.

coagulation Formation of a blood clot.

Vitamin K Needs

For women, the Adequate Intake for vitamin K is 90 µg/day; for men, it is 120 µg/day. These Adequate Intakes are based on the apparent adequacy of usual intakes and the lack of information to determine an EAR and RDA.[2] Although current intakes provide adequate vitamin K for blood clotting functions, it is not known whether increased intakes might be beneficial for other functions. The Daily Value for vitamin K is 80 µg/day.

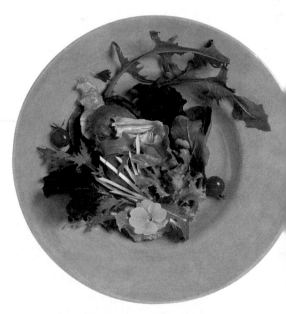

A daily salad containing dark green vegetables provides abundant vitamin K.

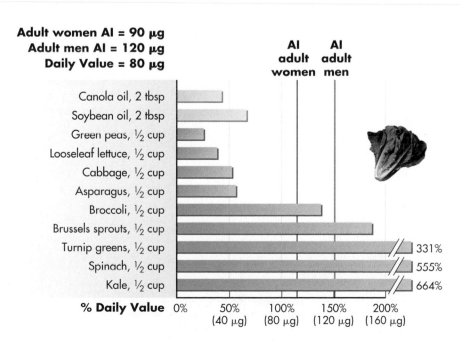

Figure 12-19 Food sources of vitamin K.

Absorption, Transport, Storage, and Excretion of Vitamin K

Approximately 80% of dietary vitamin K as phylloquinone and menaquinone is taken up by the small intestine and incorporated into chylomicrons. This process requires bile and pancreatic enzymes. The menaquinones synthesized by bacteria in the colon also are absorbed, but provide only 10% of the vitamin K we need. Vitamin K can be incorporated into the lipoproteins VLDL and LDL for transport throughout the body or for storage in the liver. Most vitamin K excretion occurs via the bile that passes out of the body in the feces, with a small amount of excretion via the urine.[33]

Functions of Vitamin K

Vitamin K is needed for the synthesis of blood-clotting factors by the liver and the conversion of preprothrombin to the active blood-clotting factor called prothrombin (Fig. 12-20). In these reactions, carbon dioxide (CO_2) is added to a glutamic acid in preprothrombin, yielding prothrombin that contains the Gla amino acid gamma-carboxyglutamic acid. (Proteins that have undergone this conversion are called Gla proteins; Gla stands for gamma-carboxyglutamic acid.) All vitamin K–dependent proteins contain Gla residues, which are needed to bind calcium and form blood clots. The conversion of preprothrombin to prothrombin depends on calcium binding with Gla to participate in the clotting reaction.[33]

In the body, vitamin K is converted to an inactive form once it has activated these clotting factors. It must then be reactivated for its biological action to persist. Drugs such as warfarin (Coumadin®), which strongly inhibit this reactivation process, act as powerful anticoagulants. People taking warfarin to lessen blood clotting should maintain a consistent dietary vitamin K intake and avoid vitamin K supplementation.[33]

Vitamin K also may play a role in bone metabolism. Three additional vitamin K–dependent Gla proteins are known to be synthesized in bone. The functions of these proteins (called osteocalcin, matrix Gla protein, and protein S) are not clearly understood. However, the synthesis of these proteins is reduced in vitamin K deficient animals and results in changes in bone health.[33] Vitamin K also may help protect the body from inflammation, thereby providing protection against cardiovascular disease and osteoporosis.[34]

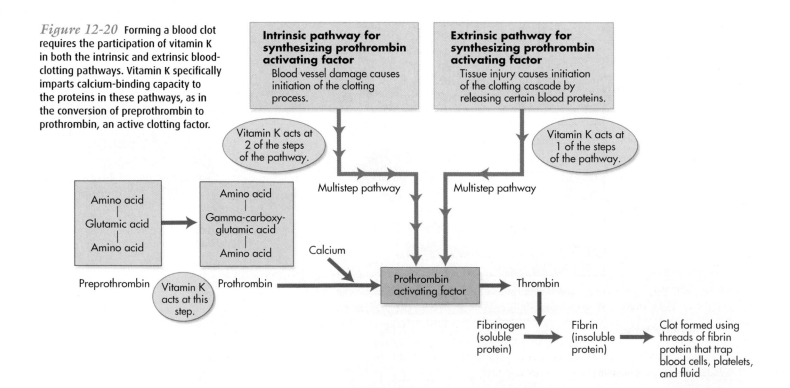

Figure 12-20 Forming a blood clot requires the participation of vitamin K in both the intrinsic and extrinsic blood-clotting pathways. Vitamin K specifically imparts calcium-binding capacity to the proteins in these pathways, as in the conversion of preprothrombin to prothrombin, an active clotting factor.

Intrinsic pathway for synthesizing prothrombin activating factor
Blood vessel damage causes initiation of the clotting process.

Extrinsic pathway for synthesizing prothrombin activating factor
Tissue injury causes initiation of the clotting cascade by releasing certain blood proteins.

Vitamin K acts at 2 of the steps of the pathway.

Vitamin K acts at 1 of the steps of the pathway.

Multistep pathway   Multistep pathway

Amino acid | Glutamic acid | Amino acid

Amino acid | Gamma-carboxy-glutamic acid | Amino acid

Calcium

Preprothrombin   Vitamin K acts at this step.   Prothrombin

Prothrombin activating factor   Thrombin

Fibrinogen (soluble protein)   Fibrin (insoluble protein)   Clot formed using threads of fibrin protein that trap blood cells, platelets, and fluid

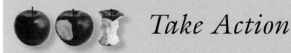 *Take Action*

Does Your Fat-Soluble Vitamin Intake Add Up?

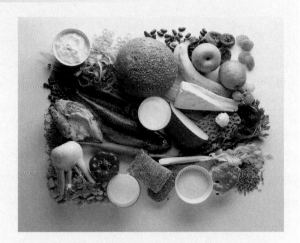

From NHANES and other dietary surveys of the American population, it's known that many individuals do not consume the recommended intakes for all the fat-soluble vitamins. Diets are often low in vitamins D and E and in carotenoid-rich fruits and vegetables. The following questions can help you determine if your dietary intake of these foods and nutrients is adequate.

1. Do you eat at least 1 cup of yellow-orange vegetables or 2 cups of dark, leafy green vegetables each day?

2. Do you consume at least 1 cup of yellow-orange fruit or juice (100% juice) each day?

3. Do you consume 2 to 3 cups of milk or yogurt, or 2 to 3 ounces of cheese, each day?

4. Do you include at least 1 teaspoon of plant oils (cottonseed, canola, sunflower, corn, or olive) in your daily diet?

5. Do you include at least ¼ cup of plant seeds or nuts in your diet each day?

6. Do you eat at least 2 to 3 servings of salmon, tuna, herring, or fish oils each week?

If you answered no to any of these questions, your diet may be lacking in essential fat-soluble vitamins, helpful phytochemicals, and other important nutrients. Review the information on food sources for each of the fat-soluble vitamins in this chapter and the guidelines provided on MyPyramid.gov to help plan a more healthful diet.

Vitamin K Deficiency

A deficiency of vitamin K is rare, but it can occur with prolonged use of antibiotics that disrupt vitamin K synthesis or with impaired fat absorption.[2] Vitamin K deficiency also can occur in newborns. Vitamin K stores are typically low at birth, so infants are at risk of defective blood clotting and hemorrhage. To prevent this possible vitamin K deficiency, newborn infants in North America are given vitamin K injections within 6 hours of delivery.

    Laboratory animal studies have shown that excessive amounts of vitamin A and vitamin E negatively affect the actions of vitamin K.[2, 35] Vitamin A is thought to interfere with the absorption of vitamin K from the intestine, whereas large doses of vitamin E can lead to a decrease in vitamin K–dependent clotting factors and increased bleeding tendency. In either case, megadose supplements of these vitamins increase the risk of vitamin K deficiency and bleeding, as noted in earlier discussions of the Upper Levels of these vitamins. Because of the risk of hemorrhaging in vitamin K-deficient individuals, physicians check a patient's vitamin K status prior to surgery.

▶ One means of detecting a vitamin K deficiency is an increase in blood-clotting time, a measure of how quickly prothrombin in the blood can form a clot.

Vitamin K Toxicity

To date, no Upper Level has been set for vitamin K.[2] Although vitamin K can be stored in the liver and bone, it is more readily excreted than other fat-soluble vitamins. When used in its natural forms of phylloquinones or menaquinones, increased amounts of vitamin K have not caused harmful effects. In contrast, high amounts of menadione, a synthetic form of vitamin K, have resulted in hemolytic anemia, excess **bilirubin** in the blood, and death in newborns.

    As you can see, the fat-soluble vitamins have numerous important functions in the body. Table 12-2 provides a summary of these vitamins.

bilirubin Bile pigment; excess in the blood causes skin and eyes to become yellow (jaundice).

Table 12-2 Summary of the Fat-Soluble Vitamins

Major Vitamin	Functions	Deficiency Symptoms	People at Risk	Sources	RDA or Adequate Intake	Toxicity Symptoms
Vitamin A						
Preformed retinoids and provitamin A carotenoids	Vision in dim light and color vision, cell differentiation, bone growth, immunity, reproduction	Poor growth, night blindness, total blindness, dry skin, xerophthalmia, hyperkeratosis, impaired immune function	Rare in U.S. but common in preschool children living in poverty in developing countries and patients with fat malabsorption syndromes	Preformed vitamin A (retinoids): liver, fortified milk, fish liver oils; Provitamin A (carotenoids): red, orange, dark green, and yellow vegetables; orange fruits	700 µg (RAE) for women and 900 µg for men	Headache, vomiting, double vision, dry mucous membranes, bone and joint pain, liver damage, hemorrhage, coma, spontaneous abortions, birth defects. Upper Level is 3000 µg of preformed vitamin A.
Vitamin D						
Cholecalciferol D$_3$ Ergocalciferol D$_2$	Maintenance of calcium and phosphorus concentrations, immune function, cell cycle regulation	Rickets in children, osteomalacia in older adults	Dark-skinned individuals, older adults with low intakes or low UV exposure, patients with fat malabsorption syndromes	Vitamin D–fortified milk, fish oils, oily fish	5–10 µg 15 µg > 70 yrs 5 µg for 19–50 yrs. 10 µg for 51–70 yrs 15 µg for > 70 yrs	Calcification of soft tissues, impaired growth, excess calcium in the blood and excretion in the urine; Upper Level is 50 µg
Vitamin E						
Tocopherols Tocotrienols	Antioxidant, prevention of free radicals damage	Hemolysis of red blood cells, degeneration of sensory neurons	Patients with fat malabsorption syndromes	Plant oils, seeds, nuts, products made from oils	15 mg alpha-tocopherol for men and women	Inhibition of vitamin K metabolism; Upper Level is 1000 mg
Vitamin K						
Phylloquinone Menaquinone	Synthesis of blood-clotting factors and bone proteins	Hemorrhage due to poor blood clotting	Those taking antibiotics for a long period of time, adults with low green vegetable intake, patients with fat malabsorption syndromes	Green vegetables, synthesis by intestinal microorganisms	90 µg for women, 120 µg for men	Rare, can cause hemolytic anemia; no Upper Level has been set

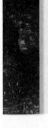

Knowledge Check

1. What are 3 foods that are rich sources of vitamin K?
2. How does vitamin K help in the formation of blood clots?
3. Why should people on the drug Coumadin® avoid taking vitamin K supplements?
4. What population groups are at increased risk of a vitamin K deficiency?

12.6 Dietary Supplements: Healthful or Harmful?

About 40% of adults in the U.S. take vitamin and/or mineral supplements on a regular basis, spending over $23 billion annually—a practice that is hotly debated.[3, 36] Opinions differ within the scientific and medical communities as to whether supplements should be widely prescribed. Some scientists and clinicians suggest that, because most Americans fail to meet dietary guidelines for the intake of fruits, vegetables, and whole grains, they may have inadequate intakes of several micronutrients. Although current evidence is insufficient to support the recommendation of multivitamin and mineral supplementation for the general population,[36] many people take supplements to reduce their susceptibility to disease, to compensate for dietary insufficiencies, to protect against age-related changes, and/or to enhance their overall well-being.

According to the Dietary Supplement Health and Education Act (DSHEA) of 1994, a supplement is defined as any product intended to supplement the diet that contains 1 or more of the following ingredients:

- A vitamin
- A mineral
- An amino acid
- An herb, a botanical, or a plant extract
- A combination of any of the above

Recall from Chapter 1 that dietary supplements are regulated differently than drugs and food additives, which the FDA tests extensively and regulates for safety, effectiveness, dose size, concerns about interactions with other substances, and health-related claims. In contrast, the FDA does not closely monitor dietary supplements, except folic acid, unless there is evidence that a supplement is dangerous or is marketed with an illegal claim. Thus, individuals need to seek advice from their physician, dietitian, or pharmacist to understand the potential health benefits and risks related to the use of dietary supplements.

Due to the limited regulation of dietary supplements, some supplement manufacturers make broad claims about the benefits of their products. Without scientific evidence, they cannot claim that their products will prevent, treat, or cure diseases. However, current laws allow them to make structure or function claims and do not prevent them from making unproved claims with regard to conditions that are not diseases. Thus, many manufacturers market their products as a means to increase energy, enhance performance, lose weight, reduce body fat, eliminate signs of aging, and relieve symptoms of menopause, fatigue, and stress. For example, a product that claims to treat menopause-related hot flashes, increase energy, enhance mood, or promote bowel health can be sold without any evidence that the product effectively does so because these conditions are not diseases. However, a product that claims to decrease the risk of cardiovascular disease by reducing blood cholesterol levels must have scientific evidence to justify this claim.

The quality, purity, and consistency of dietary supplement products also are not closely monitored by the FDA. Not surprisingly, studies of dietary supplements indicate that product quality can vary significantly. To aid consumers in purchasing supplements meeting acceptable standards, the United States Pharmacopeia (USP) designation may be listed on products that meet established USP standards for strength, quality, purity, packaging, labeling, solubility, and storage life. However, because the USP labeling of dietary supplements is voluntary, many manufacturers still use their own standards for manufacturing and quality control.

Although dietary supplements can replace specific nutrients lacking in a diet, they cannot fully correct a nutritionally poor diet. For example, most supplements do not contain fiber or phytochemicals that have health-promoting benefits. Others contain limited amounts of calcium needed for bone health and cellular functions. Supplements also

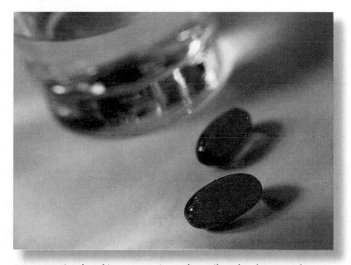

Long-term intake of just 3 to 5 times the Daily Value for some fat-soluble vitamins—particularly preformed vitamin A (retinoids)—can cause toxic effects.

Figure 12-21 Supplement savvy—a MyPyramid approach to the use of nutrient supplementation. Emphasizing the bottom portion of the pyramid is the best option. Extra benefits include fiber, numerous phytochemicals, and omega-3 fatty acids.

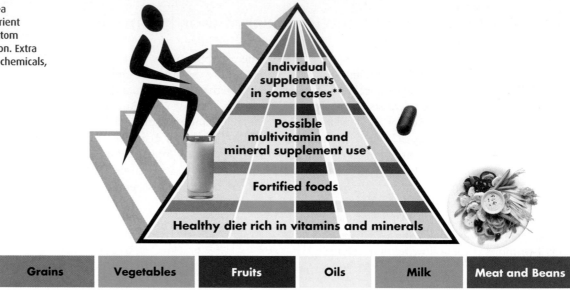

Individual supplements in some cases**

Possible multivitamin and mineral supplement use*

Fortified foods

Healthy diet rich in vitamins and minerals

| Grains | Vegetables | Fruits | Oils | Milk | Meat and Beans |

* Men and older women generally should use iron-free formulations.
** Iron and calcium supplements for younger women are examples.

may contain excess amounts of individual nutrients that can increase the risk of vitamin and mineral toxicities and nutrient interactions. For instance, a supplement with a high amount of zinc can interfere with the absorption and utilization of iron or copper; high intakes of folate can mask the symptoms of a vitamin B-12 deficiency; and excessive intakes of vitamins A and D can result in toxicity. Thus, nutrition experts suggest that the best way to meet nutritional needs is to eat a diet that includes a variety of nutrient-rich fruits, vegetables, and whole grains, with less dairy products, fish, meat and meat alternatives, nuts, and seeds. As depicted in Figure 12-21, you can use a MyPyramid approach to plan a healthful diet.

Although vitamin and mineral requirements can be met by eating a nutritionally varied diet, there may be times when the use of vitamin and/or mineral supplements is necessary:

- Women with excessive bleeding during menstruation may need iron supplements to prevent anemia.
- Women who are pregnant or breastfeeding may require iron and folate supplements to meet their needs.
- Individuals with low calorie intakes may require a multivitamin and mineral supplement to correct for limited intakes.
- Vegans may require calcium, iron, zinc, and vitamin B-12 supplements to prevent deficiencies.
- Newborn infants may need a single dose of vitamin K (as directed by a physician) to prevent bleeding problems.
- Infants and young children may need fluoride supplements to prevent dental caries.
- Individuals with limited sunlight exposure and a low intake of dairy products may need vitamin D supplements.
- Individuals with lactose intolerance or milk allergies may need calcium and vitamin D supplements.
- Individuals with specific medical conditions or those using medications that alter nutrient metabolism or nutritional status may require specific vitamin/mineral supplements.

Dietitians can assess the need for supplements in healthy people and those with disease or health risks. They also can provide guidance for choosing foods rich in specific nutrients, as well as an appropriate supplement, if one is needed. Dietitians often suggest that you start by choosing a nationally recognized brand that contains no more than

▶ These websites can help you evaluate the safety and claims of various supplements.

www.acsh.org

www.quackwatch.com

www.ncahf.org

www.eatright.org

www.dietary-supplements.info.nih.gov

www.consumerlab.com

www.complementarynutrition.org

100% of the Daily Value for the nutrients listed. Be careful that the total intake from your diet, including foods fortified with vitamins and minerals, plus your supplement does not exceed the Upper Level for any vitamin or mineral. When choosing a supplement, check for superfluous ingredients, such as bee pollen, lecithin, hesperidin complex, inositol, laetrile ("vitamin B-17"), pangamic acid, or para-aminobenzoic acid (PABA), that are not needed in our diets and often add significant expense to supplements.

CASE STUDY FOLLOW-UP

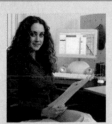

The use of Nutramega poses some health risks for Kristen. Taking 2 or 3 tablets every 3 hours would mean taking at least 16 tablets per day. This alone would provide an intake of vitamin A, vitamin C, and zinc well in excess of the Upper Levels for these nutrients. Her intake of preformed vitamin A would be 1.3 times the Upper Level; of vitamin C, 3.4 times the Upper Level; and of zinc, 3 times the Upper Level. Her intake of selenium, however, would fall well below the Upper Level set for that nutrient. This is how the math works out:

Vitamin A: 33% (0.33) times the Daily Value of 1000 µg RAE equals 330 µg RAE per tablet. Sixteen tablets yield 5280 µg RAE. The Upper Level is 3000 µg RAE for preformed vitamin A. Because 75% of the vitamin A is preformed vitamin A, this yields 3960 µg RAE of preformed vitamin A (5280 × 0.75 = 3960), or 1.3 times the Upper Level (3960 / 3000 = 1.3).

Vitamin C: 700% (7) times the Daily Value of 60 mg equals 420 mg per tablet. Sixteen tablets yield 6720 mg. The Upper Level is 2000 mg. This amount is 3.4 times the Upper Level (6720 / 2000 = 3.4).

Zinc: 50% (0.5) times the Daily Value of 15 mg equals 7.5 mg per tablet. Sixteen tablets yield 120 mg. The Upper Level is 40 mg. This amount is 3 times the Upper Level (120 / 40 = 3).

Selenium: 10% (0.1) times the Daily Value of 70 µg equals 7 µg per tablet. Sixteen tablets yield 112 µg. This is less than the Upper Level of 400 µg.

If Kristen takes the maintenance dose of 2 or 3 tablets per day, she will not be at risk of toxicities. However, Nutramega is very expensive, compared with the cost of a typical multivitamin and mineral supplement. Overall, Kristen is smart to be concerned about meeting her nutrient needs, but the stress she is under does not increase nutrient needs. A healthy diet, as shown in Table 2-10 in Chapter 2, should be her primary strategy to manage her stress and stay healthy.

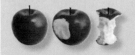 *Take Action*

A Closer Look at Supplements

With the current popularity of vitamin and mineral supplements, it is more important than ever to understand how to evaluate a supplement. Study the label of a supplement you use or one readily available from a friend or the supermarket. Then answer the following questions.

1. Based on the recommended dosage, are there any individual vitamins or minerals for which the intake is greater than 100% of the Daily Value? List these vitamins and minerals.

2. How do the suggested intakes of the vitamins and minerals in the supplement compare with the current DRIs for these nutrients?

3. Are any suggested intakes above the Upper Levels for the nutrients? List these nutrients and the Upper Level for each.

4. Are there any non-nutrient ingredients, such as herbs or botanical extracts, in the supplement? You often can find these by looking for ingredients that do not have a % of Daily Value.

5. Does at least 25 to 50% of the vitamin A in the product come from beta-carotene or other provitamin A carotenoids (to reduce the risk of vitamin A toxicity)?

6. Are there any warnings on the label for individuals who should not consume this product?

7. Are there any other signs that tip you off that this product may be more harmful than healthful?

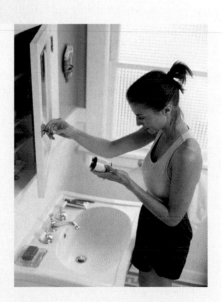

Summary

12.1 Vitamins are essential, organic compounds needed for important metabolic reactions in the body. They are not a source of energy. Instead, they promote many energy-yielding and other reactions in the body, thereby aiding in the growth, development, and maintenance of various body tissues. Vitamins cannot be synthesized in the body at all or are synthesized in insufficient amounts. Vitamins A, D, E, and K are fat soluble, whereas the B-vitamins and vitamin C are water soluble. Fat-soluble vitamins are absorbed along with dietary fat. They travel by way of the lymphatic system into general circulation, carried by chylomicrons. In disease states that limit fat digestion, fat-soluble vitamin absorption may be compromised, thereby increasing the risk of deficiency in these individuals. Fat-soluble vitamins are excreted less readily from the body than water-soluble vitamins and thus pose a potential threat for toxicity, especially of vitamins A and D. Toxicities of these fat-soluble vitamins generally occur with high doses of supplements, rather than from foods.

12.2 Vitamin A consists of a family of retinoid compounds: retinal, retinol, and retinoic acid. A plant derivative, known as beta-carotene, along with 2 other carotenoids, yields vitamin A after metabolism by the small intestine or liver. Vitamin A is found in foods of animal origin, such as liver, fish oils, and fortified milk. Carotenoids are obtained from plants and are especially plentiful in dark green and yellow-orange vegetables and fruits. Vitamin A contributes to the maintenance of vision, the normal development of cells (especially mucous-forming cells), and immune function. Preformed vitamin A can be quite toxic when taken at doses 2 to 4 times or more the RDA. Use of vitamin A supplements is especially dangerous during pregnancy because it can lead to fetal malformations.

12.3 Vitamin D can be obtained from food and it is produced by the body. The synthesis of vitamin D_3 begins with a precursor of cholesterol synthesis located in the skin and depends on ultraviolet light. With adequate sun exposure, no dietary intake of vitamin D is needed. Vitamin D food sources include fish oils and fortified milk. The provitamin, whether produced in the skin or obtained from the diet, is metabolized in the liver and kidneys to yield $1,25(OH)_2$ vitamin D_3 (or calcitriol), the active form of vitamin D.

Calcitriol is important for calcium and phosphorus absorption from the intestine and, along with other hormones, for the regulation of bone metabolism. It also is important in gene expression and immune function. Risk of vitamin D deficiency may be greater than previously observed, especially in the elderly and individuals lacking regular sunlight exposure. Vitamin D deficiency results in harmful changes in bone, a condition known as rickets in children and osteomalacia in adults. Toxicity of vitamin D can occur with excess supplementation of vitamin D, causing the deposition of calcium in the kidneys, heart, and lungs.

12.4 Vitamin E functions as an antioxidant. By donating electrons to electron-seeking or oxidizing compounds (e.g., free radicals), it neutralizes their action and prevents the widespread destruction of both cell membranes and DNA. Vitamin E is 1 of several components in the body's defense system against oxidizing agents. Vitamin E is plentiful in plant oils and food products that contain these oils. Overt vitamin E deficiency is rare. Toxicity from megadose therapy inhibits vitamin K activity and, in turn, increases the risk of hemorrhage.

12.5 Vitamin K contributes to the body's blood-clotting ability by facilitating the conversion of precursor proteins, such as prothrombin, to active clotting factors that promote blood coagulation. Vitamin K also plays a role in bone metabolism. About 10% of the vitamin K absorbed each day comes from bacterial synthesis in the intestine. Most vitamin K comes primarily from green leafy vegetables and vegetable oils in the diet. Vitamin K deficiency is rare, but it can occur in newborns. Thus, newborn infants are given vitamin K injections shortly after birth as a preventive measure.

12.6 Taking a multivitamin and mineral supplement to help meet nutrient needs is recommended by some experts, but others suggest that only some people need them. Taking many nutrient supplements can lead to nutrient-related toxicity, so their use should be considered carefully. The clearest evidence for good nutrition supports a diet rich in fruits and vegetables and whole-grain breads and cereals, rather than relying on supplements to meet nutritional needs.

Study Questions

1. Which population group is at lowest risk for fat-soluble vitamin deficiencies?

   a. low-birth-weight, premature infants
   b. very-low-income families
   c. patients with malabsorption diseases
   d. pregnant women

2. Carotenoids are a precursor form of _____.

   a. vitamin K
   b. vitamin E
   c. vitamin D
   d. vitamin A

3. Which food provides very little vitamin A?

   a. mango
   b. spinach
   c. banana
   d. liver

4. Vitamin A is involved in all of the following functions *except* _____.

   a. vision and dark adaptation
   b. hemoglobin synthesis
   c. resistance to infection
   d. cell differentiation

5. Vitamin A deficiency is associated with the symptoms of night blindness, keratinization, and increased infections.

   a. true
   b. false

6. Which of the following vitamins also can be classified as a hormone because the body can synthesize it?

   a. vitamin A
   b. vitamin D
   c. vitamin E
   d. vitamin K

7. Which of the following is a good source of vitamin D?

   a. yellow-orange vegetables
   b. salmon and sardines
   c. dark, leafy greens
   d. enriched grains

8. Which of the following is a function of vitamin D?

   a. serves as an antioxidant to protect against lipid peroxidation
   b. serves as a coenzyme in energy metabolism
   c. regulates calcium homeostasis
   d. produces blood-clotting factors

9. Vitamin D deficiency has been associated with an increased risk of diabetes, multiple sclerosis, and hypertension.

   a. true
   b. false

10. Vitamin D deficiency in children results in a condition called _____.

    a. osteomalacia
    b. beriberi
    c. rickets
    d. xerophthalmia

11. Wheat germ and vegetable oils are good sources of vitamin E.

    a. true
    b. false

12. Large doses of vitamin E have been shown to interfere with vitamin K activity and to increase the risk of bleeding.

    a. true
    b. false

13. Which of the following is the best source of vitamin K?

    a. citrus fruits
    b. dark, leafy greens
    c. enriched grains
    d. nuts and seeds

14. Which vitamin aids in blood clotting?

    a. vitamin A
    b. vitamin D
    c. vitamin E
    d. vitamin K

15. Vitamin and mineral supplements are tightly regulated by the FDA.

    a. true
    b. false

Answer Key: 1-d; 2-d; 3-c; 4-b; 5-a; 6-b; 7-b; 8-c; 9-a; 10-c; 11-a; 12-a; 13-b; 14-d; 15-b

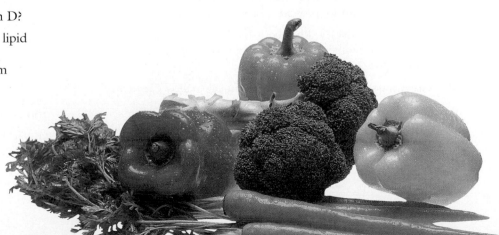

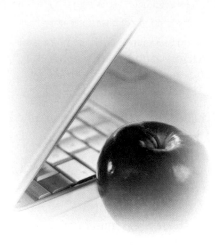

Websites

To learn more about the topics covered in this chapter, visit these websites.

Supplement Claims

www.acsh.org

www.quackwatch.com

www.ncahf.org

www.eatright.org

www.dietary-supplements.info.nih.gov

www.consumerlab.com

www.complementarynutrition.org

Micronutrient Initiative

www.micronutrient.org/home.asp

References

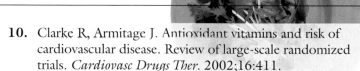

1. Food and Nutrition Board, Institute of Medicine. *Dietary Reference Intakes for vitamin C, vitamin E, selenium, and carotenoids*. Washington, DC: National Academy Press; 2000.

2. Food and Nutrition Board, Institute of Medicine. *Dietary Reference Intakes for vitamin A, vitamin K, arsenic, boron, chromium, copper, iodine, iron, manganese, molybdenum, nickel, silicon, vanadium, and zinc*. Washington, DC: National Academy Press; 2001.

3. Food and Nutrition Board, Institute of Medicine. *Dietary Reference Intakes for calcium, phosphorus, magnesium, vitamin D, and fluoride*. Washington, DC: National Academy Press; 1997.

4. Ross AC. Vitamin A and carotenoids. In: Shils ME and others, eds. *Modern nutrition in health and disease*. 10th ed. Philadelphia: Lippincott Williams & Wilkins; 2006.

5. Hak AE and others. Prospective study of plasma carotenoids and tocopherols in relation to risk of ischemic stroke. *Stroke*. 2004;35:1584.

6. Kristal AR. Vitamin A, retinoids and carotenoids as chemo-preventive agents for prostate cancer. *J Urol*. 2004;171:S54.

7. Ribaya-Mercado JD, Blumberg JB. Lutein and zeaxanthin and their potential roles in disease prevention. *J Am Coll Nutr*. 2004;23:567S.

8. Greenwald P. Cancer prevention clinical trials. *J Clin Oncol*. 2002;20:14S.

9. Kirsh VA and others. A prospective study of lycopene and tomato product intake and risk of prostate cancer. *Cancer Epidemiol Biomarkers Prev*. 2006;15:92.

10. Clarke R, Armitage J. Antioxidant vitamins and risk of cardiovascular disease. Review of large-scale randomized trials. *Cardiovasc Drugs Ther*. 2002;16:411.

11. The Micronutrient Initiative. www.micronutrient.org/home.asp.

12. Roos N and others. The role of fish in food-based strategies to combat vitamin A and mineral deficiencies in developing countries. *J Nutr*. 2007;137:1106.

13. Penniston KL, Tanumihardjo SA. The acute and chronic toxic effects of vitamin A. *Am J Clin Nutr*. 2006;83:191.

14. Rajakumar K and others. Solar ultraviolet radiation and vitamin D: A historical perspective. *Am J Pub Health*. 2006;97:1746.

15. Bischoff-Ferrari H and others. Fracture prevention with vitamin D supplementation. *JAMA*. 2005;293:2257.

16. Bischoff-Ferrari H and others. Estimation of optimal serum concentrations of 25-hydroxyvitamin D for multiple health outcomes. *Am J Clin Nutr*. 2006;84:18.

17. Dawson-Hughes B. Racial/ethnic considerations in making recommendations for vitamin D for adult and elderly men and women. *Am J Clin Nutr*. 2004;80:1763S.

18. Heaney R. Bone health. *Am J Clin Nutr*. 2007;85:3005S.

19. DeLuca H. Overview of general physiologic features and functions of Vitamin D. *Am J Clin Nutr*. 2004;80:1689S.

20. Holick MF. Vitamin D deficiency. *N Engl J Med*. 2007;357:266.

21. Mark BL, Carson JAS. Vitamin D and autoimmune disease—Implications for practice from the multiple sclerosis literature. *J Am Diet Assoc*. 2006;106:418.

22. Lappe JM and others. Vitamin D and calcium supplementation reduces cancer risk: Results of a randomized trial. *Am J Clin Nutr*. 2007;85:1586.

23. Hatun S and others. Subclinical vitamin D deficiency is increased in adolescent girls who wear concealing clothing. *J Nutr*. 2005;135:218.

24. Hypponen E, Power C. Hypovitaminosis D in British adults at age 45y: Nationwide cohort study of dietary and lifestyle predictors. *Am J Clin Nutr*. 2007;85:860.

25. Maras J and others. Intake of α-tocopherol is limited among U.S. adults. *J Am Diet Assoc*. 2004;104:567.

26. Talegawkar SA and others. Total alpha-tocopherol intakes are associated with serum alpha-tocopherol concentrations in African American adults. *J Nutr*. 2007;137:2297.

27. Traber MG. Vitamin E. In: Shils ME and others, eds. *Modern nutrition in health and disease*. 10th ed. Philadelphia: Lippincott Williams & Wilkins; 2006.

28. Meydani SN and others. Vitamin E and immune response in the aged: Molecular mechanisms and clinical implications. *Immunol Rev*. 2005;205:269.

29. Morris MC and others. Relation of the tocopherol forms to incident Alzheimer disease and to cognitive change. *Am J Clin Nutr*. 2005;81:508.

30. Murtaugh MA and others. Antioxidants, carotenoids and risk of rectal cancer. *Am J Epidemiol*. 2004;158:32.

31. Traber MG. Heart disease and single vitamin supplementation. *Am J Clin Nutr*. 2007;85:293S.

32. Bruno RS, Traber MG. Cigarette smoke alters human vitamin E requirements. *J Nutr*. 2005;135:671.

33. Suttie JW. Vitamin K. In: Shils ME and others, eds. *Modern nutrition in health and disease*. 10th ed. Philadelphia: Lippincott Williams & Wilkins; 2006.

34. Shea MK and others. Vitamin K and vitamin D status: Associations with inflammatory markers in the Framingham Offspring Study. *Am J Epidemio*. 2008;167:313.

35. Booth S and others. Effect of vitamin E supplementation on vitamin K status in adults with normal coagulation status. *Am J Clin Nutr*. 2004;80:143.

36. NIH State-of-the Science Panel. National Institutes of Health State-of-the-Science Conference statement: Multivitamin/mineral supplements and chronic disease prevention. *Am J Clin Nutr*. 2007;85:275S.

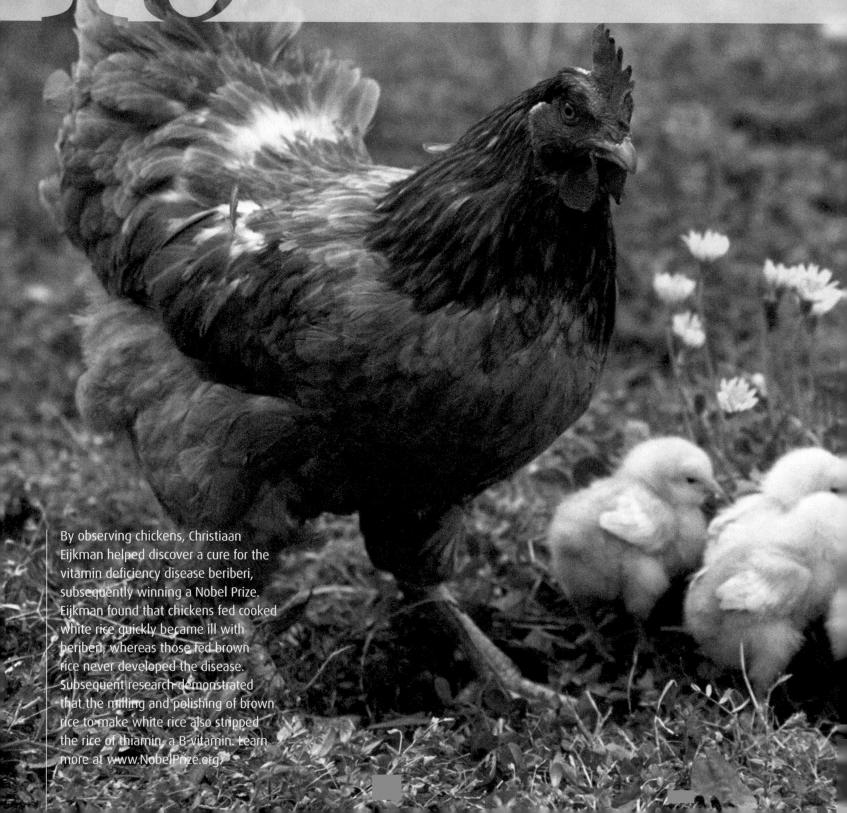

13 the Water-Soluble Vitamins

By observing chickens, Christiaan Eijkman helped discover a cure for the vitamin deficiency disease beriberi, subsequently winning a Nobel Prize. Eijkman found that chickens fed cooked white rice quickly became ill with beriberi, whereas those fed brown rice never developed the disease. Subsequent research demonstrated that the milling and polishing of brown rice to make white rice also stripped the rice of thiamin, a B-vitamin. Learn more at www.NobelPrize.org.

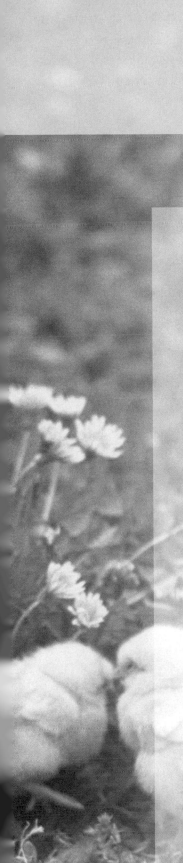

STUDENT LEARNING OUTCOMES

After studying this chapter, you will be able to:

1. Identify the water-soluble vitamins.

2. List important food sources for each water-soluble vitamin.

3. Describe how each water-soluble vitamin is absorbed, transported, stored, and excreted.

4. List the major functions of and deficiency symptoms for each water-soluble vitamin.

5. Describe the toxicity symptoms from the excess consumption of certain water-soluble vitamins.

6. Distinguish between vitamins and non-vitamins, such as carnitine and taurine.

For centuries, scurvy, pellagra, and other vitamin deficiency diseases caused enormous suffering and death. It wasn't until early in the 20th century that scientists discovered that these illnesses are caused by the absence of certain vital substances from the diet—now called vitamins.[1] Researchers discovered that restoring vitamins to the diet dramatically reversed deficiency diseases if they were supplied before significant deterioration of the body took place.

Today, vitamin deficiency diseases are rare in North America, although those with poor diets or intestinal malabsorption conditions, smokers, alcohol abusers, and the elderly may be at risk. Our typical diets contain ample and varied natural sources of vitamins, as well as many foods enriched or fortified with vitamins. In some developing countries, however, the availability of several vitamins is limited, causing vitamin deficiency diseases to be significant public health problems.

Recall from Chapter 12 that as vitamins were discovered, they were named after letters of the alphabet. The second vitamin to be discovered was water-soluble and designated "vitamin B." Although this water-soluble substance was initially thought to be a single chemical compound, subsequent research showed that "vitamin B" actually is several compounds. Numbers were added to the letter *B* to distinguish these compounds. Of the 8 B-vitamins, only 2 are still commonly referred to by letter and number: vitamin B-6 and vitamin B-12. The others now are usually referred to by the following names: thiamin (previously B-1), riboflavin (previously B-2), niacin (previously B-3), pantothenic acid, biotin, and folate. The older designations, however, are sometimes used on vitamin supplement labels. Vitamin C also is a water-soluble vitamin.

As you'll see in this chapter, the water-soluble vitamins, like the fat-soluble vitamins, work together to maintain health. The water-soluble vitamins discussed in this chapter include 8 B-vitamins, vitamin C, and a newcomer to the list of important nutrients: choline. This chapter also will briefly describe some vitamin-like compounds that may be needed in the diet under atypical circumstances. These compounds, however, currently are not classified as true vitamins because a healthy person does not require a dietary source of them and because no specific deficiency disease results when they are absent from the diet.

13.1 Water-Soluble Vitamin Overview

Like fat-soluble vitamins, water-soluble vitamins are essential organic substances needed in small amounts for the normal function, growth, and maintenance of body tissues (Fig. 13-1). For example, thiamin, riboflavin, niacin, pantothenic acid, and biotin are especially important for energy metabolism. Vitamin B-6, folate, and vitamin B-12 are important for amino acid metabolism and red blood cell synthesis.[2] Vitamin C participates in the synthesis of numerous compounds, including collagen.[3] In contrast to the fat-soluble vitamins, only small amounts of water-soluble vitamins are stored in the body. The risk of water-soluble-vitamin toxicity tends to be low because, unlike fat-soluble vitamins, water-soluble vitamins are readily removed by the kidneys and

Figure 13-1 **Vitamins and related compounds (e.g., choline) work together to maintain health.**

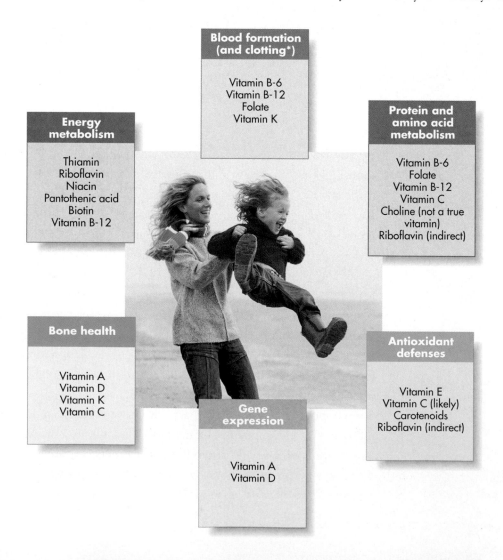

Blood formation (and clotting*)

Vitamin B-6
Vitamin B-12
Folate
Vitamin K

Energy metabolism

Thiamin
Riboflavin
Niacin
Pantothenic acid
Biotin
Vitamin B-12

Protein and amino acid metabolism

Vitamin B-6
Folate
Vitamin B-12
Vitamin C
Choline (not a true vitamin)
Riboflavin (indirect)

Bone health

Vitamin A
Vitamin D
Vitamin K
Vitamin C

Gene expression

Vitamin A
Vitamin D

Antioxidant defenses

Vitamin E
Vitamin C (likely)
Carotenoids
Riboflavin (indirect)

Table 13-1 Tips for Preserving Vitamins in Fruits and Vegetables

Preservation Methods	Why?
Keep fruits and vegetables cool until eaten.	Enzymes in fruits and vegetables begin to degrade vitamins once they are harvested. Chilling limits this process.
Refrigerate fruits and vegetables (except bananas, onions, potatoes, and tomatoes) in moisture-proof, airtight containers or in the vegetable drawer.	Nutrients keep best at temperatures near freezing, at high humidity, and away from air.
Trim, peel, and cut fruits and vegetables minimally—just enough to remove inedible parts.	Oxygen breaks down vitamins faster when more of the food surface is exposed. Whenever possible, cook fruits and vegetables in their skins.
Microwave, steam, or stir-fry vegetables.	More nutrients are retained when there is less contact with water and a shorter cooking time.
Minimize cooking time.	Prolonged cooking (slow simmering) and reheating reduce vitamin content.
Avoid adding fats to vegetables during cooking if you plan to discard the liquid.	Fat-soluble vitamins will be lost in discarded fat. If you want to add fats, do so after vegetables are fully cooked and drained.
Do not add baking soda to vegetables to enhance the green color.	Alkalinity destroys vitamin D, thiamin, and other vitamins.
Store canned and frozen fruits and vegetables carefully.	To protect canned foods, store them in a cool, dry location. To protect frozen foods, store them at 0°F (-32°C) or colder. Eat within 12 months.

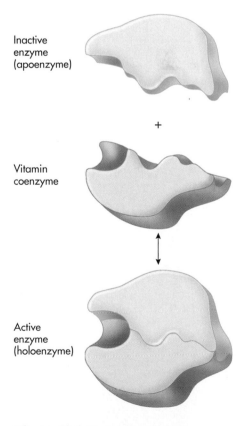

Inactive enzyme (apoenzyme)

+

Vitamin coenzyme

Active enzyme (holoenzyme)

Figure 13-2 **The enzyme-coenzyme interaction. The B-vitamins form coenzymes, which are compounds that enable specific enzymes to function.**

excreted in the urine. In fact, Tolerable Upper Intake Levels have been set for only 4 of the water-soluble vitamins and choline.

Compared with fat-soluble vitamins, water-soluble vitamins are more easily destroyed during cooking. A food's vitamin content can be decreased by exposure to heat, light, air, and alkaline substances. Water-soluble vitamins can leach into cooking water, whereas fat-soluble vitamins can leach into cooking fats and oils. Retention of the B-vitamins and vitamin C is greatest in foods that are prepared by steaming, stir-frying, and microwaving. These cooking methods limit exposure to heat and water. Fruits and vegetables are especially important sources of many vitamins; Table 13-1 lists tips for preserving their vitamin content.

Coenzymes: A Common Role of B-Vitamins

All B-vitamins form **coenzymes,** which are small, organic molecules that are a type of cofactor. Metals (e.g., zinc or magnesium) are another type of cofactor. **Cofactors** combine with inactive enzymes (called apoenzymes) to form active enzymes (called holoenzymes) that are able to catalyze specific reactions (Fig. 13-2). Table 13-2 lists examples of coenzymes formed from B-vitamins.

All 8 B-vitamins participate in energy metabolism; some also have other roles within cells. Figure 13-3 shows where the B-vitamin coenzymes function in energy metabolism. Because of the role of B-vitamins in energy metabolism, the need for many of them increases somewhat with higher amounts of physical activity. Still, this is not a major concern because the higher food intake that usually accompanies an increase in energy expenditure contributes more B-vitamins to the diet.

Table 13-2 B-Vitamins and Coenzyme Examples

B-Vitamin	Coenzyme Example*	Abbreviation
Thiamin	Thiamin pyrophosphate	TPP
Riboflavin	Flavin adenine dinucleotide	FAD
	Flavin mononucleotide	FMN
Niacin	Nicotinamide adenine dinucleotide	NAD
	Nicotinamide adenine dinucleotide phosphate	NADP
Pantothenic acid	Coenzyme A	CoA
Biotin	N-carboxylbiotinyl lysine	
Vitamin B-6	Pyridoxal phosphate	PLP
Folic acid	Tetrahydrofolic acid	THFA
Vitamin B-12	Methylcobalamin	

*Some B-vitamins form more than 1 coenzyme.

In foods, B-vitamins are present as vitamins or as coenzymes, both of which are sometimes bound to protein. Digestion frees B-vitamins from coenzymes or protein. Unbound (free) vitamins are the main form absorbed in the small intestine. Typically, about 50 to 90% of the B-vitamins in the diet are absorbed.[2] Once inside cells, the coenzyme forms of the vitamins are resynthesized. Vitamin supplements sold in the coenzyme form have no specific benefits to consumers because vitamins must be released from the coenzyme before they can be absorbed.

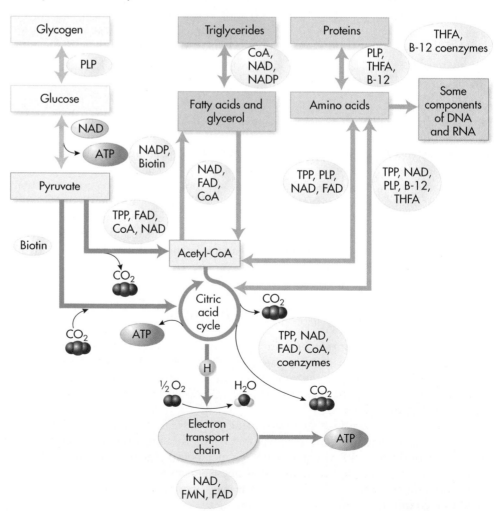

Figure 13-3 Many metabolic pathways, including those involved in energy metabolism, use coenzyme forms of the B-vitamins.

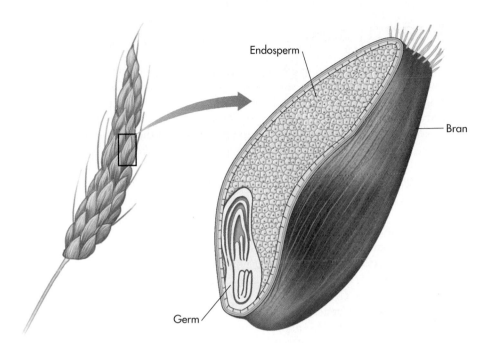

Figure 13-4 When grains are milled, the bran and germ are removed and discarded, leaving only the starch-rich endosperm.

Grains: One Important Source of B-Vitamins

Grains are an important source of many B-vitamins. However, when grains are milled, the seeds are crushed and the germ, bran, and husk layers are removed. This refining process leaves just the starch-containing endosperm, which is the only portion of the grain used to make white flour, as well as many bread and cereal products (Fig. 13-4). Because the discarded parts are rich in nutrients, milling leads to a loss of vitamins and minerals.

To counteract this nutrient loss, in the U.S., nearly all bread and cereal products made from milled grains are enriched with 4 B-vitamins—thiamin, riboflavin, niacin, and folic acid—and with the mineral iron. This enrichment program, begun in the 1940s, has helped protect Americans from the common deficiency diseases associated with a dietary lack of these nutrients. This practice, however, still leaves the products with less vitamin B-6, potassium, magnesium, zinc, fiber, and phytochemicals than in whole-grain products because whole grains contain the germ and the bran, as well as the endosperm (Fig. 13-5). Nutrition experts therefore recommend that whole-grain products, such as brown rice, oatmeal, and whole-wheat bread and pasta, be consumed daily.

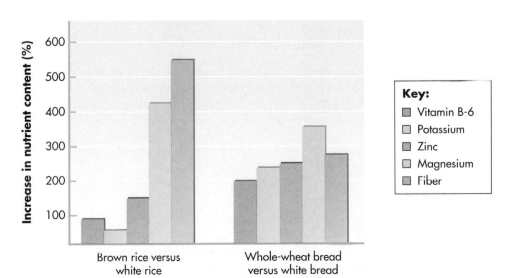

Figure 13-5 When compared with white rice, brown rice has 93% more vitamin B-6, 50% more potassium, 160% more zinc, 435% more magnesium, and 550% more fiber. Similarly, compared with white bread, whole-wheat bread has 200% more vitamin B-6, 250% more potassium, 260% more zinc, 370% more magnesium, and 285% more fiber.

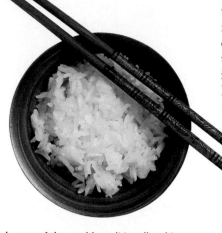

In tropical areas of the world, traditionally white rice has been favored over brown rice because it stays fresh longer. That's because, in warm climates and without refrigeration, the fat in the germ of brown rice goes rancid quickly.

🍑 13.2 Thiamin

For centuries, the devastating effects of the disease beriberi were known in Asian countries where white rice was the main (or staple) food. White rice is milled and therefore no longer contains the nutrient-rich germ. In the late 1800s, beriberi became even more common and one of the leading causes of death. This occurred because rice milling technology introduced at that time completely removed the bran and the germ, resulting in highly polished white rice but also stripping the rice grains of their thiamin content. However, scientists did not link the disease beriberi with a nutrient deficiency until early in the 1900s, when it was discovered that a vital factor in rice germ cures beriberi. That factor is the B-vitamin thiamin, also known as vitamin B-1.

Thiamin consists of a central carbon attached to a 6-member nitrogen-containing ring and a 5-member sulfur-containing ring. Its name comes from *thio*, meaning "sulfur," and *amine*, referring to the nitrogen groups in the molecule. Two phosphate groups are added (at the red dot in the thiamin's structure), to form this vitamin's coenzyme, thiamin pyrophosphate (TPP).

The chemical bond between each ring and the central carbon in thiamin (shown in red in the structure) is easily broken by prolonged exposure to heat, as can occur in cooking. When this happens, the vitamin can no longer function in the body. This destruction also occurs if food is cooked in alkaline (basic) solutions (pH ≥ 8.0). Sometimes baking soda (a base) is added to the cooking water of fresh green beans to retain their bright green color; this practice is not recommended.

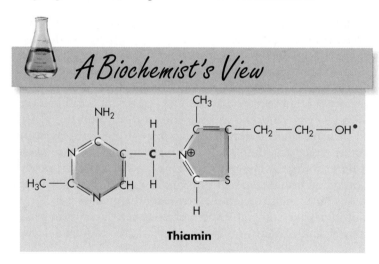

A Biochemist's View

Thiamin

Thiamin in Foods

Thiamin is found in a wide variety of foods, although generally in small amounts. As can be seen in Figure 13-6, foods rich in thiamin are pork products, sunflower seeds, and legumes. Whole and enriched grains and cereals, green peas, asparagus, organ meats (e.g., liver), peanuts, and mushrooms also are good sources. In the U.S., major contributors of thiamin are bread and rolls, ready-to-eat cereals, pasta, ham, milk, bakery products, potatoes, rice, orange juice, tomatoes, and beef.[4] Eating a variety of foods in accord with MyPyramid is a reliable way to obtain sufficient thiamin.

Thiamin Needs and Upper Level

The RDAs for thiamin are 1.2 mg per day for adult men and 1.1 mg per day for women.[2] The Daily Value on food and supplement labels is 1.5 mg. The average daily intake for thiamin in the U.S. for young men is close to 2 mg per day. For young women, it is ap-

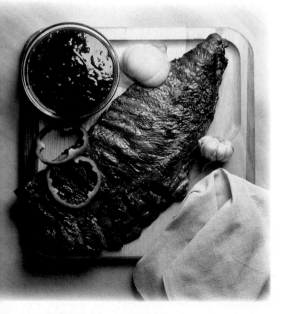

Pork is a rich source of thiamin.

Adult women RDA = 1.1 mg
Adult men RDA = 1.2 mg
Daily Value = 1.5 mg

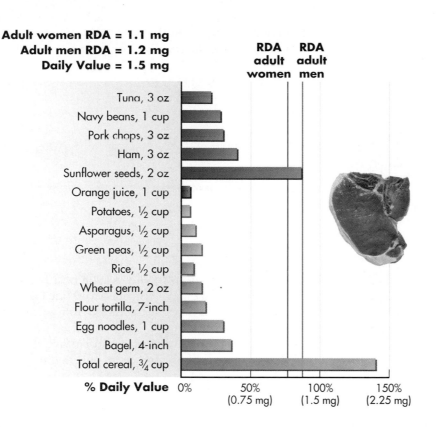

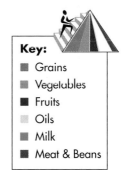

Figure 13-6 Food sources of thiamin.

Key:
■ Grains
■ Vegetables
■ Fruits
□ Oils
■ Milk
■ Meat & Beans

proximately 1.2 mg daily. There appears to be no adverse effects with excess intake of thiamin from food or supplements because it is readily excreted in the urine. Thus, no Upper Level is established for this nutrient.[2]

Absorption, Transport, Storage, and Excretion of Thiamin

Thiamin is absorbed mainly in the small intestine by a sodium-dependent active absorption process. It is transported mainly by red blood cells in its coenzyme form (thiamin pyrophosphate). Little thiamin is stored; only a small reserve is found in muscles and the liver. Any excess intake is rapidly filtered out by the kidneys and excreted in the urine.[4]

Functions of Thiamin

The coenzyme thiamin pyrophosphate (TPP) is required for the metabolism of carbohydrates and branched-chain amino acids.[5, 6] TPP is necessary for 2 different types of reactions. First, it works with specific enzymes to remove carbon dioxide (known as **decarboxylation**) from certain compounds. The conversion of pyruvate to acetyl-CoA, a critical reaction in the aerobic metabolism of glucose, is an example of the decarboxylation action of TPP.

decarboxylation Removal of 1 molecule of carbon dioxide from a compound.

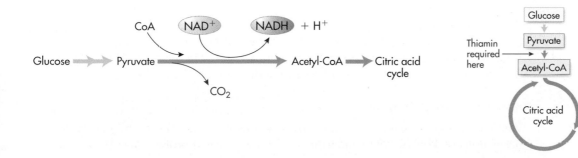

A similar decarboxylation reaction occurs in the citric acid cycle. As shown in the diagram, TPP aids in the conversion of the intermediate compound alpha-ketoglutarate to succinyl-CoA.

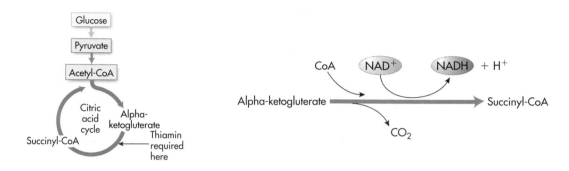

In addition to TPP, both of these reactions require 3 additional B-vitamin coenzymes: CoA (pantothenic acid), NAD (niacin), and FAD (riboflavin) (see Fig. 13-3). TPP functions in a similar manner (as a decarboxylase) in the metabolism of the branched-chain amino acids, valine, leucine, and isoleucine.

TPP also functions as a coenzyme for **transketolase**, an enzyme in the pentose phosphate pathway. In this pathway, the 6-carbon glucose is converted to the 5-carbon sugar used to form DNA and RNA.

Thiamin Deficiency

As described previously, the thiamin-deficiency disease beriberi has been associated with diets consisting mainly of white rice. For example, in the 1800s, 25 to 40% of those in the Japanese navy experienced beriberi because ship rations included white rice and little else. When meat and legumes were added to the navy rations, beriberi was eliminated. Although much less common today, beriberi still occurs among poor people in developing countries where white rice is the staple food.[7] A form of beriberi, called Wernicke-Korsakoff syndrome, is found in developed countries in some individuals with alcoholism.

Beriberi

In Sinhalese, the language of Sri Lanka, the word *beriberi* means "I can't, I can't." Those with beriberi are very weak because a deficiency of thiamin impairs the nervous, muscle, gastrointestinal, and cardiovascular systems. The symptoms of beriberi include **peripheral neuropathy** and weakness, muscle pain and tenderness, enlargement of the heart, difficulty breathing, edema, anorexia, weight loss, poor memory, and confusion.[5, 6] The nervous system is especially affected because of its reliance on glucose for energy. In thiamin deficiency, glucose metabolism is severely disrupted because pyruvate cannot be converted to acetyl-CoA, the entry compound into the citric acid cycle (see Fig. 13-3).

Beriberi often is described as either dry or wet beriberi. In dry beriberi, the main symptoms are related to the nervous and muscular systems. In wet beriberi, in addition to the neurological symptoms, the cardiovascular system is affected. The heart is enlarged, breathing may be difficult, and **congestive heart failure** may occur. Like most water-soluble vitamins, only small amounts of thiamin are stored in the body. Thus, some signs of beriberi can develop after only 14 days on a thiamin-free diet.[8]

Wernicke-Korsakoff Syndrome

Wernicke-Korsakoff syndrome (also known as cerebral beriberi) is found mainly among heavy users of alcohol. These individuals have a 3-pronged problem related to thiamin:

transketolase Enzyme whose functional component is thiamin pyrophosphate (TPP). It converts glucose to other sugars.

peripheral neuropathy Impaired sensory, motor, and reflex functions affecting arms and legs and causing calf muscle tenderness and difficulty in rising from a squatting position.

congestive heart failure Condition resulting from severely weakened heart muscle, resulting in ineffective pumping of blood. This leads to fluid retention, especially in the lungs. The symptoms include fatigue, difficulty breathing, and leg and ankle swelling.

alcohol decreases thiamin absorption, alcohol increases thiamin excretion in the urine, and alcoholics may consume a poor-quality diet without enough thiamin. Because thiamin is not readily stored in the body, the syndrome can occur rapidly. The symptoms include changes in vision (double vision, crossed eyes, rapid eye movements), **ataxia,** and impaired mental functions. The symptoms, especially those of the eye, improve with high doses of thiamin.[8]

ataxia Inability to coordinate muscle activity during voluntary movement; incoordination.

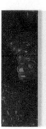

Knowledge Check

1. How is the coenzyme TPP involved in energy metabolism? What is 1 critical reaction that requires TPP?
2. What are 3 foods that are rich sources of thiamin?
3. What dietary practices are likely to lead to beriberi?

 ## 13.3 Riboflavin

Riboflavin, also known as vitamin B-2, was once called "yellow enzyme" because it has a distinctive yellow-green fluorescence. In fact, its name comes from its color (*flavin* means "yellow" in Latin). Riboflavin contains 3 linked 6-membered rings, with a sugar alcohol attached to the middle ring.

Riboflavin in Foods

Almost one-quarter of the riboflavin in our diets comes from milk products. The rest typically is supplied by enriched white bread, rolls, and crackers, as well as eggs and meat.[4] Foods rich in riboflavin are liver, mushrooms, spinach and other green leafy vegetables, broccoli, asparagus, milk, and cottage cheese (Fig. 13-7). Exposure to light (ultraviolet radiation) causes riboflavin to break down rapidly. To prevent this light-induced breakdown, paper and plastic containers—not glass—should be used as packaging for riboflavin-rich foods, such as milk, milk products, and cereals.

Riboflavin Needs and Upper Level

The RDAs for riboflavin for adult men and women are 1.3 and 1.1 mg/day, respectively. The Daily Value on food and supplement labels is 1.7 mg. North Americans have an intake of approximately 2.1 mg/day for men and 1.5 mg/day for women. There appear to be no adverse effects from consuming large amounts of riboflavin because of its limited absorption and rapid excretion via the urine, so no Upper Level has been set.[2]

Absorption, Transport, Storage, and Excretion of Riboflavin

In the stomach, hydrochloric acid (HCl) releases riboflavin from its bound forms. Free riboflavin is absorbed primarily via active transport or facilitated diffusion in the small intestine. In the blood, riboflavin is transported by protein carriers. Riboflavin is converted to its coenzyme forms in most tissues, but this occurs mainly in the small intestine, liver, heart, and kidneys. A small amount of riboflavin is stored in the

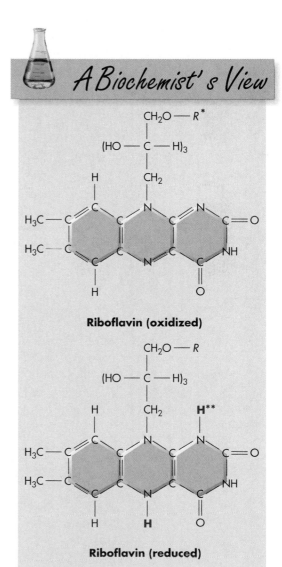

A Biochemist's View

Riboflavin (oxidized)

Riboflavin (reduced)

R* = H in free riboflavin; phosphate in the coenzyme FMN; adenine dinucleotide in the coenzyme FAD
** = Addition of 2 hydrogens (in red) in the reduced form.

Figure 13-7 Food sources of riboflavin.

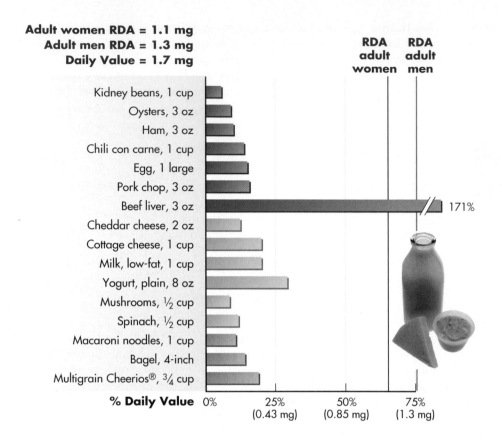

Adult women RDA = 1.1 mg
Adult men RDA = 1.3 mg
Daily Value = 1.7 mg

Kidney beans, 1 cup	
Oysters, 3 oz	
Ham, 3 oz	
Chili con carne, 1 cup	
Egg, 1 large	
Pork chop, 3 oz	
Beef liver, 3 oz	171%
Cheddar cheese, 2 oz	
Cottage cheese, 1 cup	
Milk, low-fat, 1 cup	
Yogurt, plain, 8 oz	
Mushrooms, 1/2 cup	
Spinach, 1/2 cup	
Macaroni noodles, 1 cup	
Bagel, 4-inch	
Multigrain Cheerios®, 3/4 cup	

RDA adult women | RDA adult men

% Daily Value 0%   25% (0.43 mg)   50% (0.85 mg)   75% (1.3 mg)

liver, kidneys, and heart. Any excess intake is excreted in the urine.[9] For people who take excessive amounts in supplement form, riboflavin imparts a bright yellow color to the urine that glows under a black light.

Functions of Riboflavin

Riboflavin is a component of 2 coenzymes that play key roles in energy metabolism: flavin mononucleotide (FMN) and flavin adenine dinucleotide (FAD).[9] These coenzymes, also referred to as flavins, have oxidation and reduction functions.[9] (See Section 9.1 in Chapter 9.) FAD is the oxidized form of the coenzyme. When it is reduced (gains 2 hydrogens, equivalent to 2 hydrogen ions and 2 electrons), it is known as $FADH_2$.

The riboflavin coenzymes are involved in many reactions in various metabolic pathways.[9] They are critical for energy metabolism and are involved in the formation of other compounds, including other B-vitamins and antioxidants.

Energy Metabolism

- In the citric acid cycle, the oxidation of succinate to fumarate requires the FAD-containing enzyme *succinate dehydrogenase*. The $FADH_2$ donates hydrogen to the electron transport chain.

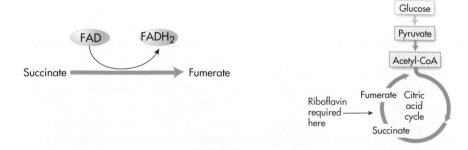

- In fatty acid breakdown (beta-oxidation) to acetyl-CoA, the enzyme *fatty acyl dehydrogenase* requires FAD (see Chapter 9).
- FMN shuttles hydrogen atoms into the electron transport chain.

Other B-Vitamin Functions

- The formation of niacin from the amino acid tryptophan requires FAD (see Section 13.4).
- The formation of the active vitamin B-6 coenzyme (pyridoxal phosphate) requires FMN.
- Riboflavin participates in folate metabolism (and, in this way, participates indirectly in homocysteine metabolism).

Antioxidant Function

- The synthesis of the antioxidant compound glutathione depends on the FAD-containing enzyme *glutathione reductase*. Recall from Chapter 12 that glutathione is an important part of the cell's antioxidant defense network.

Riboflavin Deficiency

Riboflavin deficiency, called **ariboflavinosis,** primarily affects the mouth, skin, and red blood cells. The symptoms include inflammation of the throat, mouth (stomatitis), and tongue (glossitis); cracking of the tissue around the corners of the mouth (angular cheilitis); and moist, red, scaly skin (seborrheic dermatitis) (Fig. 13-8). Anemia, fatigue, confusion, and headaches also may occur. Some of the symptoms of ariboflavinosis may result from deficiencies of other B-vitamins because they work in the same metabolic pathways as riboflavin and are often supplied by the same foods.

Ariboflavinosis develops after 2 months on a riboflavin-deficient diet and is rare in otherwise healthy people. Biochemical evidence of deficiency (low riboflavin levels in red blood cells or reduced activity of the enzyme glutathione reductase) is most often seen in adolescent girls and elderly people.[10] Diseases such as cancer, certain forms of cardiovascular disease, and diabetes can lead to or worsen a riboflavin deficiency.[2] People with alcoholism, malabsorption disorders, or very poor diets may be at risk of riboflavin deficiency. The long-term use of phenobarbital also may adversely affect riboflavin status because this drug increases the breakdown of riboflavin and other

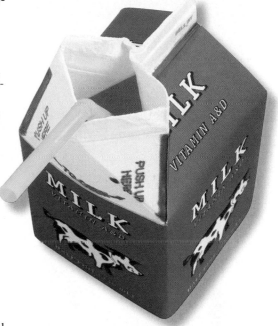

Milk products are good sources of riboflavin. Plastic and cardboard containers protect the riboflavin from UV radiation, which causes riboflavin to break down.

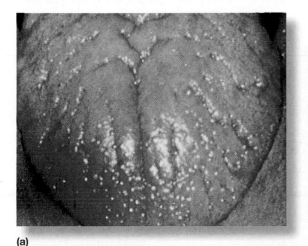

(a)

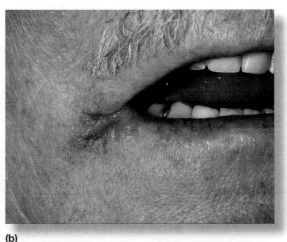

(b)

Figure 13-8 (*a*) Glossitis is a painful, inflamed tongue that can signal a deficiency of riboflavin, niacin, vitamin B-6, folate, or vitamin B-12. (*b*) Angular cheilitis, also called cheilosis or angular stomatitis, is another result of a riboflavin deficiency. It causes painful cracks at the corners of the mouth. Both glossitis and angular cheilitis can be caused by other medical conditions; thus, further evaluation is required before diagnosing a nutrient deficiency.

nutrients in the liver. Marginal riboflavin intake may occur in those who do not consume milk or milk products. Presently, little is known about the effects of a marginal riboflavin deficiency.

Knowledge Check

1. What foods are rich in riboflavin?
2. What are 3 general functions of riboflavin?
3. What are the 2 coenzymes formed from riboflavin?

 ## 13.4 Niacin

Pellagra—the deficiency disease of the B-vitamin niacin—is the only dietary deficiency disease ever to reach epidemic proportions in the U.S.[11] In the early 1900s, pellagra affected thousands in southeastern states before scientists discovered its link with niacin-poor diets. Niacin, or vitamin B-3, exists in 2 forms—nicotinic acid (niacin) and nicotinamide (niacinamide). Both forms are used to synthesize the niacin coenzymes: nicotinamide adenine dinucleotide (NAD) and nicotinamide adenine dinucleotide phosphate (NADP⁺).

Niacin in Foods

Niacin can be obtained from foods as the vitamin itself (preformed niacin) or synthesized in the body from the essential amino acid tryptophan.[12] Poultry, meat, and fish provide about 25% of the preformed niacin in North American diets. Another 11% comes from enriched bread and bread products. Coffee and tea also contribute a little preformed niacin to the diet. Figure 13-9 shows some rich sources of preformed niacin—mushrooms, wheat bran, fish, poultry, and peanuts. Protein-rich foods also are good sources of niacin because they provide tryptophan. Unlike some other water-soluble vitamins, niacin is very heat stable and little is lost in cooking.

In the synthesis of niacin from tryptophan, 60 mg of dietary tryptophan is needed to make about 1 mg of niacin.[2] Riboflavin and vitamin B-6 also are required. Protein is about 1% tryptophan, so 1 g of protein provides 10 mg of tryptophan. The overall con-

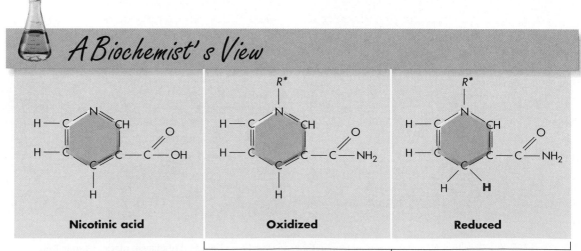

A Biochemist's View

Nicotinic acid   **Oxidized**   **Reduced**

R^* = Nicotinamide linked to adenine dinucleotide or adenine dinucleotide phosphate

Coenzyme forms using nicotinamide

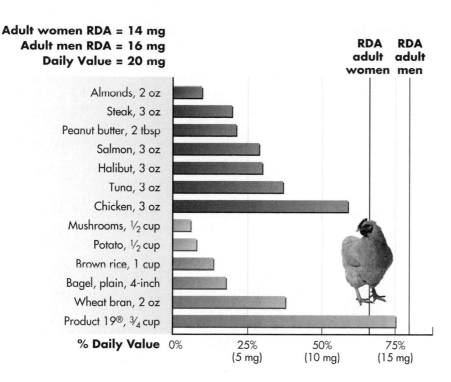

Figure 13-9 Food sources of niacin.

Adult women RDA = 14 mg
Adult men RDA = 16 mg
Daily Value = 20 mg

tribution of dietary protein to niacin can be roughly estimated as shown in the following example of a diet containing 90 g of protein.

$$1 \text{ g protein yields } 10 \text{ mg tryptophan}$$

$$60 \text{ mg tryptophan yields } 1 \text{ mg niacin}$$

$$90 \text{ g protein} \times 10 \text{ mg tryptophan/g protein} = 900 \text{ mg tryptophan}$$

$$\frac{900 \text{ mg tryptophan}}{60 \text{ mg tryptophan/mg niacin}} = 15 \text{ mg niacin}$$

A "shortcut" for this calculation is to divide protein intake (in grams) by 6. In the previous example, 90 g protein/6 yields 15 mg niacin.

To account for the direct (preformed) and indirect (from tryptophan) sources of niacin, dietary requirements and the amounts in foods are expressed as niacin equivalents (NE).[2] Thus, a diet that provides 13 mg preformed niacin and 90 g protein supplies approximately 28 NE (13 mg preformed + 15 mg from tryptophan). Individuals with an adequate protein intake meet much of their niacin requirement through tryptophan. Nutrient databases often underestimate niacin in the diet because the amount of tryptophan in many foods has not been determined yet.

Niacin Needs and Upper Level

The niacin RDA for adult men is 16 mg/day; for adult women, it is 14 mg/day. The RDA for niacin is expressed as niacin equivalents (NE) to account for preformed niacin in foods and niacin synthesized from tryptophan. Typical intakes of niacin in the U.S. exceed the RDA; in fact, tryptophan is the major source of niacin. The Daily Value for niacin on food and supplement labels is 20 mg. The Upper Level for niacin, 35 mg/day, applies only to niacin supplements and fortified foods.[2]

Absorption, Transport, Storage, and Excretion of Niacin

Nicotinic acid and nicotinamide are readily absorbed from the stomach and the small intestine by active transport and passive diffusion, so that generally almost all the niacin that

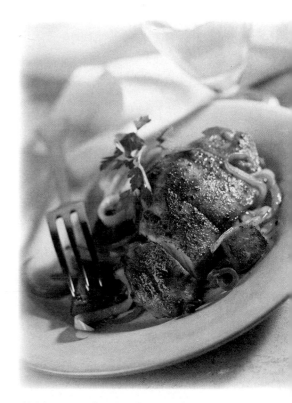

Chicken is a good source of niacin. Also, the tryptophan chicken contains can be used to synthesize niacin.

is consumed is absorbed. However, the bioavailability of niacin is low in some grains, especially corn. This is because the niacin is tightly bound to protein; thus, less than 30% can be absorbed. Niacin can be released from the protein and its bioavailability improved by soaking corn in a solution of calcium hydroxide dissolved in water (known as lime water). This practice is common among native peoples of Latin America where corn is a staple food; it protects them from niacin deficiency. After being absorbed, niacin is transported via the portal vein to the liver, where it is stored or delivered to the body's cells. Niacin is converted to its coenzyme forms in all tissues. Any excess niacin is excreted in the urine.[12]

Functions of Niacin

Like the coenzyme forms of riboflavin, the coenzyme forms of niacin, NAD^+ and $NADP^+$, are active participants in oxidation-reduction reactions.[12] The niacin coenzymes function in at least 200 reactions in cellular metabolic pathways, especially those that produce ATP. NAD^+ is required mainly for the catabolism of carbohydrates, proteins, and fats (Fig. 13-10). NAD^+ acts as an electron and hydrogen acceptor in glycolysis and the citric acid cycle. Under anaerobic conditions, NAD^+ is regenerated when pyruvate is converted to lactate. Under aerobic conditions, $NADH + H^+$ donates electrons and hydrogens to acceptor molecules in the electron transport chain, thereby contributing to ATP synthesis. Alcohol metabolism also requires niacin coenzymes (see section 9.5 in Chapter 9).

The reactions start with an oxidized form of a niacin coenzyme. However, synthetic pathways in the cell—those that make new compounds—use $NADPH + H^+$, the reduced form of the coenzyme. This coenzyme is important in the biochemical pathway for fatty-acid synthesis. Cells that synthesize a lot of fatty acids (e.g., those in the liver and female mammary glands) have higher concentrations of $NADPH + H^+$ than cells not involved in fatty-acid synthesis (e.g., muscle cells).

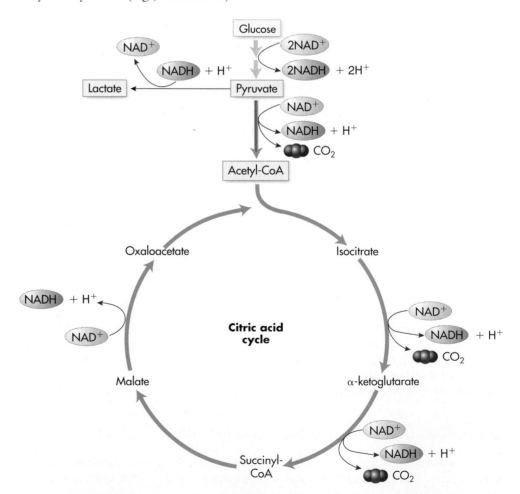

Figure 13-10 The coenzyme form of niacin, NAD^+, is required for glycolysis and the citric acid cycle. The NAD^+ is reduced to NADH. When pyruvate is reduced to form lactate, NADH is converted to NAD^+.

Niacin Deficiency

Because almost every metabolic pathway uses either NAD⁺ or NADPH ⊦ H⁺, it is not surprising that a niacin deficiency causes widespread damage in the body. The niacin deficiency disease pellagra, once a significant public health problem in the U.S., is now eradicated here, thanks to the enrichment of grains and protein-rich diets. The discovery of how pellagra develops from a poor diet, rather than a bacterial infection (as most believed until the early 1900s), is a fascinating story.

The first official record of pellagra, made in 1735 by Spanish physician Gaspar Casal, called this disease *mal de la rosa,* or "red sickness." This name referred to the rough, red rash that appears on skin exposed to sunlight, such as the forearms, backs of the hands, face, and neck (called Casal's necklace). The name *pellagra* comes from the Italian *pelle,* meaning "skin," and *agra,* mean "rough" (Fig. 13-11). Other symptoms of pellagra include diarrhea and dementia. Thus, pellagra is identified by the 3 Ds: dermatitis, diarrhea, and dementia. Death, the fourth D, can result if the disease is not treated.[12]

Pellagra has long been associated with corn-based diets. Although there is no evidence of pellagra among the native populations of North, Central, and South America, where corn (maize) has been the staple food in the diet for thousands of years, pellagra outbreaks followed the introduction of corn into Europe and Africa. As mentioned previously, the main reason for this was that the indigenous peoples of Latin America treated corn with alkali (from lime water or wood ashes), which released the niacin that is tightly bound to protein. Unfortunately, this treatment was not adopted in Europe, Africa, or the U.S. When maize became a staple food, especially among poor people who could afford few other foods, the result was a very low niacin intake, often resulting in pellagra. Scientists have since discovered another reason that corn-based diets can lead to pellagra—corn contains little of the amino acid tryptophan.

During the early 1900s, pellagra was rampant in the southeastern U.S., where corn was the staple food of poor people. More than 10,000 Americans died of pellagra in 1915. From 1918 until the end of World War II in 1945, approximately 200,000 Americans suffered from this disease. Many people had such severe dementia that they were forced to live out their lives in mental institutions. One reason that pellagra remained a problem for so long was the false belief that pellagra was an infectious disease. In the

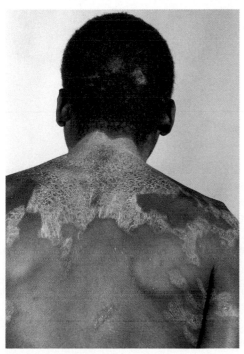
(a)

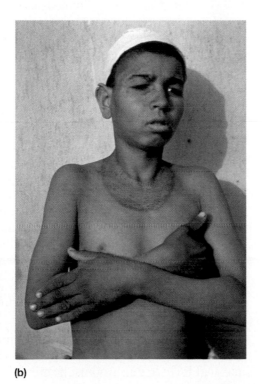
(b)

Figure 13-11 The dermatitis of pellagra. *(a)* Dermatitis on both sides (bilateral) of the body is a typical symptom of pellagra. Sun exposure worsens the condition. *(b)* The rough skin around the neck is referred to as Casal's necklace.

1910s and 1920s, Dr. Joseph Goldberger, a public health specialist, observed that institutionalized patients had pellagra but the better-fed staff did not—if pellagra was infectious, he reasoned, the staff should have "caught" it from their patients. He, his wife, and his colleagues proved that pellagra is not caused by an infectious pathogen by participating in experiments that exposed them to biological samples, such as skin, feces, and scabs, from pellagra patients. Goldberger also induced pellagra in volunteer prisoners by serving a cornmeal-only diet, then cured them by adding meat, milk, and vegetables to their diets. Finally, in 1937, researchers discovered that nicotinic acid dramatically cures a similar disease in dogs, called black tongue. Soon after, the enrichment of grain products with niacin in the U.S. virtually eliminated pellagra, although isolated cases still occur due to severe malabsorption, chronic alcoholism, or Hartnup's disease (a genetic disorder in which the tryptophan to niacin pathway is blocked). Today, pellagra still can be found in Africa, particularly when famine occurs, or in refugee camps when rations are mostly maize.[13, 14]

Pharmacological Use of Niacin

Niacin, as nicotinic acid, is sometimes prescribed by physicians to lower LDL cholesterol levels and increase HDL cholesterol levels.[15] When combined with diet, exercise, and other cholesterol-lowering medications, nicotinic acid can reduce the risk of heart attack. The dose required, 1 to 2 g daily, is more than 60 times the RDA. The most common side effect is flushing of the skin, but GI tract upset and liver damage also can occur. Although niacin is readily available in dietary supplement form, it must not be used as a substitute for the prescription formulation of niacin, which is carefully prepared to an exact dosage and has controlled time-release.[15] Recall that dietary supplements are not regulated by the FDA. The flushing seen with excess niacin intake was used to determine the Upper Level of 35 mg for niacin.[2]

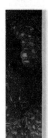

Knowledge Check

1. What are 2 metabolic pathways that require a niacin coenzyme?
2. In addition to preformed niacin in foods, what is another source of niacin in the diet?
3. Why are populations in Latin America not afflicted with pellagra, despite relying heavily on a corn-based diet?

 13.5 Pantothenic Acid

The name *pantothenic acid* was taken from the Greek word *pantothen,* meaning "from every side," because it is present in all body cells and is supplied by a wide variety of foods. Pantothenic acid is part of coenzyme A (CoA), which is used throughout the body in energy metabolism. CoA forms when pantothenic acid combines with a derivative of adenosine diphosphate (ADP) and part of the amino acid cysteine. Cysteine provides the sulfur atom, which is the functional end of the coenzyme.[16]

Pantothenic Acid in Foods

Our food supply provides ample amounts of pantothenic acid. Common sources include meat, milk, and many vegetables (Fig. 13-12). Other foods rich in pantothenic acid include mushrooms, peanuts, egg yolks, yeast, broccoli, and soy milk. In

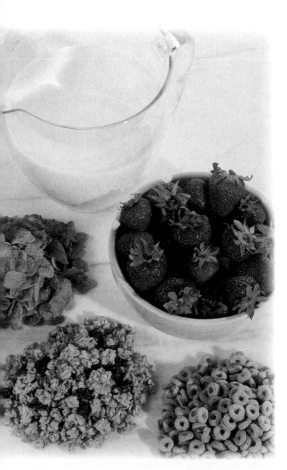

Many breakfast cereals are fortified with pantothenic acid.

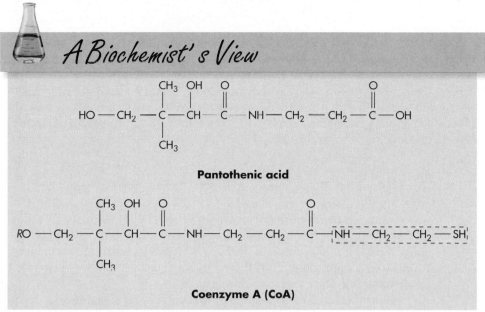

A Biochemist's View

Pantothenic acid

Coenzyme A (CoA)

Pantothenic acid is part of the coenzyme A (CoA) molecule
R = Derivative of adenosine diphosphate (ADP)
Boxed area = Part of the amino acid cysteine

general, unprocessed foods are better sources of pantothenic acid than processed foods because milling, refining, freezing, heating, and canning can reduce pantothenic acid in foods.[2]

Pantothenic Acid Needs and Upper Level

For adults, the Adequate Intake set for pantothenic acid is 5 mg/day.[2] Adults generally consume the Adequate Intake or more. The Daily Value on food and supplement labels is 10 mg. There is no known toxicity for pantothenic acid, so no Upper Level has been set.[2]

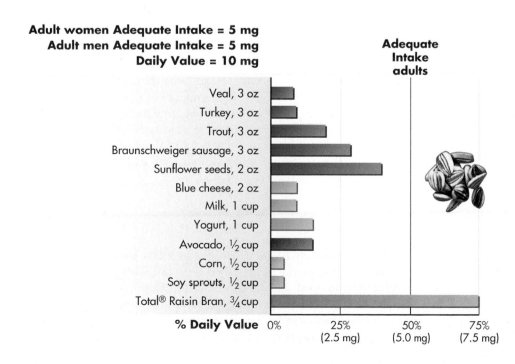

Adult women Adequate Intake = 5 mg
Adult men Adequate Intake = 5 mg
Daily Value = 10 mg

Adequate Intake adults

Veal, 3 oz
Turkey, 3 oz
Trout, 3 oz
Braunschweiger sausage, 3 oz
Sunflower seeds, 2 oz
Blue cheese, 2 oz
Milk, 1 cup
Yogurt, 1 cup
Avocado, ½ cup
Corn, ½ cup
Soy sprouts, ½ cup
Total® Raisin Bran, ¾ cup

% Daily Value 0%   25% (2.5 mg)   50% (5.0 mg)   75% (7.5 mg)

Figure 13-12 Food sources of pantothenic acid.

Absorption, Transport, Storage, and Excretion of Pantothenic Acid

The pantothenic acid portion of any coenzyme A in the diet is released during digestion in the small intestine. It is then absorbed and transported throughout the body bound to red blood cells. Storage is minimal and is in the coenzyme form. Excretion of pantothenic acid is via the urine.[16]

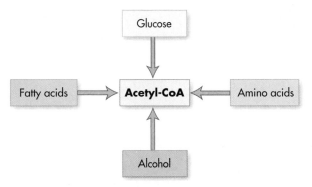

Pantothenic acid is required for the formation of coenzyme A, part of the structure of acetyl-CoA.

Functions of Pantothenic Acid

Coenzyme A is essential for the formation of acetyl-CoA from the breakdown of carbohydrate, protein, alcohol, and fat.[6] Acetyl-CoA molecules most often enter the citric acid cycle (with eventual ATP production). However, acetyl-CoA also is an important biosynthetic building block used to build fatty acids, cholesterol, bile acids, and steroid hormones.

Pantothenic acid also forms part of a compound called the acyl carrier protein. This protein attaches to fatty acids and shuttles them through the metabolic pathway designed to increase their chain length. As coenzyme A, pantothenic acid also donates fatty acids to proteins in a process that can determine their location and function within a cell.

Pantothenic Acid Deficiency

Pantothenic acid deficiency is very rare and has been observed only when a deficiency was experimentally induced.[2] Its symptoms include headache, fatigue, impaired muscle coordination, and GI tract disturbances.

Knowledge Check

1. How is pantothenic acid related to the formation of ATP?
2. What are 3 good sources of pantothenic acid?

13.6 Biotin

Biotin's discovery was linked to what researchers in the 1920s called "egg-white injury." Rats fed large amounts of raw egg whites developed severe rashes, lost their fur, and became paralyzed. These symptoms were reversed when the rats were fed yeast, liver, and other foods. These observations led to the discovery of this B-vitamin. Biotin is a coenzyme that participates in reactions that add carbon dioxide to compounds.[17]

Sources of Biotin: Food and Microbial Synthesis

Biotin is commonly found in 2 forms in foods: as a free vitamin and as the protein-bound form, called biocytin. This vitamin is widely distributed in food, but its concentration varies considerably. Good sources include whole grains, eggs, nuts, and legumes (Fig. 13-13). The biotin content of food has been determined for only a small number of foods, so nutrient databases are incomplete.

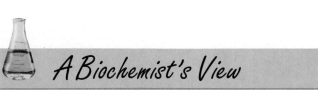

A Biochemist's View

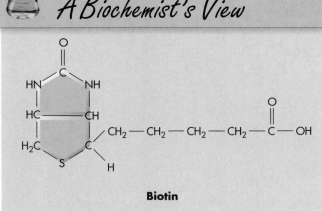

Biotin

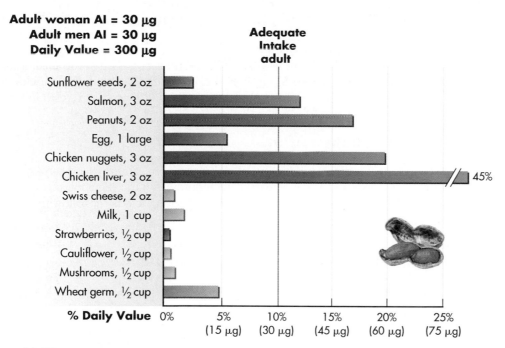

Figure 13-13 Food sources of biotin.

We excrete more biotin than we consume; thus, it appears that bacteria in the large intestine synthesize biotin. However, it is not yet known the extent to which the biotin synthesized by the flora in the large intestine is bioavailable because biotin is absorbed most efficiently from the small intestine.

Biotin Needs and Upper Level

The Adequate Intake for biotin for adults is 30 µg/day.[2] The diets of adults generally meet the Adequate Intake level. The Daily Value on food and supplement labels is 300 µg, 10 times the current estimate of needs. There is no Upper Level for biotin.[2]

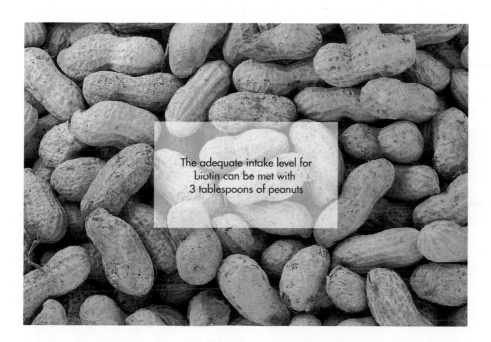

The adequate intake level for biotin can be met with 3 tablespoons of peanuts

Absorption, Transport, Storage, and Excretion of Biotin

In the small intestine, the enzyme biotinidase releases biotin from biocytin and other biotin-dependent enzymes found in foods. Free biotin is absorbed in the small intestine via a sodium-dependent carrier. Biotin is stored in small amounts in the muscles, liver, and brain, and its excretion is mostly via the urine, although some is excreted in bile.[17]

Functions of Biotin

Biotin functions as a coenzyme for several carboxylase enzymes that add carbon dioxide to various compounds.[17] These enzymes are required for the metabolism of carbohydrates, proteins, and fats. Reactions dependent on biotin include the following:

- The carboxylation of pyruvate to form oxaloacetate, a citric acid cycle intermediate. Recall that, when glucose supplies run low, oxaloacetate serves as a starting point for gluconeogenesis (see Chapter 9).

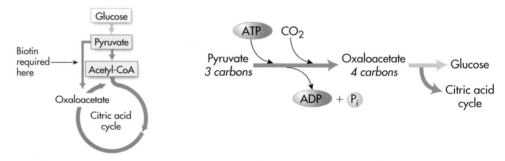

- The breakdown of the amino acids threonine, leucine, methionine, and isoleucine for use as energy.
- The carboxylation of acetyl-CoA to form malonyl-CoA, so that fatty acids can be synthesized (see Section 13.5).

Biotin Deficiency

Overall, biotin deficiencies are rare. About 1 in 112,000 infants is born with a genetic defect that results in very low amounts of the enzyme biotinidase.[18] As a result, these infants cannot break down biocytin in foods for absorption. A biotin deficiency develops, and symptoms (skin rash, hair loss, convulsions, and impaired growth) occur within a few weeks to months following birth. The affected individual is typically treated throughout life with regular doses of biotin supplements.

Biotin deficiency also has resulted from the regular ingestion of large amounts (> 12) of raw eggs each day. Raw eggs contain a protein, **avidin**, that binds biotin, limiting its absorption.[6] Cooking eggs denatures avidin, which prevents it from binding to biotin.

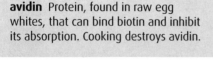

avidin Protein, found in raw egg whites, that can bind biotin and inhibit its absorption. Cooking destroys avidin.

Knowledge Check

1. Biotin is a coenzyme for several carboxylase enzymes. In general, what do these enzymes do?
2. How can a biotin deficiency occur?

13.7 Vitamin B-6

Nearly all amino acids require a vitamin B-6 coenzyme in their metabolism. Vitamin B-6 is a family of 3 compounds: pyridoxal, pyridoxine, and pyridoxamine. All 3 forms can be phosphorylated (have a phosphate group added) to become active vitamin B-6 coenzymes. The primary vitamin B-6 coenzyme is pyridoxal phosphate (PLP). Vitamin B-6 is converted to PLP by adding a phosphate group (PO_4) to its hydroxyl group. The generic name for this vitamin is B-6, or pyridoxine.[19]

Vitamin B-6 in Foods

Vitamin B-6 is stored in the muscle tissues of animals; thus, meat, fish, and poultry are some of the richest sources. Although vitamin B-6 in foods of animal origin is often more readily absorbed than that in foods of plant origin, whole grains also are good sources of vitamin B-6. However, vitamin B-6 is lost during the refining of grains, and it is not one of the vitamins added during enrichment. Most fruits and vegetables are not good vitamin B-6 sources, but there are some exceptions: carrots, potatoes, spinach, bananas, and avocados (Fig. 13-14). The leading sources of vitamin B-6 in the U.S. are fortified ready-to-eat cereals, poultry, beef, potatoes, and bananas.[4] Like many other water-soluble vitamins, vitamin B-6 can be lost when foods are exposed to heat and other processing.

Vitamin B-6 Needs and Upper Level

The RDAs for vitamin B-6 are 1.3 and 1.7 mg/day in adult women and men, respectively. The Daily Value on food and supplement labels is 2 mg. Average daily intakes of vitamin B-6 for adult men and women are somewhat above the RDA.

The Upper Level for adults is set at 100 mg/day.[2] Intakes of 2 to 6 g of vitamin B-6 daily for 2 months or more can lead to irreversible nerve damage, as can long-term intakes greater than 200 mg/day.[20] Bodybuilders and women attempting to treat themselves for premenstrual syndrome (PMS) have developed symptoms such as walking difficulties and hand and foot numbness. Some nerve damage in individual sensory neurons is probably reversible, but damage to ganglia (where many nerve fibers converge) is probably permanent.

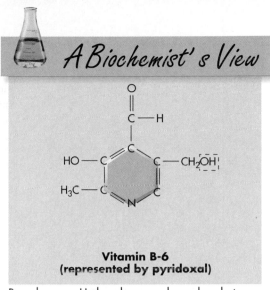

A Biochemist's View

**Vitamin B-6
(represented by pyridoxal)**

Boxed area = Hydroxyl group where phosphate is added.

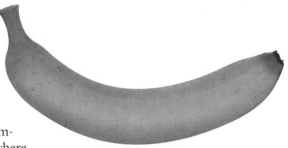

Bananas are a good plant source of vitamin B-6.

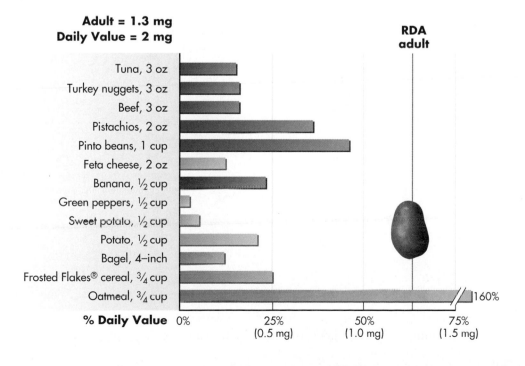

**Adult = 1.3 mg
Daily Value = 2 mg**

RDA adult

Food	% Daily Value
Tuna, 3 oz	
Turkey nuggets, 3 oz	
Beef, 3 oz	
Pistachios, 2 oz	
Pinto beans, 1 cup	
Feta cheese, 2 oz	
Banana, ½ cup	
Green peppers, ½ cup	
Sweet potato, ½ cup	
Potato, ½ cup	
Bagel, 4–inch	
Frosted Flakes® cereal, ¾ cup	
Oatmeal, ¾ cup	160%

% Daily Value   0%   25% (0.5 mg)   50% (1.0 mg)   75% (1.5 mg)

Figure 13-14 Food sources of vitamin B-6. Note that after age 51, the RDA increases (men: 1.7 mg; women: 1.5).

Absorption, Transport, Storage, and Excretion of Vitamin B-6

The absorption of vitamin B-6 is by passive diffusion. The coenzyme form is normally converted to the free vitamin form for absorption, but at high concentrations some of the coenzyme may be absorbed as such. Vitamin B-6 is transported via the portal vein to the liver, where most of it is phosphorylated. From the liver, the phosphorylated forms (mainly PLP) are released for transport in the blood bound to the transport protein albumin. Muscle tissue is the main storage site for vitamin B-6. Excess vitamin B-6 is generally excreted in the urine.[19]

Functions of Vitamin B-6

Vitamin B-6 coenzymes participate in numerous metabolic reactions. For example, PLP is a coenzyme in more than 100 enzymatic reactions, almost all of which involve nitrogen-containing compounds, such as amino groups (NH_2).

Metabolism

▶ Homocysteine is receiving a great deal of attention, especially regarding the development of brain disorders, bone disorders, and cardiovascular disease. Meeting B-vitamin (riboflavin, vitamin B-6, folate, and vitamin B-12) and choline needs allows for the metabolism of homocysteine to nutrients, such as the amino acids methionine and cysteine. This keeps homocysteine blood levels low and helps protect the body from homocysteine's potentially toxic consequences.

A major role of PLP is to participate in amino acid metabolism. A very important function of PLP is as a coenzyme for transamination reactions that transfer amino groups to allow the synthesis of non-essential amino acids (see Chapter 7). Without PLP, every amino acid would be essential because it would have to be supplied by the diet (Fig. 13-15).[19] PLP also helps convert homocysteine to the amino acid cysteine, which occurs during the metabolism of (methionine) the amino acid (see Appendix C for details on methionine and homocysteine metabolism).

PLP also is required for the release of glucose from glycogen. In this way, PLP helps maintain blood glucose concentration.[19]

Synthesis of Compounds

In the red blood cell, PLP catalyzes a step in the synthesis of heme, a nitrogen-containing ring that is inserted into certain proteins to hold iron in place. The best known of these proteins is hemoglobin, which uses iron to transport oxygen in the blood.[19]

Figure 13-15 An example of a transaminase enzyme pathway that utilizes vitamin B-6. This pathway allows cells to synthesize non-essential amino acids. In this example, pyruvate gains an amino group from glutamic acid to form the non-essential amino acid alanine.

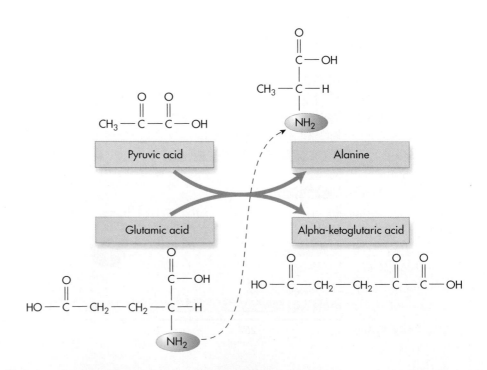

Not only are amino acids used to build proteins, but they also are used to make non-protein nitrogen-containing compounds. Many of these compounds are neurotransmitters, which are important for brain function. PLP is involved in the synthesis of several neurotransmitters: serotonin from tryptophan, dopamine (DOPA) and norepinephrine from tyrosine, histamine from histadine, and gamma-aminobutyric acid (GABA) from glutamic acid.[19]

PLP participates in vitamin formation, too. It plays an important role in the synthesis of the B-vitamin niacin from the amino acid tryptophan.[19]

Vitamin B-6 Deficiency

Vitamin B-6 deficiency is rare in North America. When a deficiency does occur, the symptoms may include seborrheic dermatitis, **microcytic hypochromic anemia** (from decreased hemoglobin synthesis), convulsions, depression, and confusion due to altered tryptophan metabolism or neurotransmitter synthesis.[19] Low blood concentrations of PLP have been observed in those with very poor diets and in alcoholics. Acetaldehyde, produced during alcohol metabolism, decreases the formation of PLP by cells and may reduce its biological activity. A number of medications can decrease the amount of PLP in the blood: L-DOPA, used to treat Parkinson's disease; isoniazid, an anti-tuberculosis medication; and theophylline, used to treat asthma. Individuals taking these medications may need vitamin B-6 supplementation.

Pharmacological Use of Vitamin B-6

Supplemental vitamin B-6 has a long history as a treatment for carpal tunnel syndrome, premenstrual syndrome, and nausea during pregnancy. Carpal tunnel syndrome, a common painful nerve disorder of the wrist and hand, has been treated with large daily doses (typically, 50 to 300 mg/day) of vitamin B-6. How vitamin B-6 might be related to carpal tunnel syndrome is unclear; theories include that it repairs damaged nerves or reduces pain perceptions. A comprehensive review of research studies in this area concluded that, despite limitations related to the quality of the research in this area, there is some support for using vitamin B-6 in the treatment of carpal tunnel syndrome.[20] This therapy should be supervised by a physician, not self-administered, especially because vitamin B-6 toxicity can worsen nerve damage.

The evidence that vitamin B-6 supplementation improves premenstrual syndrome (PMS) is weak. PMS is a multi-symptom disorder that occurs 1 to 2 weeks prior to menstruation. The symptoms include fluid retention, bloating and weight gain, breast tenderness, abdominal discomfort, headache, cravings for sugar and alcohol, mild depression, and anxiety. Most menstruating women experience 1 or more of these symptoms to some degree.[21] Because studies of vitamin B-6 and PMS have not shown significant benefit, vitamin B-6 cannot be recommended as a treatment for this disorder.[22]

Nausea is experienced by 70 to 85% of women during the first trimester of pregnancy (see Chapter 16). Sometimes physicians recommend vitamin B-6 supplementation, typically 30 to 75 mg/day, to reduce nausea. A review of the research on treating nausea during pregnancy suggests that this therapy is both safe and likely to help reduce nausea.[23] Even though vitamin B-6 supplements to treat nausea are available over the counter without a prescription, pregnant women should first discuss this treatment option with their physicians.

► In the early 1950s, some infants were accidentally fed a commercial formula in which vitamin B-6 had been destroyed by oversterilization. The infants developed abnormal electroencephalogram (EEG) readings and experienced convulsions. The reason was probably a lack of neurotransmitter synthesis in the brain. The situation was successfully treated.

microcytic hypochromic anemia Anemia characterized by small, pale red blood cells that lack sufficient hemoglobin and thus have reduced oxygen-carrying ability. It also can be caused by an iron deficiency.

Knowledge Check

1. How is the PLP coenzyme used in amino acid metabolism?
2. What are 3 good food sources of vitamin B-6?
3. What are 2 signs of vitamin B-6 toxicity?

13.8 Folate

The name of the B-vitamin folate comes from the Latin word *folium,* meaning "leaf." It was given this name because leafy green vegetables are excellent sources. *Folate* is the generic name, referring to the various forms of the vitamin found naturally in foods. The term **folic acid** refers to the synthetic form of the vitamin found in supplements and fortified foods.

Folate consists of 3 parts: pteridine, para-aminobenzoic acid (PABA), and 1 or more molecules of the amino acid glutamic acid (glutamate). If, as shown in its structure, only 1 glutamate molecule is present, it is designated folic acid (folate monoglutamate). In food, about 90% of the folate molecules have 3 or more glutamates attached to the carboxyl group (red asterisk in the structure) and are known as polyglutamates.[24]

A Biochemist's View

Pteridine | Para-aminobenzoic acid | Glutamate

Folic acid

* = In foods, additional glutamate molecules are usually linked here to the carboxyl group

Folate in Foods

The biological availability of folate in food from a mixed diet is generally thought to be about 50% of folic acid, but it may be closer to 80%.[25] Foods that have the largest amount and most bioavailable folate are liver, legumes, and leafy green vegetables (Fig. 13-16). Other, rich sources of folate include avocados and oranges. Bread and cereal products from milled grains are fortified with folic acid, making them good sources of this vitamin. Ready-to-eat cereals, bread, legumes, orange and grapefruit juice,

▶ PABA by itself is sometimes added to supplements, but there is no current scientific rationale for this.

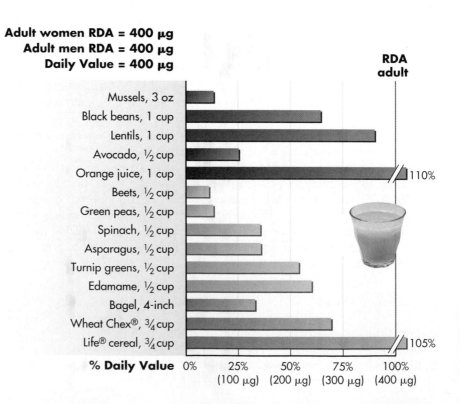

Adult women RDA = 400 µg
Adult men RDA = 400 µg
Daily Value = 400 µg

RDA adult

Mussels, 3 oz
Black beans, 1 cup
Lentils, 1 cup
Avocado, ½ cup
Orange juice, 1 cup — 110%
Beets, ½ cup
Green peas, ½ cup
Spinach, ½ cup
Asparagus, ½ cup
Turnip greens, ½ cup
Edamame, ½ cup
Bagel, 4-inch
Wheat Chex®, ¾ cup
Life® cereal, ¾ cup — 105%

% Daily Value 0% 25% 50% 75% 100%
(100 µg) (200 µg) (300 µg) (400 µg)

Figure 13-16 Food sources of folate.

lettuce, milk, and potatoes are leading sources of the vitamin in the U.S. diet. Although milk and potatoes are not particularly rich sources of folate, they are so commonly consumed that their contribution to folate intake is relatively high.

Food processing and preparation can destroy 50 to 90% of the folate in food. Folate is extremely susceptible to destruction by heat, oxidation, and ultraviolet light. (Vitamin C in foods helps protect folate from oxidative destruction.) The regular consumption of fresh or lightly cooked fruits and vegetables can help you gain the full benefits of their folate contents.

Folate Needs and Dietary Folate Equivalents

The folate RDA for adults is 400 µg/day, as is the Daily Value on food and supplement labels. The RDA is expressed as dietary folate equivalents (DFEs).[2] DFEs reflect the differences in the absorption of food folate and synthetic folic acid. The relationship between DFEs, food folate, and folic acid is as follows.

1 DFE = 1 µg food folate = 0.6 µg folic acid = 0.5 µg folic acid taken
                                        taken with food   on an empty stomach

DFEs are calculated using this equation:

$$DFE = \mu g \text{ food folate} + (\mu g \text{ folic acid} \times 1.7)$$

For example, the Daily Value for a serving of ready-to-eat breakfast cereal is listed on the label as 50%, so the amount of folic acid is 200 µg per serving (Daily Value of 400 µg × 0.50). Because this folate is mainly synthetic folic acid, the 200 µg is multiplied by 1.7, yielding 340 µg DFE. If the diet also contains 300 µg of food folate, the total DFE intake is 640 µg DFE (300 µg + 340 µg), which exceeds the adult RDA. Nutrient databases report the folate in certain foods as DFEs.

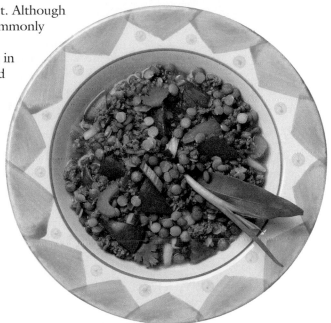

Lentils are a rich source of folate.

Upper Level for Folate

The Upper Level for synthetic folic acid is set at 1000 µg (1 mg); intakes above this level may mask a vitamin B-12 deficiency (see Section 13.9).[2] The Upper Level does not apply to folate in foods because absorption is limited. In response to the concern that high doses of folic acid might mask a vitamin B-12 deficiency, the FDA limits the amount of folic acid in non-prescription vitamin supplements. These levels are set at 400 µg for non-pregnant individuals when no statement of age is listed on the supplement label. When age-related doses are listed, there can be no more than 100 µg for infants, 300 µg for children, and 400 µg for adults. Over-the-counter prenatal supplements can contain 800 µg.

Absorption, Transport, Storage, and Excretion of Folate

To be absorbed, folate polyglutamates must be broken down (hydrolyzed) in the GI tract to the monoglutamate form. Enzymes known as folate conjugases, produced by the absorptive cells, remove the additional glutamates. The monoglutamate form is then actively transported across the intestinal wall. Very large doses of folic acid from supplements are absorbed by passive diffusion. When synthetic folic acid is consumed as a supplement and without food, it is nearly 100% bioavailable. Consumed with food, as in fortified cereal grains, absorption is slightly reduced.[2]

The portal vein delivers the monoglutamate form of folate from the small intestine to the liver, where it is converted to the polyglutamate form once inside a cell. (This change allows folate to be trapped in a cell.) Then, folate is either stored in the liver or released into the blood or bile. Folate in bile is reabsorbed by the enterohepatic circulation. Alcohol interferes with this process, which is one reason alcoholics often become folate deficient. Folate is excreted in both the urine and the feces.

▶ Some people have a genetic defect that results in reduced activity in an enzyme important in folate metabolism. This causes folate to be less biologically active and may predispose them to a higher risk of cancer or a pregnancy affected by a neural tube defect. This is currently an active area of research in folate nutrition. Testing for this defect is not yet routine, but it may be one day.

▶ THFA transfers these single-carbon groups:

Methyl (—CH$_3$)

Formyl (—CH=O)

Methylene (—CH$_2$—)

Methenyl (—CH=)

▶ Although folate deficiency can be induced to treat cancer, folate deficiency also may cause concern with regard to cancer. Because folate aids in the transfer of methyl groups for DNA synthesis, even mild folate deficiency may contribute to abnormal DNA integrity, which in turn affects certain cancer-protecting genes. A daily intake of 400 μg (the RDA) may protect against cancers, such as colorectal cancer.

Functions of Folate

Folate coenzymes are required for the synthesis and maintenance of new cells. Folate coenzymes function in metabolic pathways in which single carbon groups (listed in the margin) are exchanged. The folate coenzymes are formed from a central coenzyme form called tetrahydrofolic acid (THFA). Folate coenzymes are critical for DNA synthesis, and amino acid metabolism.[24]

DNA Synthesis

THFA is required for the synthesis of DNA, which contains 4 nitrogenous bases: cytosine and thymine (pyrimidines) and adenine and guanine (purines). The pyrimidine thymine is formed by the addition of a methylene group (CH$_2$) to the pyrimidine uracil. A folate coenzyme supplies the CH$_2$. Folate and vitamin B-12 function are closely linked. A vitamin B-12 coenzyme is required to recycle the folate coenzyme needed for DNA synthesis (see Section 13.9). Thus, folate and vitamin B-12 deficiencies can produce identical signs and symptoms.

THFA (—CH$_2$—)   THFA (free)

Uracil ▪▪▪▪▪▪▪▪▪▪▶ Thymine ▪▪▪▶ ▪▪▪▶ DNA

THFA also is needed for the synthesis of the purines (adenine and guanine) in DNA. Thus, DNA synthesis and repair may decline in a folate shortage.

The cancer drug methotrexate takes advantage of the key role of THFA in DNA synthesis. Methotrexate, referred to as a folate antagonist, interferes with THFA metabolism. This, in turn, reduces DNA synthesis throughout the body. This reduction in DNA synthesis can halt the growth of cancer cells, but it also affects other rapidly proliferating cells, such as intestinal and red blood cells. As a result, the typical side effects of methotrexate therapy are the same as for a folate deficiency (e.g., diarrhea and anemia). Methotrexate also is used to treat several immunological disorders, such as rheumatoid arthritis, psoriasis, asthma, and inflammatory bowel disease. Individuals treated with methotrexate are sometimes advised to take supplemental folic acid to reduce the drug's toxic side effects.[26] This supplementation probably does not influence the effectiveness of methotrexate.

Amino Acid Metabolism and Other Functions

THFA is important in amino acid metabolism, especially the inter-conversions of amino acids.[24] It accepts 1-carbon groups from various amino acids and is responsible for converting the amino acid glycine to the amino acid serine (the main source of methyl groups for THFA) and converting the essential amino acid histidine to the amino acid glutamic acid. THFA, along with vitamin B-12, is involved in a pathway that converts the amino acid homocysteine to the amino acid methionine.

Another key function of folate is the formation of neurotransmitters in the brain. A few studies suggest that supplementing antidepressant medications with folic acid can enhance the treatment of depression.[27] Folate also may help maintain normal blood pressure and reduce the risk of developing colon cancer.

Folate Deficiency

Folate deficiency can result from low intake, inadequate absorption (often associated with alcoholism), increased need (most commonly occurring in pregnancy), compromised utilization (typically associated with vitamin B-12 deficiency), the use of certain chemotherapy medications, and excessive excretion (linked to long-standing diarrhea).

Persons at risk for developing a folate deficiency include chronic alcoholics, those with very poor diets, and those who take certain medications, including anti-convulsants. In addition, folate deficiencies (other than neural tube defects) sometimes occur in pregnant women because pregnancy greatly increases the need for this vitamin (600 μg DFE/day).

Pregnant women require extra folate because of the increased rate of cell division, and thus of DNA synthesis, in their own bodies and in the developing fetus.[2] Prenatal care often includes prenatal multivitamin and mineral supplements fortified with folate to compensate for the extra needs associated with pregnancy.

A deficiency of folate first affects cell types that are actively synthesizing DNA because these cells have a short life span and rapid turnover rate.[24] For instance, red blood cells have a 120-day life span and are vulnerable to folate deficiency. Without folate, precursor cells in the bone marrow cannot form new DNA and therefore cannot divide normally to become mature red blood cells. The cells grow larger because there is continuous formation of RNA, leading to the increased synthesis of protein and other cell components. Hemoglobin synthesis also intensifies. However, when it is time for the cells to divide, they lack sufficient DNA for normal division.

Unlike normal mature red blood cells, these cells (called **megaloblasts**) retain their nuclei and remain in a large, immature form. Most megaloblasts do not make it out of the bone marrow. Any of these large cells that do enter the bloodstream are called **macrocytes.** Their presence results in a form of anemia called **megaloblastic,** or **macrocytic, anemia** (Fig. 13-17).

Large, immature cells also appear throughout the GI tract during chronic folate deficiency.[24] This occurs because DNA synthesis is impaired, which hinders cell division in the GI tract. This change contributes to a decreased absorptive capacity of the GI tract and persistent diarrhea. White blood cell synthesis also is disrupted by a folate deficiency because these cells are made in rapid bursts during immune challenges (e.g., infections). Thus, immune function can be diminished during a folate deficiency.

megaloblast Large, nucleated, immature red blood cell in the bone marrow, which results from the inability of a precursor cell to divide when it normally should.

macrocyte Literally, "large cell," such as a large red blood cell.

megaloblastic (macrocytic) anemia Anemia characterized by abnormally large, nucleated, immature red blood cells, which result from the inability of a precursor cell to divide normally.

Steps in Folate Deficiency

1. A decrease in blood folate concentration
2. A decrease in red cell folate
3. Defective DNA synthesis
4. A change in the structure of certain white blood cells
5. An increase in blood concentration of homocysteine (and methylmalonic acid)
6. Megaloblastic changes in bone marrow and other rapidly dividing cells
7. An increase in the size of circulating red blood cells
8. Megaloblastic (macrocytic) anemia

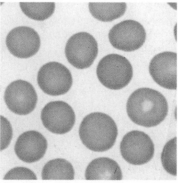

These are normal blood cells in the bloodstream. The size, shape, and color of the red blood cells show that they are normal. Mature red blood cells have lost their nuclei.

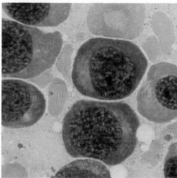

The megaloblastic blood cells seen here in the bone marrow are arrested at an immature stage of development. They still have their nuclei and are slightly larger than normal red blood cells.

Red blood cell precursor (stem cell)

Folate and vitamin B-12 adequate → Cells divide normally.

Folate or vitamin B-12 deficient → Cells are unable to divide.

Figure 13-17 Megaloblastic anemia occurs when blood cells are unable to divide, leaving large, immature red blood cells. Either a folate or vitamin B-12 deficiency may cause this condition. Measurements of blood concentrations of both vitamins are taken to help determine the cause of the anemia. Megaloblastic anemia due to folate deficiency has decreased substantially since folate fortification of grains began in 1998.

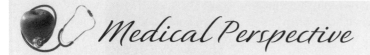

Medical Perspective

Neural Tube Defects

A maternal deficiency of folate and a genetic predisposition have been linked to the development of **neural tube defects** in the fetus (Fig. 13-18). These defects include spina bifida (a spinal cord or spinal fluid bulge through the back) and anencephaly (the absence of a brain). In both cases, there is a defect in the very early development of the neural tube, the structure that subsequently forms the brain, spinal cord, spinal nerves, and spinal column. Victims of spina bifida may exhibit paralysis, incontinence, hydrocephalus (the abnormal buildup of spinal fluid in the brain), and learning disabilities. Children born with anencephaly die shortly after birth.

Folate is critical to normal neural tube development. The neural tube forms and closes very early in pregnancy—the first 21 to 28 days after conception (see Chapter 16). During this time of critical development, many women are unaware that they are pregnant. Thus, ensuring good folate status for all women capable of becoming pregnant is critical.[28] As discussed earlier in the chapter, the folic acid fortification of refined cereals and grains was begun in the U.S. in 1998. Before fortification, about 4000 pregnancies per year were affected by a neural tube defect. Since fortification, the number of babies born with a neural tube defect has decreased by a third but the likelihood of a neural tube defect varies by race and ethnicity. The highest rates are in Hispanic women, followed by white women. The lowest rates are among Black and Asian women.[29] Some scientists are urging the government to double folic acid fortification levels to decrease further the incidence of neural tube defects, but others are concerned that higher levels may have unintended consequences, such as masking a vitamin B-12 deficiency (see Section 13.9). Currently, it is recommended that all women capable of becoming pregnant consume 400 µg of folic acid daily from supplements and fortified foods, in addition to getting folate from a varied diet. Food fortification supplies adults in the U.S. with about 200 µg/day of folic acid.

▶ Women who have had a child with a neural tube defect are advised to consume 4 mg/day of folic acid beginning at least 1 month before any future pregnancy. This must be done under strict physician supervision. For further information about neural tube defects, see the website www.sbaa.org.

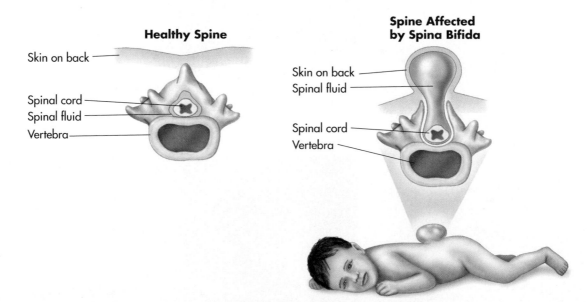

Figure 13-18 Neural tube defects result from a developmental failure affecting the spinal cord or brain in the embryo. Very early in fetal development, a ridge of neural-like tissue forms along the back of the embryo. As the fetus develops, this material differentiates into the spinal cord and body nerves at the lower end and into the brain at the upper end. At the same time, the bones that make up the vertebra gradually surround the spinal cord on all sides. If any part of this sequence of events goes awry, many defects can appear. The worst is total lack of a brain (anencephaly). Much more common is spina bifida, in which the backbones do not form a complete ring to protect the spinal cord. Deficient folate status in the mother during the beginning of pregnancy increases the risk of neural tube defects, as does a genetic predisposition.

Knowledge Check

1. How do folate in food and synthetic folic acid differ? Which form is better absorbed?
2. What are 3 foods that are good sources of folate?
3. What type of anemia signifies a folate deficiency?

CASE STUDY

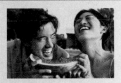

Suzanne and Ted are planning to start a family. They are especially concerned because Suzanne's sister gave birth last year to a baby with spina bifida. In preparation for her pregnancy, Suzanne takes a multivitamin supplement and eats fortified breakfast cereal most days. She also tries to include oranges, orange juice, broccoli, and spinach salads in her diet. What is spina bifida? How do Suzanne's diet and multivitamin supplement help prevent this serious disorder?

13.9 Vitamin B-12

Vitamin B-12, also known as cobalamin, is unique among the vitamins on 2 accounts. First, foods of animal origin, such as meat, poultry, fish, and dairy products, are the only reliable sources of vitamin B-12. Second, it is the only vitamin that contains a mineral (cobalt) as part of its structure.[30] Vitamin B-12 has a complex, multi-ring structure. The cyanocobalamin form of vitamin B-12 forms 2 active coenzymes (methylcobalamin and 5-deoxyadenosylcobalamin) by replacing the cyano group (shown in red) with another group, such as a methyl group or a hydroxyl group. The discovery of vitamin B-12 and how it prevents the vitamin B-12 deficiency disease, pernicious anemia, were so significant that vitamin B-12 researchers were awarded 6 Nobel prizes in the time period 1934–1965.

Vitamin B-12 in Foods

Plants do not synthesize vitamin B-12. In fact, all vitamin B-12 compounds are synthesized exclusively by microorganisms, mainly bacteria. Animals acquire vitamin B-12 from soil ingested while eating and grazing. Ruminant animals, such as cows and sheep, also synthesize vitamin B-12 from bacteria in the multiple compartments of their stomachs.

For humans, the sources of vitamin B-12 are foods of animal origin, such as meat, poultry, seafood, eggs, and dairy products. Especially rich sources of vitamin B-12 are organ meats, such as liver, kidneys, and heart, and fortified foods, such as ready-to-eat cereals (Fig. 13-19). Although algae and fermented soy products, such as tempeh and miso, are sometimes advertised as being good plant sources of vitamin B-12, vegans should not rely on them to meet vitamin B-12 requirements. These foods often contain vitamin B-12 analogs (compounds similar to vitamin B-12) that do not function as vitamin B-12 in the body.

Vitamin B-12 Needs and Upper Level

The RDA of vitamin B-12 for adults is 2.4 µg/day. The Daily Value on food and supplement labels is 6 µg. On average, adult men consume 3 times the RDA and women consume 2 times the RDA. This high intake provides the average meat-eating person with a 2 to 3 years' storage of vitamin B-12 in the liver. No adverse effects have been observed with excess vitamin B-12 intake from food or from supplements, so there is no Upper Level for this vitamin.[2]

A Biochemist's View

Vitamin B-12 (cyanocobalamin)

*CN = cyano group

Figure 13-19 Food sources of vitamin B-12.

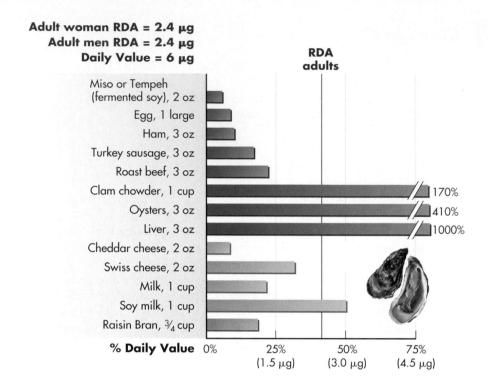

Adult woman RDA = 2.4 μg
Adult men RDA = 2.4 μg
Daily Value = 6 μg

RDA adults

Miso or Tempeh (fermented soy), 2 oz	
Egg, 1 large	
Ham, 3 oz	
Turkey sausage, 3 oz	
Roast beef, 3 oz	
Clam chowder, 1 cup	170%
Oysters, 3 oz	410%
Liver, 3 oz	1000%
Cheddar cheese, 2 oz	
Swiss cheese, 2 oz	
Milk, 1 cup	
Soy milk, 1 cup	
Raisin Bran, ¾ cup	

% Daily Value   0%   25% (1.5 μg)   50% (3.0 μg)   75% (4.5 μg)

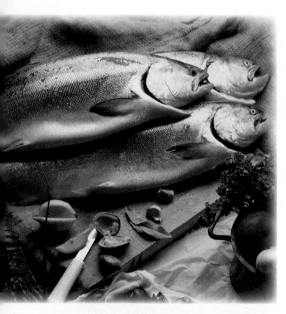

Fish, seafood, and related products are good sources of vitamin B-12.

R-protein Protein, produced by the salivary glands, that enhances the absorption of vitamin B-12, possibly by protecting the vitamin during its passage through the stomach.

intrinsic factor Substance in gastric juice that enhances vitamin B-12 absorption.

Absorption, Transport, Storage, and Excretion of Vitamin B-12

As shown in Figure 13-20, the absorption of vitamin B-12 is quite complex. In food, vitamin B-12 is bound to protein. HCl and pepsin in gastric juice release vitamin B-12 from these proteins. In the stomach, the free vitamin B-12 binds to **R-protein,** which originates in the salivary glands. In the small intestine, pancreatic protease enzymes (e.g., trypsin) release vitamin B-12 from the R-protein/vitamin B-12 complex. The free vitamin B-12 then combines with **intrinsic factor,** a proteinlike compound, produced by parietal cells in the stomach, that enhances vitamin B-12 absorption. The vitamin B-12 intrinsic factor complex travels to the ileum, where vitamin B-12 is absorbed and transferred to the blood transport protein transcobalamin II. This vitamin B-12/transcobalamin II complex enters the portal vein and is delivered to the liver.[30] The liver can store enough vitamin B-12 to last several years; this is not the case with other water-soluble vitamins. Although vitamin B-12 is continually secreted into the bile, most of it is reabsorbed by enterohepatic circulation, thereby efficiently "recycling" this vitamin. Little vitamin B-12 is excreted in the urine.

Normally, healthy adults absorb about 50% of the vitamin B-12 in foods. However, the absorption of vitamin B-12 can be disrupted by numerous defects, including the following.[2, 31]

- The absence of or defective synthesis of R-protein, pancreatic proteases, or intrinsic factor
- Defective binding of the intrinsic factor/vitamin B-12 complex to receptor cells in the ileum
- The absence (or surgical removal) of much or all of the ileum and stomach
- Diseases in the ileum, such as Crohn's disease
- Bacterial overgrowth of the small intestine
- Tapeworm infestation
- The use of certain anti-reflux medications that significantly reduce acid production by the parietal cells (e.g., omeprazole [Prilosec®])
- The use of the medication metformin to lower blood sugar in type 2 diabetes[32]
- Chronic malabsorption syndromes as may occur with various gastrointestinal disorders

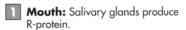

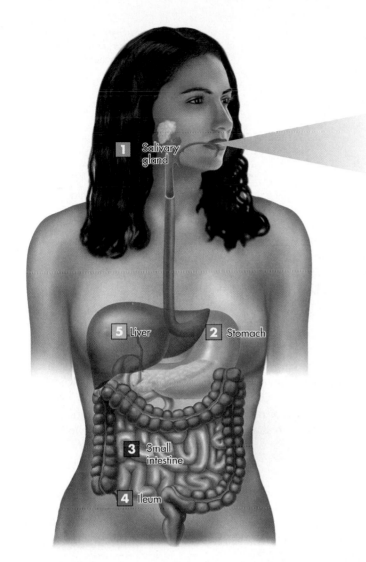

Figure 13-20 Absorption of vitamin B-12. Many factors and sites in the gastrointestinal tract participate. Defects arising in the stomach or small intestine can interfere with vitamin B-12 absorption, in turn causing pernicious anemia.

1 **Mouth:** Salivary glands produce R-protein.

2 **Stomach**
a. HCl and pepsin release vitamin B-12 bound to protein in food.
b. Free vitamin B-12 binds with R-protein
c. Parietal cells secrete intrinsic factor.

3 **Small intestine**
a. Trypsin from pancreas releases R-protein from vitamin B-12.
b. Vitamin B-12 links with intrinsic factor.

4 **Ileum:** Vitamin B-12/intrinsic factor complex is absorbed into blood and binds to transport protein transcobalamin II.

5 **Liver:** Vitamin B-12 stored in liver.

• Atrophic gastritis, which decreases the production of HCl and digestive enzymes needed to cleave the R-protein vitamin B-12 complex in foods; 10 to 30% of older adults have atrophic gastritis and, thus, are advised to eat foods fortified with vitamin B-12 and/or take a supplement because these contain free vitamin B-12 in crystalline form, which is readily absorbed.

Functions of Vitamin B-12

Vitamin B-12 is required for 2 enzymatic reactions.[30] First, the formation of the amino acid methionine from the amino acid homocysteine is catalyzed by the enzyme methionine synthase, which requires the vitamin B-12 coenzyme methylcobalamin (Fig. 13-21). Homocysteine accepts a methyl group from methylcobalamin, which forms methionine. Methionine, in turn, is the source of S-adenosyl methionine (SAM). In many reactions, SAM serves as a methyl donor. Methylation reactions are important for DNA and RNA regulation, myelin regulation, and the synthesis of many biochemical compounds. The methionine synthesis reaction also explains the close link between vitamin B-12 and folate: methylcobalamin obtains its methyl group from the folate coenzyme 5-methyl-tetrahydrofolate. When the methyl group is donated to vitamin B-12, the folate coenzyme THFA is reformed. When vitamin B-12 is lacking, THFA declines and the symptoms of folate deficiency can ensue. When either folate or vitamin B-12 is lacking, methionine and SAM synthesis decline and the amount of homocysteine in the body increases.

Figure 13-21 Interrelationships of vitamin B-12 and folate with the amino acids homocysteine and methionine. **1** One methyl group from 5-Methyl Tetrahydrofolate (5-Me-THFA) is donated to cobalamin (vitamin B-12). This reaction generates tetrahydrofolate (THFA) and methyl cobalamin (Me-Cobalamin). **2** Me-Cobalamin donates the methyl group to homocysteine. This reaction is catalyzed by the enzyme methionine synthase. This reaction generates cobalamin and methionine. When vitamin B-12 is lacking: 5-Me-THF builds up and THF decreases which slows or stops nucleic acid synthesis. Homocysteine levels also rise.

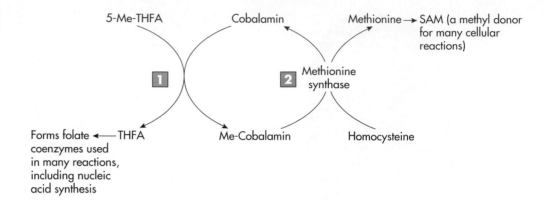

mutase Enzyme that rearranges the functional groups on a molecule.

The enzyme methylmalonyl **mutase** requires the second vitamin B-12 coenzyme, 5-deoxyadenosylcobalamine. This enzyme is needed for the metabolism of fatty acids with an odd number of carbon molecules (most fatty acids have an even number of carbon molecules). It allows these fatty acids to be oxidized in the citric acid cycle and to provide energy.

Vitamin B-12 Deficiency

Researchers in mid-19th century England noted a form of anemia that causes death within 2 to 5 years of initial diagnosis. They called this disease **pernicious anemia** (*pernicious* means "leading to death"). It is now known that this disease can result from the inadequate production of the intrinsic factor required for vitamin B-12 absorption. Poor vitamin B-12 status is still fairly common today, and impaired absorption of the vitamin B-12 found in foods is most often to blame.

Macrocytic Anemia

When a vitamin B-12 deficiency is severe enough that body stores are gone or almost gone, a megaloblastic, macrocytic anemia results. The anemia produced in vitamin B-12 deficiency is identical to that produced in a folate deficiency. Because a lack of vitamin B-12 impairs folate metabolism, normal DNA and red blood cell synthesis is disrupted, resulting in macrocytic anemia (see Fig. 13-17).

Neurological Changes

A vitamin B-12 deficiency produces nerve degeneration, which can be fatal. The neurological complications produce sensory disturbances in the legs, such as burning, tingling, prickling, and numbness (collectively referred to as **paresthesia**).[30] Walking is difficult and balance is seriously affected. Many mental problems exist as well, such as loss of concentration and memory, disorientation, and dementia. As the condition worsens, bowel and bladder control is lost. Visual disturbances are common, too. There also are numerous GI tract problems, ranging from a sore tongue to constipation. The neurological complications often precede the development of anemia.

Elevated Plasma Homocysteine Concentrations

Poor vitamin B-12, folate, and vitamin B-6 status can each result in high circulating levels of the amino acid homocysteine (see Fig. 13-21). Many studies have shown that high homocysteine levels in the blood are a risk factor for heart attacks and strokes. Other researchers have found that high levels of plasma homocysteine also are associated with cognitive dysfunction and osteoporotic fractures.[33]

Researchers have long known that supplementing the diet with folate, vitamin B-12, and vitamin B-6 can reduce blood levels of homocysteine. However, the evidence that supplementing with these vitamins can reduce the diseases associated with high blood levels of homocysteine is not strong. Several large studies that compared vitamin supplements with placebo treatments found that the supplements did not prevent heart disease, even though homocysteine levels declined.[34, 35] In addition, it appears that supplements of vitamin B-12, vitamin B-6, and folate do not improve cognitive function.[36] However, in one study, folate and vitamin B-12 supplements decreased the risk of hip fracture in a group of older Japanese patients.[33] Even though B-vitamin supplements have not been shown to decrease the risk of heart disease or improve cognition, ample B-vitamin intakes are vital for normal physiological function and good health.

Persons at Risk of Vitamin B-12 Deficiency

Poor vitamin B-12 status affects about 20% of older Americans. In the elderly, most cases are due to impaired absorption of the vitamin B-12 in foods due to atrophic gastritis. This deficiency is not usually severe enough to produce anemia, but it can cause neurological problems and elevated blood homocysteine. The consumption of crystalline vitamin B-12, either as a dietary supplement or in fortified foods (many breakfast cereals are fortified with vitamin B-12), can improve vitamin B-12 status in older persons with or without gastric atrophy.[37]

As noted earlier, those with a malabsorption syndrome of any kind have an increased need for vitamin B-12. For those diagnosed with a vitamin B-12 deficiency due to impaired absorption, 3 options are available: (1) monthly injections of vitamin B-12 to bypass the GI tract, (2) the use of a vitamin B-12 nasal gel, which also bypasses the GI tract, and (3) very high oral doses (1 to 2 mg) daily of vitamin B-12. A very small amount of vitamin B-12 can be absorbed by passive diffusion and does not require the intrinsic factor system. When very large amounts of vitamin B-12 are ingested, enough can be absorbed to meet vitamin B-12 requirements and correct vitamin B-12 deficiency.[38, 39]

Vegetarians also can become vitamin B-12 deficient. However, if a person becomes a vegetarian in adulthood, vitamin B-12 stores in the liver can delay a severe deficiency for a long time. Infants born to or breastfed by vegetarian or vegan mothers also can develop vitamin B-12 deficiency, accompanied by anemia and long-term neurological problems, such as diminished brain growth, degeneration of the spinal cord, and poor intellectual development. Vegetarians have several options for obtaining vitamin B-12. If they are not vegans, they can obtain vitamin B-12 from dairy products and eggs. In addition, vitamin B-12 supplements and food products fortified with vitamin B-12 are available.

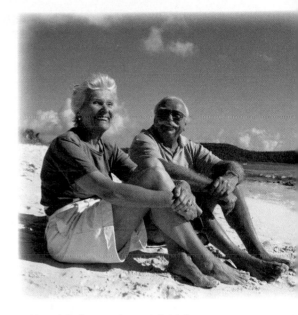

Older adults have an increased risk for poor vitamin B-12 status.

Knowledge Check

1. What roles do HCl, pepsinogen, intrinsic factor, and the ileum play in vitamin B-12 absorption?
2. How are vitamin B-12 and folate metabolism related?
3. Which foods are good sources of vitamin B-12?

 ## 13.10 Choline

For many years, choline often was included in supplements as a "supposed" B-vitamin, but most nutrition experts claimed that choline was not a vitamin at all because liver synthesis could meet the requirement for choline. However, recent research demonstrates that humans consuming choline-deficient diets develop liver and kidney problems.[40] Still, choline is not yet considered a B-vitamin. It does not have a coenzyme function and the amount of choline in the body is much greater than the amount of a typical B-vitamin.

Choline in Foods

Choline is widely distributed in foods of animal origin, mostly in the form of phosphatidylcholine (lecithin) in cell membrane and blood lipoproteins. Milk, liver, eggs, and peanuts are rich sources (Fig. 13-22). Lecithins often are added to food

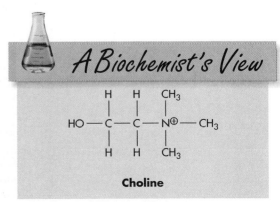

A Biochemist's View

Choline

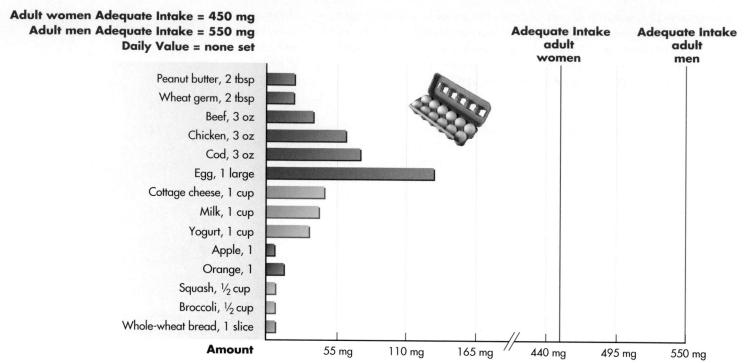

Adult women Adequate Intake = 450 mg
Adult men Adequate Intake = 550 mg
Daily Value = none set

Figure 13-22 Food sources of choline.

during processing, so this is yet another source. Data on the choline content of foods are still incomplete; however, nutrient data are increasing.[41] Because choline is so widespread in the diet, a deficiency is unlikely.

Choline Needs and Upper Level

The Adequate Intake for choline for adult men is 550 mg/day; for adult women, it is 425 mg/day. Few data exist to assess whether a dietary supply is needed at all life stages. Although Adequate Intakes are set for choline, it may be that the choline requirement can be met by body synthesis at some or all stages of life. We also consume ample choline from food, at least 700 to 1000 mg/day, so there is no need to supplement a diet with choline.[2]

The Upper Level for adults is 3.5 g/day. Very high doses of choline have been associated with a fishy body odor (arising from a breakdown product), low blood pressure, vomiting, salivation, sweating, and GI tract effects.[2]

Absorption, Transport, Storage, and Excretion of Choline

Choline is absorbed from the small intestine by way of transport proteins. The liver takes up choline rapidly from the blood delivered by the portal vein from the small intestine. All tissues contain some stores of choline. Some choline is excreted in the urine, but most of the excess is converted to a related donor (betaine) of single-carbon groups (e.g., methyl groups).

Functions of Choline

Choline is a component of phospholipids, such as phosphatidylcholine (lecithin), a major component of cell membranes and blood lipoproteins. Choline also functions as a precursor for acetylcholine, a neurotransmitter associated with attention, learning, memory, muscle control, and many other functions. Liver export of VLDL is associated with the action of choline, too. The methyl ($—CH_3$) group of choline can be used to form methionine from homocysteine,[40] and supplementation with choline in healthy men has shown to decrease homocysteine concentrations. Preliminary research suggests that high choline intakes are associated with lower plasma concentrations of a compound (C-reactive protein) that indicates inflammation.[42] Because inflammation increases the risk of cardiovascular disease, choline may offer protection against this disease.

Choline → → Betaine

$—CH_3$ → Methionine

Homocysteine

Choline-Deficiency Diseases

When humans were fed choline-deficient total parenteral nutrition solutions, they developed fatty livers and liver damage. Based on these observations, plus laboratory animal studies, choline has been deemed essential, at least in some life stages and health conditions.[40]

Knowledge Check

1. Which organs are most affected by a choline-free diet?
2. What are 3 functions of choline?

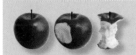 *Take Action*

B-Vitamin Supplements

B-vitamins are sometimes marketed as a way to gain energy. Consider the following common scenario. Dan, age 20, is a junior in college with a full load of classes, a part-time job, and additional campus activities. He often feels tired and stressed and attributes this to his poor eating habits. Dan frequently misses meals and fills up on fast food and snacks. One of his friends suggests that he try a B-complex vitamin supplement to boost his energy. The supplement Dan chooses is called B-complex 100. According to the label, 1 pill provides the following:

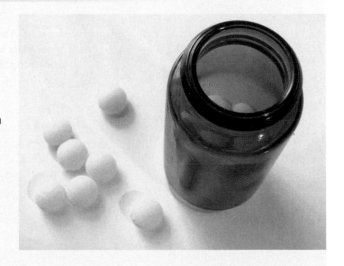

Thiamin	100 mg
Riboflavin	100 mg
Niacin	100 mg
Vitamin B-6	100 mg
Folic acid	400 µg
Vitamin B-12	100 mg
Biotin	100 µg
Pantothenic acid	100 mg
Para-aminobenzoic acid	100 mg
Choline	100 mg
Carnitine	100 mg

Compare the amounts provided in the supplement with the DRIs, including the UL for Dan. Is the B-complex 100 a good supplement for Dan? Do you think it will increase his energy? What are para-aminobenzoic acid and carnitine? What are other recommendations you might make to help Dan improve his energy and nutritional health?

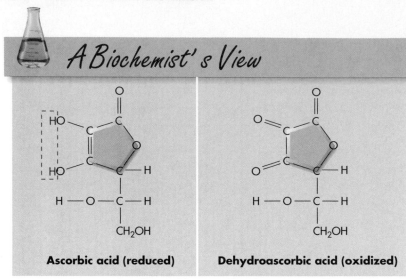

A Biochemist's View

Ascorbic acid (reduced)

Dehydroascorbic acid (oxidized)

Boxed area = Ascorbic acid (vitamin C) undergoes reversible oxidation and reduction by loss of 2 hydrogens (red).

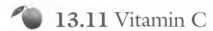

13.11 Vitamin C

Most animals are able to synthesize vitamin C and, so, do not require a dietary source. However, humans, other primates, guinea pigs, fruit bats, and a few birds and fish are unable to synthesize this water-soluble vitamin. These animals rely on their diets for a vitamin C source.[43]

Vitamin C, also known as ascorbic acid, is involved in many processes in the human body, primarily as an electron donor. The term *vitamin C* actually refers not only to ascorbic acid but also to its oxidized form, dehydroascorbic acid. By adding or losing 2 hydrogens (in the boxed area of the structure), vitamin C undergoes reversible reduction and oxidation. Both forms of vitamin C are found in the foods we eat.

Vitamin C in Foods

Most fruits and vegetables contain some vitamin C, but the richest sources are citrus fruits, peppers, and green vegetables (Fig. 13-23). Animal products and grains are generally not good sources. An intake of 5 servings per day of fruits and vegetables can provide ample vitamin C, depending on the foods chosen. However, the leading fruits and vegetables consumed in the U.S. are iceberg lettuce, tomatoes, french fries, bananas, and orange juice.[44] Of these, only orange juice is a rich vitamin C source. The major contributors of vitamin C to North American diets are oranges and orange juice, grapefruit and grapefruit juice, tomatoes and tomato juice, fortified fruit drinks, tangerines, and potatoes.

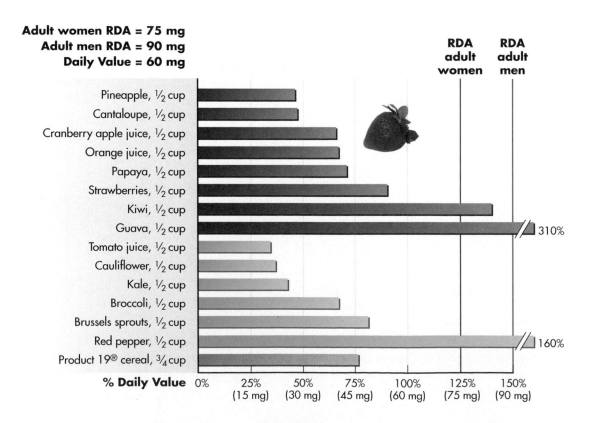

Figure 13-23 Food sources of vitamin C.

Vitamin C, the least stable vitamin, is easily lost in processing and cooking. Normal cooking can decrease vitamin C content up to 40%. This vitamin is very unstable when in contact with iron, copper, and oxygen. Juices are good foods to fortify with vitamin C because their acidity reduces vitamin C destruction.

Vitamin C Needs

The RDA for vitamin C for adult men is 90 mg/day; for adult women, it is 75 mg/day[3] and the Daily Value on food and supplement labels is 60 mg. Although average intakes in the U.S. exceed these amounts, a significant percentage of the population has low vitamin C intake and poor vitamin C status. Researchers have found that, in the U.S., 14% of men and 10% of women had serum vitamin C levels indicating vitamin C deficiency.[44] Another 34% of men and 27% of women had levels below normal but not yet in the deficiency range. Vitamin C deficiency was more common in young and middle-aged adults than in adolescents and seniors, perhaps because many teens eat fortified cereals and many seniors take vitamin supplements.

Smokers have a higher requirement for vitamin C; the RDA increases by 35 mg/day for those who smoke. Smoking creates oxidative stress, which probably increases vitamin C turnover. Currently, about 23% of the U.S. adult population are smokers. Thus, many Americans, especially smokers and poor eaters, may need more vitamin C in their diets. Vitamin C needs rise in other situations, too. Women using oral contraceptive agents may require additional vitamin C. Vitamin C needs also increase in burn and trauma patients because collagen synthesis increases greatly when rebuilding new tissue. These patients often are provided an extra 500 to 1000 mg of vitamin C per day.

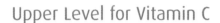

Oranges, limes, lemons, and kiwi fruit are all rich sources of vitamin C.

Upper Level for Vitamin C

The Upper Level for vitamin C is 2 g/day and is based on adverse gastrointestinal effects, such as bloating, stomach inflammation, and diarrhea.[3] High doses of vitamin C also can slightly increase the risk of kidney stone formation and of excess iron absorption, but only in those who are predisposed to form kidney stones and who have pre-existing iron absorption disorders (see Chapter 15). High doses of vitamin C can give false results in medical tests for blood in the stool. Persons taking large doses of vitamin C should discontinue the supplement before such tests. Informing your physician of your use of vitamin C and other nutrient supplements is a prudent practice.

Absorption, Transport, Storage, and Excretion of Vitamin C

The absorption of vitamin C occurs in the small intestine by active transport (for ascorbic acid) and by facilitated diffusion (for dehydroascorbic acid). The efficiency of the absorptive mechanism decreases as intake increases. About 70 to 90% of vitamin C is absorbed at daily intakes between 30 and 200 mg, whereas the rate of absorption declines substantially with doses exceeding that amount. Excretion by the kidneys rises as dietary intake increases.[43]

The amount of vitamin C stored varies widely by tissue. High concentrations are found in the pituitary and adrenal glands, white blood cells, eyes, and brain. The lowest concentrations are in the blood and saliva.

Functions of Vitamin C

Vitamin C performs a variety of important cell functions. It does so primarily by donating electrons in oxidation-reduction reactions.[43] As mentioned previously, substances that donate electrons become oxidized (lose electrons). As an electron donor, vitamin C has a cofactor role for several metalloenzymes and has antioxidant defense functions. **Metalloenzymes** contain metals, such as iron, copper, or zinc (usually as an ion), as a part of their structures. When a metalloenzyme catalyzes a reaction, the metal ion becomes oxidized. For example, reduced iron (ferrous, Fe^{2+}) is converted to its oxidized form (ferric, Fe^{3+}) during enzymatic activity. Ascorbic acid, by donating an electron to the oxidized iron, keeps the iron in its reduced ferrous form. This, in turn, allows enzymatic action to continue.

Collagen Synthesis

Collagen is the major fibrous protein that holds together the various structures of the body and gives strength to **connective tissue.** Collagen fibers are critical to the structure of bone and blood vessels, and they are essential in wound healing. A collagen molecule is like a 3-stranded rope—it consists of 3-polypeptide chains wound together to form a triple helix. Vitamin C is needed to get the 3 strands in the right shape to form the triple helix. Specifically, vitamin C helps convert the structure of 2 amino acids (lysine and proline) in collagen to hydroxylysine and hydroxyproline (Fig. 13-24). The function of vitamin C in the formation of these unusual amino acids is to interact with the metalloenzymes involved in making the conversions. Vitamin C, as a reducing agent, also keeps the iron in this metalloenzyme in the reduced Fe^{2+} form for the synthesis of other vital compounds.[43]

Synthesis of Other Vital Compounds

Vitamin C is required for the synthesis of many important biological compounds. In each case, vitamin C keeps the copper or iron in the metalloenzyme in the reduced state (as Cu^+ or Fe^{2+}). Some of the important compounds requiring vitamin C for synthesis are the amino acid tyrosine, the hormone thyroxine, the fatty acid transport compound carnitine, and the neurotransmitters norepinephrine, epinephrine, and serotonin. In addition, vitamin C is involved in the conversion of cholesterol to bile acids and biosynthesis of the hormones corticosteroids and aldosterone.

Antioxidant Activity

In vitro (in a test tube), vitamin C can be an antioxidant by donating electrons to free radicals. Recall that a free radical has an unpaired electron. A vitamin C molecule can donate electrons to free radicals so that they become stable. Researchers have proposed that vitamin C in the body's water-based fluids (e.g., blood) acts just as vitamin E does in lipid-rich environments. It also has been suggested that vitamin C can recycle vitamin E and make

connective tissue Cells and their protein products that hold different structures of the body together. Tendons and cartilage are composed largely of connective tissue. Connective tissue also forms part of bone and the non-muscular structures of arteries and veins.

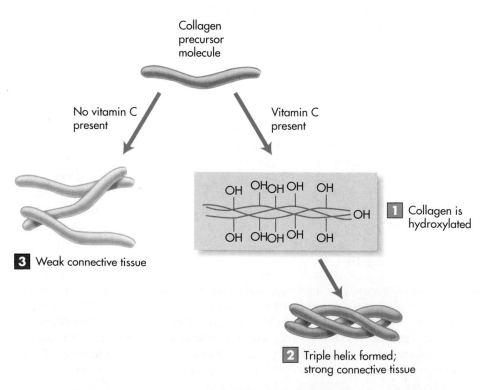

Figure 13-24 **Collagen synthesis requires Vitamin C.** ■1 Vitamin C is needed for the addition of hydroxyl groups (–OH) to the amino acid proline in collagen molecules. ■2 Collagen is unique among body proteins because it contains large amounts of the amino acid hydroxyproline, which is necessary for the formation of stable collagen fibers. ■3 Without sufficient vitamin C available to perform this task, only weak connective tissue is formed.

it function more effectively. Although these vitamin C antioxidant defense actions work well in a test tube, it's not known if vitamin C plays major or minor antioxidant roles in humans.[3] So far, some data suggest that vitamin C does have some important antioxidant effects. However, not all the results have been that positive. In fact, some research suggests that vitamin C can increase oxidative stress, such as in people with diabetes. Nonetheless, the high concentrations of vitamin C present in the eye possibly protect against photolytically generated free radicals. Likewise, high concentrations in **neutrophils**, a type of white blood cell, may be for protection against the free radicals produced during immune functions.[43]

Iron Absorption

Vitamin C with meals modestly facilitates the intestinal absorption of non-heme iron (iron that is not in hemoglobin) because of the conversion of iron in the GI tract to ferrous iron (Fe^{2+}). Vitamin C also counters the action of certain food components that inhibit iron absorption.[3]

Immune Function

White blood cells, part of the body's immune defenses, contain the highest vitamin C concentration of all body constituents. This may protect against the oxidative damage associated with cellular respiration. Free radicals generated during phagocytosis and neutrophil activation, although intended to kill bacteria or damaged tissue, also can damage the body's own immune cells. Vitamin C may reduce this self-destruction through its antioxidant defense actions. Vitamin C also may have other roles in immune function; however, supplemental vitamin C levels beyond the body's needs may not improve immune function.

Vitamin C Deficiency

A deficiency of vitamin C prevents the normal synthesis of collagen, thus causing widespread, significant changes in connective tissue throughout the body. The first signs and symptoms of scurvy, the vitamin C deficiency disease, appear after about 20 to 40 days on a diet free of vitamin C and include fatigue and pinpoint hemorrhages around hair follicles (Fig. 13-25). These hemorrhages are the most characteristic sign of scurvy. In addition, the gums and joints bleed, a classic sign of connective tissue failure. Other effects of scurvy include impaired wound healing, bone pain, fractures, and diarrhea. Psychological problems, such as depression, are common in advanced scurvy. Scurvy is fatal if not treated.[43]

Worldwide, scurvy is associated with poverty. It is especially common in infants who are fed boiled milk (all forms of milk are poor sources of vitamin C) and not given a good food source of vitamin C or a supplement. Although scurvy is considered rare in North America, poor vitamin C status is relatively common, as mentioned previously. Those with poor vitamin C status may have non-specific symptoms, including fatigue, gum bleeding, depression, and muscle pain. Alcoholics, those with poor diets, and smokers are at greatest risk.

Vitamin C, Cancer, and Heart disease

Because of its roles as an antioxidant and in promoting normal immune function, a great deal of research has examined vitamin C's ability to prevent both cancer and heart disease. For cancer, the evidence is best for cancers of the mouth, esophagus, stomach, and lung, but, not all studies are positive and it is still not known if vitamin C, either alone or in the diet, provides protection. Many researchers believe that a healthy diet, along with a healthy lifestyle, affords the best cancer prevention.

The situation is similar for vitamin C and heart disease. Many (but not all) studies suggest that good vitamin C status provides some protection against heart disease. This protection may be the result of vitamin C's role as an antioxidant. However, clinical trials of supplements of vitamins C and E (another antioxidant) have been disappointing.

▶ Although the development of scurvy in an otherwise healthy child is rare, it is possible. A 5-year-old boy developed scurvy after eating nothing but toaster pastries, cheese pizza, biscuits, and water for 5 months. The boy, who was growing and maturing normally, started to limp, his gums became swollen, and small purple spots began to appear on his skin. His baffled doctors finally diagnosed the boy as having scurvy and gave him vitamin C; his condition began to improve within a week.

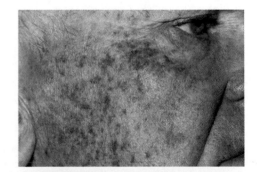
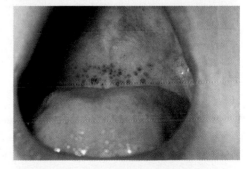

Figure 13-25 Pinpoint hemorrhages of the skin—an early symptom of scurvy. The spots on the skin are caused by slight bleeding. The person may experience poor wound healing. These are all signs of defective collagen synthesis.

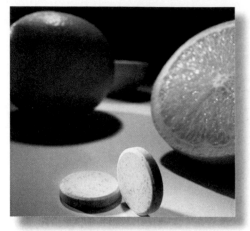

Oranges are a rich source of vitamin C. The many phytochemicals they provide are an additional benefit and are not found in vitamin C supplements.

Numerous scientific organizations, including the American Heart Association, have concluded that antioxidant supplements do not reduce the risk of heart disease.[45]

Vitamin C Intake above the RDA

Some popular authors and speakers advocate the consumption of vitamin C at amounts higher than the RDA. Surprisingly, there is little research comparing different vitamin C intake levels. If vitamin C intake is above about 100 mg/day, much of the additional vitamin C is excreted in the urine. Some research indicates that 200 mg/day is the highest amount needed to maximize the health benefits of vitamin C intake. Eating several vitamin C–rich foods each day can boost intakes to 200 mg/day.[43]

Vitamin C and the Common Cold

One aspect of high vitamin C intake (up to 1000 mg/day) that has drawn a lot of attention is its possible use for prevention or treatment of the common cold. Almost 40 studies have evaluated whether vitamin C can prevent or treat the common cold. These studies

Table 13-3 A Summary of Water-Soluble Vitamins

Vitamin	Major Functions	Deficiency Symptoms	People Most at Risk
Thiamin	Coenzyme in carbohydrate metabolism and energy release	Beriberi: anorexia, weight loss, weakness, peripheral neuropathy; Wernicke-Korsakoff syndrome	Alcoholics and people living in poverty
Riboflavin	Coenzyme in numerous oxidation-reduction reactions, including those of energy release	Ariboflavinosis: inflammation of mouth and tongue, cracks at corner of mouth	People taking certain medications if no dairy products are consumed
Niacin	Coenzyme in numerous oxidation-reduction reactions in energy metabolism, synthesis and breakdown of fatty acids	Pellagra: diarrhea, dermatitis, dementia (death)	Alcoholics and people living in poverty where corn is the dominant food
Pantothenic acid	Coenzyme in energy metabolism and fatty-acid synthesis	Weakness, fatigue, impaired muscle function, GI tract disturbances; deficiency very rare	None
Biotin	Cofactor for carboxylase enzymes that participate in fatty-acid, amino acid, and energy metabolism	Dermatitis, conjunctivitis, hair loss, nervous system abnormalities; deficiency very rare	Infants with a certain genetic defect
Vitamin B-6 (pyridoxine)	Coenzyme in amino acid metabolism, heme synthesis, lipid metabolism; homocysteine metabolism	Dermatitis, anemia, convulsions, depression, confusion	Alcoholics
Folate	Coenzyme in DNA synthesis, homocysteine metabolism	Megaloblastic (macrocytic) anemia, birth defects	Alcoholics, pregnant women, people on certain medications
Vitamin B-12 (cobalamin)	Coenzyme affecting folate metabolism, homocysteine metabolism	Megaloblastic (macrocytic) anemia, paresthesia, pernicious anemia	Older adults, vegans, patients with malabsorption syndromes
Vitamin C (ascorbic acid)	Collagen synthesis, some antioxidant capability, hormone and neurotransmitter synthesis	Scurvy: poor wound healing, pinpoint hemorrhages, bleeding gums	Alcoholics, individuals who eat few fruits and vegetables, smokers
Choline	Precursor for acetylcholine and phospholipids; homocysteine metabolism	No natural deficiency	None

suggest that any beneficial effect of vitamin C supplementation is very modest, perhaps reducing cold duration by 1 day per year in adults. Marathon runners, cross-country skiers, and soldiers training in sub-arctic environments had a slightly greater reduction in cold symptoms. At this point, despite its popularity, supplemental vitamin C cannot be recommended to prevent or treat common colds.[46]

As you can see, the water-soluble vitamins and choline play important roles in the body. Table 13-3 provides a summary of water-soluble vitamins.

CRITICAL THINKING

Carlos just saw an advertisement claiming that vitamin C will cure just about everything from colds to heart disease. How would you explain to him vitamin C's main functions in the human body?

Knowledge Check

1. How does vitamin C aid in the function of metalloenzymes in cells?
2. What are 4 good sources of vitamin C?
3. Impaired synthesis of what compound is responsible for the symptoms of scurvy, such as bleeding gums, easy bruising, and pinpoint hemorrhages?

Dietary Sources	RDA or Adequate Intake	Toxicity*
Pork and pork products, enriched and whole-grain cereals, eggs, nuts, legumes	Men: 1.2 mg/day; women: 1.1 mg/day	None recognized
Milk and milk products, mushrooms, eggs, liver, enriched grains	Men: 1.3 mg/day; women: 1.1 mg/day	None recognized
Meat, poultry, fish, enriched and whole-grain breads and cereals, tryptophan conversion to niacin	Men: 16 mg NE/day; women: 14 mg NE/day	Flushing of skin; Upper Level for adults is 35 mg/day from supplements, based on flushing of skin
Widely distributed in foods	Adequate Intake for adults: 5 mg/day	None recognized
Widely distributed in foods	Adequate Intake for adults: 30 μg/day	Unknown
Animal protein foods, potatoes, bananas, legumes, avocados	Adults 19–50: 1.3 mg/day; men over 50: 1.7 mg/day; women over 50: 1.5 mg/day	None from food but excess intake from supplements causes neuropathy, skin lesions; Upper Level is 100 mg/day, based on nerve destruction
Green vegetables, liver, enriched cereal products, legumes, oranges	400 μg/day of dietary folate equivalents	None; Upper Level for adults set at 1000 μg/day for synthetic folic acid, exclusive of food folate, based on masking vitamin B-12 deficiency
Animal foods and fortified ready-to-eat breakfast cereals	Adults 19–50: 2.4 μg/day; adults 51 and older: same, but use of fortified foods or supplements to meet needs is recommended	None recognized
Citrus fruits, papayas, strawberries, broccoli, potatoes, greens	Men: 90 mg/day; women: 75 mg/day; + additional 35 mg/day for smokers	Diarrhea and other GI tract problems; Upper Level is 2 g/day, based on development of diarrhea
Widely distributed in foods, plus self synthesis	Adequate Intake for men: 550 mg/day; women: 425 mg/day	Upper Level is 3.5 g/day, based on development of fishy body odor and reduced blood pressure

* Toxicity arises only from supplement use

13.12 Vitamin-Like Compounds

The vitamin-like compounds discussed in this section—carnitine and taurine—are necessary to maintain normal metabolism in the body. They can be synthesized by the body, but their biosynthesis often occurs at the expense of other nutrients, such as essential amino acids. The need for these compounds often increases during times of rapid tissue growth, as in preterm infants.[47] Deficiencies of these vitamin-like compounds do not exist in the average healthy adult. Nevertheless, more research is needed to clarify if metabolism is impaired or altered during certain disease states and whether the compounds should be included in infant formulas and total parenteral nutrition solutions. Currently, many manufacturers add these vitamin-like compounds to infant formulas.

Carnitine

Human needs for carnitine are met from both animal foods and biosynthesis in the liver from the amino acids lysine and methionine.[47] Meat and dairy products are the main sources of carnitine; little is found in foods of plant origin. We consume about 100 to 300 mg/day.

Within the cell, carnitine transports fatty acids from the cytosol into the mitochondria, where fatty acids are metabolized for energy. Carnitine also aids the mitochondria in removing excess organic acids produced by metabolic pathways. In addition, carnitine has displayed pharmaceutical usefulness in the removal of compounds that can build to toxic amounts in people with inborn errors of metabolism. Dosages approximately 10 times typical dietary intakes also have been shown to improve the condition of persons with progressive muscle disease and heart muscle deterioration. Although carnitine supplements have been promoted as a weight-loss or exercise aid, the research on these uses is very limited.

Adults and children who are severely malnourished or on total parenteral nutrition can have low concentrations of carnitine in their blood. Inadequate protein intake (e.g., a lack of the amino acids needed for making carnitine) leads to abnormal fatty-acid metabolism. Even though vegetarian diets are very low in carnitine, vegetarians show normal blood concentrations of carnitine. Consequently, it is doubtful that carnitine is necessary in the diets of healthy people. Carnitine may be considered a conditionally essential nutrient in times of recovery from disease and malnutrition, serious trauma, cirrhosis, kidney dialysis, or preterm birth.

Taurine

Taurine is synthesized in the body from the sulfur-containing amino acids methionine and cysteine. It is abundant in muscle, platelets, and nerve tissue. It also is attached to bile acids. Dietary sources include only foods of animal origin. North Americans consume about 40 to 400 mg/day.

Although its functions are not well understood, taurine is involved in many vital functions. It is associated with photoreceptor activity in the eye, antioxidant defense activity in white blood cells and the lungs, normal nervous system function, platelet aggregation, cardiac contraction, insulin action, and cell differentiation and growth.[47] There is no scientific evidence that taurine controls nervous system conditions (e.g., epileptic seizures, motor tics, and facial twitches) or prevents cardiovascular disease or cataracts. No clear cases of taurine deficiencies have been diagnosed in vegans, even though it is not found in plants, suggesting that synthesis by the body meets needs. Thus, it appears that healthy people need not worry about consuming taurine.

Taurine supplementation may be of benefit to children with cystic fibrosis. Some of these children experience improved growth when treated with taurine, perhaps because of increased fat absorption from the action of taurine as part of bile. Preterm infants supplemented with taurine also may exhibit improved fat absorption.

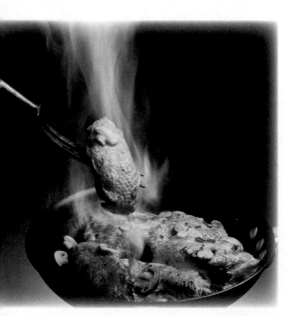

Foods of animal origin are rich in carnitine and taurine.

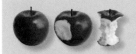

Take Action

Spotting Fraudulent Claims for Vitamins and Vitamin-Like Substances

Using your favorite search engine, search terms such as *energy boost, stress, mental acuity,* and *disease prevention,* along with *vitamin supplement.* Identify several claims for vitamin supplements that you consider fraudulent or misleading.

1. What is the cost of these supplements?

2. How do the amounts of vitamins they contain compare with the DRIs?

3. What compounds are included that are not considered essential nutrients?

4. What disclaimers or warnings are made about the products?

5. How likely is the supplement to improve a person's health?

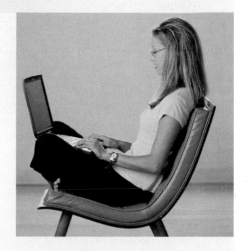

CASE STUDY FOLLOW-UP

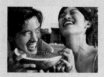

Suzanne and Ted should remember that spina bifida is caused by a failure of the spinal cord to close during the first 28 days of pregnancy, a time when neither Ted nor Suzanne may realize that Suzanne is pregnant. The B-vitamin folate must be available at the time of conception to prevent spina bifida and other birth defects. The fact that a close relative of Suzanne's has already produced a child with this birth defect should be a warning sign. Suzanne and Ted would be wise to seek the advice of a registered dietitian to ensure that Suzanne's prepregnancy diet provides enough synthetic folic acid.

Summary

13.1 The water-soluble vitamins are the 8 B-vitamins and vitamin C. A dietary source of choline also is required. The B-vitamins function as coenzymes. Deficiency symptoms typically show up in the skin, GI tract, brain, and nervous system. The water-soluble vitamins are generally stored in the body to a lesser extent than the fat-soluble vitamins. Compared with fat-soluble vitamins, water-soluble vitamins are more easily destroyed during cooking. Cereals and grains are enriched with thiamin, riboflavin, niacin, and folic acid.

13.2 Thiamin in its functional form as TPP serves as a coenzyme in energy release. Thiamin deficiency results in the disease beriberi. In North America, alcoholics are at risk of thiamin deficiency. Pork, pork products, and enriched grains are reliable sources of thiamin.

13.3 Riboflavin coenzymes, FAD and FMN, participate in a wide variety of oxidation reduction reactions, including those in numerous metabolic pathways that produce energy. A specific riboflavin deficiency is unlikely but could accompany other B-vitamin deficiencies. Dairy products and enriched grains are good dietary sources.

13.4 Niacin as NAD^+ and $NADP^+$ are coenzymes. NAD^+ is important in oxidation-reduction reactions in energy-yielding pathways. A deficiency of the vitamin produces the disease pellagra, which is seen most often in corn-based diets. Alcoholism can lead to a deficiency. Food sources of niacin are enriched cereal grains and protein foods. The body is able to synthesize the vitamin from the amino acid tryptophan. Megadoses of niacin produce a variety of toxic symptoms.

13.5 Among its functions, pantothenic acid in coenzyme form (CoA) shuttles 2 carbon fragments from the metabolism of glucose, amino acids, fatty acids, and alcohol into the citric acid cycle during energy metabolism. A deficiency of pantothenic acid is unlikely because it is widely distributed in foods.

13.6 Biotin functions as a cofactor in enzymes that add carbon dioxide to a substance. Biotin is widely distributed in foods. Intestinal bacteria also synthesize biotin. No deficiency exists in healthy people.

13.7 The vitamin B-6 coenzyme PLP participates in amino acid metabolism, especially the synthesis of non-essential amino acids. It is essential in the synthesis of heme in hemoglobin, the formation of certain neurotransmitters, and the metabolism of homocysteine. Anemia, convulsions, and decreased immune response are symptoms of a deficiency. Animal protein foods, a few fruits and vegetables, and whole-grain cereals are good sources of this vitamin. Toxic effects from excess consumption include nerve damage.

13.8 Folate in its many coenzyme forms (tetrahydrofolic acid) accepts and donates 1-carbon groups. The most notable function performed by folate is in DNA synthesis. It also participates in homocysteine metabolism. A dietary lack of this vitamin produces megaloblastic anemia and increases the risk of spina bifida. Deficiency is common among alcoholics. Folate is found in green vegetables, legumes, liver, and fortified cereal grains.

13.9 Vitamin B-12 in its coenzyme form transfers 1-carbon groups. Because of its interaction with folate, a deficiency of vitamin B-12 results in the same type of megaloblastic anemia, as well as excess homocysteine in the blood. Defective absorption of vitamin B-12 is the cause of the deficiency disease pernicious anemia. In such cases, injection of the vitamin or another pharmacological approach is necessary. Vitamin B-12 is found in animal foods, but not in plant foods. Vegans need to look for foods fortified with the vitamin or take it as part of a multivitamin and mineral supplement.

13.10 Choline is a dietary component that is available from a wide variety of foods and is synthesized in the body. Choline is required for the formation of the neurotransmitter acetylcholine and it is incorporated into phospholipids. No natural deficiency of choline has been reported.

13.11 Vitamin C functions as an electron donor in many processes, including the synthesis of collagen, a protein in connective tissue. A deficiency of vitamin C causes the disease scurvy. Fresh fruits and vegetables are reliable sources of this vitamin. Like folate, vitamin C is destroyed by heat. Among North Americans, alcoholics, smokers, and individuals who do not eat many fruits or vegetables are most likely to develop a deficiency.

13.12 Carnitine and taurine, although participating in many important biochemical reactions in the body, are not true vitamins because they can be synthesized in the body from readily available precursors. In some medical circumstances, dietary intake may be needed to augment cellular production.

Study Questions

1. When compared with whole-grain products, enriched cereals and grains provide the same or higher amounts of all of the B-vitamins.
   a. true
   b. false

2. Thiamin pyrophosphate (TPP) is required for _____.
   a. protein synthesis
   b. fatty-acid synthesis
   c. carbohydrate metabolism
   d. DNA synthesis

3. Thiamin deficiency can be found among _____.
   a. heavy users of alcohol
   b. poor people in developing countries reliant on white rice as a staple food
   c. poor people in developing countries reliant on corn as a staple food
   d. both a and b
   e. both a and c

4. Which of the following water-soluble vitamins participate in oxidation-reduction reactions?
   a. thiamin, riboflavin, niacin
   b. folate, vitamin B-12, vitamin B-6
   c. biotin, pantothenic acid, niacin
   d. vitamin C, riboflavin, niacin

5. An alcoholic who consumes no dairy products is most at risk of developing _____ deficiency.
   a. choline   c. riboflavin
   b. vitamin B-6   d. thiamin

6. Niacin can be synthesized in cells from _____.
   a. riboflavin   c. glucose
   b. fatty acids   d. tryptophan

7. Deficiencies of _____ and _____ are extremely rare.
   a. biotin; pantothenic acid   c. vitamin B-12; folate
   b. vitamin C; niacin   d. vitamin C; folate

8. Transamination reactions allow the formation of non-essential amino acids. Which vitamin is required for these reactions?

   a. folate
   b. vitamin B-12
   c. riboflavin
   d. vitamin B-6

9. The absorption of folic acid in supplements and fortified foods exceeds that of folate found in foods.

   a. true
   b. false

10. Good sources of folate include _____.

    a. lentils, spinach, asparagus, and fortified foods
    b. papayas, limes, oranges, and potatoes
    c. dairy products, fortified foods, and nuts
    d. tuna, chicken, beef, and dairy products

11. The prevention of neural tube defects is best achieved by _____.

    a. good folate status prior to becoming pregnant
    b. folic acid supplementation in the second half of pregnancy
    c. folic acid supplementation during infancy
    d. all of the above

12. Macrocytic anemia, peripheral neuropathy, and impaired cognitive function are signs of _____ deficiency.

    a. ascorbic acid
    b. niacin
    c. vitamin B-12
    d. vitamin B-6

13. Sources of vitamin B-12 include _____.

    a. whole grains, tuna, and eggs
    b. dairy products, meat, and fish
    c. citrus fruits, papayas, and bananas
    d. dairy products, whole grains, and leafy green vegetables

14. Vitamin C is required for the formation of _____, required to synthesize collagen.

    a. tryptophan
    b. serotonin
    c. hydroxyproline
    d. acetyl-CoA

15. Ingesting 1000 mg of supplemental vitamin C per day has been proven to prevent common colds.

    a. true
    b. false

Answer Key: 1-b; 2-c; 3-d; 4-d; 5-c; 6-d; 7-a; 8-d; 9-a; 10-a; 11-a; 12-c; 13-b; 14-c; 15-b

Websites

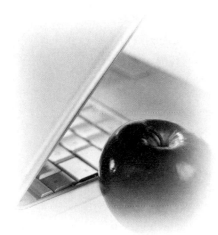

To learn more about the topics covered in this chapter, visit these websites.

Water-Soluble Vitamins

www.hsph.harvard.edu/nutritionsource/vitamins.html

www.fda.gov/consumer/updates/vitamins111907.html

lpi.oregonstate.edu/infocenter/vitamins.html

dietary-supplements.info.nih.gov/Health_Information/Vitamin_and_Mineral_Supplement_Fact_Sheets.aspx.

Beriberi

www.emedicine.com/med/topic221.htm

nobelprize.org/educational_games/medicine/vitamin_b1/eijkman.html

Scurvy

www.emedicine.com/ped/topic2073.htm

Pellagra

www.emedicine.com/ped/topic1755.htm

history.nih.gov/exhibits/Goldberger/docs/pellegra_5.htm

Pernicious Anemia

www.nhlbi.nih.gov/health/dci/Diseases/prnanmia/prnanmia_what.html

www.emedicine.com/med/topic1799.htm

Neural Tube Defects

www.sbaa.org

www.marchofdimes.com

References

1. Rosenfeld L. Vitamine-vitamin. The early years of discovery. *Clin Chem.* 1997;43:680.

2. Food and Nutrition Board, Institute of Medicine. *Dietary Reference Intakes for thiamin, riboflavin, niacin, vitamin B-6, folate, vitamin B-12, pantothenic acid, biotin and choline.* Washington, DC: National Academy Press; 1998.

3. Food and Nutrition Board, Institute of Medicine. *Dietary Reference Intakes for vitamin C, vitamin E, selenium, and carotenoids.* Washington, DC: National Academy Press; 2000.

4. Cotton PA and others. Dietary sources of nutrients among US adults, 1994 to 1996. *J Am Diet Assoc.* 2004;104:921.

5. Butterworth F. *Thiamin.* In: Shils M and others, eds. *Modern nutrition in health and disease.* 10th ed. Philadelphia: Lippincott Williams & Wilkins; 2006.

6. Gropper S and others. *Advanced nutrition and human metabolism.* Belmont, CA: Thomson Wadsworth; 2005.

7. Krishna S and others. Thiamine deficiency and malaria in adults from southeast Asia. *Lancet.* 1999;353:546.

8. U.S. National Library of Medicine, National Institutes of Health. Thiamin (thiamine), vitamin B1. 2005; http://www.nlm.nih.gov/medlineplus/druginfo/natural/patient-thiamin.html.

9. McCormick D. *Riboflavin.* In: Shils M and others, eds. *Modern nutrition in health and disease.* 10th ed. Philadelphia: Lippincott Williams & Wilkins; 2006.

10. Powers HJ. Riboflavin (vitamin B-2) and health. *Am J Clin Nutr.* 2003;77:1352.

11. Park Y and others. Effectiveness of food fortification in the United States: The case of pellagra. *Am J Publ Health.* 2000;90:727.

12. Bourgeois C and others. *Niacin.* In: Shils M and others, eds. *Modern nutrition in health and disease.* 10th ed. Philadelphia: Lippincott Williams & Wilkins; 2006.

13. Prinzo ZW. Pellagra and its prevention and control in major emergencies. 2007; http://whqlibdoc.who.int/hq/2000/WHO_NHD_00.10.pdf.

14. Seal A and others. Low and deficient niacin status and pellagra are endemic in postwar Angola. *Am J Clin Nutr.* 2007;85:218.

15. American Heart Association. Cholesterol-lowering drugs. 2008; www.americanheart.org.

16. Trumbo T. *Pantothenic acid.* In: Shils M and others, eds. *Modern nutrition in health and disease.* 10th ed. Philadelphia: Lippincott Williams & Wilkins; 2006.

17. Mock D. *Biotin.* In: Shils M and others, eds. *Modern nutrition in health and disease.* 10th ed. Philadelphia: Lippincott Williams & Wilkins; 2006.

18. Kaye CI and the Committee on Genetics. Newborn screening fact sheets. *Pediatr.* 2006;118:e934.

19. Mackey A and others. *Vitamin B6.* In: Shils M and others, eds. *Modern nutrition in health and disease.* 10th ed. Philadelphia: Lippincott Williams & Wilkins; 2006.

20. Autiero E and others. Pyridoxine hydrochloride treatment of carpal tunnel syndrome: A review. *Nutr Rev.* 2004;62:96.

21. Connolly M. Premenstrual syndrome: An update on definitions, diagnosis and management. *Adv Psychiatr Treat.* 2001;7:469.

22. Wyatt K and others. Efficacy of vitamin B-6 in the treatment of premenstrual syndrome: Systemic review. *Br J Med.* 1999;318:1375.

23. Jewell D, Young G. Interventions for nausea and vomiting in early pregnancy. *Cochrane Database of Systematic Reviews.* 2003;4:CD000145.

24. Carmel R. *Folate.* In: Shils M and others, eds. *Modern nutrition in health and disease.* 10th ed. Philadelphia: Lippincott Williams & Wilkins; 2006.

25. Winkels R and others. Bioavailability of food folates is 80% of that of folic acid. *Am J Clin Nutr.* 2007;85:465.

26. National Institutes of Health, Office of Dietary Supplements. Dietary supplement fact sheet: Folate. 2005; ods.od.nih.gov/factsheets/folate.asp.

27. Taylor MJ and others. Folate for depressive disorders. *Cochrane Database of Systematic Reviews.* 2003;2:CD003390.

28. March of Dimes. Folic acid. 2005; www.marchofdimes.com/pnhec/173_769.asp.

29. Williams LJ and others. Decline in the prevalence of spina bifida and anencephaly by race/ethnicity: 1995–2002. *Pediatr.* 2005;116:580.

30. Carmel R. *Cobalamin (vitamin B-12).* In: Shils M and others, eds. *Modern nutrition in health and disease.* 10th ed. Philadelphia: Lippincott Williams & Wilkins; 2006.

31. Wolters M and others. Cobalamin: A critical vitamin in the elderly. *Prev Med.* 2004;39:1256.

32. Ting RZ-W and others. Risk factors of vitamin B12 deficiency in patients receiving metformin. *Arch Int Med.* 2006;166:1975.

33. Sato Y and others. Effect of folate and mecobalamin on hip fractures in patients with stroke: A randomized controlled trial. *JAMA.* 2005;293:1082.

34. Loscalzo J. Homocysteine trials—Clear outcomes for complex reasons. *N Engl J Med.* 2006;354:1629.

35. Albert CM and others. Effects of folic acid and B vitamins on risk of cardiovascular events and total mortality among women at high risk for cardiovascular disease. *JAMA*. 2008; 299:2027.

36. Balk E and others. Vitamin B6, B12, and folic acid supplementation and cognitive function. A systematic review of randomized trials. *Arch Intern Med*. 2007;167:21.

37. Campbell A and others. Plasma vitamin B-12 concentrations in an elderly Latino population are predicted by serum gastrin concentrations and crystalline vitamin B-12 intake. *J Nutr*. 2003;133:2770.

38. Alpers DH. What is new in vitamin B12? *Curr Opin Gastroenterol*. 2005;21:183.

39. Nilsson M and others. Medical intelligence in Sweden. Vitamin B12: Oral compared with parenteral? *Postgrad Med J*. 2005;81:191.

40. Zeisel S, Niculescu M. *Choline and phosphaotidalcholine*. In: Shils M and others, eds. *Modern nutrition in health and disease*. 10th ed. Philadelphia: Lippincott Williams & Wilkins; 2006.

41. Patterson K and others. USDA database for the choline content of common food. Release 2. 2008; www.nal.usda.gov/fnic/foodcomp/Data/Choline/Choln02.pdf.

42. Detopoulou P and others. Dietary choline and betaine intakes in relation to concentrations of inflammatory markers in healthy adults: The ATTICA study. *Am J Clin Nutr*. 2008;87:424.

43. Levine M and others. *Vitamin C*. In: Shils M and others, eds. *Modern nutrition in health and disease*. 10th ed. Philadelphia: Lippincott Williams & Wilkins; 2006.

44. Hampl J and others. Vitamin C deficiency and depletion in the United States: The Third National Health and Nutrition Examination Survey, 1988 to 1994. *Am J Public Health*. 2004;94:870.

45. Lichtenstein A, Russell R. Essential nutrients: Food or supplements. Where should the emphasis be? *JAMA*. 2005;294:351.

46. Douglas RM and others. Vitamin C for preventing and treating the common cold. *Cochrane Database of Systematic Reviews*. 2007;3:CD000980.

47. Combs G. *Vitamins*. In: Mahan L, Escott-Stump S, eds. *Krause's food, nutrition, and diet therapy*. 11th ed. Philadelphia: WB Saunders; 2004.

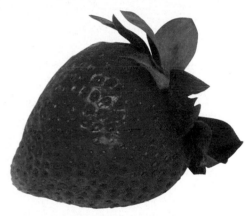

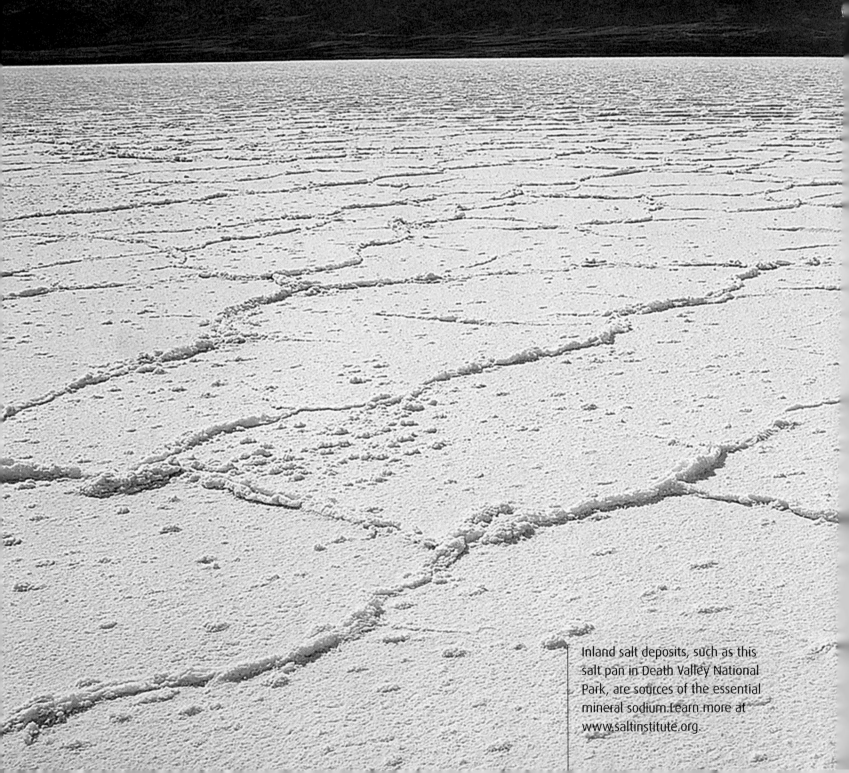

14 Water and Major Minerals

Inland salt deposits, such as this salt pan in Death Valley National Park, are sources of the essential mineral sodium. Learn more at www.saltinstitute.org.

STUDENT LEARNING OUTCOMES

After studying this chapter, you will be able to

1. Describe the factors that influence water balance and how it is maintained in the body.

2. Discuss how both dehydration and water intoxication develop and how to prevent them.

3. Identify food sources of water and major minerals.

4. Explain the functions of water and major minerals in the body.

5. Discuss the problems with low and high intakes of major minerals and how to avoid inadequate or excessive intakes.

6. Explain the role of nutrition in the prevention and treatment of hypertension.

7. Estimate and evaluate adequacy of dietary calcium intake.

8. Describe the role of nutrition in bone health and in the prevention of osteoporosis.

Pound for pound, our bodies contain more water than any other component. After oxygen, water is the most important ingredient needed for life. Without water, biological processes—and life—cease within a matter of days. Because we cannot store this crucial nutrient, we must regularly replenish the water lost from the body. Water needs vary, depending on physical activity, environmental conditions (e.g., temperature and humidity), individual characteristics, and nutrient intake, especially protein and minerals.

Many minerals also are vital to health. These inorganic substances are critical to many body functions, including cell metabolism, nerve impulse transmission, and growth and development.[1,2] Typical diets in developed countries contain sufficient amounts of most minerals, either as natural components of foods or as additives through enrichment and fortification. Although severe deficiencies of minerals are rare in developed countries, many people have lower than optimal intakes of some minerals, such as calcium, potassium, iron, and iodine, and higher than recommended intakes of others, such as sodium. Deficiencies of certain minerals remain a major public health concern in less developed countries.

Minerals often are divided into 2 categories: major and trace minerals. Major minerals are those that are present and required in larger amounts in the body. They include sodium, potassium, and chloride, which are especially important in maintaining water and ion balance in cells. The other major minerals are calcium, phosphorus, magnesium, and sulfur. As you'll see in Chapter 15, the dietary requirements for trace minerals, such as iron and zinc, are small when compared with those for major minerals. This chapter will first explore water and its roles in the body, then will continue with the major minerals and their importance in human nutrition.

483

14.1 Water

Each of the trillions of cells in the body contains and is surrounded by water (Fig. 14-1). Thus, it is no surprise that maintaining the right amount and balance of water in the body is essential to life. An adult can survive for several weeks without food, but only several days without water. This difference in survival time between food and water occurs not because water is more important than carbohydrate, fat, protein, vitamins, or minerals but, rather, because the body has no storage site for water.

Water in the Body: Intracellular and Extracellular Fluid

Water is the largest component of the human body, making up 50 to 75% of body weight, depending on age and body fat content. Water content is highest in infants and children and declines as we age. About 55% of an adult's body weight is water—that's about 10 gallons (40 liters) in a person weighing 160 pounds.[3] Lean individuals have a greater percentage of body water than those who are obese because lean tissue contains about 73% water, whereas adipose tissue is only 20% water.

Body water is found in 2 body compartments—the **intracellular** compartment, or that inside cells, and the **extracellular** compartment, or that outside cells (Fig. 14-2). Almost two-thirds of body water is found in the intracellular fluid compartment. The rest is in the extracellular fluid, where it is divided into 2 additional compartments: **interstitial fluid**, the fluid between cells, and **intravascular fluid**, the fluid in the blood and lymph.

Figure 14-1 Water and minerals are involved in many processes in the body.

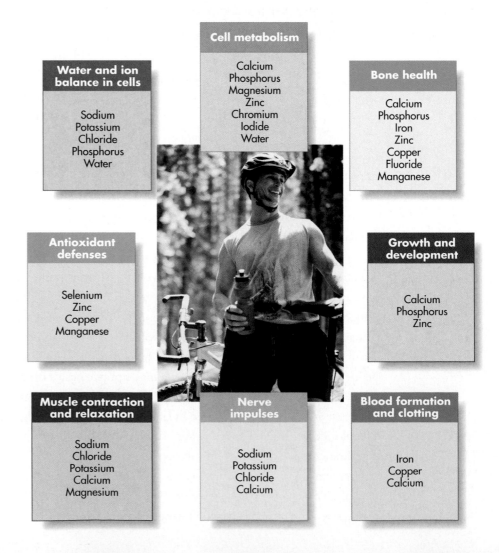

Water and ion balance in cells
Sodium
Potassium
Chloride
Phosphorus
Water

Cell metabolism
Calcium
Phosphorus
Magnesium
Zinc
Chromium
Iodide
Water

Bone health
Calcium
Phosphorus
Iron
Zinc
Copper
Fluoride
Manganese

Antioxidant defenses
Selenium
Zinc
Copper
Manganese

Growth and development
Calcium
Phosphorus
Zinc

Muscle contraction and relaxation
Sodium
Chloride
Potassium
Calcium
Magnesium

Nerve impulses
Sodium
Potassium
Chloride
Calcium

Blood formation and clotting
Iron
Copper
Calcium

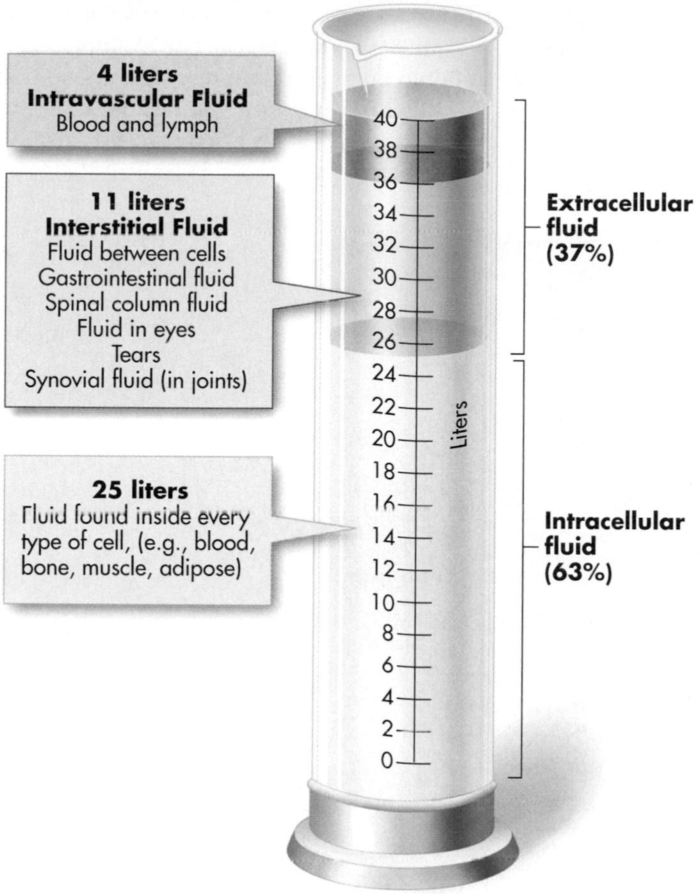
4 liters
Intravascular Fluid
Blood and lymph
11 liters
Interstitial Fluid
Fluid between cells
Gastrointestinal fluid
Spinal column fluid
Fluid in eyes
Tears
Synovial fluid (in joints)
25 liters
Fluid found inside every type of cell, (e.g., blood, bone, muscle, adipose)
40
38
36
34
32
30
28
26
24
22
20
18
16
14
12
10
8
6
4
2
0
Liters
Extracellular fluid (37%)
Intracellular fluid (63%)

Figure 14-2 **Fluid compartments in the body. Total fluid volume is about 10 gallons (40 liters).**

The fluid within these compartments is not pure water; it also contains dissolved substances known as **solutes**. The most abundant solutes are **electrolytes** that form when salts, such as sodium chloride or potassium phosphate, dissociate in solution and form **ions** (charged particles). The major positively charged electrolytes **(cations)** and the negatively charged electrolytes **(anions)** found in each fluid compartment vary (Table 14-1). Intracellular fluid contains potassium and magnesium cations, along with negatively charged phosphate anions. In extracellular fluid, positively charged sodium cations and the negatively charged chloride anions, along with bicarbonate (HCO^{3-}), predominate.

Maintenance of Water Balance

The body controls the amount of water in each compartment mainly by controlling the electrolyte concentrations in the compartments. An extremely sophisticated gatekeeping

Table 14-1 Electrolytes in Intracellular and Extracellular Fluid

Intracellular Fluid	Extracellular Fluid
Major Cations	**Major Cations**
• Potassium (K^+)	• Sodium (Na^+)
• Magnesium (Mg^{2+})	• Calcium (Ca^{2+})
Major Anions	**Major Anions**
• Phosphate*	• Chloride (Cl^-)
• Sulfate (SO^{4-})	• Bicarbonate (HCO^{3-})

*Can ionize in different forms.
Note: Organic acids and proteins also contribute positive and negative charges in body fluids.

concentration gradient Difference in the concentration of a solute from one area to another. Normally, a solute moves from where it is most concentrated to where it is least concentrated. When sodium is pumped outside the cell and potassium pumped inside the cell, they are moving instead to where each is most concentrated—that is, against the concentration gradient.

system involving pumping mechanisms keeps intra- and extracellular water volume and electrolyte concentrations within quite narrow ranges. For example, a specific protein located in the cell membrane can pump potassium ions into and sodium ions out of a cell (Fig. 14-3). Energy is used by this sodium-potassium pump to move each ion against its **concentration gradient**.

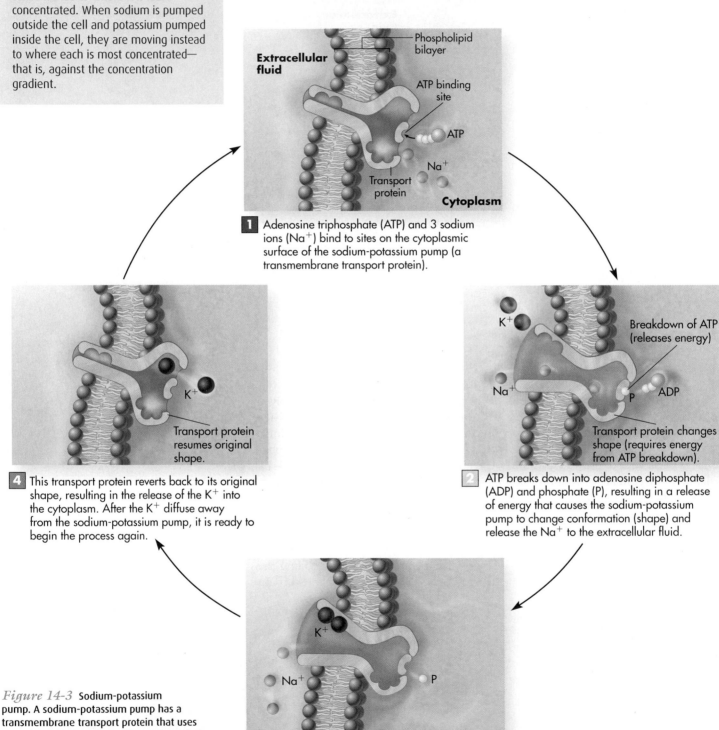

1 Adenosine triphosphate (ATP) and 3 sodium ions (Na$^+$) bind to sites on the cytoplasmic surface of the sodium-potassium pump (a transmembrane transport protein).

2 ATP breaks down into adenosine diphosphate (ADP) and phosphate (P), resulting in a release of energy that causes the sodium-potassium pump to change conformation (shape) and release the Na$^+$ to the extracellular fluid.

3 As the 3 Na$^+$ diffuse away from the sodium-potassium pump into the extracellular fluid, 2 K$^+$ from the extracellular fluid bind to sites on the extracellular surface of the sodium-potassium pump. At the same time, the phosphate produced earlier by ATP hydrolysis is released into the cytoplasm.

4 This transport protein reverts back to its original shape, resulting in the release of the K$^+$ into the cytoplasm. After the K$^+$ diffuse away from the sodium-potassium pump, it is ready to begin the process again.

Figure 14-3 Sodium-potassium pump. A sodium-potassium pump has a transmembrane transport protein that uses energy to transport Na and K ions through the membrane from a region of low concentration to a region of high concentration. This maintains a high concentration of Na$^+$ outside the cell and a high concentration of K$^+$ inside the cell. The continuous active transport can be broken into 4 steps.

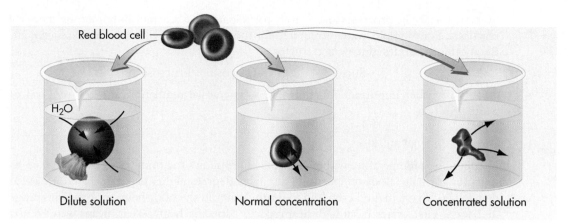

Red blood cell

H₂O

Dilute solution   Normal concentration   Concentrated solution

(a) A dilute solution with a low ion concentration results in swelling (*black arrows*) and subsequent rupture (*puff of red in the lower left part of the cell*) of a red blood cell placed into the solution.

(b) A normal concentration (a concentration of ions outside the cell equal to that inside the cell) results in a typically shaped red blood cell. Water moves into and out of the cell in equilibrium (*black arrows*), but there is no net water movement.

(c) A solution with a high ion concentration causes shrinkage of the red blood cell as water moves out of the cell and into the concentrated solution (*black arrows*).

Figure 14-4 Red blood cells affected by various ion concentrations. Osmosis causes fluid to shift in and out of the cells, depending on the ion concentration in the surrounding solution.

Water is attracted to electrolytes and other ions and thus moves via osmosis from one fluid compartment to another as the concentration of solutes change. **Osmosis** is the passive diffusion of water across a semipermeable membrane—in the body, these are cell membranes. When the concentration of solutes (mainly electrolytes) differs on the 2 sides of a cell membrane, water will move from the side with a low solute concentration to the side with the higher solute concentration. Examples of osmosis that may be familiar to you are pulling water out of strawberries by sprinkling them with sugar and crisping limp celery by placing it in water—water moves into the dehydrated celery cells.

Figure 14-4 illustrates how osmosis works. Figure 14-4*a* shows water moving from the dilute solution into the more concentrated red blood cell, which causes the cell to swell and possibly burst. In Figure 14-4*b*, there is no net movement of water because solute concentrations are equal on both sides of the cell's semipermeable membrane. However, in Figure 14-4*c*, water is drawn across the red blood cell's membrane into the concentrated solution surrounding it, causing the cell to shrink. In the body, the actual movement of water across the cell membrane is not quite as simple. Cell membranes are mainly lipid (and poorly permeable to water); thus, in many cells, water moves through water channels made from special proteins called aquaporins.

Adding water—instead of ions—to a water compartment dilutes its solute concentration, so the compartment tends to donate water by moving it via osmosis to more concentrated compartments nearby. This happens when we drink water—some of the absorbed water moves from the bloodstream into body cells, which equalizes the solute concentration in the cells with that in the bloodstream and in the interstitial fluid. Conversely, when blood loss occurs, plasma (the watery liquid part of blood) volume can be partially maintained by shifting fluid out of the intracellular compartment into the bloodstream. Tightly regulating the amount of water that enters and leaves cells is critical because large shifts in water volume in cells can disrupt cell function.

▶ Osmotic pressure is the amount of force needed to prevent dilution of the compartment containing the higher particle concentration.

Functions of Water

Because of its unique chemical and physical characteristics, water plays several key roles in the body. The maintenance of blood volume and transport of nutrients and oxygen throughout the body depend on water. Water is the basis for saliva, bile, and amniotic fluid, the fluid that surrounds a fetus growing in a woman's uterus. Water is incompressible, so it helps form lubricants in the knees and other joints. Water also serves as a solvent

At a molecular level, water is highly polar because the positive charges tend to be located near the hydrogens and the negative charges near the oxygen.

$$\delta^+ H \qquad H \delta^+$$
$$\delta^- O$$

δ denotes partial charge

This allows water molecules to form hydrogen bonds with other water molecules. The high specific heat of water results from hydrogen bonding.

specific heat Amount of heat required to raise the temperature of any substance 1°C. Water has a high specific heat, meaning that a relatively large amount of heat is required to raise its temperature. Therefore, it tends to resist large temperature fluctuations.

▶ The simplest way to determine if water intake is adequate is to observe the color of one's urine. Water intake is adequate when urine is clear or pale yellow and has little odor. Concentrated urine is very dark yellow and has a strong odor—it indicates that water intake needs to be increased (see Fig. 11-14, Chapter 11).

in many metabolic processes and actively participates as a reactant in numerous chemical reactions. For example, water is required for the hydrolysis of the disaccharide sucrose to the monosaccharides glucose and fructose.

$$\text{Sucrose} + H_2O \rightarrow \text{Glucose} + \text{Fructose}$$

Two other important functions are temperature regulation and the removal of waste products.

Temperature Regulation

Keeping body temperature within a narrow range allows the body, especially enzymes, to function normally. Body temperatures just a few degrees higher or lower than normal can damage body systems and even lead to death. Water in the body helps maintain this range in 2 ways. First, water has a high heat capacity **(specific heat).** That means water resists temperature changes, so its temperature rises slowly when it is heated. This occurs because polar water molecules are strongly attracted to one another, and a relatively large amount of heat is required to overcome this attraction. Think of heating equal amounts of oil and water in separate pans on a stove. The oil gets hot much faster than the water because the fat molecules are not strongly attracted to each other—oil has a lower specific heat.

Sweat is the second way water helps maintain normal body temperature. During exercise or hot weather, the body secretes fluids (perspiration) that evaporate through the skin pores. Heat energy is required to evaporate water, so, as perspiration evaporates, heat energy is taken from the skin, cooling it in the process. This is the main way in which the body cools itself.[2] For the most efficient cooling, perspiration must be allowed to evaporate—if it rolls off the skin or soaks into clothing, it doesn't cool us as much. Evaporation occurs most readily when humidity is low, which is why we feel more comfortable in hot, dry climates than in hot, humid ones. Of course, water lost through perspiration must be replaced, or dehydration and overheating will occur.

Waste Product Removal

Water is an important vehicle for ridding the body of waste products. Most unwanted substances in the body are water soluble and can leave the body via the urine.[2] In addition, liver metabolism converts some fat-soluble compounds, such as certain medications and potential cancer-causing substances, into water-soluble compounds that can be excreted in the urine.

A major body waste product is urea, the nitrogen-containing by-product of protein metabolism. As we eat more protein in excess of needs, more urea must be excreted in the urine. Likewise, the amount of sodium in the urine increases with higher dietary intakes of sodium.

A typical urine output of approximately 4¼ to 8½ cups (1 to 2 liters) daily can easily change in response to fluid, protein, and sodium intake.[2] The minimum urine output required to excrete usual amounts of urea and sodium waste is 2½ cups (600 ml) per day. If urine output is this low frequently, its heavy ion concentration increases the risk of kidney stone formation in susceptible people, especially men. Kidney stones are minerals and other substances that have precipitated out of the urine and accumulated in kidney tissues.

Water in Foods

Beverages and liquid foods (e.g., soups, broths) provide the greatest amount of water. Water also is abundant in fruits and vegetables, typically 75 to 95% water by weight (Fig. 14-5). Other sources that fall between 50 and 75% water are potatoes, chicken, and steak. Foods that are less than 35% water include jam, honey, crackers, and various fats in general. Vegetable oils typically contain no water.

In addition to supplying water, many beverages also provide additional energy (Table 14-2). In the U.S., soft drinks, fruit drinks, energy drinks, and other sweetened beverages are so popular that they provide 13 to 22% of total calories[4]—much higher than the 7% they provided in earlier decades.[5] In fact, soda pop is the single largest source

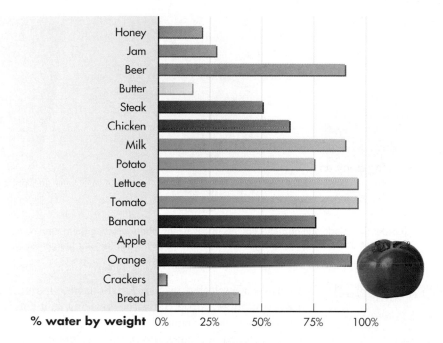

Figure 14-5 Water content of foods by weight. In addition to the MyPyramid food groups, pink is used for substances that do not fit easily into food groups (e.g., honey, candy, coffee, alcohol, and table salt).

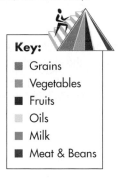

Key:
■ Grains
■ Vegetables
■ Fruits
■ Oils
■ Milk
■ Meat & Beans

Table 14-2 Calorie Content of Popular Beverages*

Beverage	Calories	Beverage	Calories
Mocha with whipped cream	250	Beer	145
Cranberry juice	200	Fat-free milk	120
Orange juice	180	Red Bull® energy drink, 8 oz	105
Regular soft drinks	160	White wine, 4 oz	90

*Amounts are 12 oz. unless otherwise noted.

of calories in the U.S. diet.[6] Nutritionists are concerned about the increasing intake of sweetened beverages because they provide little satiety and we do not compensate for the calories we drink by eating less food.[7] To prevent weight gain, the calorie content of beverages should be considered in diet planning.

Micronutrient content is another consideration for beverage choice. Soft drinks supply few micronutrients in contrast to micronutrient-rich milk and fruit juice. When

▶ The concern over excessive soft drink intake has led many school districts to eliminate or reduce students' access to soft drinks, fruit drinks, and energy drinks and to promote water as the beverage of choice.

CASE STUDY

After graduating from college, Pierre, a 24-year-old accountant, noticed he had gained 8 pounds in the past year. His employer provides free soft drinks, juice, and bottled water. Pierre decides to keep track of his food intake for a couple of days to track his calories. Just his beverage intake is provided here. To estimate his energy intake from beverages, use Table 14-2 and a nutrient database, nutrient analysis computer program, or visit this website: www.nal.usda.gov/fnic/foodcomp/search. Do you think he obtains too many calories from these beverages? What are better alternatives?

Breakfast
12 oz mocha with whipped cream
6 oz orange juice

Morning Break
12 oz cranberry juice
10 oz water

Lunch
12 oz regular cola

Afternoon Break
12 oz regular root beer or apple juice

After Work
1 or 2 12-oz beers
10 oz fat-free milk

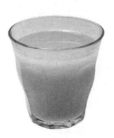
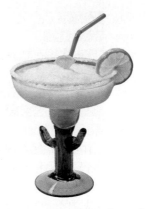
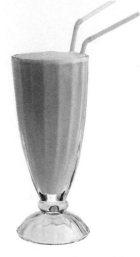

▶ It's easy to become dehydrated during air travel because the air on planes has very low humidity. This causes extra losses of water from the skin and lungs to the cabin air. Drinking extra fluid (but not alcoholic beverages), even though this means extra trips to the restroom, can prevent dehydration. Babies and children especially may need reminders to drink more.

Consider the calorie and nutrient contents of beverages when selecting them. One ounce of orange juice supplies 14 calories. A frozen margarita has 23 calories per ounce (regular margaritas have 68 calories in an ounce). Milkshakes provide 40 calories or more per ounce.

Table 14-3 Water Content of a Typical Day's Food Intake

Meals	Fluid (oz)
Breakfast	
1 cup orange juice	7.2
½ cup fat-free milk	3.6
½ cup strawberries	2.7
1 cup Cheerios®	0.4
Midmorning Snack	
1 cup water	8.0
1 banana	3.0
Lunch	
2 oz water-packed tuna	2.2
2 slices whole-wheat bread	0.9
1 large tomato	5.0
8 oz low-fat yogurt	6.8
1 cup water	8.0
1 kiwi fruit	2.6
Midafternoon Snack	
1 cup apple juice	8.0
4 fig cookies	0.5
Dinner	
2 oz baked skinless chicken	1.3
2 cups romaine lettuce	4.0
2 oz sliced red peppers	1.8
1 slice bread	1.0
1 baked potato	3.5
1 cup fat-free milk	7.0
1 tbsp oil-and-vinegar dressing	0.0
1 cup tea	8.0
Evening Snack	
12 fl oz diet soft drink	12.0
8 saltine crackers	0.03
Total	**97 (12 cups)***

*Adequate for a woman. A man should add 3 more cups of fluid.

soft drinks are selected over milk, riboflavin, vitamin D, calcium, and phosphorus intakes drop. Similarly, replacing fruit juice with sweetened beverages decreases vitamin C, vitamin A, and folate intake. Although some sweetened beverages and bottled waters are fortified with certain vitamins and minerals, they do not contain the full array of micronutrients found in more nutrient-dense beverages.

Both coffee and tea are popular beverage choices. Some websites and magazine articles advise that caffeinated beverages be disregarded as part of daily fluid intake because caffeine increases urine output. However, research studies do not support this common belief.[8, 9] Although caffeine is a mild diuretic, intakes up to 500 mg per day (the amount in about 4.5 cups of brewed coffee) do not cause dehydration or water imbalance in most people. The caffeine content of foods is given in Appendix I.

Alcoholic beverages (wine, beer, spirits) are primarily water, too. However, ethanol increases urine output by inhibiting the action of antidiuretic hormone. This hormone helps control the amount of fluid lost in the urine. When antidiuretic hormone action is blocked, dehydration can occur.

Although water is an excellent beverage choice for most of us, its source—the faucet or a bottle—deserves some thought. The U.S. is the world's leading consumer of bottled water, with an average annual consumption of 28.3 gallons (or 448 cups) per person.[10] Consumers may choose bottled water because they believe it tastes better, is more convenient, or is safer than tap water. Taste and convenience are personal views; however, bottled water is no safer than tap water in the U.S. In fact, about 40% of bottled water starts off as tap water. It also is important to consider that bottled water may not contain the fluoride needed to protect against dental caries (cavities). Further, it costs much more than tap water. Another consideration is the environmental impact of producing and disposing of the tons of plastic bottles used each year.

Water Needs

Water needs vary with factors such as body size, physical activity, environmental conditions, and dietary intake. Despite this variability, an Adequate Intake has been set to provide guidance to individuals for water intake. The Adequate Intake for total water intake per day is 15 cups (3.7 liters) for adult men and 11 cups (2.7 liters) for adult women.[2] This amount includes water from liquids (about 80%) and foods (about 20%) (Table 14-3). Getting 80% of water from fluid translates to a daily fluid intake of about 13 cups (3 liters) for men and 9 cups (2.2 liters) for women.[2] At a minimum, adults need 1 to 3 liters per day of fluid to replace daily water losses.

In addition to the fluid or water provided by foods and beverages we consume, water is generated during metabolism (recall that the oxidation of carbohydrates, proteins, and fats produces water). Water produced from metabolism is about 1 to 1½ cups (250 to 350 ml) per day.

Water output consists of sensible and insensible water losses. Sensible water losses, or those we notice, are urine output and heavy perspiration. Most of the sensible water loss is urine (600 to 1000 ml per day or more). Insensible water losses, or those we do not normally notice, include water lost through the skin (450 to 1900 ml for normal perspiration), lungs (250 to 350 ml), and feces (100 to 200 ml) (Fig. 14-6).

The intestinal tract is efficient at recycling water—about 32 cups (8000 ml) of water enters the intestinal tract daily via secretions from the mouth, stomach, intestines, pancreas, and other organs, and the diet supplies an additional 8 to 13 cups (2 to 3 liters), but only less than ½ cup to just over ¾ cup (100 to 200 ml) is lost in the feces. The kidneys also conserve water, reabsorbing about 97% of the water filtered from waste products. When recycling is impaired, such as in diarrhea or reduced ability to concentrate urine, water needs rise.

When water intake exceeds that needed to excrete waste via the urine and replace insensible losses, urine volume increases and urine becomes more dilute. Conversely, when water intake is too low to replace water losses, urine becomes more concentrated

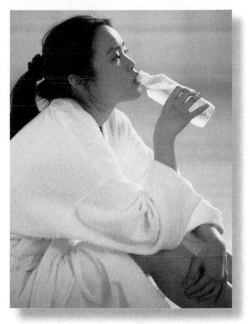

Regular intake of fluid is essential to replace daily losses.

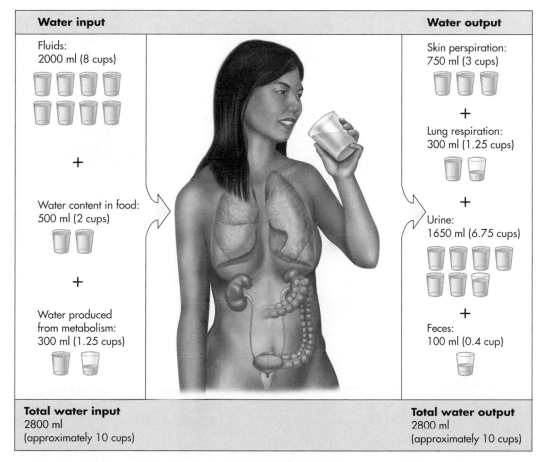

Figure 14-6 Estimate of water input vs. water output in a woman. We primarily maintain our volume of body fluids by adjusting water output to input. As you can see, most water comes from the liquids we consume. Some comes from the moisture in solid foods and the remainder is manufactured during metabolism. Water output includes losses from the lungs, urine, skin, and feces.

and less is produced. There is, however, a limit as to how concentrated urine can become. Eventually, if fluid is not consumed, the body becomes dehydrated and suffers ill effects.[2]

Dehydration

Dehydration can result from bouts of diarrhea and vomiting, fever, heavy exercise, hot weather, dry environments, or even high altitudes. In all cases of dehydration, fluid intake does not match fluid loss. Although thirst is a signal that more water is needed, the thirst mechanism does not always work well during intense exercise, illness, infancy, and old age.

Athletes and people working outside in warm and humid environments are at extra risk of dehydration, poor performance, heat exhaustion, and heat cramps. During prolonged exercise, sweat loss ranges from 3 to 8 cups (750 to 2000 ml) per hour. These individuals are advised to weigh themselves before and after practicing or working to determine their rate of weight loss and water replacement needs. Replacing at least 75% of this weight loss is advised, especially as weight loss approaches 2%. About 2.5 to 3 cups (about 750 ml) of water are recommended per pound (about 0.5 kg) of weight loss (see Chapter 11 for details on fluid use in athletics). Sick children—especially those with fever, vomiting, diarrhea, and increased perspiration—and older persons often need to be reminded to drink plenty of fluids. As Chapter 17 discusses in further detail, infants can become dehydrated easily.

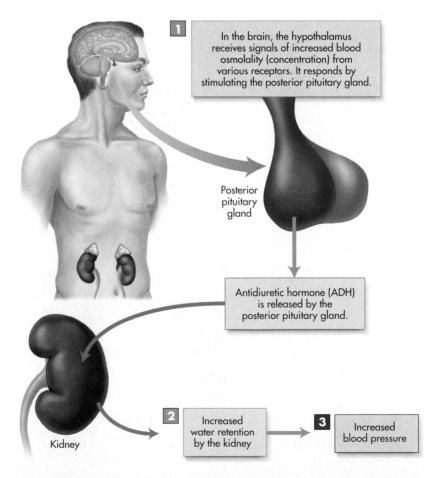

1 In the brain, the hypothalamus receives signals of increased blood osmolality (concentration) from various receptors. It responds by stimulating the posterior pituitary gland.

Posterior pituitary gland

Antidiuretic hormone (ADH) is released by the posterior pituitary gland.

Kidney

2 Increased water retention by the kidney

3 Increased blood pressure

Figure 14-7 Antidiuretic hormone is released in response to an increased concentration of blood. Antidiuretic hormone acts on the kidney to increase water retention; therefore, blood volume and, in turn, blood pressure are restored to normal values. Alcohol (ethanol) inhibits the action of antidiuretic hormone.

The signs of mild to moderate dehydration include dry mouth and skin, fatigue and muscle weakness, decreased urine output, deep yellow (concentrated) urine, headache, and dizziness. As dehydration progresses, solute concentrations in the blood rise, blood pressure decreases, and heart rate increases due to low blood volume.

The increase in the concentration of blood and decrease in blood pressure signal the body that there is a shortage of water, which triggers a series of fluid conservation measures. The pituitary gland releases **antidiuretic hormone** to signal the kidneys to conserve water by reducing urine output (Fig.14-7).[3] At the same time, falling blood pressure initiates another sequence of events beginning in the kidneys. Highly sensitive pressure receptors in the kidneys signal them to release the enzyme **renin** (Fig.14-8). Renin, in turn, activates **angiotensinogen** (a circulating blood protein made in the liver), forming angiotensin I. Angiotensin I is converted to **angiotensin II**, which, among other effects, causes blood vessels to constrict and triggers the adrenal glands to release the hormone **aldosterone**. Aldosterone, in turn, signals the kidneys to retain more sodium and chloride, and therefore more water. (Remember, water always follows electrolytes.) Thus, low blood pressure, through this roundabout sequence, causes the kidneys to increase water conservation in the body.

Despite these mechanisms to conserve water by reducing urine output, fluid continues to be lost via the insensible routes—feces, skin, and lungs. If fluid losses continue,

antidiuretic hormone Hormone secreted by the pituitary gland that signals the kidneys to decrease water excretion; also called arginine vasopressin.

renin Enzyme formed in the kidneys and released in response to low blood pressure. It acts on a blood protein called angiotensinogen to produce angiotensin I.

angiotensin II Compound, produced from angiotensin I, that increases blood vessel constriction and triggers production of the hormone aldosterone.

aldosterone Hormone, produced in the adrenal glands, that acts on the kidneys, causing them to retain sodium and, therefore, water.

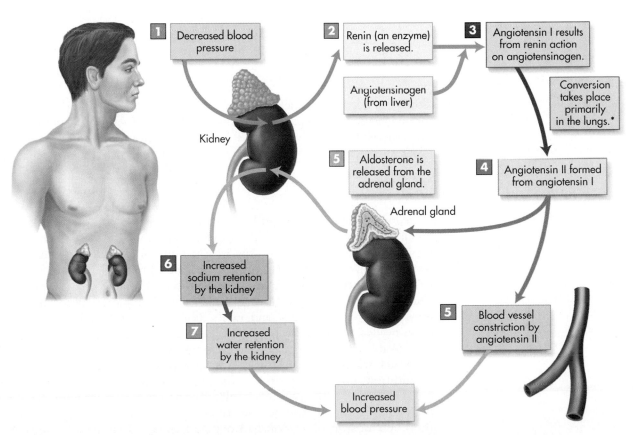

Figure 14-8 The renin-angiotensin system is one regulator of blood pressure and blood volume. A decrease in blood pressure ▮ starts the cascade of reactions (▮–▮) that restore blood pressure to the normal range. This system functions with antidiuretic hormone to control blood pressure. ▮ is listed twice because angiotensin II acts at both the adrenal gland and the blood vessels to help regulate blood pressure.
*The angiotensin-converting enzyme (ACE) inhibitors used to treat hypertension and other disorders act at this site. A new class of antihypertensive medications goes a step further to block the binding of angiotensin II to receptors in the body (e.g., in blood vessels). These are called angiotensin II receptor blockers (ARBs).

Figure 14-9 The effects of dehydration can range from thirst to death, depending on the extent of water weight lost.

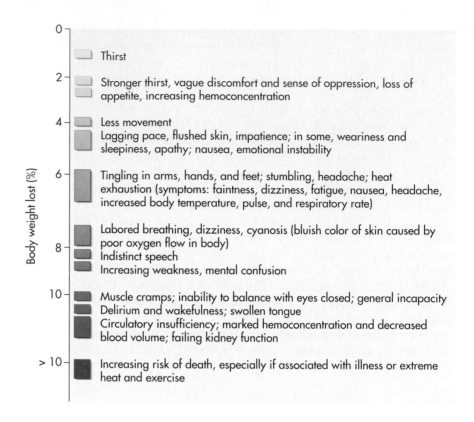

Body weight lost (%)

0 — Thirst

2 — Stronger thirst, vague discomfort and sense of oppression, loss of appetite, increasing hemoconcentration

4 — Less movement
Lagging pace, flushed skin, impatience; in some, weariness and sleepiness, apathy; nausea, emotional instability

6 — Tingling in arms, hands, and feet; stumbling, headache; heat exhaustion (symptoms: faintness, dizziness, fatigue, nausea, headache, increased body temperature, pulse, and respiratory rate)

Labored breathing, dizziness, cyanosis (bluish color of skin caused by poor oxygen flow in body)
8 — Indistinct speech
Increasing weakness, mental confusion

10 — Muscle cramps; inability to balance with eyes closed; general incapacity
Delirium and wakefulness; swollen tongue
Circulatory insufficiency; marked hemoconcentration and decreased blood volume; failing kidney function

> 10 — Increasing risk of death, especially if associated with illness or extreme heat and exercise

CRITICAL THINKING

Lily is suffering from diarrhea related to a viral infection. Why is it important for Lily to continue to drink fluids even while she is sick and has a poor appetite? Do you think that drinking fluids may help her feel better?

kidney failure, seizures, delirium, and coma can occur (Fig. 14-9). The only treatment for dehydration is to replace the lost fluids. In cases of severe dehydration, fluid replacement should be done under medical supervision. Left unchecked, severe dehydration can progress to death.

Water Toxicity

Drinking too much water can be as dangerous as consuming too little. Drinking too much water can cause a condition called water intoxication. When this occurs, the concentration of electrolytes, especially sodium, in the blood is diluted. Low serum sodium is known as **hyponatremia**. To balance intracellular and extracellular electrolyte concentrations, water from the diluted blood is pulled by osmosis into the cells. The dilution of electrolytes and the swelling of cells can cause headache, blurred vision, muscle cramps, convulsions, and, rarely, death. Many of the side effects occur when the brain swells from too much water.

Water intoxication is rare. In general, very few people are at risk of drinking too much water, but problems can occur with some diseases and mental disorders.[2] In addition, infants under 6 months of age given extra bottles of water or overdiluted formula[11] and endurance athletes who overconsume water, trying to prevent dehydration, may consume too much water. Although 13% of the finishers in the 2002 Boston Marathon had hyponatremia, fewer than 1% were at a dangerously low level of sodium.[12] Such hyponatremia can be prevented by not overdrinking and by consuming sports drinks containing at least 100 mg of sodium per 8-ounce serving, instead of plain water (Chapter 11 discusses water needs for active individuals).

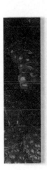

Knowledge Check

1. Which body compartment holds the largest amount of water? How much of the body's water is found there?
2. What affects the amount of water required each day?
3. What are some of the factors to consider when selecting beverages?
4. How do sensible and insensible water losses differ?
5. What are the main signs of dehydration?

CASE STUDY FOLLOW-UP

Beverages contribute 1100 to 1250 calories per day to Pierre's diet. This would be an easy place to reduce his calorie intake. He could replace the mocha with a non-fat latté; water, or a mix of half juice/half water in place of the full-strength juice; choose diet soda and lite beer; or decrease his alcohol intake.

 Global Perspective

Water for Everyone

In North America, we wash our bodies, clothes, dishes, and cars and water our plants and lawns often with little thought to the source of the water, its safety, or how much we use. According to the United Nations, the average daily per capita water use in the U.S. and Europe ranges from 52 to 160 gallons (200 to 600 liters).[13] Contrast this with the approximately 5½ gallons (20 liters) that the United Nations suggests is the minimum daily clean water need per person. In reality, water needs greatly exceed this amount because water is required for agriculture, energy production, and industry. Agriculture, primarily for irrigation, accounts for about 70% of the world's water consumption. Millions of people (farmers, herders, fishing people), especially in rural areas, rely on water for their incomes and food production.[13] Water is vital for food security and good health. When water is in short supply, incomes and economic development fall, and poverty, malnutrition, and poor health increase.

According to the United Nations, about 1 in 3 persons faces water shortages—1.2 billion live where there is not enough water (parts of the Middle East, Mexico, Pakistan, Africa, India, and China), and another 1.6 billion live where there is inadequate infrastructure to move water from its sources to where it is needed.[13] Sometimes water sources are several miles away from homes. People, often women, may walk several miles daily to the water source and then carry the water back to the home. When you consider that each gallon of water weighs more than 8 pounds, the energy needed for carrying water alone adds up to a huge calorie expenditure.

Equitable water distribution is a major challenge. Many rivers and aquifers cut across several regions and countries, which may disagree on how to manage and share water resources. Droughts and floods caused by global warming and unstable climates further increase the challenge of water management.

Equally important are basic sanitation and access to safe water. Poor water quality often is caused by a lack of basic sanitation. Water contaminated with sewage, herbicides, pesticides, and toxins, such as arsenic and lead, can cause disease, and those who are weakened from malnutrition are most likely to succumb to waterborne diseases. Diarrheal diseases, linked to a variety of pathogens in water and poor sanitation, cause 5000 deaths daily—mostly in malnourished children under the age of 5 years.[13] Other water-related diseases, such as the parasitic disease schistosomiasis which can damage organs, afflict millions more.[14] The cycle of infection continues when poor sanitation allows feces from those suffering from waterborne diseases to find their way into the water supply and infect others. Breaking the cycle of waterborne diseases depends on water purification and wastewater treatment.

Providing clean water in many areas of the world remains challenging because of a lack of technical and economic resources. Basic sanitation and simple, low-cost ways to test and clean the water (remove both particles and microbes) are needed.

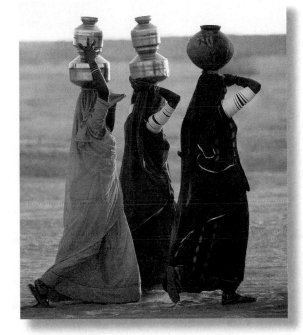

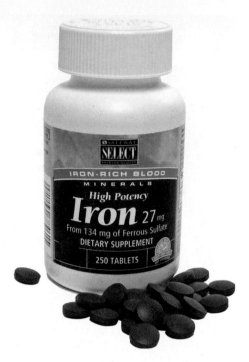

Some mineral supplements pose a high risk of toxicity. Generally, mineral intake from a supplement should not exceed 100% of the Daily Value unless supervised by a physician or registered dietitian.

bioavailability Degree to which the amount of an ingested nutrient is absorbed and is available in the body.

 14.2 Overview of Minerals

Minerals are essential inorganic elements needed in small amounts in the diet for the normal function, growth, and maintenance of body tissues. Minerals are indispensable in human diets because they are basic elements and, thus, cannot be synthesized in the body. There are far more minerals than those that are considered to be nutrients. As you know, to be recognized as a nutrient, evidence must indicate that health declines when the substance is not consumed and, if the nutrient deficiency is not in advanced stages, the deficiency and related symptoms can be alleviated by increased intake of the nutrient.

Mineral nutrients are divided into major minerals and trace minerals, depending on the amount needed each day. Generally, if we require 100 mg or more of a mineral daily, it is considered a major mineral, or macromineral; otherwise, it is considered a trace mineral, or micromineral. Major minerals are found in larger quantities in the body than trace minerals (Fig. 14-10). Using these criteria, calcium and phosphorus are examples of major minerals and iron and copper are trace minerals.

Food Sources of Minerals

Minerals in the average North American's diet come from both plant and animal sources. For some minerals, animal-based foods are the richest source and have the best **bioavailability**. For instance, dairy products are rich sources of bioavailable calcium, whereas meat is a rich source of bioavailable iron and zinc. On the other hand, potassium, magnesium, and manganese are more plentiful in plant-based than animal-based food products, but compounds in plants may diminish their bioavailability.

The quantity of minerals found in food is influenced by many agricultural factors, including genetic variations that affect the ability of plants and animals to absorb and store minerals, the mineral composition of animal feed and medications, soil and water

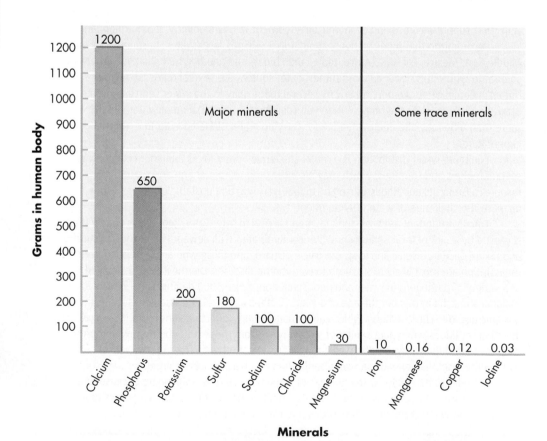

Figure 14-10 Approximate amounts of minerals present in the average human body. Some other trace minerals of nutritional importance not shown are selenium, zinc, chromium, fluoride, and molybdenum.

mineral composition, and the mineral content of fertilizers and pesticides. Food mineral content also is affected by food processing factors. For example, minerals (e.g., iron) from cooking equipment and food containers can migrate into food. Phosphorus, calcium, and other minerals are in additives used to enhance flavor, maintain texture, and preserve foods. Sanitizing solutions may leave mineral-containing residues, such as iodine, that are picked up by foods prepared in the cleaned equipment. Processing also can decrease mineral content. Typically, the more refined a plant food, the lower its mineral content. Milling grains, for instance, removes iron, selenium, zinc, copper, and other minerals.

More and more foods are being fortified with minerals. Iron has been added to milled grains since the enrichment program began in the 1940s. In the U.S., salt fortified with iodine has been available for nearly 90 years. Many products, such as orange juice, are enriched with calcium. Most breakfast cereals are fortified with a wide array of minerals.

Absorption, Transport, and Excretion of Minerals

Foods offer a plentiful supply of many minerals, but the body varies in its capacity to absorb and use them. The ability to absorb minerals from the diet depends on many factors. One significant factor is the physiological need for a mineral at the time of consumption. In general, when the need for a mineral is high, such as the need for iron in growing children, the absorption of that mineral increases. In contrast, absorption tends to decline when the body has adequate stores of the mineral.

Bioavailability is the second significant factor in the body's ability to absorb minerals. The bioavailability of minerals can be greatly influenced by the amount of minerals consumed—that's because many minerals have similar molecular weights and charges (valences). For example, magnesium, calcium, iron, and copper can each exist in the 2^+ valence state. These minerals can compete with each other for absorption, thereby affecting each other's bioavailability.[15] As an example, an excess of zinc in the diet can decrease the absorption and metabolism of the mineral copper. This competition for absorption is of little concern when minerals are supplied by a varied diet; however, individual mineral supplements can create a serious imbalance. Thus, it is safest to choose mineral supplements that contain 100% or less of the Daily Value and use individual mineral supplements only under medical supervision.

Mineral bioavailability also is strongly affected by non-mineral substances in the diet. The components of fiber, especially **phytic acid (phytate)** in wheat grain fiber, can limit the absorption of some minerals by chemically binding to them and preventing their release during digestion. As noted in Chapter 5, fiber intake greatly above the Adequate Level of 25 to 38 g/day can adversely affect mineral status. However, if grains are leavened with yeast, enzymes produced by the yeast can break some of the chemical bonds between phytic acid and minerals. Breaking these bonds increases the bioavailability of the minerals. The zinc deficiencies found among some Middle Eastern populations are attributed partly to their heavy reliance on **unleavened breads,** resulting in low bioavailability of dietary zinc.

Oxalic acid (oxalate) is another substance, found in leafy green plants, that binds minerals and makes them less bioavailable. Spinach, for example, contains plenty of calcium, but only about 5% of it can be absorbed because of the vegetable's high concentration of oxalic acid.[16] On the other hand, about 32% of the dietary calcium is absorbed from milk and milk products.

Polyphenols are a group of compounds containing at least 2 ring structures that each have at least 1 hydroxyl group (OH) attached. Polyphenols also can lower the bioavailability of minerals, especially iron and calcium. Many polyphenols occur naturally in plants, such as tea, dark chocolate (cacao beans), and wine (grapes). Some types of polyphenols, such as flavonoids and tannins, may help prevent cancer and heart disease.

Mineral bioavailability can be enhanced by some vitamins. Vitamin C can improve iron absorption when both are consumed in the same meal. The vitamin D hormone $[1,25 \, (OH)_2$ vitamin D] improves calcium, phosphorus, and magnesium absorption.[1]

phytic acid (phytate) Constituent of plant fibers that binds positive ions (e.g., zinc) to its multiple phosphate groups and decreases their bioavailability.

unleavened bread Bread that does not contain leavening agents, such as yeast or baking powder. Leavening agents cause bread dough to rise. Flat breads, such as pita bread and tortillas are unleavened. French and Italian bread, biscuits, and muffins are leavened breads.

oxalic acid (oxalate) Organic acid, found in spinach, rhubarb, and other leafy green vegetables, that can depress the absorption of certain minerals (e.g., calcium) present in the food.

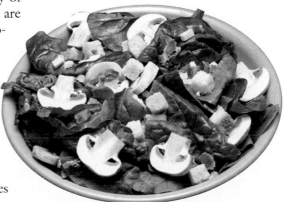

Spinach often is touted as a rich source of calcium, but little of the calcium present is bioavailable—that is, available to the body.

Gastric acidity also promotes the bioavailability of many minerals. Hydrochloric acid (HCl) in the stomach makes minerals more bioavailable by dissolving them and converting them to a form that can be more easily absorbed. For example, HCl provides an electron to ferric iron (Fe^{3+}) to yield ferrous iron (Fe^{2+}), which is better absorbed than ferric iron. Reduced stomach acid production, common in old age and with the use of antacids, can hinder mineral bioavailability.

Many factors affect the degree to which dietary and supplemental minerals are absorbed. The amount of a mineral listed in a nutrient database or on a food label does not necessarily reflect the amount that actually can be absorbed. For this reason, it is important to consider the composition of the total diet when assessing mineral intake, especially trace minerals intake, because food contains such minute amounts of these nutrients.

Once absorbed, minerals travel in the blood, either in a free form or bound to proteins. For example, calcium ions can be found free in the blood or bound to the blood protein albumin. Trace minerals in their free form are often highly reactive and are toxic if not bound. Thus, many trace minerals have specific binding proteins that transport them in the bloodstream. Many also are bound by specific cellular proteins once they are taken up by cells.

Mineral excretion takes place primarily through the urine. However, some minerals, such as copper, are secreted by the liver into the bile for excretion in the feces. When kidney function fails, mineral intake must be controlled to avoid mineral toxicity, such as with phosphorus and magnesium.[1]

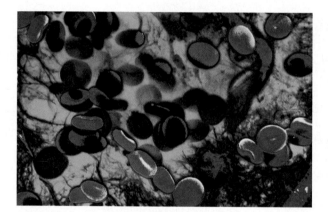

Red blood cells contain the mineral iron.

Functions of Minerals

The metabolic roles of minerals vary considerably. Water balance requires sodium, potassium, calcium, and phosphorus. Sodium, potassium, and calcium aid in the transmission of nerve impulses throughout the body. Some minerals, such as magnesium, copper, and selenium, function as cofactors and enable enzymes to carry out chemical reactions. Minerals also are components of many body compounds. For example, iron is a component of hemoglobin in red blood cells. Body growth and development also depend on certain minerals, such as calcium and phosphorus. At all levels—cellular, tissue, organ, and whole body—minerals play important roles in maintaining body functions (see Fig. 14-1).

Mineral Deficiencies

Calcium is a major mineral that is likely to be deficient in some diets. Currently, most North American girls and women, along with older men, do not meet the recommended intake for calcium.[17] Potassium and magnesium intakes also fall short of DRI recommendations. Of the trace minerals, iron, zinc, and iodine are most likely to be deficient in diets (see Chapter 15).

Mineral Toxicity

Excess mineral intake can be toxic, particularly trace minerals, such as iron and zinc. The use of mineral supplements, especially if intake will exceed the Upper Level, is best considered after consultation with a registered dietitian or physician. The potential for toxicity is not the only reason to carefully consider the use of mineral supplements. As discussed previously, high intakes of one mineral can hinder the absorption of others. Also, mineral supplements can be contaminated—with lead, for example. Selecting brands approved by the U.S. Pharmacopeia (USP) lessens this risk. The USP-approved brands are tested to assure that contaminants are not present in harmful amounts, that the ingredients listed on the label are present and will dissolve in the body, and that the supplements were made under safe and sanitary conditions.

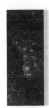

Knowledge Check

1. How are the major minerals differentiated from trace minerals?
2. What are 2 factors that can decrease bioavailability of a mineral?
3. What are 3 functions of minerals in the body?

 # 14.3 Sodium (Na)

Salt—the most important source of the essential nutrient sodium—is either mined from inland salt deposits created by ancient seas or produced by the evaporation of sea water. Salt has been highly valued as a food flavoring and preservative for thousands of years—the earliest reference being in the Book of Job written around 300 B.C. Today, many of us enjoy the flavor salt adds to food. Salt also is important in the production of many common food products, such as cheese, cured meats, pickled vegetables, and bread. Despite these attributes, many nutrition scientists believe that our intake of sodium is too high for good health.

Sodium in Foods

Salt, sodium chloride (NaCl), contributes most of the sodium to our diets (Fig. 14-11). Salt is 40% sodium and 60% chloride, which means that a teaspoon of salt (about 6 g) provides 2300 mg of sodium. However, most of the sodium we consume doesn't come from the salt shaker at home. The majority—75 to 80%—is added during food processing and at restaurants, either as salt or sodium-containing food additives. Sodium naturally present in foods provides about 10% of the sodium we consume, and the salt added in cooking and at the table provides another 10 to 15%. Other sodium sources are softened tap water and certain medicines.

▶ Salt has a colorful history. At one time, it was the custom to rub salt on newborn babies as a symbol of purity and to ensure their good health. Salt was once so scarce that it was used as money. Caesar's soldiers received part of their pay in salt. This part of their pay was known as their "salarium," and from this custom came today's word *salary*. The expression "not worth his salt" meant that a man did not earn his wages.

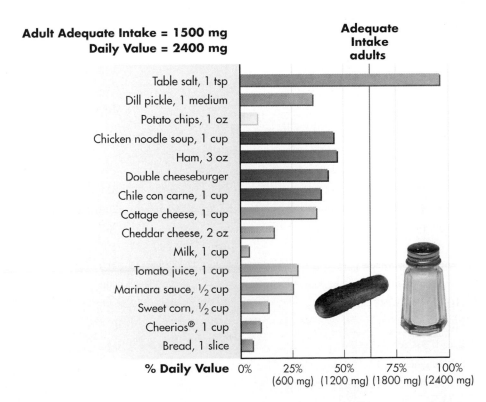

Figure 14-11 Food sources of sodium.

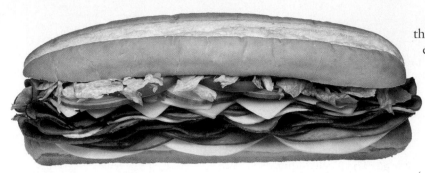

Cured meats are very high in sodium.

Almost all unprocessed foods naturally contain little sodium; the higher amount found in milk (about 100 mg/cup) is one exception. Consider that, if we ate only unprocessed foods and added no salt, daily sodium intake would be about 500 mg.[2] Comparing this with the 2300 to 4700 mg or more typically eaten by adults, it is clear that food processing contributes most of our dietary sodium. Processed foods tend to be higher in sodium because this versatile mineral is part of many compounds—flavorings (table salt), flavor enhancers (monosodium glutamate), preservatives (sodium benzoate), leavening agents (sodium bicarbonate, also called baking soda), curing agents (sodium nitrite), wetting agents for quick-cooking cereals (sodium phosphate), color preservatives (sodium bisulfite), anti-caking agents that keep powdered foods from clumping (sodium aluminum silicate), and many others. Table 14-4 shows how sodium levels change when food is processed.

The major contributors of sodium in the U.S. diet are white bread and rolls, hot dogs and lunch meats, cheese, soups, and processed foods that contain canned tomato sauce, partly because these foods are eaten so often.[18] Foods especially high in sodium include cured meats, condiments, bottled sauces (e.g., soy, barbecue, steak), gravies, pickles, mustard, seasoned rice and pasta mixes, dried and canned soups, and canned and frozen entrees. Many of these foods are now available in reduced sodium versions.

Table 14-4 Sodium Content of Foods during Processing

Food Category	Sodium (mg)
Dairy Products	
Milk, 1 cup	100
Cheddar cheese, 2 oz	350
American cheese, 2 oz	900
Meats	
Beef roast, 3 oz	60
Beef jerky, 3 oz	1880
Pork loin, 3 oz	50
Ham, fresh, 3 oz	190
Ham, cured, 3 oz	1130
Bacon, 3 slices (3 oz)	2010
Vegetables	
Fresh peas, raw, ½ cup	2
Fresh peas, cooked and salted at home, ½ cup	190
Frozen peas, ½ cup	81
Frozen peas, cooked and salted at home, ½ cup	260
Frozen peas in mushroom sauce, ½ cup	385
Canned peas, low sodium, ½ cup	2
Canned peas, ½ cup	310
Canned peas in mushroom sauce, ½ cup	490
Grain Products	
Flour, ½ cup	1
Bread, 2 slices	320
Saltine crackers, 12	470

Restaurant foods often contain excessive amounts of sodium. For example, a large order of cheese fries with ranch dressing contains more than 4000 mg of sodium, and a chicken fajita dinner may have more than 3500 mg of sodium.

Sodium Needs

The Adequate Intake for adults under age 51 is 1500 mg of sodium per day. The AI decreases to 1300 mg per day for those aged 51 to 70 years and 1200 mg per day for those older than age 70.[2] The Daily Value for sodium is 2400 mg (2.4 g). The Daily Value is very close to the Upper Level of 2300 mg per day for sodium and, so, should be regarded as the upper limit of sodium intake. These are generous amounts; only about 200 mg of sodium is needed daily to maintain normal physiological functions. In addition to supporting good health, the Adequate Intake was set above the amount needed to allow for a more varied diet, so that not all foods need to be low in sodium.[2]

Absorption, Transport, Storage, and Excretion of Sodium

Almost all the sodium consumed is absorbed in the intestinal tract. Sodium, like potassium and chloride ions, is absorbed by active transport in both the small and large intestines. Energy for the active transport of sodium is supplied by the sodium-potassium pump, shown in Figure 14-3. Most sodium in the body is found in the extracellular fluid compartment (ECF). The amount of sodium in the ECF is closely regulated. When sodium intake is high, excess sodium is excreted by the kidneys. Conversely, when the concentration of sodium in the blood is low, the hormone aldosterone inhibits sodium excretion by the kidneys (see Fig. 14-8). Sodium also is lost via the feces and perspiration.

Functions of Sodium

Sodium has 3 main functions: it helps in the absorption of glucose and some amino acids in the small intestine, it is required for normal muscle and nerve function, and it aids in water balance. Muscle contraction and nerve impulse conduction rely on the electrical charge created by the shift of both sodium and potassium ions across the cell membrane.

Because sodium is the main solute in the ECF, it regulates the ECF and plasma volumes. When the amount of sodium in the body increases, more water is retained in the body until the excess sodium is excreted. In some diseases, such as **nephrotic syndrome** and **congestive heart failure,** sodium excretion by the kidneys is faulty, causing significant fluid retention and edema. Even in healthy persons, water retention can occur, especially when standing for long periods of time in hot weather. Consuming less sodium can improve this condition.

nephrotic syndrome Type of kidney disease that results from damage to the kidney, often caused by another disease, such as diabetes. The symptoms include fluid retention, weight gain, and high blood pressure.

Sodium Deficiency

Sodium deficiency is rare because of the abundance of sodium in the food supply, coupled with relatively low requirements for sodium. Nevertheless, sodium depletion can occur when losses exceed intake, such as in excessive perspiration. However, only when weight loss from perspiration exceeds about 2% of total body weight (or about 5 to 6 lb) should sodium losses be of concern.[3] Even then, merely salting foods is sufficient to restore body sodium levels for most people. Athletes, however, may need to consume sports drinks during competition to avoid the depletion of sodium and other electrolytes (see Chapter 11). Although perspiration tastes salty on the skin, sodium is not highly concentrated in perspiration. Rather, water evaporating from the skin leaves sodium

CRITICAL THINKING

Mrs. Massa has recently seen and heard a lot about the amount of salt in foods. She has been surprised by the number of articles that advise the public to decrease the amount of salt in their food. If sodium is such a bad thing, Mrs. Massa wonders, why do you need to have any at all? How would you explain to her the need for some sodium?

behind. (Perspiration contains about two-thirds the sodium concentration found in blood.) Sodium depletion also can occur because of diarrhea or vomiting, especially in infants. Electrolyte drinks are used in such cases to replace sodium (see Chapter 17).

Low blood sodium, hyponatremia, is one sign of sodium depletion. The symptoms of hyponatremia include headache, nausea, vomiting, fatigue, and muscle cramps. Seizures, coma, and death can occur in severe cases. Hyponatremia also results from the ingestion of excess water, as discussed in Section 14.1.

Excess Sodium and Upper Level

The Upper Level for sodium for adults is 2300 mg/day (2.3 g). About 95% of North American adults have sodium intakes that exceed the Upper Level. Sodium intakes over the Upper Level can increase the chance of developing high blood pressure (hypertension), heart disease, and stroke.[19] Preliminary research suggests that the risk of heart disease can be reduced by 25% with a sodium reduction of about 1000 mg/day.[20] Section 14.6 of this chapter gives a more detailed overview of hypertension.

Concern over high sodium intake has led some major medical organizations, including the American Medical Association and the World Health Organization, to call for a 50% reduction in the sodium content of processed and restaurant foods to reduce sodium intake to less than 2400 mg/day.[21-23] Public health scientists estimate that reducing sodium intake by 50% will reduce the prevalence of hypertension by at least 20% and will reduce mortality from coronary heart disease and stroke.[22, 24]

Sodium intakes greater than 2 g per day also increase calcium loss in the urine and are of potential concern for the loss of calcium from bones. However, scientists have not been able to link high sodium intakes to osteoporosis.[25] Extra calcium in the urine can lead to the formation of calcium oxalate kidney stones, the most common type; thus,

Table 14-5 Guidelines for Decreasing the Amount of Salt (Sodium Chloride) in the Diet

Choose These Foods More Often	Choose These Foods Less Often
Grains: whole grains or enriched breads and cereals; plain rice and pasta	Packaged rice and pasta mixes
Vegetables: fresh and frozen plain (no sauce) vegetables	Canned vegetables (read the labels), tomato and pasta sauces, frozen vegetables with sauce
Fruits: fresh, canned, and frozen fruits	Commercial fruit pies, turnovers
Dairy: low-fat milk, yogurt	Cheeses, especially processed
Meats and substitutes: fresh or frozen lean meats, poultry, fish, shellfish, unsalted lean pork, eggs, tuna or salmon canned without added salt, canned and drained meat and poultry, unsalted nuts or seeds, dried peas, beans, and lentils	Salted nuts; frozen breaded meat, fish, and poultry; and processed meats, such as luncheon meats, bologna, salami, hot dogs, bacon, ham, and beef jerky
Entrees: prepared from fresh ingredients or those labeled reduced sodium	Instant and canned soups, frozen entrees and dinners, pizza, many fast-food items
Snack items: unsalted crackers, popcorn, pretzels, breadsticks	Salted crackers, popcorn, chips
Seasonings and condiments: fresh and dried herbs, lemon juice, low sodium seasoning products	Salt added during cooking, bouillon cubes, seasoning salts, soy sauce, teriyaki sauce, barbeque sauces, pickles, olives, bottled salad dressings
Softened water	Unsoftened or bottled low sodium water

reducing sodium levels is warranted for individuals prone to kidney stones.[26] In summary, reducing sodium intakes to below the Upper Level is likely to improve health for many by lowering the risk of cardiovascular disease and kidney stone formation.

As discussed in Chapter 2, Nutrition Facts labels can help you become aware of the amount of sodium in your diet. Many food processors are responding to consumer desire for less sodium by offering modified foods. The terms, such as *salt-free, sodium free,* and *low sodium,* that appear on food labels can help you quickly locate these foods. Table 14-5 provides suggestions for trimming dietary sodium intake. Note that the desire for salty taste is learned—that is, by eating salty food often, people gradually acquire a taste preference for salty foods. However, as sodium intake decreases, the preference for salty flavors declines.

Knowledge Check

1. Which foods contribute the most sodium to the diet?
2. How does the Adequate Intake (AI) of sodium compare with typical intakes in North America?
3. How is excess sodium eliminated from the body?
4. What are the 3 main functions of sodium?
5. What are some strategies for decreasing sodium in the diet?

14.4 Potassium (K)

Potassium, a silvery grey metal, was discovered in the early 1800s. Its name comes from the word *potash,* which means "extracted in a pot from the ash of burnt trees." As you might guess from the origin of its name, plant-based foods are rich sources of this mineral. However, despite its abundance in the food supply, potassium intakes are low in many parts of the world, including the U.S. and Europe.

Potassium in Foods

Potassium occurs naturally in many foods and, unlike sodium, unprocessed foods are the best sources (Fig. 14-12). Fruit, vegetables, milk, whole grains, dried beans, and meats are all good sources. The major contributors of potassium to the U.S. adult diet include milk, potatoes, coffee, beef, tomatoes, and orange juice.[18] Other sources of potassium are salt substitutes (potassium chloride) and food additives, such as acesulfame-K, an artificial sweetener; dipotassium guanylate, a flavor enhancer; potassium aluminum silicate, an anti-caking agent; and potassium propionate, a preservative.

Potassium Needs

The Adequate Intake for potassium for adults is 4700 mg (4.7 g) per day.[2] The Daily Value used on food and supplement labels is 3500 mg. Average potassium intakes for U.S. adults fall below both of these recommendations, ranging from 2100 to 3300 mg daily.[17] Thus, many people need to boost their potassium intakes, preferably by eating more fruits, vegetables, whole-grain breads and cereals, and reduced-fat milk and dairy products.[2]

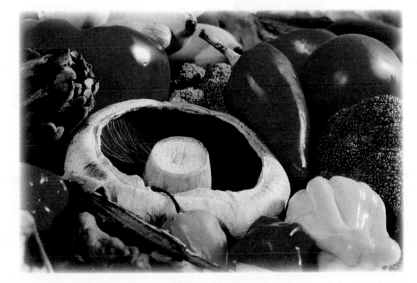

Vegetables are a rich source of potassium, as are fruits.

Figure 14-12 Food sources of potassium.

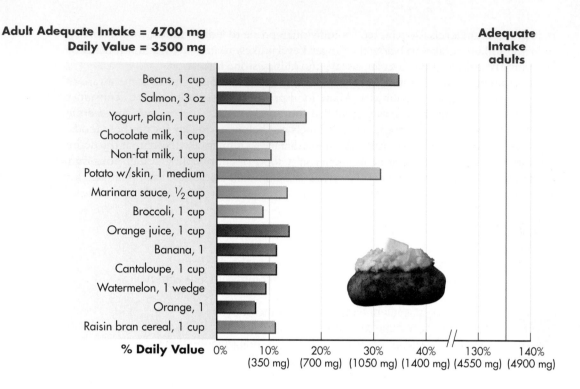

Adult Adequate Intake = 4700 mg
Daily Value = 3500 mg

Adequate Intake adults

Beans, 1 cup	
Salmon, 3 oz	
Yogurt, plain, 1 cup	
Chocolate milk, 1 cup	
Non-fat milk, 1 cup	
Potato w/skin, 1 medium	
Marinara sauce, ½ cup	
Broccoli, 1 cup	
Orange juice, 1 cup	
Banana, 1	
Cantaloupe, 1 cup	
Watermelon, 1 wedge	
Orange, 1	
Raisin bran cereal, 1 cup	

% Daily Value 0%   10%   20%   30%   40%   130%   140%
                        (350 mg) (700 mg) (1050 mg) (1400 mg) (4550 mg) (4900 mg)

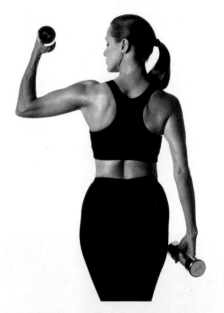

Potassium and sodium aid in muscle contraction.

Absorption, Transport, Storage, and Excretion of Potassium

The body absorbs about 90% of the potassium consumed. Like sodium, potassium is absorbed in both the small and large intestines. The potassium ion (K^+) is transported to the body's cells, where 95% of the body's potassium is found. As with sodium, potassium balance is achieved primarily through kidney excretion or retention.[3]

Functions of Potassium

Potassium is the major cation inside the cell and performs many of the same functions as sodium. Both are involved in maintaining fluid balance, transmitting nerve impulses, and contracting muscle. (Recall that muscle contraction and nerve impulse conduction rely on the electrical charge created by the shift of both potassium and sodium ions across the cell membrane.) Like sodium, potassium influences the excretion of calcium, but in the opposite direction—when dietary potassium is high, the amount of calcium excreted in the urine declines.[27]

Potassium also is thought to blunt the effects of a high salt intake and help keep blood pressure normal. High dietary potassium intake suppresses the renin-angiotensin system (see Fig. 14-8) and promotes the excretion of excess sodium and water.[2, 28] Rising rates of hypertension in the U.S. may be due, in part, to a high dietary sodium to potassium ratio.[28]

Potassium Deficiency

Low blood potassium, known as **hypokalemia,** is a life-threatening problem. The symptoms include weakness, fatigue, constipation, and an irregular heartbeat (arrhythmias) that impairs the heart's ability to pump blood. Consuming too little potassium also can raise blood pressure and the risk of stroke.[2, 29] High blood pressure and stroke are discussed further in the Medical Perspective: Hypertension and Nutrition.

The depletion of potassium from the body and low blood potassium most often are caused by excessive potassium losses via the urine or the gastrointestinal tract. Some diuretics used to treat hypertension deplete potassium from the body by increasing the amount excreted in the urine. For these people, high potassium foods are good additions to the diet, as are potassium chloride supplements if recommended by a physician. Not all diuretics increase potassium in the urine, however; some are formulated to spare potassium.

More rarely, very low dietary intake can cause low blood potassium. In persons with eating disorders, low food intake, vomiting, and laxative use, make potassium depletion and hypokalemia a common and very serious problem. Alcoholics also may have poor diets lacking in potassium. Athletes who exercise heavily may lose extra potassium in their sweat. These losses can be replaced with a healthy diet rich in high potassium foods.

Excess Potassium and Upper Level

High blood potassium, known as **hyperkalemia**, is a life-threatening problem. Hyperkalemia almost never occurs in healthy persons. Even when dietary potassium intake is extremely high, the excess is readily excreted by the kidneys. However, when kidney function is poor, potassium readily builds up in the blood and can cause irregular heartbeat and even cardiac arrest. Potassium levels can be controlled in these cases by careful attention to the potassium content of the diet.[3]

The use of potassium in supplement form to treat a deficiency or poor intake is harmless if the kidneys function normally. Thus, no Upper Level has been set.[2] However, taken in excessive amounts, potassium supplements can cause intestinal upset.

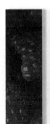

Knowledge Check

1. Which food groups are generally good sources of potassium?
2. Where is most of the potassium in the body found?
3. What are 2 serious disorders linked to low potassium intakes?
4. Why is hyperkalemia (high blood potassium) rare?

 ## 14.5 Chloride (Cl)

Chloride is an essential nutrient—it is the main anion (Cl⁻) in the extracellular fluid. The chloride ion should not be confused with the element chlorine (Cl_2). Chlorine is a strong oxidant that is widely used to purify water, disinfect swimming pools, bleach fabrics, and produce many products (e.g., paper, plastics). Chlorine, along with chlorine gas, is toxic.

Chloride in Foods

Almost all the chloride in the diet is from table salt—sodium chloride. Therefore, the same foods that provide sodium in the diet also provide most of the dietary chloride. Chloride also is found in seaweed, olives, rye, lettuce, a few fruits, and some vegetables. Salt substitutes usually contain potassium chloride.

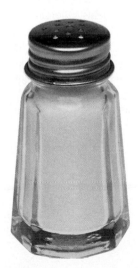

Most chloride in the diet comes from table salt—sodium chloride.

Chloride Needs

The Adequate Intake for chloride for adults is 2300 mg. This amount is based on the 40:60 ratio of sodium to chloride in salt (the Adequate Intake of 1500 mg of sodium is accompanied by 2300 mg of chloride).[2] The Daily Value used on food and supplement labels is 3400 mg. An average daily consumption of 9 g of salt yields 5.4 g (5400 mg) of chloride.

Absorption, Transport, Storage, and Excretion of Chloride

Chloride, like sodium and potassium, is almost completely absorbed in the small and large intestines. Chloride absorption follows right along with sodium absorption. This allows a balance of electrical charges between the negatively charged chloride ion (Cl^-) and the positively charged sodium ion (Na^+). Most chloride is found in the extracellular fluid, where it is associated with sodium. Like sodium and potassium, the excretion of chloride occurs mainly through the kidneys.[3]

Functions of Chloride

Chloride is the main anion (Cl^-) in the extracellular fluid, where its negative charge balances the positive charge from the sodium ion. Together, sodium and chloride help maintain extracellular fluid volume and balance. They also aid in the transmission of nerve impulses. In addition to its role as an electrolyte, chloride has other important functions. It is a component of the HCl produced in the stomach, and it is used during immune responses when white blood cells attack foreign cells. Finally, chloride helps maintain acid-base balance and dispose of carbon dioxide by way of exhaled air.

Chloride Deficiency

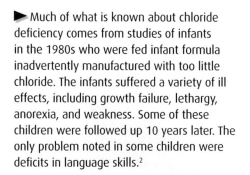

► Much of what is known about chloride deficiency comes from studies of infants in the 1980s who were fed infant formula inadvertently manufactured with too little chloride. The infants suffered a variety of ill effects, including growth failure, lethargy, anorexia, and weakness. Some of these children were followed up 10 years later. The only problem noted in some children were deficits in language skills.[2]

A chloride deficiency is generally unlikely because our dietary sodium chloride (salt) intake is so high. Frequent and lengthy bouts of vomiting—if coupled with a nutrient-poor diet—can cause a deficiency because of loss of HCl.[3] The symptoms include weakness, anorexia, and lethargy. The loss of HCl can disrupt the balance of acids and bases in the body.

Upper Level for Chloride

The Upper Level for chloride is 3.6 g/day. This amount is based on the amount of chloride that parallels the Upper Level for sodium (2300 mg/day) using the 40:60 ratio of sodium to chloride in salt.[3] As just noted, the average adult typically consumes much more than this amount. Dietary chloride has been implicated in the effects of sodium chloride on increasing blood pressure.[30] Still, as one lowers sodium intake as part of hypertension therapy, chloride intake automatically falls as well.

Knowledge Check

1. What is the source of most dietary chloride?
2. What are the functions of chloride in the body?
3. How were chloride needs and Upper Level set?

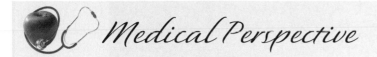

Medical Perspective

Hypertension and Nutrition

About 1 in 3 adults has high blood pressure (hypertension). Blood pressure, measured in millimeters of mercury (mm Hg), is the force of the blood against artery walls. Simply put, it measures how hard the heart is working and what condition the arteries are in. It is expressed as 2 numbers. The higher number is the systolic blood pressure—the pressure in the arteries when the heart beats. The second value is the diastolic blood pressure—the pressure in the arteries between beats when the heart relaxes. Optimal blood pressure is less than 120 over 80 mm Hg. Table 14-6 gives the blood pressure categories currently in use for adults.

Table 14-6 Classification of Blood Pressure*

Category	SBP mm Hg		DBP mm Hg
Normal	< 120	and	< 80
Prehypertension	120–139	or	80–89
Hypertension, stage 1	140–159	or	90–99
Hypertension, stage 2	≥ 160	or	≥ 100

* SBP = systolic blood pressure; DBP = diastolic blood pressure.
Source: Seventh Report of the Joint National Committee on Prevention, Detection, Evaluation and Treatment of High Blood Pressure (JNC 7), NIH Publication Number 03-5231, May 2003.

Causes of Hypertension

Diseases such as kidney disease, liver disease, and diabetes can sometimes cause a condition known as secondary hypertension. This occurs in about 5 to 10% of individuals with hypertension and is due to the underlying disease. Most individuals with hypertension, however, are classified as having primary (or essential) hypertension. Although many of the factors associated with the development of primary hypertension have been documented, the actual cause is not fully known. Primary hypertension develops over a period of years in response to changes in the arteries, kidneys, and sodium/potassium balance.[28] As we age, our arteries tend to narrow and become more rigid through a process called arteriosclerosis. Additionally, endothelial cells that line the arteries often release vasoconstrictors, substances that cause the arteries to constrict, in response to arterial damage, poor blood flow, stress, and other factors. Although these events alone can result in increased blood pressure, their additive effects on kidney function increase arterial pressure. The kidney releases increased renin, causing the formation of additional angiotensin II enzyme (see Fig. 14-8). Angiotensin II is a powerful vasoconstrictor that triggers the kidney's retention of sodium and water. Diets high in sodium and low in potassium worsen these physiological changes. Over time, the result is elevation of blood pressure.

Risk Factors for Hypertension

Age, race, obesity, and diabetes all affect the risk of high blood pressure.[31] As people increase in age, so does blood pressure; over 90% of those over age 55 will develop high blood pressure in their lifetimes. African-Americans tend to develop hypertension more often and at a younger age than whites. Obesity also increases the risk of developing high blood pressure. An increase in fat mass adds extra blood vessels, which increases the heart's workload, as well as blood pressure. Elevated blood insulin concentration associated with insulin-resistant adipose cells

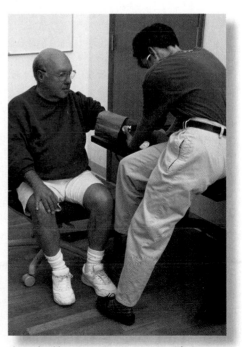

The risk of hypertension increases with age.

(continued)

Medical Perspective, continued

is another reason for this link to obesity. Insulin increases sodium retention in the body and accelerates atherosclerosis. An estimated 65% of people with diabetes also have hypertension.

Hypertension is a serious chronic disease and health hazard. Recall from Chapter 6 that the high pressure in the arteries damages the arteries over time. Eventually, this high pressure damages the "target organs" of hypertension—the heart, brain, kidney, and eyes—increasing the risk of heart attack, stroke, dementia, kidney disease, and vision loss. Recall from Chapter 1 that cardiovascular disease, stroke, and kidney failure are the first, third, and ninth leading causes of death, respectively. Unfortunately, hypertension is often a silent disease, with no warning signs or symptoms. This is why it is important to get your blood pressure checked regularly. If hypertension is detected in its early stages, treatment is often more effective.

Lifestyle Modifications to Prevent and Treat Hypertension

A healthy lifestyle (Table 14-7) is the cornerstone for preventing and treating high blood pressure and its complications.[31-34] Note that these recommendations, with the exception of the DASH dietary pattern, are already familiar from the Dietary Guidelines for Americans and MyPyramid. Following these recommendations can help keep blood pressure normal throughout life. In overweight persons, even a modest weight loss of 10 pounds can reduce blood pressure.[31, 34] Similarly, moderate physical activity can decrease blood pressure, especially in those who have been sedentary. Aerobic exercise strengthens the heart, helps keep arteries healthy, and can prevent high blood pressure. Improving insulin sensitivity, losing weight, and increasing physical activity also help prevent diabetes (and hypertension). Keeping alcohol intake and sodium under control is an additional step to help control blood pressure.

▶ Pregnancy-induced hypertension (PIH) is a type of hypertension that can occur during pregnancy. This condition can be very dangerous for the mother and growing fetus. (See Chapter 16.)

▶ Preliminary studies show a link between bone lead concentrations and increased risk of hypertension. More information is needed, but it is suspected that even small amounts of lead stored over decades may damage the kidneys and eventually result in hypertension. This is just one of the many deleterious effects of lead exposure.

Table 14-7 Lifestyle Modifications to Lower Blood Pressure

Modification	Recommendation	Average Systolic Blood Pressure Reduction Range
Weight reduction	Maintain healthy body weight (BMI 18.5–24.9 kg/m²).	5–20 mm Hg/10-kg weight reduction
DASH eating plan	Adopt a diet rich in fruits, vegetables, and low-fat dairy products with reduced content of saturated and total fat.	8–14 mm Hg
Aerobic physical activity	Engage in regular aerobic physical activity at least 30 minutes per day, most days of the week.	4–9 mm Hg
Dietary sodium reduction	Reduce dietary sodium intake to ≤ 2.4 g sodium or 6 g sodium chloride per day.	2–8 mm Hg
Limited alcohol consumption	Men should have no more than 2 drinks per day; women should have no more than 1 drink per day.	2–4 mm Hg

Source: Seventh Report of the Joint National Committee on Prevention, Detection, Evaluation and Treatment of High Blood Pressure (JNC 7). NIH Publication Number 03-5231, May 2003.

Regular moderate exercise helps control blood pressure levels.

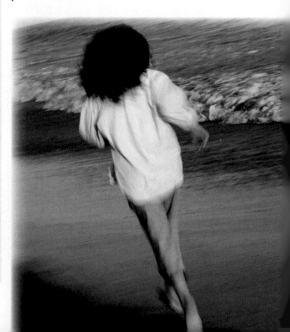

Minerals, Phytochemicals, and Hypertension

The issue of sodium restriction and its role in treating and preventing high blood pressure has been vigorously debated for years. The Intersalt study, conducted with over 10,000 people from 32 countries and often regarded as the "landmark" sodium intake and hypertension study, found that, as urinary sodium excretion increased, so did blood pressure.[35] (Urinary sodium excretion is a much more sensitive indicator of sodium intake than estimating dietary intake of sodium.) However, with higher sodium intakes, a phenomenon called "salt sensitivity" occurs. This means that only about 25 to 50% of people experience high blood pressure when they have a high salt intake. Unfortunately, there is no easy way for a person or medical provider to determine if sodium sensitivity is a problem, but it is known that African-Americans, overweight persons, those with diabetes, and the elderly are more likely to be sodium sensitive. These individuals should limit sodium to 1500 mg per day; others can aim for less than 2400 mg per day.

Diets rich in fruits and vegetables help control blood pressure.

It also appears that the amount of potassium, compared with sodium, in the diet affects blood pressure.[28] Diets high in potassium and low in sodium offer the most protection against high blood pressure.[28] Such diets are consistent with the Adequate Intake recommendations for potassium (4700 mg per day) and sodium (1500 mg per day). On the other hand, low potassium and high sodium diets, like those many people eat today, are more likely to result in high blood pressure.[28] Diets rich in calcium, magnesium, and fiber also have been linked to lower blood pressure, but individual supplements of these nutrients generally do not show beneficial effects.[36]

Chocolate and caffeine consumption also has been linked to blood pressure. Some small, short-term studies suggest that consuming dark chocolate in amounts as little as 6 grams daily can cause a modest reduction in blood pressure.[37, 38] Dark chocolate contains polyphenols, which may help improve the synthesis of compounds that cause the vasodilatation of arteries. However, more research is necessary before dark chocolate can be considered a reliable way to reduce blood pressure. On the other hand, although caffeine temporarily increases blood pressure, caffeinated beverages are not thought to cause or worsen hypertension.[39]

The DASH Diet

The DASH (Dietary Approaches to Stop Hypertension) diet was designed to test the effect of a diet low in saturated fat, total fat, and cholesterol and high in fruits, vegetables, and low-fat dairy products on blood pressure. The diet is rich in magnesium, potassium, calcium, protein, and fiber (Table 14-8). In fact, the amounts of magnesium, potassium, calcium, and fiber greatly exceed typical intakes, but without using nutritional supplements. The DASH eating plan is shown in Table 14-9.

Table 14-8 Nutrient Goals for the DASH Diets (for a 2,100-Calorie Eating Plan)

Total fat	27% of calories	Sodium	2300 mg*
Saturated fat	6% of calories	Potassium	4700 mg
Protein	18% of calories	Calcium	1250 mg
Carbohydrate	55% of calories	Magnesium	500 mg
Cholesterol	150 mg	Fiber	30 g

*1500 mg sodium was a lower goal tested and found to be even better for lowering blood pressure. It was particularly effective for middle-aged and older individuals, African-Americans, and those who already had high blood pressure.
Source: Your Guide to Lowering Your Blood Pressure with DASH. http://www.nhlbi.nih.gov/health/public/heart/hbp/dash/new_dash.pdf. NIH Publication Number 06-4082, April 2006.

(continued)

Medical Perspective, continued

Table 14-9 The DASH Eating Plan

Food Group	Daily Servings	Serving Sizes
Grains*	6–8	1 slice bread 1 oz dry cereal† ½ cup cooked rice, pasta, or cereal
Vegetables	4–5	1 cup raw leafy vegetable ½ cup cut-up raw or cooked vegetable ½ cup vegetable juice
Fruits	4–5	1 medium fruit ¼ cup dried fruit ½ cup fresh, frozen, or canned fruit ½ cup fruit juice
Fat-free or low-fat milk and milk products	2–3	1 cup milk or yogurt 1½ oz cheese
Lean meats, poultry, and fish	6 or less	1 oz cooked meats, poultry, or fish 1 egg
Nuts, seeds, and legumes	4–5 per week	⅓ cup or 1½ oz nuts 2 tbsp peanut butter 2 tbsp or ½ oz seeds ½ cup cooked legumes (dry beans and peas)
Fats and oils	2–3	1 tsp soft margarine 1 tsp vegetable oil 1 tbsp mayonnaise 2 tbsp salad dressing
Sweets and added sugars	5 or less per week	1 tbsp sugar 1 tbsp jelly or jam ½ cup sorbet, gelatin 1 cup lemonade

Source: Your Guide to Lowering Your Blood Pressure with DASH. http://www.nhlbi.nih.gov/health/public/heart/hbp/dash/new_dash.pdf. NIH Publication Number 06-4082, April 2006.
* *Whole grains are recommended for most grain servings as a good source of fiber and nutrients.*
† *Serving sizes vary between ½ cup and 1¼ cups, depending on cereal type.*

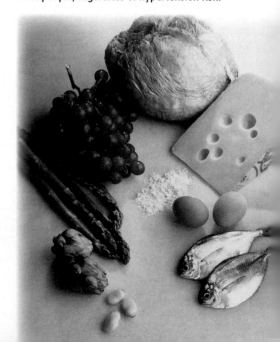

Opting for fruits, vegetables, and low-fat foods recommended by the DASH diet represents a sound approach to nutrition for most people, regardless of hypertension risk.

A careful test of the DASH diet revealed that it significantly lowered blood pressure in those with normal blood pressure, prehypertension, and hypertension (see Table 14-6). The biggest blood pressure drop occurred in those with hypertension—the diet worked about as well as some common blood pressure drugs. The DASH diet with the lowest amount of sodium (1500 mg/day) resulted in the largest decline in blood pressure.[40] The effectiveness of the DASH diet tells us that dietary choices can be as important as medications in controlling high blood pressure.

The health benefits of the DASH diet may extend beyond blood pressure reduction. In addition to nutrients, the diet's focus on fruits, vegetables, and whole grains contributes many other compounds to the diet. For instance, these foods are abundant in phytochemicals, such as polyphenols, antioxidants, and carotenoids, that can help prevent cancer and heart disease.

Drug Therapy for Hypertension

Medication usually isn't prescribed for hypertension until diastolic blood pressure measures at least 90 mm Hg and/or systolic blood pressure reaches 140 mm Hg on 3 or more occasions.[31] The following are the general classes of hypertension medications.

- Diuretics are used most frequently. They increase water and salt excretion from the body. Some diuretics also increase potassium excretion, requiring those using these medications to monitor potassium intake carefully. Examples of diuretics include furosemide (Lasix®) and hydrochlorothiazide (HydroDIURIL®).
- Beta-blockers (metropolol [Lopressor®]) slow the heart rate and force of heart contraction.
- Angiotensin-converting enzyme (ACE) inhibitors (captropril [Capoten®]) reduce the conversion of angiotensin I to angiotensin II in the lung (see Fig. 14-8), which leads to vasodilation.
- Calcium channel blockers (nifedipine [Adalat®, Procardia®]) prevent calcium from entering the cells of the heart and blood vessels, which causes vasodilation.

Knowledge Check

1. What are the risk factors for developing high blood pressure?
2. Why is the periodic measurement of blood pressure important?
3. Why is hypertension a dangerous condition?
4. What lifestyle changes can help prevent and treat hypertension?

 # 14.6 Calcium (Ca)

Calcium is an essential mineral for normal bone and tooth development. The calcium deficiency disease osteoporosis, or "porous bone," has been known since early history. Archeologists have even discovered 4000-year-old Egyptian mummies with the classic sign of osteoporosis—the dowager's hump or curved spine.[41] Calcium also has many industrial applications—one is as plaster of Paris, which was first used to set broken bones 1000 years ago.

Calcium in Foods

Dairy products, such as milk and cheese, provide a rich supply of bioavailable calcium and make up just over half the calcium in U.S. diets (Fig. 14-13).[18] White bread, rolls, crackers, and other foods made with dairy products are other contributors. Leafy greens, such as collards, kale, and turnip greens; broccoli; and calcium-fortified foods, such as fruit juices and breakfast cereals supply this mineral. The tiny soft bones present in canned fish, such as salmon and sardines, provide calcium, too. Another source of calcium is soybean curd (tofu) made using calcium carbonate.

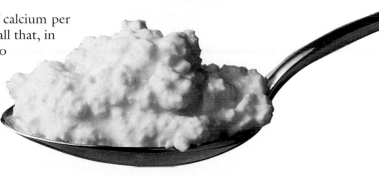

Cottage cheese contains less calcium than other dairy products because most of its calcium is lost during production.

When selecting foods as sources of calcium, both the amount of calcium per serving and the bioavailability of the calcium must be considered.[42] Recall that, in some plant foods, such as leafy greens, much of the calcium is bound to oxalic acid and is poorly absorbed.[16] As shown in Figure 14-14, the amount of calcium absorbed varies widely. For example, as little as 5% of the 250 mg of calcium in a cup of spinach is bioavailable—about 13 mg. In contrast, a third of the 300 mg of calcium in a cup of milk is absorbable, yielding nearly 100 mg for absorption. Calcium bioavailability is especially important for vegans and non-dairy users to consider.

Figure 14-13 Food sources of calcium.

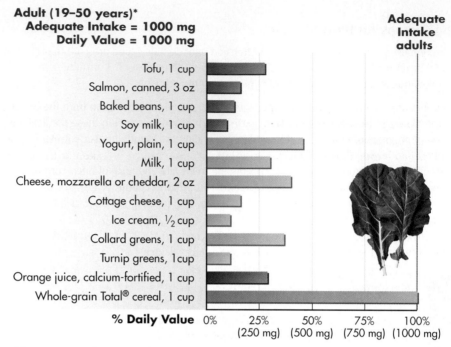

Adult (19–50 years)*
Adequate Intake = 1000 mg
Daily Value = 1000 mg

Adequate Intake adults

- Tofu, 1 cup
- Salmon, canned, 3 oz
- Baked beans, 1 cup
- Soy milk, 1 cup
- Yogurt, plain, 1 cup
- Milk, 1 cup
- Cheese, mozzarella or cheddar, 2 oz
- Cottage cheese, 1 cup
- Ice cream, ½ cup
- Collard greens, 1 cup
- Turnip greens, 1cup
- Orange juice, calcium-fortified, 1 cup
- Whole-grain Total® cereal, 1 cup

% Daily Value 0% 25% (250 mg) 50% (500 mg) 75% (750 mg) 100% (1000 mg)

*After age 51, Adequate Intake is 1200 mg.

Figure 14-14 The amount of calcium absorbed differs, depending on the food. [16, 42] Even though only about 30% of the calcium in dairy products is absorbed, these foods are rich in calcium and provide a greater total quantity of calcium than many foods containing better-absorbed calcium.

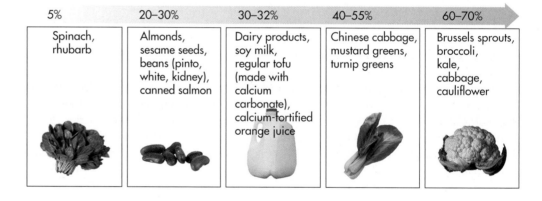

5%	20–30%	30–32%	40–55%	60–70%
Spinach, rhubarb	Almonds, sesame seeds, beans (pinto, white, kidney), canned salmon	Dairy products, soy milk, regular tofu (made with calcium carbonate), calcium-fortified orange juice	Chinese cabbage, mustard greens, turnip greens	Brussels sprouts, broccoli, kale, cabbage, cauliflower

CRITICAL THINKING

Lieu is a vegetarian. She stopped eating meat and dairy products when she was 15 years old. She does eat fish and eggs, though, along with a variety of other foods. Lieu is now 28 years old and wants to start a family. She is concerned about obtaining enough calcium from her diet to ensure her baby's health. How can she consume enough calcium to meet her own and her baby's needs?

Calcium Needs

The Adequate Intake for calcium ranges from 1000 to 1200 mg/day for adults. For adolescents between the ages of 9 and 18, the Adequate Intake is higher—1300 mg to allow for increases in bone mass during this time of rapid growth. The Daily Value used on food and supplement labels is 1000 mg.

In the U.S., average calcium intakes range from approximately 670 to 780 mg/day for women and 800 to 1100 mg/day for men.[17] Nearly one-fourth of women consume only about 500 mg per day.[17] Half of girls ages 9 to 18 consume less than 840 mg (or 65% of Adequate Intake) per day. Thus, dietary intakes of calcium by many women, especially young women, are well below the Adequate Intake amount, whereas intakes by most men are roughly equivalent to it.

Although diet is the best source, calcium supplements can be helpful, especially for individuals with low calorie intakes (such as elderly persons) and those who avoid dairy products. Supplements contain calcium salts, such as calcium carbonate (the form in calcium-based antacid tablets) and calcium citrate. The amount of calcium in a supplement depends on the form used. Calcium carbonate supplements have the highest proportion of calcium (40%), whereas those with calcium gluconate have the least (9%). The

Supplement Facts label lists the amount of elemental calcium found in each pill. To boost absorption levels, calcium supplements may contain vitamin D and other bone-building nutrients. Also, stomach acid produced during digestion improves absorption, so, for the greatest benefit, take calcium supplements in doses no higher than 500 mg and take them with or just after meals. Calcium citrate, which itself is acidic, is better absorbed by those with low stomach acid.[16]

Interactions with other minerals are important to consider when using calcium supplements. There is some evidence that calcium supplements may decrease zinc, iron, and magnesium absorption, although such effects appear to be small. To minimize the potential for mineral interactions, calcium supplements should not be taken at the same time as other mineral supplements.

Concern also exists over lead contamination of calcium supplements. Recall from Chapter 3 that lead ingestion causes an array of harmful effects on the body. In one study, nearly a quarter of the calcium supplements contained lead. The supplements made from natural sources, such as oyster shell and bone meal, were more likely to be contaminated.[43] Beginning in 2008, the FDA requires that companies test the purity and composition of their dietary supplement products.[44] Recall that buying the brands approved by the U.S. Pharmacopeia (USP) lessens the risk of purchasing contaminated supplements.

Calcium Absorption, Transport, Storage, Regulation, and Excretion

Calcium absorption occurs along the length of the intestinal tract.[16] However, absorption is most efficient in the upper part of the small intestine because its slightly acidic pH helps keep the calcium dissolved in its ionic form (Ca^{2+}). Intestinal contents become more alkaline as they pass through the intestine; thus, calcium absorption decreases at the terminal end of the small intestine and colon, although some still occurs via passive diffusion. In addition, active vitamin D hormone—$1,25\,(OH)_2$ vitamin D—promotes and regulates the active transport of calcium that occurs in the upper intestinal tract (see Chapter 12). When an individual has poor vitamin D status, calcium absorption is reduced.

Adults absorb about 25 to 30% of the calcium present in the foods they eat.[1] Several factors can affect calcium absorption. During periods of growth when the body needs extra calcium—such as infancy and pregnancy—absorption levels might reach 75%. Calcium absorption is higher when calcium sources are ingested with other foods and not on an empty stomach. Lactose, other sugars, and protein can enhance calcium absorption, too. Calcium absorption tends to decline with age, especially after age 70. Postmenopausal women generally absorb the least calcium. Other factors limiting calcium absorption include large intakes of phytic acid in fiber, oxalic acid, dietary phosphorus, and polyphenols (tannins) in tea. Vitamin D deficiency and diarrhea also inhibit calcium absorption.[1] Additionally, fat malabsorption that can occur with some intestinal disorders can lower calcium absorption because calcium binds with fatty acids, forming unabsorbable soaps in the intestinal lumen.

Calcium in the bloodstream is transported to cells either as free ionized calcium or bound to proteins. The skeleton and teeth hold more than 99% of the body's calcium. However, all cells, not just those in bone, have a crucial need for calcium.

The concentration of calcium in the bloodstream is regulated by very tight hormonal control. This means that normal blood calcium can be maintained even when calcium intake is poor, because calcium can be "withdrawn" from the bones to keep blood and cellular concentrations normal. (This situation makes blood calcium a poor measure of calcium status.) As discussed in Chapter 12, when blood calcium falls, the parathyroid gland releases parathyroid hormone (Fig. 14-15). This hormone raises blood calcium levels by working with $1,25\,(OH)_2$ vitamin D to increase the kidneys' reabsorption of calcium rather than excrete it in the urine. Parathyroid hormone also helps increase calcium

▶ No form of natural calcium, such as coral calcium or oyster shell calcium, is superior to typical supplement forms. Companies making such claims of superiority have been prosecuted by the U.S. Federal Trade Commission for false advertising.

▶ Some calcium supplements are poorly digested because they do not readily dissolve. To test for solubility, put a supplement in 6 oz of vinegar. Stir every 5 minutes. It should dissolve within 30 minutes.

▶ A 154-lb (70-kg) person has about 2.2 to 3 lb (1000 to 1400 g) of calcium stored in bones and teeth.

Ninety-nine percent of the calcium in the body is found in bones.

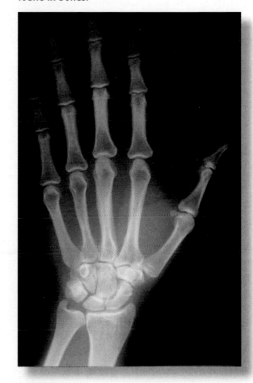

Figure 14-15 Blood parathyroid hormone and calcitonin are key factors in controlling blood calcium levels. When blood calcium rises too high **1**, the thyroid gland releases calcitonin **2**. This hormone restores blood calcium to normal levels (**2**–**5**). When blood calcium levels fall too low **6**, the thyroid gland releases parathyroid hormone **7**. This hormone restores blood calcium to normal levels (**7**–**11**). Parathyroid hormone also helps activate vitamin D hormone [1,25 $(OH)_2$ vitamin D]. On a day-to-day basis, parathyroid hormone is the most important regulator of blood calcium levels.

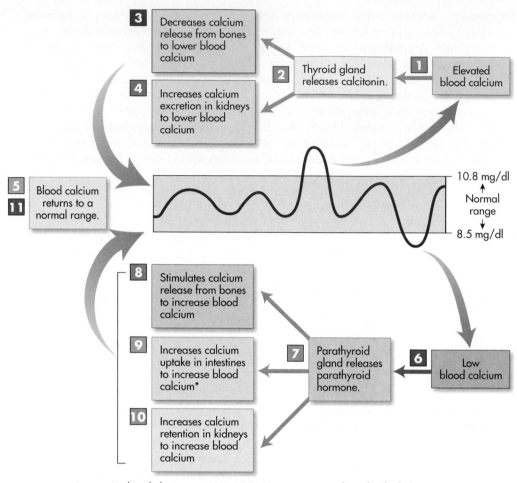

*Indirectly by increasing 1,25 $(OH)_2$ vitamin D synthesis by the kidneys.

absorption indirectly by promoting the synthesis of 1,25 $(OH)_2$ vitamin D. In addition, parathyroid hormone often works in conjunction with 1,25 $(OH)_2$ vitamin D to increase the calcium released from bones.

When blood calcium levels rise too high, the release of parathyroid hormone falls. This causes calcium excretion via the urine to increase. The synthesis of 1,25 $(OH)_2$ vitamin D also decreases, causing a drop in calcium absorption. In addition, the thyroid gland secretes the hormone calcitonin, which blocks calcium loss from bones. All these metabolic changes keep blood calcium within the normal range.

In addition to being excreted via the urine, other routes for dietary calcium excretion are the skin and the feces (Fig. 14-16). Calcium that is a part of intestinal secretions also can pass out of the body in the feces.[1]

Functions of Calcium

Developing and maintaining bones are calcium's major functions in the body. Calcium also is required for blood clotting, the transmission of nerve impulses, muscle contraction, and cell metabolism.

Bone Development and Maintenance

Bone consists of a network of protein fibers, primarily collagen, and minerals. Calcium and phosphorus, obtained from the diet, are the main minerals in bone. The diet also supplies other minerals needed for healthy bones, including magnesium, potassium, sodium, fluoride, vitamin K, and sulfur. Calcium and phosphorus form the latticelike crystal

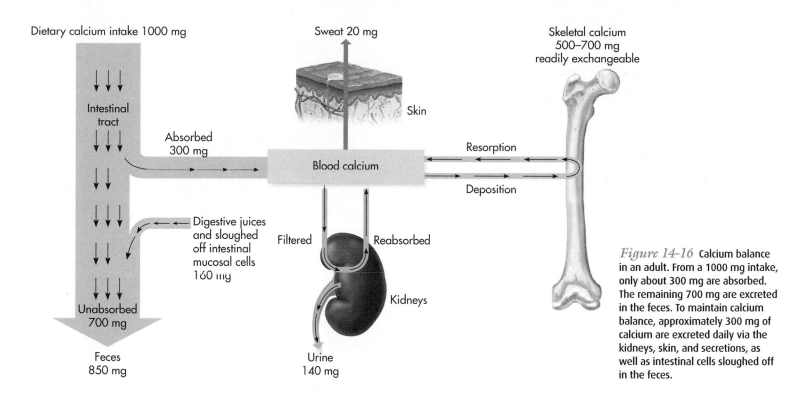

Figure 14-16 Calcium balance in an adult. From a 1000 mg intake, only about 300 mg are absorbed. The remaining 700 mg are excreted in the feces. To maintain calcium balance, approximately 300 mg of calcium are excreted daily via the kidneys, skin, and secretions, as well as intestinal cells sloughed off in the feces.

hydroxyapatite, $Ca_{10}(PO_4)6OH_2$, which binds to the collagen fibers. This combination of materials allows bone to be resilient and strong. Collagen protein allows the skeleton to absorb impact (bone does not usually break when you jump) and the hydroxyapatite crystal makes bone strong (bone does not bend or collapse when you jump).

The outer, dense shell of bone is **cortical** bone; it makes up about 75% of the skeletal mass. The remainder is **trabecular** bone, a hard, spongy network of rods, plates, and needlelike spines that add strength without much weight (Fig. 14-17). Trabecular bone is abundant at the ends of the long bones, inside the spinal vertebrae, and inside the flat bones of the pelvis. Trabecular bone also is where most minerals move into and out of bone.

Bone is continually being built, broken down, and reshaped. This process of removing and replacing bone is referred to as **remodeling**. Remodeling is vital for bone health because it allows bones to grow normally and to repair and replace damaged (e.g., very small cracks) or brittle areas. Remodeling also permits calcium and phosphorus to be "withdrawn" and used for other functions when dietary intake is insufficient. Three main types of bone cells function in bone growth and remodeling: osteoblasts, osteocytes, and osteoclasts (see Fig. 14-17). **Osteoblasts** are bone-building cells that produce collagen and add minerals to form healthy bone. Some of the fully mineralized osteoblasts mature to form osteocytes, the most numerous cells in bones. **Osteocytes** are biochemically active; they can take up calcium from the blood and release it back into the blood, as well as help bone become more dense, if needed. In contrast, **osteoclasts** are cells on the bone surface that dissolve bone (termed *bone resorption*) by releasing acid and enzymes. Their activity is stimulated by parathyroid hormone, often in conjunction with $1,25\ (OH)_2$ vitamin D. Osteoclasts are very active when a diet is deficient in calcium—they release calcium from the bone, so that it can enter the blood. Remember, a supply of calcium is vital to all cells, not just to bone cells.

During times of growth, total osteoblast activity exceeds osteoclast activity, so we make more bone than we break down. This also can occur when bone is put under high stress—a right-handed tennis player, for example, builds more bone in that arm than in the left arm. Most bone is built from infancy through the late adolescent years. Calcium recommendations are set high during these times to support this bone-building activity.

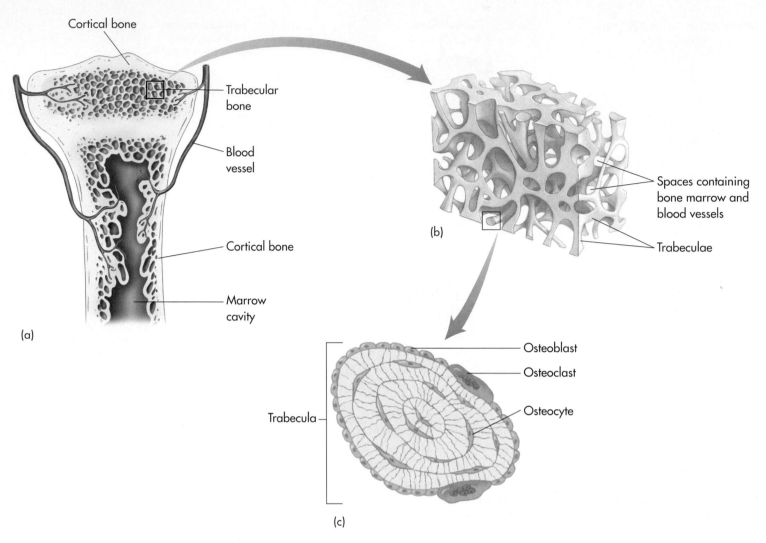

Cortical bone

Trabecular bone

Blood vessel

Cortical bone

Marrow cavity

(a)

Spaces containing bone marrow and blood vessels

Trabeculae

(b)

Osteoblast

Osteoclast

Osteocyte

Trabecula

(c)

Figure 14-17 (*a*) Cortical and trabecular bone. Cortical bone forms the shafts of bones and the outer mineral covering. (*b*) Trabecular bone supports the outer shell of cortical bone in various bones of the body and has the most metabolic activity. (*c*) Osteoblasts build new bone; osteoclasts break down or resorb bone; osteocytes form from osteoblasts and are surrounded by mineral.

▶ The tooth consists of a hard, yellowish tissue called dentin, which is covered with enamel in the crown and cementum in the root. Enamel, the hardest substance in the body, is almost entirely hydroxyapatite crystals. Produced before the tooth erupts, enamel is not a living tissue and, unlike bone, does not undergo remodeling. Enamel can be easily damaged by acids produced by bacteria in the mouth from the metabolism of sugars and carbohydrates. This damage is known as dental caries, or cavities. Repairing dental caries requires the skills of a dentist. The number of dental caries in the U.S. population has declined because of the addition of fluoride to some municipal water supplies, bottled water, and oral care products. Fluoride helps strengthen the enamel and makes it more resistant to acids. It also helps remineralize enamel in the earliest stages of damage.

Small increases in bone mass continue between 20 and 30 years of age. Genetic background controls up to 80% of the variation in the peak bone mass ultimately built.[27]

Throughout adulthood, bone remodeling is ongoing. In fact, most of the adult skeleton is replaced about every 10 years.[45] However, beginning in middle age, osteoclast activity generally becomes more dominant in both men and women. This can result in a total loss of about 25% of bone, depending on how long the person lives.[46] Women experience even greater bone loss when estrogen levels fall in menopause because estrogen inhibits bone breakdown by decreasing osteoclast activity. Women can experience an additional 20% loss of bone in the first 5 to 7 years following menopause.[46] Absent or irregular menses in younger women, which can occur because of very low body weight, eating disorders, or the female athlete triad (see Chapter 11), signal low estrogen levels and a likelihood of substantial bone loss before middle age. When the rate of bone loss exceeds the rate at which bone is rebuilt, bone mass and bone strength decline and the risk of fracture rises greatly. (Significant bone mass loss, known as osteoporosis, is discussed in the Medical Perspective: Osteoporosis later in the chapter.)

Blood Clotting

Calcium ions participate in several reactions in the cascade that leads to the formation of fibrin, the main protein component of a blood clot. (See Fig. 12-20 in Chapter 12 for more details on blood clotting.)

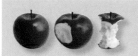

Take Action

Estimate Your Calcium Intake

Dietary Sources of Calcium	Number of Servings per Day	Calcium Content (mg per Serving)	Calcium Intake (mg per Day)
Calcium-fortified juice, 6 oz Yogurt, 8 oz		× 350	
Milk, any type, 1 cup Calcium-fortified soy milk, 1 cup Canned sardines, 3 oz Parmesan cheese, grated, 1 oz Lasagna or manicotti, 1 cup Quiche, 1 piece Tofu (processed with calcium), 4 oz		× 300	
Hard natural cheeses—Cheddar, mozzarella, Swiss, 1 oz Cheese pizza, 1 slice of 12″–pie Broccoli, 1 cup		× 200	
Soft cheeses—Ricotta or fortified cottage cheese (not regular cottage cheese), ¼ cup Calcium-fortified cereal bars and granola bar, 1 each Canned pink salmon, 3 oz Meat-topped pizza, 1 slice of 12″ pie Chinese cabbage and mustard greens, 1 cup		× 150	
Processed cheeses—American or Swiss, 1 slice Macaroni and cheese, prepared from box, 1 cup Almonds, ¼ cup		× 100	
Calcium intake from other foods; add 290 mg if you are a female or 370 mg if you are a male		+ 290 or + 370 mg	
Other calcium sources to consider: fortified cereals and vitamin and mineral supplements (check the labels)		Varies	
500 mg per serving calcium supplements: pills, calcium-fortified candies		× 500	
Total calcium intake:			

Compare your calcium intake with the AI for calcium, found on the inside cover of your textbook.

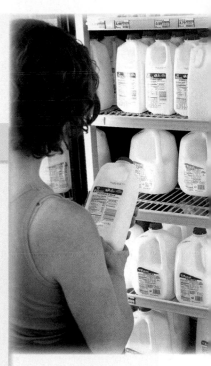

Transmission of Nerve Impulses to Target Cells

When a nerve impulse reaches its target site—such as a muscle, other nerve cells, or a gland—the impulse is transmitted across the **synapse,** the junction between the nerve and its target cells. In many nerves, the arrival of the impulse at the target site causes calcium ions from the extracellular medium to flow into the nerve. The rise in calcium ions in the nerve triggers synaptic vesicles to release their store of neurotransmitters. The released neurotransmitter then carries the impulse across the synapse to the target cells (Fig. 14-18).

In an entirely different process, nerve impulses develop spontaneously if insufficient calcium is available, leading to what is called hypocalcemic **tetany.** This condition is characterized by muscle spasms because the muscles receive continual nerve stimulation.

tetany Continuous, forceful muscle contraction without relaxation.

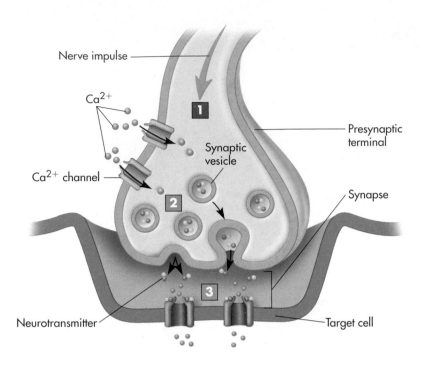

Figure 14-18 The release of a neurotransmitter. Nerve impulses, by opening Ca²⁺ channels **1**, stimulate the fusion of synaptic vesicles containing neurotransmitters with the cell membrane of the nerve terminals **2**. This leads to the release of a neurotransmitter into the synapse **3**. The neurotransmitter is carried across the synaptic to the target cells.

calmodulin Calcium-binding protein occurring in many tissues and participating in the regulation of many biochemical and physiological processes.

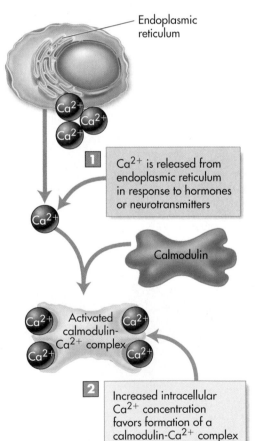

Figure 14-19 Intracellular calcium (Ca²⁺) binds to the protein calmodulin, activating it. Many intracellular enzymes require calmodulin for activity. These include enzymes required for smooth muscle contraction and to initiate the breakdown of glycogen.

Inadequate parathyroid hormone release or action is the typical cause of hypocalcemia (low blood calcium).[16]

Muscle Contraction

The critical role of calcium in muscle contraction is most easily understood in the context of skeletal muscles, but other types of muscles use calcium in a similar fashion. When a skeletal muscle fiber is stimulated by a nerve impulse from the brain, calcium ions are released from intracellular stores within the muscle cells. The resulting increase in the concentration of calcium ions in a muscle cell is one factor, along with sufficient ATP that permits the contractile proteins to slide along each other.[16] This sliding leads to muscle contraction. Then, to allow for subsequent relaxation, the calcium ions are actively transported to the intracellular storage site and the contractile proteins slide apart. (See Fig. A-4 in Appendix A.)

Cell Metabolism

Calcium ions help regulate metabolism in the cell by participating in the **calmodulin** system. Each calmodulin binds 4 calcium ions. When calcium enters a cell (often because of hormone action) and binds to the protein calmodulin, the resulting calcium-calmodulin complex activates many intracellular enzymes, including one that initiates the breakdown of glycogen (Fig. 14-19).[16]

Potential Health Benefits of Calcium

Researchers have examined links between calcium intake and the risks of a wide array of diseases. Overall, the benefits of a diet providing adequate calcium extend beyond bone health. Both calcium and dairy products may protect against the development of colon cancer.[47, 48] Dietary calcium also may protect against some forms of kidney stones and, as discussed in the Medical Perspective: Hypertension and Nutrition earlier in the chapter, a calcium-rich diet (800 to 1200 mg/day) may help decrease blood pressure.

A possible link among calcium intake, metabolism, and body weight may exist. Studies in animals, as well as epidemiological studies in people, suggest that high calcium

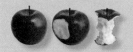 *Take Action*

Bone Health

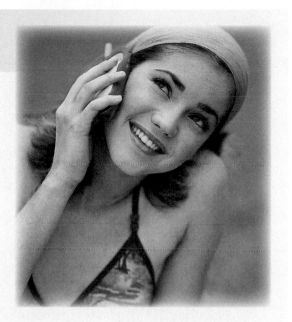

Jana, a sophomore in high school, recently gave up drinking milk to help control her weight. Jana also just started smoking and her level of physical activity is low. Jana's diet on a recent day consisted of the following items. For breakfast, she had oatmeal made with water, a banana, and a cup of fruit juice. At midmorning, she bought a snack cake from the vending machine. At lunch, she had vegetable pasta, bread with olive oil, a small salad, 1 ounce of mixed nuts, and a soft drink. For dinner, she had a hamburger, along with mixed vegetables and another soft drink. As an evening snack, she had some cookies and hot tea.

1. What factors place Jana at risk of poor bone health?

2. What changes to her current lifestyle could reduce that risk?

3. Create an eating plan that could help Jana reduce her risk of osteoporosis.

diets, especially high dairy intake, may prevent the accumulation of body fat.[49] Hormones that regulate calcium metabolism also help regulate the formation and breakdown of fat in adipose cells. However, in clinical trials of weight loss and increased calcium from either dairy foods or supplements, the extra calcium sometimes aided weight loss, but just as often did not.[50] At this point, those attempting weight loss should meet calcium requirements, but the focus for weight loss should be on the overall energy balance of the diet.

For women with a low calcium intake, supplementation with calcium may help reduce the risk of developing high blood pressure during pregnancy. However, in well-nourished women, calcium supplements probably do not help with this problem.[51, 52]

Upper Level for Calcium

The Upper Level for calcium is 2500 mg/day, which is based on evidence of increased risk of developing kidney stones at higher intakes.[1] Normally, the small intestine prevents the absorption of excess calcium. However, both **hyperparathyroidism** and the consumption of high levels of supplemental calcium can cause calcium levels in the blood to increase and lead to calcification of the kidneys and other organs. Other symptoms are irritability, headache, kidney failure, kidney stones, and decreased absorption of other minerals. Ordinarily, calcium in food and usual doses of calcium supplements do not pose a health threat because this mineral is present in relatively modest amounts.

hyperparathyroidism Overproduction of parathyroid hormone by the parathyroid gland, usually caused by a tumor. In most cases, there are no symptoms except hypercalcemia but, in more severe cases, weakness, confusion, nausea, and bone pain occur. Hypertension and kidney stones also are problems.

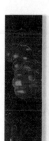 *Knowledge Check*

1. Which foods are the most bioavailable sources of calcium?
2. How do parathyroid hormone and vitamin D regulate serum calcium?
3. What are the functions of osteoblasts, osteocytes, and osteoclasts in bone?
4. Other than building bones and teeth, what are the functions of calcium in the body?

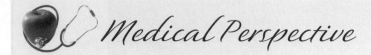

Medical Perspective

Osteoporosis

Osteoporosis is the disease most often linked to low intakes of calcium. When calcium intake is insufficient, the body withdraws calcium from bone. This action preserves the indispensable functions of calcium, such as those that keep the heart and muscles working. However, bone health is related to many factors, including several other nutritional and lifestyle factors.

Osteoporosis develops over a period of many years. A failure to maintain adequate bone mass in the body first leads to a state of osteopenia called low bone mass. Osteopenia can be caused by the vitamin D deficiency disease osteomalacia, certain medications, cancer, anorexia nervosa, or other health conditions. Osteoporosis is diagnosed when bone loss and strength decline significantly and bones become fragile and likely to break (Fig. 14-20).[45] The bones most likely to break are the hip, wrist, and vertebrae in the spine. Hip fractures are the most devastating—about 20% of those who suffer a hip fracture will die during the first year after the fracture, and those who do survive often can no longer walk without help and must move into long-term care facilities.[45, 53] Loss of bone in the spine leads to compression fractures in the vertebrae, loss of height, and eventually **kyphosis** (dowager's hump).

Osteoporosis currently affects more than 8 million women and 2 million men in the U.S. and an additional 34 million have low bone mass.[46] In the U.S., African-Americans have the lowest rates of osteoporosis, followed by those of Hispanic/Latino heritage. The highest rates are seen in Caucasians and Asians. The factors commonly associated with a higher risk of osteoporosis are listed in Table 14-10. Half of all women and a quarter of all men over age 50 living in the U.S. are likely to suffer an osteoporosis-related bone fracture in their lifetimes. Currently, osteoporosis-related costs in the U.S. equal $17 billion per year in direct medical expenses, and they will increase to $50 billion by 2040.[46] There are now good ways to diagnose, treat, and prevent osteoporosis.

kyphosis Abnormal convex curvature of the spine, resulting in a bulge at the upper back.

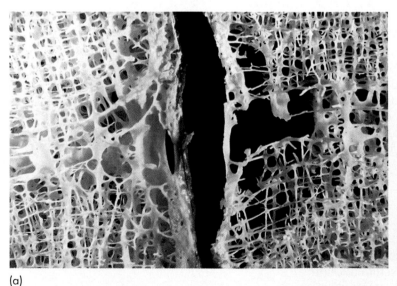
(a)

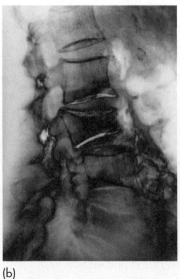
(b)

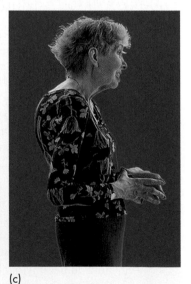
(c)

Figure 14-20 (*a*) Normal and osteoporotic trabecular bone. Note in the picture on the right how there is much less trabecular bone. Breaks in horizontal or vertical trabecular beams weaken a bone's support system and increases the risk for bone fracture. (*b*) Colorized X ray of vertebrae severely damaged by osteoporosis. (*c*) Abnormal curvature of the upper spine—kyphosis.

Table 14-10 Factors Associated with a Higher Risk of Osteoporosis

- History of osteoporotic fracture in a first-degree relative (i.e., parent or sibling)
- Small, thin skeletal frame
- Low peak bone mass
- Advancing age
- Being a Caucasian or an Asian post-menopausal woman
- Amenorrhea (cessation of normal menstrual periods; indicates insufficient estrogen)
- Oophorectomy (removal of ovaries; results in estrogen deficiency)
- Smoking (smoking can have direct toxic effects on bone and can impact the absorption and metabolism of bone-forming nutrients; smokers also are likely to be less physically active)
- Low calcium intake
- Vitamin D deficiency
- Low physical activity
- Excessive alcohol consumption
- Presence of other diseases, such as cystic fibrosis, anorexia nervosa, type 1 diabetes mellitus, inflammatory bowel disease, celiac disease, multiple sclerosis, or epilepsy (these diseases can cause impaired absorption, metabolism, and utilization of bone-forming nutrients; in some cases, nutrient excretion may be increased)
- Chronic use of some medications, especially glucocorticoids (used to treat many inflammatory and autoimmune diseases)

Source: From National Osteoporosis Foundation and the Surgeon General's Report on Bone Health and Osteoporosis.

Osteoporosis Diagnosis

A simple and very accurate test to identify osteoporosis is a dual energy X-ray absorptiometry (DEXA) bone scan.[45] DEXA scans measure bone mineral density in the spine, hip, and total body using a very low dose of X-ray radiation (about 1/10 of that received during a chest X-ray). For this test, a person lies down on his or her back on a table for 10 to 20 minutes while an imaging arm glides over the length of the body (see Fig. 10-13 in Chapter 10). The ability of a bone to block the path of radiation is used as a measure of bone mineral density at that bone site. The DEXA measurements of the observed bone density is compared with that of a person at peak bone density (Fig. 14-21). The score resulting from these comparisons indicate whether bone mineral density is normal, low (osteopenia), or very low (osteoporosis).

Peripheral DEXA and ultrasound are other ways to measure the bone density of one part of the body, such as the wrist or heel. Peripheral methods are faster than DEXA but are not as accurate because the density of one part of the body may not reflect the density of other areas susceptible to fractures, such as the spine.

Osteoporosis Prevention and Treatment

There are a variety of strategies that can help build peak bone mass, thereby preventing osteoporosis.[45, 54, 55] One very important lifelong strategy is to get ample quantities of bone-building nutrients: calcium, vitamin D, phosphorus, magnesium, and vitamin K. Mounting evidence indicates potassium also may be important to bone health.[55] The optimal amount of vitamin D needed to prevent or slow bone loss is an area of active research and discussion. Some research suggests that the Adequate Intake (5 to 15 ug/day) is not sufficient for some individuals (see Expert Perspective from the Field in Chapter 12).[56] Vitamin D intakes substantially higher than the Adequate Intake may be recommended for older adults, as well as those with osteopenia or osteoporosis.[46] Studies show that supplemental calcium, especially at a minimal dose of 1200 mg per day and vitamin D doses of 800 IU or more, may help prevent or slow bone loss and reduce osteoporotic fracture, especially in older adults and post-menopausal women with low serum levels of vitamin D.[56, 57] The Women's Health Initiative, a 7-year study of 36,282 post-menopausal women, found that those who took daily supplements of calcium (1000 mg calcium carbonate) and vitamin D (10 µg [400 IU]) throughout the entire

(continued)

Medical Perspective, continued

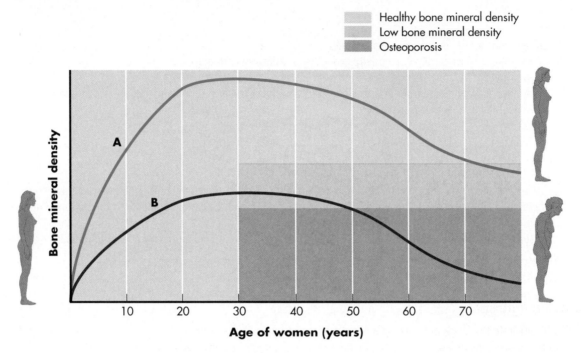

Figure 14-21 The relationship between peak bone mass and the ultimate risk of developing osteoporosis and related bone fractures.
- **Woman A** had developed a high peak bone mass by age 30. Her bone loss was slow and steady between ages 30 and 50 and sped up somewhat after age 50 because of the effects of menopause. At age 75, the woman had a healthy bone mineral density value and did not show evidence of osteoporosis.
- **Woman B** with low peak bone mass experienced the same rate of bone loss as woman A. By age 50, she already had low mineral density and by age 70 kyphosis and spinal fractures had occurred.

Given the low calcium intakes that are common among young women today, line B is a sobering reality. Following a diet and lifestyle pattern that contributes to maximal bone mineral density can help women follow line A and significantly reduce their risk of developing osteoporosis.

study period had higher hipbone densities and a 29% reduction in hip fractures than those taking a placebo.[58]

An active lifestyle that includes weight-bearing physical activity is also important to build and maintain muscle and bone mass. An added bonus is that exercise can help improve balance and strength, which reduces the risk of falling—a major cause of bone fractures in older and frail adults.

Other osteoporosis prevention strategies include smoking cessation and limited alcohol intake. In addition, moderating caffeine, sodium, and protein intake is advised because high intakes can depress calcium absorption when dietary calcium intake is low.[1]

▶ To reduce the risk of falls, older people should exercise, limit medications and alcohol that affect physical coordination, and wear corrective lenses if their visual function is impaired.

Drug Therapy for Osteoporosis Prevention

At menopause, women should discuss osteoporosis prevention strategies with their health-care providers. They also need to keep accurate measures of their height—a decrease of more than 1½ inches from pre-menopausal height is a sign that significant bone loss is taking place (Fig. 14-22). Currently, the following 5 medical therapies can be used to slow bone loss at menopause in women.

- Estrogen slows osteoclast activity, which limits bone resorption.
- Bisphosphonates bind to hydroxyapatite crystals and osteoclasts, which slows bone resorption. (Bisphosphonates are often used in lieu of estrogen because of the increased risk

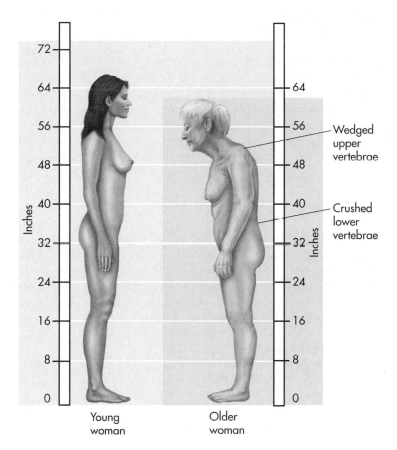

Figure 14-22 A loss of height and a distorted body shape are common signs of osteoporosis. Monitor your adult height changes to detect early osteoporosis.

Young woman

Older woman

Wedged upper vertebrae

Crushed lower vertebrae

of certain cancers and cardiovascular disease in some post-menopausal women.) Examples include alendronate (Fosamax®) and ibandronate (Boniva®).

- Selective estrogen receptor modulators (SERMs) (e.g., raloxifene [Evista®]) increase the utilization of existing estrogen in the body, which slows osteoclast activity.
- Calcitonin (Miacalcin®) inhibits osteoclast activity and bone resorption.
- Parathyroid hormone (PTH) (teriparatide [Forteo®]) stimulates osteoblast activity and new bone formation.

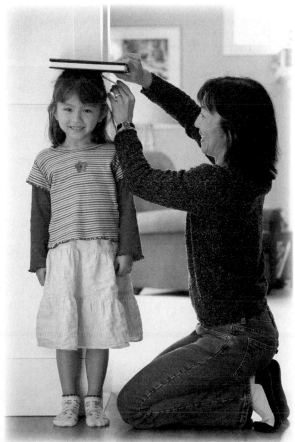

To measure height accurately at home, tape a measuring tape (preferably made of metal) to a wall that does not have a baseboard. Be sure the measuring tape starts exactly at the floor and goes straight up the wall (perpendicular to the floor). With your shoes off and your back to the wall, stand up straight in front of the measuring tape. Your heels, buttocks, shoulders, and head should touch the wall. Keep eyes parallel with the floor. To determine your height, have a friend hold a piece of rigid cardboard above your head. The cardboard should be parallel to the floor with an edge touching the measuring tape. Then, slide the cardboard down the wall until it touches the highest point of your head—this is your maximum height.

14.7 Phosphorus (P)

Phosphorus is an essential mineral required by every cell in the body. This phosphorescing (glowing) mineral wasn't discovered until the late 1600s, when Henning Brand, a merchant and amateur alchemist, distilled urine, hoping to manufacture gold! Instead, he discovered glowing white phosphorus in the bottom of the flask. Phosphorus was obtained in this way until researchers discovered that bones are another rich (and more pleasant!) source of this mineral. As you might guess from its history, this essential mineral is a major component of bone and teeth, and dietary excesses are removed by the kidneys.

Phosphorus in Foods

Milk, cheese, meat, bakery products, and cereals provide most of the phosphorus in the adult diet.[18] Bran, eggs, nuts, and fish also are sources (Fig. 14-23). Food additives, such as monosodium phosphate (emulsifier), monocalcium phosphate (jelling agent/dough conditioner), and nutrients used for fortification (e.g., iron phosphate), also contribute as much as 400 mg per day of phosphorus to the diet. Note that phosphorus from food additives may not be included in nutrient databases.[18]

Figure 14-23 Food sources of phosphorus.

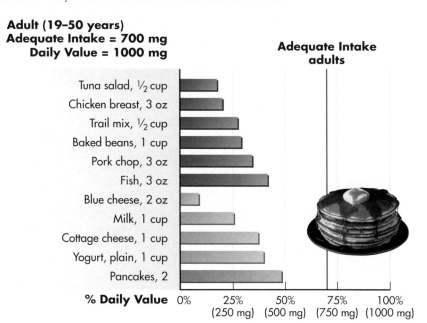

Adult (19–50 years)
Adequate Intake = 700 mg
Daily Value = 1000 mg

Adequate Intake adults

Tuna salad, 1/2 cup	
Chicken breast, 3 oz	
Trail mix, 1/2 cup	
Baked beans, 1 cup	
Pork chop, 3 oz	
Fish, 3 oz	
Blue cheese, 2 oz	
Milk, 1 cup	
Cottage cheese, 1 cup	
Yogurt, plain, 1 cup	
Pancakes, 2	

% Daily Value 0%   25% (250 mg)   50% (500 mg)   75% (750 mg)   100% (1000 mg)

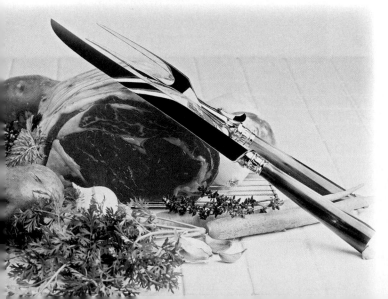

Meats are a rich source of phosphorus.

Phosphorus Needs

The RDA for both adult men and women is 700 mg/day.[1] Average intakes in adults range from 950 to 1650 mg per day.[17] Thus, a phosphorus deficiency is unlikely in healthy adults, especially because it is so efficiently absorbed. The Daily Value for phosphorus used on food and supplement labels is 1000 mg.

Absorption, Transport, Storage, and Excretion of Phosphorus

Adults absorb up to 70% of dietary phosphorus. Absorption occurs mainly in the upper small intestine and is absorbed by both active transport and diffusion. The active vitamin D hormone 1,25(OH)$_2$ vitamin D enhances absorption. Phosphorus in grains and legumes is mainly in the form of phytates and is poorly absorbed because we lack enzymes that release the phosphorus.[1] However, phosphorus in grain products prepared with yeast (e.g., bread) is better absorbed due to the breakdown of the phytate by the yeast.

Approximately 80% of the phosphorus in the body is found in bones and teeth as calcium phosphate (hydroxyapatite). The remainder of the phosphate is found in every cell in the body and in the extracellular fluid as PO_4^{2-}. Phosphorus is excreted by the kidneys. The degree of excretion is the primary mechanism by which blood phosphorus level is regulated.[59]

Functions of Phosphorus

In addition to being a major component of bones and teeth, phosphorus is critical to the function of every cell in the body. As HPO_4^{2-} or $H_2PO_4^-$, phosphorus is the main intracellular anion, similar to chloride in the extracellular fluid. As a component of ATP and creatine phosphate, phosphorus is critical to energy production and storage. This mineral also is a part of DNA and RNA, phospholipids in cell membranes, and numerous enzyme and cellular message systems. Many hormones depend on phosphorylation for their activation. Phosphorus also helps regulate acid-base balance in the body. Ample intakes of phosphorus, like that of calcium, potassium, and magnesium, may help protect against hypertension.[60]

Phosphorus Deficiency

Phosphorus deficiency is rare, but a chronic deficiency of phosphorus can contribute to bone loss, decreased growth, and poor tooth development. The symptoms of rickets may occur in phosphorus-deficient children because of insufficient bone mineralization. Other symptoms of phosphorus deficiency include anorexia, weight loss, weakness, irritability, stiff joints, and bone pain. Marginal phosphorus status can be found in preterm infants, alcoholics, older people eating nutrient-poor diets, those with long-term bouts of diarrhea and weight loss, and people who frequently use aluminum-containing antacids, which can bind phosphorus in the small intestine.[59]

Toxicity and Upper Level for Phosphorus

Like phosphorus deficiency, toxicity from phosphorus is rare. High blood concentrations of phosphorus (hyperphosphatemia) can cause calcium-phosphorus precipitates to form in body tissues. Poor kidney function is the most common cause of hyperphosphatemia.

The typical American diet often has a low calcium intake coupled with a high phosphorus intake. For many decades, nutritionists thought this ratio of calcium to phosphorus contributed to mild hyperparathyroidism and bone loss. However, it is now thought that elevated PTH and bone loss occur in response to not meeting calcium needs (as can occur when soft drinks are substituted for milk and other calcium sources), rather than to the ratio of calcium to phosphorus in the diet. The Upper Level for phosphorus in adulthood is 3 to 4 g/day, based on the risk of developing a high blood concentration.[1]

▶ People who have experienced extreme weight loss and long-term poor nutrient intake are at risk of low blood phosphorus and a related condition called refeeding syndrome. If these individuals are aggressively refed, such as in a hospital or in a famine relief setting (in the developing world), much of the small amount of phosphorus in the bloodstream will shift into cells in order to participate in essential metabolic pathways. This shift can cause blood phosphorus to be so low that respiratory failure and other critical health conditions may result. To avoid this problem, clinicians generally start by checking a starving person's blood phosphorus and correcting the deficiency (if present), then gradually refeeding while monitoring and adjusting blood phosphorus to keep it in the normal range.[59]

Knowledge Check

1. Which foods are high in phosphorus?
2. In addition to its structural roles for bones and teeth, what are 2 critical roles of phosphorus in the body?
3. What are some of the symptoms of phosphorus deficiency?

Figure 14-24 Food sources of magnesium.

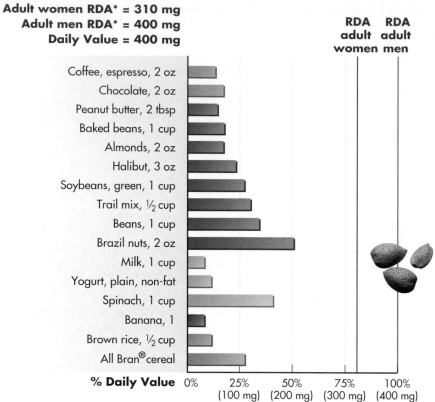

Adult women RDA* = 310 mg
Adult men RDA* = 400 mg
Daily Value = 400 mg

* After age 30, RDA is 320 mg for women and 420 mg for men.

14.8 Magnesium (Mg)

Magnesium was first discovered in Magnesia, a region of Greece. This silvery white metal is abundant in soil and in ocean water. It is an essential nutrient for both plants and animals—a wide array of foods supply us with magnesium.

Magnesium in Foods

Magnesium is found in chlorophyll. Thus, some of the richest sources of magnesium are plant products, such as green leafy vegetables, broccoli, squash, beans, nuts, seeds, whole grains, and chocolate (Fig. 14-24). Animal products, such as milk and meats, supply some magnesium, although less than the plant-based foods. Another source of magnesium is hard tap water, which contains a high mineral content (hard water also contains calcium). Refined foods generally are low in magnesium. The form of magnesium in multivitamins and mineral supplements (magnesium oxide) is not well absorbed. About 45% of dietary magnesium comes from vegetables, fruits, grains, and nuts, whereas about 30% comes from milk, meat, and eggs.

Magnesium Needs

The RDAs for magnesium are 400 mg/day for men 19 to 30 years of age and 310 mg/day for women 19 to 30 years of age.[1] Magnesium needs increase slightly (10 to 20 mg/day) beyond age 30. The Daily Value on food and supplement labels is 400 mg. Adults in the U.S. fall short on magnesium intake, with intakes averaging about 80% of the RDA.[17]

Nuts are a rich source of magnesium.

Absorption, Transport, Storage, and Excretion of Magnesium

About 40 to 60% of the magnesium consumed is absorbed, but absorption efficiency can rise to about 80% when intakes are low. Magnesium is absorbed in the small intestine by both passive and active absorption. The active vitamin D hormone 1,25 (OH)$_2$ vitamin D enhances magnesium absorption to a limited extent. About half of the magnesium is found in bones and the rest is stored in other tissues, such as muscles. The kidneys primarily regulate blood concentrations of magnesium and are able to reduce magnesium loss into the urine when blood magnesium is low.[61]

▶ Magnesium sulfate is sometimes used to treat pregnancy-induced hypertension (see Chapter 16). Magnesium likely relaxes blood vessels, leading to a fall in blood pressure.

Functions of Magnesium

Magnesium has a vital role in a range of biochemical and physiological processes. Magnesium helps stabilize ATP by binding to the phosphate groups of this molecule. In fact, magnesium is required by more than 300 enzymes that utilize ATP, including those required for energy metabolism, muscle contraction, and protein synthesis. A magnesium-dependent enzyme system pumps sodium out of cells and potassium into cells—this process seems especially sensitive to magnesium deficiency. Magnesium also is needed for DNA and RNA synthesis. Its role in calcium metabolism contributes to bone structure and mineralization. Magnesium also is important for nerve transmission, heart and smooth muscle contraction, insulin release from the pancreas, and insulin action on cells. Other possible benefits of magnesium include decreasing blood pressure by dilating arteries, preventing heart rhythm abnormalities, and protecting against gallstone formation.[61, 62]

Magnesium Deficiency

Magnesium deficiency causes an irregular heartbeat, sometimes accompanied by weakness, muscle spasms, disorientation, nausea, vomiting, and seizures. These symptoms may be related to abnormal nerve cell function caused by an impairment of sodium and potassium pumping. Magnesium deficiency also can cause a fall in PTH release, resulting in low blood calcium. The action of 1,25(OH)$_2$ vitamin D also is blunted during magnesium deficiency. Both of these factors may contribute to an increasing risk of osteoporosis in those with poor magnesium status. Low intakes of magnesium also may increase the risk of Metabolic Syndrome (see Chapter 5).[63] A magnesium deficiency develops very slowly because the body stores it readily.[1]

Excessive loss of magnesium either from the intestinal tract or the urine is responsible for most magnesium deficiencies.[61] People with GI disorders who experience prolonged bouts of diarrhea and vomiting are at risk. Those who take certain diuretics, alcoholics, and those with poorly controlled diabetes excrete more magnesium in their urine. Diets low in magnesium can worsen this situation. In addition, heavy perspiration for weeks in hot climates can increase magnesium requirements.

Upper Level for Magnesium

The Upper Level of 350 mg/day for magnesium refers to supplement and other nonfood sources only, such as certain antacids and laxatives (e.g., Milk of Magnesia®). Intakes exceeding this amount from non-food sources can lead to diarrhea.[1] Toxicity also can occur during kidney failure because the kidneys are the primary regulator of blood magnesium. High blood magnesium causes weakness, nausea, slowed breathing, eventual malaise, coma, and death. Older people are at particular risk of magnesium toxicity because kidney function tends to decline with age.

Knowledge Check

1. Which foods are good sources of magnesium?
2. What are the functions of magnesium in the diet?
3. What are the symptoms of magnesium deficiency?
4. Which groups are most likely to be magnesium deficient?

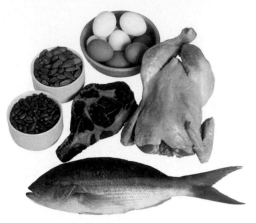

Protein-rich foods supply sulfur in the diet.

14.9 Sulfur (S)

Sulfur, a bright yellow mineral, is provided primarily by the sulfur-containing amino acids methionine and cysteine. Inorganic sulfate also is found in water and food—for example, as a preservative that protects the color of dried fruits and white wines. There is no AI or RDA established for sulfur, nor is an Upper Level established because we are able to obtain ample sulfur from protein-containing foods.[2] Sulfur is required for the synthesis of several sulfur-containing compounds, it helps stabilize the structure of proteins (e.g., collagen, hair, nails, skin), and it participates in regulating the acid-base balance in the body. No deficiency or toxicity symptoms are associated with sulfur.

As you can see, the major minerals play important roles in the body. Table 14-11 provides a summary of the major minerals.

Table 14-11 Summary of the Major Minerals

Mineral	Major Functions	RDA or Adequate Intake	Dietary Sources	Deficiency Symptoms	Toxicity Symptoms
Sodium	Major positive ion of the extracellular fluid, aids nerve impulse transmission and muscle contraction, water balance, aids glucose and amino acid absorption	*Age 19–50 years:* 1500 mg *Age 51–70 years:* 1300 mg *Age 70 years or more:* 1200 mg	Table salt, processed foods, condiments, sauces, soups, chips	Muscle cramps, headache, nausea, vomiting, fatigue	Contributes to hypertension in susceptible individuals, increases calcium loss in urine, upper Level: 2300 mg
Potassium	Major positive ion of intracellular fluid, aids nerve impulse transmission and muscle contraction, water balance	4700 mg	Potato, squash, bananas, orange juice, milk and milk products, meat, legumes, whole grains	Irregular heartbeat, loss of appetite, muscle cramps, increased risk of hypertension and stroke	Slowing of the heartbeat, as seen in kidney failure
Chloride	Major negative ion of extracellular fluid, participates in acid production in stomach, aids nerve impulse transmission, water balance	2300 mg	Table salt, some vegetables, processed foods	Convulsions in infants	Linked to hypertension in susceptible people when combined with sodium, upper Level: 3600 mg
Calcium	Bone and tooth structure, blood clotting, aids in nerve impulse transmission, muscle contractions, enzyme regulation	*Age 9–18 years:* 1300 mg *Ages greater than 18 years:* 1000–1200 mg	Milk and milk products, canned fish, leafy vegetables, tofu, fortified orange juice (and other fortified foods)	Increased risk of osteoporosis	May cause kidney stones and other problems in susceptible people; upper Level: 2500 mg
Phosphorus	Major ion of intracellular fluid, bone and tooth strength, part of ATP and other metabolic compounds, acid-base balance	*Age 9–18 years:* 1250 mg *Ages greater than 18 years:* 700 mg	Milk and milk products, processed foods, fish, soft drinks, bakery products, meats	Possibility of poor bone maintenance	Impairs bone health in people with kidney failure, poor bone mineralization if calcium intakes are low, upper Level: 3–4 g
Magnesium	Bone formation, aids enzyme function, aids nerve and heart function	*Men:* 400–420 mg *Women:* 310–320 mg	Wheat bran, green vegetables, nuts, chocolate, legumes	Weakness, muscle pain, poor heart function, seizures	Diarrhea, weakness, nausea, and malaise in people with kidney failure, upper Level of 350 mg, but refers to non-food sources (e.g., supplements) only
Sulfur	Part of vitamins and amino acids, aids in drug detoxification, acid-base balance	None	Protein foods	None observed	None likely

Summary

14.1 Water accounts for 50 to 75% of the weight of the human body. The intracellular compartment holds two-thirds of the body's water, with the balance in the extracellular compartment. Electrolytes dissolved in the body's water help maintain fluid balance. Water's unique chemical properties enable it to dissolve substances and to serve as a medium for chemical reactions, temperature regulation, and lubrication. For adults, daily fluid needs are estimated at 9 cups (women) to 13 cups (men), but temperature, physical exertion, and other factors can greatly affect water requirements. Water balance is regulated by hormones that act on the kidneys. A water deficit results in dehydration, but too much water can cause the rare condition of water intoxication and hyponatremia.

14.2 Minerals are divided into the major and trace minerals. Animal foods are the best sources of calcium, iron, and zinc. Plant foods are good sources of potassium and magnesium. The absorption of minerals can be affected by the need for the minerals, the consumption of supplements, and the presence of phytic and oxalic acids. Minerals are needed for water balance, the transmission of nerve impulses, and muscle contraction. They function as enzyme cofactors and as components of body tissues. Minerals taken in excess can be toxic.

14.3 Sodium, the major positive ion (cation) found outside cells, is vital in fluid balance and nerve impulse transmission. The North American diet provides abundant sodium through processed foods and table salt. Sodium intakes often exceed the Upper Level. A high sodium intake is linked to hypertension.

14.4 Potassium, the major positive ion (cation) found inside cells, has functions similar to those of sodium. Milk, fruits, and vegetables are good sources. Potassium intakes in the U.S. fall below the Adequate Intake. Low potassium diets increase the risk of hypertension and stroke. Too much potassium is only a problem when kidney function is poor.

14.5 Chloride is the major negative ion (anion) found outside cells. It is important in digestion as part of gastric hydrochloric acid and in immune and nerve functions. Table salt supplies most of the chloride in our diets. Hypertension is a serious health problem that afflicts 1 in 3 adults. It increases the risk of cardiovascular disease, stroke, dementia, and kidney and eye disease. The cause of hypertension is not known, but contributors are an impaired ability of the kidney to excrete sodium along with increased arterial resistance. Hypertension is higher in those who are older, African American, overweight, or have diabetes. The DASH diet, low in sodium and fat, and high in fiber, potassium, magnesium, and calcium is effective in treating hypertension. Weight

reduction, limiting alcohol, and increasing physical activity also play a role. Hypertension often is treated with medication when lifestyle measures are not adequate.

14.6 Calcium forms a vital part of bone structure and is very important in blood clotting, muscle contraction, nerve transmission, and cell metabolism. Calcium absorption is enhanced by stomach acid and the active vitamin D hormone. Milk and milk products are rich calcium sources and calcium supplements can help meet calcium needs. In addition to its role in bone formation, calcium may help reduce the risk of colon cancer. Researchers are trying to understand if calcium and dairy intake are related to body weight regulation. Osteoporosis is a disease that develops over many years and is more common in women than in men. It represents an increase of bone resorption over bone building. The prevention and treatment of osteoporosis involve consuming adequate bone-building nutrients, engaging in weight-bearing physical activity, minimizing the risk of falls, not smoking, and limiting alcohol intake. Supplemental vitamin D and calcium may help prevent a decrease in bone mineral density and fractures. Medications to treat osteopenia and osteoporosis are available.

14.7 Phosphorus is a part of ATP and other key metabolic compounds, aids the function of some enzymes, and forms part of cell membranes and bone. It is efficiently absorbed, and deficiencies are rare. Typical food sources are dairy products, bakery products, and meats.

14.8 Magnesium, a mineral found mostly in plants, is important for nerve and heart function and as a cofactor for many enzymes. Whole grains (bran portion), vegetables, nuts, seeds, milk, and meats are typical food sources. Magnesium deficiency causes irregular heartbeat, weakness, disorientation, nausea, vomiting, and seizures. This can be seen in those who abuse alcohol and take certain diuretics. The UL refers only to supplements. Intakes over the UL can cause diarrhea.

14.9 Sulfur is incorporated into certain vitamins and amino acids. Its ability to bond with other sulfur atoms enables it to stabilize protein structure. There is no AI, RDA, or UL established for sulfur.

Study Questions

1. The main electrolytes found inside the cell are _____.
   a. calcium, sodium, and chloride
   b. sulfate, potassium, and chloride
   c. potassium, magnesium, and phosphate
   d. sodium, chloride, and potassium

2. When the amount of water in the body is low, the hormones _____ and _____ signal the kidney to conserve water and salt.
   a. insulin; calcitonin
   b. antidiuretic hormone; aldosterone
   c. estrogen; angiotensin II
   d. calmodulin; aldosterone

3. Both _____ and _____ can bind to minerals and limit their absorption.
   a. phytic acid; oxalic acid
   b. vitamin C; iron
   c. sodium; potassium
   d. protein; fiber

4. Most salt in the diet comes from _____.
   a. table salt added at home
   b. processed foods
   c. restaurant foods
   d. both b and c

5. Sodium intake in the U.S. typically exceeds the Upper Level.
   a. true
   b. false

6. Low potassium intakes are associated with _____.
   a. eating disorders
   b. diets that contain little unprocessed fresh foods and high amounts of processed foods
   c. excessive alcohol intake
   d. all of the above

7. The functions of the chloride ion include _____.
   a. serving as the main anion in the intracellular fluid
   b. aiding the transmission of nerve impulses
   c. forming acid in the stomach
   d. both b and c

8. _____ potassium intake and _____ sodium intake are associated with a higher risk of high blood pressure and stroke.
   a. high; low
   b. low; high
   c. low; low
   d. high; high

9. A blood pressure of 135/90 mm Hg is classified as _____.
   a. hypertension
   b. normal blood pressure
   c. prehypertension
   d. low blood pressure

10. Important lifestyle modifications for preventing hypertension include _____.
    a. maintaining a healthy BMI
    b. eating a diet rich in potassium, calcium, and magnesium
    c. not smoking
    d. all of the above

11. Significant non-dairy sources of calcium include _____.
    a. almonds, beans, mustard greens, broccoli, and tofu
    b. meat, eggs, and fish
    c. whole-grain breads and cereals, peanuts, bananas, and spinach
    d. all of the above

12. Calcium absorption is likely to be highest in _____.
    a. post-menopausal women
    b. adults in middle age
    c. adolescent males and females
    d. both a and b

13. Which of the following is *not* a risk factor for osteoporosis?
    a. low physical activity
    b. low calcium and vitamin D intakes
    c. obesity
    d. amenorrhea

14. Phosphorus deficiency is a common problem in North America.
    a. true
    b. false

15. Over half of the magnesium in the body is found in the _____.
    a. heart
    b. liver
    c. bones
    d. brain

Answer Key: 1-c; 2-b; 3-a; 4-d; 5-a; 6-d; 7-d; 8-b; 9-c; 10-d; 11-a; 12-c; 13-c; 14-b; 15-c

Websites

To learn more about the topics covered in this chapter, visit these websites.

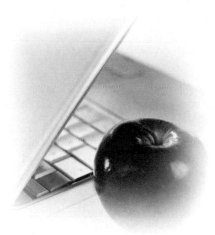

Water

www.epa.org

www.bottledwater.org

Hypertension

www.nhlbi.nih.gov/guidelines/hypertension/jnc7full.htm

www.americanheart.org

DASH Diet

www.nhlbi.nih.gov/health/public/heart/hbp/dash/new_dash.pdf

who.int/dietphysicalactivity/Salt_Report_VC_april07.pdf

Calcium

www.nationaldairycouncil.org

Osteoporosis

www.nof.org

www.osteofound.org

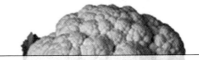

References

1. Food and Nutrition Board, Institute of Medicine. *Dietary Reference Intakes for calcium, phosphorus, magnesium, vitamin D and fluoride.* Washington, DC: National Academy Press; 1997.

2. Food and Nutrition Board, Institute of Medicine. *Dietary Reference Intakes for water, potassium, sodium, chloride and sulfate.* Washington, DC: National Academy Press; 2005.

3. Oh MS, Uribari J. Electrolytes, water and acid-base balance. In: Shils ME and others, eds. *Modern nutrition in health and disease.* 10th ed. Baltimore: Lippincott Williams & Wilkins; 2006.

4. Storey ML and others. Beverage consumption in the US population. *J Am Diet Assoc.* 2006;106:1992.

5. Neilsen S, Popkin B. Changes in beverage intake between 1977 and 2001. *Am J Prev Med.* 2004;27:205.

6. Block G. Foods contributing to energy intake in the US: Data from NHANES III and NHANES 1999–2000. *J Food Comp Anal.* 2004;17:439.

7. Mattes RD. Fluid energy—Where's the problem? *J Am Diet Assoc.* 2006;106:1956.

8. Armstrong L. Caffeine, body fluid-electrolyte balance, and exercise performance. *Int J Sport Nutr Exerc Metab.* 2002;12:189.

9. Grandjean AC and others. The effect of caffeinated, non-caffeinated, caloric and non-caloric beverages on hydration. *J Am College Nutr.* 2000;19:591.

10. International Bottled Water Association. Beverage marketings 2006 market report findings. 2007; www.bottledwater.org.

11. Bruce RC, Kliegman RM. Hyponatremic seizures secondary to oral water intoxication in infancy: Association with commercial bottled drinking water. *Pediatr.* 1997;100:e4.

12. Almond CSD and others. Hyponatremia among runners in the Boston Marathon. *New Eng J Med.* 2005;352:1550.

13. United Nations. Coping with water scarcity—Challenge of the twenty-first century. 2007; www.unwater.org/wwd07/downloads/documents/escarcity.pdf.

14. World Health Organization. Schistosomiasis. The disease and how it affects people. 200l; www.who.int/water_sanitation_health/diseases/schisto/en/.

15. Food and Nutrition Board, Institute of Medicine. *Dietary Reference Intakes for vitamin A, vitamin K, arsenic, boron, chromium, copper, iodine, iron, manganese, molybdenum, nickel, silicon, vanadium, and zinc.* Washington, DC: National Academy Press; 2001.

16. Weaver C, Heaney R. Calcium. In: Shils M and others, eds. *Modern nutrition in health and disease.* 10th ed. Baltimore: Lippincott Williams & Wilkins; 2006.

17. Moshfegh A and others. What we eat in America, NHANES 2001–2002: Usual nutrient intakes from food compared to Dietary Reference Intakes. U.S. Department of Agriculture, Agricultural Research Service; 2005.

18. Cotton PA and others. Dietary sources of nutrients among US adults, 1994 to 1996. *J Am Diet Assoc.* 2004;104:921.

19. Altun B, Arici M. Salt and blood pressure: Time to challenge. *Cardiol.* 2006;105:9.

20. Cook NR and others. Long term effects of dietary sodium reduction on cardiovascular disease outcomes: Observational follow-up of the trials of hypertension prevention (TOHP). *Br Med J.* 2007;334:885.

21. Dickinson BD and others. Promotion of healthy lifestyles I: Reducing the population burden of cardiovascular disease by reducing sodium intake. *Arch Intern Med.* 2007;167:1460.

22. Havas S and others. The urgent need to reduce sodium consumption. *JAMA.* 2007;298:1439.

23. World Health Organization. Reducing salt intake in populations. Report of WHO forum and technical meeting. 2007; who.int/dietphysicalactivity/Salt_Report_VC_april07.pdf.

24. Cook N and others. Long term effects of dietary sodium reduction on cardiovascular disease outcomes: Observational follow-up of the Trials of Hypertension Prevention (TOHP). *Br Med J.* 2007;334:885.

25. Heaney RP. Role of dietary sodium in osteoporosis. *J Am College Nutr.* 2006;25:271S.

26. Borghi L and others. Dietary therapy in idiopathic nephrolithiasis. *Nutr Rev.* 2006;64:301.

27. Heaney RP. Bone biology in health and disease. In: Shils M and others, eds. *Modern nutrition in health and disease.* Baltimore: Lippincott Williams & Wilkins; 2006.

28. Adrogué H, Madias N. Sodium and potassium in the pathogenesis of hypertension. *New Eng J Med.* 2007;356:1966.

29. Liebman B. Stroke: How to avoid a brain attack. *Nutrition Action Healthletter.* 2007;34:1.

30. Kotchen TA, Kotchen JM. Nutrition, diet and hypertension. In: Shils M and others, eds. *Modern nutrition in health and disease.* 10th ed. Baltimore: Lippincott Williams & Wilkins; 2006.

31. National Heart Lung and Blood Institute. 7th report of the Joint National Committee on Prevention, Detection, Evaluation and Treatment of High Blood Pressure. 2004; http://www.nhlbi.nih.gov/guidelines/hypertension/jnc7full.htm.

32. Appel L and others. Effects of comprehensive lifestyle modification on blood pressure control: Main results of the PREMIER clinical trial. *JAMA.* 2003;289:2083.

33. Elmer PJ and others. Effects of comprehensive lifestyle modification on diet, weight, physical fitness and blood pressure control: 18-month results of a randomized trial. *Ann Intern Med.* 2006;144:485.

34. Wexler R, Aukerman G. Nonpharmacologic strategies for managing hypertension. *Am Fam Physician.* 2006;73:1953.

35. Intersalt Cooperative Research Group. Intersalt: An international study of electrolyte excretion and blood pressure: Results for 24-hour urinary sodium and potassium excretion. *Brit Med J.* 1988;297:319.

36. Dickinson HO and others. Lifestyle interventions to reduce raised blood pressure: A systematic review of randomized controlled trials. *J Hypertension.* 2006;24:215.

37. Taubert D and others. Effects of low habitual cocoa intake on blood pressure and bioactive nitric oxide: A randomized controlled trial. *JAMA.* 2007;298:49.

38. Grassi D and others. Short-term administration of dark chocolate is followed by a significant increase in insulin sensitivity and a decrease in blood pressure in healthy persons. *Am J Clin Nutr.* 2005;81:611.

39. Winkelmayer WC and others. Habitual caffeine intake and the risk of hypertension in women. *JAMA.* 2005;294:2330.

40. Champagne C. Dietary interventions on blood pressure: The dietary approaches to stop hypertension (DASH) trials. *Nutr Rev.* 2006;64:S53.

41. Patlak M. Bone builders: The discoveries behind preventing and treating osteoporosis. *FASEB J.* 2001;15:1677e.

42. Titchenal AC, Dobbs J. A system to assess the quality of food sources of calcium. *J Food Comp Analysis.* 2007;20:717.

43. Ross EA and others. Lead content of calcium supplements. *JAMA.* 2000;284:1425.

44. FDA. Final rule for current good manufacturing practices (CGMPs) for dietary supplements. 2007; www.cfsan.fda.gov/~dms/dscgmps7.html.

45. U.S. Department of Health and Human Services. *Bone health and osteoporosis: A report of the surgeon general.* Rockville, MD: U.S. Department of Health and Human Services, Office of the Surgeon General; 2004.

46. National Osteoporosis Foundation; 2007. www.nof.org/.

47. Larsson SC and others. Calcium and dairy food intakes are inversely associated with colorectal cancer risk in the cohort of Swedish men. *Am J Clin Nutr.* 2006;83:667.

48. Park S-Y and others. Calcium and vitamin D intake and risk of colorectal cancer: the Multiethnic cohort study. *Am J Epidemio.* 2007;165:784.

49. Zemel MB. The role of dairy foods in weight management. *J Am College Nutr.* 2005;24:537S.

50. Trowman R and others. A systematic review of the effects of calcium supplementation on body weight. *Brit J Nutr.* 2006;95:1033.

51. Hofmeyr GJ. Calcium supplementation during pregnancy for preventing hypertensive disorders and related problems. *Cochrane Database of Systematic Reviews;* 2006.

52. Trumbo PR, Ellwood KC. Supplemental calcium and risk reduction of hypertension, pregnancy-induced hypertension and preeclampsia: An evidence-based review by the US Food and Drug Administration. *Nutr Rev.* 2007;65:78.

53. Lane NE. Epidemiology, etiology and diagnosis of osteoporosis. *Am J Obst Gynecol.* 2006;194:S3.

54. Dawson-Hughes B. Osteoporosis. In: Shils M and others, eds. *Modern nutrition in health and disease.* Baltimore: Lippincott Williams & Wilkins; 2006.

55. Lanham-New SA. The balance of bone health: Tipping the scales in favor of potassium-rich, bicarbonate-rich foods. *J Nutr.* 2008;137:1725.

56. Holick MF. Vitamin D deficiency. *New Eng J Med.* 2007;357:266.

57. Benjamin M and others. Use of calcium or calcium in combination with vitamin D supplementation to prevent fractures and bone loss in people aged 50 years and older: A meta-analysis. *Lancet.* 2007;370:657.

58. Jackson RD and others. Calcium plus vitamin D supplementation and the risk of fractures. *NewEng J Med.* 2006;354:669.

59. Knochel JP. Phosphorus. In: Shils M and others, eds. *Modern nutrition in health and disease.* 10th ed. Baltimore: Lippincott Williams & Wilkins; 2006.

60. Elliott P and others. Dietary phosphorus and blood pressure: International study of macro- and micro-nutrients and blood pressure. *Hypertension.* 2008;51:669.

61. Rude RK, Shils M. Magnesium. In: Shils M and others, eds. *Modern nutrition in health and disease.* Baltimore: Lippincott Williams & Wilkins; 2006.

62. Tsai CJ and others. Long-term effect of magnesium consumption on the risk of symptomatic gallstone disease among men. *Am J Gastroenterol.* 2008; 103:383.

63. He K and others. Magnesium intake and incidence of Metabolic Syndrome among young adults. *Circulation.* 2006;113:1675.

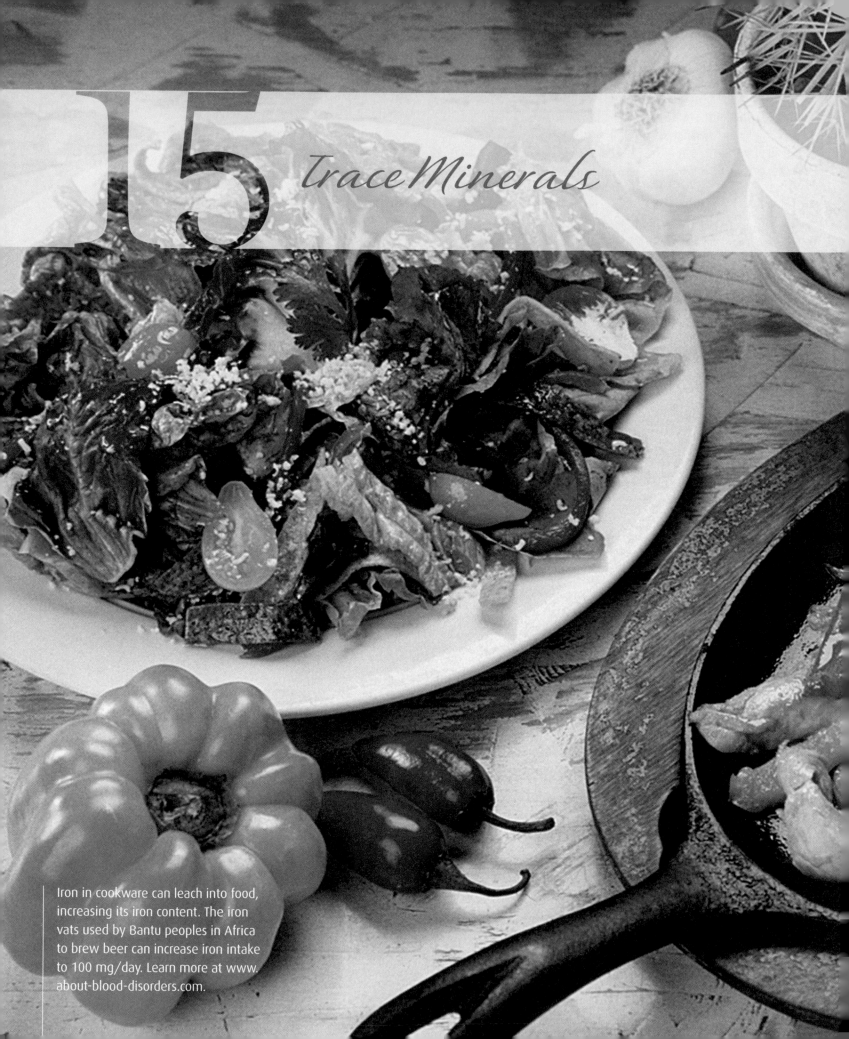

15 Trace Minerals

Iron in cookware can leach into food, increasing its iron content. The iron vats used by Bantu peoples in Africa to brew beer can increase iron intake to 100 mg/day. Learn more at www.about-blood-disorders.com.

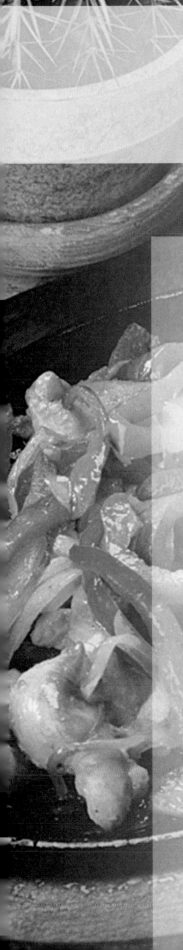

STUDENT LEARNING OUTCOMES

After studying this chapter, you will be able to:

1. Discuss the major functions of each trace mineral.

2. List 3 important food sources for each trace mineral.

3. Describe how each trace mineral is absorbed, transported, stored, and excreted.

4. Describe the deficiency symptoms of trace minerals.

5. Describe the toxicity symptoms from the excess consumption of certain trace minerals.

6. Describe the development of cancer and the effect of genetic, environmental, and dietary factors on the risk of developing cancer.

Trace minerals are essential inorganic substances needed in small quantities in the diet (less than 100 mg daily) and are found in relatively minute amounts in the body (less than 5 g). In fact, all of them combined make up less than 1% of the minerals in the body. Despite these tiny, or "trace," amounts, trace minerals are essential for normal development, function, and overall health. For example, iron is needed to build red blood cells; zinc, copper, selenium, and manganese help protect us from the damaging effects of free radicals; and iodine is needed to maintain normal metabolism.

With the exception of iron and iodine, the essentiality of trace minerals in humans has only been recognized within the last 50 years. Intensive trace mineral research began in the early 1960s with the discovery of a group of Middle Eastern adolescent boys who did not grow normally or sexually mature because they were zinc deficient.[1] Since then, scientists have discovered that many trace minerals are essential for normal body function and that physiological abnormalities occur when they are deficient in the diet.

The unique characteristics of trace minerals have presented many challenges to researchers. For example, because there are such small quantities in the body, measuring the amount in the body and changes in trace mineral concentrations is often difficult.[2] Therefore, it is hard to accurately assess trace mineral status in the body and set recommended intake levels. Evaluating the amount of trace minerals in foods also can be difficult. Many agricultural factors and food characteristics affect the amount of trace minerals in food, especially in plant-based foods. Thus, nutrient databases may not provide an accurate indication of the total amount and/or bioavailability of a trace mineral in a specific food. Despite the challenges presented by trace minerals, knowledge of these nutrients continues to expand as new scientific technologies emerge and permit the study of their roles in cellular functions and more precise measurements of their levels in the body.

535

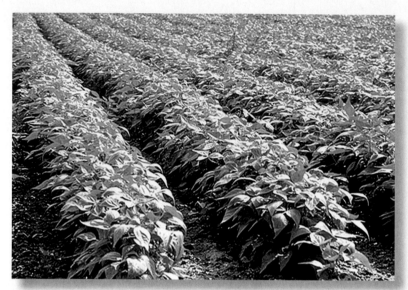

The trace mineral content of plant-based foods depends on the mineral content of the soil in which they were grown.

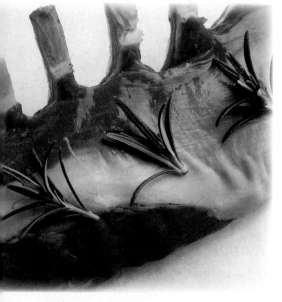

Red meat is a major source of heme iron in the North American diet.

Figure 15-1 Food sources of iron. In addition to the MyPyramid food groups, pink is used for substances that do not fit easily into food groups (e.g., honey, candy, coffee, alcohol, and table salt)

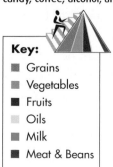

Key:
- ■ Grains
- ■ Vegetables
- ■ Fruits
- □ Oils
- ■ Milk
- ■ Meat & Beans

15.1 Iron (Fe)

The importance of iron for the maintenance of health has been recognized for centuries. In 4000 B.C., Persian physician Melampus gave iron supplements to sailors to compensate for the iron they lost from bleeding during battles. Maintaining iron status is still a problem throughout the world today. In many developing nations, almost two-thirds of all children and women of childbearing age have an iron deficiency.[3] Although iron deficiency is less prevalent in the U.S. and other industrialized countries, it is a significant public health concern in children and young women.

Iron in Foods

Dietary iron occurs in several forms. In animal flesh (beef, pork, seafood, and poultry), most of the iron is present as hemoglobin and myoglobin, which collectively is called **heme iron**. The rest of the iron present in these foods, as well as all the iron in vegetables, grains, and supplements, is called **non-heme iron**.

The richest sources of iron in North American diets are meats and seafood (Fig. 15-1). Because iron is added to refined flour as a part of the enrichment process, bakery products (e.g., bread, rolls, and crackers) provide iron as well. Relatively high amounts of iron also are found in spinach and other dark leafy greens and in kidney, garbanzo, and navy beans. However, many factors cause the iron in enriched and plant-based foods to be less bioavailable than iron from animal-based foods.

In addition to the iron in foods, iron cookware can contribute to iron intake. When foods are cooked in iron pans, small amounts of iron from the cookware are transferred to the food. Acidic food, such as tomato sauce, increases the amount of iron transferred from the cookware to the food and, in turn, increases the total iron content.

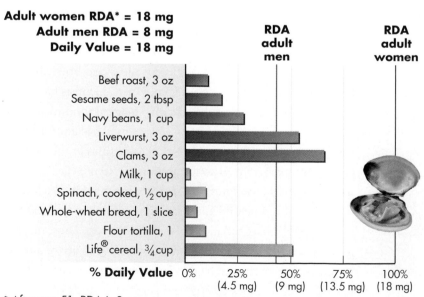

Adult women RDA* = 18 mg
Adult men RDA = 8 mg
Daily Value = 18 mg

RDA adult men

RDA adult women

- Beef roast, 3 oz
- Sesame seeds, 2 tbsp
- Navy beans, 1 cup
- Liverwurst, 3 oz
- Clams, 3 oz
- Milk, 1 cup
- Spinach, cooked, ½ cup
- Whole-wheat bread, 1 slice
- Flour tortilla, 1
- Life® cereal, ¾ cup

% Daily Value 0%   25%   50%   75%   100%
                        (4.5 mg) (9 mg)   (13.5 mg) (18 mg)

* After age 51, RDA is 8 mg.

Iron Needs

The RDA for adult women is 18 mg/day and 8 mg/day for adult men.[4] After age 51, the RDA for women drops to 8 mg/day because most women enter menopause and no longer lose iron via menstrual blood. Although iron absorption can vary considerably, the RDA values are based on the premise that approximately 18% of dietary iron is absorbed each day from typical Westernized diets, such as those eaten in most of North America.[4] The Daily Value for iron used on food labels and supplements is 18 mg.

Westernized diets typically contain about 6 mg of iron for every 1000 kcal.[4] Thus, the average 2000-kcal diet provides about 12 mg of iron. In North America, the average daily iron intake is approximately 17 mg for men and 12 mg for women.

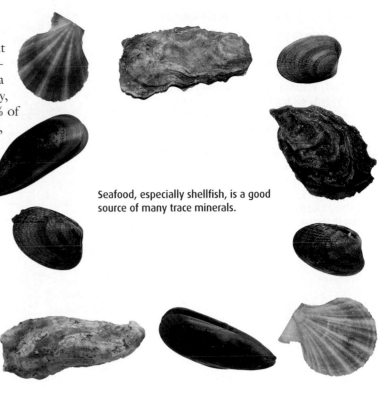

Seafood, especially shellfish, is a good source of many trace minerals.

Absorption, Transport, Storage, and Excretion of Iron

Iron is absorbed across the brush border membrane into the small intestine by carrier-mediated mechanisms. The enterocytes (intestinal absorptive cells) produce different iron-binding carrier proteins that play an important role in the absorptive process and overall regulation of iron status.[5] **Ferritin,** a key iron-binding protein produced in the enterocyte, binds and stores mucosal iron, thereby preventing it from entering the bloodstream (Fig. 15-2). The amount of mucosal ferritin produced is in proportion to body iron stores. Thus, when iron stores are low, very little ferritin is made, which allows greater amounts of iron to enter the mucosal iron pool for transport out of the enterocytes into the bloodstream. If iron stores are high or saturated, larger amounts of ferritin are made to bind iron as it enters the intestinal cells. Although a portion of this ferritin-bound iron remains in the intestinal iron pool, much of it is excreted when the intestinal cells slough off after several days. This process is called a "mucosal block" because it prevents iron from entering the bloodstream and, in effect, blocks the excess accumulation of iron. Large doses of iron, however, can overtax the mucosal block's protective ability and increase the risk of toxicity.

When iron needs are high, most of the iron absorbed into enterocytes is released into an intestinal iron pool. This iron is then transported out of the enterocytes by a protein, called ferroportin, into the interstitial fluid for release into the bloodstream and distribution to body cells.[5] To transport absorbed iron to body cells, the iron is oxidized from the ferrous (Fe^{2+}) form to the ferric (Fe^{3+}) form by a copper-containing enzyme (either hephaestin in the enterocyte or ceruloplasmin in the blood) and bound to a serum protein called transferrin.[5] Each transferrin molecule can bind 2 molecules of ferric iron for transport through the blood to body cells.

All cells have transferrin receptors, located on their surface membrane, that allow them to take in the transferrin-iron complex.[6] Cells can control the amount of iron they take in by altering the synthesis of transferrin receptors. When more iron is needed, the cell increases the number of transferrin surface receptors to enhance iron uptake. Conversely, when cellular iron need is low, the number of receptors decreases.

After transferrin binds to its surface receptor, it is engulfed into the cell by endocytosis (see Chapter 4). Within the cell **lysosomes,** iron is released from transferrin and the receptor-protein complex is returned to the cell surface for reuse. The released iron is utilized for cellular functions or stored in the form of ferritin or **hemosiderin.**

Intestinal absorption, cellular uptake, and the storage of iron are tightly regulated because the body has a limited ability to excrete iron that has been absorbed. In fact, approximately 90% of the iron used each day is recovered and recycled. Only about 10% is excreted, mainly via the small amount of bile lost in the feces. One of the proteins that

▶ The copper-containing proteins (hephaestin and ceruloplasmin) needed to oxidize iron from the ferrous (Fe^{2+}) to the ferric (Fe^{3+}) form demonstrate the close link between copper and iron metabolism.

ferritin Iron-binding protein in the intestinal mucosa that binds iron and prevents it from entering the bloodstream; also the primary storage form of iron in the liver and other tissues.

lysosome Cell organelle that digests proteins, such as transferrin, and breaks down bacteria and old or damaged cell components.

hemosiderin Iron-binding protein in the liver that stores iron when iron levels in the body exceed the storage capacity of ferritin.

Figure 15-2 Iron absorption and distribution.

1. Iron binds with a mucosal protein, called ferritin, when stored in intestinal cells.
2. If intestinal absorptive cells are sloughed off before iron is absorbed, the iron passes out of the body in the feces. This sloughing allows the body to control the absorption of iron.
3. Iron that enters the bloodstream binds to transferrin. For a detailed look at iron absorption, see the figure below.
4. Iron binds to transferrin and is then distributed to the liver, muscle, bone marrow and other body tissue.
5. The liver and spleen harvest iron from worn-out red blood cells, thereby allowing most iron in the body to be reused.

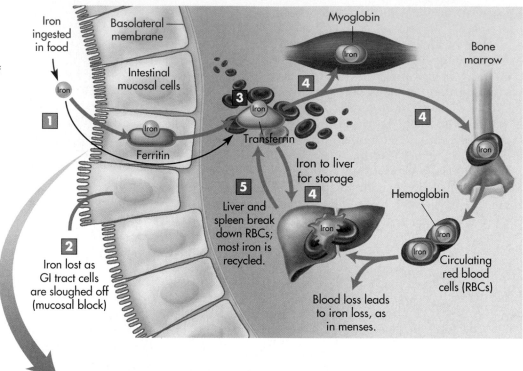

Detailed view of iron absorption.

A. Heme iron is transported across brush border and enters the same pool as non-heme iron. Dietary non-heme iron (Fe^{3+}) must be reduced for transport across the brush border.

B. Some iron is used or stored within the enterocyte in ferritin and lost when the intestinal mucosa is sloughed.

C. Ferroportin aids in export of iron out of the intestinal cell for incorporation into serum transferrin.

aids in the regulation of iron balance is called hepcidin.[7] The loss of this protein results in iron overload.

Factors Affecting Iron Absorption

The amount of iron absorbed is affected by the body's iron needs and stores and by diet composition. When iron status is adequate, approximately 14 to 18% of dietary iron is absorbed from a typical North American diet.[4] However, when iron need is high and stores are low, the small intestine absorbs up to 35 to 40% of dietary iron. In contrast, when iron need is low and stores are saturated, less than 5% of dietary iron is absorbed.

In addition to iron storage levels, iron absorption is affected by the form of iron in foods eaten, the total amount of iron present in the diet, dietary composition (food components that increase or decrease the bioavailability of iron), and the acidity of the gastric contents.

The amount of dietary iron absorbed is dependent on whether the iron is in the form of heme or non-heme iron. Heme iron is absorbed much more readily than non-heme iron and is not highly affected by dietary composition. This is one reason that meat is an efficient way to obtain iron. Additionally, meat provides greater amounts of iron than naturally occur in plant-based foods, so smaller quantities provide similar amounts of iron.

Plant-based non-heme iron absorption is hindered by several dietary factors. Phytic acid in whole grains and legumes and oxalic acid in leafy green vegetables bind non-heme iron and reduce its absorption. For this reason, whole grains and leafy green vegetables do not contribute significant amounts of iron, despite containing relatively high amounts of iron for a plant food. High intakes of dietary fiber from plant-based diets also bind non-heme iron and reduce its bioavailability.

Polyphenols, such as the tannins found in tea, and related substances in coffee are known to reduce non-heme iron absorption. Therefore, individuals trying to rebuild iron stores are advised to reduce coffee and tea consumption, particularly at meal times. Excessive intakes of other minerals, such as zinc, manganese, and possibly calcium, may interfere with non-heme iron absorption. Because of these potential mineral-mineral interactions, individuals with high iron needs should avoid taking iron supplements with foods or supplements containing significant amounts of these minerals.

The absorption of non-heme iron can be enhanced by a component of meat, called the meat protein factor (MPF). Eating even a small amount of meat with non-heme iron–containing foods can be an effective means of boosting non-heme iron absorption. Vitamin C, or other organic acids, in the diet also increase non-heme iron absorption. Vitamin C provides an electron to Fe^{3+} (ferric iron) to yield Fe^{2+} (ferrous iron), which then forms a soluble complex with vitamin C. Ferrous iron is better absorbed than ferric iron because it more readily crosses the mucosal layer of the small intestine and reaches the brush border of the intestinal absorptive cells. (Heme iron does not need to undergo this reduction reaction because the iron in heme is already in the more soluble ferrous form.)

Although no iron absorption occurs in the stomach, gastric acid plays an important role in the absorption of non-heme iron by promoting the conversion of ferric (Fe^{3+}) iron to ferrous (Fe^{2+}) iron. If the amount of gastric acid produced is low, less ferric iron is converted to ferrous iron and overall non-heme iron absorption is decreased. This is of concern in individuals who regularly take antacids or other medications to reduce gastric acidity (and symptoms of reflux) as well as in older adults, many of whom have reduced gastric acid production. These factors that affect iron absorption are summarized in Table 15-1.

Functions of Iron

Iron plays an important role in diverse functions in the body. Many of these functions are dependent on iron's ability to participate in oxidation and reduction (redox) reactions, changing Fe^{2+} (ferrous) to Fe^{3+} (ferric) iron and back. Although iron's ability to switch back and forth between Fe^{2+} and Fe^{3+} is vital, this reactivity can be harmful because iron can form free

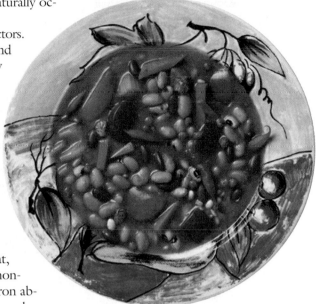

Plant-based foods, such as beans, contain compounds that can reduce the absorption of trace minerals.

CRITICAL THINKING

Nicole was diagnosed with iron deficiency anemia. Her physician advised her to take an iron supplement each day. Her friend recommended she eat extra vitamin C-rich foods daily. Nicole is confused—she thought iron deficiency anemia was caused by a lack of iron. Why would increasing her intake of vitamin C help Nicole?

Table 15-1 Factors That Affect Iron Absorption

Factors That Increase Absorption	Factors That Decrease Absorption
High body demand for red blood cells (blood loss, high altitude, physical training, pregnancy)	Low need for iron (high level of storage iron)
Low body stores of iron	Phytic acid in whole grains and legumes
Heme iron in food	Oxalic acid in leafy vegetables
Meat protein factor (MPF)	Polyphenols in tea, coffee, red wine, and oregano
Vitamin C intake	Reduced gastric acidity
Gastric acidity	Excessive intake of other minerals (zinc, manganese, calcium)

Figure 15-3 Most iron in the body is present in heme within hemoglobin and myoglobin. Iron gives hemoglobin and myoglobin the ability to carry oxygen. Hemoglobin contains 4 heme compounds whereas myoglobin contains one heme compound.

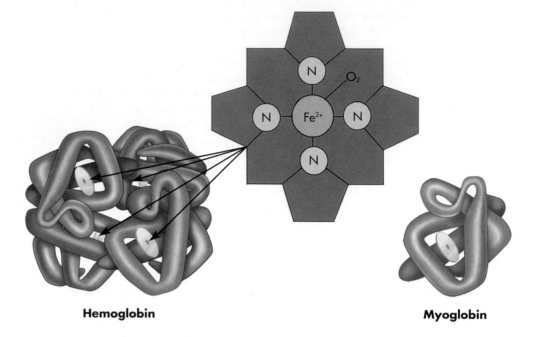

Hemoglobin

Myoglobin

Table 15-2 Iron Proteins
Iron in Functional Proteins
Hemoglobin
Myoglobin
Iron-containing enzymes
Iron in Transport Proteins
Transferrin
Ferroportin
Iron in Storage Proteins
Ferritin
Hemosiderin

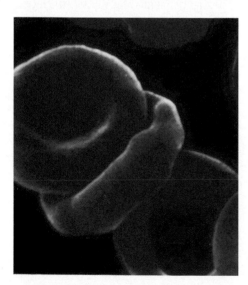

Figure 15-4 Red blood cells have a life span of about 120 days. As a red blood cell matures, its nucleus is expelled, along with its DNA. Thus, red blood cells cannot duplicate. The body recycles iron from worn-out red blood cells to help produce new red blood cells.

radical compounds that damage cell membranes and DNA. To prevent these destructive effects and preserve iron for healthful uses, very little free iron is found in the body. Instead, iron is tightly bound to transport, functional, or storage proteins (Table 15-2).

Iron is an essential part of 2 proteins, hemoglobin and myoglobin, that are involved in the transport and metabolism of oxygen. Hemoglobin, which is found in erythrocytes (red blood cells), is composed of 4 iron-containing heme compounds that each bind 1 molecule of oxygen (Fig. 15-3). As a component of hemoglobin, iron carries oxygen in the blood from the lungs to all tissues of the body. It also transports carbon dioxide back to the lungs for expiration. Because the body produces approximately 200 billion erythrocytes each day, much of the body's iron is contained in hemoglobin. If the oxygen-carrying capacity of erythrocytes declines, the kidneys produce the hormone erythropoietin, which stimulates the bone marrow to produce more red blood cells (Fig. 15-4). This, in turn, increases the body's need for iron to support hemoglobin production.

Iron has a similar oxygen-carrying role in myoglobin, a protein in muscle cells. Each myoglobin contains 1 iron molecule (attached to heme) that transports oxygen from red blood cells to skeletal and heart muscle cells. During iron deficiency, when the delivery of oxygen to these cells becomes limited, individuals often develop shortness of breath and fatigue, especially with physical activity or exertion. Thus, maintaining adequate iron status is critical to exercise and work performance.

Iron-containing enzymes play a vital role in functions such as energy metabolism, drug and alcohol transformation, and the excretion of organic compounds. Within the mitochondria, iron is a component of cytochromes that carry electrons from NADH + H$^+$ and FADH$_2$ to molecular oxygen in the electron transport chain. Iron also is required in the first step of the citric acid cycle for the conversion of citrate to subsequent compounds (Fig. 15-5). Alcohol and many drugs are metabolized in the liver by the iron-containing P-450 enzymes prior to excretion.

Iron is a cofactor for enzymes involved in the synthesis of neurotransmitters (dopamine, epinephrine, norepinephrine, and serotonin). These are important for normal early cognitive development and lifelong brain function.

The immune system requires iron for the production of lymphocyte and natural killer (NK) cells that help prevent infections. If iron status is low, the effectiveness of these cells is impaired and the likelihood of infections increases. Although iron deficiency increases infection risk, iron overload also can increase the incidence of infections because bacteria require iron to grow and proliferate. Thus, iron status must be maintained within a defined range to prevent deficiency as well as overload.

Table 15-3 Stages of Iron Deficiency

Marginal or Early Iron Deficiency →	Moderate Iron Deficiency →	Severe Iron Deficiency, Iron Deficiency Anemia
• ↓ Iron intake • ↑ Iron losses • ↓ Iron stores • ↑ Transferrin receptors • No apparent symptoms	• Depleted iron stores • ↓ Work/exercise capacity • ↓ Immune function • ↓ Iron transport	• ↓ Hemoglobin and red blood cell synthesis (anemia) • ↓ Oxygen transport • ↑ Fatigue • Poor work/exercise performance • ↑ Incidence of infection • ↓ Growth and cognitive development in children • ↑ Mortality

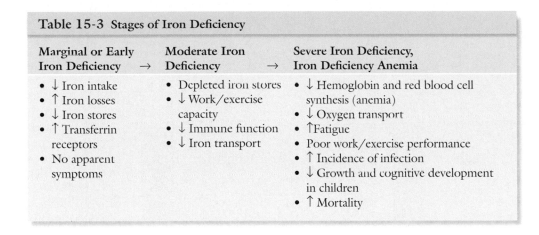

Figure 15-5 **Iron is needed to convert citrate to isocitrate.**

Iron Deficiency

Iron deficiency is the most common trace mineral deficiency worldwide.[3] In the early stages of iron deficiency (summarized in Table 15-3), symptoms may be minimal or unapparent because the body can mobilize stores of iron from ferritin (the primary iron storage protein). However, even a mild to moderate deficiency of iron can compromise immune function and work performance. As iron deficiency progresses and stores are depleted, the lack of iron for heme and hemoglobin synthesis results in the development of iron deficiency anemia. This impairs oxygen transport in the blood, causing fatigue and a decreased ability to perform normal activities. Iron deficiency anemia also compromises immune function, impairs energy metabolism, and delays cognitive development.[8-10] Iron deficiency anemia is of particular concern in young children because cognitive and developmental impairments may not be reversible.

Clinicians can, in part, diagnose anemia by viewing the erythrocytes (red blood cells) under a microscope. In iron deficiency anemia, the red blood cells are smaller than normal (called microcytic) and paler (called hypochromic) (Fig. 15-6). Clinicians also can measure blood hematocrit (percent of total blood volume comprised of red blood cells)

▶ Anemia develops when the number of red blood cells falls below normal levels. There are many causes of anemia. The lack of iron for hemoglobin synthesis and red blood cell production in severe iron deficiency is one cause of anemia.

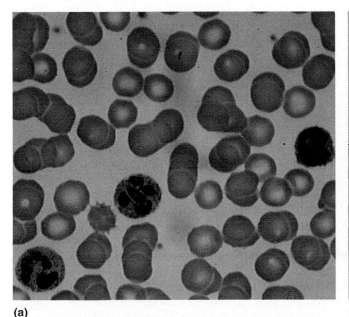

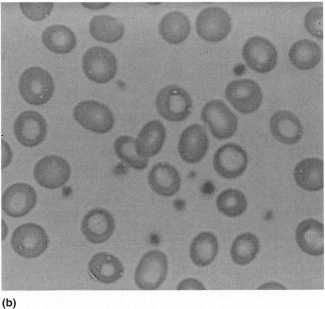

(a)   (b)

Figure 15-6 **Iron deficiency anemia.** (a) Red blood cells that are the normal size and color. (b) Iron-deficient red blood cells. They are smaller (microcytic) and paler (hypochromic) than normal. Color loss is a result of a decreased amount of the pigment hemoglobin. Hypochromic red blood cells also have a reduced capacity to carry oxygen. That is why people feel tired when they have iron deficiency anemia.

Figure 15-7 Iron deficiency reduces the number of red blood cells created. A hematocrit blood test measures the percentage of blood composed of red blood cells. The photo on the right is centrifuged whole blood. Note how red blood cells account for about 55% of the whole blood volume, which is the top of the normal range for adult males. The normal range for males is a hematocrit of 40–55% and for females is 37–47%.

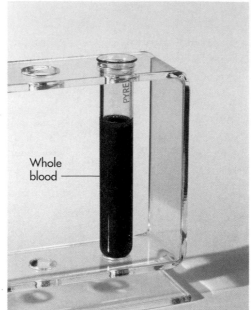
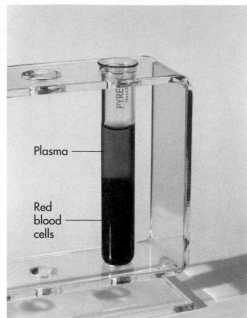

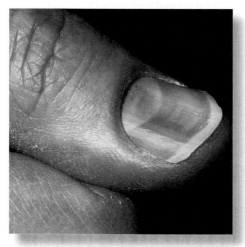

Long-standing, severe iron deficiency anemia can lead to thin, brittle, concave (spoon-shaped) nails.

▶ The consumption of soil and similar non-food substances (called pica, see Chapter 16) can lead to iron deficiency anemia because these substances bind iron in the intestinal tract and prevent absorption. Blood loss caused by intestinal or blood-borne parasite infections is another common cause of anemia in many parts of the world.

and blood hemoglobin, both of which decrease in iron deficiency anemia (Fig. 15-7). However, these are not sensitive measures of iron status because they remain unchanged in the earlier stages of iron deficiency and are affected by many factors (e.g., disease, inflammation, blood loss, deficiencies of other nutrients) other than iron status. Thus, many experts recommend using transferrin receptor number to assess iron status because it reflects cellular iron need and is unaffected by the factors that limit the use of other iron biomarkers.[6]

Many individuals are at risk of iron deficiency and iron deficiency anemia.[4] Premature infants (born before 37 weeks of pregnancy) are at increased risk because iron stores needed for the first few months of life accumulate during the last weeks of pregnancy. Thus, these infants are born with low stores, which can be depleted quickly by their high iron needs. Young children also are at risk because they are growing fast and typically have low intakes of iron-rich meat and high intakes of iron-poor cow's milk. In the U.S., iron-fortified formulas and cereals provided by the Special Supplemental Nutrition Program for Women, Infants, and Children (WIC) to children from limited-resource families who are at nutritional risk have been instrumental in decreasing rates of iron deficiency anemia. However, in less developed countries, many young children are iron deficient because iron supplementation programs frequently are not available.

Teenage girls and women of childbearing age are at risk of iron deficiency because of monthly menstrual blood losses and low intake of iron-rich foods. In the U.S. alone, approximately 3.3 million women of childbearing age have iron deficiency anemia.[11] Even though menstruation stops during pregnancy, pregnant women need to be certain to consume sufficient iron because their own blood volume (and red blood cell number) is increasing, as is that of the fetus. Vegetarians and others who lack food sources of heme iron also are at increased risk of iron deficiency.[12] Although they may have high intakes of plant-based iron foods, their diets contain many factors that decrease the bioavailability of this iron (see Table 15-1). These individuals need to include vitamin C–rich foods in their diets and consider using iron-fortified foods as well as multivitamin-mineral supplements that contain iron.

Individuals who donate blood more than 2 to 4 times a year may be at increased risk of iron deficiency. The donation of 1 pint (0.5 L) of blood represents a loss of 200 to 250 mg of iron. For most healthy individuals, it takes several months to replace this iron, although women may need a longer interval between donations to rebuild their iron stores. As a health precaution, blood banks test potential donors' blood for anemia prior to allowing blood donations.

Iron Overload and Toxicity

Although iron deficiency is a major public health concern, iron also poses a risk for toxicity. Thus, an Upper Level of 45 mg/day has been set for iron.[4] Intakes above this level, especially from supplements and highly fortified foods, can cause nausea and vomiting, stomach irritation, diarrhea, and impaired absorption of other trace minerals.

In the U.S., accidental iron overdose is the leading cause of poisoning in young children under the age of 6 years. Children are more vulnerable to iron poisoning than adults because their absorptive mechanisms cannot respond as rapidly as those of an adult. The primary cause of iron overload in children is the consumption of excess chewable, iron-containing supplements. The FDA has ruled that all iron supplements must carry a warning about toxicity. As an added precaution, supplements that contain 30 mg or more per tablet must be individually wrapped.

In adults, iron overload is most commonly the result of **hemochromatosis,** a genetic condition that affects about 1 person in every 200 to 500. In hemochromatosis, the mucosal block that usually protects the body from excess iron absorption is ineffective.[13] Due to a defect in the normal degradation cycle of the transport protein ferroportin, higher than normal amounts of iron are absorbed and transported across the enterocyte for binding to transferrin and distribution to tissues.[7] Because the body lacks a mechanism for eliminating this excess iron, iron accumulates in the body, leading to iron overload and tissue injury. This causes saturation of iron-binding proteins and, over time, results in iron deposits in the liver, the heart, and other organs. Left untreated, this eventually can lead to liver disease and heart failure.

Adult iron overload also may result from excess supplementation, and frequent blood transfusions. The iron introduced into the body through repeated blood transfusion also bypasses the protective mucosal block and can result in dangerously high iron stores in the body if not monitored closely.[4]

The treatment of iron toxicity depends on the underlying cause. For individuals using excess supplemental iron, supplement use should be stopped. In hemochromatosis, treatment consists of periodic blood removal (a procedure similar to that used for obtaining blood donations).[13] Another treatment approach is to administer a chelator drug that binds iron and increases its excretion. However, chelator drugs also bind other trace minerals, causing possible secondary trace mineral deficiencies.

hemochromatosis Genetic disorder characterized by increased absorption of iron, saturation of iron-binding proteins, and iron deposits in the liver, heart, pancreas, joints, and pituitary gland.

▶ Hemosiderosis is the storage of excess iron in the form of hemosiderin. It does not cause organ damage the way hemochromatosis does because, in hemosiderosis, excess iron is stored in normal iron storage proteins. In hemochromatosis, however, the storage proteins are saturated with iron and iron accumulates in the liver, the heart, and other organs.

Knowledge Check

1. How is iron involved in the metabolism of oxygen within the body?
2. Why are heme-containing foods a more efficient means of obtaining dietary iron than non-heme-containing foods?
3. What factors increase and decrease iron absorption?
4. What are the symptoms of iron deficiency and iron deficiency anemia?
5. What population groups are at greatest risk of iron deficiency anemia?
6. Why are children at risk of iron toxicity?

15.2 Zinc (Zn)

Zinc has been recognized as an essential nutrient in animals since the 1930s. However, it was 30 years later before it became apparent from studies in the Middle East that zinc is essential in humans for normal growth and development.[1] Since that time, scientists have learned that almost all the cells of the body contain zinc, as it is required for many different functions within cells.

Figure 15-8 Food sources of zinc.

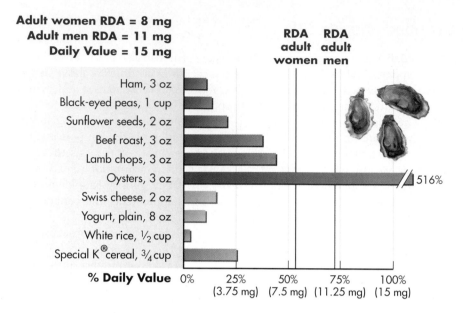

Adult women RDA = 8 mg
Adult men RDA = 11 mg
Daily Value = 15 mg

	RDA adult women	RDA adult men

Ham, 3 oz
Black-eyed peas, 1 cup
Sunflower seeds, 2 oz
Beef roast, 3 oz
Lamb chops, 3 oz
Oysters, 3 oz — 516%
Swiss cheese, 2 oz
Yogurt, plain, 8 oz
White rice, ½ cup
Special K® cereal, ¾ cup

% Daily Value 0%   25% (3.75 mg)   50% (7.5 mg)   75% (11.25 mg)   100% (15 mg)

metallothionein Protein involved in the binding and release of zinc and copper in intestinal and liver cells.

Zinc in Foods

Protein-rich meat and seafood are usually good sources of zinc (Fig. 15-8). North Americans obtain about 70% of their dietary zinc from animal-based foods, such as beef, lamb, and pork. Plant-based foods, such as nuts, beans, wheat germ, and whole grains, also can contribute significant amounts of zinc to our diets. Although some breakfast cereals are fortified with zinc, it is not included in the enrichment process of flour. Therefore, refined flour products are poor sources of zinc.

Whole-grain breads and cereals can contribute significant amounts of zinc to the diet; however, unleavened whole-grain bread is very high in phytic acid and other factors that decrease zinc bioavailability. Yeast fermentation (used in the preparation of yeast-leavened breads) reduces the effect of phytic acid up to tenfold and thus increases zinc absorption. The high intake of unleavened breads in traditional Middle Eastern diets, combined with the relatively low zinc intakes, resulted in the symptoms of zinc deficiency in adolescent boys (Fig. 15-9) that led scientists to recognize zinc as an essential nutrient in humans.

Dietary Needs for Zinc

The RDAs for zinc are 11 mg/day for adult men and 8 mg/day for adult women.[4] The RDAs are based on the average amount needed to replace the daily losses in feces, urine, and sweat and on an estimated dietary absorption of 40%. The Daily Value for zinc is 15 mg. Data from NHANES surveys indicate that mean zinc intakes for many adults in the U.S. currently meet RDA guidelines.[14]

Absorption, Transport, Storage, and Excretion of Zinc

Zinc is absorbed throughout the small intestine by simple diffusion and active transport. When zinc is absorbed into intestinal cells, it induces the synthesis of **metallothionein**, a protein that binds zinc in much the same way that mucosal ferritin binds iron. The regulation of zinc absorption may be, in part, related to the synthesis of metallothionein because it hinders the movement of zinc from intestinal cells.[15] If zinc is not transported out of the intestinal absorptive cell into the bloodstream before the intestinal cells are sloughed off, it passes out

Figure 15-9 On the right, an Egyptian farm boy, age 16 years old and 49 inches tall, with limited growth and sexual development associated with zinc deficiency.

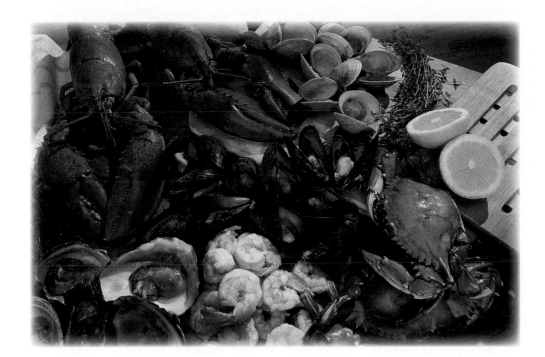

Shellfish, such as lobster, crabs, and oysters, are excellent zinc (and copper) sources.

of the body in the feces. Thus, a mucosal block, similar to that for iron, decreases excess absorption of zinc. However, large doses of zinc can override the mucosal block.

Like iron, the absorption of zinc is affected by diet composition and the body's need for the mineral. As summarized in Table 15-4, zinc absorption increases when zinc intake is low or marginal, when animal protein intake is high, and when body needs for zinc are elevated. In contrast, zinc absorption decreases when zinc or non-heme iron intake is excessive, dietary fiber and phytic acid intake is high, and zinc status is adequate.

Zinc absorbed into the bloodstream binds to blood proteins, such as albumin, for transport to the liver. The liver repackages and releases zinc into the blood bound to alpha-2-macroglobulin, albumin, and other proteins. Although there is no storage site for zinc, the body maintains an exchangeable pool of zinc in the liver, bone, pancreas, kidney, and blood.[16] This allows the body to recycle zinc and maintain zinc status when intake is low.

Fortunately, excess zinc (unlike iron) is readily excreted through the feces, thus decreasing the risk of toxicity. Small amounts also are excreted in urine and sweat.

Functions of Zinc

As many as 300 different enzymes in the body require zinc.[17] In fact, it is hard to name a body process or body structure that isn't affected either directly or indirectly by zinc. Zinc contributes to DNA and RNA synthesis, alcohol metabolism, heme synthesis, bone formation, acid-base balance, immune function, reproduction, growth and development, and the antioxidant defense network (as a part of the Cu/Zn superoxide dismutase

CRITICAL THINKING

Before class last week, Shane heard his friends talking about taking zinc lozenges to prevent colds and flu. He wasn't sure that this was effective, but knew his friends hadn't been sick lately, so he starting taking 50 mg daily. Is this a safe level of intake? What recommendations would you give Shane?

Table 15-4 Factors That Affect Zinc Absorption

Factors That Increase Absorption	Factors That Decrease Absorption
Low to moderate zinc intake	Phytic acid and fiber in whole grains
Zinc deficiency	Excessive zinc intake
Animal protein intake	High non-heme iron intake
Increased need for zinc	Good zinc status

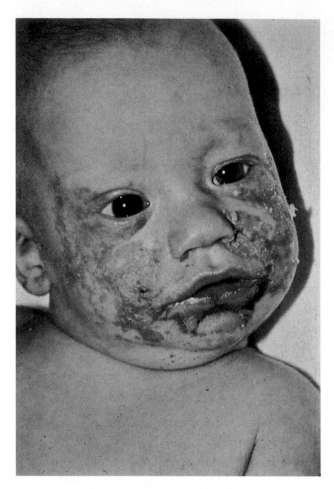

Figure 15-10 This preterm infant's zinc deficiency was caused by low zinc stores at birth and below normal levels of zinc in his mother's breast milk.

[SOD] enzyme). In addition, zinc stabilizes the structures of cell membrane proteins, gene transcription fingers (known as "zinc fingers"), and receptor proteins for vitamin A, vitamin D, and thyroid hormone.[17]

Zinc also may play a role in shortening the duration of common colds.[18] However, because studies have not consistently shown that zinc supplementation is effective in decreasing the length of colds, more research is needed.

Zinc Deficiency

In many parts of the world where poverty limits food choices, zinc deficiency is a major health concern today.[3, 19] The symptoms include loss of appetite, delayed growth and sexual maturation, dermatitis, impaired vitamin A function, alopecia, decreased taste sensitivity, poor wound healing, immune dysfunction, severe diarrhea, birth defects, and increased infant mortality (see Fig. 15-9; Fig. 15-10). Compromised zinc status also impairs the integrity of zinc-containing structural proteins in cell membranes, zinc fingers, and protein receptors. As a result, these proteins can no longer perform their functions.[17]

In North America, overt zinc deficiencies were first observed in the early 1970s in hospitalized patients receiving total parenteral nutrition. Zinc was not added to the original parenteral solutions because the protein source in these solutions contained zinc. When the composition of these solutions was changed to provide isolated amino acids (lacking zinc) as the primary protein source, zinc deficiency symptoms quickly developed.

In North America, overt zinc deficiency is uncommon. Mild zinc deficiencies have been reported in young children, individuals with Crohn's disease and other malabsorptive diseases, those on kidney dialysis, and individuals who restrict their intake of animal-based foods.[17] Other individuals also may be at risk of mild or marginal deficiencies.[20] However, it is difficult to detect marginal deficiencies because assessment measures that reflect changes in zinc status are lacking. In addition, marginal zinc deficiencies are likely to go undetected because they do not typically result in specific physical symptoms. Much attention is being devoted to finding more sensitive ways of measuring mild zinc deficiency.[2]

Severe zinc deficiency can result from a rare genetic condition called acrodermatitis enteropathica. This condition develops after weaning and results in impaired intestinal zinc absorption. Treatment with supplemental zinc is effective in restoring zinc status.[17]

Zinc Toxicity

Signs of zinc toxicity have been reported with supplemental intakes of zinc at 5 or more times the RDA. Thus, the Upper Level is set at 40 mg/day.[4] The symptoms include loss of appetite, nausea, vomiting, intestinal cramps, and diarrhea. Toxicities also have been reported to impair immune function and reduce copper absorption and the activity of copper-containing enzymes.[17] Individuals taking zinc supplements and/or zinc lozenges (for the relief of cold symptoms) should do so cautiously and with the guidance of a dietitian to avoid toxicity symptoms and potential mineral-mineral interactions.

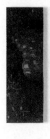

Knowledge Check

1. What functions in the body are dependent on zinc?
2. What are good dietary sources of zinc?
3. What are the symptoms of zinc deficiency?
4. Why are mild zinc deficiencies difficult to detect?

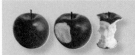

Take Action

Iron and Zinc Intake in a Sample Vegan Diet

Two months ago, Steve decided to become a vegan to improve his diet and overall health. He has asked you to evaluate his diet. His food and beverage intake yesterday is listed below. Does Steve's diet pose any nutritional risks? Is he meeting his needs for iron and zinc?

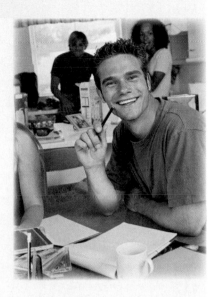

Breakfast
Soy milk, 1 cup
Raisin Bran cereal, 1 cup
Banana, 1
Black coffee, 12 oz

Lunch
Sandwich:
    Whole-wheat bread, 2 slices
    Tomato, 1 small
    Bean sprouts, ¼ cup
    Mayonnaise, 2 tbsp
Granola bar, 1
Orange, 1
Water, 12 oz

Snack
Oatmeal cookies, 3 small
Apple juice, 12 oz

Dinner
Salad:
    Romaine lettuce, 1½ cups
    Carrot, shredded, 1
    Cucumber, ½ sliced
    Mushrooms, ⅓ cup
    French dressing, 3 tbsp
White bean soup, 2 cups
Whole-wheat crackers, 8
Soy cheese, 1 oz
Hot tea, 12 oz

Snack
Popcorn, 3 cups
Root beer, 12 oz

Start by analyzing Steve's iron and zinc intake using a nutrient database, nutrient analysis software, or a website (www.nal.usda.gov/fnic/foodcomp/search). What is your conclusion? Does Steve's diet appear to be a healthy way to eat? What other nutrient intakes may be of concern?

15.3 Copper (Cu)

The use of copper to treat disease dates back to around 400 B.C. However, the essentiality of copper was not fully recognized until 1964, when conclusive evidence of human copper deficiency was reported. Copper has vital functions as a part of many important proteins and enzymes in the body.

Copper in Foods

Copper is found in a variety of foods (Fig. 15-11). Good sources of copper include liver, shellfish, nuts, seeds, mushrooms, soy products, and dark chocolate. Legumes, whole-grain products, and the tap water in many communities also are important sources. Although meat is only a marginal source of copper, it may promote copper absorption from other foods, as it does for iron.

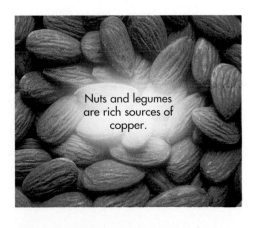

Nuts and legumes are rich sources of copper.

Dietary Needs for Copper

The adult RDA for copper is 900 μg/day.[4] This allowance is based on the amount needed for the normal activity of copper-containing enzymes and proteins in the body. The average adult intake in North America ranges from about 1000 to 1600 μg/day. The Daily Value on food and supplement labels is 2 mg.

Figure 15-11 Food sources of copper.

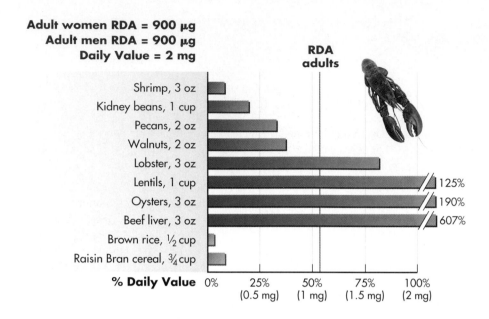

Absorption, Transport, Storage, and Excretion of Copper

Copper absorption occurs primarily in the small intestine. Like zinc, copper is absorbed by simple diffusion and active transport into intestinal absorptive cells and then transported out of the mucosal cells into the bloodstream.[21] In the blood, copper is bound to albumin and other proteins and moves rapidly to the liver (the main storage site) and kidneys. Copper is transported from the liver to other tissues bound primarily to the protein ceruloplasmin. Within the tissues, ceruloplasmin binds to specific receptors, which release copper to transporters within the cells.[21]

Very little copper is stored in the body. However, excess copper can bind to intestinal metallothionein, which may increase the short-term availability of copper.[15, 21] Copper is excreted mainly through the bile into the GI tract for fecal elimination.

Copper absorption is the primary means of regulating copper balance. Thus, absorption can vary from approximately 12 to 70% of dietary intake. The factors affecting copper absorption have not been as fully studied as those for iron and zinc. However, copper absorption is known to increase when dietary copper is low and to decrease when intakes of copper, iron, and/or zinc are excessive.

Functions of Copper

Like iron, copper is an important component of many enzymes because of its ability to alternate between 2 oxidation states (Cu^{1+} and Cu^{2+}). Copper-containing enzymes have many functions in metabolism.[21] For example, 1 enzyme, ceruloplasmin (also called ferroxidase I) is involved in oxidizing ferrous (Fe^{2+}) iron to ferric (Fe^{3+}) iron for incorporation into transferrin and subsequent transport from the liver to body cells. One effect of low ceruloplasmin levels is that little iron is transported from storage, resulting in decreased hemoglobin synthesis and the development of anemia. Thus, copper and iron metabolism are closely linked.[21]

In combination with zinc, copper also functions as a part of a family of enzymes known as **superoxide dismutase (SOD)** enzymes. These enzymes eliminate superoxide free radicals, which prevents oxidative damage to cell membranes. Another copper-containing enzyme, cytochrome C oxidase, catalyzes the last step of the electron transport chain in energy metabolism. Copper is involved in the regulation of neurotransmitters (serotonin, tyrosine, dopamine, and norepinephrine) via the enzyme monoamine oxidase. In addition, copper also has an important role in connective tissue formation as a component of lysyl oxidase. Lysyl oxidase cross-links the

superoxide dismutase (SOD) Enzyme that deactivates a superoxide free radical ($O^{2 \cdot -}$). SOD can contain the trace minerals copper and zinc or manganese.

strands in 2 structural proteins (elastin and collagen) that give tensile strength to connective tissues in the lungs, blood vessels, skin, teeth, and bones.

Copper Deficiency

Severe copper deficiency is relatively rare in humans. Deficiencies have been reported in premature infants fed milk-based formulas, in infants recovering from malnutrition, in patients on long-term total parenteral nutrition without added copper, and in individuals with the genetic disorder Menkes disease.[22] The symptoms of copper deficiency include anemia, decreased white blood cell counts (leukopenia and neutropenia), and skeletal abnormalities (osteopenia).

Recent studies suggest that copper deficiency may increase the risk of neurological disorders, such as amyotrophic lateral sclerosis (Lou Gehrig's disease) and Alzheimer's disease. However, further studies are needed to determine the possible role of copper deficiency in the etiology of these disorders.[23]

Researchers also have become concerned about the possible effects of mild copper deficiencies resulting from prolonged marginal intakes of copper. Unfortunately, detecting marginal copper deficiency can be challenging due to a lack of reliable indicators. As with zinc, analyses of copper levels in tissues and blood may not fully reflect changes in copper status and can be affected by various diseases.[23] The symptoms associated with marginal intakes include suboptimal immune function, glucose intolerance, increased serum cholesterol, and cardiac abnormalities.[21]

Copper Toxicity

Although copper toxicity is not common in humans, it has been reported in children taking accidental overdoses, in individuals consuming copper-contaminated food or water, and in Wilson's disease (a genetic disorder resulting in excess copper storage) (Fig. 15-12). The symptoms of toxicity include abdominal pain, nausea, vomiting, and diarrhea. In severe cases, an accumulation of copper in the liver and the brain causes cirrhosis and neurological damage, respectively. The Upper Level for copper is set at 10 mg/day because higher intakes increase the risk of liver damage.[4]

Knowledge Check

1. Which enzymes require copper for functioning?
2. What are 3 rich sources of copper?
3. Why do many individuals with copper deficiency develop iron deficiency anemia?

▶ Deficiencies of many micronutrients can cause anemia.
- Vitamin E deficiency can lead to hemolytic anemia (see Chapter 12).
- Vitamin K deficiency, especially coupled with the use of certain antibiotics, can lead to blood loss and hemorrhagic anemia (see Chapter 12).
- Vitamin B-6 deficiency can lead to microcytic hypochromic anemia (see Chapter 13).
- Folate deficiency can lead to megaloblastic (or macrocytic) anemia (see Chapter 13).
- Vitamin B-12 malabsorption can lead to macrocytic anemia (see Chapter 13).
- Iron deficiency can lead to microcytic hypochromic anemia.
- Copper deficiency can lead to iron deficiency anemia.

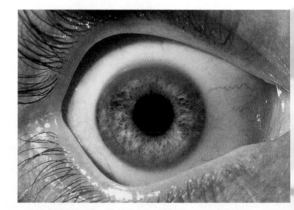

Figure 15-12 Individuals with Wilson's disease deposit copper in the outer edges of the cornea. The ring is a golden to greenish-brown color.

15.4 Manganese (Mn)

Manganese has been recognized as an essential trace mineral since the early 1930s. However, much less is known about manganese than iron, zinc, and copper. As scientists develop more sensitive measures of trace mineral status and function, they will have a clearer picture of the role of manganese in health and disease.

Manganese in Foods

Whole-grain cereals, nuts, legumes, and tea are the best sources of manganese (Fig. 15-13). Meat and dairy products contribute very little manganese to the diet. Based on dietary surveys, the North American diet provides between 2 and 6 mg/day.

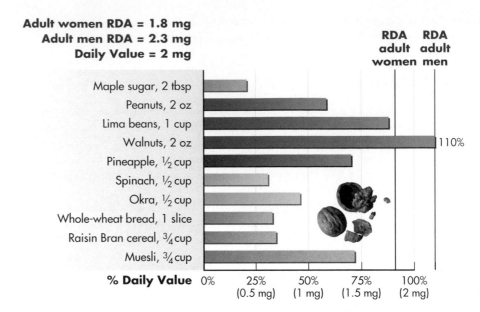

Adult women RDA = 1.8 mg
Adult men RDA = 2.3 mg
Daily Value = 2 mg

	RDA adult women	RDA adult men

Maple sugar, 2 tbsp
Peanuts, 2 oz
Lima beans, 1 cup
Walnuts, 2 oz — 110%
Pineapple, ½ cup
Spinach, ½ cup
Okra, ½ cup
Whole-wheat bread, 1 slice
Raisin Bran cereal, ¾ cup
Muesli, ¾ cup

% Daily Value   0%   25% (0.5 mg)   50% (1 mg)   75% (1.5 mg)   100% (2 mg)

Figure 15-13 **Food sources of manganese.**

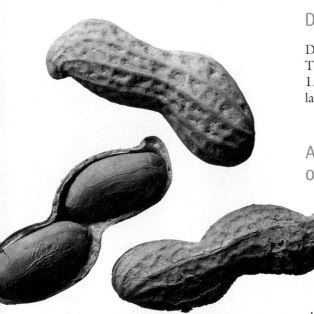

Manganese is found in peanuts and other legumes.

Dietary Needs for Manganese

Data are currently insufficient to determine the dietary requirement for manganese. Thus, an Adequate Intake (AI) for manganese was set at 2.3 mg/day for adult men and 1.8 mg/day for adult women.[4] The Daily Value for manganese on food and supplement labels is 2 mg.

Absorption, Transport, Storage, and Excretion of Manganese

Manganese is absorbed in the small intestine via simple diffusion and active transport. Following absorption, manganese is bound to transferrin and alpha-2-macroglobulin for transport to the liver and subsequent delivery to other tissues, such as the pancreas, kidneys, and bone (a possible storage site). Excretion occurs mainly via bile and is the primary means of regulating manganese levels in the body.[21]

Approximately 10% of the manganese in food is absorbed. Absorption is affected by the amount of manganese in the diet and by iron status. Absorption is increased by low manganese intake and adequate iron status and is decreased by high intakes of manganese and possibly calcium, iron, and phytates.

Functions of Manganese

Manganese shares some functional similarities with zinc and copper.[21] For example, like zinc and copper, it serves as a cofactor for many enzymes in the body. Manganese-dependent enzymes have important functions in nitrogen and carbohydrate metabolism, in cholesterol and urea synthesis, in cartilage formation, and in the antioxidant defense network (as Mn superoxide dismutase). Like copper, manganese can alternate between different oxidation states (Mn^{2+}, Mn^{3+}, and Mn^{7+}). This enables it to participate in various metabolic reactions.

Manganese Deficiency and Toxicity

Manganese deficiency has not been well documented in humans. In fact, only a few cases have ever been reported. The symptoms associated with deficiency include poor growth, skeletal abnormalities, impaired glucose metabolism, and abnormal reproductive function.[21]

Although manganese is considered to be less toxic than most trace minerals, toxicities have been reported in several children receiving long-term parenteral nutrition and from the inhalation of airborne industrial and automobile emissions.[21] Toxicity causes severe neurological impairment and the development of symptoms similar to those seen in Parkinson's disease (muscle stiffness, tremors). Thus, an Upper Level of 11 mg/day was set for manganese to prevent possible damage to the nervous system.[4]

Knowledge Check

1. What are 3 rich sources of manganese?
2. How is manganese function similar to that of zinc and copper?
3. How is manganese status regulated in the body?

 15.5 Iodine (I)

Iodine (I_2), present in food as iodide (I^-) and other non-elemental forms, is unique in many ways from other trace minerals. It is the heaviest element needed for human health and is responsible for only 1 function in the body, the synthesis of thyroid hormones.[24]

Iodine in Foods

The natural iodine content of most foods is relatively low. Saltwater seafood, seaweed, iodized salt, molasses, and dairy products are the best sources of iodine (Fig. 15-14). Dairy products are not naturally good sources of iodine, but they often provide significant amounts because iodide is added to cattle feeds and sanitizing solutions used in dairy

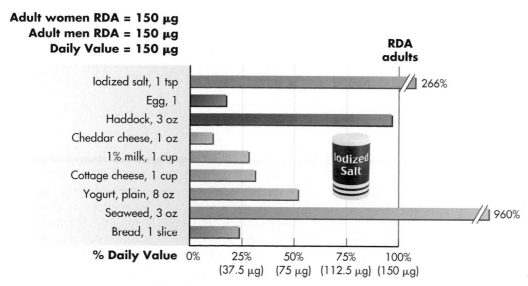

Figure 15-14 Food sources of iodine.

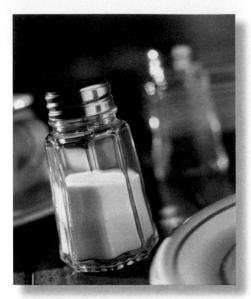

A small amount of iodized salt in one's diet meets iodine needs.

processing. Breads and cereals also may contribute dietary iodine if they are prepared with iodized salt and/or dough conditioners (compounds that strengthen dough and improve bread volume and texture).

Plant-based foods also may provide iodine if the soil in which they were grown was rich in this mineral. However, soil content can vary significantly from region to region, resulting in great differences in iodine content. Iodine-rich soil tends to be near oceans because seawater is naturally high in iodine. When seawater evaporates, the iodine in the air falls on nearby soil.

For many Americans, iodized salt used in cooking and at the table provides most of their iodine. Iodized salt contains 76 µg of iodine per gram of salt. In practical terms, this means that about a half teaspoon (about 2 g) of salt supplies the adult RDA for iodine. Although many Americans also have a significant salt intake from processed foods, non-iodized salt is typically used in processed foods. Many specialty salts, including sea salts, also are non-iodized, so it is important to read labels when purchasing different types of salt.

The bioavailability of iodine is decreased by compounds, called goitrogens, found in raw vegetables such as turnips, cabbage, Brussels sprouts, cauliflower, broccoli, rutabagas, potatoes, and cassava, as well as peanuts, soy, peaches, and strawberries. **Goitrogens** decrease iodine absorption and inhibit iodine use by the thyroid gland. The risk of iodine deficiency is elevated in less developed parts of the world where raw vegetable intake is high and iodine intake low. Goitrogens are of little concern in developed countries because these foods are typically cooked (which helps destroy goitrogen activity) and iodine-rich foods are widely available.

Dietary Needs for Iodine

The adult RDA for iodine is 150 µg/day.[4] This recommendation is based on the amount needed to maintain adequate uptake and turnover by the thyroid gland. In the U.S., usual dietary iodine intakes range between 190 and 300 µg/day. This does not account for amounts provided by iodized salt sprinkled on foods at the table. The Daily Value for iodine used on food and supplement labels is 150 µg.

Absorption, Transport, Storage, and Excretion of Iodine

Most of the iodine present in foods is in the form of iodide and, to a lesser extent, iodates. These forms are very efficiently absorbed in the small intestine. After absorption, most of the iodine (the general term used for the mineral) is transported to the thyroid gland. The thyroid gland actively accumulates iodine, in essence "trapping" it to support thyroid hormone synthesis. Excess iodine is excreted primarily via the kidneys into the urine.[24]

A Biochemist's View

Thyroxine (T_4). Triiodothyronine (T_3) has a similar structure but lacks 1 iodine (I), indicated in this figure with a red asterisk.

Functions of Iodine

Iodine is an essential component of the thyroid hormones thyroxine (T_4) and triiodothyronine (T_3). Most of the circulating thyroid hormone in the body is in the form of T_4. Within body cells, T_4 loses an iodine molecule and is converted to T_3, the active form of the hormone. The enzymes involved in this conversion (called deiodinase enzymes) all require the trace mineral selenium. Thus, a selenium deficiency can limit the activity of deiodinase enzymes, resulting in decreased T_3 levels.

Although iodine has a singular function, this function has widespread consequences because of the vital role that thyroid hormones play in maintaining normal metabolism. As a component of T_3, iodine is involved in the regulation of many important metabolic and developmental functions. This includes the regulation of basal energy expenditure, macronutrient metabolism, growth, brain development, and organ maturation.[24]

Iodine Deficiency Disorders (IDD)

Iodine deficiency disorders, the collective name for **endemic** goiter and endemic cretinism, occur when dietary iodine intake is insufficient. When iodine availability decreases and plasma levels of T_4 hormone drop, the pituitary gland secretes thyroid-stimulating hormone (TSH). In response to increased TSH levels, the thyroid gland enlarges in an attempt to increase its efficiency at trapping iodine. The characteristic enlargement of the thyroid gland that occurs is called a **goiter**. This early adaptive response allows the thyroid gland to temporarily maintain thyroid hormone synthesis. Although a goiter is a painless condition, it can cause pressure on the esophagus and trachea and impair their function. If the underlying iodine deficiency is not corrected, decreased T_4 synthesis, slowed metabolism, and more serious complications can develop.[24]

Iodine deficiency is of particular concern during pregnancy because of the adverse effects it can have on the developing offspring.[25, 26] These include congenital abnormalities, low birth weight, neurological disorders, impaired mental function, poor physical development, and death. The resulting restriction of brain development and growth, called **cretinism** (Fig. 15-15), is characterized by severe mental retardation, loss of hearing and speech abilities, short stature, and muscle spasticity.

Descriptions of goiter have been documented for many centuries in China and other parts of the world. Prior to World War I, goiter was very common in the Great Lakes region of the U.S., where the soil and lake waters are very low in iodine. Cretinism also was common in parts of the U.S. Today, approximately one-third of the world's population remains at risk of iodine deficiency.[11, 26] Almost every country in the world still has iodine-deficient areas. The highest incidence of iodine deficiency disorders occurs in South America, Asia, Africa, and the Middle East.

The discovery in the early 1920s, by scientists in the U.S. and Switzerland, that iodine can prevent the development of goiter resulted in the fortification of table salt in the United

endemic Habitual presence of a disease within a given geographic area.

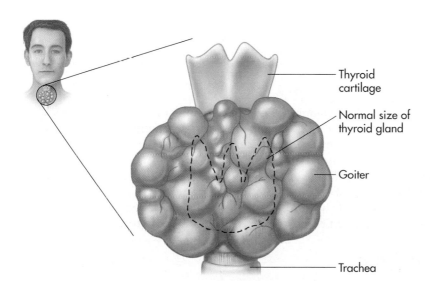

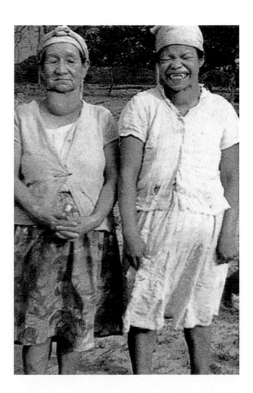

Figure 15-15 **The mother (left) has a goiter. The daughter also has a goiter, as well as many characteristics of cretinism (mental retardation, deaf, mute).**

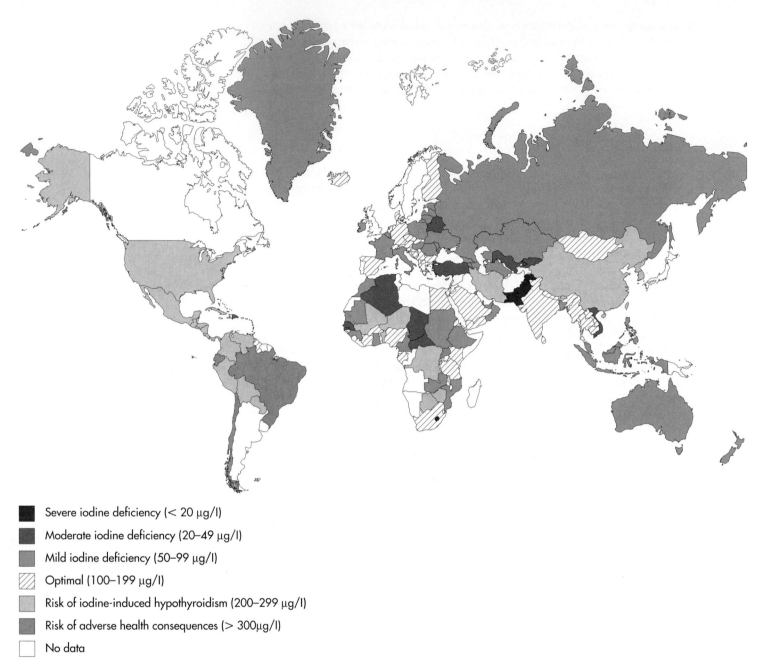

Severe iodine deficiency (< 20 µg/l)

Moderate iodine deficiency (20–49 µg/l)

Mild iodine deficiency (50–99 µg/l)

Optimal (100–199 µg/l)

Risk of iodine-induced hypothyroidism (200–299 µg/l)

Risk of adverse health consequences (> 300µg/l)

No data

Figure 15-16 Iodine deficiency disorders are moderate to severe in many areas of the world. Adverse health consequences can occur from excessive dietary iodine as well.

Courtesy of the World Health Organization, *Iodine Status Worldwide, WHO Global Database on Iodine Deficiency.*

States and many other countries. Using a small amount of iodized salt has eradicated endemic iodine deficiency in these areas. Unfortunately, many countries have yet to adopt iodine fortification programs. Consequently, iodine deficiency remains an international public health problem.[27] In fact, approximately 50% of the world's population live in countries where iodine deficiency is still a significant concern (Fig. 15-16). The World Health Organization (WHO) believes that iodine deficiency is the "greatest single cause of preventable brain damage and mental retardation" and has set a goal of eliminating this deficiency within the next decade by increasing the use of fortified salt, oil, milk, and other food products.[26]

Iodine Toxicity

The Upper Level is set at 1100 µg/day for adult men and women to prevent health-related risks.[4] Like iodine deficiency, iodine toxicity can cause enlargement of the thyroid gland and decreased thyroid hormone synthesis.[28] Toxicities have been reported in Japan, due to high intakes of iodine-rich seaweed, and in Chile, due to high levels of environmental iodine, increased iodine use in water purification, and excessive fortification of salt. Although hypothyroidism is the most common result of iodine toxicity, excess iodine intakes also may increase the risk of autoimmune thyroid disease and thyroid cancer.

Knowledge Check

1. What are 3 rich sources of iodine?
2. What is the main function of iodine?
3. Why is iodine deficiency still prevalent in many areas of the world?
4. What are the symptoms of iodine deficiency?

CASE STUDY

At a recent family reunion, Gina learned that an aunt was currently undergoing treatment for colon cancer. Her grandmother explained that 2 other family members had died of the disease before Gina was born. After the reunion, Gina decided to learn more about colon cancer and how her family history of the disease might affect her. Gina learned that 150,000 Americans are diagnosed with colon cancer each year and that her family history increases her chances of developing the disease. While searching online, she came across a site that recommended taking 200 mg/day of the trace mineral selenium to prevent the disease. She then went to her local supermarket and found that 100 selenium tablets containing 200 mg each cost only $7.50 a bottle. Gina figured this supplement was cheap "insurance" against developing the disease and, so, began taking 200 mg of selenium a day. Is Gina's practice harmful? Are there other dietary practices she should consider to help protect her from developing colon cancer?

15.6 Selenium (Se)

The essentiality of selenium in human health was not recognized until 1979, when Chinese scientists noted that a cardiac condition in children and young women living in Keshan province could be prevented by selenium. Scientists' understanding of the role of selenium in Keshan disease and other aspects of human health has developed rapidly since that time.[29]

Selenium in Foods

The selenium content of food varies significantly in relation to the soil content where the plant was grown or the animal raised.[30] For example, the selenium content of grains grown in selenium-rich soil will be greater than that of grains grown in low selenium soil. In general, the best sources of selenium are seafood, meats, cereals, grains, and nuts (Fig. 15-17).

Dietary Needs for Selenium

The adult RDA for selenium is 55 µg/day.[31] The RDA is based on the amount of selenium needed to maximize glutathione peroxidase activity in the blood. In North America, daily intakes of selenium are typically above the RDA. The Daily Value on food and supplement labels is 70 µg.

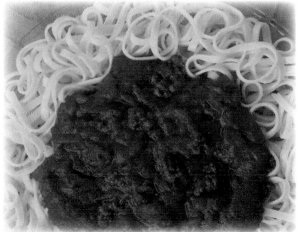

Pasta made from wheat grown in most parts of North America is a good source of selenium.

Figure 15-17 Food sources of selenium.

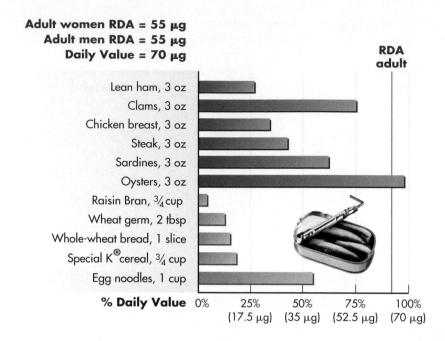

Absorption, Transport, Storage, and Excretion of Selenium

Most of the selenium in foods is bound to the amino acids methionine (as selenomethionine) and cysteine (as selenocysteine). Both forms are well absorbed in the small intestine, with absorption ranging from 50 to 100% of dietary intake. Unlike many of the other trace minerals, absorption is not affected by the body's selenium stores and absorption does not play a role in maintaining homeostasis. Selenium balance is achieved primarily through urinary excretion, rather than intestinal absorption.

Little is known about the transport of selenium across membranes. After absorption, selenium is distributed to target tissues with the highest concentrations found in the blood, liver, muscle, kidneys, and skeleton. Within tissues, selenomethionine provides a "storage pool" of selenium, whereas selenocysteine serves as the biologically active form of the mineral.

Functions of Selenium

Selenium is a component of at least 25 different enzymes and proteins in the body.[29] One of its most recognized functions is in the antioxidant defense network, as a part of glutathione peroxidase (GPX) enzymes, thioredoxin reductase enzymes, and selenoprotein P (Fig. 15-18). As part of the antioxidant defense network, selenium helps prevent lipid peroxidation and cell membrane damage. Its ability to destroy highly reactive peroxyl free radicals spares vitamin E for use in other antioxidant functions. Another important function of selenium is in thyroid metabolism as a part of iodothyronine deiodinase enzymes. Recall from the discussion of iodine that the deiodinase enzymes that convert thyroxine (T_4) to triiodothyronine (T_3) require selenium.

It is likely that selenium also plays an important role in immune function.[29] Scientists believe that selenium may prevent Keshan disease by inactivating a virus linked to its development. Additionally, selenium may decrease the risk of prostate, lung, or other cancers, although recent studies have provided conflicting results.[29, 32, 33] Further research is needed to understand more clearly the role of selenium in the prevention of chronic disease.

Selenium Deficiency

Inadequate selenium intake is not known to cause a specific deficiency disease. As mentioned previously, selenium deficiency is associated with changes in thyroid hormone metabolism and a possible increased risk of certain cancers. Selenium deficiency also is

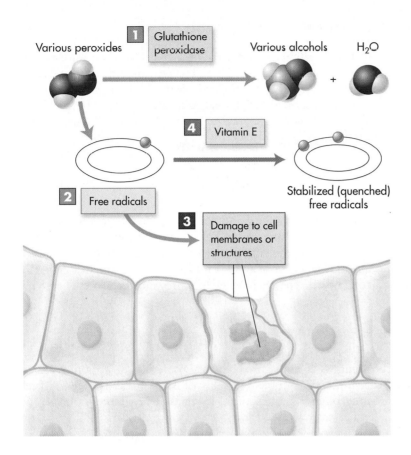

Figure 15-18 Selenium is part of the glutathione perioxidase system, **1** which breaks down peroxides, such as hydrogen peroxide (H_2O_2), to water (H_2O) before they can form free radicals **2** and damage cells **3**. This breakdown of peroxides, in turn, spares some people of the need for vitamin E **4**, which is a major free radical scavenger.

associated with the development of Keshan disease, a disease characterized by insufficient cardiac function. This disease was first observed in the Keshan province of China where the soil is almost devoid of selenium. It has since been diagnosed in other regions, including New Zealand and Finland. Although Keshan disease can be prevented through selenium supplementation, the related cardiac disorders are not corrected by selenium once the disease has developed.

Selenium Toxicity

Excess supplementation of selenium can result in toxicity. In fact, selenium toxicity has been observed in intakes as low as 1 to 3 mg daily taken over many months. The symptoms of toxicity include nausea, diarrhea, fatigue, hair loss, changes in nails, and skin rashes. The Upper Level for selenium is 400 µg/day.[31]

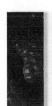

Knowledge Check

1. What are 3 rich sources of selenium?
2. How is selenium function linked to iodine metabolism?
3. What diseases are associated with selenium deficiency?

15.7 Chromium (Cr)

The importance of chromium in the diet has been recognized only in recent years. Like many trace minerals, the functions of this nutrient are emerging with advances in research technology.

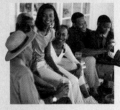

CASE STUDY FOLLOW-UP

Gina's supplement dose of 200 µg/day, plus a typical dietary intake of 105 µg/day, is below the Upper Level of 400 µg/day. Therefore, her practice is probably safe. Whether it will be helpful in reducing colon cancer risk awaits further research. Until further information is available, the widespread use of such a high dose of selenium is not recommended.

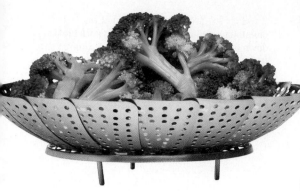

Broccoli is a good source of chromium.

Chromium in Foods

Chromium is widely distributed in a variety of foods. However, information regarding the chromium content of foods is lacking. Thus, many nutrient databases do not yet include values for chromium. Processed meats, liver, eggs, whole-grain products, broccoli, mushrooms, dried beans, nuts, and dark chocolate tend to be good sources of the mineral. Chromium is used to manufacture steel; thus, small amounts of chromium are transferred to food via food processing equipment.

Dietary Needs for Chromium

The Adequate Intakes for chromium in adults aged 19 to 50 years are 35 μg/day for men and 25 μg/day for women.[4] After age 50, the Adequate Intake decreases to 30 μg/day for men and 20 μg/day for women. The Adequate Intake is based on the amounts typically found in nutritious diets. The average intake in North America generally meets the Adequate Intake standard. The Daily Value for chromium is 120 μg.

Absorption, Transport, Storage, and Excretion of Chromium

Very little chromium is absorbed from dietary sources. Absorption appears to increase when intakes are low, although bioavailability of the mineral has been difficult to assess. Once absorbed, chromium is transported by transferrin via the bloodstream and accumulates in the bones, liver, kidneys, and spleen. Concentrations in human tissues are very low because most dietary chromium is excreted in the feces.

Functions of Chromium

The functions of chromium are not fully known. Chromium may enhance insulin action, promote glucose uptake into cells, and normalize blood sugar levels.[34] However, chromium supplementation in patients with type 2 diabetes has not been shown to be effective in controlling blood glucose.[35] Many athletes use chromium supplements to enhance muscle mass and strength, despite a lack of research evidence supporting its effectiveness.

Chromium Deficiency and Toxicity

Chromium deficiency has been difficult to assess due to the lack of sensitive measures of chromium status. Several cases of chromium deficiency have been reported in individuals receiving chromium-free parenteral solutions. The symptoms included weight loss, glucose intolerance, and nerve damage.

Few serious effects have been reported from excess dietary chromium intake. Thus, an Upper Level has not been set.[4] Nutritionists have expressed concern about the safety of high doses of chromium supplements used by many athletes and have recommended continued monitoring for possible toxicities.

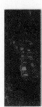

Knowledge Check

1. What are the proposed functions of chromium?
2. What are rich food sources of chromium?
3. What are the symptoms of chromium deficiency?

15.8 Fluoride (F)

Fluoride, the ionic form of fluorine, may not be an essential nutrient because all basic body functions can occur without it. However, in the early 1930s, it was observed that individuals living in the southwestern U.S., where the water naturally contained high concentrations of fluoride, had fewer dental caries (cavities). Many people in these areas also had small spots on their teeth (known as mottling, or fluorosis) due to excess fluoride (Fig. 15-19). Although discolored, the mottled teeth were virtually free of dental caries. This discovery led to research studies confirming this mineral's ability to reduce cavities and the start of controlled water fluoridation in parts of the U.S.

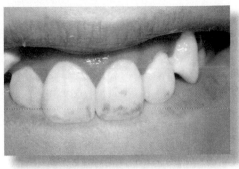

Figure 15-19 Fluorosis, or mottled enamel, caused by overexposure to fluoride.

Fluoride in Foods

Today, in North America, the major source of fluoride is fluoridated water. Typically, fluoridated water contains about 0.2 mg of fluoride per 8 ounces, or 0.7 to 1.2 mg/liter.[36] However, not all public or private water sources are fluoridated (Fig. 15-20).

In addition to fluoridated water, tea, seafood, and seaweed provide the greatest amounts of dietary fluoride. The use of fluoridated toothpastes and mouth rinses and fluoride treatments provides non-dietary ways of obtaining fluoride. The prevalence of these non-dietary sources has caused considerable debate as to whether water fluoridation should be continued and whether individuals are now at greater health risks from possible excess fluoride exposure.[36]

▶ To determine if your water supply is fluoridated, contact your local water supplier or have the water in your home analyzed for fluoride content. Your dentist can help you decide the best means for obtaining sufficient fluoride.

Dietary Needs for Fluoride

The Adequate Intakes for fluoride are 3 mg/day for adult women and 4 mg/day for adult men.[37] For infants up to 6 months of age, the Adequate Intake is 0.01 mg/day.

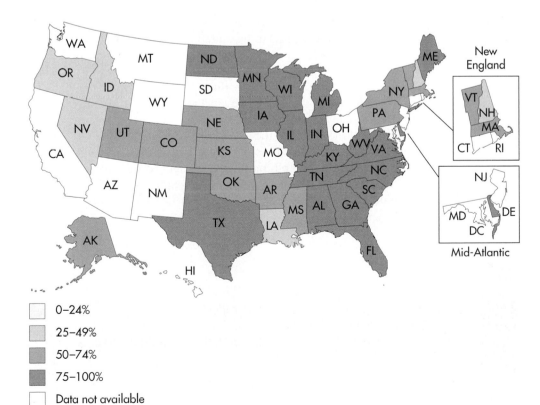

0–24%
25–49%
50–74%
75–100%
Data not available

Figure 15-20 Percentage of state populations served by public water systems with fluoridated water.

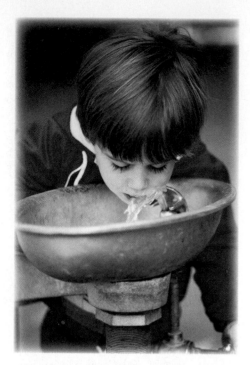

Following the fluoridation of water in 1945 in many North American cities, the incidence of dental caries decreased dramatically.

This increases to 0.5 mg/day for infants 6 to 12 months of age and ranges from 0.7 to 3 mg/day for young children and adolescents. The Adequate Intake recommendations are based on the amount needed to provide resistance to dental caries without causing mottling of the tooth enamel.[37]

Absorption, Transport, Storage, and Excretion of Fluoride

The absorption of dietary fluoride occurs rapidly in the stomach and small intestine via passive diffusion. Overall, approximately 80 to 90% of fluoride consumed is absorbed. Absorbed fluoride is transported in the bloodstream and concentrated in teeth and the skeleton. The amount of fluoride deposited in the teeth and bones is greatest during infancy, childhood, and adolescence. Calcified tissue deposition and urinary excretion are the major means for removing fluoride from the circulation.

Functions of Fluoride

Although a truly essential function for fluoride has not been described, fluoride is recognized for its beneficial role in supporting the deposition of calcium and phosphorus in teeth and bones and in protecting against the development of dental caries.[36] Fluoride works in several ways to prevent caries. During the development of teeth and bones, fluoride forms hydroxyfluorapatite crystals. These crystals provide greater resistance (than typical hydroxyapatite crystals) to bacteria and acids in the mouth that can erode tooth enamel. Fluoride in the blood contributes to fluoride in the saliva, which promotes the remineralization of enamel lesions and reduces the net loss of minerals from tooth enamel.

Fluoride Deficiency and Toxicity

A lack of fluoride is associated with an increased incidence of dental caries. However, no specific deficiency disorder or disease appears to be caused by insufficient fluoride intake. In contrast, fluoride toxicity has been reported in young children who have swallowed fluoride tablets or solutions. Although rare, acute toxicity can occur rapidly and be life-threatening. Thus, fluoridated toothpastes, mouth rinses, and supplements need to be kept out of the reach of children. The signs of toxicity include nausea, vomiting, diarrhea, sweating, spasms, convulsions, and coma.

Mottling, or fluorosis, of the enamel is the result of chronic intake of excess fluoride during tooth development. Dental fluorosis is not associated with any health risk but does result in discoloration and possible pitting of the enamel. To minimize the risk of fluorosis, an Upper Level has been set at 0.1 mg/kg body weight/day (0.7 to 2.2 mg/day) for infants and children up to 8 years of age. The Upper Level for children over age 8 and for adults is 10 mg/day.[37]

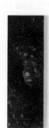

Knowledge Check

1. How does fluoride help prevent dental caries?
2. What are rich sources of fluoride?
3. Why should fluoridated toothpastes, mouth rinses, and supplements be kept out of the reach of children?

Table 15-5 Key Trace Mineral Summary

Mineral	Major Functions	Deficiency Symptoms	Individuals at Risk	Adult RDA or Adequate Intake	Good Dietary Sources	Toxicity Symptoms
Iron	Functional component of hemoglobin and other key compounds used in respiration; immune function; cognitive development; energy metabolism	Fatigue on exertion; poor immune function; anemia	Infants; preschool children; women in childbearing years	Males: 8 mg Females: 18 mg	Meats; seafood; enriched breads; fortified cereals; eggs	Gastrointestinal upset; Upper Level is 45 mg/day
Zinc	Required for many enzymes; immune function; growth and development; stabilizes cell membranes and body proteins	Skin rash; diarrhea; decreased appetite and sense of taste; hair loss; poor growth and development	Vegetarians; elderly people; people with alcoholism; malnourished populations	Males: 11 mg Females: 8 mg	Seafoods; meats; whole grains	Decreased copper absorption, diarrhea, nausea, cramps, depressed immune function; Upper Level is 40 mg/day
Copper	Aids in iron metabolism; works in antioxidant enzymes and those involved in connective tissue metabolism	Anemia; low white blood cell count; poor growth	People using excessive zinc supplementation	900 µg	Liver; cocoa; nuts; whole grains; shellfish; legumes	Excessive supplement use can cause vomiting, nausea, diarrhea, and nervous system and liver disorders; Upper Level is 10 mg/day
Selenium	Part of an antioxidant system as glutathione peroxidase; activates thyroid hormones	Keshan disease; reduced thyroid hormone	People in areas of the world with low selenium content in the soil	55 µg	Meats; eggs; fish; seafoods; whole grains; nuts	Nausea, vomiting, hair loss, diarrhea, changes in nails; Upper Level is 400 mg/day
Iodine	Component of thyroid hormones that regulates basal metabolism, growth, and development	Goiter; cretinism	Major problem in parts of the world where soil iodine is low and fortified foods are not available	150 µg	Iodized salt; saltwater fish; dairy products	Inhibition of function of the thyroid gland; Upper Level is 1.1 mg/day
Fluoride	Increases resistance of tooth enamel to dental caries; mineralization of bones and teeth	Although not a true deficiency symptom, dental caries is a risk	Areas where water is not fluoridated	Males: 4 mg Females: 3 mg	Fluoridated water; toothpaste; dental treatments; tea; seaweed	Fluorosis, or mottling (staining) of tooth enamel; acute toxicity can be fatal; Upper Level is 10 mg/day
Chromium	Enhances insulin action	Glucose intolerance	Rare	Females: 20–25 µg Males: 30–35 µg	Eggs; liver; whole grains; nuts; mushrooms; processed meats	No report of dietary toxicity; No Upper Level set
Manganese	Cofactor of several enzymes; involved in carbohydrate metabolism and antioxidant protection	Poor growth; skeletal abnormalities	Rare	Females: 1.8 mg Males: 2.3 mg	Nuts; tea; legumes; whole-grain cereals	Nervous system disorders; Upper Level is 11 mg/day
Molybdenum*	Cofactor for several enzymes	Not known in humans	Rare	45 µg	Grains; nuts; legumes	Poor growth in laboratory animals; Upper Level is 2 mg/day

*Often classified as an ultratrace mineral, but unlike other ultratrace minerals it has an established RDA.

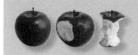

Take Action

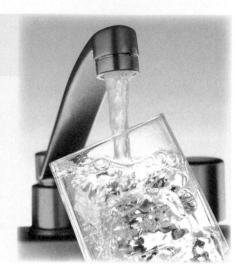

Is Your Local Water Supply Fluoridated?

Healthy People 2010 set a goal that 75% of the people in the U.S. will be served by community water systems that add sufficient fluoride. Today, only about 60% of Americans have access to naturally or artificially fluoridated water. Do you know if your community water supply is fluoridated? To find the answer, check with your local water department. Is the water naturally rich in fluoride, or is this mineral added to the water supply? What amount of fluoride is in the drinking water? If it is added to the water supply, how long has this procedure been in operation? If the water supply does not supply fluoride, how could you obtain sufficient fluoride?

 ## 15.9 Molybdenum (Mo) and Ultratrace Minerals

Molybdenum is often classified as an ultratrace mineral. Although it is needed in "ultratrace" amounts, experts recognize that molybdenum, like many trace minerals, is essential for the activity of several enzymes. Molybdenum is obtained from plant-based foods, such as grains, legumes, and nuts. Like iodine and selenium, the molybdenum content of foods can vary, depending on the soil in which the plant was grown. The RDA for molybdenum is very small (45 µg/day) and is based on its role as a cofactor required for the activity of several enzymes.[4] The dietary intakes in North America typically meet or exceed the RDA. The Daily Value used on food and supplement labels is 75 µg. Deficiencies of molybdenum are very rare, as are toxicities. However, an Upper Level of 2000 µg/day for adults was set to prevent harmful consequences noted in animal studies.[4]

The body contains other minerals in extremely small, or "ultratrace," amounts that do not yet have clearly defined, essential physiological functions. The minerals arsenic,

Table 15-6 **Ultratrace Mineral Summary**

Mineral	Proposed Functions	Typical Intake by Adults	Estimated Daily Need	Upper Intake Level	Dietary Sources
Boron	Cell membrane function (ion transport), steroid hormone metabolism	0.75–1.35 mg	1–13 mg	20 mg	Legumes, fruits, vegetables, potatoes, wine
Nickel	Metabolism of amino acids, fatty acids, vitamin B-12, and folic acid	69–162 µg	25–35 µg	1 mg	Chocolate, nuts, legumes, whole grains
Silicon	Bone formation	19–40 mg	35–40 µg	None set	Root vegetables, whole grains
Arsenic	Amino acid metabolism, DNA function	30 µg	12–25 µg	None set*	Fish, grains, cereals
Vanadium	Mimics insulin action	6–18 µg	10 µg	1.8 mg	Shellfish, mushrooms, parsley, dill

*Although an Upper Level has not been set, the addition of this mineral to food is not recommended.

boron, nickel, silicon, and vanadium fall within this classification (Table 15-6). It is likely that these ultratrace minerals function as cofactors for specific enzymes or compounds, promote normal growth and development, and/or decrease the risk of certain diseases. However, further research is needed to define their specific roles in the body and to set RDAs or Adequate Intakes. Deficiency symptoms for these elements are not yet known. An Upper Level has been established for boron, nickel, and vanadium because of toxicity concerns associated with increased exposure to these minerals.[4]

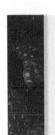

Knowledge Check

1. What are good sources of molybdenum?
2. What is the function of molybdenum?
3. Why are arsenic, boron, nickel, silicon, and vanadium classified as ultratrace minerals?
4. Which of the ultratrace minerals have an established Upper Level?

Global Perspective

The Micronutrient Initiative

Millions of children die needlessly every year from measles, diarrhea, and other illnesses because deficiencies of vitamin A and zinc compromise their ability to fight infections.[3,11] Over half of the young children in developing countries are at risk of poor physical and mental development due to deficiencies of iron and iodine.[11]

The Micronutrient Initiative is an international organization, formed in 1990, that is dedicated to eliminating worldwide vitamin and mineral deficiencies. The Canadian-based network is comprised of nutritional scientists, practitioners, and policy makers who work together to utilize basic research knowledge to find solutions for ending micronutrient malnutrition. The focus of the Micronutrient Initiative has been to develop local food fortification programs and cultivate working partnerships with governments, food industries, international agencies, and the private sector to provide a sustained impact on improving the health and well-being of our world's population.[11]

The Micronutrient Initiative has been actively involved in nutritional programs in 75 countries. Some of the key achievements of the network include these.

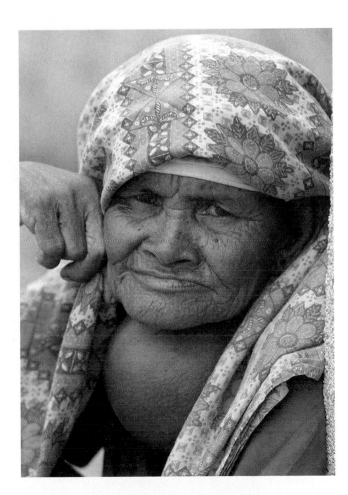

- Iron and folic acid fortification of flour in the Middle East and North Africa
- Marketing of complementary foods in South Asia
- Expansion of universal salt iodization
- Partnerships with private foundations to develop global food fortification coalitions
- Establishment of the Global Vitamin A Initiative to provide vitamin A supplements to 1.5 billion children in 70 countries

To learn more about the Micronutrient Initiative, visit its website: www.micronutrient.org/home.asp.

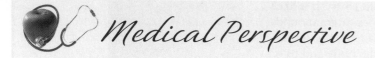

Medical Perspective

Nutrients, Diet, and Cancer

Cancer is the second leading cause of death for North American adults. Many dietary factors, such as antioxidant nutrients (e.g., selenium and vitamin C), calcium, and other nutrients may help protect against cancer. On the other hand, dietary factors, such as excessive fat and calorie intake, may increase cancer risk.

What Is Cancer?

Cancer is not a single disease. It occurs in many forms in different organs and types of cells in the body (Fig. 15-21). In fact, even in the same organ or tissue, cancers may be quite different in nature. Lung, prostate, breast, and colorectal cancers account for slightly over half of all cancers in North America and are the leading cause of cancer-related death for all racial and ethnic groups. While these statistics are unsettling, the recent decline in cancer rates and cancer-related deaths is encouraging. Early screening programs, new detection methods and more effective cancer therapies have helped improve the prognosis for many cancers.

In general, cancer is characterized by the abnormal and uncontrolled division of altered cells. As these altered cells multiply, they often form tumors, which can be benign or malignant.

Benign tumors are non-cancerous because they are enclosed in a membrane that prevents them from spreading. They are harmful only if they interfere with normal function. For instance, a benign brain tumor can cause complications and death if it blocks blood flow in the brain. Unlike benign tumors, **malignant** tumors are capable of invading surrounding structures and spreading to other areas of the body. They can **metastasize** (spread) to distant parts of the body via the blood and/or lymph and can form invasive tumors in almost any area.

Most cancers are classified as carcinomas, sarcomas, lymphomas, or leukemias. Carcinomas constitute about 80 to 90% of all cancers. They develop from epithelial cells that cover external and internal areas (or surfaces) of the body and affect secretory organs, such as the breast. Sarcomas are cancers of connective tissues, such as in bone. Lymphomas, such as Hodgkin's and non-Hodgkin's lymphomas, are malignant tumors in the lymph nodes and lymphoid tissues. Leukemias are cancers of precursor white blood cells formed in the bone marrow. Although leukemias do not produce a tumor as other cancers do, they exhibit the basic characteristics of rapid and uncontrolled cell growth that can spread to other areas of the body. Therefore, they are still classified as cancers.

Estimated % of Cancer Deaths		
Male		**Female**
< 1%	Brain	2%
4%	Esophagus and stomach	< 1%
31%	Lung	26%
	Breast	15%
4%	Liver	< 1%
6%	Pancreas	6%
7%	Leukemia and lymphomas	7%
10%	Colon and rectum	10%
6%	Urinary	
	Ovary	6%
9%	Prostate	
	Uterus and cervix	3%
23%	All others (e.g., oral and skin) (e.g., oral, skin, and bladder)	24%

Figure 15-21 **Cancer can affect numerous types of cells and organs.**

Development of Cancer

Most cells exist in a balanced cycle between turning cell replication on and turning it off. This cell cycle is controlled by the genes in DNA that promote cell replication (called protooncogenes) and prevent replication (called tumor suppressor genes). Cancer often results from a lack of suppressor genes or the overactivity of protooncogenes. The cancer gene (oncogene) is like an out-of-control protooncogene—it makes hundreds of copies of itself without any constraints. Normally, tumor suppressor genes act as braking mechanisms within the cell to prevent uncontrolled growth. When something goes wrong with these genes, the oncogenes are free to promote rapid cell growth. Within a cell, repair mechanisms constantly look for errors in DNA replication and make corrections. However, sometimes the repair mechanisms fail, resulting in an inherited defect, or a DNA mutation.

Early defects that are not caught and repaired predispose the cell to additional errors, which increase the risk of cancer.

Carcinogenesis, the development of cancer, is a 3-step process (Fig. 15-22).

- Step 1 is the exposure of a cell to a carcinogen (cancer-causing agent) that triggers the initiation of cancer. Initiation can develop spontaneously or be induced by carcinogens such as tobacco, radiation (e.g., sun exposure), alcohol, occupational toxins, viruses, food contaminants (e.g., aflatoxin mold), dietary factors, and drugs. The initiation stage of carcinogenesis, during which DNA is altered, is relatively short, ranging from minutes to days.

- Step 2 is the promotion state, which may last for months or even years. During this period, the mutation is locked into the genetic material of the cell. Compounds that increase cell division, called promoters,

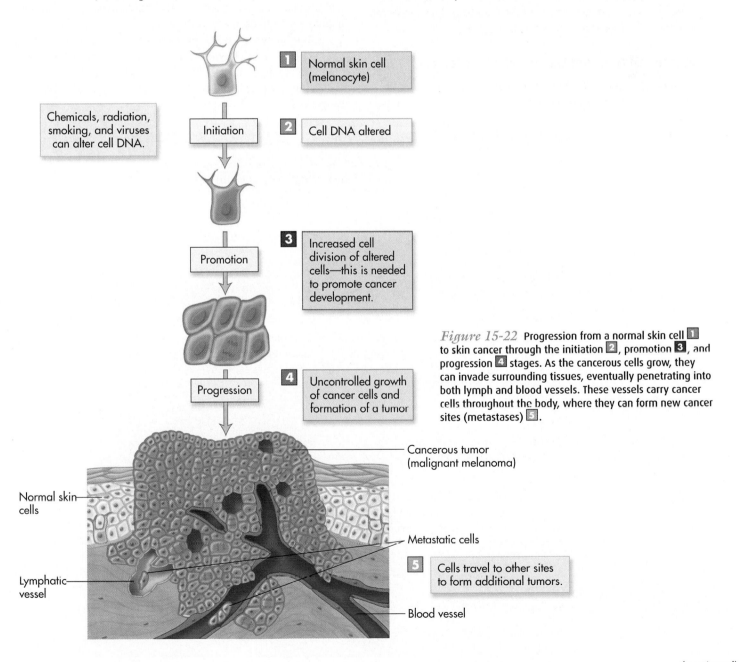

Chemicals, radiation, smoking, and viruses can alter cell DNA.

Initiation

Promotion

Progression

1 | Normal skin cell (melanocyte)

2 | Cell DNA altered

3 | Increased cell division of altered cells—this is needed to promote cancer development.

4 | Uncontrolled growth of cancer cells and formation of a tumor

5 | Cells travel to other sites to form additional tumors.

Normal skin cells

Lymphatic vessel

Cancerous tumor (malignant melanoma)

Metastatic cells

Blood vessel

Figure 15-22 Progression from a normal skin cell 1 to skin cancer through the initiation 2, promotion 3, and progression 4 stages. As the cancerous cells grow, they can invade surrounding tissues, eventually penetrating into both lymph and blood vessels. These vessels carry cancer cells throughout the body, where they can form new cancer sites (metastases) 5.

(continued)

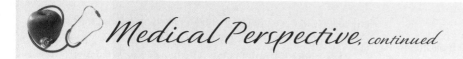

Medical Perspective, continued

encourage uncontrolled replication of the altered DNA. Promoters may reduce the time available for repair mechanisms to enhance the replication of altered DNA cells. Excess alcohol, estrogen, and *Helicobacter pylori* bacteria in the stomach may all act as promoters.

- Step 3, cancer progression, begins with the appearance of cells that grow autonomously (out of control). During the progression phase, these malignant cells proliferate, invade surrounding tissue, and metastasize to other sites. Early in this stage, the immune system may find the altered cells and destroy them. Alternately, the cancer cells may become so defective that their DNA prevents their growth. However, if nothing stops cancer cell growth, 1 or more tumors eventually develop.

Genetic, Environmental, and Dietary Factors

Although our genetic makeup may contribute to a risk of certain cancers, such as colorectal, breast, and prostate cancer, genetic factors account for only about 1 to 15% of the incidence of all cancers. This does not explain the dramatic differences in cancer types and rates noted in different parts of the world. For example, in poorer countries, cancers of the stomach, liver, mouth, esophagus, and uterus are most common. In affluent countries, cancers of the lung, colon and rectum, breast, and prostate gland predominate. Because of these differences, many experts believe that environmental factors, such as exposure to radiation, chemicals, and air and water pollutants; smoking; lack of physical activity; obesity; and diet play a greater role in cancer initiation and development. The menu in Table 15-7 provides an example of a dietary plan to decrease cancer risk.

The following are the primary dietary factors associated with cancer risk.[38-42] However, much of the evidence is based on epidemiologic studies which cannot show cause and effect. Further research is needed to confirm how diet affects cancer risk.

Table 15-7   Example of a Diet Intended to Limit the Risk for Cancer—Low in Fat and High in Fruits, Vegetables, and Antioxidants

Breakfast

4 oz calcium-fortified orange juice
1 cup ready-to-eat whole-grain breakfast cereal
1 cup 1% milk
1 cup fresh blueberries
1 slice whole-wheat toast, jelly, soft margarine
Hot green tea

Lunch

Sandwich: ½ cup curried chicken salad served on 1 whole-wheat bagel
Assorted raw vegetables: carrots, celery, broccoli, cucumber, green pepper
1 cup 1% milk
Fresh fruit cup with strawberries, melon, grapes, apple
2 fig cookies

Snack

¼ cup mixed nuts and raisins
4 oz apple-blueberry juice

Dinner

3 oz grilled salmon (or other fish)
Baked potato topped with shredded mozzarella cheese (¼ cup) and green onions
Roasted corn on the cob, soft margarine
Fresh garden salad with low-fat Italian dressing
1 whole-wheat dinner roll
1 scoop sherbet with fresh raspberries
Hot raspberry tea

Snack

6 oz cranberry juice
2 cups popcorn

- *Fruits and vegetables.* Diets low in fruits and vegetables (rich sources of antioxidant nutrients, such as selenium, vitamin A, vitamin C, and vitamin E and phytochemicals) have been associated with an increased incidence of certain cancers. However, a dietary pattern high in fruits and vegetables may not offer a protective effect against the development of, the recurrence of, or survival in certain types of cancer.[43,44]

- *Excessive energy intake and obesity.* Excessive energy intake and obesity have been associated with an increased risk of breast cancer. This relationship may occur because obesity increases the production of hormones such as estrogen and insulin. Additionally, cancer cells may multiply more readily when excess energy is available to support their growth.

- *Meat.* High intakes of meats, especially red meat and grilled meat, are associated with an increased risk of colorectal, kidney, pancreatic, and stomach cancers. The saturated fat content of red meat, and the production of polyaromatic hydrocarbons (e.g., benzopyrene) when meats are charbroiled, may increase the risk of cancers. Nitrosamine compounds found in processed meats such as sausage, hot dogs, and bacon also may increase cancer risk.

- *Fried foods.* In addition to increasing calories and fat content, fried foods also contain acrylamide, which can increase cancer risk. Acrylamide is not naturally found in these foods but is produced when potatoes and other starches are fried at high temperatures.

- *Alcohol.* Excess alcohol intake increases the risk of cancers of the mouth, throat, esophagus, breast, and colon. Alcohol abuse also severely damages the liver and other tissues in the body, which may predispose them to cancer development.

- *Vitamin D and calcium.* Some evidence suggests that low intakes of calcium and vitamin D may increase the risk of colorectal cancer. Calcium may bind free fatty acids and bile acids in the colon and prevent them from interacting with potential cancer cells. Vitamin D may inhibit the progression of cancer growth from malignant polyps in the colon.

Based on current knowledge of diet and cancer risk, the American Institute for Cancer Research has provided guidelines for reducing cancer risk (Table 15-8). Additional information can also be found on the following websites:

www.cancer.org (American Cancer Society)

www.aicr.org (American Institute for Cancer Research)

www.icic.nci.nih.gov (CancerNet)

www.cancer.med.upenn.edu (Oncolink)

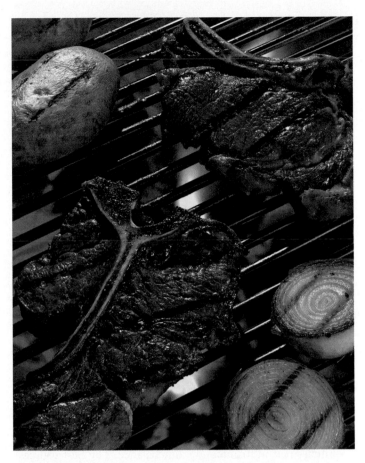

High intakes of grilled meats and seafood may increase the risk of some cancers.

Table 15-8 American Institute for Cancer Research Diet and Health Guidelines for Cancer Prevention

1. Choose a diet rich in a variety of plant-based foods.
2. Eat plenty of vegetables and fruits.
3. Maintain a healthy weight and be physically active.
4. Drink alcohol only in moderation, if at all.
5. Select foods low in fat and salt.
6. Prepare and store food safely.

And always remember . . . do not use tobacco in any form.

Summary

15.1 The absorption of iron depends on the body's need for iron and on the form of iron in food (heme vs. non-heme). Heme iron (from animal-based foods) is better absorbed than non-heme iron (primarily from plant-based foods). Liver, beef, and seafood are the best sources of dietary iron. The iron in plant foods is poorly absorbed. The body cannot readily excrete excess iron. Thus, the body regulates iron absorption and iron storage to maintain iron homeostasis. Iron is a critical component of hemoglobin, myoglobin, and many enzyme systems. Two-thirds of the body's iron is contained in hemoglobin, where it helps transport oxygen from the lungs to the tissues. In the early stages, iron deficiency does not result in obvious physical symptoms because iron stores can be mobilized to temporarily maintain many of iron's functions. As stores are depleted, iron deficiency anemia develops, causing fatigue, weakness, increased infection rate, delayed growth, and impaired brain development. Accidental iron overdose is the leading cause of poisoning in toddlers and young children. In adults, iron toxicity usually occurs from excess supplementation or from a genetic disorder, called hemochromatosis, that causes an overabsorption of iron.

15.2 Like iron, zinc absorption is affected by the need for the mineral and the amount in the diet. Absorption also plays a primary role in maintaining zinc balance. The best sources of zinc are oysters, meat, nuts, legumes, and whole grains. Zinc functions as a component of proteins and enzymes involved in stabilizing the structures of cell membrane proteins, reproduction, growth and development, immune function, and antioxidant defense (with copper as Cu/Zn SOD enzymes). Zinc deficiency causes impairments in taste, appetite, immune function, growth, sexual development, and reproduction. In many parts of the world, zinc deficiency (like iron deficiency) is still a serious public health concern. Zinc toxicity also is of concern in populations where zinc supplementation has become more common.

15.3 The best dietary sources of copper are liver, legumes, whole grains, and dark chocolate. Copper is involved in the mobilization of iron from body stores, in the cross-linking of proteins in connective tissue formation, and as a part of antioxidant defense. Although copper deficiency and toxicity are rare in humans, RDA and UL guidelines have been established to promote intakes within safe ranges.

15.4 Manganese is found in whole grains, nuts, legumes, and tea. Manganese functions in antioxidant defense and as a component of different metabolic enzymes. Manganese deficiency and toxicity rarely have been reported in humans.

15.5 Iodine is an essential part of the thyroid hormones thyroxine (T_4) and triiodothyronine (T_3) and thus plays a role in many metabolic and developmental functions in the body. The iodine content of the soil in which a plant was grown determines the iodine content of the plant food. The iodine content of most foods is low; thus, many populations obtain iodine from iodized salt. Iodination has eradicated endemic iodine deficiency in these areas. In countries where the iodination of salt, oil, or other food products is not available, iodine deficiency is a serious health concern. Iodine deficiency results in enlargement of the thyroid gland (goiter) and severe growth and mental impairment (cretinism).

15.6 Selenium acts as a cofactor for glutathione peroxidase, which prevents the oxidative destruction of cell membranes by hydrogen peroxide and free radicals. Selenium also aids in the conversion of the thyroid hormone T_4 to T_3. The selenium content of the soil in an area greatly affects the amount of selenium in the foods from that area. In general, meat, eggs, seafood, grains, and seeds are the best sources of selenium. In areas where the soil lacks selenium, deficiencies are more prevalent. Selenium deficiency increases the risk of Keshan disease and possibly of certain cancers. Because selenium has a narrower range of safety for intake than most other trace minerals, selenium supplementation can cause symptoms of toxicity at lower levels of intake.

15.7 The functions of chromium are not fully known. Chromium may enhance the action of insulin and promote the uptake of glucose into cells. Chromium is widely distributed in a variety of foods. Chromium deficiency and toxicity have not been well documented in humans.

15.8 Although fluoride is not truly classified as an essential trace mineral, it is beneficial in decreasing the incidence of dental caries. Most North Americans obtain fluoride from fluoridated drinking water, toothpaste, mouth rinses, and dental treatments. Excess fluoride causes discoloration of the teeth, known as enamel mottling or fluorosis.

15.9 The best dietary sources of molybdenum are legumes, grains, and nuts. Molybdenum is a component of several enzymes involved in nitrogen metabolism. Reports of molybdenum deficiency and toxicity are very rare. Boron, nickel, silicon, vanadium, and arsenic are classified as ultratrace minerals. Further research is needed to determine their functions in the body. Cancer is a disease that develops from uncontrolled replication of mutated cells. It begins by exposure to cancer-causing agents (carcinogens) such as tobacco, radiation, viruses, and certain dietary factors. Low intakes of fruits and vegetables, antioxidants, calcium, and vitamin D and excessive intakes of energy, red meats, fried foods, alcohol, and dietary fat have been associated with increased risk of cancer.

Study Questions

1. Trace mineral status often is difficult to evaluate due to the relatively small amounts of minerals contained in blood and tissues and the lack of sensitive measures that reflect body mineral content.

    a. true   b. false

2. Which of the following decreases iron absorption?

    a. increased need
    b. decreased intake
    c. meat protein factor
    d. phytic acid

3. Which of the following minerals is a component of hemoglobin and myoglobin?

    a. zinc
    b. copper
    c. iron
    d. manganese

4. Which of the following groups is at greatest risk of iron deficiency anemia?

    a. college students
    b. middle-aged males
    c. well-trained athletes
    d. adolescent girls

5. Accidental iron overdose is the leading cause of poisoning in young children.

    a. true   b. false

6. Which of the following is a good source of zinc?

    a. oysters
    b. blueberries
    c. low-fat yogurt
    d. lean bacon

7. Which of the following is a symptom of zinc deficiency?

    a. microcytic anemia
    b. poor growth
    c. goiter
    d. cardiomyopathy

8. Which of the following proteins/enzymes contains copper?

    a. glutathione peroxidase
    b. deiodinase
    c. thyroxine
    d. lysyl oxidase

9. Manganese is involved in the body's antioxidant defense network as a component of the enzyme manganese superoxide dismutase.

    a. true   b. false

10. Which of the following is a function of iodine?

    a. acts as a component of superoxide dismutase enzyme
    b. aids in thyroid hormone metabolism
    c. functions in antioxidant defense
    d. enhances insulin activity

11. Which of the following is associated with the development of cretinism?

    a. iron deficiency
    b. zinc deficiency
    c. iodine deficiency
    d. selenium deficiency

12. Selenium deficiency can cause impaired iodine metabolism.

    a. true   b. false

13. Which of the following helps protect against dental caries?

    a. iodine
    b. managanese
    c. fluoride
    d. chromium

14. Which of the following is *not* classified as an ultratrace mineral?

    a. arsenic
    b. boron
    c. iodine
    d. vanadium

15. Low intakes of calcium and vitamin D have been associated with increased risk of cancer.

    a. true   b. false

Answer Key: 1-a; 2-d; 3-c; 4-d; 5-a; 6-a; 7-b; 8-d; 9-a; 10-b; 11-c; 12-a; 13-c; 14-c; 15-a

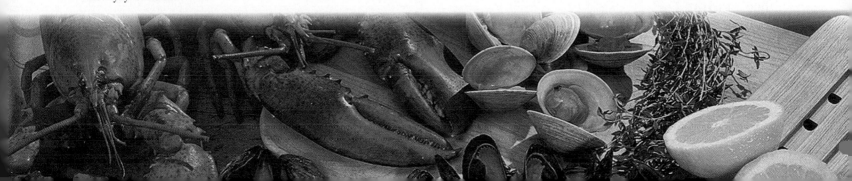

Websites

To learn more about the topics covered in this chapter, visit these websites.

Trace Minerals

www.eatright.org

www.ironoverload.org

www.healthfinder.org

Nutrient Composition

www.nal.usda.gov/fnic/foodcomp/search

Micronutrient Initiative

www.micronutrient.org/home.asp

Cancer

www.cancer.org

www.aicr.org

www.icic.nci.nih.gov

www.cancer.med.upenn.edu

References

1. Prasad AS. Zinc deficiency. *Br Med J.* 2003;326:409.

2. Hambidge KM. Biomarkers of trace mineral intake and status. *J Nutr.* 2003;133:948S.

3. Muller O, Krawinkel M. Malnutrition and health in developing countries. *Can Med Assoc J.* 2005;173:279.

4. Food and Nutrition Board, Institute of Medicine. *Dietary Reference Intakes for vitamin A, vitamin K, arsenic, boron, chromium, copper, iodine, iron, manganese, molybdenum, nickel, silicon, vanadium and zinc.* Washington, DC: National Academy Press; 2001.

5. Donovan A and others. The ins and outs of iron homeostasis. *Physiology.* 2005;21:115.

6. Souminen P and others. Single values of serum transferrin receptor and transferrin receptor ferritin index can be used to detect true and functional iron deficiency in rheumatoid arthritis patients with anemia. *Arthritis Rheum.* 2000;43:1016.

7. Neweth E, Ganz T. Regulation of iron metabolism by hepcidin. *Ann Rev Nutr.* 2006;26:323.

8. Beard JL. Iron biology in immune function, muscle metabolism and neuronal functioning. *J Nutr.* 2001;131:568.

9. Ekiz C and others. The effect of iron deficiency anemia on the function of the immune system. *Hematol J.* 2005;5:579.

10. Murray-Kolb LE, Beard JL. Iron treatment normalizes cognitive functioning in young women. *Am J Clin Nutr.* 2007;85:778.

11. Mason JB and others. *The micronutrient report:Current progress and trends in the control of vitamin A, iron, and iodine deficiencies.* Ottawa, Ontario: The Micronutrient Initiative; 2001.

12. ADA Reports. Position of the American Dietetic Association and Dietitians of Canada: Vegetarian diets. *J Am Diet Assoc.* 2003;103:748.

13. Franchini M, Veneri D. Hereditary hemochromatosis. *Hematology.* 2005;10:145.

14. Food Surveys Research Group. What we eat in America, NHANES 2001–2002. 2007; www.ars.usda.gov/foodsurvey.

15. Kang YJ. Metallothionein redox cycle and function. *Exp Biol Med.* 2006;231:1459.

16. Miller LV and others. Development of a compartmental model of human zinc metabolism: Identifiability and multiple studies analyses. *Am J Physiol Regul Integr Comp Physiol.* 2000;279:R1671.

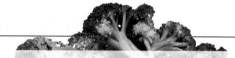

17. King JC, Cousins RJ. Zinc. In: Shils ME and others, eds. *Modern nutrition in health and disease.* 10th ed. Philadelphia: Lippincott Williams & Wilkins; 2006.

18. Turner RB, Citnarowski WE. Effect of treatment with zinc gluconate or zinc acetate on experimental and natural colds. *Clin Infect Dis.* 2000;31:1202.

19. Hambidge KM. Human zinc deficiency. *J Nutr.* 2000;130:S1344.

20. Wood RJ. Assessment of marginal zinc status in humans. *J Nutr.* 2000;130:S1350.

21. Grider A. Zinc, copper and manganese. In: Stipanuk MH, ed. *Biochemical, physiological, molecular aspects of human nutrition.* 2nd ed. St. Louis: Saunders; 2006.

22. Beshgetoor D, Hambidge KM. Clinical conditions altering copper metabolism in humans. *Am J Clin Nutr.* 1998;67:1007S.

23. Zatta P, Frank A. Copper deficiency and neurological disorders in man and animals. *Brain Res Rev.* 2007;54:19.

24. Freake HC. Iodine. In: Stipanuk MH, ed. *Biochemical, physiological, molecular aspects of human nutrition.* 2nd ed. St. Louis: Saunders; 2006.

25. Dunn JT, Delange F. Damaged reproduction: The most important consequence of iodine deficiency. *J Clin Endocrinol Metab.* 2001;86:2360.

26. World Health Organization. Micronutrient deficiencies: Iodine deficiency disorders. 2008; www.who.int/nutrition/topics/idd/.

27. Zimmerman MB. Assessing iodine status and monitoring progress of iodized salt programs. *J Nutr.* 2004;134:1673.

28. Teng W and others. Effect of iodine intake on thyroid diseases in China. *N Engl J Med.* 2006;354:2783.

29. Papp LV and others. From selenium to selenoproteins: Synthesis, identity and their role in human health. *Antioxid Redox Signal.* 2007;9:775.

30. Finley JW. Selenium accumulation in plant foods. *Nutr Rev.* 2005;63:196.

31. Food and Nutrition Board, Institute of Medicine. *Dietary Reference Intakes for vitamin C, vitamin E, selenium and carotenoids.* Washington, DC: National Academy Press; 2000.

32. Combs G. Current evidence and research needs to support a health claim for selenium and cancer prevention. *J Nutr.* 2005;135:343.

33. Vogt TM and others. Racial differences in serum selenium concentration: Analysis of US population data from NHANES III. *Am J Epidemiol.* 2007;166:280.

34. Althuis MD and others. Glucose and insulin responses to dietary chromium supplements: A meta-analysis. *Am J Clin Nutr.* 2002;76:148.

35. Kleefstra N and others. Chromium treatment has no effect in patients with type 2 diabetes in a Western population: A randomized, double-blind, placebo-controlled trial. *Diabetes Care.* 2007;30:1092.

36. ADA Reports. Position of the American Dietetic Association: The impact of fluoride on health. *J Am Diet Assoc.* 2005;105:1620.

37. Food and Nutrition Board, Institute of Medicine. *Dietary Reference Intakes for calcium, phosphorus, magnesium, vitamin D and fluoride.* Washington, DC: National Academy Press; 1997.

38. Chao A and others. Meat consumption and risk of colorectal cancer. *JAMA.* 2005;293:172.

39. Pan MH and others. Food bioactives, apoptosis, and cancer. *Mol Nutr Food Res.* 2008;52:43.

40. Meyerhardt JA and others. Association of dietary patterns with cancer recurrence and survival in patients with stage III colon cancer. *JAMA.* 2007;298:754.

41. Campbell and others. Dietary patterns and risk of incident gastric adenocarcinoma. *Am J Epidemiol.* 2008;167:295.

42. Stacewicz-Sapuntzakis M and others. Correlations of dietary patterns with prostate health. *Mol Nutr Food Res.* 2008;52:114.

43. Pierce JP and others. Influence of a diet very high in vegetables, fruit and fiber, and low in fat on prognosis following treatment for breast cancer. *JAMA.* 2007;298:289.

44. Travis RC and others. A prospective study of vegetarianism and isoflavone intake in relation to breast cancer risk in British women. *Int J Cancer.* 2008;122:705.

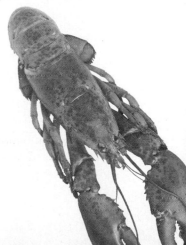

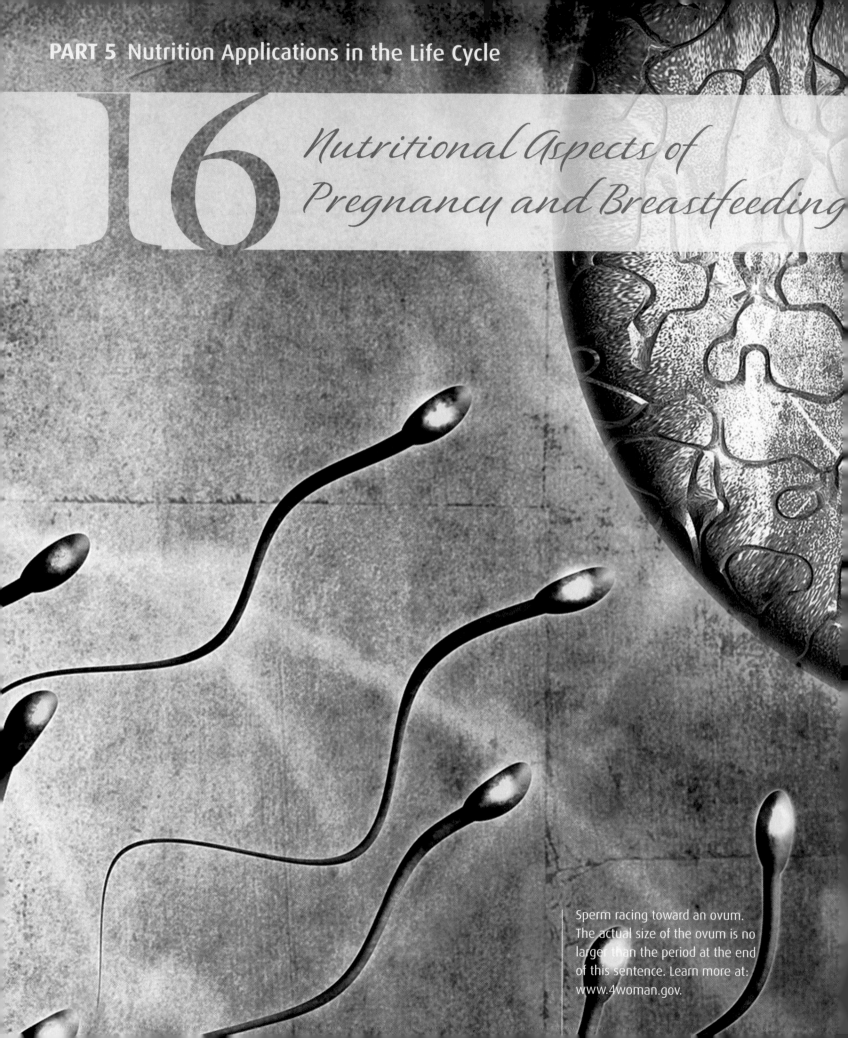

16

Nutritional Aspects of Pregnancy and Breastfeeding

Sperm racing toward an ovum. The actual size of the ovum is no larger than the period at the end of this sentence. Learn more at: www.4woman.gov.

STUDENT LEARNING OUTCOMES

After studying this chapter, you will be able to:

1. Describe factors that predict a successful pregnancy outcome.

2. List major physiological changes that occur in the body during pregnancy and describe how nutrient needs are altered.

3. Specify the optimal weight gain during pregnancy for adult women.

4. Describe the special nutritional needs of pregnant and lactating women, summarize factors that put them at risk for nutrient deficiencies, and plan a nutritious diet for them.

5. Identify nutrients that often need to be supplemented during pregnancy and lactation and explain the reason for each.

6. Discuss potential nutrition-related problems that occur during pregnancy and suggest techniques for coping with these problems.

7. List substances and practices to avoid during pregnancy and lactation and describe why they are harmful.

8. Describe the physiological process of breastfeeding.

Pregnancy is a very special time. Parents-to-be often feel a strong desire to produce a healthy baby, which can arouse new interest in nutrition and health information. Most want to do everything possible to maximize their chances of having a robust, lively newborn. Ideally, women begin improving their health and nutrient intake (especially folic acid) as well as eliminating potentially harmful habits long before becoming pregnant.

Despite these intentions, the number of infants who die in North America is higher than in many other industrialized nations. In Canada, about 4.7 of every 1000 infants per year die before their first birthday and, in the U.S., the rate is 6.4. Comparing these numbers with Sweden, which has a rate of about 2.8 of every 1000 infants, indicates there is room for improvement.

Although some genetic and environmental factors that affect fetal and newborn health are beyond her control,[1] a woman's conscious decisions about health and nutrition can significantly affect both her own and her baby's lifelong health.[2] This chapter will examine how a woman who eats nutritiously before and during pregnancy and while breastfeeding can help her baby have a healthy start in life.

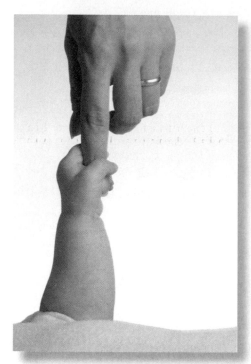

The time to begin thinking about prenatal nutrition is before becoming pregnant. This includes making sure folic acid intake is adequate (400 μg of synthetic folic acid per day) and that any supplemental use of preformed vitamin A does not exceed 100% of the Daily Value.

▶ In the U.S., 7% of births are low birth weight babies—many of these are from multiple births. Most are premature and a third experience prenatal growth retardation.

▶ A goal of *Healthy People 2010* is to reduce low birth weight and preterm births by one-third.

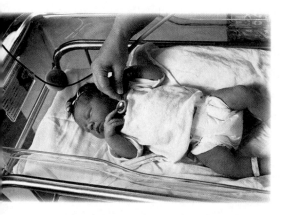

A healthy full-term newborn usually weighs about 7.5 pounds and is 20 inches long.

🍑 16.1 Pregnancy

Pregnancy, or **gestation,** may be the most sensitive stage of the life cycle—nutrient and calorie supplies at this time impact the final outcome.[3] To help ensure the optimal health of both the mother and her offspring, adequate nutrition is vital both before and during pregnancy. Researchers often define a **favorable pregnancy outcome** as a full-term gestation period (longer than 37 weeks) that results in a live, healthy infant weighing more than 5.5 pounds (2.5 kg)[1, 3] and permits the mother to return to her prepregnancy health status.

An infant's chances of survival depend greatly on both gestation length and birth weight.[3] The closer the gestation period comes to full-term, the greater the physical maturation and birth weight. Many **preterm** (born before 37 weeks) infants have numerous medical problems, including those that complicate nutritional care, such as poor sucking and swallowing abilities and **low birth weight** (weighing less than 5.5 pounds, or 2500 grams). A healthy full-term newborn usually weighs about 7.5 lb. Low birth weight babies are 40 times more likely to die during the first 4 weeks of life than a heavier infant. Those who survive are more likely to be ill and handicapped than heavier babies.

Suboptimal maternal nutrient and calorie intakes are linked with low birth weights. Although low birth weight is most commonly associated with being born preterm, infants who suffer prenatal growth retardation weigh less than expected for their gestational age—these infants are **small for gestational age**. Thus, a full-term infant weighing less than 5.5 lb at birth is small for gestational age. In contrast, a preterm infant is almost always low birth weight but may not be small for gestational age.

Low birth weight infants are more likely than normal weight infants to have medical and nutritional complications, including problems with blood glucose control, temperature regulation, growth, and development in the early weeks after birth. These babies also are at risk of developing more body fat and less lean body mass in childhood, thereby increasing their risk of chronic disease in adulthood.[4] The long-term consequences of prenatal growth retardation are much more profound than previously imagined—sometimes fetal health is harmed to the extent that its own future offspring also will be affected.[5] By eating a nutritious diet, pregnant women promote adequate growth and development throughout gestation and help ensure that the baby is born healthy, on time, and with the mental, physical, and physiological capabilities to grow and develop normally. A nutritious diet also helps protect the mother's health.

Prenatal Developmental Stages: Conception, Zygotic, Embryonic, and Fetal

The first stage of gestation begins at conception, when a sperm unites with an egg **(ovum)** (Fig. 16-1). About 30 hours after conception, the **zygote,** as the fertilized egg is called, begins the lifelong process of cell division. This cluster of cells drifts down the fallopian tube to the woman's uterus and, within a week after conception, it has nestled deeply into the uterine lining and firmly attached itself there. The second stage begins 2 weeks after conception; the zygote is now called an **embryo.**

When the embryonic stage begins, the cells have already separated into a stack of 3 thin layers (Fig. 16-2). One layer of cells, called the endoderm, will develop into the digestive system, liver, and pancreas. Another layer, the mesoderm, provides the cells targeted to become the skeleton, muscles, heart, and blood vessels. From the last cell layer, the ectoderm, will come the skin, nervous system, and sensory organs. When this stage ends after week 8, the embryo is quite complex, yet it is no larger than a pea (approximately 3/8 inch, or 8 mm, long). The major organs are in place and some, such as the heart and liver, have begun to function.

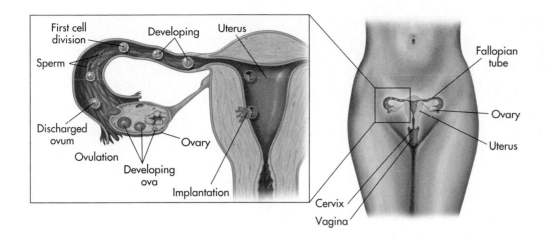

Figure 16-1 After release from an ovary (ovulation), the ovum enters the abdominal cavity and finds its way into the fallopian tube. Receptor molecules on the ovum surface attract and "trap" sperm cells "swimming" up the fallopian tube. As soon as 1 sperm enters the ovum, complex mechanisms in the egg are activated to block the entry of another sperm. The 23 chromosomes from the sperm combine with the 23 chromosomes already in the ovum to make up the 46 chromosomes of the developing offspring.

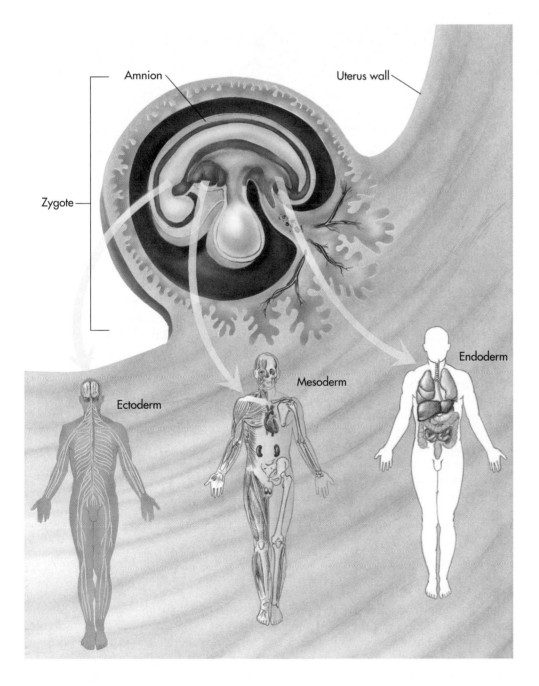

Figure 16-2 The body systems that develop from the zygote's 3 cell layers.

Figure 16-3 Body proportions change significantly during fetal development and continue until adulthood.

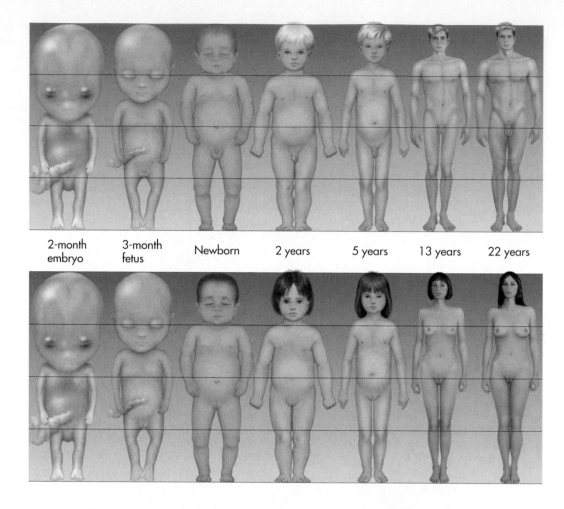

| 2-month embryo | 3-month fetus | Newborn | 2 years | 5 years | 13 years | 22 years |

After the eighth week until birth, the developing offspring is known as a **fetus.** The fetal stage is when the most rapid growth occurs. In fact, about 90% of all fetal growth occurs in the last 20 weeks of gestation. During the fetal stage, length increases 20 times or more to an average of 20 to 22 inches (51–56 cm). Weight skyrockets, increasing about 3500 times, to an average weight of 7 to 8 pounds (3.2–3.6 kg). Body proportions change rapidly, too. When this stage begins, the head and the body are nearly the same size (Fig. 16-3). Between 21 and 30 weeks, body proportions shift to be similar to those of newborn infants, although the fetus is still quite slim and has loose, baggy skin. Body fat rises from less than 1% at 20 weeks to 16% by 38 weeks. The stored subcutaneous fat smoothes and tightens the skin and, most importantly, insulates the body. Infants born prematurely have difficulty regulating body temperature, which greatly affects their nutrient and calorie needs.

Premature infants also are at risk of nutrient deficiencies because nutrient stores do not accumulate appreciably until the last 4 to 6 weeks of gestation. By 38 to 40 weeks, a healthy fetus has built substantial nutrient stores and developed sufficiently to thrive outside the uterus.

Critical Periods

For purposes of discussion, pregnancy is often divided into 3 periods called **trimesters.** Figure 16-4 describes the major developmental milestones of gestation during each trimester. This complicated developmental process must occur precisely on schedule. That is, there is a finite window of opportunity, called a **critical period,** for cells to develop into a particular tissue or organ. As you can see, most critical periods occur during the first trimester. For instance, critical heart development occurs during the third to sixth weeks. Critical tooth development happens during the sixth to eighth weeks of gestation. Nutrient deficiencies or exposure to nutrient excesses, certain pathogens, trauma,

trimester Three 13- to 14-week periods into which the normal pregnancy is somewhat arbitrarily divided for purposes of discussion and analysis (the length of a normal pregnancy is about 40 weeks, measured from the first day of the woman's last menstrual period).

radiation, tobacco smoke, and toxins (e.g., drugs and alcohol) during a critical period can interfere with normal development, causing effects ranging from severe physical or mental abnormalities to **spontaneous abortion** (a naturally occurring premature termination of a pregnancy prior to 20 weeks of gestation)[6] (Table 16-1). Early spontaneous abortions, also called miscarriages, usually result from a genetic defect or fatal error in fetal development. About half or more of all pregnancies end in this way, often so early that a woman does not realize she was pregnant. An additional 15 to 20% are lost before normal delivery.

Although the greatest risk is in the first trimester, a detrimental prenatal environment during the fetal stage also can adversely affect development; however, the damage often has less catastrophic consequences. Nonetheless, maternal nutrient deficiencies or exposure to toxins can cause low nutrient stores, retarded growth, abnormal organ function, mental abnormalities, and/or a shorter than normal gestation period. Often, nutrient deficits during fetal life can be partly reversed by adequate nutrition after birth.

> ### CRITICAL THINKING
>
> Alexandra wants to have a baby. She has read that it is very important for women to be healthy during pregnancy. However, Jane, her sister, tells her that the time to begin to assess her nutritional and health status is before she becomes pregnant. What additional information should Jane give Alexandra?

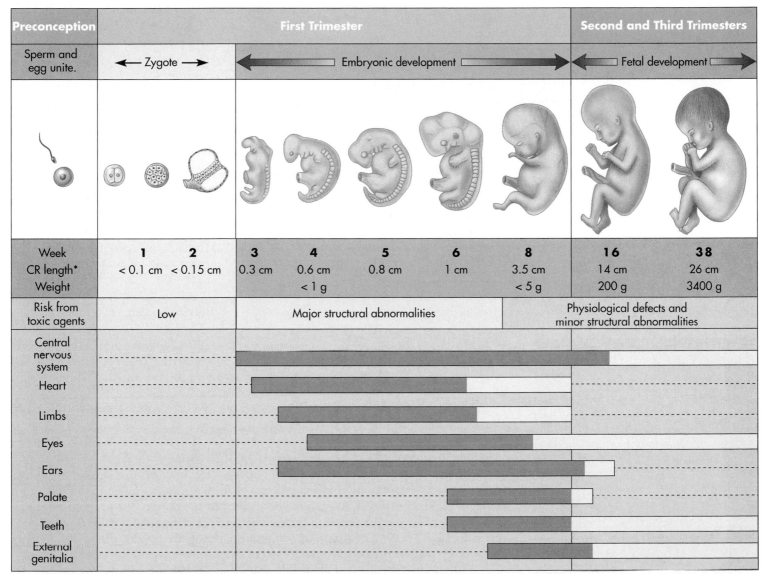

*Body length is customarily expressed as crown-to-rump length (CRL), which is measured from the crown of the head to the curve of the buttocks and does not include the lower limbs. Recall that 2.54 cm = 1 in.

Figure 16-4 Critical periods of development are indicated with orange bars. The orange shading indicates when the effects of malnutrition and/or exposure to toxins, such as alcohol and drugs, are likely to be most severe. As the white bars in the chart show, however, damage to the eyes, brain, and genitals also can occur during the last months of pregnancy.

Table 16-1 Potential Effects of Maternal Calorie and Nutrient Deficiencies and Excesses on Developing Offspring

Food Component	Potential Effect of a Deficiency	Potential Effect of an Excess
Calories	Growth retardation Low birth weight	High birth weight Complications during labor and delivery
Protein	Reduced head circumference Fewer cells than normal, impact particularly severe in the brain	If high consumption is coupled with low carbohydrate intake, may lower glucose availability and restrict energy available to the fetus
Vitamin C	Premature birth	Sudden drop in vitamin C after birth may cause vitamin C deficiency symptoms
Folate	Spontaneous abortion Fluid accumulation in the skull, leading to brain damage Growth retardation Premature birth Neural tube defects	May inhibit maternal absorption of other nutrients Hinders diagnosis of maternal vitamin B-12 deficiency
Vitamin A	Premature birth Eye abnormalities and impaired vision Maternal death	Birth defects that affect the nervous and cardiovascular systems Facial deformities
Vitamin D	Low birth weight Rickets Lack of enamel on teeth	Calcification of soft tissues, such as the kidneys Mental retardation Growth retardation
Calcium	Decreased bone density	May hinder maternal absorption of minerals, such as iron and zinc
Iron	Low birth weight Premature birth Increased risk of fetal or infant death	May hinder maternal absorption of minerals, such as zinc and calcium
Iodine	Cretinism (mental and physical growth retardation)	Thyroid disorders
Zinc	Nervous system malformations Growth retardation Birth defects that affect the brain and bones	May hinder maternal absorption of minerals, such as copper and iron

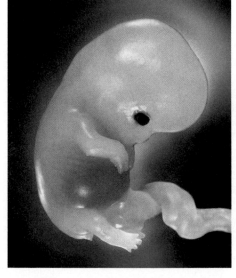

The umbilical cord is the pipeline that delivers nutrients and oxygen to and removes waste from the developing offspring.

Nourishing the Zygote, Embryo, and Fetus

A zygote nourishes itself by absorbing secretions from glands in the uterus and digesting some of the uterine lining. As a zygote develops into an embryo, the placenta begins to form inside the mother's uterus. The placenta takes over the role of delivering nourishment to the developing organism throughout the remainder of pregnancy. The placenta is a spongy, pancake-shaped, temporary organ that taps into the mother's blood supply.

The umbilical cord is the pipeline that connects the placenta to the fetus. Fetal blood travels from the fetal heart to the placenta by way of 2 umbilical arteries and returns (nutrient-enriched and waste-free) to the fetus by means of 1 umbilical vein. As shown in Figure 16-5, the placenta contains both maternal and fetal blood vessels. Although these vessels are not directly connected, they are so close together that nutrients and oxygen pass easily from the mother to the fetus, and fetal wastes are shuttled

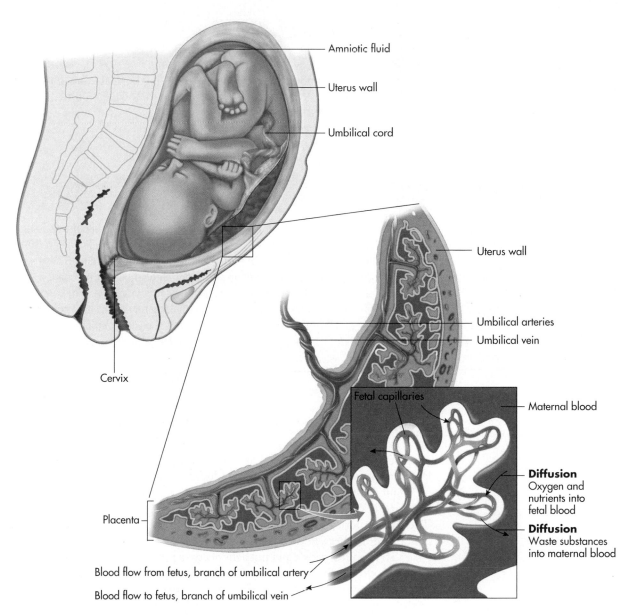

Figure 16-5 The placenta is the organ through which nourishment flows to the fetus. The inset shows how the blood circulatory systems of the mother and fetus work together to provide the fetus with oxygen and nutrients while removing fetal waste products.

from the fetus to the mother for excretion. To accomplish these tasks, the placenta uses all the absorption mechanisms employed by the GI tract (see Chapter 4). The placenta also synthesizes fatty acids, cholesterol, and the fetus's main fuel—glycogen. In addition, the placenta produces hormones that help direct maternal nutrients to the fetus, control fetal metabolism, promote the changes in the mother's body that support pregnancy, and cause nausea.[7, 8]

The placenta grows throughout pregnancy to keep up with the increasing demands of the developing fetus. At birth, a healthy placenta weighs about 1.5 lb (0.7 kg) and is about 6 to 8 inches in diameter and 1 inch thick. It has about 13 square meters of contact between maternal and fetal circulation.

The placenta's size and ability to support optimal fetal growth depend on the mother's nutritional status. Poorly nourished women tend to have smaller placentas with fewer blood vessels and smaller cells than those of well-nourished mothers. If the placenta is smaller than normal, the area of contact between the mother and fetus is reduced, which decreases the placenta's capacity to deliver nutrients and remove wastes. Small placentas may hinder optimal fetal growth and development.

▶ The 13 square meters that exists between maternal and fetal circulation is equal to the sleeping area of 3 king-size beds.

CASE STUDY

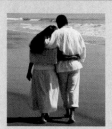

Tracey and her husband have decided that they are ready to have a child. Tracey has been reading everything she can find on pregnancy because she knows that her prepregnancy health is important to the success of her pregnancy. She has just turned 25 and avoids alcohol, does not smoke, does not take any medications, and limits her coffee intake to 4 cups a day and her soft drink intake to 3 colas per day. She has decided to breastfeed her infant and has already inquired about childbirth classes. She has modified her diet to include some extra protein, along with more fruits and vegetables. Recently, she started swimming 5 days a week and plans to continue swimming throughout her pregnancy. She also has started taking an over-the-counter vitamin and mineral supplement. Tracey and her husband think that they have covered all the key areas of prepregnancy care. List a few positive attributes of her current practices. What are some potential problem areas and information they may have missed?

 ## 16.2 Nutrient Needs of Pregnant Women

Pregnancy is one of the most nutritionally demanding stages of the life cycle.[9] In just 9 months or so, a mother's body provides all the calories and nutrients needed to produce an infant 5000 times larger than the fertilized egg. To accomplish this, a pregnant woman needs additional calories and more of almost every nutrient than a non-pregnant woman. The extra calories and nutrients support the growth and development of the fetus, placenta, and mother's body, as well as increased maternal metabolism.

To meet her calorie and nutrient needs, a pregnant woman should eat more nutrient-dense food. Metabolic adjustments that allow pregnant women to use some nutrients more efficiently (e.g., protein), absorb some better (e.g., calcium, iron), and/or excrete less of others (e.g., zinc, riboflavin) also help meet the calorie and nutrient demands of pregnancy. Sufficient quantities of calories and all nutrients are needed for a favorable pregnancy outcome; however, only calories and the nutrients of particular importance during pregnancy are discussed in this chapter.

Energy Needs

A pregnant woman needs extra calories to support the growth of her own tissues, as well as those of the fetus. Additional calories also are needed to fuel the extra metabolic workload pregnancy puts on a woman's heart, lungs, and other organs. Few, if any, of these extra calories are needed during the first trimester of pregnancy, when the developing offspring gains little weight. During the second trimester, a daily increase of about 350 calories is recommended. And, in the third trimester, a daily increase of approximately 450 calories is recommended.[10] Women who begin pregnancy overweight or obese should aim for a somewhat smaller increase in calories. Those who are in their teens, underweight, or physically active likely will need more calories. In fact, underweight women who increase their energy intake are more likely to give birth to healthier babies and experience fewer infant deaths than those who do not increase energy intake. Women who are physically active during pregnancy may need to increase their intake by more than 350 to 450 calories because greater body weight requires more energy for activity.

Infants born to women who consumed insufficient calories are small and more likely to die soon after birth. Those who survive are likely to experience severe, lifelong consequences. There is substantial evidence that individuals who suffered calorie restrictions during fetal life develop the capacity to use calories in a "thrifty" manner. That is, throughout their lives they need fewer calories to maintain their bodies and support physical activity. Although this thrifty calorie usage promotes survival when the food supply is restricted, it elevates the risk of obesity and type 2 diabetes when food is abundant. Infants who are born small also have a greater risk of developing heart disease, high blood cholesterol levels, diabetes, and high blood pressure and experiencing impaired immune function.

Recall that the mineral iodine is used to make thyroid hormone (the primary energy use regulator). Sufficient iodine is needed during pregnancy to ensure that adequate amounts of thyroid hormone are produced. Using iodized salt can easily meet the need for this mineral. As you learned in Chapter 15, iodine deficiency during pregnancy can lead to severe birth defects.

Nutrients Needed for Building New Cells

Cells grow and develop at a rapid rate during fetal life. Over the course of gestation, a single cell zygote will divide millions of times, creating trillions of cells. Although every nutrient plays an important role in manufacturing these new cells, the roles of protein, essential fatty acids, zinc, folate, vitamin B-12, and iron are especially noteworthy during pregnancy.

Protein intake recommendations for pregnant women are more than 50% above that of non-pregnant women. Even with this substantial increase, insufficient intakes of protein are uncommon in the U.S. and Canada because this nutrient is so plentiful that women, pregnant or not, consume amounts exceeding the RDA. Protein supplements are neither needed nor recommended during pregnancy.

Essential fatty acids are required for normal fetal growth and development, particularly of the brain and eyes. Sufficient intakes, especially of the omega-3 fat docosahexaenoic acid (DHA), may improve gestation duration and infant birth weight, length, and head circumference. Many women need to increase the amount of omega-3 fats in comparison to the amount of omega-6 fats they consume. In addition, they should minimize their *trans* fatty acid intake during pregnancy.

Zinc intake by both pregnant and non-pregnant women often is less than the RDA; however, deficiencies are uncommon. Severe zinc deficiency may cause birth defects, fetal growth retardation, premature birth, and spontaneous abortion.[11, 12] Pregnant women may experience prolonged labor, bleeding, infections, and serious complications, such as pregnancy-induced hypertension and preeclampsia, discussed later in this chapter. Those who eat zinc-poor diets and have a high fiber or iron intake (which impairs zinc absorption), need to pay particular attention to zinc intake. Certain medications, cigarette smoking, alcohol abuse, and strenuous exercise may prevent the placenta from transferring adequate zinc to the fetus.

Folate and vitamin B-12 are critical for the synthesis of DNA and fetal and maternal cells. For instance, red blood cell formation, which requires folate, increases during pregnancy. When folate intake is insufficient, fewer red blood cells are synthesized, causing folate-related anemia. Insufficient folate intake also may cause premature birth, low birth weight, fetal growth retardation, spontaneous abortion, poor placenta development, and other pregnancy complications.

Folate deficiencies in the very early stages of pregnancy also can cause neural tube defects (see Chapter 13). The neural tube is tissue that develops into the brain and spinal cord (Fig. 16-6). It starts as a shallow groove running down the back of the embryo that, at 28 days of gestation, folds in on itself to create a tube. If it fails to close at the top, the brain will not develop fully and death occurs soon after birth. The spine is incompletely formed when the tube does not seal at the bottom, causing spina bifida. Depending on the severity of spina bifida, children may be paralyzed or have curvature of the spine, dislocated hips, or other physical handicaps. There is some evidence that poor folate status also may play a role in the development of heart defects, Down syndrome, and other birth defects.[1]

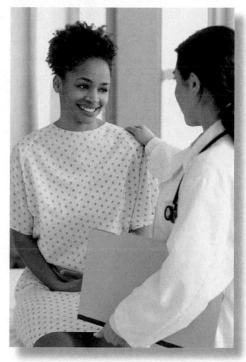

To ensure optimal health and rapid treatment of medical conditions that develop during pregnancy, a pregnant woman should consult with her health-care provider on a regular basis. Ideally, this consultation should begin before she becomes pregnant.

▶ A goal of *Healthy People 2010* is to increase to 80% the number of pregnancies that begin with optimal folate status in an effort to reduce the occurrence of neural tube defects.

▶ Heart defects affect 1 in 110 newborns and account for a third or more of infant deaths due to birth defects, more than for any other congenital anomaly. Taking multivitamins containing folic acid during early pregnancy is associated with a significant reduction in risk of heart defects.

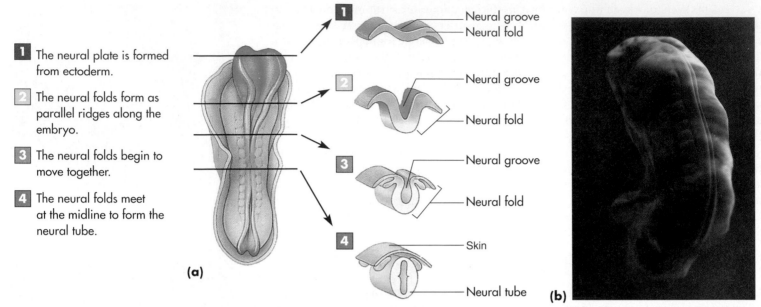

1 | The neural plate is formed from ectoderm.

2 | The neural folds form as parallel ridges along the embryo.

3 | The neural folds begin to move together.

4 | The neural folds meet at the midline to form the neural tube.

(a)

1 — Neural groove, Neural fold

2 — Neural groove, Neural fold

3 — Neural groove, Neural fold

4 — Skin, Neural tube

(b)

Figure 16-6 (*a*) The formation of the neural tube. (*b*) The neural tube of a 23-day-old embryo that is beginning to fuse.

▶ Women who have previously given birth to an infant with a neural tube defect, such as spina bifida, should consult their physicians about the need for folic acid supplementation. A daily intake of 4 mg of synthetic folic acid at least 1 month prior to conception is recommended, but it must be taken under a physician's supervision.

Folic acid, the synthetic form of folate used in supplements and fortified foods, can prevent half or more of all neural tube defects. Folic acid is absorbed almost twice as well as the folate that naturally occurs in foods. Thus, experts recommend that all women who have the potential to become pregnant take folate supplements or eat folate-fortified foods in addition to eating a folate-rich diet. This recommendation extends to all these women because a significant proportion of pregnancies are unplanned and neural tube defects occur in the first month of pregnancy—before many realize they are pregnant. Women who have previously delivered an infant with a neural tube defect may need to consume more folate than the RDA. However, before exceeding the Upper Level of folate, women should consult a health-care provider because large doses of folate can make it difficult to diagnose a vitamin B-12 deficiency.

Insufficient intake of vitamin B-12 also may contribute to the development of neural tube defects. Women who eat animal products usually consume sufficient amounts of vitamin B-12; however, vegans will need a vitamin B-12 supplement.

Prior to 1998, when the FDA began requiring folate fortification of grains and cereals, only 10% of women met the folate RDA. Almost 1 in every 1000 babies born in the U.S. had a neural tube defect. Since folate fortification began, the number of babies born with neural tube defects has declined by 17%.[13]

Iron needs rise significantly during pregnancy, mainly because of the increasing number of maternal red blood cells and accumulating fetal iron stores. The increased demand for iron puts many pregnant women at a greater risk of iron deficiency anemia than individuals in any other stage of the life cycle. Iron stored prior to pregnancy can supply some of the extra iron; however, most women enter pregnancy with poor iron stores. To help meet iron demands, maternal iron absorption increases up to 3 times and this mineral is conserved because menstruation stops during pregnancy. Even with these adaptations and a carefully planned diet, it is very difficult to meet the need for iron.

Many experts recommend that pregnant women take a low-dose iron supplement (30 mg/daily). However, because iron can interfere with zinc and copper absorption and utilization, women taking iron supplements also may need a zinc and copper supplement.[3] Iron supplements can decrease appetite and cause nausea and constipation; taking them between meals or just before going to bed can minimize these problems. Coffee or tea should not be consumed with an iron supplement because these beverages contain substances that interfere with iron absorption. Eating foods rich in vitamin C along with iron supplements or foods that contain heme iron helps boost iron absorption.

Recall that individuals with iron deficiency anemia have fewer red blood cells than normal; consequently, they have a reduced capacity to deliver oxygen to their body cells. In pregnancy, iron deficiency anemia means that less than optimal amounts of oxygen may reach the fetus. Iron deficiency anemia causes low birth weight, premature birth, and infant death, and it may result in low iron stores in the infant. In addition, pregnant women with this condition may experience preeclampsia, labor and delivery complications, and an increased risk of death.[1]

Iron deficiency anemia, which is a dangerous condition, should not be confused with a normal change called the anemia of pregnancy. During pregnancy, the number of maternal red blood cells increases 20 to 30%, but the liquid portion of the blood (plasma) expands 50%. Thus, there is a lower ratio of red blood cells to total blood volume. This hemodilution, known as **physiological anemia,** is a common, expected condition during pregnancy and does not pose a danger to the health of the mother or the fetus.

Nutrients Needed for Bone and Tooth Development

The fetus needs large quantities of vitamin D, calcium, phosphorus, magnesium, and fluoride for normal bone and tooth development. Of these, calcium and vitamin D need particular attention.

Even though a full-term fetus stores about 30,000 mg of calcium, the recommended intake of this mineral does not rise during pregnancy. That's because, early in pregnancy, the mother's body adjusts to absorb calcium much more efficiently. The calcium is stockpiled in her bones, to be drawn on during late pregnancy and lactation.[14] However, many women, pregnant or not, fail to consume the AI for calcium, putting themselves at increased risk of osteoporosis later in life. Too little vitamin D may cause mothers to develop the vitamin D deficiency disease osteomalacia and their fetuses to develop rickets, to grow poorly, and to inadequately calcify bones and teeth.

Vegans, pregnant teens, women at risk of pregnancy-induced hypertension, and those who do not consume dairy products are at risk of consuming insufficient calcium. Those who do not consume milk, which is fortified with vitamin D, or have limited exposure to sunlight also risk getting too little vitamin D. These women should choose foods fortified with calcium and vitamin D and discuss using a supplement with their healthcare providers. A vitamin D supplement is particularly important during the winter in northern latitudes (see Chapter 12).

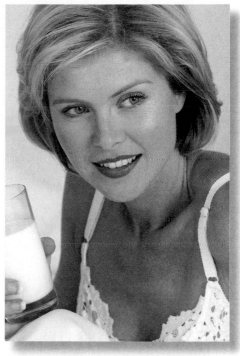

Milk and other dairy products supply the calcium pregnant women need to support optimal fetal development as well as protect their own bones.

Pregnant Women Do Not Have an Instinctive Drive to Consume More Nutrients

It is a common myth that women instinctively know what to eat during pregnancy and that, by responding to "cravings," they get the nutrients they need. Many women report craving some foods or beverages during pregnancy. Cravings range from the unusual (clay and rubber bands) to the ordinary (ice cream, pickles, and chocolate). In addition to cravings, many pregnant women experience aversions to certain odors and flavors, such as alcohol, eggs, coffee, fried foods, meat, and tomato sauce. The cause of cravings and aversions remains a mystery; they may be related to hormonal changes in the mother or family traditions. There is no evidence that cravings and aversions are the result of nutrient deficiencies.

The desire to eat or avoid certain foods or combinations of foods won't affect a woman's health as long as her overall diet provides adequate nutrients and calories. To cope with strong cravings for ordinary food items, a pregnant woman should eat small amounts of the desired food along with regular meals or snacks. When craved foods dominate the diet to the extent that variety is limited or when aversions severely inhibit food intake, malnutrition may occur.

Some women also practice **pica,** the eating of non-food substances, such as laundry starch, coal, clay, and tire inner tubes, over a sustained period of time. Abnormal cravings for certain food items, such as baking soda and cornstarch, also are

Expert Perspective *from the Field*

Grains and Folic Acid Fortification

Early in the 1990s, several research groups published studies showing that women who took folic acid supplements both before becoming pregnant and during their pregnancies were less likely to have babies affected by neural tube defects. Careful consideration of this research led to the 1992 recommendation by the Public Health Service that all women of childbearing age consume 400 µg of folic acid daily to reduce their risk of having a pregnancy affected by a neural tube defect. The most common neural tube defects are spina bifida and anencephaly (see Chapter 13).

Although it's not yet known exactly how folic acid protects against neural tube defects, developing neural tissue has a high need for folate. In this tissue, folate is required for DNA synthesis, cell division, and the normal transformation of amino acids into components that form neural tissue. In addition, folate helps coordinate cell differentiation. Research suggests that, when folate intake is low, neural tissue does not develop normally and neural tube defects may occur. An insufficient supply of folate may be the result of a low dietary intake; some women have a genetically determined inefficient use of folic acid and thus have an increased need for this vitamin.

Many women consume insufficient amounts of folate-rich foods (e.g., spinach and turnip greens, dried beans and peas, avocados, bananas, and asparagus) and do not meet the RDA. In response to this shortfall, in 1998 the FDA mandated that enriched grains be fortified with folic acid. According to Judi Adams,* at the fortification level required, 2 slices of bread provide over 10% of the RDA. Because whole grains are not fortified, they provide less than 5% of the daily folic acid RDA. Breakfast cereals are the only food permitted to be fortified with 100% of the folate RDA (i.e., 400 µg) per serving. Few women are aware that enriched grain products are good sources of folic acid.

Adams notes that, although the Dietary Guidelines for Americans recommend consuming at least half of the recommended grain servings as whole grains, enriched cereals and grains can contribute significantly more folic acid to the diet. By including both whole-grain and enriched grains in their diets at the levels recommended by MyPyramid, women can obtain substantial amounts of folate. To ensure sufficient folic acid for neural tube defect reduction, the

March of Dimes Birth Defects Foundation also recommends that all women of childbearing years exceed the RDA of 400 µg folic acid per day by eating a folate-rich diet and taking a multivitamin supplement that supplies 400 µg folic acid. However, less than half of women take a daily folic acid supplement.

Since the fortification of grains with folic acid began, neural tube defects have declined, sparing 1000 babies per year from a neural tube defect. (This decline cannot, however, be attributed entirely to folic acid fortification.) Despite this improvement, there are still about 3000 babies born in the U.S. each year with a neural tube defect. In some regions of the country (e.g., the Southeast) and among some racial groups (e.g., Hispanics), rates of neural tube defects are higher than average. According to Adams, these groups may not be benefiting fully from folic acid enrichment of grains. For example, grits, which are made from corn, are popular in the southeastern U.S. and usually are not fortified with folic acid. Likewise, corn tortillas are not always fortified with folic acid. Adams also notes that specialty grains, such as amaranth and quinoa which are served as whole-grains, are not enriched.

Reading ingredient labels and Nutrition Facts panels is the only way to know if a grain product has been fortified with folic acid. It is especially important for women who follow gluten-free diets (and therefore do not consume wheat) to check grain labels for fortification.

To learn more about folic acid and neural tube defects, visit www.marchofdimes.com. To learn more about the Folic Acid for a Healthy Pregnancy campaign and the seal that identifies grain products fortified with folic acid, go to www.grainpower.org.

Judi Adams, MS, RD, President, Grain Foods Foundation (www.grainpower.org). Ms. Adams has been with the Grain Foods Foundation since 2004. Her previous work in nutrition education, spanning a period of 35 years included positions with the North Dakota State University Extension Service, North Dakota Wheat Commission, National Sunflower Association, and Wheat Foods Council. She also served as the Director of Marketing for the Wyoming Department of Agriculture. In addition, Ms. Adams has published and spoken extensively on the importance of grains and whole grains in a healthful diet.

considered pica.[1] Pica is not unique to any one group. It is practiced by both sexes and many racial and ethnic groups. Pica is especially common among women who, during childhood, observed family members eating non-food items. It seems to be more frequently practiced during pregnancy than other times.

The potential dangers posed by pica far outweigh any perceived benefits. Some non-food substances, such as mothballs, toilet bowl freshener blocks, and chalk, may

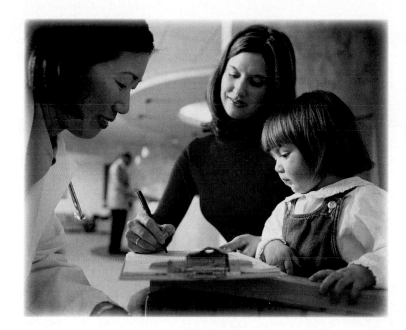

Humans cannot rely on cravings to meet nutrient needs. Nutrition advice from experts is much more reliable.

contain dangerously high levels of toxins, such as lead. Clay can block the intestines and may contain parasites and pathogens that impair mineral absorption. Laundry starch is high in calories (1800 calories per pound) but lacks all other nutrients, except carbohydrate, and can lead to malnutrition and obesity. Pica can have dire consequences for the pregnant woman (e.g., malnutrition, anemia, and death) and her fetus (e.g., premature birth, low birth weight, poor nutrient stores, and death).

Knowledge Check

1. What effect can eating too few calories during pregnancy have on offspring?
2. What nutrients are needed to build cells during fetal growth? What effect will consuming insufficient amounts of these nutrients during pregnancy have on offspring?
3. Why is it important to ensure an adequate folate intake before pregnancy?
4. How do iron deficiency anemia and physiological anemia differ?
5. How might practicing pica during pregnancy affect the pregnancy outcome?

16.3 Diet and Exercise Plan for Pregnancy

A pregnant woman's nutrient needs increase dramatically, whereas her calorie needs increase only a small amount. Selecting low-fat foods helps keep calories in line and increases the nutrient density of her diet. By choosing carefully, the woman can meet the increased nutrient demands of pregnancy and facilitate optimal fetal growth without consuming excessive calories.

The recommended daily increase of 350 to 450 calories doesn't sound like much, but the usefulness of this increase depends on how the woman decides to "spend" those calories. Two soft drinks or a chocolate candy bar supplies nearly the number of extra calories daily a woman needs in the second and third trimesters—and provides almost no nutrients. On the other hand, 2 glasses of fat-free milk, a small spinach salad, and a bowl of strawberries will meet two-thirds the calcium and vitamin A, one-fourth the folate, and exceed the vitamin C needs for 1 day, all for less than 350 calories.

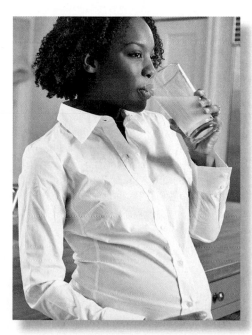

Pregnancy leads to increased nutrient needs for the mother. Meeting these needs is an important step toward a successful pregnancy.

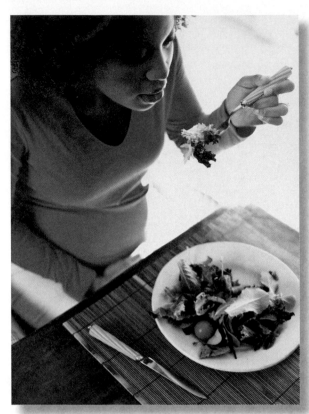

A salad each day provides many nutrients for the prenatal diet.

One approach to a diet plan that supports a successful pregnancy outcome is based on MyPyramid. For an active adult woman in the first trimester, about 2200 kcal are recommended. The plan should include the following.

- Milk Group: 3 cups of calcium-rich, low-fat or fat-free foods to supply protein, calcium, and carbohydrate, as well as other nutrients; calcium-fortified foods from other food groups can make up for gaps between calcium intake and need
- Meat and Beans Group: 6 ounce-equivalents to deliver needed iron and zinc
- Vegetables Group: 3 cups to provide vitamins and minerals; 1 cup should be rich in vitamin C and 1 cup should be rich in folate
- Fruit Group: 2 cups to supply vitamins and minerals
- Grains Group: 7 ounce-equivalents emphasizing whole-grain and enriched foods
- Oils Group: 6 teaspoons of vegetable oil, especially oils that provide essential fatty acids
- Discretionary Calories: up to 300 calories for weight maintenance

In the second and third trimesters, the plan recommends slight increases in almost every food group. In specific, the plan should include about 2600 kcal, divided like this:

- Milk Group: 3 cups
- Meat and Beans Group: 6½ ounce-equivalents
- Vegetables Group: 3½ cups
- Fruit Group: 2 cups
- Grains Group: 8 ounce-equivalents
- Oils Group: 7 teaspoons of vegetable oil
- Discretionary Calories: up to 400 calories for gradual weight gain

Table 16-2 illustrates a daily menu based on the basic diet plan for women in the second and third trimesters. This menu meets the extra nutrient needs associated with pregnancy. Women who need to consume more than 2600 kcal—and some do for various reasons—should incorporate additional fruits, vegetables, and whole-grain breads and cereals, not poor nutrient sources, such as desserts and regular soft drinks.

Prenatal Vitamin and Mineral Supplements

Special supplements formulated for pregnancy are prescribed routinely for pregnant women by most physicians. Some are sold over the counter, whereas others are dispensed by prescription because of their high synthetic folic acid content (1000 µg), which could pose problems for others, such as older people (see Chapter 13). Prenatal supplements also are high in iron. It is important not to exceed the recommended dose because megadoses of vitamin and mineral supplements can be dangerous for both the pregnant woman and the fetus. For example, iron, zinc, selenium, and vitamins A, B-6, C, and D can exert toxic effects when taken in large doses.[3] Supplemental preformed vitamin A is especially important to keep under control; it should not exceed 3000 µg RAE/day (15,000 IU per day) because higher levels are linked with **teratogenic** birth defects (see Chapter 12), mainly during the first trimester.

Many health professionals believe a pregnant woman should take nutrient supplements only when there is evidence that her usual diet is likely to limit maternal or fetal growth and development. For many pregnant women, the only supplement needed is iron during the last 2 trimesters. A multivitamin and mineral supplement is recommended for women who have a history of frequent dieting; are teenagers or vegans; have a low income; are underweight; smoke or abuse alcohol or illegal drugs; are carrying multiple fetuses; and/or are eating a diet restricted in variety. Supplements of specific nutrients may be recommended in circumstances where these nutrients are inadequate. For instance, vegans may need a vitamin B-12 supplement.

CRITICAL THINKING

Hannah, a 16-year-old high school student, has just discovered that she is pregnant. At 5'3" and 105 lb, she is underweight and her typical diet lacks many essential nutrients. For breakfast, she has coffee and a doughnut, if anything at all. She often skips lunch or eats chips from the vending machine. She then eats a well-rounded dinner with her family. What risks do you see in this situation for Hannah and her baby?

▶ To help pregnant and lactating women personalize MyPyramid, the USDA has created this website especially for these women: www.mypyramid.gov/mypyramidmoms/index.html.

Table 16-2 Sample 2600 kcal Daily Menu That Meets the Nutritional Needs of Most Pregnant and Breastfeeding Women

Breakfast	Amount
Fortified whole-grain breakfast cereal	1 cup
Orange juice	1 cup
Fat-free milk	1 cup
Calories	**420**
Morning Snack	
Whole-wheat toast	1 slice
Plain low-fat yogurt	1 cup
Tangerine and blueberries	½ cup
Calories	**240**
Lunch	
Spinach salad	2 cups
Italian dressing	2 tablespoons
Sweet red pepper	½ pepper
Hard-cooked egg	1 egg
Whole-wheat bread	1 slice
Peanut butter	2 tablespoons
Calories	**450**
Afternoon Snack	
Whole-wheat crackers	6 crackers
Tomato juice	1 cup
Cheddar cheese	1½ ounces
Calories	**290**
Dinner	
Grilled chicken breast, skinless**	3½ ounces
Brown rice	1 cup
Broccoli	1 cup
Calories	**425**
Evening Snack	
Granola bar	1-ounce bar
Raisins	1 ounce
Sunflower seeds	1 ounce
Calories	**375**
Discretionary Calories	Up to 400 kcal*
Total Calories for the Day	**2600**

Total intake of fluids, such as water, should be 10 cups or so per day.

*Amount of discretionary calories will vary based on the actual food choices made within each MyPyramid group.

**Substituting a veggie burger for the chicken breast makes this menu a practical guide for a vegetarian.

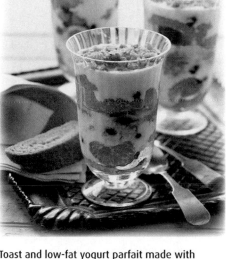

Toast and low-fat yogurt parfait made with fresh fruit add important nutrients to a pregnant woman's diet.

Pregnancy, in particular, is not a time to self-prescribe medications or vitamin and mineral supplements. For example, although vitamin A is a routine component of prenatal vitamins, it is important to note that intakes over 3 times the RDA can have toxic effects on the fetus.

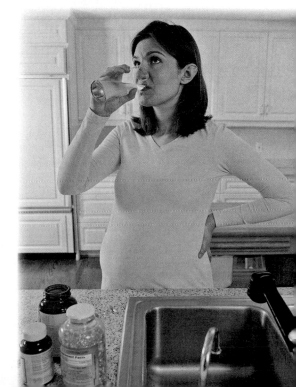

Physical Activity during Pregnancy

A low- or moderate-intensity exercise program can offer physical and psychological benefits to a woman experiencing a normal, healthy pregnancy. Benefits include improved cardiovascular function, an easier and less complicated labor, and an improved attitude and mental state.[15] Exercise also can help prevent or treat gestational diabetes. Infants born to women who exercise tend to be leaner and more neurologically mature than babies born to non-exercisers. Women with high-risk pregnancies, such as those experiencing premature labor contractions, may need to restrict their physical activity.

To ensure optimal health for both herself and her infant, a pregnant woman should first consult her health-care provider before beginning or continuing with an exercise program. The following recommendations for exercise during pregnancy can be used to plan a safe exercise program.

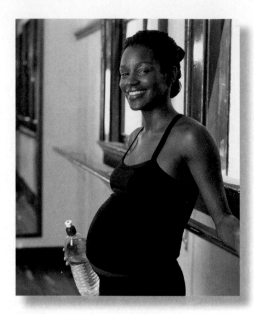

Health-care providers typically encourage healthy, well-nourished pregnant women to engage in moderate exercise as long as increased energy and nutrient needs are met.

- Exercise moderately for about 30 minutes daily on most days of the week.
- Drink plenty of liquids to maintain normal fluid and electrolyte balance and avoid dehydration.
- Keep heart rate below 140 beats per minute to maintain adequate blood (and oxygen) flow to the fetus.
- Include a cooldown period at the end of exercise sessions, so that heart rate can gradually return to normal.
- After about the fourth month, avoid exercises that are done while lying down because the enlarged uterus compresses blood vessels and cuts down blood flow to the fetus.
- Avoid deep flexing (e.g., deep knee bends), joint extensions (e.g., leg stretches), and activities that jar the joints (e.g., jumping) because connective tissue that has become more elastic to facilitate normal childbirth can be damaged if overstressed in exercise.
- Prevent increases in body temperature by not exercising in hot, humid weather or engaging in strenuous activities for more than 15 minutes. High body temperatures can damage enzymes that regulate fetal development.
- Stop exercising immediately if discomfort occurs—aches and pains are a warning that something may be wrong.
- Avoid strenuous or endurance activities because they can cause lower than normal birth weights.
- Avoid activities that could cause abdominal trauma (e.g., horseback riding, martial arts), that involve rapid shifts in balance or body position that may cause accidental falls (e.g., basketball, skiing, hockey), or that compress the uterus (e.g., scuba diving).
- Avoid becoming overly tired.

Global Nutrition

Pregnancy and Malnutrition

Prolonged undernutrition is detrimental at any life stage, but its effects are particularly profound during pregnancy and fetal life. About 500,000 women worldwide die each year from complications of pregnancy and childbirth—most are in developing countries. In Africa, for example, women give birth, on average, to more than 6 live babies. Coupled with chronic undernutrition, these high birth rates result in a 1 in 20 chance that a woman will die from pregnancy-related causes. In contrast, North American women face a risk of only 1 death from pregnancy-related causes in about 8000 births. Pregnancy-related death is the social indicator that differs most between the developing and industrialized worlds.

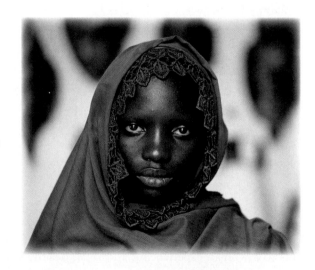

The fetus also faces major health risks from undernutrition during gestation. When nutrient needs are not met, the infant is often born prematurely and, as a result, has reduced lung function and a weakened immune system. These conditions not only compromise health but also increase the likelihood of premature death. Long-term problems in growth and development can result if the infant survives. In extreme cases, low birth weight infants face 5 to 10 times the normal risk of dying before the age of 1 year. Worldwide, more than 30 million infants are born each year with low birth weight.

Although it is difficult to specify the extent to which poor nutrition will affect each pregnancy, a daily diet containing only 1000 kcal has been shown to greatly restrict fetal growth and development.[16] Increased maternal and infant death rates seen in famine-stricken areas of Africa and wartime observations provide further evidence. For example, during World War II, food supplies in Holland were extremely restricted for about 6 months. Babies conceived before the food shortage and delivered during or after the shortage were only slightly shorter and lighter in weight than normal. They were less likely to be spontaneously aborted, stillborn, or premature; to have birth defects; or to develop mental disorders later in life than were babies conceived near the end of the food shortage, when maternal nutrient stores and body weight were depleted. Similar outcomes were seen among women who became pregnant during the siege of Leningrad, when food was extremely limited.

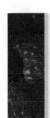

Knowledge Check

1. How many servings from each food group should pregnant women consume in the last 2 trimesters?
2. Nutrient supplements during pregnancy are recommended for which groups of women?
3. What types of physical activities should pregnant women avoid?

 16.4 Nutrition-Related Factors Affecting Pregnancy Outcome

Evidence shows that a nutritious diet before pregnancy as well as during pregnancy can have a profound effect on both the mother's health and that of her child. The factors in Table 16-3 are associated with less than optimal nutritional status and put women at great risk of a poor pregnancy outcome.

Table 16-3 Maternal Factors That Increase Risk of Nutrient Deficiencies and Poor Pregnancy Outcome

Factor	Condition Increasing Risk of Nutrient Deficiencies
Body weight	
Prepregnancy	BMI less than 19.8 or greater than 26
During pregnancy	Inadequate or excessive weight gain Inappropriate pattern of weight gain
Age	Young age
Eating patterns	Regular omission of foods from 1 or more major food groups (e.g., vegan diets)
	Excessive consumption of a single type of food
	Fasting and weight-loss diets
	Special diets to control maternal health conditions, such as heart disease, kidney disease, diabetes, and genetic disorders (e.g., phenylketonuria)
	Eating disorders
	Food cravings, aversions, and pica
Health	Pregnancies spaced less than 12 to 18 months apart
	More than 3 previous pregnancies if under age 20, more than 4 if over age 20
	Carrying more than 1 fetus
	Inadequate prenatal health care
	Diseases such as HIV/AIDS and diabetes
	Onset of gestational diabetes mellitus
	Onset of pregnancy-induced hypertension, preeclampsia, and/or eclampsia
Sociocultural factors	Low income
	Limited educational achievement
	Lack of family or social support
Food supply	Food contaminants (e.g., mercury, lead, PCBs, pesticides)
	Foodborne illness pathogens
	High caffeine intake
Lifestyle choices	Use of alcohol, drugs, tobacco, or herbal and botanical products

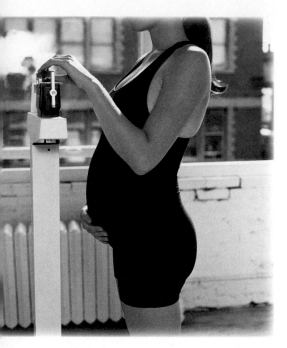

Following weight gain recommendations during pregnancy helps increase the chances of a successful outcome.

Maternal Prepregnancy Weight

An infant's birth weight is closely related not only to length of gestation but also to the woman's prepregnancy weight and the amount of weight she gains during pregnancy.[1, 17] Infants born to women who began pregnancy substantially above or below a healthy weight are more likely to experience problems than women who began pregnancy at a normal weight. For instance, babies born to obese women are at increased risk of having birth defects, such as neural tube defects, death in the first few weeks after birth, and obesity in childhood.[18] Many obese pregnant women experience high blood pressure, gestational diabetes, and difficult deliveries. Obese women can reduce these risks by losing weight *before* becoming pregnant.

Women who begin pregnancy underweight (BMI < 19.8) are more likely to have infants who are low birth weight and premature than women at a normal weight.[1] These differences may be because underweight women tend to have lighter placentas and lower nutrient stores, especially iron, than heavier women, which can affect fetal growth negatively. An underweight woman can improve her nutrient stores and pregnancy outcome by gaining weight before pregnancy or gaining extra weight during pregnancy.

Prepregnancy weight and nutrient stores not only affect pregnancy outcome but also affect the woman's ability to become pregnant. Many underweight women experience amenorrhea, which may reduce their ability to ovulate. The chances of ovulating and becoming pregnant improve when body fat increases to a healthy level. Low nutrient intakes also affect a man's ability to produce enough viable sperm. When the number of sperm is low and/or the sperm's ability to propel itself is reduced, fertilization is unlikely to occur. Zinc, folate, and vitamin C affect the quality of sperm; when these nutrients are in short supply, men may experience fertility problems.[19]

Maternal Weight Gain

The weight a woman gains during pregnancy allows the fetus to grow and her body to accommodate it, as well as prepare for lactation. Figure 16-7 illustrates how the weight

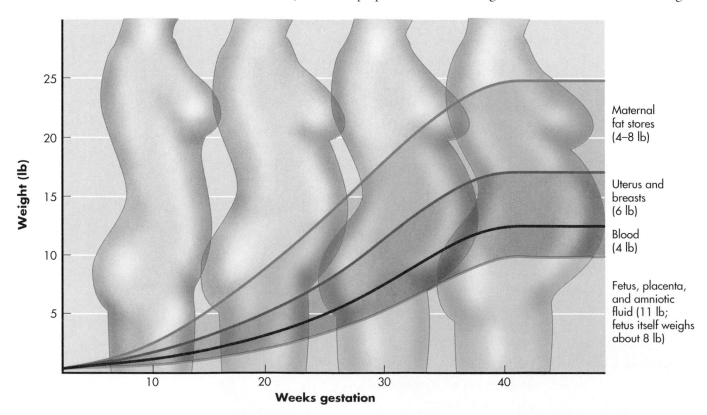

Figure 16-7 Components of weight gain in pregnancy. A weight gain of 25 to 35 lb is recommended for most women. Note that the various components total about 25 lb.

Table 16-4 Recommended Weight Gain in Pregnancy Based on Prepregnancy Body Mass Index (BMI)

Prepregnancy BMI Category	Total Weight Gain* (lb)	Total Weight Gain* (kg)
Low (BMI less than 19.8)	28 to 40	12.5 to 18
Normal (BMI 19.8 to 25.9)	25 to 35	11.5 to 16
High (BMI 26 to 29)	15 to 25	7 to 11.5
Obese (BMI greater than 29)	15 (or more)	7 (or more)

*The listed values are for pregnancies with 1 fetus. Short women (less than 62 in.) should strive for gains at the lower end of the ranges. For women of normal BMI who are carrying twins, the range is 35 to 45 lb (16 to 20 kg). Adolescents within 2 years of their first menstrual period should strive for gains at the upper end of the ranges.
Reprinted with permission from *Nutrition during Pregnancy and Lactation*, Copyright 1992 by the National Academy of Sciences. Courtesy of the National Academy Press, Washington, DC.

gained during pregnancy is divided. The recommendations for prenatal weight gain have steadily increased in the last 60 years from 15 to 16 pounds in the 1950s to 25 to 35 pounds in the 1990s for women of normal prepregnancy weight. Studies have shown repeatedly that gaining the amount of weight currently recommended by the National Academy of Science's Institute of Medicine improves the chances of optimal health for both mother and fetus if gestation lasts at least 38 weeks.

As shown in Table 16-4, a healthy goal for total weight gain for a woman of normal BMI averages about 25 to 35 lb (11.5 to 16 kg). For women with a low BMI (< 19.8), the goal increases to 28 to 40 lb (12.5 to 18 kg). The goal decreases to 15 to 25 lb (7 to 11.5 kg) for women at a high BMI (26 to 29) and 15 lb (7 kg) or more for an obese woman (BMI > 29). The weight gain recommendations are given as ranges to allow for differences within each BMI group. Women who are better off aiming for the lower end of the range are short (under 62 inches tall) or were malnourished during childhood and experienced growth retardation. These women may have difficulty delivering a normal-size infant. Those who should aim for the upper end of the range include adolescents because they tend to have smaller babies than older women who gain the same amount of weight during pregnancy. Women carrying more than 1 fetus will need to gain more weight to support optimal growth of all the fetuses. For example, women carrying twins should gain 35 to 45 lb, and those carrying triplets should gain 50 lb (23 kg). African-American women have an increased risk of delivering low birth weight infants; however, recent evidence indicates that these women may not need to aim for the upper end of the weight gain range.

The weight gain recommendations in Table 16-4 promote optimal fetal growth while minimizing the risks of complications at delivery, postpartum maternal weight retention, and the infant's chances of developing chronic disease later in life. Unfortunately, many women do not gain the recommended amounts. Women who gain less than the amount recommended have an increased risk of giving birth to a baby that is premature, is small for gestational age,

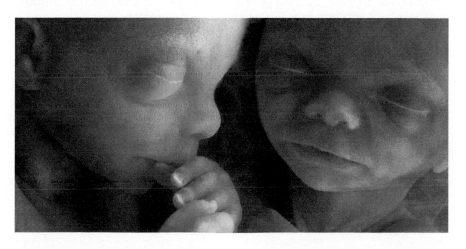

The nutrient needs of a woman carrying multiple fetuses are higher than those of a woman carrying a single fetus.

and/or dies soon after birth.[16] In contrast, women who gain excessively higher amounts than the recommendations typically give birth to very large babies and experience an increase in complications at delivery, infant mortality, and weight retention postpartum.

Pattern of Maternal Weight Gain

The pattern the woman's weight gain follows is as important as the amount she gains. During the first trimester, most women should gain about 2 to 4 pounds (0.9 to 1.8 kg), most of which is accounted for by the enlarging breasts and uterus. After that, a woman who starts at a normal weight should gain about 1 pound (0.4 kg) a week at a slow, steady rate. Underweight women should gain a bit more than a pound (0.5 kg), and overweight women should gain about three-quarters of a pound (0.3 kg) weekly. In the second trimester, weight gain is divided between mother and fetus. In the third trimester, weight gain is almost all fetal tissue. Low weight gain in either of the last 2 trimesters increases the chances of prenatal growth retardation. Low weight gain in the last trimester raises the risk of premature birth.

If a woman deviates from the desirable weight gain pattern, she should work with her health-care provider to make appropriate adjustments. For example, if a woman begins to gain too much weight during her pregnancy, she should not try to lose weight. Instead, she should minimize her intake of foods that provide unnecessary calories. Even if a woman gains 35 lb in the first 7 months of pregnancy, she must still gain more during the last 2 months to have an optimal outcome. However, she should slow the increase in weight to parallel the rise on the prenatal weight gain chart. Alternately, if a woman has not gained the desired weight by a given point in pregnancy, she should not try to gain the needed weight rapidly. Instead, she should slowly gain a little more weight than the typical pattern to meet the goal by the end of the pregnancy.

A sudden change in weight (up or down) may signal health problems for the mother. For instance, a sudden, erratic gain may be caused by fluid retention. This may indicate that the mother has pregnancy-induced hypertension, a potentially life-threatening condition.

Young Maternal Age

Teenage pregnancy poses special nutrition and health challenges for both the mother and the developing offspring. Young women continue maturing physically for about 5 years after the onset of menstruation **(menarche).** Because the average age for menarche is 13 years in the U.S., most women younger than 18 years are not as physically ready to be pregnant as they will be later. In addition, the teen years are a period of high nutrient needs, and teens' nutrient intakes frequently are below recommended amounts. It is difficult for a pregnant adolescent to consume adequate amounts of nutrients to support her own growth. It is even more difficult to meet the additional needs to support fetal growth. Many teens enter pregnancy underweight and gain too little weight during pregnancy. In addition, many teens do not receive adequate prenatal care. For all of these reasons, babies born to teens are at greater risk of premature birth, prenatal growth retardation, and death soon after birth. Teens also have more stillbirths and spontaneous abortions than older women.

Maternal Eating Patterns

Pregnant women with diets that deviate greatly from the recommended diet either by restricting dietary intake or eating excessive quantities of a limited number of foods risk getting too few nutrients and a poor pregnancy outcome.[20] Ketosis can result from restricting carbohydrate intake or fasting and is not desirable for the growing fetus. Ketone bodies are thought to be poorly used by the fetal brain and may slow its development. Pregnant women can develop significant amounts of ketones after only 20 hours of fasting, so eating regular meals and avoiding fasting for more than 12 hours is important. In addition, weight-loss diets should never be attempted during pregnancy, regardless of prepregnancy weight or weight gain during pregnancy because of the rise in ketones that can occur. Including at least 175 g of carbohydrate in the diet every day helps prevent ketosis.

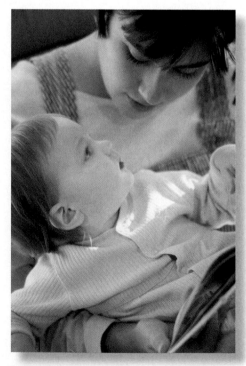

Healthy nutrition, prenatal care starting before pregnancy, and the avoidance of unsafe behaviors, such as smoking and taking drugs, are key factors in promoting a successful pregnancy outcome. Very young mothers often are ill prepared to cope with the physiological, emotional, and societal pressures of pregnancy. These factors contribute to the added risks they face.

Women who have eating disorders or other nutrition-related health conditions, such as diabetes or phenylketonuria, need to work with health-care providers to be certain their diets meet both their own as well as fetal needs. As mentioned previously, food cravings, aversions, and pica also can affect dietary quality and pregnancy outcome.

Lacto-ovo-vegetarians and lacto-vegetarians generally do not face special difficulties in meeting nutritional needs during pregnancy. On the other hand, for a vegan, careful diet planning before and during pregnancy is crucial to ensure sufficient intakes of protein, vitamin D (or sufficient sun exposure), vitamin B-6, iron, calcium, zinc, and especially vitamin B-12.[21] The basic vegan diet listed in Chapter 7 should be modified to include more grains, beans, nuts, and seeds to supply the necessary extra amounts of some of these nutrients. The use of a prenatal multivitamin and mineral supplement is generally advocated to help fill micronutrient gaps. However, supplements are not high in calcium (200 mg per pill). If iron and calcium supplements are used, they should not be taken together, to avoid possible competition for absorption.

Maternal Health

Women with conditions that affect their psychological or physical health may not consume an adequate diet and have less than optimal nutrient stores.

Pregnancy History

Numerous previous pregnancies and/or closely spaced pregnancies (less than 1 year apart) may deplete a woman's nutrient stores, which increases the risk that a subsequent pregnancy will result in a preterm birth, low birth weight infant, or small for gestational age infant. Carrying more than 1 fetus also increases nutrient needs and makes it difficult to consume sufficient calories and nutrients to support optimal growth of the fetuses.

Prenatal Care

If prenatal care is inadequate, delayed, or absent, untreated maternal nutritional deficiencies can deprive a developing fetus of needed nutrients.[6] In addition, untreated chronic diseases, such as hypertension or diabetes, increase the risk of fetal damage. Without prenatal care, a woman is 3 times more likely to deliver a low birth weight baby. Although the ideal time to start prenatal care is before conception, about 20% of women in the U.S. receive no prenatal care throughout the first trimester—a critical time to positively influence pregnancy outcome.

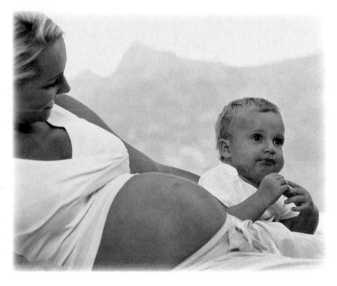

Closely spaced pregnancies increase the risk that the woman's nutrient stores will become depleted.

Acquired Immune Deficiency Syndrome

Individuals infected with human immunodeficiency virus (HIV) or who have acquired immune deficiency syndrome (AIDS) have increased needs for energy and some vitamins and minerals. Supplements of some nutrients, such as vitamin A, zinc, and iron, may adversely affect those who are HIV-positive.[22] Thus, careful dietary planning is needed by women with HIV or AIDS. In addition, women may pass HIV to the fetus during pregnancy or the birth process. About 1 in 3 infected newborns will develop AIDS symptoms and die within a few years. Studies show that the odds of mother-infant transmission can be cut significantly if the woman begins taking the drug azidothymidine (AZT) and other related AIDS medications by the fourteenth week of pregnancy. Providing these medications just before birth is helpful as well. Thus, some experts advocate screening pregnant women for HIV and AIDS and treating those with AIDS using AZT.[23]

Pregnancy-Induced Hypertension

It is normal to see an elevation in blood pressure during pregnancy; however, pregnancy-induced hypertension causes it to rise abnormally high. Pregnancy-induced hypertension impairs the delivery of oxygen and nutrients to the fetus; thus, the fetus may experience retarded growth and premature birth. Pregnancy-induced hypertension can escalate into potentially deadly conditions called preeclampsia and eclampsia (formerly called toxemia). **Preeclampsia** is high blood pressure accompanied by protein in the urine, headaches, blurred vision, changes in blood clotting, nervous system disorders, and edema throughout the body. It can progress to **eclampsia,** which causes maternal convulsions and coma. Blood pressure may climb so high that the kidneys and liver are damaged, and both the mother and her fetus may die. In fact, eclampsia is the leading cause of maternal and newborn death in the U.S.

Certain proteins, including some produced by the placenta, appear to be involved in the development of preeclampsia.[24] Preeclampsia and eclampsia are most common among women who have a high BMI, are pregnant for the first time or have multiple-birth pregnancies, are younger than 20 or older than 35 years, or had hypertension before pregnancy.[1] In addition, women who experienced pregnancy-induced hypertension, preeclampsia, and/or eclampsia in a previous pregnancy or who have a family history of these conditions are at increased risk of developing these conditions.[1]

Some evidence indicates that inadequate nutrient intakes may contribute to the development of preeclampsia. However, in well-nourished women, calcium supplements probably do not help with this problem.[25, 26] In addition, recent evidence indicates that fish oil supplements, as well as sodium restriction, are not effective in reducing the risk of preeclampsia.[24, 27] Pregnancy-induced hypertension resolves itself when the pregnancy ends. However, because the problem often begins well before the normal end of gestation, treatment may be necessary to prevent the worsening of the disorder. Bed rest and magnesium sulfate are the most effective treatment methods, although their effectiveness varies.[28] Magnesium likely acts to relax blood vessels and, so, leads to a fall in blood pressure. Several other treatments, such as various anti-seizure and anti-hypertensive medications, are under study.

Diabetes Mellitus

Women with poorly controlled type 1 or type 2 diabetes are at great risk of a poor pregnancy outcome. If blood glucose levels are elevated, the embryo or fetus is likely to have major birth defects that lead to spontaneous abortion, infant death, or serious infant illness. To prevent these consequences, women with diabetes need to work closely with their health-care providers to bring their diabetes under control before pregnancy and keep their blood glucose at normal levels throughout pregnancy.

During pregnancy, another type of diabetes, gestational diabetes, develops in approximately 4% of women who entered pregnancy without diabetes, with the number increasing to 7% in the Caucasian population. Hormones synthesized by the placenta decrease the efficiency of insulin and lead to a mild increase in blood glucose. An excessive rise in blood glucose can lead to gestational diabetes, often beginning in weeks 20 to 28. Gestational diabetes is particularly prevalent in women who have a family history of diabetes, are obese, are older than 25, or had gestational diabetes in a prior pregnancy. Pregnant women often are screened for gestational diabetes between 24 to 28 weeks of pregnancy.

Exercise and a diet that distributes low glycemic load carbohydrates throughout the day are important for keeping gestational diabetes under control. Some women also may need insulin therapy.[29] Untreated gestational diabetes can severely deplete fetal iron stores. In addition, uncontrolled diabetes can cause the fetus to grow quite large.[30] The oversupply of glucose from maternal circulation signals the fetus to increase insulin production, which causes fetal tissues to readily use glucose for growth. Another threat is that the infant may have low blood glucose at birth because of the tendency to produce extra insulin that began during gestation. Other concerns are the potential for preterm delivery and increased risk of birth trauma and malformations. The abnormally high blood glucose levels caused by gestational diabetes often return to normal after giving birth; however, the mother's risk of developing diabetes later in life rises, especially if she is obese. Infants born to mothers with gestational diabetes also may have higher risks of developing obesity and type 2 diabetes as they grow to adulthood.

Maternal Sociocultural Factors

Women with limited income or educational achievement and those who lack social support networks tend to have inadequate diets. Thus, to help women of low socioeconomic status procure the foods and nutrition education they need, the U.S. Department of Ag-

---

Dietary Recommendations for Gestational Diabetes

1. Get approximately 50 to 60% of calories from complex carbohydrates.
2. Consume approximately 12 to 20% of calories from protein.
3. Consume approximately 20 to 30% of calories from fat.
4. Divide calorie intake among 3 meals and 3 snacks. The bedtime snack is especially important because it helps prevent low blood sugar levels during the night. This snack should include both protein and complex carbohydrate.

riculture funds the Expanded Food and Nutrition Program (EFNEP), the Food Stamp Program, and the Women, Infants, and Children (WIC) program.

EFNEP and the Food Stamp Program provide nutrition education for those with limited resources. Program participants learn about good nutrition, meal planning, and techniques for stretching food dollars. The Food Stamp Program also provides foods for those with limited financial resources. WIC provides nutritious foods specifically to low-income pregnant, postpartum, and breastfeeding women, as well as infants and children up to age 5 who are at nutritional risk. WIC participants receive milk, cheese, eggs, fruit or vegetable juice, iron-fortified cereal, beans, peanut butter, and other nutritious foods that supply nutrients often lacking in their diets, such as vitamins A and C, folate, iron, calcium, and protein. They attend nutrition education classes and are encouraged to seek and maintain appropriate medical care. This combination of supplemental foods, nutrition education, and health-care referrals has helped improve the nutrition-related health conditions of WIC participants. In addition, participation in WIC is linked to higher birth weights, fewer infant deaths, and lower medical costs after birth.

Maternal Food Supply

The food supply in the U.S. and Canada can provide all of the nutrients needed for a successful pregnancy outcome. However, intakes of the compounds found in some foods should be limited during pregnancy.

Environmental contaminants can enter food through food containers, polluted water, and farming and food preparation practices. As described in Chapter 3, common food contaminants that pose dangers to the pregnant woman and her fetus include lead, mercury, polychlorinated biphenyls (PCBs), and pesticides. Lead can leach into food from lead crystal glasses, some dishes, and the solder used to seal copper water pipes. Fish are the food source most likely to be contaminated with mercury, PCBs, and other pollutants that were dumped into waterways and accumulated in the fish living there. To minimize pregnant women's exposure to mercury, the FDA and Environmental Protection Agency (EPA) advise pregnant women to avoid swordfish, shark, king mackerel, and tilefish and keep their intake of other fish and shellfish to 12 ounces (no more than 6 ounces from albacore tuna) per week. The effect of pesticide residues on humans is largely unknown. However, everyone, including pregnant women, can minimize exposure to pesticides by thoroughly washing all fruits and vegetables.

Foodborne illness risk increases during pregnancy. Thus, as noted in Chapter 3, pregnant women should avoid foods frequently found to be contaminated with pathogens, such as raw sprouts, unpasteurized milk and juices, and raw or undercooked meat and eggs. Exposure to the bacterium that causes the foodborne illness listeriosis (*Listeria monocytogenes*) is especially dangerous during pregnancy; it can cause spontaneous abortion, premature delivery, stillbirth, and infections in the newborn. Contaminated soft cheeses, such as Mexican-style cheese, feta, Brie, Camembert, and blue-veined cheeses (e.g., Roquefort) are often the cause of listeriosis. Thus, pregnant women are advised to avoid these cheeses. In addition, they are advised to cook leftovers and processed meats (e.g., hot dogs, deli meats) until steaming hot.

Maternal exposure to the parasite that causes toxoplasmosis can lead to infant death or brain damage. This parasite is found in cat feces, bird feces, and the soil. Raw meat can be contaminated with this parasite. To avoid toxoplasmosis, pregnant women should avoid litter boxes, kittens, and birds; carefully wash all produce to remove any soil; and thoroughly cook all meat.

Caffeine is a stimulant and diuretic found in coffee, tea, some soft drinks, and chocolate products. It also is a common additive in many medications, including headache and cold remedies. High caffeine intake (more than 500 mg daily) may hinder a woman's ability to become pregnant. During pregnancy, caffeine can affect fetal heart rate and breathing and decrease blood flow through the placenta. In addition, the fetus is unable to detoxify caffeine. Caffeine also may decrease the absorption of certain nutrients, such as calcium, iron, and zinc.[3] Heavy caffeine use during pregnancy may lead to caffeine withdrawal symptoms in the newborn. However, the evidence that caffeine consumption during pregnancy exerts a lasting adverse effect on the fetus is limited and very unclear. Nevertheless, many experts agree that it is sensible

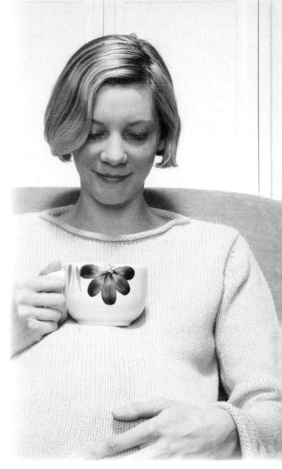

Pregnant women should limit caffeine intake during pregnancy.

▶ Other lifestyle choices unrelated to nutrition that can harm the developing fetus include:

- Exposure to hot temperatures in hot tubs and saunas
- X-ray exposure, including dental X-rays
- Job- and hobby-related hazards, such as chemicals and toxins used in manufacturing, hairdressing, and artwork

▶ Alcohol is found in beer, wine, and hard liquor, as well as in many mouthwashes and cough syrups.

▶ Head circumference of a child from birth until about age 3 years is an indicator of brain growth and development. The smaller the head in proportion to the body, the more likely the brain has suffered irreversible growth retardation.

▶ For more information about fetal alcohol syndrome, visit the website www.cdc.gov/ncbdd/fas.

▶ A goal of *Healthy People 2010* is 100% abstinence from alcohol, cigarettes, and illicit drugs by pregnant women.

to limit caffeine intake during pregnancy to around 300 mg daily, which is about 3 cups of coffee or 4 cups of caffeinated soft drinks (see Appendix I).

Food additives, such as phenylalanine (a component of the non-caloric sweetener aspartame in NutraSweet® and Equal®), cause concern in some pregnant women. Recall from Chapter 3 that, in the U.S., the safety of food additives must be demonstrated before they are approved for use in food. High amounts of phenylalanine in maternal blood disrupt fetal brain development if the mother has the genetic disease phenylketonuria (see Chapter 9). If the mother does not have this condition, it is unlikely that the baby will be affected by moderate aspartame use.

Maternal Lifestyle

Lifestyle choices can have an important impact on pregnancy outcome. Alcohol, drugs, herbal and botanical products, and smoking are lifestyle choices that increase the risk of a poor pregnancy outcome. A woman should avoid substances that can harm the developing offspring, especially during the first trimester. This caution holds true, as well, for the time when a woman is trying to become pregnant. As previously mentioned, a woman is unlikely to be aware of her pregnancy for at least a few weeks.

Alcohol is consumed by more than half of all women in the U.S. of childbearing age. Alcohol intake can impair the ability to become pregnant. During pregnancy, alcohol may displace nutrient-dense foods in the mother's diet. Alcohol also slows nutrient and oxygen delivery to the embryo or fetus, retarding growth and development. Although the most severe damage occurs during the embryo stage, a time with many critical periods, consuming alcohol at any time during pregnancy can cause damage to the embryo or fetus that lasts a lifetime.

Of every 1000 babies born in the U.S. each year, as many as 30 have alcohol-related defects.[31] Recall from Chapter 8 that the main features of fetal alcohol syndrome are facial malformations, growth retardation, and central nervous system defects, including profound mental retardation and a small brain size. These children are among the smallest in height, weight, and head circumference for their age. Prenatal exposure to alcohol also may cause somewhat lesser effects, known as fetal alcohol effects. These children may experience lifelong learning difficulties, short attention spans, and hyperactivity. Some also have the physical birth defects associated with exposure to alcohol.

It is not clear how alcohol causes these malformations and disabilities. However, alcohol freely crosses the placenta. Within minutes of its consumption, alcohol is present in the amniotic fluid, where the alcohol's intensity is magnified by the small size of the embryo or fetus. It addition, the effects of the alcohol are prolonged because the developing offspring is unable to metabolize the alcohol. It must wait for maternal blood to slowly carry the alcohol away.

No one is sure how much alcohol it takes to cause developmental problems. However, consuming as little as 1 ounce per day has resulted in mental and physical defects. The more alcohol consumed during pregnancy, the worse the effects are likely to be. Until a safe level of alcohol consumption during pregnancy is known, experts recommend that pregnant women drink no alcohol. Because of the potentially deleterious effect on the embryo early in pregnancy, experts recommend that women planning a pregnancy avoid alcohol in case they do become pregnant and that women who drink alcohol avoid becoming pregnant.

Drugs, whether over-the-counter, prescription, or illegal, have the potential to cause detrimental effects on a pregnant woman's nutrition status and pregnancy outcome. Common drugs that can cause problems during pregnancy include aspirin (especially when used heavily), hormone ointments, nose drops, cold medications, rectal suppositories, weight-control pills, medications prescribed for previous illnesses, marijuana, and cocaine. They may deplete nutrient stores, alter nutrient absorption, and decrease the desire to eat. In addition, drugs may reduce blood flow to the fetus, which deprives it of oxygen and nutrients. A prescription drug that deserves special attention is Accutane® (isotretenoin), a form of vitamin A commonly used to treat severe acne. Babies born to mothers who take high doses of vitamin A, whether it is from isotretenoin or supplements, may experience severe birth defects, including nervous system abnormalities and facial and cardiovascular deformities. Prior to taking any drug, a pregnant woman should discuss its use with her health-care provider.

Herbal and botanical products can exert potent druglike effects on both the mother and the fetus. Until the safety of these products can be verified, experts recommend that pregnant women use all herbal and botanical products—including herbal tea—with caution and under the guidance of a health-care professional.

Nicotine and carbon monoxide affect the fetus when the pregnant woman smokes or is exposed to second-hand cigarette or cigar smoke. Smoking restricts blood flow, reducing the amount of oxygen and nutrients, especially zinc, that reaches the fetus, which, in turn, impairs growth. Smokers' babies are more likely to be premature, experience prenatal growth retardation, and die soon after birth than are non-smokers' babies. They also have an increased risk of birth defects, childhood cancer, and sudden infant death. Contributing to the smaller birth size is the fact that smokers are likely to have a lower prepregnancy weight and to gain less weight during pregnancy. Plus, many smokers' diets are less nutritious than those of non-smokers.

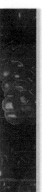

Knowledge Check

1. How does maternal prepregnancy weight and weight gain during pregnancy affect pregnancy outcome?
2. What are the maternal weight gain recommendations for underweight, normal-weight, and overweight women?
3. What are the symptoms of pregnancy-induced hypertension?
4. Why is it important to keep blood glucose levels under control during pregnancy?
5. What precautions should pregnant women take to avoid foods that might contain environmental contaminants or foodborne disease pathogens?
6. What effects can lifestyle choices related to alcohol, drugs, herbal and botanical products, and smoking have on pregnancy outcome?

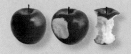 *Take Action*

Healthy Diets for Pregnant Women

A college friend, Angie, tells you that she is newly pregnant. You are aware that she usually likes to eat the following foods for her meals.

Breakfast

Skips this meal or eats a granola bar
Coffee

Lunch

Sweetened yogurt, 1 cup
Small bagel with ¼ cup cream cheese
Occasional piece of fruit
Regular caffeinated soda, 12 oz

Snack

Chocolate candy bar or 2 slices of bologna

Dinner

2 slices of pizza, fried shrimp dinner, or 2 eggs with 2 slices of toast
Seldom eats a salad or vegetable
Regular caffeinated soda, 12 oz

Snacks

Pretzels or chips, 1 oz
Regular caffeinated soda, 12 oz

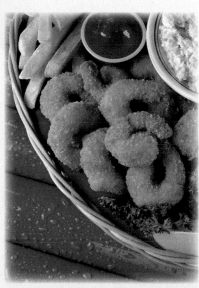

1. Evaluate Angie's diet for protein, carbohydrate, iron, vitamin B-6, folate, and zinc. How does her intake compare with the recommended amounts for pregnancy?

2. Now redesign Angie's diet and make sure that her intake meets pregnancy needs for protein, carbohydrate, iron, vitamin B-6, folate, and zinc. (Hint: Fortified foods, such as breakfast cereals, are usually nutrient-rich foods that can help individuals meet their nutrient needs.)

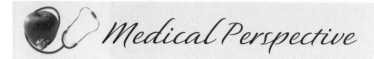

Medical Perspective

Nutrition-Related Physiological Changes of Concern during Pregnancy

The intense physical and hormonal changes that affect almost every aspect of the woman's body begin soon after the egg is fertilized. As the pregnancy progresses, the physical changes become more pronounced and the growing fetus places an increasing burden on the mother. Although the woman's body adapts well to this burden, she may experience some nutrition-related problems, such as heartburn, constipation, morning sickness, and edema. Usually, these difficulties are relatively minor and easy to remedy with diet and lifestyle changes. However, if the problems continue and prevent the woman from eating a nutritious diet, she should contact her health-care provider.

Heartburn

During pregnancy, the expanding uterus crowds abdominal organs and compresses them (Fig. 16-8). Crowding the stomach reduces its ability to stretch enough to accommodate a normal-size meal. Consequently, stomach acid and partially digested food may be pushed upward out of the stomach into the esophagus, causing a burning sensation commonly called heartburn (see Chapter 4). Hormones (e.g., progesterone) that slow the speed of digestion and relax sphincters in the gastrointestinal tract also can contribute to heartburn.[1]

Women usually can ease heartburn by eating several small meals instead of a few large ones, avoiding spicy and fatty foods, and limiting caffeine and chocolate intake. Women also should consume liquids mostly between meals to decrease the volume of food in the stomach after meals and thus relieve some of the pressure that encourages reflux. To keep acid from backing up into the esophagus, women should wait a couple of hours after eating to lie down and should sleep with their heads elevated slightly. Antacids contain certain minerals that may cause constipation, excessive sodium intake, and other problems, so they should be used only on the recommendation of a health-care provider.

Constipation

Hormones relax the intestinal muscles, which slows digestion and permits increased nutrient absorption. This slowdown also causes more water than usual to be re-absorbed, which leads to hard, dry stools. In addition, iron supplements may cause hard, dry stools.[1] Such stools are difficult to excrete, especially late in pregnancy as the fetus compresses the GI tract. Straining to excrete hard, dry stools may cause hemorrhoids (see Chapter 4).

Pregnant women often can avoid both constipation and hemorrhoids by consuming high fiber foods, drinking more fluids, and exercising. The Adequate Intake for fiber in pregnancy is 28 g/day, slightly more than for the non-pregnant woman. Fluid needs are 10 cups/day. Iron supplement dosage also may need adjustment. Stool softeners and laxatives may contain substances that can harm the fetus or cause dehydration; thus, they should be used only on the advice of a health-care provider.

Figure 16-8 **The growing fetus crowds and compresses abdominal organs.**

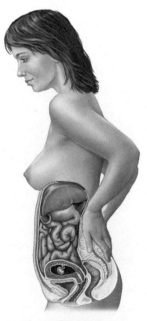

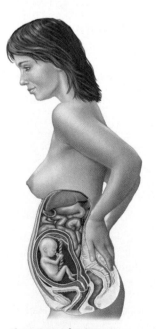

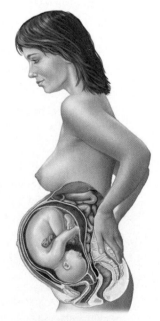

(a) First trimester   **(b) Second trimester**   **(c) Third trimester**

Nausea and Vomiting

During the first few months of pregnancy, about 70 to 85% of women experience frequent bouts of nausea and vomiting. This nausea may be related to the increased sense of smell induced by pregnancy-related hormones circulating in the bloodstream. This is commonly called morning sickness, although it can occur at any time of the day and persist all day. It is often the first signal to a woman that she is pregnant. Mild cases often can be treated by breathing cool, fresh air; avoiding offensive odors; avoiding large fluid intakes early in the morning; avoiding an empty stomach; and eating specific foods that ease symptoms. The iron in prenatal supplements may trigger nausea in some women; changing the type of supplement used or postponing iron supplements until the second trimester may provide relief. If a woman thinks her prenatal supplement is related to morning sickness, she should discuss switching to another brand with her physician. Some women find that starchy, bland foods, such as dry toast, crackers, or cereal, relieve feelings of nausea better than high-fat or high-protein foods. Sweets, such as hard candy, popsicles, and carbonated beverages, help other women cope. Women need to learn from experience which foods help quell queasy feelings and have them readily available.[1]

Usually, nausea stops after the first trimester; however, in about 10 to 20% of cases, it continues throughout the pregnancy. Severe nausea and vomiting that continues beyond 14 weeks of gestation, known as **hyperemesis gravidarium,** is a serious condition that may require hospitalization. Left untreated, it can result in dehydration, malnutrition, and electrolyte or metabolic disturbances that adversely affect both maternal and fetal health.

Edema

Placental hormones cause various body tissues to retain fluid during pregnancy. Blood volume also greatly expands during pregnancy. The extra fluid normally causes some swelling (edema). Plus, the enlarging uterus compresses blood vessels in the legs, which slows down blood circulation and the removal of waste products (including water). As a result, edema in the lower legs, especially around the ankles, is expected to a certain degree in late pregnancy. Edema in the lower legs is of concern only when accompanied by high blood pressure, protein in the urine, or the failure of the edema to subside when a woman elevates her feet. The presence of any of these factors may signal pregnancy-induced hypertension.

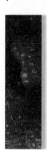

Knowledge Check

1. Why are heartburn and constipation common in pregnancy?
2. What are some practices that can help women cope with nausea during pregnancy?
3. Edema accompanied by which factors may signal pregnancy-induced hypertension?

CRITICAL THINKING

Sandy, who is 4 months pregnant, has been having heartburn after meals, constipation, and difficult bowel movements. What remedies might you suggest to Sandy to relieve her problems?

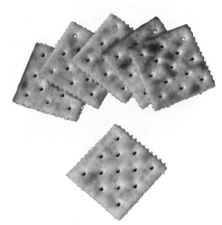

A few crackers on waking or between meals can help relieve the nausea of morning sickness.

► To prevent and treat nausea and vomiting during pregnancy, the American College of Obstetricians and Gynecologists recommends that women begin taking supplements prior to conception and use vitamin B-6 alone (see Chapter 13) or with the antihistamine doxylamine. Ginger also may help relieve nausea.

CASE STUDY FOLLOW-UP

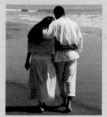

From a dietary standpoint, Tracey is smart to take a close look at her protein intake because her needs will increase somewhat during pregnancy. More fruits and vegetables supply extra folate, and her use of an over-the-counter vitamin and mineral supplement helps ensure that she will have an ample amount. Still, she should schedule an appointment with her physician to discuss her plans to become pregnant and learn more about vitamin and mineral supplements. She would probably eventually benefit more from a prenatal supplement because it will have more iron than over-the-counter multivitamin and mineral supplements. Her diet may not have enough calcium, so she should pay as much attention to consuming extra calcium as she does to consuming protein. Avoiding alcohol and tobacco is a smart move. Many experts would say that Tracey is consuming too much caffeine and would be wise to cut back on coffee and caffeine-containing soft drinks to a total of 3 or fewer servings per day. Swimming is an excellent choice for exercise, as long as it is not too vigorous. Brisk walking and stationary biking (spinning) are also good choices.

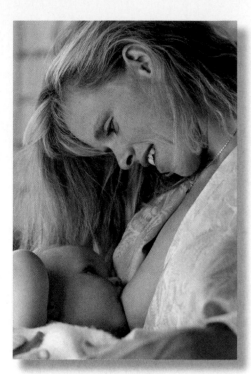

Breastfeeding is the preferred way to feed an infant.

16.5 Lactation

Lactation (breastfeeding) is a natural physiological process of female mammals that occurs in the postpartum period when the mother's breast secretes milk and suckles the offspring. Preparation for lactation begins when a young girl enters puberty. Hormones, particularly estrogen, secreted during puberty stimulate the growth and development of the mammary glands. The most obvious change in the breasts is their size, which is due to the deposition of fat (Table 16-5). Less visible changes include the growth and development of the milk-producing/storage cells (lobules) and the network of ducts that connect the glands to the nipple (Fig. 16-9). Malnutrition during adolescence can impair breast development and limit a woman's future ability to provide adequate nourishment for a growing baby.

Once developed, the mammary glands are fairly inactive until early in pregnancy. At that time, hormones secreted by the placenta cause the milk-producing glands to mature and the lactiferous ducts to branch more.

Table 16-5 Mammary Gland Development

Puberty: Ovarian hormones stimulate the development of the milk-producing cells (lobules) and ducts.

During pregnancy: Placental hormones stimulate lobules to mature and ducts to grow and branch.

Following childbirth: Pituitary hormones cause the breasts to begin producing milk (the hormone prolactin) and releasing milk (the hormone oxytocin). Suckling stimulates the pituitary to continue releasing prolactin. If the nipple is not suckled regularly, milk production ceases.

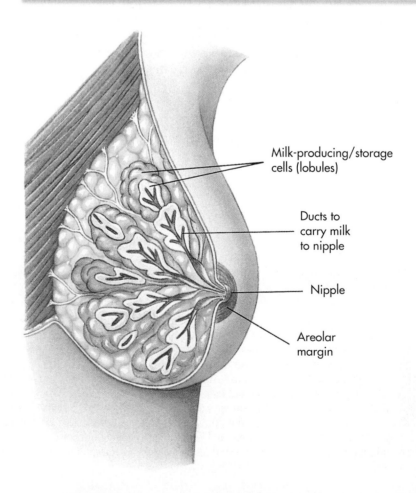

Milk-producing/storage cells (lobules)

Ducts to carry milk to nipple

Nipple

Areolar margin

Figure 16-9 Many types of cells form a coordinated network to produce and secrete human milk.

Milk Production

The manufacture and secretion of **prolactin,** the principal hormone that promotes milk production, are stimulated by the birth of the baby and by suckling. When the baby suckles at the breast, nerve signals stimulate the pituitary gland in the brain, causing it to release prolactin. The prolactin travels in the blood to the milk-producing glands in the breast and stimulates them to synthesize milk. If suckling stops (or never occurred after delivery), prolactin is not released and milk secretion usually stops in a few days. The breasts gradually return to their prepregnancy state.

During the earliest days of life, sucking is strongest in the first hour or so after birth; thus, this is the best time for the first feeding.[32] In the first few days after delivery, the baby should suckle often (at least every 2 or 3 hours for 15 to 20 minutes on each breast) to promote the establishment of lactation. After a few weeks, nursing sessions can become less frequent. As long as the mother breastfeeds her baby regularly, milk production will continue and can theoretically go on for years.

Throughout lactation, the amount of milk produced closely parallels infant demand. That is, the more an infant suckles, the more milk that is produced. This is what makes it possible for a woman to adequately breastfeed even twins and triplets. To **wean** a child, it is best to gradually stop breastfeeding, usually by eliminating 1 daily feeding each week. Abruptly stopping causes the breast to become painfully engorged with milk for several days.

wean To gradually accustom an infant to discontinuation of breast- or bottle-feeding by offering liquids from a cup and food from a spoon.

Release of the Milk from the Breast

An important brain-breast connection—commonly called the **let-down reflex**—is necessary for breastfeeding (Fig. 16-10). The pituitary gland releases the hormone **oxytocin,** which causes the musclelike cells in the breast tissues to contract and release (let down) the milk from the lobules. The milk then travels through the ducts to the nipple area.

During the first few weeks after delivery, this reflex must be triggered by the infant suckling the mother's breasts. Once lactation is established, the let-down reflex becomes automatic. It can be triggered just by thinking about her infant or hearing a baby cry. It generally takes 2 to

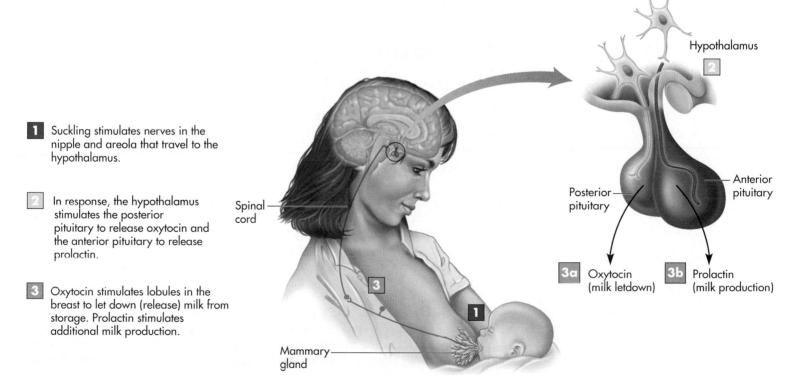

1 Suckling stimulates nerves in the nipple and areola that travel to the hypothalamus.

2 In response, the hypothalamus stimulates the posterior pituitary to release oxytocin and the anterior pituitary to release prolactin.

3 Oxytocin stimulates lobules in the breast to let down (release) milk from storage. Prolactin stimulates additional milk production.

Hypothalamus

Posterior pituitary

Anterior pituitary

Spinal cord

3a Oxytocin (milk letdown)

3b Prolactin (milk production)

Mammary gland

Figure 16-10 Suckling sets in motion the sequence of events that triggers milk production and the let-down reflex. This reflex releases milk from the milk-producing lobules into the ducts that carry the milk to the nipple.

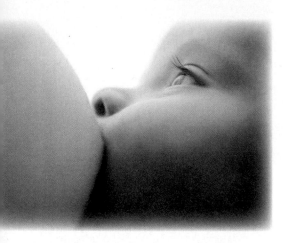

Before the let-down reflex becomes automatic, the infant must suck hard to cause the milk to be released. This vigorous suckling makes nipples sore. Health-care providers can help pregnant women prepare their nipples to minimize soreness. Most women find that nipple soreness is not a problem after about 2 or 3 weeks of breastfeeding.

3 weeks to fully establish a feeding routine in which both the infant and mother feel comfortable, the milk supply meets infant demand, and initial nipple soreness disappears. Establishing the breastfeeding routine requires patience, but the rewards are great.

The let-down reflex is easily inhibited by nervous tension, a lack of confidence, and fatigue. If the let-down reflex does not occur, the baby will be able to obtain only the small amount of milk that trickles out of the lobules between feedings. This will lead to a hungry, fussy baby, which likely will increase the mother's stressful, tense feelings—a vicious cycle. Women have a much better chance of successfully establishing lactation if they are in a relaxed, supportive environment and understand the process of lactation.[32] Careful monitoring during the first week of lactation by a physician or lactation consultant also helps ensure that breastfeeding and infant weight gain are proceeding normally.

Milk Types and Composition

Colostrum, transitional milk, and mature milk are the successive types of milk produced while lactation is being established. **Colostrum—** thin, yellowish, "immature" milk—may first appear anytime from late pregnancy to several days postpartum. This early milk is richer in protein, minerals, and vitamin A than later milk, but it has less carbohydrate (i.e., lactose) and slightly fewer calories. It also contains antibodies and immune system cells, some of which pass unaltered through the infant's immature GI tract into the bloodstream and provide the infant with a defense against some diseases during the first few months of life when the immune system is very immature.[33] (The first few months of life are the only time when we can readily absorb whole proteins across the GI tract.) One component of colostrum, the *Lactobacillus bifidus* **factor,** encourages the growth of *Lactobacillus bifidus* bacteria, which limits the growth of potentially toxic bacteria in the infant's intestine. In addition, colostrum contains a potent laxative, which helps the infant excrete the fecal matter that collected in the intestinal tract during fetal life.

The colostrum gradually changes in the early days after delivery to become transitional milk. Transitional milk contains more fat, lactose, water-soluble vitamins, and calories than colostrum. Within a week or so, transitional milk is replaced by mature milk. Mature human milk is thin and almost watery in appearance and often has a slightly bluish tinge. It provides about 20 calories per ounce and, with the possible exceptions of vitamin D and iron,[32] meets all the nutrients the growing baby needs (see Chapter 17).

Knowledge Check

1. What is the role of prolactin?
2. How is oxytocin involved in the let-down reflex?
3. How does colostrum differ from mature milk?

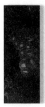 16.6 Nutrient Needs of Breastfeeding Women

The nutrient and calorie demands of lactation on the mother are tremendous, in some cases exceeding those of pregnancy. The quantities of nutrients needed during lactation are not so surprising when you consider that the milk secreted by a lactating woman can fulfill her infant's entire nutrient and calorie needs for approximately the first 6 months of life—the time when the infant's growth rate and nutrient needs per pound of body weight are at a lifetime high.

The lactating woman's Dietary Reference Intakes (DRIs) are based on the quantity of milk produced by the average mother, its nutrient content, and the amounts of her nutrient stores used to produce milk. The RDA value for iron is lower than that of both a pregnant and non-pregnant woman because human milk contains only a small amount of iron and because women who exclusively breastfeed their infants often do not resume menstruating for 6 months or so, thereby conserving iron. However, when a lactating woman begins menstruating again, her iron RDA returns to that of non-pregnant women.

Maternal Nutritional Status

The "recipe" for human milk is set by nature. The "ingredients" (i.e., nutrients) are drawn from the mother's diet, with deficits of some nutrients being made up by the mother's stores. These 2 sources of nutrients keep the composition and volume of the milk at fairly constant levels. If the mother's diet is poor for a prolonged period and she has depleted nutrient stores, the quantity of milk may decline. Maternal malnutrition must be extremely severe before the quality of milk produced drops.

At the other end of the spectrum lie maternal diets that contain nutrients in amounts exceeding recommended intakes. In the case of macronutrients and water, excess amounts usually have no effect on milk composition or volume, although the proportions of different fatty acids in the milk vary with maternal intake. If vitamin and mineral intakes exceed the recommendations, increased levels of these nutrients may appear in the milk. Doses several times greater than the RDA or Adequate Intakes may cause vitamin or mineral levels in human milk to be so high that they cause druglike effects.

An adequate intake of all nutrients by the mother is vital during lactation. Many lactating women consume calcium, magnesium, zinc, folate, and vitamin B-6 in amounts less than recommended. Adequate calcium intake is especially important because women who breastfeed their babies for 6 months or more lose significant amounts of calcium from their bones. Fortunately, with adequate calcium intake, bone density begins to return to normal within a few months after the baby is weaned. Adequate water and calorie intakes are particularly important.

Water is the main component of human milk, like other milk. Inadequate water intake can alter milk composition, decrease the amount of milk produced, and lead to maternal dehydration. To keep herself well hydrated, a breastfeeding woman should drink to satisfy her thirst. Most need an extra 32 ounces of fluid daily, in addition to the 72 ounces recommended for non-pregnant women. Some women, especially those breastfeeding more than 1 baby, need to consume even greater quantities.

Calorie needs can be met by eating the same number of servings from each food group as recommended for a pregnant woman in the last 2 trimesters (see Table 16-2). The average breastfeeding woman uses about 800 calories per day during the first 6 months of lactation to produce 750 ml of milk daily. Approximately 400 to 500 calories should come from her diet, with the remainder supplied by the fat stored during pregnancy.[10] Relying on stored fat to meet part of her calorie need helps the lactating woman gradually lose the extra body fat accumulated during pregnancy, especially if breastfeeding is continued for 6 months or more and the woman performs some physical activity.[34] Overweight women appear to be able to rely on stored fat to meet their entire daily calorie need for lactation without adversely affecting the growth of their infants. However, severe calorie restrictions and weight loss greater than 1 to 4 pounds per month likely will reduce the total amount of milk produced.

After 6 months of breastfeeding, all of these extra calories likely will need to come from the woman's diet if she has returned to her prepregnancy weight. Inadequate calorie intakes will cause her body weight to continue to drop and, if BMI is substantially below 18.5, she may become unable to produce enough milk for her growing child.

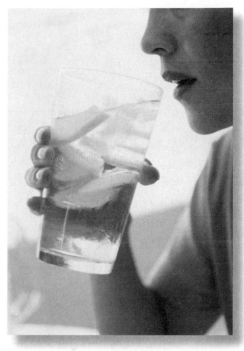
Water needs rise during lactation.

Food Choices during Lactation

Lactating women can enjoy all foods in moderation. Although single food items that a mother eats have very little bearing on her milk's nutritional quality or the amount she manufacturers, many cultures believe that certain foods, such as garlic and beer, boost the amount of milk produced. There is no scientific evidence that any food in particular promotes milk production or alters its nutrient composition, but, as discussed later in this chapter, there is some very good evidence that certain substances in food may affect the infant.

As in pregnancy, a serving of a fortified ready-to-eat breakfast cereal or a multivitamin and mineral supplement is advised to help meet extra nutrient needs. Like pregnant women, breastfeeding mothers should consume sufficient amounts of omega-3 fatty acids because they are secreted into breast milk and are important for the development of the

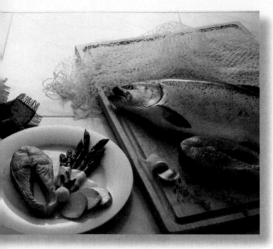

Eating fish at least twice a week will help breastfeeding women ensure that their infants receive important omega-3 fatty acids. It is important, however, to avoid fish that are likely contaminated with mercury (see Chapter 3).

infant's nervous system. Fish and supplements can provide these fatty acids. The FDA and EPA recommendations related to fish intake during pregnancy also apply during breastfeeding (see Chapter 3). Breastfeeding women may want to avoid eating peanuts or peanut butter because several studies have shown that peanut allergens pass into breast milk, potentially increasing the infant's risk of peanut allergy (see Chapter 7). However, the benefits of restricting the lactating mother's diet appear to be limited to infants at high risk of developing allergies (i.e., infants with a parent or sibling with food allergies).[35]

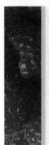

Knowledge Check

1. What effect does maternal nutritional status have on the quality and quantity of the breast milk she produces?
2. What are the calorie intake recommendations for lactating women?
3. What steps can lactating women take to ensure they consume an adequate amount of nutrients?
4. What is the basic food plan suitable for breastfeeding women?

16.7 Factors Affecting Lactation

Breastfeeding offers nutritional, immunological, and psychological benefits to the infant. Breastfeeding mothers, too, may gain health benefits, including a lower risk of ovarian and premenopausal breast cancer, bone remineralization to levels exceeding those before lactation, weight loss, quicker return of the uterus to its prepregnancy state, and less post-partum bleeding (Table 16-6). Although breastfeeding confers many advantages to both the mother and the child, several factors may affect milk quality and/or safety: maternal weight, age, and eating patterns; maternal and infant health; sociocultural factors; and maternal food supply and lifestyle choices.

Maternal Weight

Women who were obese prior to pregnancy often have greater difficulty initiating and continuing breastfeeding. These women may need to supplement human milk with infant formula until they develop a sufficient milk supply.

Maternal Age

Infants breastfed by adolescent mothers may grow more slowly than infants of older mothers. Teens can successfully breastfeed their offspring, but they need to work with their health-care providers to ensure that their own as well as their infant's nutrient needs are adequately met.

Table 16-6 Advantages of Breastfeeding for Mothers*

- Earlier recovery from pregnancy due to the action of hormones that promote a quicker return of the uterus to its prepregnancy state
- Decreased risk of ovarian and premenopausal breast cancer
- Potential for quicker return to prepregnancy weight
- Potential for delayed ovulation and therefore reduced chances of pregnancy (a short-term benefit, however)
- Potential bone remineralization to levels exceeding those before lactation
- Less postpartum bleeding
- Reduced risk of Metabolic Syndrome later in life[36]

*See Table 17-1 (Chapter 17) for a summary of advantages to infants provided by human milk.

Maternal Eating Patterns

A nutritious diet is the best choice for both the breastfeeding mother and her infant. However, an occasional day of poor intake is not a cause for concern—nutrient and/or calorie inadequacies usually can be made up using the mother's nutrient stores. It is only when a mother's diet is poor for several weeks or months that maternal nutrient stores may become depleted and her milk supply negatively affected.

Maternal and Infant Health

Breastfeeding may be ruled out by certain medical conditions in either the infant or the mother. For example, breastfeeding may be detrimental to infants with the inborn error of metabolism phenylketonuria or galactosemia (see Chapter 9). The high concentration of phenylalanine and galactose in human milk may overwhelm the impaired ability of these infants to metabolize these nutrients, leading to serious illness and even death.

Infectious or chronic diseases and their compatibility with breastfeeding need to be carefully considered by the mother and her health-care provider because medications and infectious agents can be transmitted to the baby via the mother's milk. A minor disease, such as a cold, is not a reason to stop breastfeeding. The baby is likely to catch the disease, anyway, because he or she was exposed before the mother's symptoms were apparent. Also, the immune factors in human milk may provide some protection for the breastfed baby against the minor disease. However, serious infectious diseases, such as tuberculosis and hepatitis C, can be life-threatening, so it may be safer for women with such diseases to feed their babies infant formula.

Medical advances have made it possible for women with several serious chronic diseases, such as diabetes, multiple sclerosis, lupus, phenylketonuria, and cystic fibrosis, to safely breastfeed their infants. Chronic diseases that are incompatible with breastfeeding are cancer being treated with chemotherapy medications and human immunodeficiency virus (HIV). HIV can be transmitted to the baby via human milk; thus, HIV-infected women are advised not to breastfeed. However, in regions of the world where infectious disease and malnutrition are the primary causes of infant death, the risk of not breastfeeding may outweigh the risk of possible transmission of HIV infection.[22, 37] Widespread lack of basic sanitation (e.g., lack of clean water and soap) may make it more dangerous to feed the baby infant formula because formula prepared with polluted water and placed in a dirty bottle frequently causes diarrhea—the number 1 killer of infants in developing countries (see Chapter 4).

Breast surgery may affect a woman's ability to produce milk and/or secrete it. Many women who have had breast implants are able to breastfeed. Women who have had breast reduction surgery may not be able to breastfeed if the milk-producing glands have been removed or their connection to the lactiferous ducts has been disrupted.

Sociocultural Factors

Overall, breastfeeding is a learned skill, and mothers need knowledge to breastfeed safely, especially with their first child. Women are more likely to decide to breastfeed and continue to do so if they know the advantages of breastfeeding, how to breastfeed their babies, what problems to expect, and how to cope with those problems; receive support from their partners; deliver their babies in a hospital that supports breastfeeding; and have health-care providers and experienced friends who are knowledgeable and able to lend needed support. Lack of information, low self-confidence, a lack of role models, and/or an inadequate support system may limit breastfeeding success.

The widespread increase in availability of lactation consultants over the past several years has helped increase access to accurate information, role models, and social support. In almost every community, a group called La Leche League offers classes in breastfeeding and advises women who have difficulties with it.

▶ For more information on breastfeeding, visit the following websites.

www.lalecheleague.org
www.breastfeeding.com
www.nal.usda.gov/wicworks

▶ *Healthy People 2010* has set a goal of 75% of women breastfeeding their infants at the time of hospital discharge, 50% breastfeeding for 6 months, and 25% still breastfeeding at 1 year.

▶ Males shouldn't be left out of the breastfeeding educational opportunities. This is because the single most important influence on a woman's decision to breastfeed or bottle-feed her baby is her partner's attitude.

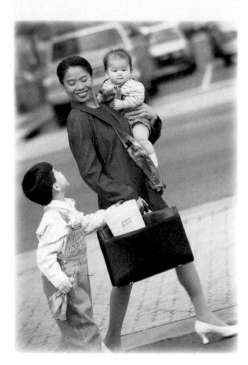

Breastfeeding a baby after returning to work is possible, but it requires planning.

Misinformation or a lack of information deters many women from attempting breastfeeding and causes many others to abandon it after only a few weeks. The following are some points that are important to know about breastfeeding.

- Practically all women are physically able to breastfeed their children.
- Women with anatomical problems in the breast (e.g., flat or inverted nipples) usually can have those problems corrected prior to pregnancy and subsequently breastfeed successfully.
- Women with small breasts can produce all the milk their babies need; there is no relationship between breast size and quantity of milk produced.
- Even after returning to work or school, many women can continue to breastfeed. They may alternate breastfeeding with bottle-feeding by other caregivers, express breast milk into a bottle that can be given by others, or breastfeed during breaks if the baby is nearby. Mothers can use a breast pump to express milk into a sterile bottle and then store it in a refrigerator or freezer. A schedule of expressing milk and using supplemental formula feedings is most successful if begun after 1 to 2 months of exclusive breastfeeding.
- Many modest women find that breastfeeding in public can be done discreetly with the breast covered by a loose-fitting blouse or baby blanket. To the casual observer, it appears that the woman is simply holding her infant closely.
- In the U.S., no state or territory has a law prohibiting breastfeeding. However, indecent exposure (including the exposure of women's breasts) has long been a common law or statutory offense. During the 1990s, some states, such as Florida and North Carolina, began to clarify the right to breastfeed and decriminalized public breastfeeding. Since then, several other states have passed similar laws.
- A breastfeeding mother can tell whether her baby is getting enough milk if the baby has 6 or more wet diapers each day and shows normal growth.
- Breastfeeding women can become pregnant. It's true that, when babies are exclusively breastfed, ovulation is delayed and the chances of becoming pregnant during the first 6 months after a birth are low. However, there is no guarantee that a lactating woman won't ovulate and get pregnant, so a reliable birth control method should be used.
- In many cases, mothers can breastfeed a premature and/or low birth weight infant. If the infant is unable to suckle, the mother can express milk and feed it to the infant. This type of feeding demands great maternal dedication; however, recent evidence indicates that human milk aids mental development in premature infants.[38] The fortification of human milk with certain nutrients (calcium, phosphorus, sodium, and protein) is often necessary to match the preterm infant's rapid growth.

Maternal Food Supply

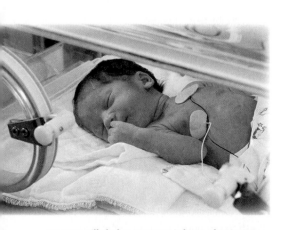

Human milk fed to preterm infants often must be fortified with certain nutrients to match their unique nutrient needs.

Compounds in the food that the mother eats can be secreted into her milk. Environmental contaminants, such as pollutants and pesticides, can appear in human milk. The risks of these substances are largely unknown. However, the benefits of human milk are well established and the effect of environmental contaminants on the breastfed infant have been seen mostly when the mother herself was suffering from the effects of the contaminants. A few measures a woman can take to counteract some known contaminants are to avoid freshwater fish from polluted waters, to carefully wash and peel fruits and vegetables, and to remove the fatty parts of meat, because pesticides concentrate in fat. In addition, a woman should not try to lose weight rapidly while nursing (no more than ¾ to 1 lb/week) because contaminants stored in her fat tissue might then enter her bloodstream and affect her milk. If a woman questions whether her milk is safe, especially if she has lived in an area known to have a high concentration of toxic wastes or environmental pollutants, she should consult her local health department.

Caffeine may make infants irritable, tense, and unable to sleep. Lactating women can prevent these adverse effects by avoiding caffeine-containing foods or medications or limiting intake to 1 or 2 cups of coffee, tea, or cola daily.

Certain foods or compounds in foods (e.g., cabbage, chocolate) may cause some infants to become upset or not want to eat. Some foods can impart flavors to milk that may affect an infant's desire to eat. For instance, in one study, when milk smelled of garlic, babies spent more time suckling. When it smelled of alcohol, they suckled less. If a woman notices a connection between her diet and the baby's fussiness or unwillingness to eat, she should avoid the offending food. It's a good idea to experiment to see if eating the food causes feeding problems again because the irritability or unwillingness may not be related to the mother's diet at all.

Maternal Lifestyle Choices

Substances related to lifestyle choices (e.g., alcohol, drugs, herbal and botanical products, nicotine) also are secreted into breast milk. The amount secreted is usually small (1 to 2% of the mother's dose) but may be a potent and harmful dose for a baby.

Alcohol, especially beer or wine, was recommended for centuries as a way for new mothers to relax and allow babies to nurse longer. However, research shows that consuming alcohol actually reduces milk output and causes babies to drink less and have disrupted sleep patterns. And infants are not as efficient as adults at breaking down alcohol, so the effects linger longer. The safest route for mothers and babies is to avoid alcohol altogether. However, lactating women who want to drink alcohol (beer, wine, or liquor) are advised to limit their intake and wait 3 to 4 hours before nursing again. The amount of alcohol in breast milk peaks about 30 to 60 minutes after the mother ingests it, then declines.

Medication use should be carefully considered by the lactating woman and her health-care provider. If a drug is necessary, she and the health-care provider need to decide whether the drug and lactation are compatible. If so, they can work out a plan for taking the drug and observing the infant's response. If the medication will be taken for a short time, the woman can express her milk by hand or with a breast pump and discard it. The baby can be fed formula until the mother is finished taking the medication. All illegal drugs should be avoided during lactation. The most commonly used illegal drugs, marijuana and cocaine, depress milk production and pass easily into breast milk. Marijuana in human milk slows infant development, and cocaine in milk causes babies to vomit and have tremors, breathing difficulties, and convulsions. Drug addicts should not breastfeed their infants.

Many herbal and botanical products contain druglike compounds that may appear in milk.[39] All herbal and botanical products should be used cautiously during lactation.

Smoking also affects breastfeeding success and safety. In comparison with non-smokers, women who smoke or breathe secondhand smoke produce less milk and their babies gain less weight. They also secrete nicotine in their milk, which can cause vomiting, slow breathing, increased blood pressure, and apathy in the infant. Lactating women, like pregnant women, are advised not to smoke. However, those who are smokers are advised to breastfeed because the benefits of breast milk outweigh the risk of nicotine exposure.

Breastfeeding may not be the optimal choice for some women. Alternatives to breastfeeding, along with the nutritional needs of infants, children, adolescents, and adults, are explored in Chapter 17.

Knowledge Check

1. How does maternal prepregnancy weight and age affect breastfeeding success?
2. What diseases are incompatible with breastfeeding?
3. What steps can pregnant and lactating women take to overcome common sociocultural factors that affect breastfeeding success?
4. What effects can lifestyle choices related to alcohol, drugs, herbal and botanical products, and smoking have on breastfed infants?

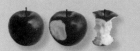 *Take Action*

Investigating Breastfeeding

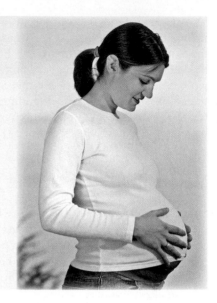

Maggie is 8 months pregnant and considering breastfeeding her baby. She doesn't know anyone who has breastfed and isn't sure that it is the best choice.

1. What additional information would you provide Maggie to help her make the most informed decision?

2. Where can Maggie get additional accurate information to help her decide?

3. If Maggie decides to breastfeed, what can Maggie do now to improve her chances of success?

Summary

16.1 A favorable pregnancy outcome is one lasting the full-term gestation period that results in a live, healthy infant weighing more than 5.5 pounds and permits the mother to return to her prepregnancy health status. Low birth weight babies weigh less than 5.5 pounds and have a high infant mortality rate. Low birth weight often is associated with premature birth. Full-term and preterm infants who weigh less than the expected weight for their duration of gestation are described as small for gestational age. A critical period is the specific time during embryonic or fetal life when cells develop into a particular tissue or organ. Nutrient deficiencies or excesses can interfere with normal development and cause physical or mental abnormalities. The zygote nourishes itself by absorbing secretions from glands in the uterus and digesting some of the uterine lining. Then, the placenta takes over the role of delivering nourishment to the developing offspring. The placenta contains both maternal and fetal blood vessels, which are so close together that nutrients and oxygen pass easily from the mother to the fetus and fetal wastes are shuttled from the fetus to the mother for excretion.

16.2 A pregnant woman needs additional calories and more of almost every nutrient than a non-pregnant woman to support the growth and development of the fetus, placenta, and mother's body. Pica, the eating of non-food substances, can have dire consequences for the pregnant woman and her fetus.

16.3 A pregnant woman's meal plan should include nutrient-dense foods from every food group. Special vitamin and mineral supplements formulated for pregnancy are prescribed routinely for pregnant women by most physicians. A low- or moderate-intensity exercise program offers physical and psychological benefits to a woman experiencing a normal, healthy pregnancy.

16.4 An infant's birth weight is closely related to length of gestation, the mother's prepregnancy weight, and the amount of weight she gains during pregnancy. The physical and hormonal changes that affect almost every aspect of the woman's body begin soon after the egg is fertilized and may cause nutrition-related problems, such as heartburn, constipation, morning sickness, and edema.

16.5 Lactation (breastfeeding) is a natural physiological process that occurs in the postpartum period, when the mother's breast secretes milk and suckles the offspring. Prolactin is the principal hormone that promotes milk production. The let-down reflex occurs when oxytocin causes milk to be released from the milk-producing lobules. The let-down reflex is easily inhibited by nervous tension, a lack of confidence, and fatigue. Colostrum is a thin, yellowish, "immature" milk that appears anytime from late pregnancy to several days postpartum. Mature human milk is thin and almost watery in appearance; with the possible exceptions of vitamin D and iron, it supplies all the nutrients the growing baby needs.

16.6 A lactating woman's DRI is based on the quantity of milk produced by the average mother, its nutrient content, and the amounts of her nutrient stores used to produce milk. If the mother's diet is poor for a prolonged period and she has depleted nutrient stores, the quantity of milk produced may decline. Maternal malnutrition must be extremely severe before the quality of milk produced drops. The average breastfeeding woman uses about 800 calories per day during the first 6 months of lactation to produce 750 ml of milk daily. Approximately 400 to 500 calories should come from her diet, with the remainder supplied by the fat stored during pregnancy. Breastfeeding offers benefits to the infant and mother.

16.7 Maternal factors that can negatively affect breastfeeding success include high prepregnancy weight, young age, long-term poor nutrient intake, certain diseases, lack of information and role models, and an inadequate support system. Compounds in the food that the mother eats, including contaminants, caffeine, alcohol, drugs, and nicotine, can be secreted into her milk.

Study Questions

1. Which of the following is true of a favorable pregnancy outcome?
   a. lasts longer than 37 weeks
   b. results in an infant weighing more than 5.5 pounds
   c. permits the mother to return to her prepregnancy health status
   d. all of the above

2. Iron needs rise significantly during pregnancy because _____.
   a. the fetus is building iron stores.
   b. the number of red blood cells increase in the mother
   c. the fetus breaks down red blood cells rapidly
   d. all of the above
   e. both a and b

3. A woman who begins pregnancy at a healthy weight should gain _____.
   a. 15 pounds or less
   b. 25 to 35 pounds
   c. 28 to 40 pounds
   d. none of the above

4. If development does not occur during a critical period, the embryo can make up for this development later when more nutrients are available.
   a. true
   b. false

5. The placenta delivers nutrients and oxygen to the fetus.
   a. true
   b. false

6. Compared with non-pregnant women, during the third trimester pregnant women need to increase calorie intake by about _____.
   a. 200 kcal
   b. 250 kcal
   c. 450 kcal
   d. 800 kcal

7. Prescription prenatal supplements often contain higher levels of which nutrient than those that can be purchased over the counter?
   a. vitamin A
   b. vitamin B-6
   c. calcium
   d. folic acid

8. Which of the following is *not* likely to increase the risk of poor pregnancy outcome?
   a. weight gain of less than 15 pounds
   b. a pregnancy within 12 months of a previous pregnancy
   c. a maternal age of 20 to 25 years
   d. limited educational achievement
   e. both c and d

9. Hormonal changes during pregnancy may cause _____.
   a. heartburn
   b. diarrhea
   c. edema
   d. both a and c

10. To cope with morning sickness, many women find relief by drinking a large glass of water on awakening in the morning.
    a. true
    b. false

11. Which of the following hormones promotes milk production?
    a. oxytocin
    b. prolactin
    c. estrogen
    d. placental hormone

12. The let-down reflex is triggered by _____.
    a. a baby suckling at the breast
    b. a baby crying
    c. thoughts about a baby
    d. all of the above

13. If a lactating woman's vitamin and mineral intakes exceed the RDA, increased levels of these nutrients may appear in the milk.

    a. true
    b. false

14. The thin, yellowish milk secreted in the first few days after birth is rich in antibodies and immune system cells.

    a. true
    b. false

15. Which of the following compounds can be secreted into human milk?

    a. alcohol
    b. food flavors
    c. drugs
    d. caffeine
    e. all of the above

Answer Key: 1-d; 2-e; 3-b; 4-b; 5-a; 6-c; 7-d; 8-c; 9-d; 10-b; 11-b; 12-d; 13-a; 14-a; 15-e

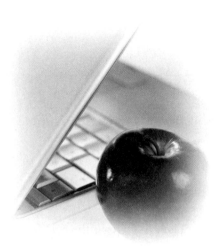

Websites

To learn more about the topics covered in this chapter, visit these websites.

Pregnancy

MarchofDimes.com

www.nlm.nih.gov/medlineplus/pregnancy.htm

health.discovery.com/centers/pregnancy/pregnancy.html

www.nichd.nih.gov/health/topics/pregnancy.cfm

www.mypyramid.gov/mypyramidmoms/index.html

fnic.nal.usda.gov

Fetal Alcohol Syndrome

www.cdc.gov/ncbddd/fas/default.htm

Breastfeeding

www.lalecheleague.org

www.breastfeeding.com

www.nal.usda.gov/wicworks

References

1. Kaiser LL, Allen LH. Position of the American Dietetic Association: Nutrition and lifestyle for a healthy pregnancy outcome. *J Am Diet Assoc*. 2002;102:1479.

2. Brundage S. Preconception health care. *American Family Physician*. 2002;65:2507.

3. National Academy of Science, Institute of Medicine, Food and Nutrition Board. *Nutrition during pregnancy*. Washington, DC: National Academy Press; 1990.

4. Hediger ML, Overpeck MD, Kuczmarski RJ, McGlynn A, Maurer KR, Davis WW. Muscularity and fatness of infants and young children born small- or large-for-gestational-age. *Pediatrics*. 1998;102:e60.

5. Prentice AM, Goldberg GR. Energy adaptations in human pregnancy: Limits and long-term consequences. *Am J Clin Nutr*. 2000;71:1226S.

6. Brundage S. Preconception health care. *Am Fam Physician*. 2002;65:2507.

7. King JC. Physiology of pregnancy and nutrient metabolism. *Am J Clin Nutr*. 2000;71:1218S.

8. Huxley RR. Nausea and vomiting in early pregnancy: Its role in placental development. *Ob Gyn*. 2000;95(5):779.

9. Allen L. Multiple micronutrients in pregnancy and lactation: An overview. *Am J Clin Nutr*. 2005;81:1206S.

10. Institute of Medicine, Food and Nutrition Board. *Dietary Reference Intakes for energy, carbohydrate, fiber, fat, fatty acids, cholesterol, protein, and amino acids*. Washington, DC: National Academy Press; 2002.

11. Institute of Medicine, Food and Nutrition Board. *Dietary Reference Intakes for vitamin A, vitamin K, arsenic, boron, chromium, copper, iodine, iron, manganese, molybdenum,*

nickel, silicon, vanadium, and zinc. Washington, DC: National Academy Press; 2001.

12. King JC. Determinants of maternal zinc status during pregnancy. *Am J Clin Nutr.* 2000;71:1334S.

13. Tamura T, Picciano M. Folate and human reproduction. *Am J Clin Nutr.* 2006;83:993.

14. Institute of Medicine, Food and Nutrition Board. *Dietary Reference Intakes for calcium, phosphorus, magnesium, vitamin D, and fluoride.* Washington, DC: National Academy Press; 1997.

15. Kelly A. Practical exercise advice during pregnancy. *Physician Sport Med.* 2005;33:24.

16. Hulsey T and others. Maternal prepregnant body mass index and weight gain related to low birth weight in South Carolina. *Southern Med J.* 2005;98:411.

17. Kabiru K, Raynor B. Obstetric outcomes associated with increase in BMI category during pregnancy. *Am J Ob Gyn.* 2004;191:928.

18. Galtier-Dereure F and others. Obesity and pregnancy: Complications and cost. *Am J Clin Nutr.* 2000;71:1242S.

19. Wong WY and others. Effects of folic acid and zinc sulfate on male factor subfertility: A double-blind, randomized, placebo-controlled trial. *Fertil Steril.* 2002;77:491.

20. Keen K and others. The plausibility of micronutrient deficiencies being a significant contributing factor to the occurrence of pregnancy complications. *J Nutr.* 2003;133:1597S.

21. Koebnick C and others. Long-term ovo-lacto vegetarian diet impairs vitamin B-12 status in pregnant women. *J Nutr.* 2004;134:3319.

22. World Health Organization. *Nutrient requirements for people living with HIV/AIDS.* Geneva, Switzerland: World Health Organization; 2003.

23. Patterson KB and others. Frequent detection of acute HIV infection in pregnant women. *AIDS.* 2007; 21:2303.

24. Levine R and others. Soluble endoglin and other circulating antiangiogenic factors in preeclampsia. *New Eng J Med.* 2006;355:992.

25. Hofmeyr G. Calcium supplementation during pregnancy for preventing hypertensive disorders and related problems. *Cochrane Database of Systematic Reviews.* 2006.

26. Trumbo P, Ellwood K. Supplemental calcium and risk reduction of hypertension, pregnancy-induced hypertension and preeclampsia: An evidence-based review by the US Food and Drug Administration. *Nutr Rev.* 2007;65:78.

27. Makrides M, Gibson RA. Long-chain polyunsaturated fatty acid requirements during pregnancy and lactation. *Am J Clin Nutr.* 2000;71:307.

28. Wagner L. Diagnosis and managements of preeclampsia. *Am Fam Physician.* 2004;70:2317.

29. Crowther C and others. Effect of treatment of gestational diabetes mellitus on pregnancy outcomes. *New Eng J Med.* 2005;352:2477.

30. Rosenburg T and others. Maternal obesity and diabetes as risk factors for adverse pregnancy outcomes: Differences among four racial/ethnic groups. *Am J Publ Health.* 2005;95:1545.

31. Eustace L and others. Fetal alcohol syndrome: A growing concern for health care professionals. *J Ob Gyn Neonat Nurs.* 2003;32:215.

32. Work Group on Breastfeeding, American Academy of Pediatrics. Breastfeeding and the use of human milk. *Pediatrics.* 1997;100:1035.

33. Field C. The immunological components of human milk and their effect on immune development in infants. *J Nutr.* 2005;135:1.

34. American Dietetic Association. Position of the American Dietetic Association: Promoting and supporting breastfeeding. *J Am Diet Assoc.* 2005;105:810.

35. Greer FR and others. Effects of early nutritional interventions on the development of atopic disease in infants and children: The role of maternal dietary restriction, breatfeeding, time of introduction of complementary foods, and hydrolyzed formulas. *Pediatrics.* 2008;121:183.

36. Ram KT and others. Duration of lactation is associated with lower prevalence of the Metabolic Syndrome in midlife—SWAN, the Study of Women's Health across the Nation. *Am J Obstet Gynecol.* 2008;198:268.

37. Department of Health and Human Services, Office on Women's Health. *HHS blueprint for action on breastfeeding.* Washington, DC: USDHHS; 2000.

38. Vohr B and others. Persistent beneficial effects of breast milk ingested in the neonatal intensive care unit on outcomes of extremely low birth weight infants at 30 months of age. *Pediatrics.* 2007;120:e953.

39. Seely D and others. Safety and efficacy of panax giseng during pregnancy and lactation. *Can J Clin Pharmacol.* 2008;15:e87

17 *Nutrition during the Growing Years*

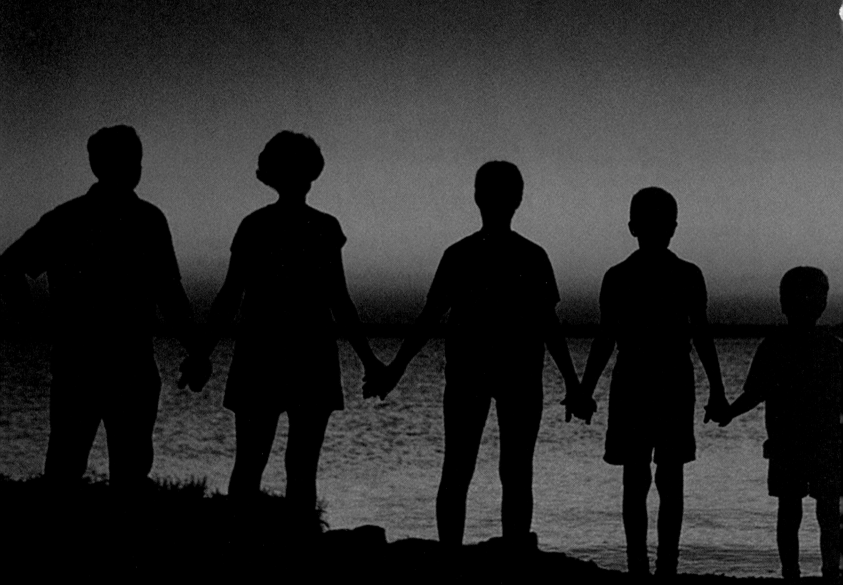

A nutritious diet supports normal growth and development throughout the growing years. Learn more at www.cdc.gov.

STUDENT LEARNING OUTCOMES

After studying this chapter, you will be able to:

1. Describe normal growth and development during infancy, childhood, and adolescence and the effect of nutrition on growth and development.

2. Describe the calorie and nutrient needs of infants, children, and adolescents.

3. Compare the nutritional qualities of human milk and infant formula.

4. Explain the rationale—from the standpoints of both nutrition and physical development—for the delay in feeding infants solid foods until 4 to 6 months of age.

5. Describe the recommended rate and sequence for introducing solid foods into an infant's diet.

6. Discuss the factors that affect the food intake of children and adolescents.

7. Plan nutritious diets for infants, children, and adolescents using MyPyramid.

8. Describe the potential nutrition-related problems that may occur during the growing years and their impact on future health.

In the span of less than 2 decades, a helpless human newborn grows and develops into an independent, physically mature adult. This transformation is guided by genetic endowment and is highly dependent on an adequate supply of energy and nutrients. More than 14 million calories, 430 pounds of protein, 14 pounds of calcium, and vast quantities of every other nutrient are needed over the course of the growing years to develop into a healthy adult.[1,2]

Current trends in nutrition and overall health among children and adolescents in North America indicate that more children are receiving vaccinations than ever before, fewer teenagers are giving birth, and fewer children and teens are living in poverty. In contrast to this good news, the percent of children and teenagers who are obese, have Metabolic Syndrome and type 2 diabetes, and are not getting enough sleep is rising. In addition, physical activity is dropping as "screen time" (use of computers, television, and videos) increases. Milk intake is down and soft drink consumption is up. Whole grains, fruits, and vegetables also are in short supply in children's diets.

This chapter will explore the effect of nutrition, from the beginning of infancy to the end of adolescence, on growth, development, and health. Because of the critical importance of adequate nutrition in infancy and the difficulties encountered in feeding some infants, a special emphasis is placed on this developmental stage.

🍑 17.1 Growing Up

As humans move from infancy to adulthood, height and weight increase. Body composition changes and organs mature. Normal growth and development are highly dependent on calorie and nutrient intake. Insufficient calories and nutrients, along with too little sleep and lack of loving care, can impair one's ability to thrive (grow and develop to the fullest physical and mental genetic potential).

When nutrients are missing at critical developmental phases, growth slows and may even stop. As with the fetus, the effects of poor dietary intake in infancy, childhood, and adolescence depend on its severity, timing, and duration. Overall, eating a poor diet during the growing years hampers the cell division that occurs at critical stages. Consuming an adequate diet later usually cannot compensate for lost growth because the hormonal and other conditions needed for growth likely will not be present. Once the time for growth ceases, a sufficient nutrient intake helps maintain health and weight but cannot make up for lost growth.

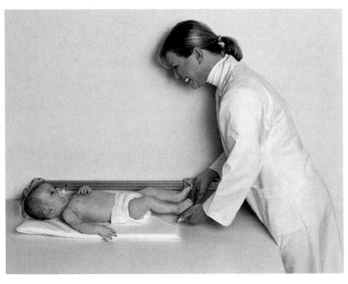

The term *length* is used in place of *height* when referring to children less than 2 to 3 years old because young children are measured lying on their backs with their body straight and legs extended.

▶ The rapid weight gain during adolescence is difficult for many adolescent girls to accept because they fear they are becoming fat. Consequently, they may restrict calories and impair their bodies' chances to "grow up."

Height and Weight

Physical growth rate is at its peak velocity during infancy, which causes nutrient needs, per unit of body weight, to be at their lifetime highest level. Most babies have doubled their birth weight by 4 to 6 months of age. By their first birthdays, they have tripled their birth weight and increased in length by 50%.[3]

In contrast to the rapid and usually smooth increases in height and weight of the first year, the physical growth rate of childhood is much slower and occurs in bursts.[2] In fact, it is normal for weight and height to remain unchanged for weeks, then suddenly spurt up. Nutrient and calorie needs, as well as the child's appetite, tend to rise and fall in response to these normal growth fluctuations. Healthy children grow a few inches taller each year. As you can see in Figure 17-1, they gain 4 to 6 pounds (2 to 3 kg) or so yearly until age 8 or 9; then the rate of weight gain increases to about 8 to 10 pounds annually until just before puberty, when many children normally store a few pounds of extra body fat.

Adolescence, the transition from childhood to adulthood, is one of the most rapid phases of physical growth. One-third of all the growth in a lifetime occurs during this stage. Adolescence starts with the onset of **puberty,** which, on the average, begins between the ages of 10 and 13 in girls and approximately 2 years later in boys. Puberty ends about 8 to 10 years after it starts, when the person is physically mature and capable of reproduction. Early-maturing girls may begin their growth spurt as early as age 7 to 8, whereas early-maturing boys may begin their growth spurt by age 9 to 10.[4]

When puberty begins, height and weight increase rapidly and the extra fat stored just before puberty usually decreases if the child did not enter puberty obese. The rate of growth in height peaks about 18 months after puberty begins, and then it slows down. For most females, height increases at its fastest rate at age 11, then slowly decelerates until they reach their adult height at about age 14 or 15. Girls usually begin menstruating during this growth spurt, and they gain little additional height 2 years after menarche. Most males experience peak velocity in height increases at age 13 years and attain their adult height around age 18. Both males and females may continue growing taller into their twenties. During adolescence, females grow about 10 inches (25 cm) in height and boys gain about 12 inches (30 cm). When they finish growing, teens will have gained about 15% of their adult height and weigh 45 to 85% more than when they entered this stage.

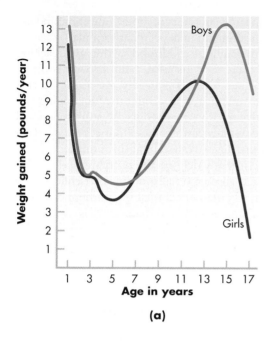

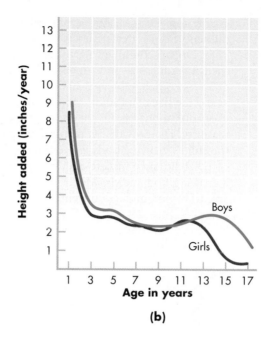

Figure 17-1 Growth rates for height and weight. The higher the line in any year, the greater the amount of annual gain compared with other years. Large weight gains occur in both infancy and puberty, whereas the very high length gain in infancy is never reached again. If graphs such as these were plotted in smaller time segments, they would appear as zigzag lines, rather than smooth lines, reflecting short, periodic spurts and plateaus in growth that occur from infancy to the end of adolescence.

Body Composition

As males and females move through the growing years, body composition changes, too. As you'll see later in this chapter, these changes affect nutrient needs in many ways. The proportion of body water declines during the first 2 or 3 years of life, at which point it achieves levels similar to those of adults.

The proportion of lean body tissue increases as infants and children grow older. Males and females enter adolescence with similar percentages of lean body tissue; however, during adolescence males secrete testosterone, which causes them to gain more muscle mass, develop a heavier skeleton, and build a greater quantity of red blood cells than females. By the end of adolescence, females have two-thirds as much lean body tissue as males.

The proportion of body fat rises from birth to age 1, then declines slowly until age 7, at which point it begins gradually to increase again. During adolescence, body fat continues to rise in females, but it declines in males. This is because females secrete estrogen, which stimulates the accumulation of subcutaneous fat. This body fat is essential for sexual maturation.[5] When a female's body fat equals about 16 to 17% of body weight and her body weight reaches about 100 pounds (46 kg), menstrual periods begin and become regular once body fat reaches approximately 22%. The increasing regularity of the menstrual periods indicates that a female is nearing adult levels of body fat and is ending her growth. When adolescence ends, females have twice as much body fat as males.

Researchers once speculated that overfeeding during infancy may increase adipose tissue cell numbers. Today, it is known that the number of adipose cells also can increase even in adulthood. Still, if energy intake is limited during infancy to keep down the number of adipose cells, the growth and development of other organ systems, especially the brain and nervous system, also may be severely restricted. In addition, most obese infants become normal-weight preschoolers without excessive diet restrictions. The risk of stunted growth and development makes it unwise to greatly restrict dietary intake of infants, as well as that of children and teens.

Body Organs and Systems

In addition to the obvious outward changes in weight and height, babies, children, and teens are maturing inside. For instance, during infancy the kidneys double in size and begin to eliminate waste more efficiently. The stomach gradually increases its capacity and begins secreting digestive enzymes. By about age 4 to 6 months, the digestive tract has matured greatly, too. These changes enable infants to eat larger amounts of food at mealtime and use nutrients from a greater variety of foods than just human milk or infant formula.

Organs continue to grow and develop throughout childhood, with many reaching their full adult size and function during this stage. For instance, brain growth is three-quarters complete by age 2 and is finished by age 6 to 10 years. By age 9, the heart is nearly the size of an adult's and the respiratory system is approaching the functioning level of adulthood. By late childhood, the digestive tract has reached its full adult functional maturity. The growth and maturation of these systems permits them to meet the needs of the child's growing body. For example, a mature digestive system absorbs nutrients more completely, and a mature circulatory system efficiently delivers the nutrients and oxygen a growing body needs. More complete nutrient absorption also means that children are able to begin building nutrient stores that can help them meet the high nutrient demands of adolescence. During adolescence, any remaining growth and maturation is completed. The most obvious changes during adolescence are the maturation of the reproductive system and the development of secondary sexual characteristics.

Knowledge Check

1. Approximately how much would you expect a baby born weighing 8 pounds to weigh at his or her first birthday?
2. At which stage of the growing years (infancy, childhood, adolescence) is growth the fastest?
3. How does body composition differ between males and females at the beginning and end of adolescence?
4. How does a mature digestive system help support growth?

17.2 Physical Growth

The single best indicator of a child's nutritional status is growth. Thus, health-care professionals use growth charts matched to the child's gender to determine if growth is progressing normally. Figure 17-2 shows sample growth charts. They have several **percentile** curves (shown in blue) because children grow at different rates—many of which can be considered normal. The percentile curve a specific child follows depends on dietary intake and genetic potential. For example, a child who is adequately nourished and has tall parents may fall in the 90th percentile for stature-for-age and 75th percentile for weight-for-age. Also, by having several percentile curves, health-care professionals can compare one child's growth with the growth of others of the same age. For instance, if a boy's stature-for-age falls at the 25th percentile, he is shorter than 75% of the other boys of the same age. If a girl's weight-for-age is at the 95th percentile, she is heavier than all but 5% of girls of the same age. If a child's BMI-for-age is at the 50th percentile, the child has a lower BMI than half of all children of the same age.

Tracking Growth

Growth should be tracked over time to identify a child's growth percentile and determine if growth is progressing normally. It takes 1 to 3 years for an infant to establish his or her own percentile. (Preterm infants may move up several percentiles—especially in length-for-age—because they usually experience "catch-up" growth and grow to the size they would have been had they been full-term.) Once growth percentiles are established, a healthy child who is eating a nutritious diet will maintain about the same percentile curves from year to year (shown in green on Fig. 17-2). Small growth spurts and lags are expected, but a sudden jump up or down 2 or more percentile curves may signal that a child is experiencing growth problems caused by calorie excesses or deficits, nutrient in-

percentile Classification of a measurement of a unit into divisions of 100 units—for example, an individual's rank in a group of others of the same age and gender.

▶ For ages ranging from birth to 36 months, growth chart options include weight-for-age, length-for-age, weight-for-length, and head circumference-for-age. For ages 2 to 20 years, growth charts are available for weight-for-age, stature-for-age, and body mass index (BMI)-for-age.

▶ BMI has fixed cutoff points (e.g., a BMI of 25 for an adult is considered overweight). As Figure 17-2 shows, this is not true for children, for whom BMI is both gender- and age-specific.

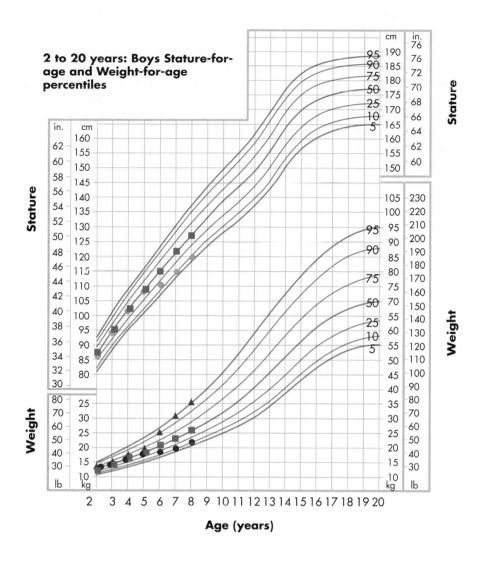

2 to 20 years: Boys Stature-for-age and Weight-for-age percentiles

Age (years)

Figure 17-2 These growth charts are used to track the growth of males between the ages of 2 and 20. This growth chart depicts the gains in weight and stature that are expected as males increase in age. A certain weight and stature (height) correspond to a percentile value, which is a ranking of the person among 100 peers. The green squares represent a boy who is adequately nourished and growing normally. Notice how this boy continues along the same percentile curve from year to year. He is in the 50th percentile for weight from ages 2 to 8. The purple triangles show what might happen to his weight if the boy begins overeating. The red dots illustrate how weight is affected if the boy's access to food is restricted. The orange dots indicate how height can be affected if food restrictions are prolonged and severe. Growth charts for all age groups and genders are available at www.cdc.gov/growthcharts and in Appendix K.

adequacies, illness, or psychosocial problems.[4] If, for example, a child begins overeating, BMI-for-age may jump several percentile curves (shown in purple on Fig. 17-2). When BMI-for-age reaches the 85th percentile, the child is overweight; when it reaches the 95th percentile, the child is obese.[6] At the 95th percentile, the diagnosis of obesity can be established if a physical exam indicates the child is truly overfat, which is generally the case at this percentile.

If a child's access to food is restricted, BMI-for-age may drop to a lower percentile (shown in red on Fig. 17-2). A child is underweight when BMI-for-age drops below the 5th percentile. If food restriction is prolonged and severe, stature-for-age also may drop to a lower percentile (shown in orange on Fig. 17-2). Unless the child has short parents, he or she is likely experiencing growth stunting if stature-for-age drops below the 5th percentile. Special growth charts that include the 3rd and 97th percentiles are available for medical specialists to use when caring for children growing at the outer percentiles.

In early physical checkups, a health professional usually measures the head circumference as another means of assessing growth, especially brain growth. The brain grows faster in infancy than at any other time of life, with this rapid growth ending at about 18 months of age. How nutritional status affects brain development and intelligence quotient (IQ) is difficult to measure because scientists haven't figured out how to separate the effects of nature from those of nurture. However, several studies have determined that breastfed infants have higher IQs than infants fed with infant formula.[4] At the same time, studies from Central America suggest that IQ after age 5 years relates more closely to the amount of schooling a child receives than to nutritional intake during childhood.

Indicators of Nutritional Status

At Risk of Developmental Problems
Birth to 2 years: head circumference-for-age < 5th percentile or > 95th percentile

Stunted Growth
Birth to 2 years: length-for-age < 5th percentile

2 to 20 years: stature-for-age < 5th percentile

Underweight
Birth to 2 years: weight-for-length < 5th percentile

2 to 20 Years: BMI-for-age <5th percentile

Overweight
Birth to 2 years: weight-for-length > 95th percentile

2 to 20 years: BMI-for-age ≥85th < 95th percentile

Obese
2 to 20 years: BMI-for-age ≥ 95th percentile or BMI ≥30, whichever is smaller

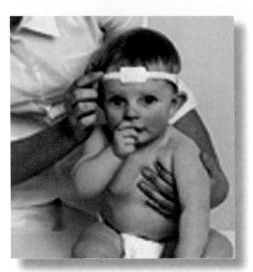

Brain growth is faster in infancy than in any other stage of life. Head circumference measurements can help determine if growth is proceeding as expected.

epiphyses End segments of long bones (called the epiphyseal plate or growth plate) that contain a thin area of active bone growth. Once this growth stops, adult height is attained and no further significant growth in height can occur.

Using Growth Chart Information

A child's growth rate reflects calorie and nutrient intake.[2] BMI-for-age (or weight-for-length for children younger than 2 years old) is a good indicator of recent nutritional status. An insufficient diet in the immediate past causes a drop in BMI because weight decreases while height stays relatively the same. Excessive calorie intake results in a rise in BMI because weight increases without a corresponding increase in height. Stature-for-age is a good indicator of long-term nutritional status because undernutrition usually must be prolonged before stature is affected noticeably.

Infants and young children who do not grow at the expected rate for several months and are dramatically smaller or shorter than other children the same age, especially those who fall below the 5th percentile, are said to experience **failure to thrive**. Although physical abnormalities (e.g., heart defects, cleft palate), infections, intestinal problems, and hard to diagnose inborn errors of metabolism cause some cases of failure to thrive, nutrition or feeding problems are the cause of many cases. Nutrition problems include a lack of access to sufficient and/or appropriate food caused by poverty, and parents who do not know how to meet a child's nutrient needs. Feeding problems may occur as a result of physical problems (e.g., the child has a weak sucking ability), poor feeding techniques (e.g., the parents limit feeding time), mental depression in the mother, and/or negative socialization factors (e.g., poor parent:infant relations).[6,7] Infants not only need food; they also need to be cuddled, hear voices, and have eye contact, especially at feeding times. In all cases, a physician should determine the actual cause of failure to thrive and work with parents to treat the problem.[4]

The long-term effects of failure to thrive caused by nutrition and food problems depend on the severity and length of time the child is malnourished. Continually receiving minimal quantities of food may permanently and irreversibly stunt growth and development. However, if dietary restrictions are followed by an adequate diet and positive social stimulation, children of all ages are likely to experience a faster than expected growth rate and "catch up" to where they would have been, had malnutrition not occurred.[8]

Growth in height ceases when the growth plates at the ends of the bones, called **epiphyses,** fuse. This process begins at around 14 years of age in girls and 15 years of age in boys and ends at about 5 years later. For these reasons, a 16-year-old undernourished girl who is 4 feet 8 inches tall cannot attain her full adult height simply by eating better. She will be able to increase the diameter of her muscles, but overall muscle growth will be limited by the length of her bones.[4] Catch-up growth is possible even when growth retardation has been severe and prolonged, if the epiphyses have not closed.

CASE STUDY

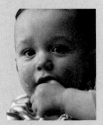

Damon is a 7-month-old boy who was taken into a clinic for a routine checkup. On examination, he seemed thin, and he plotted on the growth chart at the 25th percentile for weight and the 50th percentile for length. His physician scheduled a follow-up appointment in 3 months. At the 10-month-visit, Damon appeared sluggish. He was again plotted on the growth chart and was now at the 5th percentile for weight, but still at the 50th percentile for length. A registered dietitian interviewed Damon's 16-year-old mother to collect information on his dietary intake. The 24-hour diet recall consisted of 2 bottles of infant formula, 3 bottles of Kool-Aid®, and a hot dog. However, the mother was still in school, and at night she often left Damon with a neighbor so that she could go out for a few hours. Thus, she was not aware of all that he ate. What problems do you think are present in Damon's diet? What potential dangers await Damon if his health status continues along this current growth trend?

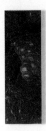

Knowledge Check

1. What factors affect the percentile growth curve a child follows?
2. Why are growth charts used to track growth over time?
3. What factors contribute to failure to thrive?
4. When is it no longer possible to grow taller?

17.3 Nutrient Needs

All of the changes that occur during the growing years influence energy and nutrient intakes and needs, but growth rate has the greatest effect. The faster the growth rate, the greater the nutrient and calorie needs per pound of body weight. Thus, the greatest needs, pound for pound, occur during infancy, when growth is at its peak velocity. Although calorie and nutrient needs per pound of body weight steadily decline after infancy, the total quantity of calories and nutrients needed rises throughout childhood because the body grows larger. During puberty, nutrient needs, like growth rate, increase sharply and gender differences in nutrient needs become more obvious (Fig. 17-3). The total quantities of nutrients and calories required are greater during adolescence than any other time except pregnancy and lactation. Males need more of many nutrients than females do because males are larger, develop more muscle mass and bone density, and have a longer, more intense growth period.

Energy

The rapid growth and high metabolic rate of infants and toddlers cause their calorie needs, pound for pound, to be 2 to 4 times greater than adults'. Calorie needs for metabolic rate are high mainly because an infant's body has a large surface area, which allows a great deal of body heat to be lost. Thus, many calories are used to keep the body warm. Newborns need approximately 50 calories per pound each day to support their rapid growth and high basal metabolic rate. After 2 to 3 months of age, calorie needs drop to approximately 43 calories per pound daily and remain at about this level until age 3 years or so. The slower growth of childhood in comparison with infancy translates into a gradual reduction in calorie needs per pound of body weight. For example, calorie needs per

▶ From birth until age 2 years, basal metabolic rate continues to rise rapidly. After age 2, it rises slowly until puberty, when it increases dramatically. After puberty, basal metabolic rate rises slowly until about age 30; then it gradually decreases throughout life.

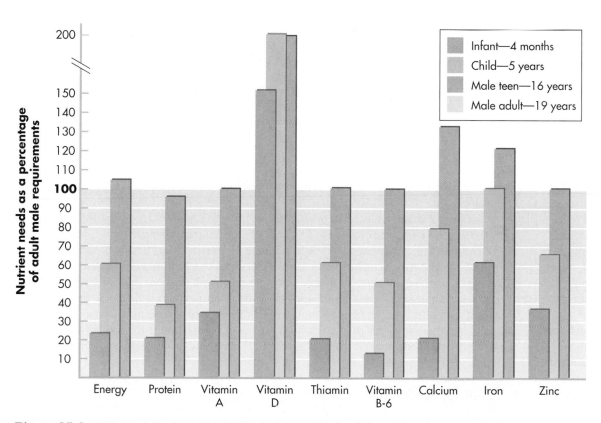

Figure 17-3 Compared with adults, infants' relative energy needs are lower than their needs for other nutrients, as illustrated by the different heights of the orange bars. Thus, infants need to obtain relatively larger amounts of nutrients from a smaller intake of food than adults. This also is true for young children (blue bars), but to a lesser extent.

pound decrease to 32 by age 5 and drop to about half that amount by age 15. Although calorie needs *per pound* decrease during the growing years, total calorie needs rise steadily and peak for females at about age 15 or 16 and for males around age 18.[2]

Protein

▶ The American Academy of Pediatrics recently indicated that reduced fat milk is appropriate for children aged 12 months to 2 years for whom overweight is a concern or who have a family history of obesity, high blood cholesterol levels, or cardiovascular disease. Parents are advised to consult with a registered dietitian to ensure low fat diets for children at risk for heart disease adequately meet dietary needs.[37]

Daily protein needs in infancy are roughly 1.5 g/kg of body weight daily to support their rapid rate of tissue synthesis—that is nearly twice as much protein per pound of body weight as adults. However, extra protein can be a problem for babies. Recall that the nitrogen from protein consumed in excess of need must be removed and excreted via the kidneys. Thus, large intakes of protein, as well as minerals, may overtax infants' immature kidneys and cause dehydration. Young infants need all the essential amino acids that adults do, as well as some others that are also considered essential for infants.

During childhood and early adolescence, protein needs per pound of body weight are lower than during infancy but are 20 to 40% higher than in adulthood.[2] Children's protein needs are affected greatly by the growth and maturation of body organs. The protein needs for children 1 to 3 years is 1.1 g/kg of body weight/day, dropping to 0.95 g/kg of body weight/day (34 to 52 g/day) for older children. Protein needs in adolescence are slightly higher than in adulthood because teens are increasing their lean body mass.

Protein malnutrition during the growing years can have profound, lifelong consequences. Physical development will be impaired if protein intake is inadequate or if calories are restricted to the point that protein must be used for energy. Inadequate protein intakes are uncommon in technologically developed countries, such as the U.S. and Canada; only excessive dilution of infant formula with water or severely restricted food intake is likely to lead to low protein intake. Dietary protein inadequacies, however, are a leading contributor to childhood illness, delayed or stunted growth, and death in developing countries.

Fat

▶ The National Cholesterol Education Program (NCEP) is designed to decrease heart disease by reducing the number of Americans with high blood cholesterol. To achieve this goal, the NCEP, American Academy of Pediatrics, and American Heart Association recommend screening children over the age of 2 years who have a parent with high blood cholesterol or a parent or grandparent with heart disease before age 55. Children and teens with other risk factors, such as high blood cholesterol levels, obesity, high blood pressure, diabetes mellitus, a sedentary lifestyle, or cigarette smoking, also should be screened. Those with elevated total cholesterol and/or low-density lipoprotein (LDL) cholesterol levels should reduce dietary saturated fat and cholesterol. If after dietary intervention LDL levels remain very high in children over age 8, medication is indicated.[37] Visit www.nhlbi. nih.gov/about/ncep/index.htm to learn more about the NCEP.

Fat is an important part of infants' diets. It provides constituents such as cholesterol and essential fatty acids. In addition, because it contains many calories in a small volume, fat can meet infants' high calorie demands without overfilling their small stomachs.

Total fat should account for about 40 to 55% of a baby's calorie intake.[2] Infants, as well as children and teens, need at least 5 grams of essential fatty acids each day. In infancy, the fatty acids arachidonic acid and docosahexaenoic acid have especially important roles—the eyes and nervous system, especially the brain, depend on them for normal development.

Heart disease has its roots in childhood. However, dietary recommendations meant to reduce the risk of heart disease do *not* apply to children younger than 2 years old unless children are at increased risk for heart disease. In fact, many health experts, including those from the American Academy of Pediatrics and the National Cholesterol Education Program, warn against low-fat diets before age 2 because they can deprive young children of nutrients and calories and impair growth. Most health experts believe it is wise to reduce fat intake gradually between ages 2 and 5 until children are getting an average of 30 to 35% of their calories from fat. As fat intake declines, children should replace fat calories with nutrient-rich foods, such as fruits, vegetables, lean meats, and low-fat dairy products.

Carbohydrate

Lactose is the primary carbohydrate in the diets of most infants.[2] Starch intake increases when solid foods, such as baby cereals and vegetables, are added to an infant's diet. Once the diet includes foods other than human milk or infant formula, children should slowly increase their starch intake to equal about half their total calorie intake and limit simple carbohydrate intake. Many children and teens consume much larger amounts of simple carbohydrates than recommended.

Fiber intake recommendations for children less than age 1 are not yet set. However, after age 1, the daily Adequate Intake is 14 grams of total fiber per 1000 calories eaten.[2] Many children in the U.S. do not consume sufficient fiber.[2] High fiber diets are not recommended for children because they tend to be high in bulk and inadequate in calories. In addition, they may bind minerals and block absorption to the extent that deficiencies occur.

Water

Water is of critical importance throughout the life cycle. But this nutrient is of special importance for babies because their need for water, per pound of body weight, is greater than that of older humans. One reason babies need more water is that their body surface area per pound of weight is about 3 times greater than adults'; thus, babies lose much more of their body water through the skin. A second reason is that infants have proportionately more body water than adults and turn over body water 7 times faster than adults. A third reason is that the high metabolic rate of infants (about twice that of adults) produces a greater quantity of wastes that need to be excreted by the kidneys and lungs. A final reason is that a newborn's kidneys are only about half as efficient as adult kidneys. As a result, infants use much more water than adults use to wash away the same amount of waste in the urine.

A young baby's need for water is usually met by human milk or formula. However, infants need supplementary water when they have diarrhea, vomiting, or fever or when the weather is hot. Infants also need supplementary water once they begin eating foods other than human milk and formula because the amount of waste that must be filtered out by the kidneys and excreted in the urine increases. Feeding cow milk to infants who are less than 1 year old is not recommended for many reasons, one reason being it produces a greater amount of waste than either human milk or infant formula.[9]

Giving infants too much water can be harmful, too, because it can lead to water intoxication. Overdiluting infant formula and feeding water instead of formula or human milk are the most common causes of water intoxication. Overall, it is best to limit supplemental fluids to about 4 ounces (120 ml) per day, unless a physician thinks a greater need exists because of disease or other conditions. In cases of disease, a physician likely will recommend special fluid-replacement formulas containing electrolytes, such as sodium and potassium. Fluid-replacement formulas are available in supermarkets and pharmacies to treat dehydration; they should not be confused with bottled water.

Vitamins and Minerals

All vitamins and minerals play an important role in supporting normal growth, but some are of particular concern during the growing years. For example, throughout the growing years, iron deficiency anemia is common. Children and adolescents also consume too little calcium, zinc, folate, and vitamins A and C. Many newborns have low stores of fluoride, vitamin K, and vitamin D.

Iron

Healthy full-term infants are born with internal iron stores. However, by the time birth weight doubles, usually by 4 to 6 months of age, iron stores are depleted. If the mother was iron-deficient during pregnancy, these iron stores will be exhausted even sooner. To maintain a desirable iron status, the American Academy of Pediatrics recommends that breastfed infants receive iron supplementation and formula-fed infants be given an iron-fortified formula starting at birth.[4] Low iron infant formulas are sometimes prescribed to treat infants with various intestinal problems, but their use is discouraged. In addition, infants need solid foods to supply extra iron by about 6 months of age. In fact, this need for iron is a major consideration in deciding when to introduce solid foods.

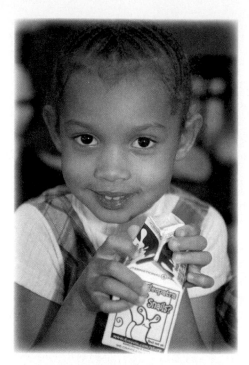

Getting sufficient calcium during childhood is difficult if milk is excluded from the diet. However, overconsumption of milk can displace other foods and lead to nutrition-related problems, such as iron deficiency anemia.

CRITICAL THINKING

Tatiana has been breastfeeding her baby exclusively since he was born 7 months ago. When she and her husband took the baby for his checkup, they were told that he was anemic. They were very surprised because they thought that human milk contained all the nutrients the baby needed for the first year of life. How might you explain the baby's anemia?

Children 1 to 2 years old are particularly vulnerable to iron deficiency anemia because their diets often are dominated by milk, a low iron food, and most are no longer receiving iron-fortified formula. In addition, they typically do not like meat or have difficulty chewing it. In some cases, intestinal parasites contribute to iron deficiency. Iron-fortified cereal and easily chewed meats (e.g., ground beef) can help children boost iron intake; serving iron-rich food with vitamin C–rich food increases the absorption of this mineral.

Teens also are vulnerable to iron deficiency anemia because their need increases by about 40% for males and nearly 90% for females during this life stage.[10] Much of the increase, especially in males, results from expanding lean body mass, which directly incorporates substantial quantities of iron. As the body grows, blood volume also increases, including red blood cells, which contain iron. In addition, with the onset of menstrual periods, adolescent females need additional iron to replace the blood lost. About 10% of teenagers have low iron stores or iron deficiency anemia. Iron deficiency anemia sometimes occurs in girls after they start menstruating (particularly those with heavy menstrual flows) and in boys during their growth spurt when they are building large amounts of lean body tissue.

If anemia does develop, iron supplements are used under a physician's guidance. Fortunately, childhood anemia is less common today in North America, probably because of children's use of iron-fortified breakfast cereals and the Special Supplemental Nutrition Program for Women, Infants, and Children (WIC). WIC emphasizes the importance of iron-fortified formulas and cereals and distributes them to low-income parents of infants and preschool children considered to be at nutritional risk.

Calcium

Optimum calcium intake and weight-bearing exercise throughout the growing years are important to forming strong bones. Calcium needs rise sharply starting around age 9 years and remain high until the end of adolescence, largely because bones are growing longer and denser. In fact, the majority of bone formation occurs between the ages of 9 and 18. Less than optimal calcium intakes may lead to decreased bone density and a greater risk of osteoporosis later in life. Unfortunately, teens' calcium intake usually falls well below the RDA, although males are more likely to have adequate calcium intake than females. Many teenage females replace calcium-rich milk, which they perceive to be "fattening," with calcium-poor soft drinks.

Fluoride

Both the American Dental Association and the American Academy of Pediatrics recommend fluoride supplements for those between the ages of 6 months and 16 years whose drinking water is low in fluoride.[1] Parents should consult their dentist for advice on meeting their children's need for fluoride.

Zinc

Although zinc deficiency does not appear to be a problem, many children and teens in the U.S. may be consuming too little. Low intakes occur because children consume small portions of rich sources, such as meat. In addition, because the *2005 Dietary Guidelines for Americans* suggests that children over age 2 years follow a diet low in saturated fat and cholesterol, rich sources of zinc as well as iron may be lacking in their diets. Low zinc intake during the growing years may impair growth. Breakfast cereal fortified with zinc can help provide this mineral.

Folate

The diets of many older children and teenagers are low in folate.[11] This is probably because vegetable intake tends to be less than recommended. Also, during the teenage years, meals frequently are eaten away from home—compared with foods prepared at home, cafeteria and restaurant foods tend to be lower in folate, as well as vitamins A and C. Insufficient intakes of these vitamins may impair normal growth. The low folate intake of teenage girls is of particular concern as they reach childbearing age because folate deficiency can lead to neural tube defects in their offspring.

Vitamin D

Vitamin D is of special importance during the growing years because of its role in normal bone development.[12] A lack of vitamin D will lead to the bone deformations seen in rickets (see Chapter 12). Ample vitamin D is provided by brief exposure to sunlight daily. When sunlight exposure is limited, as is often the case in northern latitudes, dietary vitamin D is needed. Infant formula supplies vitamin D to infants. The American Academy of Pediatrics recommends that breastfed infants born to vitamin D deficient women or infants not exposed to sufficient sunlight receive a 200 IU vitamin D supplement daily.[13]

Vitamin K

Infants are at risk of vitamin K deficiency because they are born with little or no vitamin K stores and they have sterile intestines. The vitamin K–producing bacteria that thrive in the intestines begin to grow when a baby is fed for the first time. However, it may take several weeks for the bacteria to multiply to a level that can provide the infant with adequate vitamin K. In the meantime, infants have low vitamin K levels and may experience slowed blood clotting and unchecked bleeding.[10] To prevent these problems, the American Academy of Pediatrics recommends that all infants receive a dose of vitamin K at birth, and some state laws require it.

Vitamin and Mineral Supplements

With the exception of a vitamin K supplement for newborns, an iron supplement for breastfed infants, a vitamin B-12 supplement for breastfed infants of vegan mothers, a vitamin D supplement for some infants, and a fluoride supplement for infants, children, and teens with an unfluoridated water supply, routine nutrient supplementation is not needed by healthy children and teens.[14] However, supplements may be recommended for children and teens who are poor eaters, vegans, pregnant, on programs to manage obesity, and/or deprived, neglected, or abused. The American Academy of Pediatrics suggests that these children and teens may benefit from a children's multivitamin and mineral supplement not exceeding 100% of the RDA or Adequate Intakes. Still, as mentioned previously, supplements are not a substitute for a healthy diet.

▶ The warning given to parents to keep medicines (including vitamin and mineral supplements) out of the reach of children and not treat them as candy cannot be overemphasized. The most common cause of poisoning in children is overdoses of supplements, especially those containing iron. Just 6 high-potency iron pills can be fatal for a 1-year-old. Iron poisoning causes bloody diarrhea, shock, liver damage, coma, and even death. Immediate medical care is essential because once the iron is absorbed into the body it is very difficult (if not impossible) to remove.

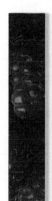

Knowledge Check

1. Why do adolescent males need more of many nutrients than females?
2. Why are the calorie and protein needs of infants, per pound of body weight, higher than adults'?
3. What are the recommended fat intake levels for infants and young children?
4. Why is the need for water of critical importance during infancy?
5. Why are children 1 to 2 years old vulnerable to iron deficiency anemia?
6. Why do calcium needs rise sharply during adolescence?
7. What vitamin and mineral supplements are recommended for infants, children, and teens?

17.4 Feeding Babies: Human Milk and Formula

Parents of a new baby have a thousand things to do, but menu planning isn't one of them. With few exceptions, human milk or iron-fortified infant formula coupled with the internal nutrient stores the baby built during fetal life should meet an infant's nutrient needs at least until age 4 to 6 months. The decision to breastfeed, formula-feed, or feed a baby a combination of these is a personal one. There are many valid reasons for selecting either, and both will enable babies to grow normally.

Nutritional Qualities of Human Milk

According to the American Academy of Pediatrics and American Dietetic Association, human milk is the most ideal and desirable source of nutrients for infants, including premature and sick newborns.[15] Both of these organizations recommend breastfeeding exclusively for the first 6 months of life, with the continued combination of breastfeeding and infant foods until age 1 year.[16] The World Health Organization goes beyond that to recommend breastfeeding (with appropriate solid food introduction) for at least 2 years. However, surveys show that only about 70% of North American mothers begin to breastfeed their infants in the hospital, and at 6 months only 33% are still breastfeeding their infants.[17] Breastfeeding for the recommended length of time is best, but breastfeeding for even just the first few weeks is beneficial.

Human milk may share many similarities with the milk from other mammals, but its nutrient composition and bioavailability are uniquely engineered by nature for human babies, just as cow milk is designed for calves and sheep milk is designed for lambs. Unless altered, milk from cows or other animals should never be fed to infants younger than 12 months old. Except in cases of severe maternal malnutrition or other special cases, human milk contains ample supplies of all the nutrients needed for the first 6 months of life, except possibly for vitamin D, iron, and fluoride.[12, 15]

The protein in human milk is mostly synthesized by breast tissue. Some proteins, such as immune factors (e.g., antibodies) and enzymes, enter the milk directly from the mother's bloodstream. The major proteins in human milk (lactalbumin and other whey proteins) are easier for the infant to digest and less stressful to the immature kidneys than is the protein in cow milk (casein). Also, the proteins in human milk are not likely to cause allergic reactions in infants; thus, breastfed babies are less likely to develop allergies and food intolerances than formula-fed ones.

Another human milk protein, lactoferrin, increases the rate of iron absorption by the infant. As a result, more iron is absorbed from human milk than infant formula or milk from other animals, even though human milk contains less iron than these foods. Immune factor proteins and other compounds, such as bifidus factor, work against harmful viruses, bacteria, and parasites. Because the immune system is not fully mature until age 2, these proteins and compounds offer a distinct advantage not found in infant formula. In fact, breastfed babies have fewer infections, fewer and less severe bouts with diarrhea, and better survival rates than those fed formula.

The fats in human milk come from the mother's diet and are synthesized by breast tissue. The mother's current and long-term dietary intake of fat affects the profile of fatty acids of her breast milk. Human milk is high in cholesterol and linoleic acid, both of which are required for normal brain growth and development. It also contains omega-3 fatty acids, such as docohexaenoic acid, which are needed for normal development of the retina in the eye and nervous system tissue.[18] The lipids in human milk also promote efficient digestion. The amount of fat in human milk changes during a feeding session. In the early part of a feeding session (first 5 to 10 minutes on a breast), the baby receives foremilk. Foremilk is watery and contains less fat and fewer calories than hind milk, which is released after the foremilk. Infants need to breastfeed long enough (a total of 20 or more minutes) to get the calories in the fat-rich hind milk to be satisfied between feedings and to grow well.

Lactose is the main carbohydrate in human milk. The sugar galactose is synthesized in the breast, whereas glucose enters from the mother's bloodstream.[4] Human milk composition provides adequate water for the infant when the baby is exclusively breastfed.[18]

Nutritional Qualities of Infant Formula

Commercial iron-fortified infant formulas provide a safe nutritious alternative to human milk in areas of the world where high standards for water purity and cleanliness are common. Only formulas that are commercially made specifically for infants are safe to use. It is important to note that milk (e.g., cow, goat, soy), sweetened condensed milk,

Comparison of Human Milk and Cow Milk (mg/L)		
Nutrient	Human Milk	Cow Milk
Total protein	10.6	30.9
Fat	45.4	38
Lactose	71	47
Calcium	344 mg	1370 mg
Phosphorus	141 mg	910 mg

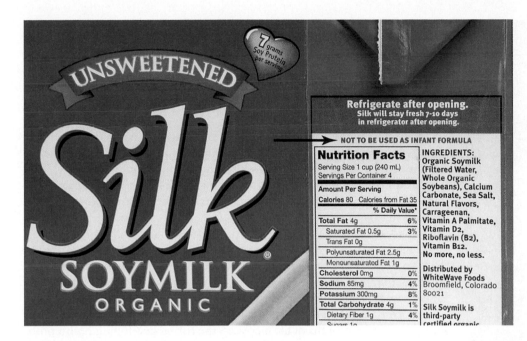

Nutrition Facts

Serving Size 1 cup (240 mL)
Servings Per Container 4

Amount Per Serving

Calories 80   Calories from Fat 35

	% Daily Value*
Total Fat 4g	6%
Saturated Fat 0.5g	3%
Trans Fat 0g	
Polyunsaturated Fat 2.5g	
Monounsaturated Fat 1g	
Cholesterol 0mg	0%
Sodium 85mg	4%
Potassium 300mg	8%
Total Carbohydrate 4g	1%
Dietary Fiber 1g	4%
Sugars 1g	

INGREDIENTS: Organic Soymilk (Filtered Water, Whole Organic Soybeans), Calcium Carbonate, Sea Salt, Natural Flavors, Carrageenan, Vitamin A Palmitate, Vitamin D2, Riboflavin (B2), Vitamin B12. No more, no less.

Distributed by WhiteWave Foods Broomfield, Colorado 80021

Silk Soymilk is third-party certified organic

Figure 17-4 Soy beverages are sometimes incorrectly called "soy milk." They should not be confused with soy-based infant formula—they do not meet an infant's nutrient needs. Soy beverages used in place of infant formula or human milk can cause serious health problems. To help prevent confusion, many soy beverage manufacturers print a warning on their beverages similar to this, "Do Not Use as Infant Formula."

evaporated milk, and homemade formulas are inappropriate choices for infants—they do not conform to strict federal guidelines for calorie content, nutrient composition, and sanitation and, as a result, can cause life-threatening problems (Fig. 17-4). For example, goat milk is too low in folate, iron, and vitamin C. Cow milk is a poor source of vitamin C, vitamin E, copper, iron, and linoleic acid. Its high protein and mineral content overtaxes an infant's immature kidneys and increases the risk of dehydration.[19] Its calcium is so high that it can cause bleeding in the stomach and intestine. The protein in cow milk is difficult for infants to digest and absorb. In addition, cow milk contains many potentially allergy-causing proteins.

In the U.S., the nutrient content of commercial infant formulas is regulated by the Infant Formula Act of 1980, which requires that they meet standards set by the American Academy of Pediatrics. These standards are set to match the nutrient composition of human milk as closely as possible. Although laboratory analysis procedures are quite sophisticated, the exact composition of human milk is not totally known. Thus, formulas only closely approximate the nutrient composition of human milk. Formulas, however, do not duplicate the immunological protection of human milk.

Infant formulas generally contain lactose and/or sucrose for carbohydrate, vegetable oils for fat, and modified proteins from cow milk, soy, or meat. Sometimes infant formulas must be switched several times before the best one for the infant is found. A wide variety of commercial infant formulas are sold to meet the various health needs of infants. For example, soy-based infant formulas are available for infants who can't tolerate lactose or proteins in formulas made with cow milk. Infant formula made with protein that has been "predigested" (broken down into peptides and amino acids) can help infants with digestive problems. Formulas that address the special nutrient needs of preterm infants are available. Other, more specialized formulas also are made for specific medical conditions, such as phenylketonuria. In any case, parents should consult a physician when choosing or changing their infant's formula. It is important to use an iron-fortified formula unless a physician recommends otherwise.

Transitional formulas/beverages have been introduced by some manufacturers for older infants and toddlers. Some of these products are for use after 6 months of age, whereas others are intended only for toddlers. These transitional products have less fat than human milk or standard infant formulas and a mineral content more like human milk than cow milk. According to the manufacturers, the advantages of

▶ There are substantial differences in the nutrient composition of the milk of mothers who deliver prematurely and those who deliver at term. Researchers don't know why these differences exist, but they hypothesize that the preterm milk may be designed to meet the specific nutrient and immunological needs of the premature infant, which are different from the needs of a baby born at term.

Formula-fed infants should remain on infant formula until age 1 year.

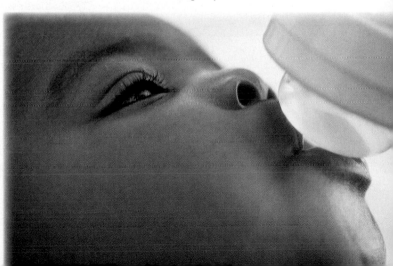

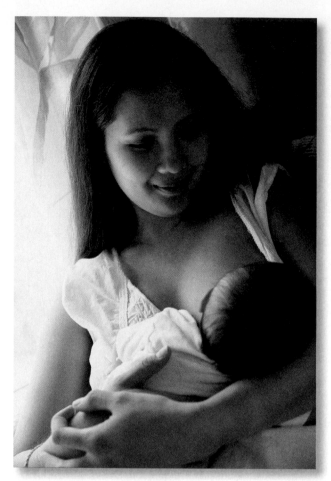

Breastfed infants tend to have fewer ear infections (otitis media) because they do not sleep with a bottle in their mouths.

these transitional formulas/beverages over standard infant formulas include lower cost and better flavor. As stated previously, before making any formula change, parents should seek advice from their child's physician.[4]

Comparing Human Milk and Infant Formula

In addition to the nutritional and immunological differences described previously, human milk and commercial formula also differ in terms of health benefits, cost, convenience, and possibly mother-child bonding (Table 17-1). The health benefits of human milk for infants are not limited to its nutritional contributions. Factors in human milk promote the maturation of the immune system and intestinal tract. Breastfed infants also have a reduced risk of childhood asthma, leukemia, obesity, diabetes, chronic intestinal diseases, misaligned teeth, ear infections, and respiratory infections. They also are less likely to be obese in childhood and adolescence than formula-fed peers. In addition, there is evidence that children who were breastfed have significantly higher visual acuity and cognitive development scores than those who received no maternal milk. As the amount of human milk an infant receives during the first 6 months of life increases, the risk of developing health problems decreases. In addition, the longer the children are breastfed, the more their cognitive development scores rise.

Human milk is almost always less expensive than formula, even after accounting for the costs of breast pump equipment and the slight increase in food required by the mother. Whether breastfeeding is more or less convenient than formula-feeding depends greatly on the circumstances. Preparing formula requires considerable time, careful sanitation, and exact measurements. Thus, human milk, which requires no preparation, is much more convenient to prepare. However, if the mother wants to feed her child human milk during times she is away from the child, she will need to express her milk and store it in bottles. The preparation time and sanitation measures needed for this are similar to that needed to prepare formula.

Mother-child bonding is one benefit frequently attributed to breastfeeding. It is true that breastfeeding requires an intimate physical relationship between mother and child that helps form a strong emotional bond. However, bonding depends more on close physical contact than on method of feeding. Formula-fed babies and their mothers also can develop a strong bond if the babies are held during feeding.

Table 17-1 Advantages to Infants Provided by Human Milk*

- Provides nutrients that are easily digestible and highly bioavailable and in amounts matched to needs
- Reduces risk of food allergies and intolerances, as well as some other allergies[36]
- Provides immune factor proteins (antibodies) and other compounds (*Lactobacillus bifidus*) that reduce the risk of infections and diarrhea while the immune system is still immature
- Contributes to maturation of the GI tract and immune system
- Reduces risk of childhood asthma, leukemia, obesity, diabetes, chronic intestinal diseases, misaligned teeth, ear infections, and respiratory infections
- May enhance visual acuity, nervous system development, and learning ability by providing the fatty acid docohexaenoic acid
- Establishes the habit of eating in moderation, thus decreasing the possibility of obesity later in life by about 20%
- Contributes to normal development of jaws and teeth for better speech development
- Is bacteriologically safe
- Is always fresh and ready

* For a summary of the advantages of breastfeeding for mothers, see Table 16-6 (Chapter 16).

Feeding Technique

Newborn infants usually need 2 or 3 ounces of human milk or commercial formula every 2 to 4 hours. They need to be fed often because their stomachs hold only about 3 ounces, so they fill up and empty rapidly. As infants mature, the frequency of feeding decreases because the quantity of milk consumed at one time increases.

Breastfed infants must be followed closely over the first week of life to ensure that feeding and weight gain are proceeding normally. Monitoring by a physician or lactation consultant is especially important with a mother's first child because the mother will be inexperienced with the technique of breastfeeding.

Parents may erroneously believe that encouraging a baby to eat more than desired will lengthen the time between feedings. However, this encouragement teaches them to overeat and causes physical pain when the stomach is overfilled. It is better to feed babies amounts they can easily accommodate often, rather than feeding larger amounts less frequently. Overfeeding can be avoided by watching for signs that the infant is full and terminating feeding at that time, even if some milk is left in the bottle (Table 17-2). Common signals that a bottle-feeding or breastfeeding infant has had enough include turning the head away, being inattentive, falling asleep, and becoming playful. Generally,

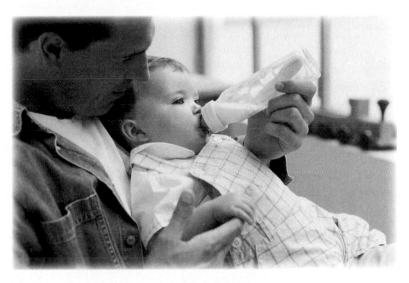

Bottle-feeding allows caregivers other than the mother to participate and may promote closer bonding with the father.

Table 17-2 Summary of Physical and Eating Skills, Hunger and Fullness Cues, and Appropriate Food for Children 0 to 24 Months of Age

Age	Skills and Developmental Signs*	Hunger Signs	Satiety Signals	Age-Appropriate New Foods to Introduce
Birth to 4 months	• Finds nipple through rooting reflex • Tongue moves up and down • Needs burping • Little head and neck control • Strong extrusion reflex	• Cries until fed • Hands form fists • Body is tense • Roots and sucks until fed • Needs 8 to 10 feedings daily	• Removes mouth from nipple • Falls asleep • Relief of body tension	• Human milk or commercial infant formula
4 to 6 months	• Can swallow non-liquids • Tongue protrudes in anticipation of nipple • Tongue moves back and forth • Learns to move food from the front of the tongue to the back • Extrusion reflex diminishes and disappears • Gaining control of head and neck • Grasps items with entire hand and brings them to the mouth • Teeth begin to erupt • Near 6 months, sits with support	• Eagerly anticipates eating • Opens mouth when sees bottle or breast • Grasps and draws bottle or breast to mouth • Needs 5 or 6 feedings daily	• Tosses head back or turns away • Covers mouth with hands • Spits out food • Becomes playful or interested in surroundings • Protests (fusses or cries)	• Iron-fortified infant cereal • Diluted fruit juices, strained fruits and vegetables

(continued)

Table 17-2 Continued

Age	Skills and Developmental Signs*	Hunger Signs	Satiety Signals	Age-Appropriate New Foods to Introduce
7 to 9 months	• Tries to grasp feeding spoon • Can form lips to rim of a cup and drink from a cup with help • Holds bottle alone • Develops pincher grasp (can pick items up with the thumb and index finger) • Brings fist to mouth and feeds self finger foods • Sits up alone, rolls over from back to front • Jaw begins to move up and down • Begins to chew and bite	• Reaches for food • Looks for food when dish is removed • Reacts to food preparation sounds • Vocalizes hunger (cries or babbles)	• Changes body position • Clamps mouth shut or puts hands in mouth • Shakes head • Says "no" • Becomes playful (throws or plays with utensils or food) • Pushes utensils or food away	• Fruit juice and fruits • Vegetables • Strained protein-rich foods (meat, fish, poultry, egg yolk, yogurt, cheese, tofu, beans) • Finger foods (teething biscuit, crackers, toast, fruit slices, thin vegetable strips)
10 to 12 months	• Is able to chew • Increases skill in biting, chewing, and swallowing • Tongue is used to lick lips • Demands to self-feed	• Grasps eating utensils • Vocalizes hunger rather than cries • Points to food	• Shakes head • Says "no" • Pushes food away • Fidgets • Grasps feeder's hand to control food intake	• Chopped, mashed table foods or commercial junior foods • Grains (pasta, rice, etc.)
12 to 24 months	• Holds cup and drinks unassisted • Uses spoon to feed self • Becomes skilled self-feeder • Food patterns become more individualized	• Vocalizes hunger, perhaps by asking for food or banging, waving, or dropping spoon • Points to food or leads adult to the refrigerator	• Shakes head • Says "no" • Fidgets	• Same as for 10- to 12-month old child with amounts determined by the child's appetite • Whole milk, egg white, orange juice, table food

*This timeline is just an estimate; skills/developmental signs of individual infants may vary by several months from the ages given. A pediatrician should be consulted if caregivers are concerned about an infant's development.

the infant's appetite is a better guide than standardized recommendations concerning feeding amounts. By carefully observing infants while feeding them and responding to their cues appropriately, caregivers can be assured that the infants' energy needs are being met and can foster trust and responsiveness.[3]

Because a mother cannot measure the amount of milk a breastfed infant takes in, the mother may fear that she is not adequately nourishing the infant. As a rule, a well-nourished breastfed infant should (1) have 6 or more wet diapers per day after the second day of life, (2) show a normal weight gain, and (3) pass at least 1 or 2 stools per day that look like lumpy mustard. In addition, softening of the breast during a feeding session helps indicate that enough milk is being consumed. Parents who sense that their infant is not consuming enough milk should consult a physician immediately because dehydration can develop rapidly.

Infants swallow a lot of air as they ingest either formula or human milk, so it's important to burp them after either 10 minutes of feeding or 1 to 2 oz (30 to 60 ml) from a bottle and again at the end of feeding. Spitting up a bit of milk is normal at this time. Once fed, infants should be placed on their backs. Infants should not be placed on their stomachs because this sleeping position has been linked to sudden infant death syndrome (SIDS). The Back to Sleep campaign, started in 1994 in the U.S., has reduced SIDS by 40%; however, plagiocephaly (flat-head syndrome) has increased as a result. To avoid flat-head syndrome, the American Academy of Pediatrics recommends periodically repositioning an infant's head while asleep and providing time on his or her stomach while awake.

Preparing Bottles

Stored human milk, as well as infant formula, is fed to infants using bottles. All equipment and utensils used to prepare, store, and/or feed infant formula or human milk should be thoroughly washed and rinsed. This includes breast pumps, bottles, nipples, measuring spoons, and the like.

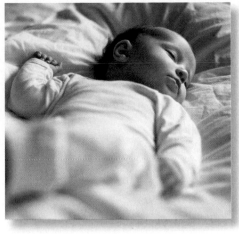

The Back to Sleep campaign advises that infants be placed on their backs for sleeping.

It is important to prepare formula by exactly following instructions on the label of powdered and concentrated formulas—adding too much or too little water can be very dangerous for infants. Only clean, cold water should be used—hot water from the faucet poses a risk of high lead content (see Chapter 3). If well water is used, it should be boiled before making formula for at least the infant's first 3 months of life. In addition, it should be analyzed for naturally occurring nitrates—excessive nitrates can cause a severe form of anemia. If municipal water systems are high in nitrates, consumers will be warned (e.g., in local newspapers) not to use the water in infant formula. If water contaminants are a concern, formula can be mixed with bottled nursery water sold in most supermarkets.

Prepared formula and expressed human milk can be fed immediately or refrigerated for up to 1 day. Human milk can be frozen for several weeks. Most infants accept room temperature formula. To warm a cold bottle of formula or stored human milk, run hot water over the bottle or place it briefly in a pan of simmering water. Infant formula and human milk fed from a bottle should not be heated in a microwave oven because hot spots may develop, which can burn the infant's mouth and esophagus. Discard any leftovers in the bottle—they are contaminated by bacteria and enzymes from the infant's saliva.

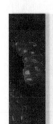

Knowledge Check

1. Why is human milk better suited to infants than cow or goat milk?
2. How do foremilk and hind milk differ?
3. What are 5 benefits of breastfeeding?
4. How might an infant signal he or she has had enough to eat?
5. How can a breastfeeding mother judge whether her infant is receiving enough nourishment?

 ## 17.5 Feeding Babies: Adding Solid Foods

As babies grow, the nutrient reserves they had at birth become depleted and human milk alone can no longer meet all their nutrient needs. Slowly, they need to begin getting some of their nutrients from **solid foods** (i.e., any food other than human milk or infant formula). Although iron-fortified commercial infant formulas can meet the nutrient needs of infants 6 to 12 months old, infants older than 6 months of age rarely are fed just infant formulas. Plus, adding solid foods helps ensure that any as yet unknown nutrient needs are met. An added bonus to exposing babies and children to a wide variety of food is helping them develop a willingness to taste new foods and learn to eat a widely varied diet. The

Figure 17-5 Dietary guidelines for infant feeding.

The American Academy of Pediatrics has issued the following guidelines.

Build to a variety of foods. For the first months of life, human milk is all an infant needs. When the infant is ready, start adding new foods, 1 at a time. During the first year, the goal is to teach an infant to enjoy a variety of nutritious foods. A lifetime of healthy eating habits begins with this important first step.

Pay attention to your infant's appetite to avoid overfeeding or underfeeding. Feed infants when they are hungry. Never force an infant to finish an unwanted serving of food. Watch for signs that indicate hunger or fullness.

Infants need fat. Although fat is the cause of many adult health problems, it's an essential source of energy for growing infants. Fat also helps the nervous system develop.

Choose fruits, vegetables, and grains, but don't overdo high-fiber foods. Although many adults benefit from higher-fiber diets, they are not good for infants. They are bulky, filling, and often low in energy. The natural amounts of fiber and nutrients in fruits, vegetables, and grains are appropriate as part of a healthy infant diet.

Infants need sugars in moderation. Sugars are an additional source of energy for active, rapidly growing infants. Foods such as human milk, fruits, and juices are natural sources of sugars and other nutrients as well. Foods that contain artificial sweeteners should be avoided; they don't provide the energy that growing infants need.

Infants need sodium in moderation. Sodium is a necessary mineral found naturally in almost all foods. As part of a healthy diet, infants need sodium for their bodies to work properly.

Choose foods containing iron, zinc, and calcium. Infants need good sources of iron, zinc and calcium for optimum growth in the first 2 years. These minerals are important for healthy blood, proper growth, and strong bones.

In the early stages of solid food introduction, these foods complement rather than replace human milk or infant formula.

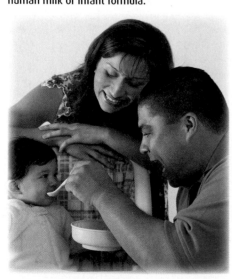

more varied one's diet is, the more nutritious it is likely to be. The American Academy of Pediatrics has issued guidelines to help parents feed their babies nutritiously (Fig. 17-5).

Deciding When to Introduce Solid Foods

The recommended age for introducing solid foods has changed as scientific knowledge has grown. In the early 1900s, solid foods were not introduced until a baby's first birthday. The age for adding solid foods decreased steadily until, by the 1950s, babies 2 and 3 weeks old were being fed cereal. Health-care experts currently agree that most babies are not ready for solid food until they are 6 months old.

The time to introduce solid foods into an infant's diet hinges on these important factors:[4]

- **Nutritional need.** The nutrient stores a baby had at birth are exhausted by the time an infant has doubled his or her birth weight and weighs at least 13 pounds. A breastfed infant needs solid foods when he or she demands to be fed more than 8 to 10 times each day. A formula-fed baby needs solids when he or she drinks 8 ounces of formula and is hungry in less than 4 hours or consumes more than a quart of formula each day and still seems hungry. This description applies to most 6-month-old infants and a few 4-month-old infants. If solid foods are delayed much past the point a baby has a nutritional need for them, growth will slow.

- **Physiological capabilities.** Kidney function is quite limited until about 4 to 6 weeks of age. Until then, waste products from excessive amounts of dietary protein or minerals can cause so much urine output that dehydration occurs. An infant's intestinal tract is immature and cannot readily digest starch before 3 months. Because infants can easily absorb whole proteins until 4 to 5 months of age, exposing them to many different proteins before age 6 months—especially those in unaltered cow milk and egg whites—may predispose a child to future allergies and other health problems. For this reason, it's best to minimize the types of proteins in a young infant's diet by focusing exclusively on human milk or infant formula as a nutrient source.

- **Physical ability.** There are 3 signs that babies are developmentally ready for solid foods. These abilities usually occur around 4 to 6 months of age, but they vary with each infant.

  - They can control head movements well and sit alone with support. These skills enable them to show interest in food by moving forward and indicate satiety by turning away. A sitting position also provides a clear passageway for food to travel from the mouth to the stomach.
  - The extrusion reflex weakens and they are able to move food from the tip of the tongue to the back of the mouth. The **extrusion reflex** (also called tongue thrusting) helps a baby express milk from the nipple, but it also causes an infant to push objects placed on the tip of the tongue, such as a spoon or food, out of the mouth.
  - They can make a chewing motion. At birth, babies have a poorly developed lower jaw and large fat pads in the cheeks that enable them to suck well. As the infant matures, the jaw line changes and the fat pads diminish—these changes allow the infant to chew and swallow, rather than just suck.

There is no advantage to introducing solid foods before an infant needs them or is ready for them. In addition to the strain that solid food puts on a young infant's organs, introducing food too early may lead to feeding problems and food dislikes. Also, the child is likely to eat far more calories than are needed. If solid food takes the place of human milk or formula, reduced nutrient intake (especially calcium) may occur. Some mistakenly believe that adding solid food early will help infants sleep through the night. Actually, this achievement is a developmental milestone not affected by the amount of food consumed. Although it is possible to force feed infants who are not developmentally ready for solid foods by putting the food in a feeder (a giant syringe) or mixing it with formula and putting it in a bottle, this practice is nutritionally unnecessary and possibly dangerous for the infant because it increases the risk of choking or inhaling food into the lungs when crying.

Rate and Sequence for Introducing Solid Foods

Between 6 and 12 months of age, human milk or formula intake gradually decreases while solid food intake slowly increases. At first, solid foods are a very small addition (1 to 2 teaspoons) to human milk or formula (Table 17-3). As the baby's first birthday approaches, calories should be evenly divided between human milk or formula and a variety of foods from all the major food groups.

Experts recommend slowly adding foods with just 1 ingredient and waiting several days before offering another new food. This method makes it easy to identify food sensitivities and allergies by watching for reactions, such as gas, diarrhea, vomiting, rash, or breathing problems

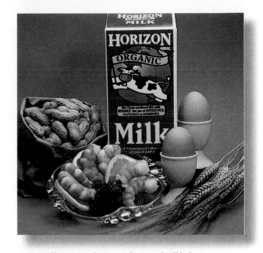

Cow milk, egg whites, wheat, shellfish, peanuts, and tree nuts (e.g., walnuts and pecans) should not be introduced until children are at least 1 year old. Delaying these foods until then can help reduce the risk of food allergies.

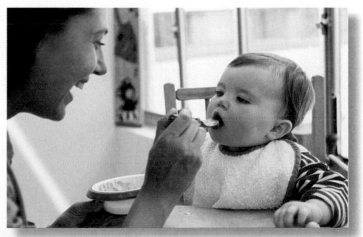

Infants show signs that they are ready for solid foods: they are able to sit up with support, the extrusion reflex weakens, and they can make a chewing motion.

CRITICAL THINKING

Irena and Chris had a baby 11 months ago. At the last checkup, the doctor told them to start feeding the baby some new solid foods. After 5 days of eating a new food, the baby woke up with a runny nose and vomiting. The doctor told them to stop giving the baby that food. How can the doctor justify her recommendation?

▶ Some experts recommend introducing vegetables before fruits because, if fruits are offered first, the infant may prefer their sweet taste and resist vegetables.

Typical Solid Food Progression Starting at 6 Months of Age*

Week 1: Rice cereal

Week 2: Add strained carrots

Week 3: Add applesauce

Week 4: Add oat cereal

Week 5: Add cooked egg yolk

Week 6: Add strained chicken

Week 7: Add strained peas

Week 8: Add strained plums

*Extending the rice cereal step for a month or so is advised if solid food introduction begins at 4 months of age. If at any point signs of allergy or intolerance develop, substitute another, similar food item.

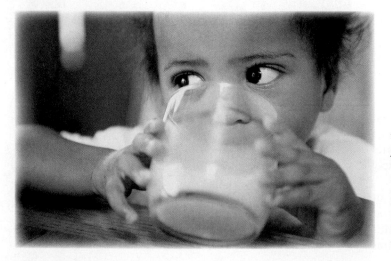

Table 17-3 Tips for Introducing Solid Foods

1. Start with teaspoon amounts of a single-ingredient food item, such as rice cereal, and increase the serving size gradually.

2. Offer solid foods after some breastfeeding or formula-feeding, when the edge has been taken off the infant's hunger.

3. Always feed solid foods from a spoon (a baby spoon [small spoon with a long handle] is best).

• Spoon feeding is a skill babies need to learn.

• Do not mix solid foods with a liquid and feed from a bottle because babies may choke. Also, eating baby foods from a bottle leads to poor eating habits and may cause children to be unwilling to try new foods and accept new textures.

4. Hold the infant comfortably on the lap, as for breastfeeding or bottle-feeding, but a little more upright to ease swallowing.

• Put a small dab of food on the spoon tip and gently place it on the infant's tongue.

• Be calm and go slowly enough to give the infant time to get used to food.

• Expect the infant to take only 2 or 3 bites of the first meals.

• Let infants decide when they are hungry and when they have had enough to eat.

(e.g., wheezing). If the baby is fed new foods too often or is fed a food with several ingredients before each ingredient has been offered alone, there is no way to tell which has caused the problem. If a symptom appears, the suspected problem food should be avoided for several weeks and then reintroduced in a small quantity. If the problem continues, a physician should be consulted. Many babies outgrow food sensitivities in childhood. Some foods that commonly cause an allergic response in infants are egg whites, chocolate, nuts, and cow milk. It's best not to introduce these foods during infancy.

The recommended sequence for introducing solid foods is designed to respond to the physical maturation and increasing nutrient needs of infants. Iron and vitamin C are the first nutrients needed by infants in quantities larger than those supplied by human milk. Thus, the first "solid" food generally recommended is iron-fortified baby cereal. Juices and pureed fruits and vegetables are the second foods usually added. In fact, fruit juice is often introduced at about the same time as cereal. Cereals and fruit juices marketed especially for babies are the preferred choice because they have no added salt, sugar, or monosodium glutamate (a flavor enhancer). Plus, the iron in infant cereals is much more absorbable than that found in adult cereals. Baby juices are fortified with vitamin C, which promotes iron absorption. Rice usually is the first cereal introduced because it is least likely to cause allergies. Wheat, the cereal most likely to cause allergies, usually is introduced last. Orange juice may be too acidic for infants and is not recommended until age 1.

Protein-rich foods, such as pureed meat, fish, chicken, beans, yogurt, egg yolk, and tofu, are introduced around age 6 to 8 months. These foods help supply the increasing amount of protein needed by the rapidly growing infant. It's best to wait until the child is a year old before serving egg whites and unaltered cow milk because they frequently cause allergic reactions in younger babies. Once cow milk is added to a child's diet, the American Academy of Pediatrics recommends that the child receive whole

There is considerable concern that some young children are consuming more fruit juice than is healthful. Excessive juice intake can cause diarrhea, gas, abdominal bloating, and tooth decay. Large amounts of juice also displace formula or human milk in the diet, causing the infant to receive inadequate amounts of calcium and other nutrients. Excessive fruit juice intake is associated with failure to thrive, GI tract complications, obesity, and short stature. The American Academy of Pediatrics advises parents not to introduce juices before age 6 months. Then, they should limit daily fruit juice intake to 4 to 6 ounces daily for children ages 1 to 6 years and 8 to 12 ounces for children 7 to 18 years old.

milk until age 2 years or older. Children who receive reduced-fat milk before age 2 years have difficulty meeting their calorie needs without exceeding their protein needs. After age 2 years, parents should consult with the child's health-care provider before switching to reduced-fat milk.

As teeth begin to appear, babies are ready for foods with more texture, such as lumpy or chopped foods (e.g., cottage cheese, cooked vegetables). By about 9 months, many babies can pick up finger foods (e.g., crackers) and begin feeding themselves. By 1 year, most can eat table foods that were cooked until tender. Parents should aim to introduce infants to a variety of foods, so that by the first birthday the infant is consuming many different foods from all food groups and the diet begins to resemble a balanced diet (Table 17-4).[3] Presenting new foods for several consecutive days can aid in an infant's acceptance of that food.

A wide variety of infant foods are sold in supermarkets. Single-food items are more desirable than mixed dinners and desserts, which are less nutrient-dense. Grinding plain, unseasoned cooked foods and serving them fresh or freezing in ice-cube-size portions for serving later is an alternative to commercial infant food. Careful attention to cleanliness is necessary when making baby food at home.

Weaning from the Breast or Bottle

When juices are added to an infant's diet around age 6 months, they should be offered in a sippy (spill-proof) cup with a wide, flat bottom. Drinking from a cup helps begin weaning. To prevent feeding problems and the overconsumption of milk, juice, or other sweetened beverages, babies should be completely weaned off bottles by age 18 months. Using a cup also helps prevent early childhood dental caries. If an infant drinks continually from a bottle, the carbohydrate-rich fluid bathes the teeth, providing an ideal growth medium for bacteria. Bacteria on the teeth then make acids, which dissolve tooth enamel. Infants should never be put to bed with a bottle or placed in an infant seat with a bottle propped up because fluid (even milk) pools around the teeth, increasing the likelihood of dental caries and ear infections.

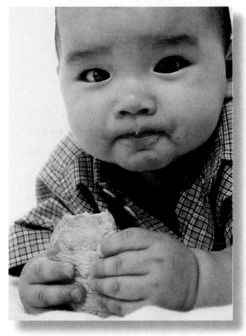

Older infants enjoy finger feeding.

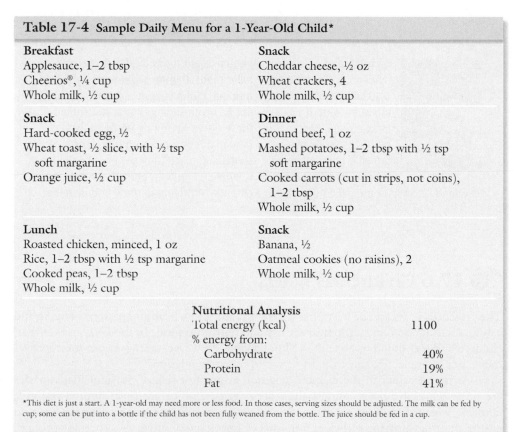

Table 17-4 Sample Daily Menu for a 1-Year-Old Child*

Breakfast	**Snack**
Applesauce, 1–2 tbsp	Cheddar cheese, ½ oz
Cheerios®, ¼ cup	Wheat crackers, 4
Whole milk, ½ cup	Whole milk, ½ cup

Snack	**Dinner**
Hard-cooked egg, ½	Ground beef, 1 oz
Wheat toast, ½ slice, with ½ tsp soft margarine	Mashed potatoes, 1–2 tbsp with ½ tsp soft margarine
Orange juice, ½ cup	Cooked carrots (cut in strips, not coins), 1–2 tbsp
	Whole milk, ½ cup

Lunch	**Snack**
Roasted chicken, minced, 1 oz	Banana, ½
Rice, 1–2 tbsp with ½ tsp margarine	Oatmeal cookies (no raisins), 2
Cooked peas, 1–2 tbsp	Whole milk, ½ cup
Whole milk, ½ cup	

Nutritional Analysis	
Total energy (kcal)	1100
% energy from:	
Carbohydrate	40%
Protein	19%
Fat	41%

*This diet is just a start. A 1-year-old may need more or less food. In those cases, serving sizes should be adjusted. The milk can be fed by cup; some can be put into a bottle if the child has not been fully weaned from the bottle. The juice should be fed in a cup.

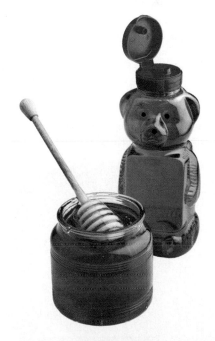

Honey should not be given to children until they are a year old because honey often contains *Clostridium botulinum* spores, which can grow and produce the deadly botulism toxin in an infant's digestive tract.

Infant Feeding Summary

Breastfed Infants

- Breastfeed for 6 months or longer, if possible. Then introduce iron-fortified infant formula when breastfeeding declines or ceases.
- Provide a vitamin D supplement (200 IU/day) (until at least 500 ml of formula is consumed).
- Consult a physician about the need for fluoride, vitamin B-12, and iron supplements.

Formula-Fed Infants

- Use an iron-fortified infant formula for the first year of life.
- Consult a physician about the need for a fluoride supplement.

All Infants

- Provide a variety of basic, soft foods after 6 months of age, progressing slowly to a varied diet.
- Add iron-fortified infant cereal at about 6 months of age.

What Not to Feed Infants

- Honey
- Very salty and very sweet foods
- Excessive amounts of infant formula or human milk. About 24 to 32 oz (750–1000 mL) of human milk or formula daily is ideal after 6 months, with food supplying the rest of the infant's energy needs.
- Cow milk before age 1 year and reduced-fat cow milk before age 2 years
- Large amounts of fruit juice

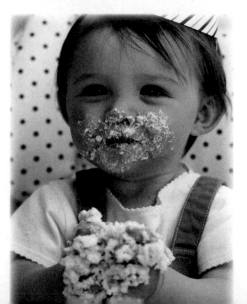

Early self-feeding attempts should be encouraged, even though they are messy.

Learning to Self-Feed

Infants begin to learn to feed themselves in late infancy and continue to develop these skills into the preschool years. Self-feeding skills require coordination and can develop only if the infant is allowed to practice and experiment. It's important that parents be patient and supportive, even though self-feeding is inefficient and very messy. Infants are solely finger feeders and don't always hit the "target" of their mouths. By the end of the first year, finger feeding becomes more efficient and chewing is easier as more teeth erupt. In addition, by age 1 year, children drink from a cup without help, which makes fewer bottle and/or breastfeedings necessary. By age 2, children can manage lifting, tilting, and lowering a cup quite well. In addition, they are fairly accomplished spoon users. Young children continue to be interested in the feel of foods, so they often engage in finger feeding or filling the spoon with their fingers. They begin using a fork by age 3 or 4 and a knife to cut soft foods by age 4 or 5.

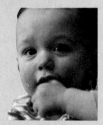

Knowledge Check

1. What physical ability signs indicate babies are developmentally ready for solid foods?
2. Why do babies need solid foods at around 6 months of age?
3. How can you determine whether a particular food has caused a sensitivity or an allergy in an infant?
4. Which foods commonly cause an allergic response and should not be introduced in infancy?
5. Why should juice be served in a cup?

CASE STUDY FOLLOW-UP

Damon's diet is inadequate for a 10-month-old infant because it lacks enough of the nutritious foods his growing body needs to support weight gain. These foods include iron-fortified cereal, pureed infant foods, and appropriate table foods. Damon should stay on infant formula until 1 year of age and should not be given sugary drinks, nor should these drinks be fed by bottle, if used. Damon needs a more energy dense diet containing a healthful variety of solid foods to provide him with enough energy and essential nutrients to grow and develop.

17.6 Children as Eaters

The preschool years are the best time for children to start a healthful pattern of living and eating, focusing on regular physical activity and nutritious food. In the U.S. and Canada, children and teens tend to be fairly well nourished. However, there is room for improvement. For example, few meet the MyPyramid recommendations.[20]

As noted earlier in the chapter, children at greatest risk of nutrient inadequacies are those who have poor eating habits, are vegans, and/or are from limited resource families. Vegan diets must be planned carefully, especially during the growing years to ensure that they provide sufficient amounts of calories and nutrients, especially protein, calcium, iron, zinc, riboflavin, vitamin B-12, and vitamin D (if sun exposure is limited) to support normal growth.[21] The Special Supplemental Nutrition Program for Women, Infants, and Children (WIC) program can help limited-resource children up to age 5 years who are at nutritional risk get the nutrients they need. In addition, encouraging school-age children and teens, especially those from limited-resource families, to participate in the U.S. Department of Agriculture administered School Breakfast Program and National School Lunch Program can help them improve their nutrient intake. School breakfasts include 4 food items (milk, grain, protein food, and vegetable or fruit), and lunch includes 5 items (milk, protein food, grain, and 2 or more vegetables and/or fruits). School breakfast participants tend to perform better in school than those who don't participate. School lunch participants can obtain 33 to 50% of their total daily nutrient intake from the meal.

Appetites

Compared with babies, children tend to have erratic appetites. Before and during a period of rapid growth, children have good appetites. When growth slows or plateaus, appetite drops off significantly. Appetite fluctuations are considered a problem only when low or high intakes occur for extended periods or the child exhibits signs of undernutrition (e.g., fatigue, increased susceptibility to infection, underweight, or failure to thrive) or overnutrition (e.g., obesity).

Caregivers who do not understand that appetite lulls are to be expected and that healthy, normal weight children have built-in feeding mechanisms that regulate food intake to match needs may resort to bribes, forcing, teasing, or trickery to get children to eat. Bribing children to eat a new food (e.g., "Eat 3 bites of carrots and you can have dessert") may achieve the parent's immediate goal, but it often has negative results in the long run. Research studies show that, when children must clear an arbitrary hurdle (e.g., 3 bites of carrots) to receive a reward (e.g., dessert), preference for the reward rises, whereas preference for the hurdle decreases. In subsequent meals when the reward is removed, children eat less of the hurdle food.[22] Bribing children to eat also teaches them that food is an appropriate reward. At the other end of the spectrum lie parents who are so excessively concerned that their children will become obese that they restrict their children's food intake. In some cases, caregivers restrict food intake so severely that the children become underweight and fail to thrive.[23]

Pressuring a child to eat more or less than is desired tells the child not to trust his or her own hunger and satiety signals—this can lead to a lifetime battle with weight problems. Teaching a child to use food to fulfill emotional needs (e.g., as a reward) can have the same effect. Successful child feeding depends on a division of responsibility between parents and children. Parents are responsible for providing appropriate, nutritious, appealing, regular meals and snacks. Children are responsible for deciding how much to eat. If the division of responsibility is respected, a normal, healthy child will eat adequate amounts with minimal fuss. Problems often arise when parents don't fulfill their responsibilities and/or take over the child's responsibilities.[23] A goal should be to make mealtime a happy, social time, sharing enjoyment of healthful foods.

When, What, and How Much to Serve

Children have small stomachs. Offering them 6 or so small meals succeeds better than limiting them to 3 meals each day. Sticking to 3 meals a day offers no special nutritional advantages; it's just a social custom. When we eat isn't nearly as important as what we eat. Frequent meals and snacks help children meet their nutrient

▶ Choking is a possible but very preventable hazard for infants and young children. Avoid choking hazards by:

- Setting a good example at the table by taking small bites and chewing foods thoroughly
- Insisting that children sit at the table, take their time, and focus on the food during meals and snacks
- Avoid giving infants and children any foods that are round, firm, sticky, or cut into large chunks; foods that can cause choking include hot dogs (unless finely cut into sticks, not coin shapes), candy, nuts, grapes, popcorn, peanut butter, coarsely cut meats, and hard pieces of fruits or vegetables (e.g., raw carrots)

During infancy, a child's attitudes toward foods and the whole eating process begin to take shape. If parents and other caregivers practice good nutrition and are flexible, they can lead a child into lifelong healthful food habits.

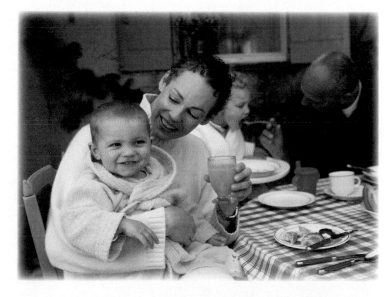

and calorie needs, as well as keep their blood glucose levels high enough to support the activity of their rapidly developing brain and nervous system. Breakfast and snacks are especially important. Children who eat breakfast or a nourishing morning snack have a greater daily intake of several vitamins and minerals than children who skip breakfast.[18, 24] Also, breakfast eaters may perform better in school and have a longer attention span than breakfast skippers. Snacks provide about 25% of the total calorie intake of many children. Nutritious snacks can add significant amounts of nutrients to the diet. However, many children are consuming high-calorie, high-fat snacks instead of healthy snacks.

From the first birthday onward, children, like adults, need several servings from each of the major food groups every day. However, the size of each serving and the number of servings are different. A serving size for children is equal to about 1 tablespoon per year of age, depending on the child's appetite. For example, a 2-year-old's dinner might contain 2 tablespoons each of ground beef, pasta, and peas (Table 17-5). Serving sizes increase gradually until late childhood, when they become the same as those for adults.

MyPyramid for children (Fig. 17-6) is a useful meal planning tool.[20] Because of the reduced appetite of preschool children, providing nutrient-dense foods is particularly important. There is no need to decrease fat or simple sugar intake severely, but fatty and sweet food choices should not overwhelm more nutritious ones.[20] An overemphasis on fat-reduced diets during childhood has been linked to an increase in eating disorders and encourages an inappropriate "good food, bad food" attitude. When planning menus, also keep in mind that children tend to like foods with crisp textures and mild flavors, as well as familiar foods. Because their taste buds are more sensitive than those of adults, preschool children often refuse to eat strongly flavored foods. In addition, young children are especially sensitive to hot-temperature foods and tend to reject them. Children also may object to having foods mixed, as in stews and casseroles, even if they like the ingredients separately.

Food Preferences

Food preferences begin to be established during fetal life and continue to develop in the years spanning infancy and adolescence. In the early childhood years, the family usually has the greatest influence on the development of food preferences and habits.[25] As children grow older, peers and teachers begin to provide new ideas about food, eating, and nutrition. Television programming and advertising also present strong lessons about food and eating.

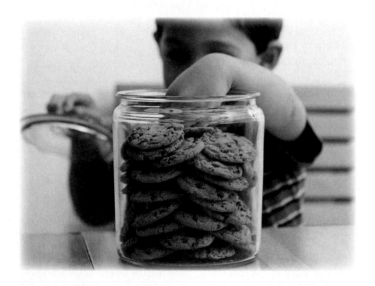

Sweets should be consumed in moderation during childhood, but they do not have to be avoided completely.

Table 17-5 Food Plan for Preschool and School-Age Children Based on MyPyramid Approximate Number of Servings[a]

Food Group	Serving Size	Age 2[b]	Age 5[c]	Age 8[c]	Age 12[c, d]
Grains	Ounce	3	5	5	6–7
Vegetables	Cup	1	1.5	2	2.5–3
Fruits	Cup	1	1.5	1.5	2
Milk	Cup	2	2	3	3
Meat and beans	Ounce	2	4	5	5.5–6
Oils	Teaspoon	3	4	5	6
Discretionary calories	Kcal	Up to 165	Up to 170	Up to 130	Up to 265–290

[a]Log on to mypyramid.gov for other ages and other activity levels.
[b]Based on less than 30 minutes of physical activity.
[c]Based on 30–60 minutes of physical activity.
[d]The lower amounts refer to girls.

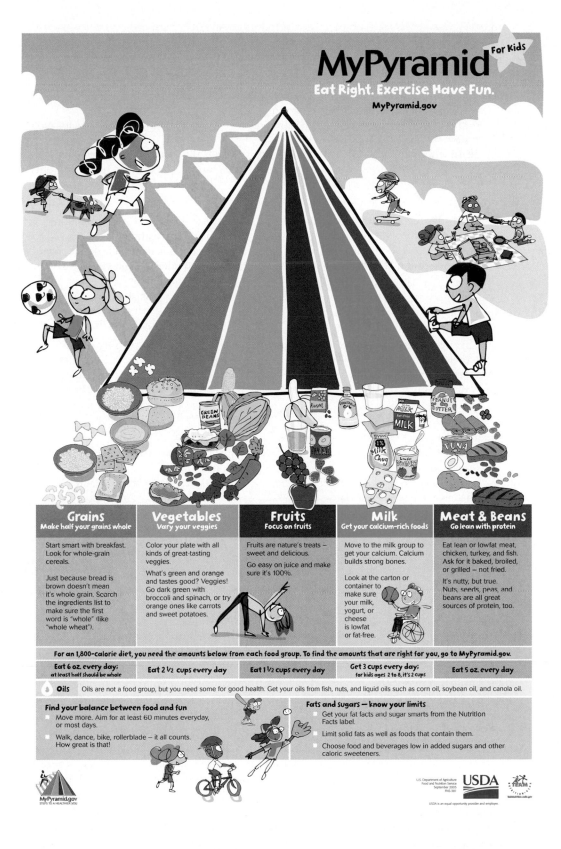

Figure 17-6 **The USDA has created a version of MyPyramid for children. The accompanying website (mypyramid.gov/kids/index.html) also features kid-friendly activities designed to encourage children to make healthier eating and activity choices.**

Steering children toward healthful foods is likely to be more successful if parents understand the eating behaviors of young children (Table 17-6) and expose children to nutrition education. Because children spend much of their younger years in school, it is a great place to learn about positive, healthy eating habits.[25] Such education can help children understand why eating a nutritious diet will make them feel more energetic, look

Table 17-6 Observed Emotional Traits, Eating Behavior, and Food-Related Skills of Preschoolers

Age (Years)	Emotional Traits	Eating Behavior	Food-Related Skills
1–2	• Fears new things • Sharing difficult • Requires constant supervision • Enjoys helping but can't be left alone • Curious • Often defiant • Eager for attention	• "Finicky" eater • Holds food in mouth without swallowing • May insist on eating the same food at meal after meal (called a food jag)	• Uses spoon with some skill (especially if hungry) • Can begin to tear, break, snap, and dip foods • Has good control of cup—lifts, drinks, sets it down, holds with one hand • Helps self-feed
3	• The "me too" age—wants to be included in everything • Responds well to options rather than demands • Sharing still difficult • Somewhat rigid about the "right" way to do things	• Eats most foods, except for certain vegetables • Dawdles over food when not hungry • Comments on how foods are served	• Uses spoon in semiadult fashion; may spear with fork • Medium hand muscle development • Feeds self independently, especially if hungry • Can pour milk and juice and serve individual portions from a serving dish if given instructions
4	• Shares well • Needs adult approval and attention—shows off • Understands; needs limits • Follows rules most of the time • Still rigid about the "right" way to do things	• Eating and talking get in the way—prefers to talk • Strong food likes and dislikes • Refuses to eat, to the point of tears	• Uses all eating utensils • Small-finger muscle development • Can wipe, wash, set table and pour premeasured ingredients • Can peel, spread, cut, roll, and mash foods; cracks eggs
5	• Helpful and cooperative with family chores and routines • Still somewhat rigid about the "right" way to do things • Very attached to parent, home, and family	• Likes familiar foods; prefers most vegetables raw • Latches on to food dislikes of family members and declares these as own	• Fine coordination in fingers and hands • Makes simple breakfast and lunch • Can measure, cut, grind, and grate with some supervision

Modified from M. Sigman-Grant, "Feeding Preschoolers: Balancing Nutritional and Developmental Needs," *Nutrition Today*, July/August 1992, p. 13. Used with permission.

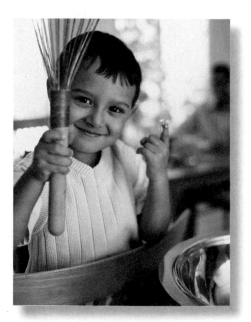
Interest in food starts early in life.

better, and work more efficiently. Regular family meals daily—whether breakfast, lunch, or dinner—helps children apply what they learn via nutrition education and build good eating habits.

The most important nutrition lessons for children of all ages involve expanding their familiarity with new foods and helping them develop a willingness to accept new foods. Teaching these lessons is challenging because children tend to reject unfamiliar foods, but the nutritional rewards of a varied diet are worth the effort. Children become familiar with new foods and are more willing to try them when they look attractive and are served in a social setting by calm, supportive, approving adults who are eating the food. If a child observes adults and older children eating and enjoying a food, there's a good chance that he or she eventually will accept it. One possible policy is the 1-bite rule: within reason, children should take at least 1 bite or taste of the foods presented to them. Giving children opportunities to make food decisions also can encourage them to try new foods. For example, parents can select several acceptable snack choices and let children choose the snack they want. Involving children in preparing a new food and serving small amounts of a new food at the beginning of the meal, when the child is most hungry, helps increase his or her acceptance of the food, too. As many as 15 to 20 exposures to a new food may be needed before the child accepts it. There may be some foods that a child will never accept—keep in mind that no one food is a dietary "essential" and children are entitled to their own likes and dislikes.

Mealtime Challenges

Many preschool children go through periods of unpredictable and unusual eating behavior. One of the most common is food jags—demanding the same meal 3 times a day for a week or more. Food jags can be monotonous (e.g., eating only green foods or only peanut butter and jelly sandwiches) but generally don't present a nutritional problem unless the food demanded is excessively high in sugar, fat, or sodium or if the jag lasts for more than a few weeks. The best way to handle most food jags is to serve the food demanded while keeping in mind that the food jag will soon pass.

Sometimes children refuse to eat. When they do, it's best not to overreact. Doing so may give the child the idea that eating is a means of getting attention or manipulating a situation. Children rarely starve themselves to any point approaching physical harm. When children refuse to eat, parents should have them sit at the table for a while; if they still aren't interested in eating, the parents can remove the food and wait until the next scheduled meal or snack. Hunger is still the best means for getting a child to eat. A sudden loss of appetite, however, may be reason for concern because it may indicate the child is ill.

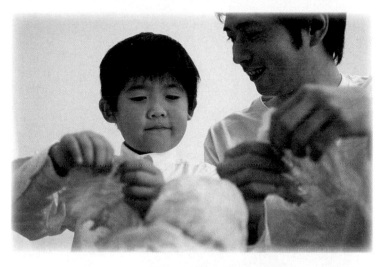

Getting children involved with food preparation can help them accept new foods.

Many parents describe their preschoolers as "picky" eaters. Picky eating is usually just another method children use to express their strong desire for independence. Nagging, forcing, or bribing children to eat reinforces picky-eating behaviors because of the extra attention. Overall, parents should focus on offering a variety of healthy foods and let the child exert some autonomy over specific types of food and the amounts eaten.

Tensions between parents, or between parents and children, especially during mealtime, often contribute to eating problems. Getting to the root of family problems and creating a more harmonious family atmosphere are important steps toward resolving many childhood feeding issues. In addition, many parents need to learn what to expect of children and appropriate food-related goals to set.

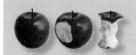 *Take Action*

Getting Young Bill to Eat

Bill is 3 years old, and his mother is worried about his eating habits. He absolutely refuses to eat vegetables, meat, and dinner in general. Some days he eats very little food. He wants to eat snacks most of the time. His mother wants him to eat a sit-down lunch and dinner to make sure he gets all the nutrients he needs. Mealtime is a battle because Bill says he isn't hungry, but his mother wants him to eat everything served on his plate. He drinks 5 or 6 glasses of whole milk per day because that is the 1 food he likes.

When his mother prepares dinner, she makes plenty of vegetables, boiling them until they are soft, hoping this will appeal to Bill. Bill's dad waits to eat his vegetables last, regularly telling the family that he eats them only because he has to. He also regularly complains about how dinner has been prepared.

Bill saves his vegetables until last and usually gags when his mother orders him to eat them. Bill has been known to sit at the dinner table for an hour until the war of wills ends. Bill's mother

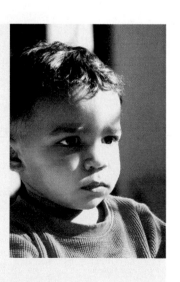

serves casseroles and stews regularly because they are convenient. Bill likes to eat breakfast cereal, fruit, and cheese and regularly requests these foods for snacks. However, his mother tries to deny his requests, so that he will have an appetite for dinner. Bill's mother asks you what she should do to get Bill to eat.

Analysis

1. List 4 mistakes Bill's parents are making that contribute to Bill's poor eating habits.
2. List 4 strategies Bill's parents might try to promote good eating habits for Bill.

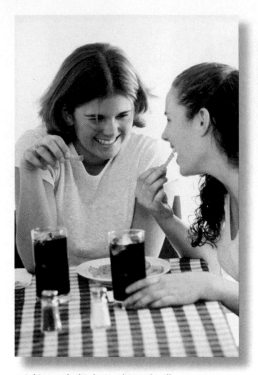

Drinking soft drinks in place of milk causes many teenagers to have inadequate calcium intake. This practice is linked to decreased bone mass and increased bone fractures in this age group. Figure 2-3 in Chapter 2 shows the stark contrast between milk and soft drinks with respect to calcium and other nutrients. If dairy products are not consumed, alternative calcium sources need to be included in the diet.

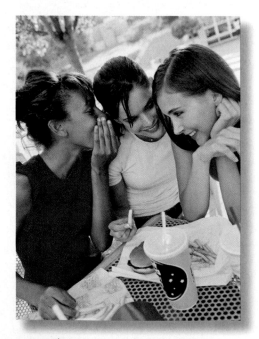

As teens become more independent, they make more and more decisions on their own, especially decisions about what, when, where, and with whom they will eat.

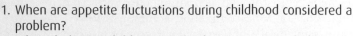

Knowledge Check

1. When are appetite fluctuations during childhood considered a problem?
2. Why is bribing a child to eat a food not recommended?
3. What are some steps caregivers can take to help children accept new foods?
4. What is the best way to handle children who go on food jags or refuse to eat?

17.7 Teenage Eating Patterns

As the teenage growth spurt begins, teenagers begin to eat more. The types and amounts of foods recommended for teenagers are the same as those for adults, except that teens have a greater need for calcium-rich foods. Adolescents in the U.S. and Canada are relatively well nourished, but they are more likely to have poor nutrient intake than those in other life stages. Teens generally eat less than the recommended amounts of fruits and vegetables. They also tend to choose foods that are higher in cholesterol, sugar, fat, saturated fat, *trans* fat, protein, and sodium than recommended. Some consume excess amounts of alcohol, too.

In comparison with teenage females, the diets of teenage males are better (but not totally adequate), mainly because boys eat 700 to 1000 calories more each day than girls.[11] (The more calories you eat, the more opportunity you have to increase nutrient intake.) A particular problem with teenage girls is that many replace milk with soft drinks, so they may not consume enough calcium to allow for maximum mineralization of bones, which increases their risk of osteoporosis later on. The Adequate Intake for calcium for both males and females between ages 9 and 18 years is 1300 mg per day, compared with only 800 mg per day for younger children.

The diets of teens are less than optimal because they frequently eat out, skip meals, and snack. As teens get older, they tend to eat more and more meals and snacks away from home. Many of these meals and snacks are purchased from vending machines, convenience stores, and fast-food restaurants. The main concern with these foods is that they often are higher in calories, fat, sugar, and sodium and lower in vitamin A, vitamin C, folate, calcium, iron, and zinc than foods served at home.

Meal skipping, especially by females and older teens, is common. Breakfast is the meal skipped most often, with more than a quarter of all teens skipping it most of the time. Snacking is very common, too—9 out of 10 teens report snacking. Overall, snacks account for about 25% of a teen's total calorie intake and, depending on the foods selected, can provide substantial nutrient contributions and even make up for nutrients missed when meals are skipped. However, most of the popular snacks among teens (e.g., potato and corn chips, ice cream, candy, cookies, cake, crackers, popcorn, presweetened breakfast drinks) are of limited nutritional value and are high in calories, fat, and/or sugar. Snacks as well as meals purchased away from home, with careful selection, can be rich in nutrients while keeping calories under control.

Nutrition experts agree that one way to get teens to eat more nutritiously is to make sure that, when teens do eat at home, they find nutritious foods, such as fruits, vegetables, milk, and fruit juice instead of soft drinks, high-fat snacks, and sugary foods.[26] Another technique for helping teens eat nutritiously is to plan family meals at least a few times a week.

Factors Affecting Teens' Food Choices

Teenagers face a variety of challenges. The struggle to establish independence and individual identity, gain peer acceptance, and cope with their heightened concern about physical appearance has profound effects on almost every aspect of teenagers' lives, including their food choices.[27] For instance, as they become more independent, teens begin making more decisions on their own, especially decisions regarding what, when, where, and with whom they will eat. As they forge their individual identities, they may participate in activities (e.g., clubs, sports, and part-time jobs) that change their lifestyles and cause them to miss many meals at home. Other factors that affect teens' food choices are their perceived and desired body images, their participation in athletics, and substance use.

Body Image

Teens are very concerned and sensitive about their appearance. The physical changes of adolescence, peer pressure, messages from the media, and the struggle to develop self-identity cause many teens to be dissatisfied with their bodies and become vulnerable to body image problems. Boys report wanting to gain weight to look stronger and more muscular. Thus, they may opt for high protein diets or supplements, both of which can impair their health without producing the desired physique. Girls frequently perceive themselves as being larger than they really are and want to lose weight, even when they are within or below the average range. The fear of obesity and a distorted body image can cause children and teens to adopt fad diets, use diet pills, set weight goals that are unrealistic and unhealthy, severely restrict food intake, and develop eating disorders[28] (see Chapter 10).

Athletics and Physical Performance

Many teenagers become involved in athletic activities. Often, their diets do not include the additional calories and nutrients they need to maintain normal growth and maturation and support their physical activity. Some athletes turn to restricted or unbalanced diets in the hope of improving performance or adhering to weight limits for their sport. For example, as described in Chapters 10 and 11, some participants in sports such as gymnastics, cheerleading, wrestling, and dancing dangerously restrict calories and/or water intake to keep their weight down. Football players and bodybuilders may overemphasize dietary protein and use protein supplements in hopes of building muscle. Endurance athletes may practice carbohydrate loading.

Diets that restrict or overemphasize any nutrient to the exclusion of other nutrients can detrimentally affect physical growth. For example, physical activity can help young people increase bone density and build a stronger skeleton. However, if calorie intake is so low that it leads to diminished body fat, which causes hormonal changes that result in irregular menstrual periods or amenorrhea, the effect on bone density is negative. The effect of these hormonal changes, which are frequently coupled with low calcium intakes at a time of increased need, can leave teenage women more susceptible to stress fractures now and osteoporosis later in life. Female athletes who experience irregular menstrual periods or amenorrhea because they are underweight need to gain weight and perhaps take a vitamin and mineral supplement (see Chapter 11). Coaches, with the help of dietitians, can encourage and teach teenage athletes to choose diets that help them grow, develop, and perform optimally.

Substance Use

Substance use among adolescents is common. Substance users tend to have poor diets, a reduced interest in food and eating, and poor nutritional status. The diets of alcohol abusers are poor because alcohol, an empty-calorie food, displaces nutritious foods (see

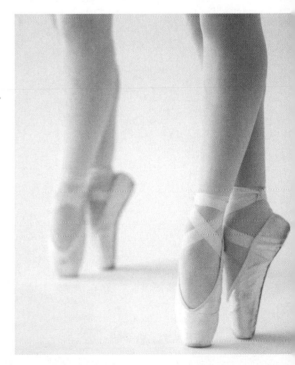

Females most at risk for irregular menstrual periods or amenorrhea are those who train many hours each day and those involved in endurance sports (e.g., marathon running) or sports that emphasize slimness (e.g., ballet, gymnastics).

Table 17-7 Food Plan for Teenagers Based on MyPyramid[a, b]

Food Group	Serving Size	Approximate Number of Servings		
		Age 13	Age 16	Age 18
Grains	Ounce	6–7	6–10	6–10
Vegetables	Cup	2.5–3	2.5–3.5	2.5–3.5
Fruits	Cup	2	2–2.5	2–2.5
Milk	Cup	3	3	3
Meat and beans	Ounce	5.5–6	5.5–7	5.5–7
Oils	Teaspoon	6	6–8	6–8
Discretionary calories	Kcal	Up to 265–290	Up to 265–425	Up to 265–425

[a] Assumes 30–60 minutes of physical activity per day. Log on to mypyramid.gov for other ages and levels of physical activity.
[b] Larger amounts refer to boys.

Chapter 8). Alcohol also alters metabolism and increases the need for and/or excretion of nutrients. Malnutrition and growth stunting can result from excessive alcohol use. Cocaine abusers tend to lose interest in food because their desire for cocaine overrides hunger sensations. As a result, they frequently lose significant amounts of weight, are malnourished, and develop eating disorders. (When rats are given unlimited cocaine and food, they choose the cocaine over food until they starve to death.) Nicotine suppresses hunger, which can lead to inadequate food intake and weight loss. In addition, the diets of smokers tend to be lower in fiber, vitamins, and minerals than those of non-smokers, and their need for vitamin C is nearly twice that of non-smokers. Marijuana distorts the appetite and creates a desire in many users to snack on foods that are high in carbohydrates, fat, and calories.

Helping Teens Eat More Nutritious Foods

Because psychological, social, and physical changes occur so rapidly during adolescence, it may be difficult to help teenagers see the value of healthy diets and exercise. In addition, many teens have a hard time relating today's actions to tomorrow's health outcomes. Therefore, it's more effective to focus on the benefits they can reap right now than to talk about health hazards that may or may not happen later. One strategy for working with teenage boys is to stress the importance of nutrition and physical activity for physical development—especially muscular development—and for fitness, vigor, and health. With teenage girls, one approach is to help them understand how choosing nutrient-dense foods and enjoyable physical activities will lead to better health and a healthy weight. Teens also need to know that healthful food habits don't mean giving up favorite foods. Small portions of fatty or sweet foods can complement larger portions of reduced-fat dairy products, lean meats, fruits, vegetables, and whole-grain products.[29] MyPyramid is a useful tool for teenage meal plans (Table 17-7).

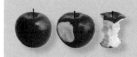

Take Action

Evaluating a Teen Lunch

These are 2 typical teen lunches and nutritional information for each.

Meal 1

2 slices pepperoni pizza
1 chocolate candy bar
20 oz cola

Meal 2

1 large hamburger
30 french fries
20 oz cola

	Meal 1	Meal 2	Nutrient Needs for Teens
Energy (kcal)	1100	1000	Males: 3000
			Females: 2200
Protein	32	20	Males: 59
			Females: 44
Vitamin C (mg)	5	18	Both genders: 45 to 75
Vitamin A (g RAE)	300	10	Males: 900
			Females: 700
Iron (mg)	3	4	Males: 11
			Females: 15
Calcium (mg)	545	100	Both genders: 1300

1. Keeping in mind that meals should meet about one-third of nutrient needs, what are the shortcomings and excesses of these meals? That is, given the nutritional information, compare these meals with one-third the RDA for protein, vitamin C, vitamin A, and iron and the Adequate Intake for calcium.

2. How would you change these meals to improve balance and meet nutrient needs?

3. Reflect on your food choices as a teenager. Do you think your meal choices were balanced and varied? Why or why not? What could you have done to improve your nutritional habits at that time? How do your nutritional habits differ now?

Knowledge Check

1. Which factors affect the quality of teenagers' diets as they get older?
2. What steps can caregivers take to help teens eat more nutritiously?
3. What effects can diminished body fat have on the bones of teenage girls?
4. What effects can substance use have on nutritional status?

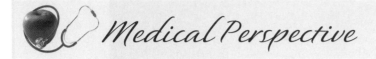

Medical Perspective

Potential Nutrition-Related Problems of the Growing Years

Parents, other caregivers, and clinicians should be on the alert for a variety of health problems related to nutrition that can occur as children move through the growing years. Typically, these problems can be prevented, or, in most cases, treated effectively with dietary modifications and/or medical intervention. Iron deficiency anemia, one common nutrition-related problem, was described earlier in this chapter. Some people consider the health problems that some children and teens experience, such as hyperactivity and acne, to be diet-related, even though scientific evidence indicates otherwise. Parents and other caregivers usually need to consult a physician when dealing with many nutrition-related health conditions. The website of the American Academy of Pediatrics (www.aap.org) also provides useful information.

Colic

Colic is sharp abdominal pain in otherwise healthy infants. The infants have repeated crying episodes, lasting 3 or more hours, that don't respond to typical remedies—such as feeding, holding, or changing diapers. Colic affects about 10 to 30% of all infants, starting at about 2 to 6 weeks of age and lasting until about 3 months of age. Crying episodes typically occur in the late afternoon and early evening. Nighttime sleeping also is usually disturbed by crying spells. Many colicky infants have flatulence, clench their fists, hold their bodies straight, draw up their legs, and want to be held.

The cause of colic is not known. It generally occurs in the absence of any physical problem in the infant. It tends to be most common in "temperamental" infants—those who are more sensitive, irritable, and intense and less adaptable and consolable than average for their age. Some researchers have speculated that an immature nervous system may cause colic. In addition, a lack of harmonious interaction between parents and the infant may contribute to the problem.

To help reduce excessive crying, parents should check to see whether the infant is tired, is bored, or wants to suckle. Holding the infant snugly to the shoulder causes many babies to become quiet and alert. Some infants can be calmed with pacifiers or by rhythmic sounds or movement.

Breastfeeding of colicky infants should continue. Mothers can try decreasing or stopping their consumption of milk and milk products, caffeine, chocolate, and strongly flavored vegetables to see if it helps reduce colic. Formula-fed infants with severe colic are sometimes helped by changing to soy-based or predigested protein formula. In addition, physicians may prescribe medication to calm colicky infants and reduce gas buildup.[4]

Coping with repeated crying spells can be challenging. Most parents benefit from the support of other adults and advice from those who have been through similar experiences. To optimize their ability to be sensitive and responsive to their infants, parents need to be well rested and set aside some time for themselves.

Gastroesophageal Reflux

Many infants develop gastroesophageal reflux (GER), more commonly known as "spitting up," during their first year of life. In most cases, GER develops before age 2 to 3 months and usually resolves on its own by the infant's first birthday. The problem occurs because the lower esophageal sphincter does not close completely, which allows milk or food in the infant's stomach to move back up into the esophagus. This can cause a painful burning sensation. In most cases, GER poses no serious medical concerns. In very rare cases, surgery may be required to remedy the problem.[4]

Milk Allergy

Cow milk contains more than 40 proteins that can cause allergic reactions in infants. Although some of these proteins are inactivated by heating (scalding) milk, others are not. A true milk allergy develops in about 1 to 3% of formula-fed infants. These infants

Colic causes inconsolable crying and can make parents feel frustrated and helpless.

(continued)

may experience vomiting, diarrhea, blood in the stool, constipation, and other symptoms. If milk allergy is suspected, a formula-fed infant can be switched to a soy-based formula. However, in 20 to 50% of cases, infants also develop a soy protein allergy. In such cases, a predigested protein formula is necessary. A breastfeeding mother can experiment by eliminating cow milk from her diet. Fortunately, milk allergies seldom last beyond 3 years of age.[4]

Constipation

Many children have bouts with constipation; for some it is a chronic problem. The most common cause is eating too little fiber, drinking too little water, drinking too much milk, and/or not responding promptly to urges to defecate. Children who have been constipated may hold in feces because they fear they will have a painful bowel movement—this can create a cycle that makes constipation worse. To prevent constipation, children over the age of 1 year need to consume 14 grams of fiber per 1000 kcal, drink plenty of water, and keep their milk intake to about 16 to 24 ounces daily. The treatment of constipation may involve the use of stool softeners, laxatives, or enemas; parents should consult a physician before using these. (Chapter 4 covers constipation in more detail.)

Diarrhea

In the U.S., about 500 infants die each year of simple dehydration resulting from diarrhea, and about 210,000 are hospitalized for this problem. Typical symptoms of dehydration include dry mouth or tongue, few or no tears when crying, no wet diapers for 3 hours or more, irritability and listlessness, and sunken eyes and cheeks. To prevent dehydration, infants with diarrhea should be given plenty of fluids, under the advice of a physician. Specialized electrolyte-replacement fluids, such as Pedialyte®, may be recommended.[4] Once diarrhea subsides, a bottle-fed infant may be switched to a soy-based, lactose-free formula for a few days to allow time for the intestine to produce sufficient lactase enzyme. A breastfed infant should continue to be breastfed for the duration of the diarrhea (see Chapter 4).

Ear Infections (Otitis Media)

When a baby sleeps with a bottle filled with formula, milk, juice, or a sweetened drink, liquids dripping from the nipple pool in the mouth and back up in the throat and tubes leading to the ears. This backup can cause bacterial growth, which can result in painful ear infections and possibly hearing loss. Many ear infections can be prevented by never allowing a child to take a bottle to bed.

Dental Caries

After the common cold, dental caries (cavities) are the most common childhood disease. Cavities form when bacteria in the mouth metabolize sugars and starch and form acids that erode tooth enamel. **Early childhood caries** (formerly called nursing bottle syndrome or baby bottle tooth decay) is a likely consequence when

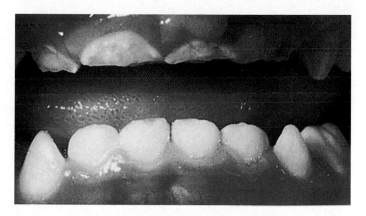

Figure 17-7 Early childhood dental caries are the result of sleeping with a bottle in the mouth.

babies and children sleep with a bottle in the mouth (Fig. 17-7). The liquid from the dripping nipple spreads over the top teeth and rear bottom teeth. (The tongue covers the front bottom teeth.) Saliva normally washes the liquid from the bottle off the teeth, but during sleep the saliva flow stops. This gives bacteria in the mouth the opportunity to metabolize the sugar in the liquid and produce acids that eat away tooth enamel.

The prevalence of dental caries in the U.S. has dropped significantly because of the increased use of fluoride-containing toothpaste, school-based dental care programs, fluoride in community water, professional fluoride treatments, and tooth sealants (a plasticlike material applied to teeth). Restricting carbohydrate intake is not an appropriate method for preventing tooth decay. However, brushing after sticky, high sugar snacks and, if gum is chewed, selecting sugarless gum help prevent caries.

Obesity

In the U.S., about 15% of school-age children are overweight. The number of cases is increasing, especially in minority populations. As indicated earlier in this chapter, obesity is generally diagnosed when a child reaches the 95th percentile for BMI and a physical exam indicates the child is truly overfat. The main consequences of obesity include ridicule, embarrassment, possible depression, and short stature linked to early puberty. These early maturers tend to be shorter and fatter throughout life than later maturers. Other significant health problems associated with obesity, such as cardiovascular disease, type 2 diabetes, and hypertension, usually appear in adulthood. However, an increase in these health-related complications has been noted in children.

The likelihood that obesity and its problems will follow children and teens into adulthood is great.[30] Although overweight infants seldom become obese children, approximately 40% of all obese children and 80% of obese teens will become obese adults and face an increased risk of several chronic diseases. Significant weight gain generally begins between ages 5 and 7, during puberty, or during the teenage years.[31]

(continued)

Medical Perspective, continued

Numerous factors, including heredity, environment, and dietary and activity behaviors, influence the development of obesity in children. In terms of heredity, the risk of obesity increases with parental obesity. Although the genetic potential of children born to one or more obese parents is high, the actual development is largely determined by whether the young person's environment promotes overeating and inactivity. Diet is an important factor, but inactivity is a key contributor to excess weight gain. One environmental factor, in particular, is of concern: inactivity caused by frequent television watching. Children watch TV for an average of 24 hours a week; many spend another 10 hours or so playing computer and video games. The American Academy of Pediatrics recommends a limit of 14 hours of TV and video time per week.[4] In addition, excessive snacking, over-reliance on fast-food restaurants, parental neglect, the media, a lack of safe areas to play, and easy availability of high-fat/high-energy food choices also contribute to childhood obesity.

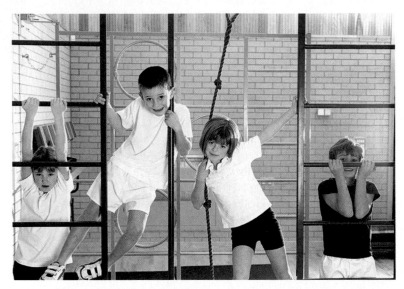

Children and teens should get 60 minutes or more of moderate to intense physical activity every day.

The best approach to obesity in children is to prevent it from occurring by offering a nutritious diet and plenty of opportunities for physical exercise (Fig. 17-8).[31, 32] However, if the precursors to obesity (inactivity and overeating) begin to appear, prevention efforts are needed immediately (more activity and fewer high-calorie foods, such as soft drinks, chips, and whole milk). If a child is already obese, the first step is to assess how much physical activity he or she engages in. If a child spends much free time in sedentary activities, more physical activities should be encouraged.

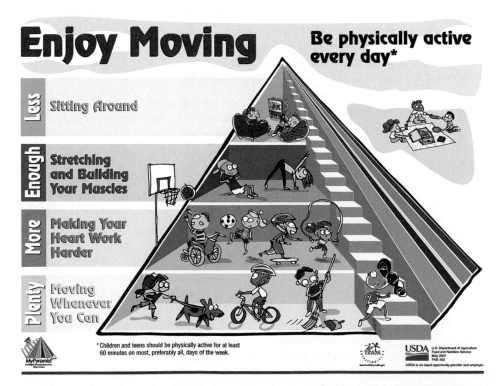

Figure 17-8 The USDA developed the "backside" of MyPyramid to describe the types of activities children should engage in and how often.

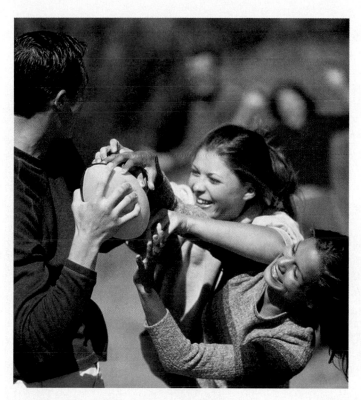

An active lifestyle coupled with a healthy diet should be part of the growing years. Lack of exercise can lead to weight problems and high blood cholesterol.

Both the U.S. government and health professionals recommend 60 minutes or more of moderate to intense physical activity per day for children and adolescents. An overall active lifestyle will help children not only attain a healthy body weight but also keep a healthy body weight later in life and reduce the risk of obesity-related diseases. An increase in physical activity won't just happen; parents and other caregivers need to plan for it. Two good ideas are getting the family together for a brisk walk after dinner and finding an after-school sport the child enjoys.

Obese children often need to find a new way to relate to foods, especially snack foods. An important family rule might be that children are allowed to eat only while sitting at the dining table or in the kitchen. This rule can stop mindless snacking in front of the television and make all family members more conscious of when they are eating. It also might be helpful to put portions of snack foods on plates rather than to allow unlimited amounts of snacks, as often happens when children eat directly from a full box of crackers or cookies.

Obese children also need support, admiration, and encouragement to bring their weight under control. A child's self-esteem is extremely fragile. Obesity itself often affects the child's psyche and mental outlook (e.g., depression). Humiliation doesn't work; it only makes the child feel worse.

Resorting to a weight-loss diet is usually not necessary. Children have an advantage over adults in dealing with obesity; their bodies can use stored energy for growth. Thus, if weight gain can

be moderated, their normal increases in height help bring weight under control. That is, growing taller while controlling weight gain lets the child "grow into" his or her weight. Low-calorie diets that result in rapid weight loss are not recommended for children and teens because they can stunt growth, cause micronutrient deficiencies, and adversely affect eating behaviors and parent-child relationships. In children younger than 2 years of age, energy-restricted diets are not recommended because insufficient fatty acid and micronutrient intake may impair brain development.[2]

Teens who remain obese after attaining their full adult height may need a weight-loss program. Still, weight loss should be gradual, perhaps 1 lb/week, and should generally follow the advice in Chapter 10. Weight-loss medications and/or surgery may be indicated for some older children and teens.[32] Using a weight-loss diet at any time during childhood or adolescence requires careful supervision by physicians and registered dietitians.

Finally, it is important to remember that not all children are designed to be tall and slender. In other words, some children simply weigh more than others. A healthy lifestyle with plenty of physical activity and nutritious foods remains the goal. (For a complete discussion of obesity, see Chapter 10.)

Hyperactivity

Hyperactivity is a medical condition characterized by distractibility, impulsiveness, disruptive behavior, and overactivity. The specific cause of hyperactivity is not known; however, a variety of diet-related causes have been proposed, such as food allergies, food additives, and/or consumption of large amounts of sugar. However, numerous carefully controlled research studies offer little scientific evidence to support claims that dietary factors cause hyperactivity or that eliminating certain dietary constituents will "cure" hyperactivity, a recent well-controlled study indicates food additives did increase hyperactivity in children. [35] Thus, it may be wise to limit food additive intake by decreasing the consumption of highly processed foods. Providing megadoses of vitamins will not "cure" hyperactivity or attention disorders and can cause liver damage and intestinal upset.

Acne

Acne is a common teen concern—about 80% of teens experience it. Although it's popularly believed that eating nuts, chocolate, and pizza can make acne worse, scientific studies have failed to show a strong link between any dietary factor and acne. Actually, acne develops when excess oily secretions block glands in the skin. Large doses of vitamins or minerals will not cure acne and can be toxic. As described in Chapter 12, physicians can prescribe a form of vitamin A (isotretinoin [Accutane® and Retin-A®]) to treat severe cases of acne. Although these treatments can be quite effective, close supervision by a physician is crucial because these vitamin A analogs can be toxic. Vitamin A itself is no help in treating acne and excess amounts of vitamin A or related analogs can cause birth defects. Thus, females taking these vitamin A medications must not become pregnant.

(continued)

Medical Perspective, continued

Teenage Pregnancy

The nutritional demands of pregnancy superimposed on the nutritional demands of adolescence can make it difficult for teens to consume a diet that can support their own growth and fetal growth. In an attempt to hide their pregnancy or retain a slim figure, pregnant teens may resort to excessive dieting. This practice, coupled with typical teenage eating patterns, lack of early prenatal care, and socioeconomic problems (e.g., incomplete education, lack of financial and emotional support), makes it even more difficult to meet nutritional demands.

A female who becomes pregnant within 2 years of menarche is at greatest nutritional risk because she is physically immature and her chances of developing complications (e.g., anemia, pregnancy-induced hypertension, spontaneous abortion, premature birth, low birth weight infant) are much greater than for a female who becomes pregnant at a later point in her physical development. In addition, mothers less than 15 years old are much more likely to die as a direct result of pregnancy complications than those who are older. (For a more complete discussion of pregnancy, refer to Chapter 16.)

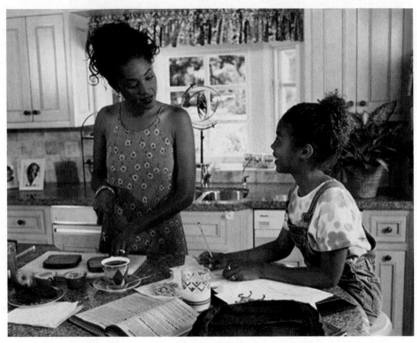

Opportunities to learn about good nutrition at home and at school help prepare children and teens to make lifelong healthy food choices.

Inadequate Nutrition Knowledge

Although children and teenagers are increasingly knowledgeable in many health areas, including nutrition, a large proportion are not exposed to nutrition education in any depth. Teaching children and teens about nutrition is important because those who do not have accurate nutrition knowledge cannot make informed food choices. In addition, learning how to select a nutritious diet can help them establish healthy eating habits early in life, and these eating habits tend to carry over into the adult years.

School-based nutrition education programs can help children and teens become more informed decision makers. Informed decision makers are able to make the best food choices for themselves at present, as well as safeguard their own health and the health of those for whom they are responsible (e.g., children, aging parents) throughout the adult years.

Modifications of Child and Teen Diets to Reduce Future Disease Risk

Parents sometimes wonder whether dietary modifications during childhood can help reduce future risks of cardiovascular disease, hypertension, and type 2 diabetes. Recall that the development

of atherosclerosis often begins in childhood.[29] As a result, many experts recommend screening for elevated blood cholesterol in children whose families have histories of early development of cardiovascular disease or high blood cholesterol and treating children with high blood cholesterol with appropriate dietary changes and possibly medication (see Chapter 6).[29] In general, it's unnecessary to discourage children and teens from consuming nutrient-dense foods, such as milk and animal proteins, just because they contain some animal fat. The overriding message is moderation in these and other fat sources, with a focus on limiting saturated fat, *trans* fat, and cholesterol intake.

Scientific data neither confirm nor refute the idea that eating less salt (sodium) reduces the risk of future hypertension. However, moderation in salt intake does help build good health habits for the future. If children become accustomed to less salt, they'll be less inclined to eat very salty foods as adults. Children with hypertension can benefit from dietary modifications, such as the DASH diet (see Chapter 6), that lower sodium intake and increase fruit, vegetable, and reduced-fat dairy food.[33] However, if a child with hypertension does not respond to diet and lifestyle therapy, medications may be prescribed.

Type 2 diabetes is generally thought of as an adult condition. In recent years, it has become more common in children and teenagers, primarily due to the rise in obesity in this age group. Up to 85% of children with type 2 diabetes are overweight at diagnosis. Experts are currently recommending that at-risk children be screened for this disease every 2 years, starting at age 10 or at the onset of puberty. Besides obesity and a sedentary lifestyle, other risk factors include having a close relative with the disease and belonging to a non-white population.[4, 34] Appropriate diet and lifestyle intervention should be implemented, along with the use of medications when necessary. A focus on low glycemic load fruits, vegetables, and whole-grain breads and cereals is especially important (see Chapter 5).

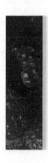

Knowledge Check

1. What advice would you give to help parents calm a colicky infant?
2. How does sleeping with a bottle contribute to early dental caries and ear infections?
3. Why is a weight-loss diet usually not necessary for children?
4. What risks do overweight children face?
5 What family characteristics indicate a child should be screened for elevated cholesterol?

Summary

17.1 Normal growth and development are highly dependent on calorie and nutrient intake. Physical growth rate is at its peak velocity during infancy, slows during childhood, then increases again during adolescence. During the growing years, height and weight increase, body composition changes, and body organs and systems mature.

17.2 The single best indicator of a child's nutritional status is growth. Growth charts matched to a child's gender are used to track physical growth over time to identify a child's growth percentile curves and determine if growth is progressing normally. BMI-for-age (or weight-for-length for children younger than 2 years old) is a good indicator of recent nutritional status. Stature-for-age is a good indicator of long-term nutritional status. Infants and young children who do not grow at the expected rate for several months and are dramatically smaller or shorter than other children the same age, especially those who fall below the 5th percentile, experience failure to thrive. Continually receiving minimal quantities of food may permanently and irreversibly stunt growth and development. Growth in height ceases when the growth plates at the ends of the bones fuse.

17.3 The greatest calorie and nutrient needs, pound for pound, occur during infancy. The total quantity of calories and nutrients needed rises throughout childhood. The total quantities of nutrients and calories needed are greater during adolescence than at any other time, except pregnancy and lactation. Adolescent males need more of many nutrients than females because males are larger, develop more muscle mass and bone density, and have a longer, more intense growth period. Total fat should account for about 40 to 55% of a baby's calorie intake. It is wise to reduce fat intake gradually between ages 2 and 5 years until children are getting an average of 30 to 35% of their calories from fat. Dietary recommendations meant to reduce the risk of heart disease do *not* apply to children younger than 2 years old. Water is of special importance for babies because they have a large body surface area per pound of weight, turn over body water quickly, produce a large quantity of wastes, and have inefficient kidneys. A young baby's need for water is usually met by human milk or formula. However, giving infants too much water can lead to water intoxication. Newborns frequently have low stores of fluoride, vitamin K, and vitamin D. Many children and adolescents consume too little calcium, zinc, folate, and vitamins A and C.

17.4 With few exceptions, human milk or iron-fortified infant formula and the baby's internal nutrient stores meet an infant's nutrient needs at least until age 4 to 6 months. Human milk is the most ideal and desirable source of nutrients for infants. Commercial iron-fortified infant formulas provide a safe, nutritious alternative to human milk. Breastfed infants must be followed closely over the first week of life to ensure that feeding and weight gain are proceeding normally. All equipment and utensils used to prepare, store, and/or feed infant formula or human milk should be thoroughly washed and rinsed.

17.5 When to introduce solid foods into an infant's diet hinges on the infant's nutritional needs, physiological capabilities, and physical ability. Between 6 and 12 months of age, human milk or formula intake gradually decreases while solid food intake slowly increases. The recommended sequence for introducing solid foods is iron-fortified baby cereal, juices and pureed fruits and vegetables, protein-rich foods, finger foods, and table foods. Parents should wait until the child is a year old before serving egg whites and unaltered cow milk because they frequently cause allergic reactions in younger babies. Infants should never be put to bed with a bottle or placed in an infant seat with a bottle propped up.

17.6 Compared with babies, children tend to have erratic appetites. Pressuring a child to eat more or less than desired tells the child not to trust his or her own hunger and satiety signals—this can lead to a lifetime battle with weight problems. Offering children 6 or so small meals succeeds better than limiting them to 3 meals daily. A serving size for children is equal to about 1 tablespoon per year of age, depending on the child's appetite. MyPyramid for children is a useful meal planning tool. The most important nutrition lessons for children of all ages involve expanding their familiarity with new foods and helping them develop

a willingness to accept new foods. Many preschool children go through periods of unpredictable and unusual eating behavior, such as going on food jags, refusing to eat, and being a picky eater. The best way to handle most of these behaviors is to not overreact, offer a variety of healthy foods, and let the child exert some autonomy over the specific types of food and amounts eaten.

17.7 The types and amounts of foods recommended for teenagers are the same as those for adults, except that teens have a greater need for calcium. The diets of teens are less than optimal because teens frequently eat out, skip meals, and snack. The struggle to establish independence and individual identity, gain peer acceptance, and cope with their heightened concern about physical appearance affects teens' food choices. Other factors that affect their food choices are perceived and desired body image, participation in athletics, and substance use. MyPyramid is a useful tool for teenage meal plans. Common nutrition-related health problems during the growing years are iron deficiency anemia, colic, gastroesophageal reflux, milk allergy, constipation, diarrhea, ear infections, dental caries, and obesity. Parents usually need to consult a physician when dealing with many nutrition-related conditions. Children from families with histories of early development of cardiovascular disease or high blood cholesterol should be screened for high blood cholesterol levels and, if necessary, treated with appropriate dietary changes and possibly medication.

Study Questions

1. At age 1 year, a 7-pound, 20-inch-long newborn growing normally would be _____.

   a. 14 pounds, 25 inches
   b. 18 pounds, 30 inches
   c. 21 pounds, 30 inches
   d. 28 pounds, 40 inches

2. When adolescence ends, females have _____.

   a. twice as much body fat as males
   b. two-thirds as much lean body mass as males
   c. one-tenth more body water than males
   d. all of the above
   e. both a and b

3. The percentile growth curve a child follows depends mostly on _____.

   a. dietary intake
   b. genetic endowment
   c. gender
   d. age
   e. both a and b

4. Children are likely experiencing growth stunting if their _____.

   a. stature-for-age falls below the 5th percentile
   b. BMI-for-age falls below the 25th percentile
   c. weight-for-length rises above the 75th percentile
   d. head circumference-for-age exceeds the 95th percentile

5. A good indicator of long-term nutritional status is stature-for-age.

   a. true   b. false

6. Pound for pound, which age group needs the most calories?

   a. newborns   c. 1-year-olds
   b. 6-month-olds   d. 3-year-olds

7. One reason water is of critical importance to infants is because they have _____.

   a. less body surface area per pound of body weight than adults
   b. a slow metabolic rate
   c. very efficient kidneys
   d. proportionately more body water than adults

8. To maintain a desirable iron status, breastfed infants should receive iron supplementation.

   a. true   b. false

9. More iron is absorbed from human milk than infant formula.

   a. true   b. false

10. Which of the following is *not* true of proteins in human milk?

    a. They are easier to digest than those in cow milk.
    b. They increase the rate of iron absorption by the infant.
    c. They protect the infant from harmful pathogens.
    d. They often lead to allergies.

11. One sign that babies are developmentally ready for solid foods is that they _____.

    a. are 3 months old
    b. can control head movements
    c. have a strong extrusion reflex
    d. have more than 6 wet diapers per day

12. Which of the following commonly causes an allergic response in infants?

    a. egg whites   c. carrots
    b. peaches   d. egg yolk

13. Bribing a child to eat a food increases the child's desire for the food.

    a. true
    b. false

14. To help children accept new foods, caregivers should _____.

    a. serve the new food at the end of the meal
    b. give the child a reward for trying it
    c. make the child stay at the table until he or she tries it
    d. involve the child in preparing the food

15. Which of the following is true of infants with colic?

    a. They should not be breastfed.
    b. They cry for several hours each day.
    c. They stop crying after being fed or having their diapers changed.
    d. They sleep without waking during the night.
    e. All of the above are true.

Answer Key: 1-c; 2-c; 3-c; 4-a; 5-a; 6-a; 7-d; 8-b; 9-a; 10-d; 11-b; 12-a; 13-b; 14-d; 15-b

Websites

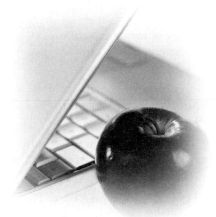

To learn more about the topics covered in this chapter, visit these websites.

American Academy of Pediatrics

www.aap.org

Life Cycle Nutrition

fnic.nal.usda.gov

www.kidshealth.org

www.ific.org

MyPyramid for Kids

mypyramid.gov/kids/index.html

teamnutrition.usda.gov/Resources/enjoymovingflyer.html

National Cholesterol Education Program

www.nhlbi.nih.gov/about/ncep/index.htm

Growth Charts

www.cdc.gov/growthcharts

References

1. Institute of Medicine, Food and Nutrition Board. *Dietary Reference Intakes for calcium, phosphorus, magnesium, vitamin D, and fluoride.* Washington, DC: National Academy Press; 1997.

2. Institute of Medicine, Food and Nutrition Board. *Dietary Reference Intakes for energy, carbohydrate, fiber, fat, fatty acids, cholesterol, protein, and amino acids.* Washington, DC: National Academy Press; 2002.

3. Butte NF and others. Body composition during the first two years of life: An updated reference. *Pediatr Res.* 2000;47:578.

4. Kleinman R, ed. *Pediatric nutrition handbook.* Chicago: American Academy of *Pediatrics*; 2004.

5. Lin-Su K and others. Body mass index and age at menarche in an adolescent clinic population. *Clinl Pediatr.* 2002;41:501.

6. Barlow SE and others. Expert committee recommendations regarding the prevention, assessment, and treatment of child and adolescent overweight and obesity: Summary report. *Pediatrics.* 2007;120:S164.

7. Whitehead R. Growth in weight and length. *Acta Paediatr.* 2003;92:406.

8. Brandt I and others. Catch-up growth of head circumference of very low birth weight, small for gestational age preterm infants and mental development to adulthood. *J Pediatr.* 2003;142:463.

9. Heird WC. Nutritional requirements during infancy. In: Bowman BA, Russell RM, eds. *Present knowledge in nutrition.* 8th ed. Washington, DC: ILSI Press; 2001:416–425.

10. Institute of Medicine, Food and Nutrition Board. *Dietary Reference Intakes for vitamin A, vitamin K, arsenic, boron, chromium, copper, iodine, iron, manganese, molybdenum, nickel, silicon, vanadium, and zinc.* Washington, DC: National Academy Press; 2001.

11. Centers for Disease Control and Prevention, National Center for Health Statistics. *Dietary intake of macronutrients, micronutrients, and other dietary constituents: United States, 1988–1994.* Washington, DC: U.S. Department of Health and Human Services; 2002.

12. Hatun S and others. Vitamin D deficiency in early infancy. *J Nutr.* 2005;135:279.

13. American Academy of Pediatrics Committee on Nutrition. Prevention of rickets and vitamin D deficiency: New guidelines for vitamin D intake. *Pediatrics.* 2003;111:908.

14. Briefel R and others. Feeding infants and toddlers study: Do vitamin and mineral supplements contribute to nutrient adequacy or excess among US infants and toddlers? *J Am Diet Assoc.* 2006;106:S52.

15. American Academy of Pediatrics, Section on Breastfeeding. Breastfeeding and the use of human milk (RE9729). *Pediatrics.* 2005;115:496.

16. American Dietetic Association. The start healthy feeding guidelines for infants and toddlers. *J Am Diet Assoc.* 2004;104:442.

17. Ryan A and others. Breast-feeding continues to increase into the new millennium. *Pediatrics.* 2002;110:1103.

18. Affenito S and others. Breakfast consumption by African-American and white adolescent girls correlates positively with calcium and fiber intake and negatively with body mass index. *J Am Diet Assoc.* 2005;105:938.

19. Dobson B, Murtaugh MA. Position of the American Dietetic Association: Breaking the barriers to breastfeeding. *J Am Diet Assoc.* 2001;101:1213.

20. American Dietetic Association. Position of the American Dietetic Association: Dietary guidance for healthy children ages 2 to 11 years. *J Am Diet Assoc.* 2004;104:660.

21. Mangels A and others. Position of the American Dietetic Association and Dietitians of Canada: Vegetarian diets. *J Am Diet Assoc.* 2003;103:748.

22. Savage JF and others. Parental influence on eating behavior: Conception to adolescence. *J Law Med Ethics.* 2007;35:22.

23. Satter E. *Child of mine. Feeding with love and good sense.* Palo Alto, CA: Bull Publishing Co.; 2000.

24. Kleinman R and others. Diet, breakfast, and academic performance in children. *Ann Nutr Metab.* 2002;46 (suppl 1):24.

25. Patrick H, Nicklas T. A review of family and social determinants of children's eating patterns and diet quality. *J Am Coll Nutr.* 2005;24:83.

26. Zabinski M and others. Psychosocial correlates of fruit, vegetable, and dietary fat intake among adolescent boys and girls. *J Am Diet Assoc.* 2006;106:814.

27. Henry B. Importance of the where as well as what and how much in food patterns of adolescents. *J Am Diet Assoc.* 2006;106:373.

28. Neumark-Sztainer D and others. Obesity, disordered eating, and eating disorders in a longitudinal study of adolescents: How do dieters fare 5 years later? *J Am Diet Assoc.* 2006;106:559.

29. American Heart Association. AHA scientific statement: Dietary recommendations for children and adolescents: a guide for practitioners. *Circulation.* 2005;112:1994.

30. Ferraro K and others. The life course of severe obesity: Does childhood overweight matter? *J Gerontol. Series B: Psychological Sciences and Social Sciences.* 2003;58:S110.

31. Klopan J and others. Preventing childhood obesity: Health in the balance—Executive summary. *J Am Diet Assoc.* 2005;105:131.

32. Kirk S and others. Pediatric obesity epidemics: Treatment options. *J Am Diet Assoc.* 2005;105:S44.

33. Couch SC and others. The efficacy of a clinic-based behavioral nutrition intervention emphasizing a DASH-type diet for adolescents with elevated blood pressure. *J Pedatr.* 2008;152:494.

34. Jones KL. Role of obesity in complicating and confusing the diagnosis and treatment of diabetes in children. *Pediatrics.* 2008;121:361.

35. McCann D and others. Food additives and hyperactive behavior behavior in 3-year-old and 8/9-year-old children in the community: a randomized, double-blinded, placebo-controlled trial. *Lancet.* 2007; 370(9598):1560.

36. Greer FR and others. Effects of early nutritional intervention on the development of atopic disease in infants and children: the role of maternal dietary restriction, breastfeeding, timing of introduction of complementary foods, and hydrolyzed formulas. *Pediatrics.* 2008; 121:183.

37. Daniels SR and others. Lipid screening and cardiovascular health in childhood. *Pediatrics.* 2008; 122:198.

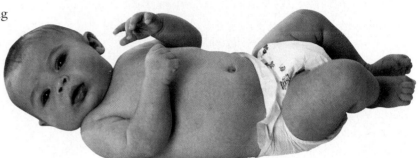

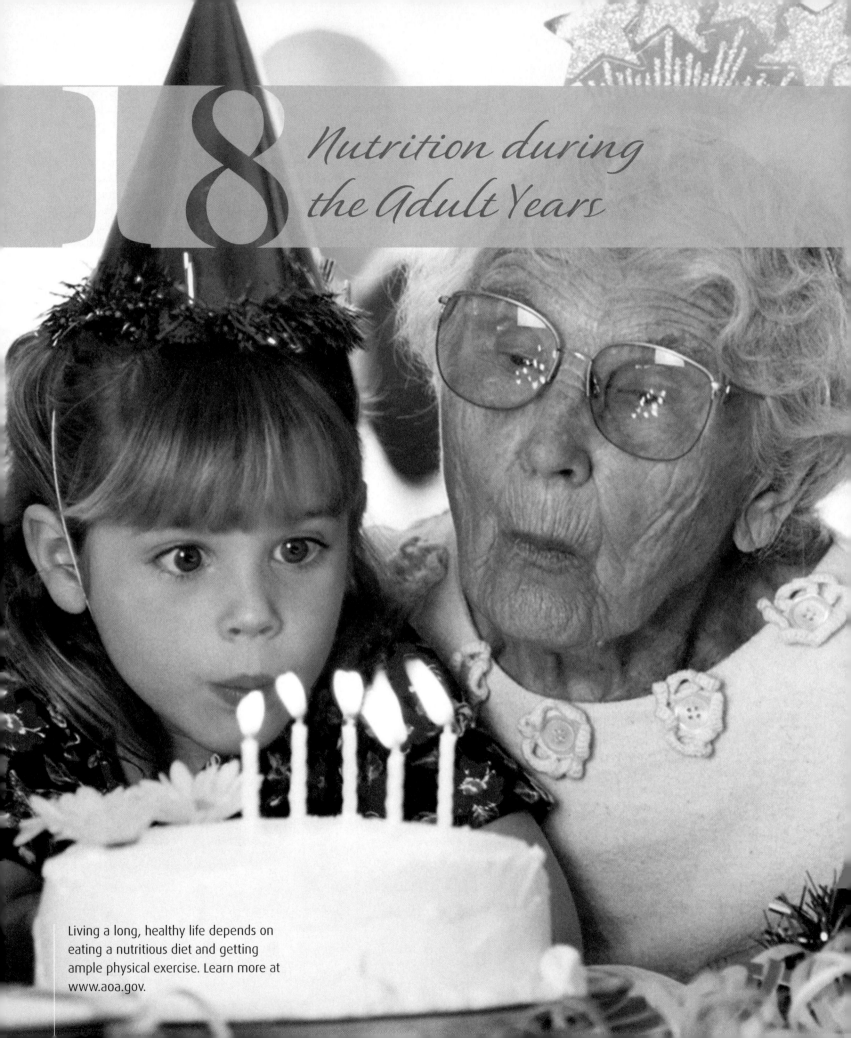

18

Nutrition during the Adult Years

Living a long, healthy life depends on eating a nutritious diet and getting ample physical exercise. Learn more at www.aoa.gov.

STUDENT LEARNING OUTCOMES

After studying this chapter, you will be able to:

1. Describe the hypotheses about the causes of aging.

2. Discuss the factors that affect the rate of aging.

3. Explain how the basic concepts that underlie the 2005 Dietary Guidelines for Americans relate to adult health.

4. Describe how physical and physiological changes that occur during adulthood affect nutritional needs.

5. Compare the dietary intake of adults with the current recommendations.

6. Discuss the effects of physical, physiological, psychosocial, and economic factors on the food intake and nutrient needs of adults.

7. Describe community nutrition services for older persons.

8. Identify nutrition-related health issues of the adult years and describe the prevention and treatment of these health problems.

9. List the potential benefits and risks associated with the use of complementary and alternative medicine practices.

A long and healthy adult life—that's what most people wish for. Thanks to a more abundant and nutritious food supply, a higher standard of living, and advances in medical technology, this wish can come true. In fact, it's already coming true. In the last century, the life expectancy for individuals born in the U.S. jumped more than 30 years. Babies born today can expect to live about 77 years—many will live even longer, and some will live the full life span possible for humans. The maximum life span for humans is generally accepted to be about 115 to 120 years.

More Americans may be living longer than before, but many are not living as healthfully (and perhaps not as long) as they could be. That is, their span of "healthy years" doesn't always correlate with the revolutionary increase in life expectancy that has occurred. Fewer than 1 in 5 people who live to age 65 or beyond are fully functional in their last year of life. For example, many suffer from diet-related chronic diseases, such as coronary heart disease, certain cancers, and osteoporosis, that impair their health. Older adults often are fatter than when they were young, their body systems have slowed appreciably, and it takes longer for the body systems to restore balance. Even though old age is often equated with "going downhill," it doesn't have to be that way. Evidence is mounting that dietary practices, exercise habits, and other lifestyle choices play a major role in determining how long a person will live and the number of years a person will maintain a fully functioning body and mind.[1]

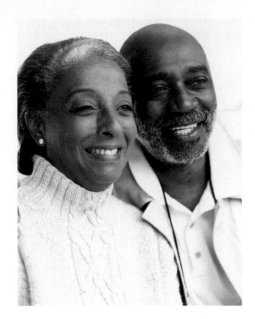

The increase in life expectancy has resulted in a phenomenon that is popularly referred to as "the graying of North America." That is, the proportion of people over age 65 is growing faster than any other segment of the population. A hundred years ago, only 1 person in 25 was 65 years or older. Today, this proportion has risen to 1 person in 8 and, in less than 40 years, people 65 years or older will account for 1 in every 5 people.

reserve capacity Extent to which an organ can preserve essentially normal function despite decreasing cell number or cell activity.

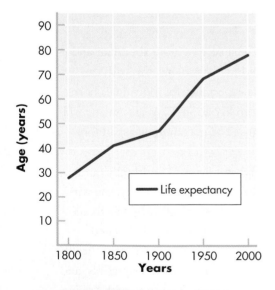

Figure 18-1 Revolutionary advances that we now take for granted—more nutritious diets, antibiotics, sewer systems, and women giving birth in hospitals—are responsible for increasing life expectancy in the 20th century.

This chapter will describe the physical and physiological changes that occur during adulthood and their impact on nutrient needs and food intake. It also will explore how dietary choices can help people keep their bodies performing efficiently and delay, prevent, or manage the declines associated with aging. That is, you'll discover how dietary practices, as well as exercise habits, can help you control the rate of aging and make the most of all the years of your life. Age quickly or slowly—it is partly your choice.

18.1 Physical and Physiological Changes during Adulthood

Adulthood, the longest stage of the life cycle, begins when an adolescent completes his or her physical growth. Unlike earlier stages of the life cycle, nutrients are used primarily to maintain the body rather than support physical growth. (Pregnancy is the only time during adulthood when substantial amounts of nutrients are used for growth.) As adults get older, nutrient needs change. For example, vitamin D needs are higher for persons in older stages of adulthood. Based on the needs for various nutrients, the Food and Nutrition Board divided the adult years into 4 stages: ages 19 to 30, 31 to 50, 51 to 70, and beyond 70 years of age. The intervals encompassing ages 19 through 50 are often referred to as young adulthood, 51 to 70 as middle adulthood, and beyond 70 years of age as older adulthood.

Adulthood is characterized by body maintenance and gradual physical and physiological transitions, often referred to as aging. **Aging** can be defined as the time-dependent physical and physiological changes in body structure and function that occur normally and progressively throughout adulthood as humans mature and become older (Fig. 18-1). From the beginning of adulthood until age 30 or so, body systems are at their peak efficiency rate. Stature, stamina, strength, endurance, efficiency, and health are at their lifetime highs. The rates of cell synthesis and breakdown are balanced in most tissues. Then, after about age 30, the rate of cell breakdown slowly begins to exceed the rate of cell renewal, leading to a gradual decline in organ size and efficiency.

As the years progress, the cumulative effects of tissue breakdown lead to an erosion of the body's efficiency in functioning—these losses occur so slowly that it usually is decades before any great differences are obvious (Fig. 18-2). Even then, body systems and organs usually retain enough **reserve capacity** to handle normal, everyday demands throughout one's entire lifetime. Problems caused by diminished capacity typically don't arise unless severe demands are placed on the aging body. For example, alcohol intake can overtax an aging liver. The stress of shoveling a snow-covered sidewalk can exceed the capacity of the heart and lungs. Coping with an illness also can push an older body beyond its capacity.

The causes of aging remain a mystery. Most likely, the physiological changes of aging are the sum of automatic cellular changes, lifestyle practices, and environmental influences, as listed in Table 18-1.[2-5] Even with the most supportive environment and healthy lifestyle, cell structure and function inevitably change over time. Eventually, cells lose their ability to regenerate vital internal parts and they die. This unavoidable dying of deteriorating cells is actually beneficial because it likely prevents diseases such as cancer. Unfortunately, there are negative consequences to this natural cell progression because, as more and more cells in an organ system die, organ function decreases. For example, kidney structures that filter blood to remove waste and reabsorb water, glucose, amino acids, and other nutrients (nephrons) are continually lost as we age. In some people, this loss exhausts the kidneys' reserve capacity and ultimately leads to kidney failure.

The diseases and physical and physiological degeneration commonly observed in older people have long been assumed to be unavoidable consequences of aging. Certainly, some of the declines we blame on aging may be inevitable, such as gradual reductions in tissue and organ cell numbers, graying hair, and reduced lung capacity. However, many of the so-called usual or degenerative age-related changes can, in fact, be minimized, prevented,

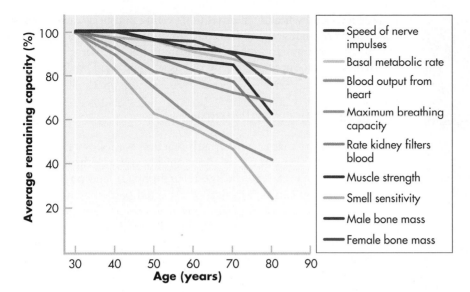

Figure 18-2 Physiological functions typically decline with age. However, when compared with the average of younger adults, some older people show minimal or no losses. The physiological changes shown here likely are more reflective of those experiencing usual aging instead of successful aging.

CRITICAL THINKING

Alexis has read several books supporting the idea that reducing typical energy intake by 30% can significantly extend one's life. Because she wants to do what is best for her 2 preschool children, she is thinking about adjusting her family's dietary habits to match this calorie restriction. What should you discuss with Alexis before she proceeds?

Table 18-1 Current Hypotheses about the Causes of Aging

Errors occur in copying the genetic blueprint (DNA).

Once sufficient errors in DNA copying accumulate, a cell can no longer synthesize the major proteins needed to function and it dies. Damage to DNA in the mitochondria also contributes to the aging process.

Connective tissue stiffens.

Parallel protein strands, found mostly in connective tissue, cross-link to each other. This decreases flexibility in key body components.

Electron-seeking compounds damage cell parts.

Electron-seeking free radicals can break down cell membranes and proteins. DNA in mitochondria typically shows this type of damage, and this damage is linked to the aging process. One way to prevent this free radical damage throughout the body is to consume adequate amounts of antioxidants.

Hormone function changes.

The blood concentration of many hormones, such as testosterone in men, falls during the aging process. Replacement of this and other hormones is possible, but the resulting risks and benefits are largely unknown.

The immune system loses some efficiency.

The immune system is most efficient during childhood and young adulthood, but, with advancing age, it is less able to recognize and counteract foreign substances, such as viruses, that enter the body. Nutrient deficiencies can impair immune function.

Autoimmunity develops.

Autoimmune reactions occur when white blood cells and other immune system components begin to attack body tissues. Many diseases, including some forms of arthritis, involve this autoimmune response.

Glycosylation of proteins occurs.

Blood glucose, when chronically elevated, attaches to (glycates) various blood and body proteins. This action decreases protein function and can encourage the immune system to attack these altered proteins.

Death is programmed into the cell.

Each human cell can divide about 50 times. Once this total number of divisions occurs, the cell dies.

Excess energy intake speeds body breakdown.

Underfed animals, such as spiders, mice, and rats, live longer than those that are well fed. Usual energy intake must be reduced by about 30% to see this effect. Currently, this approach is the only proven way to substantially slow the aging process.

and/or reversed by healthy lifestyles (e.g., eating nutritious diets, exercising regularly, getting enough sleep) and avoiding adverse environmental factors (e.g., avoiding excessive exposure to sunlight and cigarette smoke). These discoveries have led researchers to introduce the concepts of "usual aging" and "successful aging."[6]

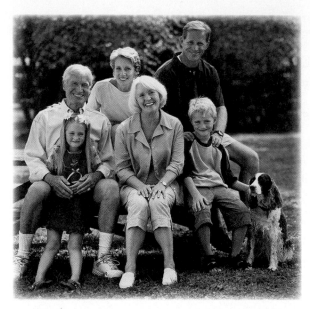

A healthy diet throughout life promotes successful aging.

Usual and Successful Aging

Body cells age, no matter what health practices we follow. However, to a considerable extent, you can choose how quickly you age throughout your adult years. *Usual aging* refers to the age-related physical and physiological changes commonly thought to be a typical or expected part of aging, such as increasing body fatness, decreasing lean body mass, rising blood pressure, declining bone mass, and increasingly poor health. Researchers point out that many of these changes really represent the aging process accelerated by unhealthy lifestyle choices, adverse environmental exposures, and/or chronic disease.[6] For instance, blood pressure does not tend to rise with age among people whose diets are traditionally low in sodium. Also, lean body mass is maintained much better in older people who exercise than in those who don't.

Successful aging, on the other hand, describes physical and physiological function declines that occur only because one grows older, not because lifestyle choices, environmental exposures, and chronic disease have aggravated or sped up the rate of aging. Those who are successful agers experience age-related declines at a slower rate and the onset of chronic disease symptoms at a later age than usual agers.[6] Striving to have the greatest number of healthy years and the fewest years of illness is often referred to as **compression of morbidity.** In other words, a person tries to delay the onset of disabilities caused by chronic disease and to compress significant sickness related to aging into the last few years—or months—of life. An example of this concept is illustrated for cardiovascular disease in Figure 18-3.

The line on the top of Figure 18-3 depicts rapid deterioration in health; symptoms of cardiovascular disease appear by about age 40, symptoms and disability occur between ages 40 and 60 years, and death occurs at about age 60. A healthier lifestyle follows the middle line. Here, cardiovascular disease is postponed, so that the first symptoms are not apparent until age 60, severe symptoms are delayed until age 80, and death follows a few years later. The line on the bottom is ideal. Disease progresses so slowly that symptoms do not appear during a person's lifetime, so the disease never impedes activities. Scientists don't yet know all of the factors that promote successful aging, but, as you'll see later in this chapter, numerous nutrition-related and lifestyle factors are known or thought to play a role in slowing the aging process and increasing health span and life expectancy.

Factors Affecting the Rate of Aging

The rate at which one ages is individual; it is determined by heredity, lifestyle, and environment. With the exception of heredity, most of the factors that influence the rate of aging are directly linked to choices that are under our control.

Heredity

Heredity defines who you are biochemically and, to some extent, it defines how long you will live (longevity).[1] Living to an old age tends to run in some families. If your parents and grandparents lived a long time, you are likely to have the potential to live to an old age,

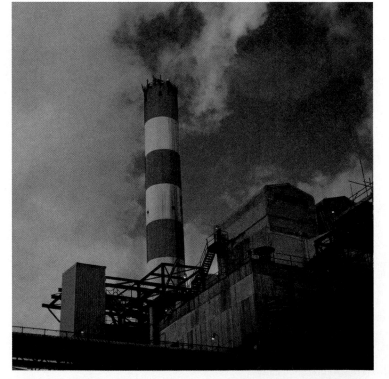

Even very healthy people have a shortened life expectancy if they are exposed to sufficient environmental stress, such as radiation and certain chemical agents (e.g., industrial solvents). Because cell aging and diseases such as cancer are aggravated by environmental factors, it makes good sense to avoid risks such as excessive sunlight exposure, hazardous chemicals, and environmental pollutants.

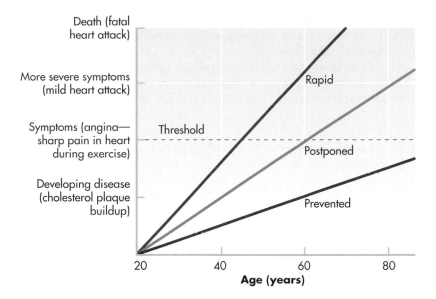

Figure 18-3 Compression of morbidity with cardiovascular disease as an example.

too. One of the most obvious genetic characteristics influencing longevity is gender. In the case of humans, as well as most other species, females tend to live longer than males.

Another genetic characteristic that can influence longevity is metabolic efficiency. Individuals with a "thrifty metabolism" require fewer calories for metabolic processes and are able to store body fat more easily than those with faster metabolic rates. Throughout history, it was the individuals with thrifty metabolism who tended to live the longest because they efficiently stored fat during times of plenty and thus had the energy stores needed to survive frequent periods of food scarcity. However, today people with a thrifty metabolism living in technologically advanced countries where food is abundant and periods of scarcity are virtually non-existent may find that their thrifty metabolism actually reduces longevity. Thrifty metabolism may enable them to store excessive amounts of body fat, which increases their risk of developing health problems that can shorten their lives (e.g., heart disease, hypertension, certain cancers). Yet another example of a genetic characteristic that may influence longevity is the rate of HDL cholesterol production. Individuals who inherit an increased ability to produce abundant HDL cholesterol may

▶ Besides having other long-lived family members, people who live to 100 years generally

- Do not smoke and do not drink heavily
- Gain little weight in adulthood
- Eat many fruits and vegetables
- Perform daily physical activity
- Challenge their minds
- Have a positive outlook
- Maintain close friendships
- Are (or were) married (especially true for men)
- Have a healthy rate of HDL cholesterol production

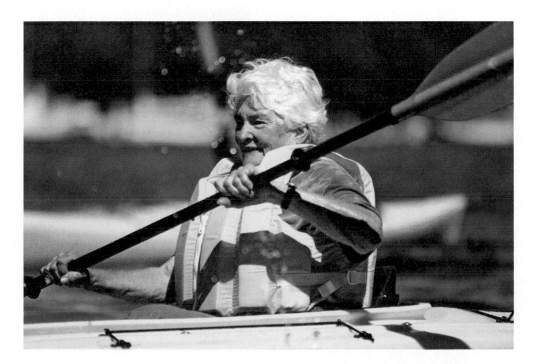

Regular exercise can lead to a healthier, more energetic, and perhaps longer life. When regular exercisers and non-exercisers of the same age are compared, death rates are significantly higher among those who don't exercise. One reason for this difference in death rate may be that inactivity increases the risk of chronic diseases. Another reason may be that inactivity is responsible for many of the physiological changes seen in usual aging that gradually weaken the body.

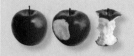

CRITICAL THINKING

The "fountain of youth" remains a mystery. Many people believe a source exists that can stop the aging process, allowing youth to remain. However, your friend asserts that the fountain of youth is not a place or a particular thing but, rather, a combination of diet and lifestyle. How can she justify this claim?

have a decreased risk of cardiovascular disease and a longer life. In contrast, those who inherit a reduced ability to produce HDL cholesterol have a greater risk of premature heart disease and a shorter life.[1]

As you know, heredity is largely unchangeable. However, heredity is not necessarily destiny—individuals can exert some control over the expression of their genetic potential. Lifestyle and environment both can modify the expression of genetic potential.

Lifestyle

Lifestyle is one's pattern of living—it includes food choices, exercise patterns, and substance use (e.g., alcohol, drugs, tobacco). Lifestyle choices can have a major impact on health and longevity,[1] as well as on the expression of genetic potential. If individuals

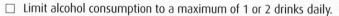

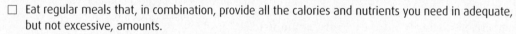

Take Action

Stop the Clock! Are You Aging Healthfully?

Americans spend several billion dollars every year on potions, gadgets, and books that are purported to extend life expectancy and stave off aging. None of these products live up to their promises; consequently, the quest for the fountain of youth remains alive. There is no surefire elixir that will stop aging in its tracks, but there are many things you can do to control the rate of aging.

If you want to stay younger longer, the following tips can help. Studies have found that adults who follow all of these suggestions have a physical health status comparable to people 30 years younger who follow few of these tips. How closely are you (or a parent or another older relative) following such a plan?

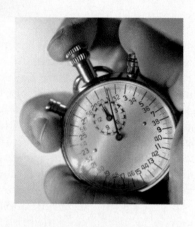

☐ Eat regular meals that, in combination, provide all the calories and nutrients you need in adequate, but not excessive, amounts.

☐ Limit alcohol consumption to a maximum of 1 or 2 drinks daily.

☐ Keep your body weight at a desirable level. Severe underweight and extreme overweight greatly reduce life expectancy.

☐ Exercise at least 3 or 4 times each week for an hour or more. But don't overdo exercise to the point that you become too thin, are physically injured, or menstruation ceases.

☐ Sleep about 7 or 8 hours each day.

☐ Do not use any tobacco products or street drugs.

☐ Limit exposure to direct sunlight to no more than 15 minutes each day.

☐ Have regular medical and dental checkups. Seek health care as soon as it is needed and follow the instructions of your health-care provider.

☐ Take responsibility for maintaining your own health—don't leave everything in the hands of your health-care provider.

☐ Protect yourself from environmental pollutants.

☐ Minimize emotional stress, adjust to the causes of stress, or learn constructive techniques for dealing with, relieving, or managing it (e.g., meditation, massage, relaxation techniques, time management, or exercise).

☐ Develop close, sustained, supportive friendships.

☐ Have an optimistic outlook and find ways to add meaning to your life. Laugh and relax regularly.

☐ Continue to learn and challenge your mind.

How many of the tips do you follow? If there are any you don't follow, it's probably a good idea to find ways to make them part of your lifestyle. Remember, you may not be able to turn back the clock, but you can keep it from ticking faster than it should.

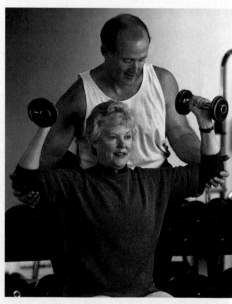

Strength training helps older adults maintain muscle mass.

have a family history of premature heart disease, they can adjust their diet, exercise, and tobacco use patterns to slow the progression of the disease, get the medical care needed, and possibly extend their lifetime. The converse is true, too. That is, lifestyle choices (e.g., high-fat diet and couch potato attitude) can increase susceptibility to diseases that hasten the rate of aging, ultimately shortening life expectancy, even if a person's genetic potential is for a very long life.

Environment

Some aspects of the environment that exert a powerful influence on the rate of aging are income, education level, health care, shelter, and psychosocial factors. For instance, incomes that enable individuals to purchase the nutritious foods, quality health care, and safe housing help decrease the rate of aging. Having the education needed to earn a sufficient income, as well as the knowledge required to select a nutritious diet and make wise lifestyle choices, also can slow the aging process. In addition, the willingness to seek health care promptly when it is needed, the capacity to follow the instructions of a health-care provider, and the desire to accept the responsibility for maintaining one's own health can slow the rate of aging. Likewise, shelter that protects individuals from physical danger, climatic extremes, and solar radiation helps slow the aging process. Allowing people to make at least some decisions for themselves and control their own activities (autonomy) and providing psychosocial support (informational and emotional resources) promote successful aging and psychological well-being. In contrast, the body may be physically stressed and aging accelerated if any or all of the converse (i.e., insufficient income, low education level, lack of health care, inadequate shelter, and/or lack of autonomy and psychosocial support) are true.

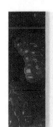

Knowledge Check

1. Why is an organ's reserve capacity important as one ages?
2. What factors contribute to successful aging?
3. What does compression of morbidity mean?
4. What effects can lifestyle have on heredity?

18.2 Nutrient Needs during Adulthood

The challenge of the adult years is to maintain the body, preserve its function, and avoid chronic disease—that is, to age successfully. A healthy diet can help achieve this goal. One blueprint for a healthy diet comes from the 2005 Dietary Guidelines for Americans, discussed in Chapter 2. Its advice can be summarized into 3 main points.

1. Consume a variety of nutrient-dense foods and beverages from the basic food groups of MyPyramid that result in a diet low in saturated and *trans* fats, cholesterol, added sugars, salt, and alcohol (if used). Foods to emphasize are vegetables, fruits, beans, whole-grain breads and cereals, reduced-fat milk or milk products, and water.
2. Maintain body weight in a healthy range by balancing energy intake with energy expended. Engage in at least 30 minutes of moderate-intensity physical activity, above usual activity, at work or home on most days of the week.
3. Practice safe food handling when preparing food. Clean hands, food contact surfaces, and fruits and vegetables before preparation, and cook foods to a safe temperature to kill microorganisms.

Appendix D reviews diet planning guidelines issued by Health Canada for Canadians. In addition, Chapter 1 discussed *Healthy People 2010*, a U.S. federal agenda aimed at disease prevention and health promotion.

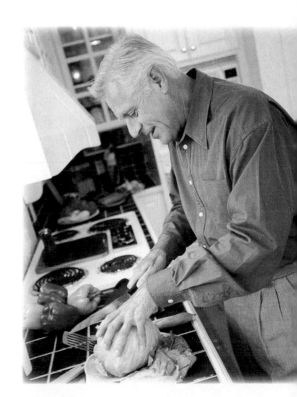

As we age, our nutrient needs change, but not the need to follow a healthy diet.

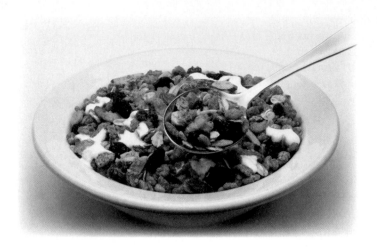

A daily serving of a whole-grain breakfast cereal is a rich source of vitamins, minerals, and fiber and, so, contributes to healthy aging.

menopause Permanent cessation of the menstrual cycle and end of fertility in women, usually occurring between the ages of 48 and 52.

▶ The Nutrition Screening Initiative uses the acronym "DETERMINE" to help identify older people whose health needs require extra attention:

· **D**isease
· **E**ating poorly
· **T**ooth loss or mouth pain
· **E**conomic hardship
· **R**educed social contact and interaction
· **M**ultiple medications
· **I**nvoluntary weight loss or gain
· **N**eed for assistance with self-care
· **E**lder at an advanced age

Overall, good nutrition benefits adults in many ways. Meeting nutrient needs delays the onset of certain diseases; improves the management of some existing diseases; speeds recovery from many illnesses; increases mental, physical, and social well-being; and often decreases the need for and length of hospitalization.[1] As you know, American adults are fairly well nourished, although some dietary excesses and inadequacies do exist. For instance, common dietary excesses are calories, fat, sodium, and, for some, alcohol. The diets of adult women tend to fall short of the recommended amounts of vitamins D and E, folate, magnesium, calcium, zinc, and fiber.[8] The diets of adult men tend be low in the same nutrients, except vitamin D, which does not become problematic until age 50. The iron intake of most women during their childbearing years (19 to 50) is insufficient to meet their needs; however, due to a reduced iron need after **menopause,** older women do get enough iron.[8]

People age 65 and up, particularly those in long-term care facilities and hospitals, are the single largest group at risk of malnutrition. They may become underweight and show signs of numerous micronutrient deficiencies (e.g., vitamins B-6 and B-12 and folate). Friends, relatives, and health-care personnel should look for poor nutrient intake in all older people, including those who live in nursing home settings. Family members have a unique opportunity to make sure nutrient needs are met by looking for weight maintenance based on regular, healthful meal patterns. To pinpoint those over age 65 at risk of nutrient deficiencies, the American Academy of Family Physicians, the American Dietetic Association, and the National Council on Aging developed the Nutrition Screening Initiative checklist (Fig. 18-4). Older Americans, family members, and health-care providers can use the checklist to identify those at nutritional risk *before* health deteriorates significantly. If problems arise in consuming a healthful diet, registered dietitians can offer professional and personalized advice.

Defining Nutrient Needs

The DRIs for adults are divided by gender into 4 age groups to reflect how nutrient needs change as adults grow older. These changes in nutrient needs take into consideration aging-related physiological alterations in body composition, metabolism, and organ function. For example, the calcium and vitamin D recommendations for older adult age groups exceed those of the youngest group to help offset changes such as reductions in the ability to absorb calcium and synthesize vitamin D in the skin.[9] In contrast to the rising need for calcium and vitamin D, the iron RDA for women declines in older age groups to reflect the decrease after menopause.[10]

Calories

After age 30 or so, total calorie needs of physically inactive adults fall steadily throughout adulthood. This is caused by a gradual decline in basal metabolism. To a great extent, adults can exert considerable control over this reduction in calorie need by exercising. Exercise can halt, slow, and even reverse reductions in lean body mass and subsequent declines in calorie need. Also, keeping calorie needs high makes it easier to meet one's nutrient needs and avoid becoming overweight.

Protein

The protein intake of adults of all ages in the U.S. and Canada tends to exceed current recommended levels. However, some recent studies indicate that consuming protein in amounts slightly higher than the RDA may help preserve muscle and bone mass. Adults who have limited food budgets, have difficulty chewing meat, or are lactose intolerant may not get enough protein. Recall that any protein consumed in excess of that needed for the maintenance of body tissue will be broken down and used as energy or stored as fat. The

A Nutrition Test for Older Adults

Here's a nutrition check for anyone over age 65. Circle the number of points for each statement that applies. Then compute the total and check it against the nutritional score.

	Points	
	2	1. The person has a chronic illness or current condition that has changed the kind or amount of food eaten.
	3	2. The person eats fewer than 2 full meals per day.
	2	3. The person eats few fruits, vegetables, or milk products.
	2	4. The person drinks 3 or more servings of beer, liquor, or wine almost every day.
	2	5. The person has tooth or mouth problems that make eating difficult.
	4	6. The person does not have enough money for food.
	1	7. The person eats alone most of the time.
	1	8. The person takes 3 or more different prescription or over-the-counter drugs each day.
	2	9. The person has unintentionally lost or gained 10 pounds within the last 6 months.
	2	10. The person cannot always shop, cook, or feed himself or herself.
Total		

Nutritional Score

0–2: Good. Recheck in 6 months.

3–5: Marginal. A local agency on aging has information about nutrition programs for the elderly. The National Association of Area Agencies on Aging can assist in finding help; call (800) 677-1116. Recheck in 6 months.

6 or more: High risk. A doctor should review this test and suggest how to improve nutritional health.

Figure 18-4 There is more variation in health status among adults over age 50 than in any other age group. Among people age 70 and over, some are independent, healthy people, whereas others are frail and require almost total care. This means that chronological age is not useful in predicting physical health status (physiological age) or nutritional risk. This checklist can be used by older Americans themselves, family members, and health-care providers to identify those at nutritional risk *before* health deteriorates significantly. People at marginal risk should look for ways to avoid reaching the high-risk category. Those at high risk should discuss their responses to the checklist with a health professional to identify ways to improve their nutritional health.

waste products produced when protein is used for energy or stored as fat must be removed by the kidneys; excessive protein intake may accelerate kidney function decline.

Fat

The fat intake of adults of all ages is often at or above the recommendations. It's a good idea for almost all adults to reduce their fat intake because of the strong link between high-fat diets and obesity, heart disease, and certain cancers. In addition, reducing fat intake "frees up" some calories that can be better "spent" on complex carbohydrates.

Carbohydrates

The total carbohydrate intake of adults of all ages in the U.S. and Canada is often lower than recommended. In addition, many adults need to shift the carbohydrate composition of their diets to emphasize complex carbohydrates more and sugary, simple carbohydrates less. A diet richer in complex carbohydrates makes it easier to meet nutrient needs and stay within calorie bounds because many highly sweetened foods are low in nutrients and high in calories. Substituting foods rich in complex carbohydrates for sweets also makes it easier for the body to control blood glucose levels—a function that becomes less efficient as the increases in body fatness and inactivity associated with usual aging occur. Declines in carbohydrate metabolism are so common that 20% of those age 65 years or older have diabetes. A diet rich in fiber helps adults reduce their risk of colon cancer and heart disease, lower their blood cholesterol levels, and avoid constipation. The typical American adult gets slightly more than half the recommended amount of dietary fiber.[8, 11]

Water

Many adults, especially those in the later years, fail to consume adequate quantities of water. In fact, many are in a constant state of mild dehydration and at risk of electrolyte imbalances. Low fluid intakes in older adults may be caused by a fading sensitivity to thirst sensations, chronic diseases, and/or conscious reductions in fluid intake in order to reduce the frequency of urination.[1] Some also may have increased fluid output because they are taking certain medications (i.e., diuretics and laxatives), have an **ostomy,** and/or experience an age-related decline in the kidneys' ability to concentrate urine. Dehydration is very dangerous and, among other symptoms, can cause disorientation and mental confusion, constipation, impacted fecal matter, and death.

Minerals and Vitamins

Adequate intake of all vitamins and minerals is important throughout the adult years. The micronutrients that need special attention because they tend to be present in less than optimal amounts in the diets of many adults are calcium, vitamin D, iron, zinc, magnesium, folate, and vitamins B-6, B-12, and E. Adults with impaired absorption or who are unable to consume a nutritious diet may benefit from mineral or vitamin supplements matched with their needs. In fact, many nutrition experts recommend a daily balanced multivitamin and mineral supplement for older adults, especially for those 70 years of age and older. Supplements or fortified foods can be especially helpful when it comes to meeting vitamin D and vitamin B-12 needs.

Calcium and Vitamin D These bone-building nutrients tend to be low in the diets of all adults. They become particularly problematic after age 50.[12] Inadequate intake of these nutrients, coupled with their reduced absorption, the reduced synthesis of vitamin D in the skin, and the kidneys' decreased ability to put vitamin D in its active form, greatly contributes to the development of osteoporosis.[9] Getting enough of these nutrients is a challenge for many older adults because food sources of vitamin D are limited in the North American diet, and the major sources—fatty fish and fortified milk—are not widely consumed by older adults. Plus, with increasing age, lactase production frequently decreases. As you know, one of the richest and most absorbable source of these nutrients, milk, contains lactose. To get the vitamin D and calcium needed, many with lactose intolerance can consume small amounts of milk at mealtime with no ill effects. Calcium-fortified foods, cheese, yogurt, fish eaten with bones (e.g., canned sardines or salmon), and dark green leafy vegetables can help those with lactose intolerance meet calcium needs—but these foods often do not provide vitamin D. Just 10 to 15 minutes per day of sunlight can make a large difference in vitamin D status.

Iron Iron deficiency anemia, the most common type of malnutrition during the adult years, is found most frequently in women in their reproductive years because their diets do not provide enough iron to compensate for the iron lost monthly during menstruation. Other common causes of iron deficiency in adults of all ages include digestive tract injuries that cause bleeding (i.e., bleeding ulcers or hemorrhoids) and the use of medicines, such as aspirin, that cause blood loss. Impaired iron absorption due to age-related declines in stomach acid production may contribute to iron deficiency in older adults.

Zinc In addition to less than optimal dietary zinc intake during adulthood, zinc absorption declines as stomach acid production

ostomy Surgically created short circuit in intestinal flow where the end point usually opens from the abdominal cavity rather than the anus—for example, a colostomy. Short circuiting the intestinal flow means more water is lost in fecal matter than would be if the intestinal tract were intact.

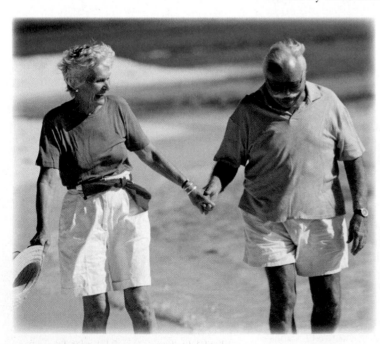

Sun exposure can help older adults meet their increased vitamin D need.

diminishes with age. Poor zinc status may contribute to the taste sensation losses, mental lethargy, and delayed wound healing many elderly adults experience.[10]

Magnesium This mineral tends to be low in adults' diets. Inadequate magnesium intakes may contribute to the loss of bone strength, muscular weakness, and mental confusion seen in some elderly adults. It also can lead to sudden death from poor heart rhythm and is linked to cardiovascular disease, osteoporosis, and diabetes. The best source of magnesium is the diet; supplements can cause loose stools and diarrhea.

Folate and Vitamins B-6 and B-12 Sufficient quantities of folate, because of its neural tube prevention qualities, are very important to women during the childbearing years. In later years, folate and vitamins B-6 and B-12 are especially important because they are required to clear homocysteine from the bloodstream; elevated blood concentrations of homocysteine are associated with increased risk of the cardiovascular disease, stroke, bone fracture, and neurological decline seen in some elderly people.[13, 14] Vitamin B-12 is a particular problem for the older population because a deficiency may exist even when intake appears to be adequate. As people age, the stomach slows its production of acid and intrinsic factor, which leads to poor absorption of vitamin B-12 and eventually pernicious anemia. Adults age 51 years and older need to meet vitamin B-12 needs with foods or supplements fortified with synthetic vitamin B-12.[15]

Vitamin E The dietary intake of most of the population falls short of recommendations for vitamin E. Low vitamin E intake means the body has a reduced supply of antioxidants, which may increase the degree of cell damage caused by free radicals, promote the progression of chronic diseases and cataracts, and speed aging. In addition, low vitamin E levels can lead to declines in physical abilities.[16]

Carotenoids

Dietary intakes of certain carotenoids have been shown to have a variety of important anti-aging and health protective effects. Specifically, lutein and zeaxanthin have been linked with the prevention of cataracts and age-related macular degeneration. Diets high in fruit and vegetables, the major sources of carotenoids and other beneficial phytochemicals, are consistently shown to be protective of a wide variety of age-related conditions.

Knowledge Check

1. What are some examples of how a healthy diet can benefit adults?
2. Which nutrients tend to be too low in the diets of adults?
3. What are 3 signs that an older person's health needs extra attention?

 ## 18.3 Factors Influencing Food Intake and Nutrient Needs

Like those of other age groups, the food choices and nutritional adequacy of adults' diets depend on the interplay of physical, physiological, psychosocial, and economic factors. Alterations in any 1 of these factors, such as age-related changes in body organs and systems or diminished psychological well-being, social interaction, or financial status, can result in deteriorations in the quality of dietary intake, nutritional status, and health.

Physical and Physiological Factors

The implications of many of the physical and physiological changes that occur during adulthood on dietary intake and nutrient needs are summarized in Table 18-2. Some of the changes listed (e.g., tooth loss, loss in taste and smell perceptions) can influence

► The relationship between nutrition and chronic disease and/or the need for medications is a 2-way street. That is, food intake and nutrient needs are influenced by chronic diseases and the need for medications. However, food and nutrient intake influence the onset of chronic diseases and reduce the amount of medication needed in the early stages of chronic disease. A nutritious diet is probably one of the most important factors in helping delay the onset of chronic disease and need for medication.

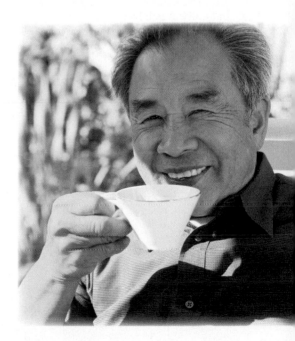
The goal of adulthood is to preserve health as late into life as possible.

Table 18-2 Nutritional Implications of Physical and Physiological Changes That Occur after about Age 30

Usual Changes	Nutritional Implications of the Changes	Ways to Minimize the Changes and Promote Successful Aging
Body Composition		
Gradual, steady decline in lean body mass (sarcopenia) and body water Slow increase in fatty tissue; redistribution of body fat from the limbs to the torso	Loss of lean body mass decreases metabolic rate, causing calorie needs to drop. Adequate fluid intake is important because a decrease in total body water elevates the risk of dehydration and decreases the body's ability to regulate its internal temperature. Excessive increases in fatty tissue raise the risk of developing conditions (e.g., high blood pressure, high blood glucose levels, type 2 diabetes, heart disease, and certain cancers) that may alter nutrient needs.	• Eating a nutritious diet that meets but does not exceed calorie needs, coupled with getting regular exercise (including strength training), helps minimize increases in body fat and maintains, or even re-builds, lean body tissue and muscular strength, which keeps basal metabolic rate up.
Skeletal System		
Slow, steady loss of bone minerals; in women, loss rises greatly in the first 5 to 10 years after menopause; may lead to osteoporosis	Adequate calcium and vitamin D during young adulthood helps build bone density and in the remainder of adulthood maintain and, perhaps, even increase bone mass. If osteoporosis causes adults to limit physical exercise, calorie needs will drop.	• Eating a diet rich in calcium and vitamin D, combined with participation in weight-bearing exercises, can help build bone mass until bones stop increasing in density (usually around age 35) and then can preserve bone minerals. Some older adults may benefit from medications that help preserve and rebuild bone. • Keeping weight at a healthy level can help preserve bone mass. • Avoiding smoking and chronic alcohol intake can help preserve bone mass because engaging in these behaviors increases the risk for osteoporosis.
Cardiovascular and Respiratory Systems		
Gradual decrease in the ability of the heart and lungs to deliver oxygen and nutrient rich blood to body cells (aerobic capacity) and remove metabolic wastes; rise in blood pressure	Reductions in cardiovascular and respiratory systems negatively affect the function of other organs (e.g., kidney, brain) and decrease their function, thus lowering calorie needs and possibly altering nutrient needs. If cardiovascular and respiratory system declines cause adults to limit physical exercise, calorie needs will drop further.	• Eating a low-fat diet rich in antioxidant nutrients, maintaining a healthy weight, avoiding cigarette smoke, and exercising regularly help minimize atherosclerotic plaque and reduce the risk of heart disease, which is responsible for many of the common age-related changes in the cardiovascular and respiratory systems. • Exercising regularly helps maintain a high level of heart and lung fitness (aerobic capacity), raises blood levels of HDL cholesterol, and keeps blood pressure under control. • Lowering sodium intake, eating less animal protein, and maintaining a healthy weight may delay the onset of age-related rises in blood pressure. • Monitoring and treating high blood lipids and hypertension helps minimize damage to the cardiovascular system. • Eating an antioxidant-rich diet and avoiding polluted air and cigarette smoke help protect the lungs. • A change that probably cannot be avoided is the decrease in lung capacity that occurs with aging: lungs shrink about 40% between the ages of 20 and 80.

Usual Changes	Nutritional Implications of the Changes	Ways to Minimize the Changes and Promote Successful Aging
Digestive System		
Diminished chewing ability if gum disease occurs and leads to tooth loss or poor fitting dentures; decline in efficiency of digestion and nutrient absorption due to reduced secretions of HCl and gastric, pancreatic, and intestinal digestive enzymes; decline in vitamin B-12 absorption due to decreased secretion of intrinsic factor; decline in the liver's ability to metabolize alcohol and drugs; slowdown in the movement of chyme through the intestines	Chewing problems may result in reduced intake of crisp or chewy foods, such as raw fruits and vegetables, whole grains, and meats. Low HCl levels may impair absorption of iron, calcium, folate, vitamin B-6, and protein. Low HCl levels also may allow larger than normal numbers of bacteria to survive and establish colonies in the small intestine, where they may impair fat and fat-soluble vitamin absorption, compete for B-vitamins, and lead to weight loss and vitamin deficiencies. Diminished secretions of HCl and intrinsic factor virtually halt vitamin B-12 absorption. Reduced secretions of digestive enzymes may impair digestion and absorption of macronutrients; however, digestion is relatively complete and malabsorption does not seem to be a problem in most older adults. Decline in liver function slows detoxification of alcohol and drugs; thus, safe intake levels of these may drop.	• Consuming a diet rich in vitamin C (to maintain gums), calcium, and vitamin D (to maintain bone surrounding teeth) and practicing good dental health habits help prevent gum disease. • Eating several smaller meals each day instead of a few larger ones may maximize digestion and absorption. • Making dietary modifications and/or getting treatment to improve malabsorption problems caused by conditions such as celiac disease, diverticulitis, and excessive bacterial growth in the small intestine helps ensure nutrient needs are met. • Consuming alcohol in moderation, if at all, helps avoid overtaxing the liver's capacity for detoxifying alcohol. • Avoiding megadoses of vitamins and minerals helps prevent imbalances in nutrient absorption and the possibility of nutrient toxicities. • Eating a fiber-rich diet, drinking plenty of fluids, and exercising regularly help prevent constipation.
Urinary System		
Decreased efficiency of kidneys in filtering out metabolic wastes, concentrating urine, and putting vitamin D synthesized in the skin in its active form; progressive weakening of muscles that control urination	Diminished kidney function may impair reabsorption of glucose, amino acids, and vitamin C and impair vitamin D status. Excessive intakes of protein, electrolytes, water-soluble vitamins, and other substances that must be filtered out by the kidneys should be avoided. Vitamin D–rich foods need to be emphasized or supplements may be needed. Reductions in the ability to concentrate urine increase the need for fluid.	Reductions in kidney filtration efficiency are not necessarily an inevitable part of aging; however, the factors that work to preserve filtration efficiency are not yet known. • Avoiding excessive intakes of nutrients and other substances that must be filtered out by the kidneys throughout life may help preserve kidney function. • Engaging in practices that maintain cardiovascular health (so that the blood supply to the kidneys is sufficient) and prevent hypertension (which can damage the kidneys) can help preserve kidney function. • In those experiencing reduced kidney function, limiting protein and electrolyte intake may restore some kidney function. • Doing muscular exercises and using behavior modification and medications can help improve functioning of the muscles that control urination.

(continued)

Table 18-2 Nutritional Implications of Physical and Physiological Changes That Occur after about Age 30, *Continued*

Usual Changes	Nutritional Implications of the Changes	Ways to Minimize the Changes and Promote Successful Aging
Nervous System		
Gradual decline in number of cells that transmit nerve signals, which may result in decreased sensory perceptions (e.g., taste and smell), slowed reaction times, and impaired neuromuscular coordination, reasoning, and memory	Loss in taste and smell may reduce desire to eat, leading to weight loss. Diminished sensory perceptions may decrease secretions from the salivary glands, stomach, and pancreas and result in impaired digestion and blood glucose regulation. Neuromuscular coordination losses may make it difficult to cook or feed oneself. Reduced reasoning abilities can result in an inability to choose a nutritious diet, and memory losses may result in forgetting to eat altogether.	At present, there is no known way to prevent reductions in nerve cells. Studies suggest that smell and taste perception losses and decreases in intellectual performance are small in healthy older people. Losses appear greater in those with arteriosclerosis. • Engaging in practices that promote a healthy cardiovascular system (exercise, low-fat diet) may help preserve nerve function. • Experimenting with herbs, spices, and flavorings can boost the taste and smell of foods. • Drinking enough fluids to prevent dehydration, engaging in lifelong learning, and getting enough sleep can help avoid mental confusion. • Keeping blood pressure under control and consuming an omega-3 rich diet may help preserve mental functioning.[30, 31]
Immune System		
Progressive decline in efficiency that increases susceptibility to infection and disease	Calorie and nutrient needs rise during infection and disease.	Reductions in immune system functioning may not be necessarily an inevitable part of aging; however, all the factors that preserve functioning are not yet known. • Eating a diet that meets nutrient needs and prevents obesity can help lower the risk of immune dysfunction. • Exercising regularly may improve immune function. • Avoiding prolonged emotional stress helps preserve immune function.
Endocrine System		
Gradual decrease in hormone synthesis, hormone release, or sensitivity to hormones	Decrease in sensitivity to insulin means that it takes longer for blood glucose levels to return to normal after a meal. Reduction in thyroid hormone slows metabolic rate and decreases calorie need. Decline in growth hormone leads to loss of lean body tissue and an increase in adipose tissue, both of which decrease metabolic rate and calorie need. Growth hormone reductions also cause the thinning of skin.	Eating a nutritious diet may influence endocrine activity by providing ample quantities of the compounds necessary for hormone synthesis and transport. • Maintaining a healthy weight, getting physical exercise, and eating a low-fat, high fiber diet can slow, prevent, and perhaps even reverse, decreased sensitivity to insulin. • Maintaining lean body mass helps keep thyroid hormone level steady. • Getting injections of growth hormone may lead to increases in lean body mass, decreases in body fat, and thicker skin; however, long-term safety and usefulness are not known.
Reproductive System		
Females: few changes until menopause (menopause is characterized by diminishing estrogen secretions and cessation of ovulation); males: slow decline in testosterone after age 60	In females, iron needs drop when menopause occurs. Healthy diets and exercise are important after menopause because the decline in estrogen causes the risk of heart disease and osteoporosis to soar. In males, the reduction in testosterone may contribute to the loss of lean body tissue, which diminishes calorie needs.	Age-related changes in the reproductive system currently appear to be unalterable.

dietary intake. Other changes (e.g., menopause, loss of lean body tissue) can alter nutrient and/or calorie needs. Still other changes (e.g., reduced stomach acidity, diminished kidney function) can cause changes in nutrient utilization. Chronic diseases and the need for medications are additional physiological changes many adults experience that can influence food intake and nutrient needs.

Body Composition

The primary changes in body composition that occur as the adult years progress are diminished lean body mass, increased fat stores, and decreased body water. Some muscle cells shrink and others are lost as muscles age; some muscles lose their elasticity as they accumulate fat and collagen. Loss of muscle mass leads to a decrease in basal metabolism, muscle strength, and energy needs. Less muscle mass also leads to lower physical activity, which makes the prognosis for maintaining muscle even worse. Clearly, it is best to avoid this vicious cycle.

Lifestyle greatly determines the rate of muscle mass deterioration. As you might predict, an active lifestyle helps maintain muscle mass, whereas an inactive one encourages its loss. In fact, much of what we associate with old age is due to a lifetime of physical inactivity. Ideally, an active lifestyle should be maintained throughout life and include both aerobic and strength training (Table 18-3). Physical activity increases muscle strength and mobility, improves balance and decreases the risk of falling, eases daily tasks that require some strength, improves sleep, slows bone loss, and increases joint movement, thus reducing injuries. It also has a positive impact on a person's mental outlook.[17] Strength training (resistance) helps reverse some of the decline in daily function associated with the muscle loss typically seen in older adulthood.

As lean tissue declines with age, body fat often increases. Much of this increase results from overeating and limited physical activity, although even athletic men and lean women typically gain some degree of midsection fat after age 50. A small fat gain in adulthood may not compromise health, but large gains are problematic. Recall that obesity can raise blood pressure and blood glucose and make walking and performing daily tasks more difficult.

Decreases in body weight are common in adults age 70 and older. Weight loss is a problem for older people in particular because it increases the risk of nutrition-related illness and death. It may indicate illness, reduced tolerance to medication, or withdrawal from life.[18, 19] Weight loss also may indicate that nervous system and hormonal factors are depressing feelings of hunger (see Chapter 10). The effects of current medication, as well as changes in taste and smell, may inhibit appetite, too. In addition, many older people live alone, a circumstance associated with depressed appetite.

Skeletal System

Recall from Chapter 14 that bone loss in women occurs primarily after menopause. Bone loss in men is slow and steady from middle age throughout later life. Many older people may suffer from undiagnosed osteomalacia, a condition primarily caused

▶ Researchers believe that maintaining lean muscle mass may be the most important strategy for successful aging. This is because maintaining lean muscle mass:

- Maintains basal metabolic rate, which helps decrease the risk of obesity
- Keeps body fat low, which helps control blood cholesterol levels and helps avoid the onset of type 2 diabetes
- Maintains body water, which decreases the risk of dehydration and improves body temperature regulation

Loss of muscle mass (sarcopenia) is very prevalent in elderly individuals and greatly increases their risk of illness and death.

▶ Older people should work with their physicians to develop a plan for limiting falls. Many falls are caused by neuromuscular coordination losses, impaired vision, walking and balance disorders, lack of regular physical activity, side effects of medication, and environmental hazards.

Exercise Guidelines for Adults

Aerobic Exercise: moderate intensity for 30 minutes daily on 5 days weekly or vigorous intensity for 20 minutes daily for 3 days weekly

Strength Training: 8 to 10 exercises 2 to 3 times weekly

Balance Exercises: For those over age 65 who are at risk for falling

Learn more at: www.ascm.org

Table 18-3 Strength Training Recommendations for Older Adults

- Exercise at least 2 days per week.
- If weights are used, start with 1 to 2 lb and gradually increase this amount over time.
- Perform exercises that involve the major muscle groups (e.g., arms, shoulders, chest, abdomen, back, hips, and legs) and exercises that build grip strength.
- Perform 8 to 15 repetitions of each exercise; then perform a second set.
- Rest between sets of exercises.
- Avoid locking joints in arms and legs.
- Stretch after completing all exercises.
- Stop exercising if pain begins.
- Breathe during strength exercises.

Source: National Institute on Aging.

▶ One in 5 older people has trouble walking, shopping, and cooking food.[29]

by insufficient vitamin D. Osteoporosis can limit the ability of older people to move about, shop, prepare food, and live normally. Consuming adequate vitamin D, calcium, and protein and not smoking, drinking alcohol moderately or not at all, and engaging in weight-bearing exercises can help preserve bone mass. Medications also can help lessen bone loss.

Cardiovascular System

The heart often pumps blood less efficiently in older people, usually because of insufficient physical activity. However, the decline in the heart's ability to pump blood is not inevitable with aging and does not occur among older people who remain physically active. In fact, it is thought that inactive lifestyles may contribute as much to the risk of cardiovascular disease as does smoking a pack of cigarettes per day. Exercising regularly, not smoking, and eating a low-fat diet rich in nutrients and moderate in sodium can help protect the cardiovascular system (see Chapter 6).

Respiratory System

Lung efficiency declines somewhat with age and is especially pronounced in older people who have smoked or continue to smoke tobacco products. Breathing becomes shallower, faster, and more difficult as the amount of active lung tissue decreases. Smoking often leads to emphysema and lung cancer. The decrease in lung efficiency contributes to a general downward spiral in body function; breathing difficulties limit physical activity and endurance and frequently discourage eating. Besides not smoking, eating an antioxidant-rich diet and being physically active help preserve lung function.

Digestive System

As mentioned previously, the production of HCl, intrinsic factor, and lactase declines with advancing age and, as a result, impairs the absorption of several nutrients. Constipation is the main intestinal problem for older people. To prevent constipation, older people should meet fiber needs, drink enough fluids, and exercise. Fiber medications are generally unnecessary but may be useful when total energy consumption does not allow for enough fiber intake. Because some medications can cause constipation, a physician should be consulted to determine if a laxative or stool softener is needed.

In addition to changes in the GI tract, the functions of the accessory organs decline as we age. For instance, the liver functions less efficiently. A history of significant alcohol consumption or liver disease will cause the liver to function even less efficiently. As liver efficiency declines, its ability to detoxify many substances, including medications, alcohol, and vitamin and mineral supplements, drops (see Chapter 8). The possibility for vitamin toxicity increases.

The gallbladder also functions less efficiently in later years. Gallstones can block the flow of bile out of the gallbladder into the small intestine, thereby interfering with fat digestion. Obesity is a major risk factor for gallbladder disease, especially in older women. A low-fat diet or surgery to remove the gallbladder may be necessary.

Although pancreatic function may decline with age, this organ has a large reserve capacity. One sign of a failing pancreas is high blood glucose, although this can occur as the result of several conditions. The pancreas may be secreting less insulin, or cells may be resisting insulin action (as is commonly seen in obese people with upper-body fat storage). Where appropriate, improved nutrient intake, regular physical activity, and weight loss (when needed) can improve insulin action and blood glucose regulation.[1]

Poor dental health contributes to food intake and digestive problems. About 30% or more of older people in North America have lost all their teeth. Attention to dental hygiene and care throughout life greatly lowers this risk. Periodontal (gum) disease commonly causes tooth loss. Replacement dentures enable some people to chew normally, but many older adults—especially men—have denture problems. When people have problems chewing, serving softer, easier-to-chew foods and allowing extra time for chewing and swallowing encourage more eating.

Urinary System

Over time, the kidneys filter wastes more slowly as they lose nephrons. The deterioration significantly decreases the kidneys' ability to excrete the products of protein breakdown, such as urea. As a result, individuals often need to avoid excess protein and keep intake at the RDA or slightly below.

Incontinence, the inability to control the muscle responsible for holding urine in the bladder, affects up to 20% of older adults living at home and about 75% of those in nursing homes. The fear of being unable to control one's bladder or the embarrassment of having to wear diapers causes many to restrict fluid intake (resulting in dehydration and constipation) and become socially isolated.

Nervous System

A gradual loss of nerve cells that transmit signals may decrease taste and smell perceptions and impair neuromuscular coordination, reasoning, and memory. Both hearing and vision decline with age. Hearing impairment is greatest in those who have been exposed constantly to loud noises, such as urban traffic, aircraft noise, and music. Because they cannot hear well, older people may avoid social contacts, which increases their risk of poor dietary intake.

Declining eyesight, frequently caused by retina degeneration and cataracts, can affect a person's abilities to grocery shop, locate desired foods, read labels for nutritional content, and prepare foods at home. Vision losses also may cause people to curtail social contacts, reduce physical activity, and not practice daily personal health and grooming routines. Macular degeneration, one form of failing eyesight in old age, is quite common, affecting about 1.75 million adults in the U.S. A major risk factor is cigarette smoking. Diets rich in carotenoids help reduce the risk of macular degeneration. The risk of developing cataracts is decreased by consuming a diet rich in fruits and vegetables.

Neuromuscular coordination losses may make it difficult to shop for and prepare food. Physical tasks as simple as opening food packages can become so difficult that individuals restrict dietary intake to foods that require little preparation and depend on others to provide food that is ready to eat. Eating may become difficult, too. Loss of coordination makes it a challenge to grasp cup handles and manipulate eating utensils. As a result, older adults may avoid foods that can be easily spilled (e.g., soups and juices) or that need to be cut (e.g., meats, large vegetable pieces) and restrict food intake to easy-to-eat finger foods. Some may even withdraw from social interaction and eat alone, which can lead to inadequate nutrient intake.

Immune System

With age, the immune system often operates less efficiently. Consuming adequate protein, vitamins (especially folate and vitamins A, D, and E), iron, and zinc helps maximize immune system function. Recurrent sicknesses and poor wound healing are warning signs that a deficient diet (especially protein and zinc) may be hindering the function of the immune system.[18] On the other hand, overnutrition appears to be equally harmful to the immune system. For example, obesity and excessive fat, iron, and zinc intake can suppress immune function.

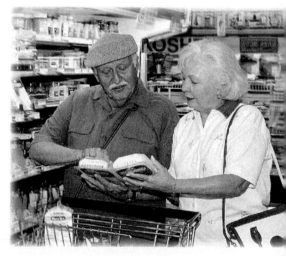

Grocery shopping can become more difficult in one's older years. Assistance from others is often very helpful.

Endocrine System

As adulthood progresses, the rate of hormone synthesis and release can slow. A decrease in insulin release or sensitivity to insulin, for instance, means that it takes longer for blood glucose levels to return to normal after a meal. Maintaining a healthy weight, exercising regularly, eating a diet low in fat and high in fiber, and avoiding foods with a high glycemic index can enhance the body's ability to use insulin and restore elevated blood glucose levels to normal after a meal.

Reproductive System

When menopause occurs, iron needs decline. A diet rich in vitamin D and calcium can help stave off the rapid loss of bone minerals that occurs after menopause. Testosterone production may decline as men age, leading to a loss of lean body mass, which results in a decreased metabolic rate and lowered caloric needs.

Chronic Disease

The prevalence of obesity, heart disease, osteoporosis, cancer, hypertension, and diabetes rises with age.[1, 6] More than 8 out of every 10 elderly people have 1 of these chronic and potentially debilitating diseases. Half of all elderly people have at least 2 chronic conditions.[20] Chronic diseases may have a strong impact on dietary intake. For instance, excessive fatness, heart disease, and osteoporosis may impair physical mobility to the extent that victims are unable to shop for and prepare food. Chronic disease also can influence nutrient and calorie needs. Cancer, for example, boosts both nutrient and calorie needs. Hypertension may indicate a need to lower sodium intake. Nutrient utilization can be affected by chronic disease, too. For instance, diabetes alters the body's ability to utilize glucose. In addition, the effects of heart disease on the kidneys may impair their ability to reabsorb glucose, amino acids, and vitamin C.

Medications

Older adults are major consumers of medications (prescription and over-the-counter) and nutrient supplements. Half of all people over age 65 take several medicines each day. The rate of supplement use increases throughout adulthood, until by age 50 approximately half of all adults are using supplements daily. Physiological declines that occur during aging (e.g., reduced body water, reduced liver and kidney function) cause the effects of medications and nutrient supplements to be exaggerated and persist longer in older adults.

Medications can improve health and quality of life, but some also adversely affect nutritional status, particularly of those who are older and/or take many different medications. For instance, some medications depress taste and smell acuity or cause anorexia or nausea that can blunt interest in eating and lead to reduced dietary intake. Some medications alter nutrient needs. Aspirin, for example, increases the likelihood of stomach bleeding, so long-term use may elevate the need for iron, as well as other nutrients. Antibiotics may deplete the body of vitamin K. Some medications may impair nutrient utilization—diuretics and laxatives may cause excessive excretion of water and minerals. Even vitamin and mineral supplements can affect nutritional status. Iron supplements taken in large doses can interfere with the functioning of zinc and copper. Folate supplements can mask vitamin B-12 deficiencies. People who must take medications should eat nutrient-dense foods and avoid any specific food or supplement that interferes with the function of the medication. For example, vitamin K can reduce the action of oral anticoagulants, aged cheese can interfere with certain drugs used to treat hypertension and depression, and grapefruit can interfere with medications such as tranquilizers and those that lower cholesterol levels (Table 18-4). A physician and pharmacist should be consulted about any restrictions on food and/or supplements.

Psychosocial Factors

A positive outlook on life and intact support networks help make food and eating interesting and satisfying. In contrast, apathy and depression caused by feelings of social isolation, grief, or change in lifestyle can lead to losses in appetite and interest in food, as well as disability. About 15% of persons 65 years old or older experience depression. Left untreated, depression can lead to a continual decline in appetite, which results in weakness, poor nutrition, mental confusion, and increased feelings of isolation and loneliness (Fig. 18-5). Sometimes people cope by overeating, which can lead to obesity and its associated problems. As many as 15% of depression cases may end in suicide. Depression is often treatable with medication, social support, and psychological intervention.[19]

Worries about possible embarrassment caused by deteriorating physical capabilities may cause older adults to withdraw from social interaction and eat alone rather than with others. Those who eat alone, regardless of the reason, seldom eat as much or as nutritiously as they should. Both young and old people who eat without companionship tend to feel unmotivated to shop for or prepare foods. Many develop an apathetic attitude toward life, which over time causes health and nutritional status to decline.[1] As you'll see

▶ Obtaining enough food may be difficult for some older persons, especially if they are unable to drive and do not have friends or relatives close by to help with cooking or shopping. Older people may equate a request for help with a loss of independence. Pride or the fear of being victimized by those they hire may stand in the way of much needed help.

▶ Pharmaceutical companies have begun to market liquid meal-replacement formulas to older adults. Previously, these products were primarily used in hospitals and nursing homes. Many of these products have an unusual taste because of the vitamins and types of proteins that have been added. Older adults can decide if the convenience, cost, and taste make this a wise diet choice.

Table 18-4 Potential Drug-Nutrient Interactions for Commonly Used Drugs

Drugs	Uses	Nutrients Affected	Potential Mechanism
Antacids (Maalox®)	Reduce stomach acidity	Calcium, vitamin B-12, and iron	Decreased absorption due to altered gastrointestinal pH
Anticoagulants (Coumadin®)	Prevent blood clots	Vitamin K	Interference with utilization
Aspirin	Is an anti-inflammatory; reduces pain	Iron	Anemia from blood loss
Cathartics (laxatives)	Induce bowel movement	Calcium and potassium	Poor absorption
Cholestyramine	Reduces blood cholesterol	Vitamins A, D, E, and K	Poor absorption
Cimetidine (Tagamet®)	Treats ulcers	Vitamin B-12	Poor absorption
Colchicine	Treats gout	Vitamin B-12, carotenoids, and magnesium	Decreased absorption due to damaged intestinal mucosa
Corticosteroids (prednisone)	Are an anti-inflammatory	Zinc Calcium	Poor absorption Poor utilization
Furosemide (Lasix®)	Decreases blood pressure; is a potassium-wasting diuretic	Potassium and sodium	Increased loss
Hydrochlorothiazide	Decreases blood pressure; is a diuretic	Potassium and magnesium	Increased loss; decreased absorption
MAO inhibitors (Parnate®)	Are an antidepressant	Tyramine (in cheese, wine, and other aged foods)	High blood pressure caused by limited tyramine metabolism
Tricyclic antidepressants (Elavil®)	Are an antidepressant	—	Weight gain from appetite stimulation

later in the chapter, in the U.S. several nutrition assistance programs can help older people obtain the food and social support needed for good health. The guidelines in Table 18-5 provide some practical suggestions to help older adults eat nutritiously.

Economic Factors

The amount of money available for purchasing food can have a great impact on the types and amounts of food one eats. Unemployment, underemployment, retirement, or anything else that limits income makes it difficult to get the best, most healthful foods and can diminish nutritional status and health. Insufficient income is a particular problem among those

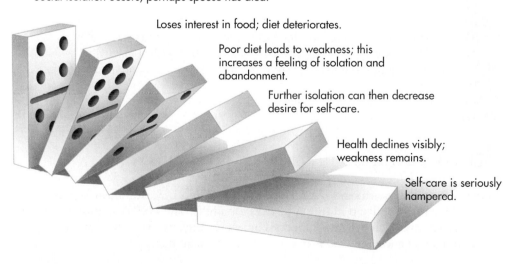

Social isolation occurs; perhaps spouse has died.

Loses interest in food; diet deteriorates.

Poor diet leads to weakness; this increases a feeling of isolation and abandonment.

Further isolation can then decrease desire for self-care.

Health declines visibly; weakness remains.

Self-care is seriously hampered.

Figure 18-5 The decline in health often seen in older adults needs to be prevented whenever possible.

Table 18-5 Guidelines for Healthful Eating in Later Years

- Eat regularly; small, frequent meals may be best. Use nutrient-dense foods as a basis for menus.
- Eat often with friends, with relatives, or at a senior center.
- Eat in a well-lit or sunny area; serve meals attractively; use foods with different flavors, colors, shapes, textures, and smells.
- If possible, take a walk before eating to stimulate appetite.
- Arrange kitchen and eating area so that food preparation and cleanup are easier.
- Use labor-saving equipment and foods (e.g., precut salad mix, canned beans, and frozen fruit).
- Try new foods, new seasonings, and new ways of preparing foods.
- Keep easy-to-prepare foods on hand for times when you feel tired.
- Share cooking responsibilities with a neighbor.
- Keep a box of dry milk handy to add nutrients to recipes for baked foods, casseroles, and meat loaf.
- If you have a freezer, cook larger amounts, divide them into small portions, and freeze.
- When necessary, chop, grind, or blend hard-to-chew foods. Softer protein-rich foods can be substituted for meat when poor dental health limits normal food intake. Prepare soups, stews, cooked whole-grain cereals, and casseroles.
- If your arm or hand movements are limited, cut the food ahead of time, use utensils with deep sides or handles, and obtain specialized utensils if needed.
- Use community resources for help in obtaining meals (e.g., the Congregate Meal Program), shopping for groceries, and meeting other daily personal or household care needs.
- Buy only what you can use; small containers may be expensive, but letting food spoil also is costly.
- Ask the grocer to break family-sized packages of wrapped meat or fresh vegetables into smaller units.
- Buy several pieces of fruit—a ripe one, a medium-ripe one, and an unripe one—so that the fruit can be eaten over a period of several days.
- Consider buying meal-replacement bars or liquid formulas for occasional snacks or meals.
- Stay physically active.

ages 65 and up and, as a result, they frequently have trouble making sure they remain well nourished. The Commodity Foods Program and Food Stamp Program are two federal U.S. programs that can help low-income individuals of all ages procure the foods they need.

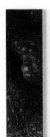

Knowledge Check

1. How does body composition tend to change as people age?
2. What body systems are adversely affected by physical inactivity?
3. How might the nervous system changes caused by aging affect dietary intake?
4. What are the risks of eating alone?

 18.4 Nutrition Assistance Programs

In the U.S., U.S. Department of Agriculture (USDA) and U.S. Administration on Aging programs provide food and nutrition services for adults. The USDA administers the following programs. Each program functions independently, has its own eligibility requirements and target audience, and may not be available in all states.

- The *Commodity Supplemental Food Program* distributes, free of charge, surplus agricultural products (e.g., cheese, peanut butter, canned foods) produced by U.S. farmers to low-income households. The foods provided vary, depending on the farm products available at the time.
- The *Food Stamp Program* provides nutrition education and supplements the food budgets of low-income households, so that participants can purchase a greater quantity of food than they could afford to buy on their food budgets alone. Food stamps can be used like money to purchase foods, food-producing plants and seeds, hot meals in group homes and shelters, and, in some areas, hot meals in certain authorized restaurants. Food Stamps cannot be used to purchase alcohol or non-food items (e.g., soap, paper goods).
- The *Child and Adult Care Food Program* provides nutritious meals and snacks to low-income children enrolled in child-care centers or residing in emergency shelters, as well as adults who are functionally impaired or ages 60 and older in non-residential adult day-care centers.
- The *Senior Farmers' Market Nutrition Program* helps provide low-income older adults with coupons that can be exchanged for fresh fruits, vegetables, and herbs at farmers' markets, roadside stands, and other community-support agriculture programs.

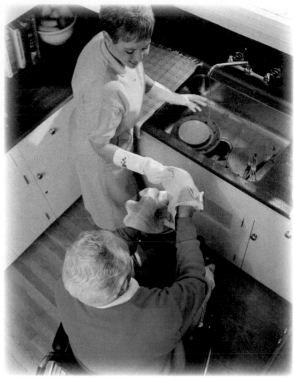

In many communities, programs assist older adults with daily tasks, which helps them meet their nutrient needs.

The U.S. Administration on Aging administers the Older Americans Act. This act is designed to help adults ages 60 years and older remain living independently in their homes and communities. Each community decides which programs and services will be provided. Community-based nutrition, health, and supportive services may include adult day care, senior center activities, transportation, information and counseling services, and health and physical activity programs. In-home care can include health and personal care, home maintenance assistance, and caregiver support services, such as nutrition advice and help with coordinating care needs.

The Elderly Nutrition Program, an important aspect of the Older Americans Act, provides nutrition services through the Congregate Meal Program and Home Delivered Meal Program (often referred to as Meals-on-Wheels). Anyone ages 60 and older can participate; however, priority usually is given to those with the greatest economic, social, and health needs. Both meal programs can help older people obtain some of the food needed for good health. Each meal meets at least one-third of the daily recommendations. The social aspect of the Congregate Meal Program provides opportunities for socialization that often improve appetite and general outlook on life. These programs also may provide shopping assistance, counseling, nutrition education, and referral to other social, rehabilitative, and transportation services.

▶ To learn about meal programs for senior citizens in your area, visit www.aoa.gov.

CASE STUDY

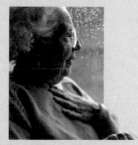

Frances is an 84-year-old woman who suffers from macular degeneration, osteoporosis, and arthritis. Since her husband died a year ago, she has moved from their family house to a small apartment. Her eyesight is progressively getting worse, making it hard to go to the grocery store or even to cook (for fear of burning herself). She is often lonely. Her only son lives 1 hour away and works 2 jobs, but he visits her as often as he can. Frances has lost her appetite and, as a result, often skips meals during the week. She has resorted to eating mostly cold foods, which are simple to prepare but are seriously limiting variety and palatability in her diet. She is slowly losing weight as a result of her dietary changes and loss of appetite. Her typical diet usually consists of a breakfast that may include a slice of wheat toast with margarine, honey, and cinnamon and a cup of hot tea. If she has lunch, she normally has a small can of peaches, half of a turkey and cheese sandwich, and a small glass of water. For dinner, she might have half of a tuna salad sandwich made with mayonnaise and a glass of iced tea. She usually eats 2 cookies at bedtime. What are the potential consequences of such a poor dietary pattern? What services are available that could help Frances improve her diet and possibly increase her appetite? What other easy-to-prepare foods could be included in her diet to make it more healthful and more varied?

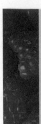

 18.5 Nutrition-Related Health Issues of the Adult Years

Diet is one of the main factors directly involved in the development of several health conditions during adulthood. The effects of diet and nutrients on many of these conditions, including atherosclerosis, cancer, constipation, diabetes, diverticular disease, heartburn, hypertension, obesity, and osteoporosis, were discussed in earlier chapters. In addition to these conditions, those discussed in this section are important to consider during adulthood. A slowing in the restoration of internal balance of the body (homeostasis) is at least partially diet-related. Other health problems, such as arthritis and Alzheimer's disease, are considered by some to be diet-related, even though scientific evidence currently indicates otherwise.

Alcohol Use

The consequences of alcohol use, especially alcohol abuse, rise with advancing age. Older adults become intoxicated on a smaller amount of alcohol than when younger because they metabolize alcohol more slowly and have lower amounts of body water to dilute the alcohol. Both men and women over the age of 65 should limit alcohol consumption to no more than 1 drink per day. (Recall from Chapter 8 that 1 drink per day is 5 ounces of wine, 12 ounces of beer, or 1.5 ounces of 80-proof liquor.) Even small amounts of alcohol can react negatively with common medications many older persons take. In addition to having adverse effects on the liver, large amounts of alcohol increase the risk of stroke and may aggravate hypertension in older adults.

Alcohol abuse is a problem among a small but significant group of older individuals who may continue this pattern from earlier in life or develop heavy drinking patterns and alcoholism in later life. Later development of this problem sometimes arises from the loneliness and social isolation caused by retirement or the loss of a spouse. Some symptoms of alcoholism in older persons include trembling hands, sleep problems, memory loss, and unsteady gait; these symptoms may be easily disregarded because they also are common symptoms of old age in general.

Slowed Restoration of Homeostasis

As body tissues and systems age and their functioning diminishes, the body takes longer and longer to restore homeostasis. For example, it takes twice as long for the kidneys to remove wastes and restore blood levels to normal after eating excess protein in a person age 80 than in a person age 30. Similarly, it takes older people longer to break down alcohol, drugs, and nutrient supplements. Consequently, blood levels of these substances rise higher and have a stronger and longer effect in older adults than younger people.

Even though the return to homeostasis is slowed, this slowdown usually is not a major problem unless disease strikes and stresses the body's capabilities. This slowdown makes an elderly person more vulnerable to illness and death. In the absence of disease, the slowed restoration of homeostasis usually is not a major problem until the end of the life span approaches. Prudent lifestyle choices may make it possible to keep the rate at

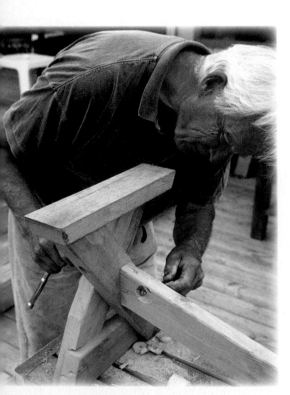

Learning new skills throughout life helps preserve cognitive function.

which the body restores homeostasis high. Taking steps to avoid stressing the body's capabilities also can help preserve optimal function of body tissues and systems (e.g., get flu shots, avoid excessive protein intake). Getting prompt medical attention when the body's capabilities are stressed by illness helps preserve optimal functioning, too. In the case of already damaged tissues and systems, avoiding stressful practices helps prevent pushing an aging body beyond its capabilities.

Alzheimer's Disease

Alzheimer's disease is an irreversible, abnormal, progressive deterioration of the brain that causes victims to steadily lose the ability to remember, reason, and comprehend. Alzheimer's disease often takes a terrible toll on the mental and eventual physical health of older people. About 4.5 million adults in the U.S. have the disease.

The 10 warning signs of Alzheimer's disease are listed in the margin. No one is sure exactly what causes this disease, but scientists have proposed various causes, including alterations in cell development or protein production in the brain, strokes, altered blood lipoprotein composition, obesity, poor blood glucose regulation (e.g., diabetes), high blood pressure, high blood cholesterol, and high free radical levels.

Preventive measures for Alzheimer's disease focus on maintaining brain activity through lifelong learning, eating a diet rich in fruits and vegetables, and taking ibuprofen.[21] The role of nutrition in preventing or minimizing the risk of this disease is being investigated.[22] Getting enough antioxidant nutrients, such as vitamins C and E, helps protect the body from the damaging effects of free radicals. Adequate intakes of folate and vitamins B-6 and B-12 are especially important because elevated blood homocysteine is also a risk factor. Dietary fats, too, may play a role in keeping this disease at bay. Individuals with diets rich in omega-3 and omega-6 foods and low in saturated and *trans* fatty acids seem to have a reduced risk of Alzheimer's disease.[23]

The dietary intakes of those with Alzheimer's disease are poor, compared with those of a similar age without this disease.[24] Caregivers of those who have Alzheimer's disease need to monitor the patient's weight to ensure maintenance of a healthy weight and nutritional state. Other tips are serving omega-3 rich fish in meals twice per week and making sure eating habits do not pose a health risk (e.g., holding food in one's mouth or forgetting to swallow). Regular physical activity has also been shown to improve mental status in people afflicted with this disease.

Arthritis

There are over 100 forms of arthritis, a disease that causes the degeneration and roughening of the once smooth cartilage that covers and cushions the bone joints and/or the formation of calcium deposits (spurs). These changes in the joints cause them to ache and become inflamed and painful to move. Osteoarthritis becomes more common with age and, by age 80, almost everyone has this condition—it is the leading cause of disability among older persons. Rheumatoid arthritis, which is not as common, is more prevalent in younger adults.

Although it is not known what causes or cures arthritis, many unproven "remedies" have been publicized. Unusual diets, food restrictions, and nutrient supplements are some of the more popular "remedies." However, no special diet, food, or nutrient has ever been proven to prevent, relieve, or cure arthritis in humans.[25] The only diet-related treatment known to offer some relief is to maintain a healthy weight. This is because excess body weight adds extra stress to the already painful arthritic joints. Although those with arthritis are not likely to benefit from dietary changes, they could experiment with their diets, provided they avoid practices that will result in inadequate, unbalanced, or excessive nutrient intakes, to see if such changes provide relief. It is important to keep in mind, though, that altering dietary practices may work for some, but no dietary changes have been found to be of help to all arthritis sufferers.[26]

10 Warning Signs of Alzheimer's Disease

1. Recent memory loss that affects job performance
2. Difficulty performing familiar tasks
3. Problems with language
4. Disorientation to time and place
5. Faulty or decreased judgment
6. Problems with abstract thinking
7. Tendency to misplace things
8. Changes in mood or behavior
9. Changes in personality
10. Loss of initiative

▶ To find out more about Alzheimer's disease, visit www.alz.org or www.nia.nih.gov/alzheimers.

▶ Glucosamine and chondroitin sulfate may stimulate the production of new cartilage in humans, so they may help the body rebuild damaged cartilage. Although currently there is no convincing proof that these supplements can repair cartilage in humans, some people do experience a reduction in the pain. Also, individuals who take higher levels of beta carotene or vitamins C, D, or E may slow the progression of osteoarthritis, but more research is needed to confirm the effectiveness of these vitamins.

CRITICAL THINKING

Jamilla is 68 years old. She has heart disease and takes several medications. She went to her local pharmacy yesterday to look for a product to help her sleep through the night. On the shelves, she found an herbal supplement claiming to be a remedy for sleeplessness. She thought that, because a pharmacy carried the product, it should be safe and should work as indicated on the label. Is she correct in these assumptions? Are there specific risks associated with taking such herbal remedies? What should Jamilla do before taking the supplement?

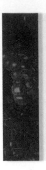

Knowledge Check

1. Why might even small amounts of alcohol be problematic for older adults?
2. What are some steps an older adult can take to minimize the effects of slowed restoration of homeostasis?
3. Which nutrients may provide protection against Alzheimer's disease?
4. How does maintaining a healthy weight help those with arthritis?

CASE STUDY FOLLOW-UP

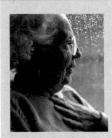

Frances could contact a local government office that offers Congregate Meal Programs and inquire about where meals are served and the transportation available to the site. This meal program would give her social contact with other older persons, which is probably an important element that is missing in her life and could help alleviate her loneliness. She also could request home-delivered meals (if available in her area) to provide 1 meal each day, which may be just what she needs to help stimulate her appetite. She also could have groceries delivered to her home if her budget could handle the extra cost. Convenience foods that could improve her diet are milk, peanut butter, breakfast cereals, chicken or tuna in a can or pouch, yogurt, sliced cheese, cottage cheese, calcium-fortified orange juice, canned or frozen fruits and vegetables, and some fresh fruits and vegetables that do not require preparation, such as bananas and pre-washed salad greens. A further possibility is eating a nutrition bar or a liquid nutritional supplement each day. The resulting increase in her nutrient intake would help prevent disease in the future and increase her sense of well-being.

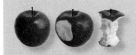 *Take Action*

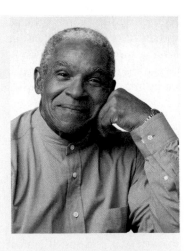

Helping Older Adults Eat Better

During their lifetimes, most people usually eat meals with families or loved ones. As people reach older ages, many are faced with living and eating alone. In a study of the diets of 4400 older adults in the U.S., 1 man in every 5 living alone who was over age 55 ate poorly. One in 4 women between the ages of 55 and 64 years had a low-quality diet. These poor diets can contribute to deteriorating mental and physical health. Consider the following example of the living situation of an older adult.

Neal, a 70-year-old man, lives alone in a home in a local suburban area. His wife died a year ago. He doesn't have many friends; his wife was his primary confidante. His neighbors across the street and next door are friendly, and Neal used to help them with yard projects in his spare time. Neal's health has been good, but he has had trouble with his teeth recently. His diet has been poor, and in the past 3 months his physical and mental vigor have deteriorated. He has been slowly lapsing into depression and, so, keeps the shades drawn and rarely leaves his house. Neal keeps very little food in the house because his wife did most of the cooking and shopping, and he just isn't that interested in food.

If you were one of Neal's friends or relatives and learned of his situation, what are 6 things you could do or suggest to help improve his nutritional status and mental outlook?

1.
2.
3.
4.
5.
6.

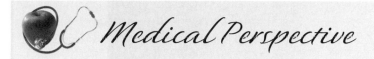
Medical Perspective

Complementary and Alternative Medicine Practices

Many adults, especially older adults, use complementary and alternative medicine (CAM) (also called complementary care and integrative medicine). CAM is defined as any medical or health-care system, practice, or product not presently part of conventional medicine. CAM can be grouped into 5 domains, some of which overlap:

1. *Biologically based practices*: using substances found in nature, such as pharmacological agents, foods, special diets, vitamins (in doses greater than used in conventional medicine), and herbs to treat or prevent disease. An herb is any plant or part of a plant used primarily for medicinal purposes. Dosage forms include capsules, tablets, extracts or tinctures, powders, dried herbs, teas, creams, ointments, and vapors (aromatherapy). Some herbal products are effective for treating specific medical problems. The best advice is to use these substances only under strict supervision of a physician. The FDA requires herbal supplement labels to include the herb name, quantity, dosage per day, and ingredients (Fig. 18-6).

2. *Mind-body interventions:* using mind techniques (e.g., hypnosis, meditation, biofeedback, yoga), creative therapies (e.g., art therapy, music therapy), patient support groups, meditation, yoga, and/or prayer to enhance physical health. Ayurveda is a natural healing process from India that includes eating healthy, fresh foods and taking medicinal herbs suited to one's particular mind-body type.

3. *Energy medicine:* using energy fields, such as magnetic fields, pulsed fields, alternating- or direct-current fields, or "biofields" (energy fields some believe surround and penetrate the body) to promote healing, such as electrical currents to help heal broken bones.

4. *Manipulative and body-based practices:* using hands to promote healing, such as chiropractic or osteopathic manipulation or massage. Other examples are qi gong (a component of traditional Chinese medicine), Reiki therapy, and therapeutic touch therapy. The FDA recognizes the effectiveness of chiropractic care in treating acute low back pain.

5. *Alternative systems of medical practice:* using alternative medicine systems like Ayurveda, naturopathy, homeopathy, or techniques from traditional medicine from another culture, such as acupuncture from Chinese medicine. Acupuncture may be effective for treating pain, nausea, and vomiting following surgery or chemotherapy, nausea during pregnancy, and recovery from a drug addiction. The FDA supports the use

▶ Studies indicate that the following herbs may be especially dangerous: germander, pokeroot, sassafras, mandrake, pennyroyal, comfrey, chaparral, yohimbe, lobelia, jin bu huan, kava kava, products containing stephanie and magnolia, senna, hai gen fen, paraguay tea, kombucha tea, tung shueh (Chinese black balls), and willow bark.

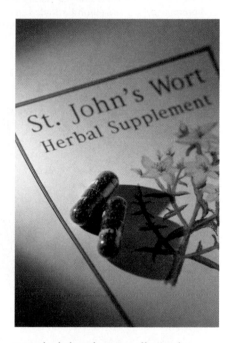

Some herbal products are effective for treating specific medical problems. To be safe, follow label instructions carefully, note potential side effects, and use them under the supervision of a physician.

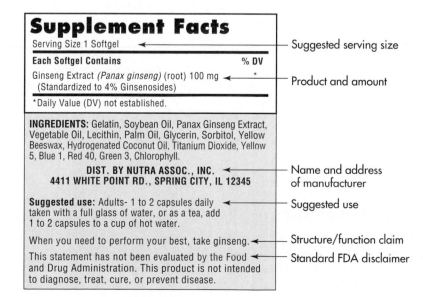

Figure 18-6 A standardized Supplement Facts label is required on herbs and other related supplements. These labels must list the ingredients, the % Daily Value (if applicable), the common name of the plant, the part of the plant used, how much is present in each dose, and a suggested daily dose.

(continued)

Medical Perspective, continued

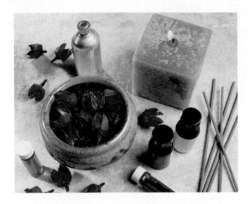

Aromatherapy is often used to help relieve stress and promote relaxation. Currently, there is no scientific evidence that aromatherapy effectively treats or prevents disease.

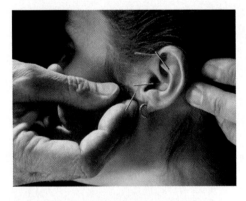

Acupuncture may offer relief from nausea after surgery or chemotherapy.

▶ Supplement labels can claim a benefit related to a classic nutrient-deficiency disease, describe how the supplement affects body structure or function (i.e., structure/function claim), and state that general well-being results from consumption of the ingredient or ingredients. A supplement label cannot claim that the product treats, cures, or prevents a disease not completely related to a given nutrient deficiency. For example, an herbal product label can claim that it may help brain function, but not that it cures Alzheimer's disease. The latter would constitute a drug claim.

of acupuncture for these purposes if delivered by a certified practitioner using single-use sterile needles made from nonreactive materials. Typically, a course of treatments should end after 10 sessions if no improvements occur.

Many consumers are interested in CAM. Some types of CAM (e.g., acupuncture and chiropractic therapies) show promise in the treatment of certain conditions.[27] However, unlike conventional medicine, most alternative therapies have little or no scientific evidence to support them, either because they do not work or because few studies have been conducted.

If treatments don't work or haven't been proven to work, why do people use them? One reason is that some people assume that natural substances are gentler forms of therapy than pharmacological medicines. Others use CAM because standard medical treatments didn't work or had too many adverse effects. Many who use alternative medicines have illnesses for which conventional medicine cannot currently offer a cure, such as arthritis, terminal stages of AIDS or cancer, and stress-related conditions. To cope with health conditions such as these, sufferers may resort to almost anything. Another reason unproven remedies remain popular is that they appear to relieve symptoms in a few people. This relief may be caused by a placebo effect, or it may be the result of the natural ups-and-downs of symptoms, remission of disease, or the possibility that the remedy contains a medicine not listed on the label. If improvement happens to coincide with the use of a remedy, a person may mistakenly believe that the remedy worked.

The possibility that an unproven remedy itself actually caused the relief does exist. For example, a person with arthritis may find that restricting a certain food eliminates an unknown food allergy that irritates the joints. Alternatively, dietary changes may improve the nutritional status of a person who is in such poor nutritional health that the immune system is unable to respond effectively to the joint inflammation causing arthritis pain. Experimenting with CAM may help some individuals find relief from health conditions.

A rational approach for someone wanting to try CAM is to keep a diary of symptoms, follow only one therapy at a time, check with his or her physician first before discontinuing a medication or medical treatment, and find out if the alternative practitioner has experience with the medical problem to be treated. Interested consumers also might see if they can enroll in a study investigating the effectiveness of the substance or procedure in question. If adverse side effects occur from an alternative therapy, consumers should contact a physician right away. Physicians are encouraged to report such adverse effects to the FDA and state and local health departments and consumer protection agencies.

When considering whether to use CAM, keep these points in mind:

- We often tend to believe what we hear or what close acquaintances tell us. This well-meaning advice is not a substitute for scientific proof of safety and effectiveness when it comes to health practices.
- The U.S. government provides little regulation of nutrient or herbal supplements or remedies (see Chapter 1).[28] Another concern is that the actual content of the active ingredients in herbal supplements may be less or more than stated on the label. "Let the buyer beware" is prudent advice when using these products.
- Fraudulent claims for diet- and health-related remedies always have been a part of our culture. Carefully scrutinize the credentials and motives of anyone providing medical or health advice. Phony credentials and bogus practitioners are common.
- If it sounds too good to be true, it probably is. The medical community gains nothing by holding back effective cures from the public, despite what the alternative practitioners may say.

A Closer Look at Herbal Therapy

Throughout history, healers have gone to the garden, forest, and sea to seek herbal remedies. Some natural products may be harmless, others are potentially toxic, and still others may be effective for some problems but dangerous when taken in the wrong dose or by people with certain medical conditions (Table 18-6). Interactions between alternative therapies and

Table 18-6 Popular Herbal Remedies, Nutrient Supplements, and Hormones

Substances	Potential Effects	Side Effects	Who Should Avoid Them
Black cohosh	May reduce postmenopausal symptoms	Nausea, fall in blood pressure	Women taking estrogen, hypertension medications, or aspirin and related drugs
Coenzyme Q-10	Fat-soluble vitamin-like substance with antioxidant properties; some people with chronic conditions, such as heart failure, have low amounts in the body and so may benefit from use	Mild gastrointestinal distress	No specific persons are at risk
Echinacea	May stimulate the immune system and shorten the duration of flulike illnesses; current studies show little or no effect	Nausea, skin irritation, allergic reactions	Anyone with an autoimmune disease or who has allergic reactions to daisies
Feverfew	May reduce the pain and frequency of migraines	Abdominal pain, mouth sores, skin rash	Anyone allergic to ragweed or taking anti-inflammatory drugs, such as aspirin
Garlic	May have antibiotic properties and slightly lower blood cholesterol and blood pressure	In large amounts, burning of the mouth, nausea, sweating, stomach irritation, lightheadedness, reduced blood clotting	Anyone taking anti-coagulant medications, such as warfarin, for cardiovascular disease or AIDS medicines
Ginger	May prevent motion sickness and nausea related to surgery and pregnancy	Gastrointestinal (GI) tract discomfort with high doses on an empty stomach	People with a history of gallstones
Ginkgo biloba	May increase the circulation of blood in the body, especially to the brain and lower extremities; evidence is very weak	GI tract upset, headache, irritability, reduced blood clotting	Anyone taking anti-inflammatory or anti-coagulant medications, including vitamin E and aspirin; anyone who has had a stroke or is prone to them
Ginseng	May decrease weakness and fatigue and increase the body's resistance to stress; studies have not confirmed any benefit	Hypertension, asthma attacks, irregular heart beat, insomnia, headache, nervousness, GI tract upset, reduced blood clotting	Anyone taking anti-coagulant medications, such as warfarin; women on hormone therapy; anyone with a chronic GI tract disease; anyone with diabetes
Glucosamine	May decrease joint inflammation and pain associated with osteoarthritis, but a recent large-scale trial showed no such benefit	GI tract discomfort, which may disappear after 2 weeks	May disrupt blood glucose regulation in people with diabetes
Milk thistle	May have a protective effect on the liver, thought to be due in part to its ability to prevent toxins from contaminating liver cell membranes	Diarrhea	No specific persons are at risk
SAMe	May promote cartilage formation and decreases joint inflammation and pain associated with osteoarthritis; may also act as a mild antidepressant (active ingredient is S-adenosylmethionine)	Mild headaches, which last for short periods of time	Anyone with cardiovascular disease, obsessive compulsive disorder, bipolar disorder, or addictive tendencies
St. John's wort	Mild antidepressant effect that may work by inhibiting monoamine oxidase (an enzyme in the brain that destroys "feel-good" hormones, such as serotonin, epinephrine, and dopamine)	Nausea, fatigue, dry mouth, dizziness, photosensitivity; increases metabolism and removal of many prescription drugs from the body	People taking medications to control depression, HIV, epilepsy, cardiovascular disease, and asthma or to suppress the immune system to keep the body from rejecting a transplanted organ

(continued)

Medical Perspective, continued

Table 18-6 Continued

Substances	Potential Effects	Side Effects	Who Should Avoid Them
Saw palmetto	May reduce symptoms of enlarged prostate gland (otherwise known as BPH, or benign prostatic hyperplasia) by increasing urinary flow and easing urination; some studies show moderate evidence of effectiveness, whereas other studies have shown little or no benefit with such use	Generally uncommon; when taken in large doses: headache, GI tract upset	People taking medication to treat enlarged prostate or BPH; anyone with a chronic GI tract disease
Valerian	May alleviate restlessness and other sleeping disorders that stem from nervous conditions	Headache, morning grogginess, irregular heartbeat, GI tract upset (also has a disagreeable odor)	Anyone taking central nervous system depressants, such as sedatives; anyone who drinks alcohol
Hormones			
DHEA	Hormone that when taken orally turns to estrogen and testosterone in the body; few, if any, benefits of supplementation are proven, such as an aid to weight loss or to treat depression; research is ongoing	Masculinization of women, acne, irritability, decreased HDL cholesterol, possible prostate or breast cancer	Women, due to possible irreversible masculinization qualities
Growth hormone	Hormone that stimulates cell synthesis, such as muscle cells, and overall body growth in children; may be useful in adults who fail to make enough of the hormone	Carpal tunnel syndrome; breast development in men; swollen ankles and legs, hypertension, diabetes, cancer	Only available by prescription; requires close physician scrutiny (very expensive)
Melatonin	Hormone that may help people fall asleep faster and reduce jet lag	Reduced ovulation in women, drowsiness, confusion, headache or morning grogginess	Anyone with cardiovascular disease and anyone of childbearing age
Testosterone	Hormone that affects muscle mass and strength; can reduce menopausal symptoms in women and possibly depression in older men	Masculinization of women; decreased HDL cholesterol, prostate gland enlargement in men (and possibly increased prostate cancer risk)	Only available by prescription; requires close physician scrutiny; risky in men showing prostate gland enlargement

Note that pregnant or lactating women, children under 2 years old, those over 65 years old, and anyone with a chronic disease should never take herbal remedies or supplements unless under the guidance of a physician.

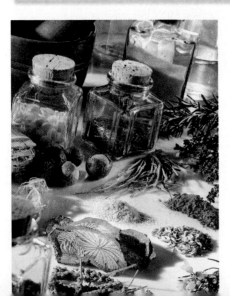

pharmaceutical drugs can be drastic and include complications such as delirium, clotting abnormalities, rapid heartbeat, and even death.

Another important risk to consider is that traditional herbal products may be mislabeled, adulterated with prescription drugs or contaminants (e.g., lead), or vary greatly in potency. Chinese combination herbs always should be avoided because of the reported cases of adverse health effects and adulteration. These questions can help you evaluate a company's herbal products:

· What analyses are done to ensure quality, quantity, and reproducibility of the ingredients in individual doses as labeled?

· Is the product labeled with Latin botanical names?

Simply because herbal remedies come from natural sources does not mean they are without health risks. Even those that have been used for centuries may cause harmful effects.

· Does the label have expiration dates and lot numbers? How are expiration dates determined?

· Does the manufacturer offer a certificate of analysis for each product?

· Has the manufacturer been in business for at least 5 years? Does it nationally distribute the product?

Overall, herbal products should be used with great caution and in consultation with a person's primary physician. Otherwise, potential side effects may go undiagnosed, dangerous herb-medicine interactions may occur, or serious complications during surgery may develop. Pregnant and nursing women, anyone with a chronic disease, and children under 2 years of age should not take herbal supplements unless their physicians consent to the practice and monitor them for potential complications.

Some herbalists claim that natural herbs cannot harm people. Scientific evidence strongly contradicts this claim. Indeed, if there is one thing experts agree on, it's this: an herb that has the ability to heal also has the ability, if misused, to harm. In addition, many conditions for which herbs are recommended (e.g., diabetes and arthritis) are not suitable for self-treatment.

For a balanced discussion of herbal medicine, visit

Alternative Medicine Foundation
www.amfoundation.org

National Institutes of Health Office of Alternative Medicine
nccam.nih.gov

American Botanical Council
www.herbalgram.org

National Institutes of Health Office of Alternative Medicine
altmed.od.nih.gov

Natural Medicine Comprehensive Database
www.naturaldatabase.com

Medline
medlineplus.nlm.nih.gov/medlineplus/complementaryandalternativemedicine.html

Knowledge Check

1. What are the 5 domains of CAM?
2. What are some tips you might give a person who is considering using an alternative therapy?
3. What are some risks associated with herbal therapies?
4. How can the risks associated with using herbal therapies be minimized?

Summary

18.1 During adulthood, nutrients are used primarily to maintain the body rather than support physical growth. As adults get older, nutrient needs change. Adulthood is characterized by body maintenance and gradual physical and physiological transitions, often referred to as "aging." The physiological changes of aging are the sum of cellular changes, lifestyle practices, and environmental influences. Many of these changes can be minimized, prevented, and/or reversed by healthy lifestyles. Usual aging refers to the age-related physical and physiological changes that are commonly thought to be a typical or expected part of aging. Successful aging describes the declines in physical and physiological function that occur because one grows older. Striving to have the greatest number of healthy years and the fewest years of illness is referred to as compression of morbidity. The rate at which one ages is individual; it is determined by heredity, lifestyle, and environment.

18.2 A healthy diet based on the 2005 Dietary Guidelines for Americans can help people preserve the body's function, avoid chronic disease, and age successfully. American adults are fairly well nourished, although common dietary excesses are calories, fat, sodium, and, for some, alcohol. Common dietary inadequacies include vitamins D and E, folate, magnesium, calcium, zinc, and fiber. People ages

65 and up, particularly those in long-term care facilities and hospitals, are the single largest group at risk of malnutrition. The Nutrition Screening Initiative checklist can help identify older adults at risk of nutrient deficiencies. The DRIs for adults are divided by gender and age to reflect how nutrient needs change as adults grow older. These changes in nutrient needs take into consideration aging-related physiological alterations in body composition, metabolism, and organ function.

18.3 The food choices and nutritional adequacy of adults' diets depend on physical, physiological, psychosocial, and economic factors. Alterations in any 1 of these factors can result in deteriorations in the quality of dietary intake, nutritional status, and health. The physical and physiological changes in body composition and body systems that occur during adulthood can influence dietary intake, alter nutrient and/or caloric needs, and/or alter nutrient utilization. The use of medications and supplements can improve health and quality of life, but some also can adversely affect nutritional status. Psychosocial status can affect food intake and health. Economic factors can have a great impact on the types and amounts of food one eats.

18.4 Programs publicly funded by the U.S. Department of Agriculture (USDA) and U.S. Administration on Aging provide food and nutrition services for adults. The USDA administers food and nutrition assistance programs, including the Commodity Foods Program, Food Stamp Program, Child and Adult Care Food Program, and Senior Farmers' Market Nutrition Program. The U.S. Administration on Aging administers the Older Americans Act, which provides community-based nutrition, health, and supportive services and may include adult day care, senior center activities, transportation, information and counseling services, and health and physical activity programs. The Congregate Meal Program and Home Delivered Meal Program can help older people obtain some of the food needed for good health.

18.5 Diet is a primary factor directly involved in the development of several health conditions during adulthood, including atherosclerosis, cancer, constipation, diabetes, diverticular disease, heartburn, hypertension, obesity,

osteoporosis, and periodontal disease. The consequences of alcohol use, especially alcohol abuse, rise with advancing age. A slowdown in the restoration of the internal balance of the body (homeostasis) is at least partially diet-related. Arthritis and Alzheimer's disease are considered by some to be diet-related, even though scientific evidence currently indicates otherwise. Complementary and alternative medicine (CAM) is any medical or health-care system, practice, or product not presently part of conventional medicine. The CAM categories are biological treatments, mind-body interventions, energy medicine, manipulative and body-based practices, and alternative systems of medical practices. Most alternative therapies have little or no scientific evidence to support them. Some herbal products may be harmless, others are potentially toxic, and still others may be effective for some problems but dangerous when taken in the wrong dose or by people with certain medical conditions. Herbal products should be used with great caution.

Study Questions

1. During adulthood, nutrients are used primarily to maintain the body.

   a. true   b. false

2. _____ is the time-dependent physical and physiological changes in body structure and function that occur normally and progressively throughout adulthood as humans mature and become older.

   a. Aging
   b. Successful aging
   c. Usual aging
   d. Graying

3. Compression of mortality is the extent to which an organ can preserve essentially normal function despite decreasing cell number or cell activity.

   a. true   b. false

4. Which of the following is *not* considered a cause of aging?

   a. Errors occur in the copying of DNA.
   b. Hormone function changes.
   c. Body system reserve capacity declines.
   d. Death is programmed into cells.

5. Physical and physiological changes associated with usual aging include _____.

   a. increasing body fatness
   b. decreasing lean body mass
   c. rising blood pressure
   d. declining bone mass
   e. all of the above

6. The rate at which one ages is determined _____.

   a. by heredity, lifestyle choices, and environment
   b. mostly by heredity, education level, and access to health care
   c. mostly by lifestyle, diet quality, and environment
   d. mostly by diet quality and exercise pattern
   e. by heredity only

7. The impact lifestyle choices can have on the expression of genetic potential is _____.

   a. none
   b. minor
   c. major

8. The diets of adults tend to be low in _____.

   a. vitamin E
   b. calcium
   c. zinc
   d. fiber
   e. all of the above

9. The DRIs for adults do not take into account aging-related changes in body composition.

   a. true   b. false

10. Which of the following is a sign that an older person's health needs extra attention?

    a. The person eats fewer than 2 meals daily.
    b. The person drinks 3 or more servings of alcohol often.
    c. The person eats alone often.
    d. All of the above are signs.
    e. Only a and b are signs.

11. Which of the following changes commonly occurs as one ages but does not influence nutrient utilization?

    a. loss in taste and smell perceptions
    b. reduced stomach acidity
    c. diminished kidney function
    d. presence of chronic disease

12. A change that tends to occur as the adult years progress is _____.

    a. increased body water
    b. decreased lung efficiency
    c. increased intrinsic factor
    d. decreased hormone synthesis and release
    e. both b and d

13. Which publicly funded programs distributes, free of charge, surplus agricultural products to low-income households?

    a. Food Stamp Program
    b. Commodity Foods Program

    c. Child and Adult Care Food Program
    d. Congregate Meal Program

14. Diet is not directly involved in the development of _____.

    a. atherosclerosis
    b. cancer
    c. diverticular disease
    d. arthritis

15. A potential risk associated with herbal products is _____.

    a. they can interact with medicines
    b. they may vary in potency
    c. they may be contaminated
    d. all of the above
    e. none of the above

Answer Key: 1-a; 2-a; 3-b; 4-c; 5-e; 6-a; 7-c; 8-e; 9-b; 10-d; 11-a; 12-c; 13-b; 14-d; 15-d

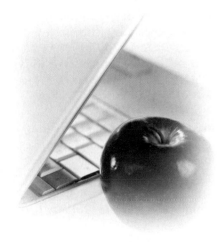

Websites

To learn more about the topics covered in this chapter, visit these websites.

Meal Programs for Older Adults

www.aoa.gov

Aging

www.nih.gov/nia

www.americangeriatrics.org

www.aoa.dhhs.gov

www.ilcusa.org

www.aging-institute.org

Nutrition for Seniors

fnic.nal.usda.gov

www.nlm.nih.gov/medlineplus/nutritionforseniors.html

Alzheimer's disease

www.alz.org

www.nia.nih.gov/alzheimers

Complementary and Alternative Medicine

www.amfoundation.org

nccam.nih.gov

www.herbalgram.org

altmed.od.nih.gov

www.naturaldatabase.com

References

1. Kuczmarski M, Weddle D. Position paper of the American Dietetic Association: Nutrition across the spectrum of aging. *J Am Diet Assoc.* 2005;105:616.

2. Moeller S and others. Overall adherence to the Dietary Guidelines for Americans is associated with reduced prevalence of early age-related nuclear lens opacities in women. *J Nutr.* 2004;134:1812.

3. Tucker K and others. The combination of high fruit and vegetables and low saturated fat intakes is more protective against mortality in aging men than is either alone: The Baltimore longitudinal study of aging. *J Nutr.* 2005;135:556.

4. Trichopoulou A and others. Modified Mediterranean diet and survival: EPIC-elderly prospective cohort study. *Br Med J.* 2005;330:991.

5. Trumbo R. Hormone changes in aging adults probed. *JAMA.* 2005;294:663.

6. Yates LB and others. Exceptional longevity in men. Modifiable factors associated with survival and function to age 90 years. *Arch Intern Med.* 2008; 168:284.

7. Gaudreau P and others. Nutrition as a determinant of successful aging: description of the Quebec longitudinal study Nuage and results from cross-sectional pilot studies. *Rejuventation Res.* 2008; 10:377.

8. Centers for Disease Control and Prevention, National Center for Health Statistics. *Dietary intake of macronutrients, micronutrients, and other dietary constituents: United States, 1988–1994.* Washington, DC: U.S. Department of Health and Human Services; 2002.

9. Institute of Medicine, Food and Nutrition Board. *Dietary Reference Intakes for calcium, phosphorus, magnesium, vitamin D, and fluoride.* Washington, DC: National Academy Press; 1997.

10. Institute of Medicine, Food and Nutrition Board. *Dietary Reference Intakes for vitamin A, vitamin K, arsenic, boron, chromium, copper, iodine, iron, manganese, molybdenum, nickel, silicon, vanadium, and zinc.* Washington, DC: National Academy Press; 2001.

11. Maurer Abbot J, Byrd-Bredbenner C. The state of the American diet. How can we cope? *Topics Clin Nutr.* 2007;3:202.

12. Linnebur S and others. Prevalence of vitamin D insufficiency in elderly ambulatory outpatients in Denver, Colorado. *Am J Geriatr Pharmacother.* 2007;5:1.

13. Kruman II and others. Folic acid deficiency and homocysteine impair DNA repair in hippocampal neurons and sensitize them to amyloid toxicity in experimental models of Alzheimer's disease. *J Neurosci.* 2002;22:1752.

14. Sesdradri S and others. Plasma homocysteine as a risk factor for dementia and Alzheimer's disease. *New Eng J Med.* 2002;346:476.

15. Institute of Medicine, Food and Nutrition Board. *Dietary Reference Intakes for thiamin, riboflavin, niacin, vitamin B6, folate, vitamin B12, pantothenic acid, biotin, and choline.* Washington, DC: National Academy Press; 1998.

16. Bertali B and others. Serum micronutrient concentrations and decline in physical function among older adults. *JAMA.* 2008;299:308.

17. Rao S. Prevention of falls in older persons. *Am Fam Physician.* 2005;72:81.

18. Robertson R, Montagnini M. Geriatric failure to thrive. *Am Fam Physician.* 2004;70:343.

19. DiMaria-Ghalili R, Amella E. Nutrition in older adults. *Am J Nurs.* 2005;105:40.

20. Goulding M and others. Public health and aging: Trends in aging—United States and worldwide. *MMWR.* 2003;52:101.

21. Getting smart about Alzheimer's. *Tufts University Health and Nutrition Letter.* 2005;23(3):1.

22. Burgener SC and others. Evidence supporting nutritional interventions for persons in early stage Alzheimer's disease (AD) *J Nutr Health Aging.* 2008;12:18.

23. Morris MC and others. Consumption of fish and n-3 fatty acids and risk of incident Alzheimer disease. *Arch Neurol.* 2003;60:940.

24. Shatenstein B and others. Poor nutrient intakes during 1-year follow-up with community-dwelling older adults with early-stage Alzheimer dementia compared to cognitively intact matched controls. *J Am Diet Assoc.* 2007;107:2091.

25. National Institutes of Health, National Institute of Arthritis and Musculoskeletal and Skin Diseases. *Health topics, handout on health: Osteoarthritis.* Washington, DC: www. niams.nih.gov; 2006.

26. Niedert K and others. Position of the American Dietetic Association: Liberalization of the diet prescription improves quality of life for older adults in long-term care. *J Am Diet Assoc.* 2005;107:1955.

27. Clarke JO and Mullin GE. A review of complementary and alternative approaches to immunomodulation. *Nutr in Clin Pract.* 2008;23:49.

28. Van Breemen RB and others. Ensuring the safety of botanical dietary supplements. *Am J Clin Nutr.* 2008;87:509S.

29. American Academy of Family Physicians. *Nutrition Screening Initiative.* Washington, DC: American Academy of Family Physicians; 2003.

30. Obisesan TO and others. High blood pressure, hypertension, and high pulse pressure are associated with poorer cognitive function in persons aged 60 and older: The Third National Health and Nutrition Examination Survey. *J Am Geriatr Soc.* 2008;56:501.

31. Beydoun MA and others. n-3 fatty acids, hypertension and risk of cognitive decline among older adults in the Atherosclerosis Risk in Communities (ARIC) study. *Pub Health Nutr.* 2008;11:17

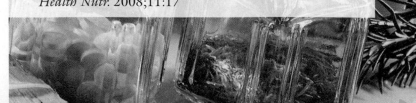

Appendix A

HUMAN PHYSIOLOGY: A TOOL FOR UNDERSTANDING NUTRITION

This appendix explores the various systems in the body beyond the digestive system, focusing specifically on how these systems relate to the study of human nutrition. This focus will set the stage for investigating the various nutrients associated with human nutrition. Before that process can begin, however, it is important to review the processes taking place in a human cell.

The Cell: Structure and Function

The cell is the basic structural and functional unit of life. Living organisms are made of many different kinds of cells specialized to perform particular functions, and all cells are derived from pre-existing cells. In the human body, the trillions of cells all have certain basic characteristics that are alike. All cells have compartments, particles, or filaments that perform specialized functions; these structures are called organelles. There are at least 15 different organelles, but this section discusses only 8. The numbers preceding the names of the cell structures correspond to the structures illustrated in Figure A-1.

1 Cell (Plasma) Membrane

There is an outside and inside to every cell, as defined by the cell (plasma) membrane. This membrane holds in the cellular contents and regulates the direction and flow of substances into and out of the cell. Cell-to-cell communication also occurs by way of this membrane. Some cells can even penetrate another cell membrane and, so, invade that cell.

The cell membrane is a lipid bilayer (or double membrane) of **phospholipids** with their water-soluble (polar) heads facing into the interior of the cell or out to the exterior of the cell. The water-insoluble (non-polar) tails are tucked into the interior of the cell membrane (Chapter 6 reviews phospholipids in detail and Appendix B reviews the concept of polar and non-polar compounds).

Cholesterol is a fat-soluble component of the membrane, so it is embedded within the bilayer. This cholesterol provides rigidity and thus stability to the membrane.

There also are various proteins embedded in the membrane. Proteins provide structural support, act as transport vehicles, and function as enzymes that affect chemical processes within the membrane. Some proteins are open channels that allow water-soluble substances to pass into and out of the cell. Proteins on the outside surface of the membrane act as receptors, snagging essential substances the cell needs and drawing them into the cell. Other proteins act as gates, opening and closing to control the flow of various particles into and out of the cell.

In addition to the lipid and protein, the membrane also contains carbohydrates that mark the exterior of the cell, called the **glycocalyx.** These carbohydrates are combined with either proteins or fats and provide a delivery service for messages to the cell's organelles. The structures also provide distinct identification for a cell. In addition, they detect invaders and initiate defensive actions. In sum, these carbohydrates provide tags that are important to cellular identity and interaction.

phospholipid Class of fat-related substances that contain phosphorus, fatty acids, and a nitrogen-containing base. Phospholipids are an essential part of every cell.

glycocalyx Projections of proteins on the microvilli. They contain enzymes to digest protein and carbohydrate.

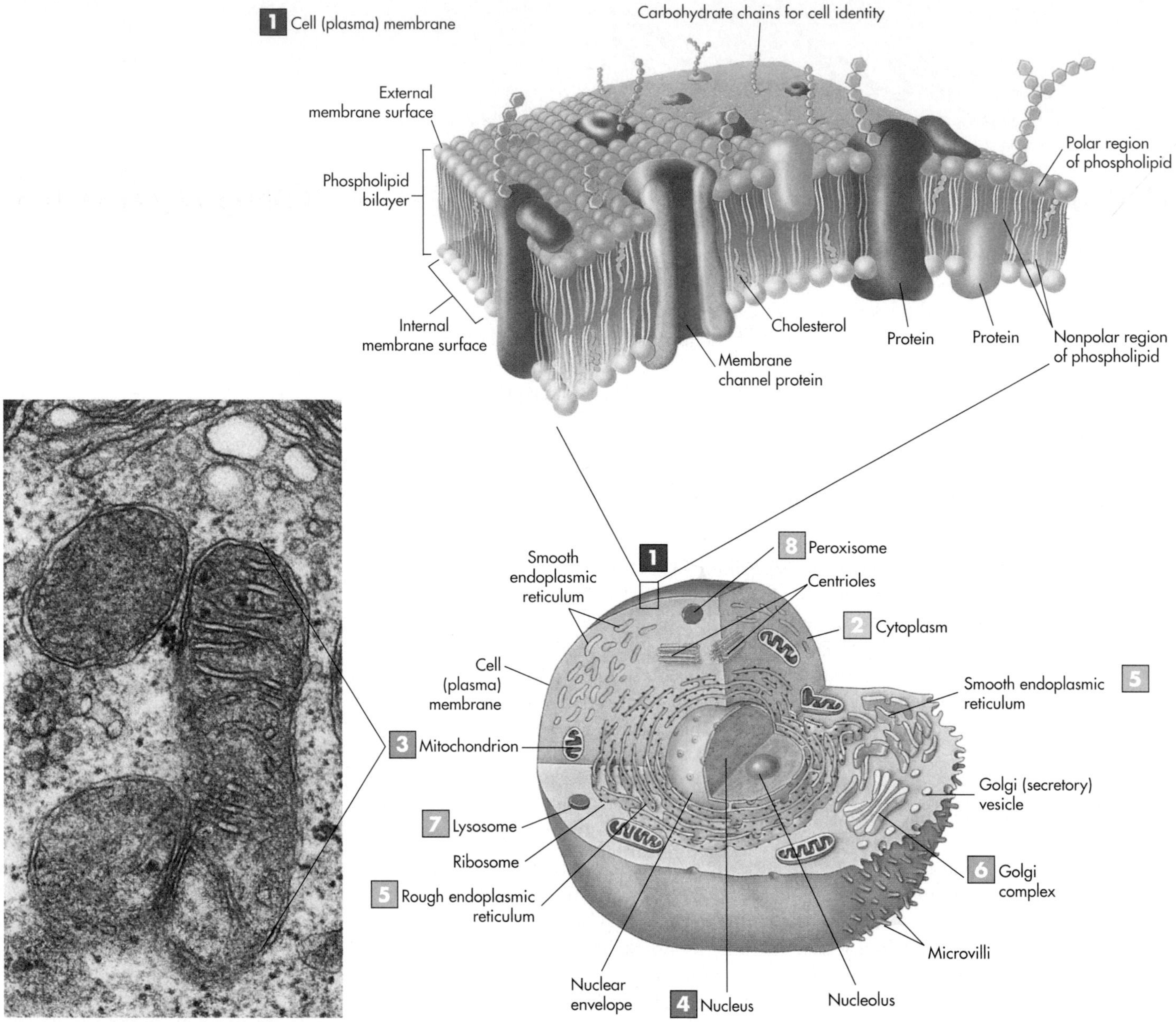

Figure A-1 An animal cell. Almost all human cells contain these various organelles. Shown in greater detail are mitochondria and the cell membrane. Note: not all cells have microvilli. The nuclear envelope encloses the nucleus. The centrioles participate in cell division.

organelles Compartments, particles, or filaments that perform specialized functions within a cell.

cytoplasm Fluid and organelles (except the nucleus) in a cell.

cytosol Water-based phase of the cytoplasm; excludes organelles, such as mitochondria.

Included within the cell membrane are **organelles.** They carry out vital roles in cell functions. Some structures allow the cell to replicate itself, others provide energy, and others destroy the cell when it is worn out. Still other organelles produce and secrete products destined for other cells.

Cytoplasm

The **cytoplasm** is the fluid material and organelles within the cell, not including the nucleus. (The **cytosol** is the fluid surrounding the organelles.) A small amount of ATP energy for use by the cell can be produced by glycolysis reactions that occur in the cytoplasm. This contributes to our survival, because it is the key process in red blood cell energy metabolism; it is called anaerobic metabolism because it doesn't require oxygen.

3 Mitochondria

Mitochondria are sometimes called "power plants," or the powerhouses of cells. These organelles are capable of converting the energy in our energy yielding nutrients (carbohydrate, protein, and fat) to a form that cells can use, ATP. This is an aerobic process that uses the oxygen we inhale, and water, enzymes, and other compounds (see Chapter 9 for details). With the exception of red blood cells, all cells contain mitochondria; only the sizes, shapes, and numbers vary.

Mitochondria have a double membrane, and this characteristic is key to overall mitochondrial function. Within the inner membrane, the electron transport chain and ATP synthesis take place. In the inner matrix of the mitochondria, the citric acid cycle, the beta-oxidation of fatty acids, and the transition reaction involving pyruvate take place.

The biochemical pathways that operate in the mitochondrial matrix also are capable of synthesizing cell components, such as the **carbon skeletons** needed to produce amino acids. These will eventually become cellular protein.

mitochondria Main sites of energy production in a cell. They also contain the pathway for oxidizing fat for fuel, among other metabolic pathways.

carbon skeleton Remains of an amino acid after the amino group has been removed.

4 Cell Nucleus

The **cell nucleus** is surrounded by its own double membrane. The nucleus controls actions that occur in the cell, using the hereditary material deoxyribonucleic acid (DNA). DNA is the "code book" that contains directions for making substances the cell needs. It consists of genes on **chromosomes.** This code book remains in the nucleus of the cell, but it conveys its information to other cell organelles by way of a similar molecule called **ribonucleic acid (RNA).** RNA is responsible for *transcribing* the information of the DNA and moving out through pores in the nuclear membrane to the cytoplasm. The RNA then carries the code to protein-synthesizing sites called **ribosomes.** There, the RNA code is *translated* into a specific protein (see Chapter 7 for details on protein synthesis). With the exception of the red blood cell, all cells have 1 or more nuclei.

The **nucleoli** are areas within the nucleus of the cell containing a combination of protein and RNA. This is where RNA is produced for export to the cytoplasm.

DNA has the secondary task of cell replication. DNA is a double-stranded molecule; when the cell begins to divide, each strand is separated and an identical copy of each is made. Thus, each new DNA molecule contains 1 new strand of DNA and 1 strand from the original DNA. In this way, the genetic code is preserved from 1 cell generation to the next. The mitochondria contain their own DNA, so they reproduce themselves independently of the nucleus.

The transport of proteins, vitamins, and other material from the cytoplasm to the nucleus also occurs through pores in the nuclear membrane, as just mentioned. These small molecules serve a variety of functions, including the activation (or inactivation) of certain parts of the DNA.

cell nucleus Organelle bound by its own double membrane and containing chromosomes; the genetic information for cell protein synthesis.

chromosome Single, large DNA molecule and its associated proteins containing many genes; stores and transmits genetic information.

ribonucleic acid (RNA) Single-stranded nucleic acid involved in the transcription of genetic information and translation of that information into protein structure.

ribosome Cytoplasmic particle that mediates the linking together of amino acids to form proteins; attached to endoplasmic reticulum as a bound ribosome or suspended in cytoplasm as a free ribosome.

nucleolus Center for ribosome production within the cell nucleus.

5 Endoplasmic Reticulum (ER)

The outer membrane of the cell nucleus is continuous with a network of tubes called the **endoplasmic reticulum (ER).** The ER is found in 2 types: rough and smooth. The rough endoplasmic reticulum has ribosomes bound to it, whereas the smooth does not. As noted earlier, ribosomes are sites of protein synthesis. Many of these proteins play a central role in human nutrition. Smooth ER is involved in lipid synthesis, the detoxification of toxic substances, and calcium storage and release in the cell.

endoplasmic reticulum (ER) Organelle in the cytoplasm composed of a network of canals running through the cytoplasm. Rough ER contains ribosomes. Smooth ER contains no ribosomes.

Golgi complex Cell organelle near the nucleus that processes newly synthesized protein for secretion or distribution to other organelles.

6 Golgi Complex

The **Golgi complex** is a packaging site for proteins and lipids that are used in the cytoplasm or are exported from the cell. The Golgi complex consists of sacs within the

secretory vesicle Membrane-bound vesicle produced by the Golgi complex; contains proteins and other compounds to be secreted by the cell.

lysosome Cell organelle that contains digestive enzymes for use inside the cell for turnover of cell parts.

apoptosis Process that occurs over time in which enzymes in a cell set off a series of events that disable numerous cell functions, eventually leading to cell death.

peroxisome Cell organelle that uses oxygen to remove hydrogens from compounds. This produces hydrogen peroxide (H_2O_2), which breaks down into O_2 and H_2O.

cytoplasm in which products of the rough endoplasmic reticulum are received, processed, separated according to function and destination, and "packaged" in **secretory vesicles** for secretion by the cell.

7 Lysosomes

Lysosomes are the cell's digestive system. They are sacs that contain enzymes for the digestion of foreign material. Sometimes known as "suicide bags," they are responsible for digesting worn-out or damaged cells. They carry out **apoptosis,** or programmed cell death, which occurs naturally or is associated with illness or infection. Certain cells that are associated with immunity contain many lysosomes.

8 Peroxisomes

Peroxisomes contain enzymes that detoxify harmful chemicals. **Hydrogen peroxide** (H_2O_2) is formed as a result of such enzyme action. Peroxisomes contain a protective enzyme called *catalase,* which prevents excessive accumulation of hydrogen peroxide in the cell, which would be very damaging. Peroxisomes also play a minor role in metabolizing one possible source of energy for cells—alcohol.

The remainder of this appendix looks at the body systems. Keep in mind that these systems depend on the cell functions just discussed.

Integumentary System

integumentary Having to do with the skin, hair, glands, and nails.

epidermis Outermost layer of the skin, composed of epithelial layers.

dermis Second, or deep, layer of the skin, under the epidermis.

decubitus ulcer Chronic ulcer (also called bedsore) that appears in pressure areas of the skin over a body prominence. These sores develop when people are confined to bed or otherwise immobilized.

The first system to examine is the one you are most familiar with, the **integumentary** system, which is made up of dissimilar elements, such as the skin, hair, various glands, and nails. The largest organ in the body, the skin, consists of 2 principal layers, the **epidermis** and the **dermis** (Fig. A-2). The epidermis is the layer of skin composed largely of dead cells, which are used for protection from environmental pathogens, toxins, injury, and water. We don't want to absorb water through the skin, nor do we want water to readily escape the body.

The dermis is a deeper and thicker layer of skin, with an extensive network of blood vessels, sweat glands, oil-secreting glands, nerve endings, and hair follicles. When people are confined to bed for long periods of time, **decubitus ulcers,** also called bedsores, may develop because of restricted blood flow to the dermis. This lack of blood causes cells to die and open wounds to develop—a potentially life-threatening situation. Adequate intakes of protein, vitamin A, vitamin C, and zinc may help prevent this problem.

The appearance of the skin, hair, and nails is clinically important because it can indicate nutritional deficiencies. For instance, hot, dry skin is an obvious sign of dehydration due to inadequate water intake. (Other signs and symptoms of nutrient deficiencies, as manifested by the skin, are described in Chapters 5, 6, 7, 12, 13, 14, and 15 as the functions of individual nutrients are explained.)

The skin plays a vital role in temperature regulation. Heat produced by the body's metabolic processes, especially the processes that occur in muscle, must be removed before cells are damaged. Heat is removed from the body through the skin. When we are cold, we warm ourselves by shivering because muscle contractions generate heat.

An important nutrient, vitamin D, can be obtained from our diet, but the skin can also make it from a cholesterol derivative in the skin. There is more detail about this process in Chapter 12.

The sweat glands produce perspiration, or sweat, which helps evaporate fluids to cool the body and excrete certain wastes. Mammary glands within the breasts are modified sweat glands designed to secrete milk to feed a newborn.

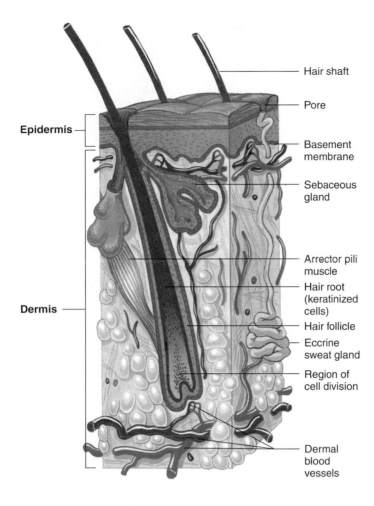

Figure A-2 Cross section of the skin. This is the major organ of the integumentary system.

Hair shaft

Pore

Epidermis

Basement membrane

Sebaceous gland

Arrector pili muscle

Hair root (keratinized cells)

Dermis

Hair follicle

Eccrine sweat gland

Region of cell division

Dermal blood vessels

Skeletal System

Approximately 206 bones make up the skeletal system; this is the rigid framework to which the soft tissues and organs of the body are attached. Each bone is an organ that participates in the overall functioning of the skeleton. Bones that make up the skull and vertebral column protect the brain and spinal cord from injury. Likewise, the rib cage protects the heart, lungs, liver, and spleen from external damage. Bones have attachment sites for skeletal muscles, ligaments, and tendons. (Bones attached to muscles allow body movement when muscles contract.) Blood cell formation, known as **hematopoiesis,** takes place within the marrow of some bones. Bones also are a storehouse for minerals, such as calcium, phosphorus, magnesium, sodium, and fluoride. Bones are metabolically active and constantly adapting to a changing environment.

Long bones, such as those in the arms and legs, consist of 2 types of body tissue: cortical and trabecular (Fig. A-3). **Cortical bone** is hard and dense. It forms a protective shell on the exterior of the bone. **Trabecular bone** is found within the cortical bone at the ends of long bones and in the vertebrae. The shaft of the long bones is a cylinder of cortical bone surrounding a central cavity containing the marrow (see Chapter 14).

At the end of the long bone is the **epiphysis,** consisting of trabecular bone covered by cortical bone. The epiphysis is strong and allows for the attachment of tendons and ligaments. Red bone marrow is made of trabecular bone and is the source of red blood cells, as well as white blood cells and platelets. In children, just behind the epiphysis is the **epiphyseal plate.** This area of bone is responsible for linear growth. When linear growth is complete, an **epiphyseal line** replaces the plate.

hematopoiesis Production of blood cells.

cortical bone Dense, compact bone that constitutes the outer surface and shafts of bone; also called compact bone. Cortical bone makes up 75 to 80% of total bone mass.

trabecular bone Spongy, inner matrix of bone found primarily in the spine, pelvis, and ends of bones; also called cancellous bone. Trabecular bone makes up 20 to 25% of total bone mass.

epiphysis End of a long bone. The epiphyseal plate—sometimes referred to as the growth plate—is made of cartilage and allows bone to grow. During childhood, the cartilage cells multiply and absorb calcium to develop into bone.

epiphyseal plate Cartilage-like layer in the long bone. It functions in linear growth.

epiphyseal line Line that replaces the epiphyseal plate when bone growth is complete.

Figure A-3 Diagram of a long bone. The epiphysis, consisting of trabecular bone, is surrounded by a layer of cortical bone. The epiphyseal line indicates that the bone has completed growth. The production of blood cells occurs in the porous chambers of trabecular bone. The collagen material, the structural material of bone, is observed by the open flap. The skeletal system provides a reserve of calcium and phosphorus for day-to-day needs when dietary intake is inadequate.

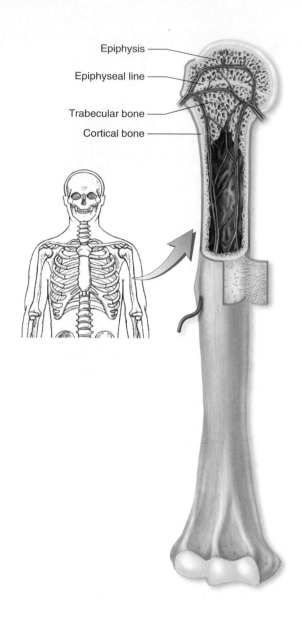

Epiphysis

Epiphyseal line

Trabecular bone

Cortical bone

collagen Major protein of the material that holds together the various structures of the body.

hydroxyapatite Compound, composed primarily of calcium and phosphate, that is deposited into the bone protein matrix to give bone strength and rigidity ($Ca_{10}[PO_4]_6OH_2$).

remodeling Constant building and breakdown of bone throughout life.

resorption Loss of a substance by physiological or pathological means.

osteoblasts Cells in bone that secrete mineral and bone matrix.

osteoclasts Bone cells that arise originally from a type of white blood cell. Osteoclasts secrete substances that lead to bone erosion. This erosion can set the stage for subsequent bone mineralization.

Bones are constructed from several types of cells under the influence of a variety of growth factors. These factors stimulate the formation of **collagen,** a type of flexible protein matrix , which forms the basic shape of bone. Minerals—principally, calcium and phosphorus—are embedded in the matrix, which give the bone strength. **Hydroxyapatite,** the calcium phosphorus salt deposited in the protein matrix, constitutes about 85% of the minerals in bone and makes it possible for the bone to resist compression and bending.

Calcification (also called ossification) of bone varies from bone to bone, but most bones mature (are ossified) by ages 17 to 25. However, some bones, such as the sternum (breastbone), may not complete growth until age 30-plus years.

Bone is constantly **remodeled** throughout life. Formation and **resorption** of bone occur because of the continual activity of **osteoblasts** and **osteoclasts.** Osteoblasts are bone-building cells and osteoclasts are bone-resorbing cells. In the first 20 or so years of life, bone formation is greater than resorption. By age 50 or 60, resorption is greater than deposition and bone diseases are likely to occur. Exercise promotes bone deposition, whereas a lack of exercise results in bone loss.

Bone deposition (ossification) and bone resorption (dissolution) also maintain homeostasis of calcium and phosphorus in the blood. Three hormones control the process: the vitamin D hormone ($1,25(OH)_2$ vitamin D, or calcitriol), calcitonin, and parathyroid hormone (PTH).

Other hormones are involved in bone maintenance, such as growth hormone; thyroid hormones; sex hormones, especially estrogen; and adrenocorticoid hormones. In addition, vitamins A, K, and C perform important jobs in bone metabolism. More information about bones can be found in Chapters 11 through 15, which cover exercise, vitamins, and minerals.

Muscular System

The functions of the muscular system are to provide movement and to generate body heat. Most of the energy released by a muscle cell during physical exercise is in the form of heat. **Muscle fibers** respond when stimulated by motor **neurons** (nerve cells). A muscle cell converts the chemical energy in ATP into the mechanical energy of muscle contraction.

There are 3 types of muscle tissue: **smooth, cardiac,** and **skeletal muscle.** Smooth muscle fibers have a single nucleus and function in involuntary movements within internal organs. Cardiac muscle fiber is striated (striped) with a single nucleus. The stripes in muscle fibers are caused by the arrangement of alternating dark and light contractile proteins (**myosin** and **actin**). This type of muscle performs the involuntary rhythmic contractions of the heart. Skeletal muscle, also containing striated muscle fibers, has several nuclei and is involved in voluntary movements. Skeletal muscle is attached to bone by **tendons.** (Note that Chapter 11 also discusses some specific muscle fiber types.)

Skeletal Muscle

Skeletal muscle fibers are actually long cells with the same organelles that are in other cells. However, unlike most other cells, skeletal muscle cells possess an excellent supply of fuel in the form of glycogen, the body's storage form of the sugar glucose.

Skeletal muscles contract when stimulated by motor neurons. Motor neurons can stimulate several muscle fibers simultaneously. A single muscle fiber is not very efficient. The activation of numerous muscle fibers by multiple motor neurons results in increased muscle strength as the number of fibers stimulated by neurons increases.

Muscle Contraction

As previously mentioned, within muscle fibers are the dark and light stripes called striations. Each muscle cell, when viewed in the electron microscope, contains subunits called **myofibrils.** The myofibrils are the source of the light and dark bands, or stripes. The importance of these structures is the presence of the unique proteins actin and myosin. The functioning structure of the myofibril is the **sarcomere,** the contracting unit.

When a muscle fiber is stimulated by a neuron to contract, one of the first events to occur is the release of large amounts of calcium from storage in the smooth endoplasmic reticulum (also called the sarcoplasmic reticulum). This is the "on" switch. The presence of calcium allows the 2 main proteins, myosin and actin, to get ready to slide into each other and set the **power stroke** in motion. Of course, energy is required to carry out the muscle contraction. Here is where ATP plays the key role (Fig. A-4).

Another ATP is needed to release the actin from the myosin. This is the end of the contraction. As the muscle moves to the "off" position, the calcium is transported back to storage, the muscle fiber relaxes, and it gets ready for another contraction.

The factor that allows muscle action to occur at all is the essential nutrient calcium. When the muscle is relaxed, there is very little calcium in the cytoplasm of the muscle cell because calcium is in storage. However, when the muscle is ready to go to work, as directed by the motor neuron, calcium is moved out of storage, which sets the stage

muscle fiber Component of a muscle cell.

neuron Structural and functional unit of the nervous system, consisting of cell body, dendrites, and axon.

smooth muscle Muscle tissue under involuntary control; found in the GI tract, artery walls, respiratory passages, urinary tract, and reproductive tract.

cardiac muscle Muscle tissue that makes up the walls of the heart; produces rhythmical, involuntary contractions.

skeletal muscle Muscle tissue responsible for voluntary body movements.

myosin Thick filament protein that connects with actin to cause a muscle contraction.

actin Protein in muscle fiber that, together with myosin, is responsible for contraction.

tendon Dense connective tissue that attaches a muscle to a bone.

myofibril Bundle of contractile fibers within a muscle cell.

sarcomere Portion of a muscle fiber that is considered the functional unit of a myofibril.

power stroke Movement of the thick filament alongside the thin filament in a muscle cell, causing muscle contraction.

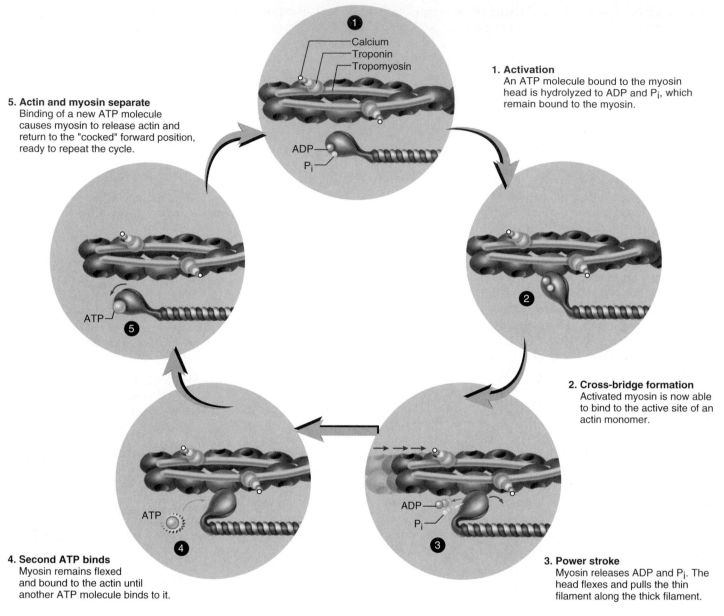

5. Actin and myosin separate
Binding of a new ATP molecule
causes myosin to release actin and
return to the "cocked" forward position,
ready to repeat the cycle.

1. Activation
An ATP molecule bound to the myosin
head is hydrolyzed to ADP and P_i, which
remain bound to the myosin.

Calcium
Troponin
Tropomyosin

ADP
P_i

ATP

ATP

4. Second ATP binds
Myosin remains flexed
and bound to the actin until
another ATP molecule binds to it.

ADP
P_i

2. Cross-bridge formation
Activated myosin is now able
to bind to the active site of an
actin monomer.

3. Power stroke
Myosin releases ADP and P_i. The
head flexes and pulls the thin
filament along the thick filament.

Figure A-4 Muscle contraction. In Step 1, or activation, an ATP is bound to the myosin head (purple) and is split into ADP and P_i. Troponin and tropomyosin
are proteins that participate in this process. During Step 2, the activated myosin can now bind to the actin (the red beads). In Step 3, the myosin head releases the
ADP and P_i. The head flexes and pulls the thin filament along the thick filament. This is the *power stroke*. In Step 4, the myosin remains bound to the actin until
another ATP binds to the myosin. The new ATP causes the myosin to release the actin, so that it can get ready for another cycle, Step 5. Actin and myosin separate,
which leads to muscle relaxation. The white dot in this figure is calcium, a nutrient required for muscle action.

for the power stroke. And, when the contraction ends, the calcium is released from the
muscle fibers and goes back into storage.

Cardiac and Smooth Muscle

Cardiac muscle and smooth muscle, although similar in many ways to skeletal muscle in their
use of calcium as an off/on switch, operate under involuntary control. In cardiac muscle, the
stimulation occurs automatically by a group of muscle cells. These cells initiate the heartbeat
and set the heart rate under control of the brain and the influence of certain hormones.

Smooth muscles are found in the lungs, blood vessels, GI tract, and other internal organs. In the GI tract, they produce important contractions in peristalsis (see Chapter 4 for details).

▶ A unique feature of smooth muscle is its ability to stretch. By the end of pregnancy, the smooth muscle in the uterus can be stretched up to 8 times its prepregnant length.

Circulatory System

The circulatory system is made up of 2 separate systems: the cardiovascular system and the lymphatic system. The cardiovascular system consists of the heart and blood vessels. The lymphatic system consists of lymphatic vessels, lymph, and a number of lymph tissues.

One organ vital to our existence is the heart, a 4-chambered pump that keeps blood continuously circulating around the body. It takes about 1 minute for blood to leave the heart, circulate to all tissues in the body, and return to the heart. When we are exercising strenuously, the blood can circulate at a rate of 6 times per minute.

The cells that make up the tissues of the body need a constant supply of water, oxygen, and nutrients. In addition, the body needs ATP energy, which comes from the breakdown of energy nutrients within the cells. The blood carries oxygen from the lungs to all organs in the body. The blood also carries nutrients from the digestive tract to all tissues and to storage sites when nutrients are not needed immediately for energy, growth, or repair. Waste materials produced by cells must be removed by way of the skin, lungs, kidneys, and digestive tract. This, too, is a function of the cardiovascular system. The delivery of hormones to their target cells, the maintenance of a constant body temperature, and the distribution of white blood cells to protect against invading pathogens are all performed by the blood and circulatory systems without our being aware of any specific action. The circulatory system has chemical means to prevent excessive blood loss from damaged vessels using the clotting process (see Chapter 12).

Blood Constituents

Red blood cells, known as **erythrocytes,** carry oxygen to all tissues and play a role in the return of carbon dioxide to the lungs. The white blood cells, known as **leukocytes,** function as part of the immune system. They protect the body from invading pathogens. The blood is able to clot because of platelets and other clotting factors. The liquid part of blood is known as **plasma.** In contrast, **serum** is the fluid that results after the blood is first allowed to clot before being centrifuged; it does not contain the blood-clotting factors.

Heart Structure

The heart has 2 sides, left and right. The right side is closest to your right arm; likewise, the left side is closest to your left arm. The upper part of the heart has left and right **atria,** which empty simultaneously into the lower part of the heart, consisting of the left and right **ventricles.**

Blood travels in blood vessels from the left side of the heart through the **aorta** to major **arteries.** Arteries become smaller and smaller until they are so tiny they are classified as **arterioles.** The blood flows from the arterioles into microscopic, weblike structures called **capillaries.** Capillaries are just 1 cell layer thick and have pores that allow oxygen, water, and other nutrients to leave the blood for surrounding cells and that allow waste and other products of cellular metabolism to enter the blood. There are few cells in the body that aren't close to a capillary. Larger blood vessels are not porous, so blood cannot escape these vessels. Only in the capillaries can the blood discharge and recover substances associated with nearby cells.

erythrocyte Mature red blood cell. It has no nucleus and a life span of about 120 days; contains hemoglobin, which transports oxygen and carbon dioxide.

leukocyte White blood cell.

plasma Fluid, non-cellular portion of the circulating blood. This includes the blood serum plus all blood-clotting factors. In contrast, serum is the fluid that results after the blood is first allowed to clot before being centrifuged; this does not contain the blood-clotting factors.

serum Portion of the blood fluid remaining after (1) the blood is allowed to clot and (2) the red and white blood cells and other solid matter are removed by centrifugation.

atria Two upper chambers of the heart, which receive venous blood.

ventricles Two lower chambers of the heart, which contain blood to be pumped from the heart.

aorta Major blood vessel leaving from the left ventricle.

artery Blood vessel that carries blood away from the heart.

arteriole Small artery.

capillary Microscopic blood vessel that connects an arteriole and a venule; the functional unit of the circulatory system.

venule Tiny vessel that carries blood from the capillary to a vein.

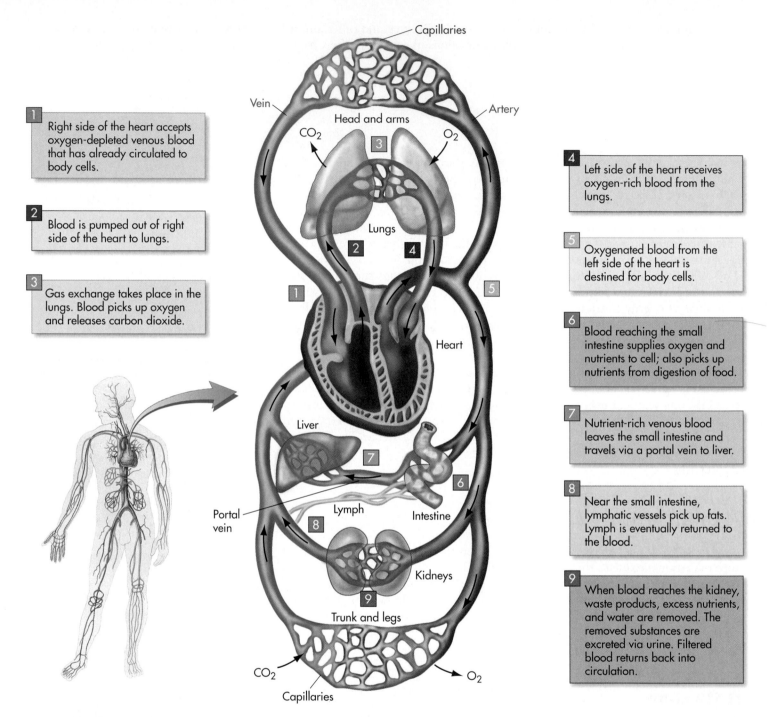

1. Right side of the heart accepts oxygen-depleted venous blood that has already circulated to body cells.

2. Blood is pumped out of right side of the heart to lungs.

3. Gas exchange takes place in the lungs. Blood picks up oxygen and releases carbon dioxide.

4. Left side of the heart receives oxygen-rich blood from the lungs.

5. Oxygenated blood from the left side of the heart is destined for body cells.

6. Blood reaching the small intestine supplies oxygen and nutrients to cell; also picks up nutrients from digestion of food.

7. Nutrient-rich venous blood leaves the small intestine and travels via a portal vein to liver.

8. Near the small intestine, lymphatic vessels pick up fats. Lymph is eventually returned to the blood.

9. When blood reaches the kidney, waste products, excess nutrients, and water are removed. The removed substances are excreted via urine. Filtered blood returns back into circulation.

Figure A-5 Blood circulation through the body. This figure shows the paths that blood takes from the heart to the lungs (Steps 1–3), back to the heart (Step 4), and through the rest of the body (Steps 5–9). The red color indicates blood that is richer in oxygen; blue is for blood carrying more carbon dioxide. Arteries and veins go to all parts of the body.

vein Blood vessel that conveys blood to the heart.

systemic circuit Part of the circulatory system concerned with the flow of blood from the left ventricle to the body and back to the right atrium.

As the blood exits the capillaries, it flows into tiny **venules,** which enlarge and become **veins,** returning the blood to the right side of the heart. The route from the left side of the heart to the capillaries and then back to the right side of the heart is called the **systemic circuit** of blood (Figs. A-5, A-6, and A-7).

The flow of blood through the circulatory system is measured by pressure in millimeters of mercury. The average arterial (artery) pressure is about 100 mm Hg, whereas the average venous pressure is only 2 mm Hg. To guarantee return flow to the heart, blood is moved through the veins by the contraction of skeletal muscles. Also, valves in the veins prevent a backflow of blood.

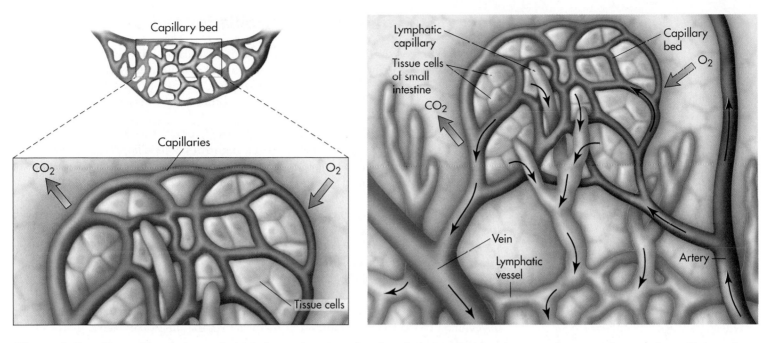

Figure A-6 **Capillary and lymphatic vessels.** (*a*) Exchange of oxygen and nutrients for carbon dioxide and waste products occurs between the capillaries and the surrounding tissue cells. (*b*) Lymphatic vessels are also present in capillary beds, such as in the small intestine. Lymphatic vessels in the small intestine are also called *lacteals*. Note that the lymphatic vessels are blind-ended.

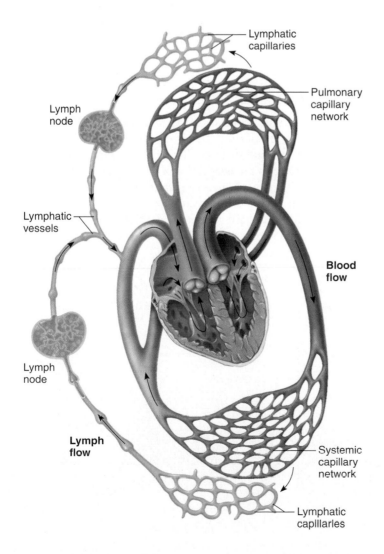

Figure A-7 **Lymph.** As lymph moves through the lymphatic system, it encounters lymph nodes containing immune cells that destroy invading pathogens. Lymph also carries dietary fat and fat-soluble nutrients from the digestive tract to the blood, using the thoracic duct.

Flow of Materials between Capillaries and Cells

extracellular fluid (ECF) Fluid present outside the cells. It includes intravascular and interstitial fluids; represents about one-third of all body fluid.

lymphatic vessel Vessel that carries lymph.

pulmonary circulation System of blood vessels from the right ventricle of the heart to the lungs and back to the left atrium of the heart.

portal system Veins in the GI tract that convey blood from capillaries in the intestines and portions of the stomach to the liver; also called hepatic portal system.

portal vein Large vein that leaves from the intestines and stomach and connects to the liver.

As the blood flows from the arterioles into the capillaries, the hydrostatic pressure generated by the force of the heart's contraction causes fluid to flow into spaces around the surrounding cells, called the **extracellular fluid (ECF)** (Fig. A-8). Some of this fluid returns to the capillaries and some enters another nearby vessel called a **lymphatic vessel.**

Oxygen and nutrients leave the capillaries, enter the ECF, and are then delivered to cells by 1 of the mechanisms mentioned in Chapter 4: passive and facilitated diffusion, active transport, and pinocytosis. Cellular products plus waste substances are collected in the ECF and are either released to the capillaries that connect to the venules or channeled into the lymphatic vessels. Oxygen travels to the cell by diffusing from the blood into the extracellular fluid and then in through the cell membrane. Carbon dioxide exits the cell and goes to the blood in the same way. This is 1 of 2 important gas exchange activities in the body and is often referred to as internal respiration.

The right atrium of the heart receives dark red venous blood from the body, which is then pumped into the right ventricle. The right ventricle pumps blood through the pulmonary arteries to the capillaries in the lungs. The lungs then return the freshly oxygenated blood to the left atrium of the heart via the pulmonary veins. This route is known as **pulmonary circulation.**

As the blood moves through the pulmonary capillaries, carbon dioxide is released for expiration, and the inhaled oxygen is taken up by the blood. This is the other site for gas exchange in the body, often referred to as external respiration. The oxygenated blood (now a bright red) in the atrium is pumped to the left ventricle. The blood is pumped out of the left ventricle and through the aorta to the systemic circuit.

Other Circulatory Systems

One capillary bed does not send blood back to the heart but rather directs it toward the liver. This is the **portal system** of the GI tract composed of veins draining blood from the capillaries of the intestines and stomach. These veins empty into a large **portal vein,** which acts as a direct pipeline to the liver. (The brain also has a portal system.)

The heart also has its own circulatory system. Coronary vessels supply blood to meet cardiac needs. These arteries are particularly susceptible to damage by deposits of cholesterol and other lipids in the artery wall. This accumulation of cholesterol can lead to coronary heart disease. (There is more about this disease in Chapter 6.)

Figure A-8 **Distribution of body fluids.** The intracellular compartment contains fluid in the cell, which is free to move into the extracellular compartment. The extracellular compartment contains the fluid between the cell and the capillary, called interstitial fluid. The extracellular fluid also includes the fluid within blood and lymphatic vessels. This figure shows the fluid (plasma) from the blood moving freely between cells and capillaries through the interstitial fluid.

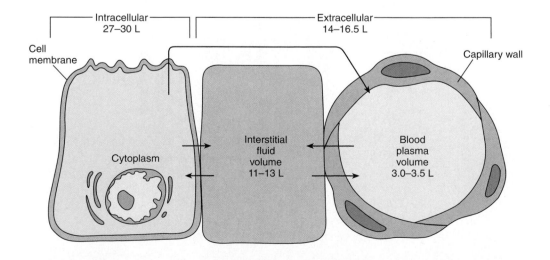

Lymphatic System

The lymphatic system is closely related to the immune system in that both defend us against pathogenic invaders. As the lymphatic system collects fluid from tissues, it picks up microorganisms as well. The fluid passes through many **lymph nodes** as it makes its way back to the bloodstream. In the nodes is an abundant collection of white blood cells ready to detect pathogens in the lymph fluid and quickly destroy them. The lymphatic system consists of lymphatic vessels, lymph fluid, lymph nodes, and lymphatic tissue, with its population of immune cells.

The interstitial, or extracellular, fluid (fluid surrounding the cell) contains many components that are too large to pass through holes in the capillaries, so they are blocked from returning directly to the bloodstream. Therefore, they take an indirect route via the lymphatic system back to general circulation (see Fig. A-7).

Lymph also serves as the passageway by which fat-soluble nutrients are absorbed from the GI tract and carried into the bloodstream. Lymph also contains bacteria, viruses, cellular trash, and cancer cells on their way to invade some distant site. Lymph generates immune cells, called **lymphocytes,** that combat these invaders (see the section "Immune System").

At the terminal end of the capillaries, the amount of fluid released from the capillaries into the venules is less than the amount of fluid entering the capillaries from the arterioles. The missing 15% of fluid represents the extracellular fluid that is returned to the vascular system via the lymphatic system. This fluid is subsequently delivered to the lymphatic system by way of specialized capillaries called lymphatic capillaries. Blood plasma and fluid in the tissues are constantly being interchanged. The fluid, which is now called **lymph,** enters these porous vessels and consists of extracellular fluid and proteins too large to squeeze back into the capillaries.

In addition to microorganisms, the lymph contains absorbed dietary fat. The absorption of fats occurs only in the **lacteals,** which are lymphatic capillaries of the small intestine, not the portal vein. From the lacteals, lymph is directed into larger vessels, called **lymph ducts,** and is moved toward the heart by the action of skeletal muscle contractions and other body movements.

As the lymph makes its way back to the heart, it encounters clusters of lymph nodes containing phagocytic cells, lymphocytes, and mobile **macrophages,** which help destroy invading pathogens and filter the lymph. **T lymphocytes** and **B lymphocytes** are found in these nodes and are major players in immunity (see the section "Immune System"). When you are ill and seek medical attention, do you ever wonder why your physician checks the lymph glands in your neck for swelling? Swelling means the lymph nodes are in combat against an invading pathogen.

The spleen, thymus gland, and tonsils are considered lymphoid organs. The spleen contains phagocytes, which filter out foreign substances and destroy worn-out red blood cells. The thymus gland is important in immunity during childhood. Tonsils protect against invaders that are inhaled or eaten.

Eventually, the lymph empties into the thoracic duct and the right lymph duct, then into veins that enter the right atrium of the heart, and finally into general circulation (see Fig. A-7). (There is further discussion of transport of lipid substances in the lymph system in Chapter 6.)

Immune System

The cells that carry out immune functions are known collectively as the immune system. Unlike other systems in the body, they do not exist as anatomically connected organs but, rather, as separate collections of cells throughout the body. They defend against invading pathogens—microorganisms or substances capable of producing disease. They

---

lymph node Small structure located along the course of the lymphatic vessels.

lymphocyte Class of white blood cells involved in the immune system, generally comprising about 25% of all white blood cells. There are several types of lymphocytes with diverse functions, including antibody production, allergic reaction, graft rejection, tumor control, and regulation of the immune system.

lymph Clear, plasmalike fluid that flows through lymphatic vessels.

lacteal Small lymph duct within a villus of the small intestine.

lymph duct Large lymphatic vessel that empties lymph into the circulatory system.

macrophage Any large, mononuclear phagocytic cell in the tissues and derived from a monocyte in the blood. Besides functioning as important phagocytes, macrophages secrete numerous cytokines and act as antigen-presenting cells.

T lymphocyte Type of white blood cell that recognizes intracellular antigens (e.g., viral antigens in infected cells), fragments of which move to the cell surface. T lymphocytes originate in the bone marrow but must mature in the thymus gland.

B lymphocyte Type of white blood cell that recognizes antigens (e.g., bacteria) present in extracellular sites in the body and is responsible for antibody-mediated immunity. B lymphocytes originate and mature in the bone marrow and are released into the blood and lymph.

discriminate between "self" and "non-self." They are very sensitive indicators of the body's nutritional status. The most numerous of the immune system cells are the leukocytes.

Our bodies constantly wage war against disease-producing microorganisms, such as bacteria, viruses, fungi, and parasites, against substances capable of producing disease, such as toxins from snake venom; and against allergens, which trigger allergic reactions via **antigen** release (see Chapter 7) or cancer cells (Fig. A-9). The most common invaders are bacteria, which are 1-cell organisms with a cell wall in addition to a cell membrane, and viruses, which are nucleic acids surrounded by a protein coat. Viruses can't multiply by themselves because they lack ribosomes for protein synthesis, so they survive by taking over host cells and instructing them to produce the proteins and energy the viruses need for survival.

antigen Foreign substance, generally large, that induces a state of sensitivity and/or resistance to microbes or toxic substances after a lag period; substance that stimulates a specific aspect of the immune system.

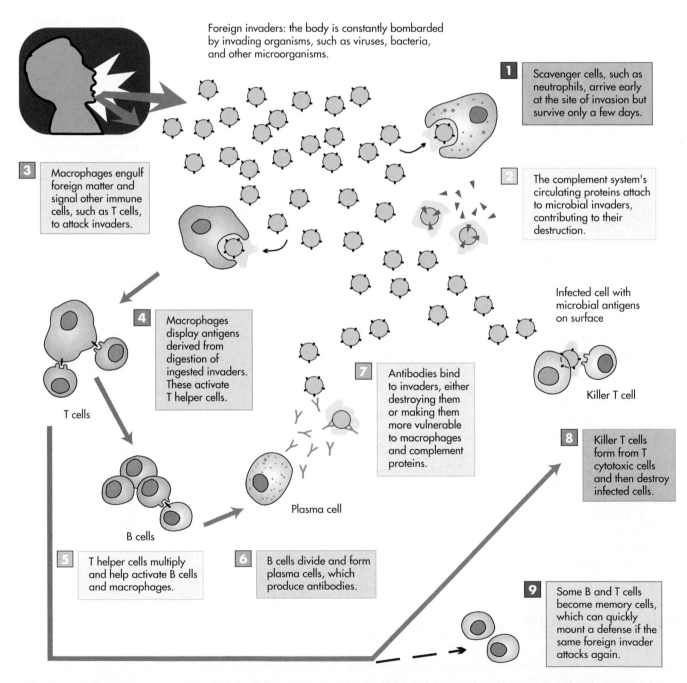

Foreign invaders: the body is constantly bombarded by invading organisms, such as viruses, bacteria, and other microorganisms.

1 Scavenger cells, such as neutrophils, arrive early at the site of invasion but survive only a few days.

3 Macrophages engulf foreign matter and signal other immune cells, such as T cells, to attack invaders.

2 The complement system's circulating proteins attach to microbial invaders, contributing to their destruction.

Infected cell with microbial antigens on surface

4 Macrophages display antigens derived from digestion of ingested invaders. These activate T helper cells.

T cells

Killer T cell

7 Antibodies bind to invaders, either destroying them or making them more vulnerable to macrophages and complement proteins.

8 Killer T cells form from T cytotoxic cells and then destroy infected cells.

Plasma cell

B cells

5 T helper cells multiply and help activate B cells and macrophages.

6 B cells divide and form plasma cells, which produce antibodies.

9 Some B and T cells become memory cells, which can quickly mount a defense if the same foreign invader attacks again.

Figure A-9 Biological warfare. The body commands a wide assortment of defenders to reduce the danger of infection and help guard against repeated microbial infections. The ultimate target of the immune response is an antigen—commonly, a foreign protein from a bacterium or another microbe.

Table A-1 Types and Functions of Leukocytes

Leukocyte	Function
Neutrophil	Phagocytizes bacteria; forms highly toxic compounds that destroy bacteria
Eosinophil	Phagocytizes antigen-antibody complex, allergy-causing antigens, inflammatory chemicals; attacks parasites, such as worms
Basophil	Secretes histamine, a vasodilator, thus increasing blood flow to tissues; secretes heparin, which prevents blood clotting
Lymphocyte	Natural killer cell that attacks cells infected with viruses or that have turned cancerous; B lymphocytes present antigens and activate other cells of the immune system; can become plasma cells that secrete antibodies; serve as memory cells in humoral immunity; T lymphocytes destroy foreign cells, regulate the immune response, and serve as memory cells in cellular immunity
Monocyte	Differentiates into numerous types of macrophages; macrophages phagocytize pathogens, dead neutrophils, and cellular debris; they present antigens and activate other cells of the immune system

Leukocytes and Macrophages

Leukocytes, also known as white blood cells, are produced in the bone marrow and may undergo further development in tissues outside the marrow. They travel via the blood and enter tissues where they function. They are classified by their structure and their affinity for certain types of dye. For example, a monocyte has a single, prominent nucleus. Another type of immune cell takes up the red dye eosin and, so, is called an eosinophil. There are 5 general types of leukocytes, which are listed in Table A-1, along with a brief description of their functions.

Macrophages are found in almost all tissues of the body. They are derived from 1 kind of leukocyte, the monocyte. When a monocyte leaves the blood and enters a tissue, it is transformed into a macrophage. At birth, a baby is already supplied with macrophages, which continue to develop throughout life. They are strategically located throughout the body to phagocytize foreign material.

Mast cells are produced in the bone marrow and exist in almost all tissues and organs. They release histamine and the other chemicals involved in inflammation.

Other participants in the immune system are **cytokines,** a complicated group of protein messengers produced by various cells throughout the body. They regulate the host cells' function and growth.

There are 2 types of immunity: nonspecific, or natural, immunity and specific, or acquired, immunity. Nonspecific immunity protects against foreign invaders without having to recognize the specific appearance of the invaders, whereas specific immunity is acquired.

Nonspecific Immunity

Nonspecific immunity is an array of mechanisms that are present at birth and do not require any activation. They are barriers such as the skin and the **mucous membranes** of the GI tract, reproductive system, urinary tract, and respiratory tract. The **mucus** produced by these tissues traps invaders. Internally, another form of nonspecific immunity is phagocytic cells, which can swallow bacteria and other harmful substances and ultimately destroy them. Acid produced by the stomach (HCl) can destroy ingested pathogens. Inflammation is a local response to infection or injury. The purpose is to destroy or inactivate foreign invaders and begin the process of repair. Fever is also an internal defense mechanism. It seems to aid in the recovery process by reducing the amount of iron in the

mast cell Tissue cell that releases histamine and other chemicals involved in inflammation.

cytokine Protein secreted by a cell that regulates the activity of neighboring cells.

nonspecific immunity Defenses that stop the invasion of pathogens; requires no previous encounter with a pathogen.

mucous membrane Membrane that lines passageways open to the exterior environment; also called mucosae.

mucus Thick fluid secreted by glands throughout the body. It contains a compound that has both a carbohydrate and a protein nature. It acts as both a lubricant and a means of protection for cells.

interferon Group of proteins released by virus-infected cells that binds to other cells, stimulating synthesis of antiviral proteins that in turn inhibits viral multiplication.

specific immunity Function of lymphocytes directed at specific antigens.

antibody-mediated immunity Specific immunity provided by B lymphocytes; also known as humoral immunity.

antibody Blood protein that inactivates foreign proteins in the body. This helps prevent and control infections.

immunoglobulin Protein in the blood that is responsible for antibody-mediated immunity and that binds specifically to antigens; also called *antibody.* Immunoglobulins are produced by certain white blood cells in response to a foreign substance (antigen) in the bloodstream.

plasma cell B lymphocyte that produces about 2000 antibodies per second.

memory cell B lymphocyte that remains after an infection to convey long-lasting or permanent immunity.

complement Series of blood proteins that participate in a complex reaction cascade following stimulation by an antigen-antibody complex on the surface of a bacterial cell. Various activated complement proteins can enhance phagocytosis, contribute to inflammation, and destroy bacteria.

cell-mediated immunity Process in which T lymphocytes come in contact with invading cells in order to destroy them.

cytotoxic T cell T cell that interacts with the infected host cell through receptor sites on the T cell surface.

helper T cell T cell that interacts with macrophages and secretes substances to signal an invading pathogen; stimulates B lymphocytes to proliferate.

blood, which reduces bacterial activity. Fever also seems to be associated with an increase in **interferons.** Viral infections are subject to short-term control by this group of proteins released by infected cells. Interferons are receiving a lot of attention as potent weapons against cancers, hepatitis C, and other diseases.

Specific Immunity

Antibody-mediated immunity is directed at specific molecules. When non-specific immunological defenses fail to halt an invasion by pathogens or by toxins produced by pathogens, the antibody—mediated immunity mechanism comes into action. This mechanism is based on the action of antibodies, lymphocytes, and other cells of the immune system.

Recall that antigens are molecules that are generally large in size and foreign to the body. A given molecule can have a number of antigenic determinant sites that stimulate the production of various antibodies. When we successfully fight off an invader, chemicals called **antibodies** are in action. Antibodies are highly specific proteins produced by B lymphocytes in response to antigens. Antigens are detected as dangerous intruders. They are detected because the immune system can identify "self" from "non-self" molecules. (Recall that 1 role of the carbohydrates on the cell membrane is to identify "self.")

The lymphocytes that produce antibodies, designated B lymphocytes, are produced in the bone marrow. These B lymphocytes wage war against bacterial infections, as well as some viral infections and even a few parasites. B lymphocytes (or B cells) and antibodies, also known as **immunoglobulins,** come in 5 major classifications. These bind to the antigen on the invader and begin a process of attack. This antibody-antigen interaction soon produces **plasma cells,** resulting in the production of more antibody proteins to continue the attack. A person can produce as many different antibodies as there are exposures to specific antigens. It is estimated that there are 100 million trillion antibody molecules per person, representing a few million species of antigens.

Memory cells are then produced by B cells and provide active immunity. Once you have been exposed to an antigen, you develop active immunity. Obviously, this is the basis of vaccinations; an inactivated pathogen is injected and the body develops immunity to that pathogen.

The blood also contains a group of proteins called **complement** proteins. Complement proteins are released into the area of infection and attach to the target pathogen to be destroyed. The antibody-antigen combination does not cause the destruction of the pathogenic invaders, but it does identify them, so that they can be attacked by nonspecific immune processes, such as the complement proteins. Complement proteins attach to the pathogenic invader and drill holes in its membrane, thus leading to its destruction. (The hole in the wall allows water to flow into the cell, causing the cell to burst.)

T lymphocytes (T cells) directly attack and destroy specific cells, which are identified by specific antigens on the cell surface. T lymphocytes produce **cell-mediated immunity** because they are in contact with the enemy cell. T cells must be first activated in the thymus gland.

The T lymphocytes that are killers are known as **cytotoxic T cells.** They recognize the infected cell and attach themselves through a CD8 receptor. There are also **helper T cells.** They attach to an infected cell through a CD4 receptor. They promote phagocytic activity. Together, the cytotoxic and helper T cells bind to the infected cell and lead to the cell's destruction. You may have heard of CD4 cells because they are markers for AIDS. When the disease progresses, the CD4 count decreases as the virus attacks helper T cells (and macrophages).

Most information concerning the relationship of nutrition to immunity comes from studies in poor countries of the developing world, where children die of infectious diseases secondary to malnutrition. Protein-energy malnutrition deficiencies of vitamins and minerals and an inadequate intake of certain fatty acids seriously alter immune function. (There is more information about how individual nutrients make it possible to support an immune response in Chapters 12 through 15.)

Allergies are types of immune responses. One type of allergic response is almost immediate. The symptoms are produced by B lymphocytes exposed to an allergen, as demonstrated by a runny nose, red eyes, and itchy skin (dermatitis). The culprit is **histamine,** an altered form of the common amino acid histidine. This type of immune response can be treated by antihistamine drugs. (Allergies are further discussed in Chapter 7.)

Delayed hypersensitivity, an abnormal T cell response, can occur as late as 72 hours after exposure. The best-known example of this type of immune response is contact dermatitis caused by contact with poison ivy, poison oak, or poison sumac.

A final type of immunity is known as autoimmunity. Here the immune system fails to recognize "self," thinking a normal cell is an antigen. The immune system then goes on the attack by activating T lymphocytes and the production of antibodies by B lymphocytes, which kills the cell. In other words, the defense mechanisms are confused and attack the body rather than invaders. There are at least 40 autoimmune diseases. Some well-known examples are rheumatoid arthritis, type 1 diabetes, and multiple sclerosis.

histamine Breakdown product of the amino acid histidine that stimulates acid secretion by the stomach and has other effects on the body, such as contraction of smooth muscles, increased nasal secretions, relaxation of blood vessels, and changes in constriction of airways.

Respiratory System

To produce sufficient energy to meet body needs, there must be oxygen present to help convert food energy into ATP. When oxygen is supplied to the tissues, carbon dioxide is produced and removed from the body by the combined actions of the cardiovascular and respiratory systems.

The organs of the respiratory system are the nose, pharynx, larynx, trachea, bronchi, and lungs. *Respiration* refers to breathing and to the exchange of gases between the blood and other tissues. The respiratory tract features the **alveoli** (plural) in the lungs. These are tiny structures where a form of gas exchange takes place, described previously as external respiration (Fig. A-10). The **alveolus** (singular), the basic functional unit of respiration,

alveoli, alveolus Basic functional unit of the lungs.

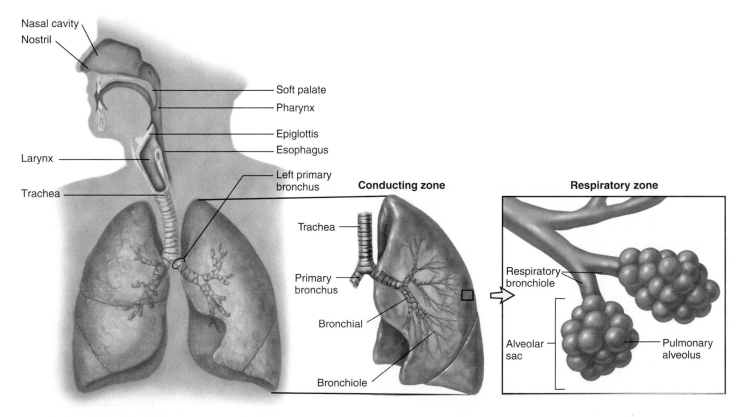

Figure A-10 **Anatomy of the respiratory system. Air enters through the nose and mouth and is conducted into the bronchioles of the lungs. Gas exchange occurs in the alveoli.**

recovers oxygen from inhaled air and loads it onto red blood cells for transport to target tissues throughout the body. Simultaneously, carbon dioxide in the blood is released into the lungs and ultimately is exhaled into the air.

Air reaches the lungs from the nasal cavity and the mouth by first passing through the **pharynx** to the **larynx.** The larynx is open to the trachea during breathing but closes during swallowing. The **trachea** is the tube that connects the larynx to the **bronchial tree.** The bronchial tree, located in the lungs, looks like a tree with branches. The branches on this tree get smaller and smaller the farther out they go from the tree trunk (the trachea) into lung tissue until finally they turn into **bronchioles,** the location of the pulmonary alveoli.

The distance across the alveoli is 2 cells thick—1 cell for the alveoli plus 1 cell for the pulmonary capillaries. Gas exchange allows CO_2 and O_2 to diffuse easily between the blood and lungs. There are approximately 300 million alveoli in the lungs, providing a tremendous surface area for the diffusion of gases.

Another aspect of respiration is the discharge of water through the lungs. This process is obvious on a cold day when the breath we exhale turns to ice crystals, and we can see vapor forming around the mouth and nose. Of course, such water loss is much more extensive during hot, humid weather when the body loses heat via the lungs.

Nervous System

The nervous system is a regulatory system controlling a variety of body functions. It can detect changes in various organs and take corrective action when needed to maintain the constancy of the internal environment, **homeostasis.** The nervous system regulates activities that occur almost instantaneously, such as muscle contractions and perception of danger.

The nervous system consists of the **central nervous system (CNS)** and the **peripheral nervous system (PNS).** The central nervous system contains the brain and spinal cord. The peripheral nervous system, with its nerves coming from the central nervous system, branch out to all organs of the body.

The basic structural and functional unit of the nervous system is the neuron—a cell that responds to electrical and chemical signals, conducts electrical impulses, and releases chemical regulators (Fig. A-11). Neurons allow us to perceive what is occurring in our environment, engage in learning, store vital information in memory, and control the body's voluntary actions. Incoming information depends on sensory receptors, such as visual, auditory, smell, and tactile receptors.

pharynx Organ of the digestive tract and respiratory tract located at the back of the oral and nasal cavities.

larynx Structure between the pharynx and trachea that contains the vocal cords.

trachea Airway leading from the larynx to the bronchi.

bronchial tree Bronchi and the branches that stem out to bronchioles.

bronchioles Smallest division of the bronchi.

homeostasis Series of adjustments that prevent change in the body's internal environment.

central nervous system (CNS) Brain and spinal cord portions of the nervous system.

peripheral nervous system (PNS) Nerves of the central nervous system that lie outside the brain and spinal cord.

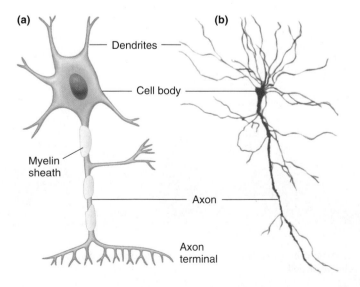

Figure A-11 (*a*) An illustration of a neuron, or nerve cell, showing the cell body with dendrites and the axon. The axon releases the neurotransmitters. (*b*) How a neuron looks under a light microscope.

(a)

Dendrites

Cell body

Myelin sheath

Axon

Axon terminal

(b)

Neurons can't produce new cells, although some can regenerate parts of their structures. Loss of nerve tissue causes loss of important functions. A spinal cord injury is likely to cause permanent paralysis.

Neuroglia (glial cells) protect neurons and aid in their function. They are far more abundant than neurons. For example, 1 group of neuroglia wraps nerves in a protective myelin sheath, a job associated with vitamin B-12 (see Fig. A-11). This sheath acts as an insulating material, isolating 1 nerve conduction pathway from the others. Another group of neuroglia phagocytizes pathogens and disposes of cellular debris in the CNS.

Each neuron contains a cell body with a nucleus and rough endoplasmic reticulum, **dendrites,** and an **axon.** Information (electrical or chemical stimuli) enters the cell through the dendrites and/or the cell body, and the output of electrical impulses leaves by way of the axon.

You may be wondering about the term *nerve.* A **nerve** is a bundle of axons located outside the CNS. Nerves contain axons of both sensory and motor neurons.

Axons end close to, or may be in physical contact with, the next neuron. In most cases, however, the electrical signal at the end of the axon is converted to a chemical signal, called a **neurotransmitter,** that is released into the gap (Fig. A-12). The transmission from neuron to neuron or from neuron to muscle cell is by way of these neurotransmitters. The space between 1 neuron and the next is known as a **synapse.** Neurotransmitters that bridge the gap are derived from common nutrients found in foods (see Chapter 7 for more details). There are a variety of neurotransmitters—**dopamine, norepinephrine, acetylcholine,** and **serotonin** are just a few.

The body's fight or flight mechanism—the ability to survive a threat—depends on the **adrenergic** effect provided by adrenergic neurons secreting **epinephrine** and norepinephrine. The adrenergic effect stimulates the heart to beat faster, constricts blood vessels to raise blood pressure, increases breathing, and promotes the breakdown of glycogen in the liver. These changes are essential to survival because they make it possible to provide plenty of glucose, our basic muscle fuel, instantly when there is an emergency and muscles need to respond quickly. **Cholinergic** effects usually produce the opposite response of adrenergic effects.

The brain has a tremendous metabolic rate; the blood it requires accounts for 20% of the total cardiac output. This translates into 750 ml of blood per minute being pumped through the brain, yielding a steady supply of oxygen and glucose. Any interruption in the supply of these 2 substances is life-threatening. The brain also generates waste materials, which are promptly removed by this high blood flow rate.

All the structures that make up the nervous system are related to nutritional status. For example, most of the axons of the CNS and PNS are covered by myelin. Vitamin B-12 plays a key role in the formation of myelin.

The transmission of information through the nervous system depends on nutrients obtained from the diet: calcium, sodium, and potassium. The sodium ion (Na^+) (mostly extracellular) and the potassium ion (K^+) (mostly intracellular) located on either side of the axon membrane exchange places as they flow through ion channels in response to electrical stimulation. This is how an electrical signal is transmitted. They are later pumped back to their previous location.

---

neuroglia (glial cells) Specialized support cells of the central nervous system.

dendrite Relatively short, highly branched nerve cell process that carries electrical activity to the main body of a nerve cell.

axon Part of a nerve cell that conducts impulses away from the main body of the cell.

nerve Bundle of nerve cells outside the central nervous system.

neurotransmitter Compound, made by a nerve cell, that allows for communication between a nerve cell and other cells.

synapse Space between the end of 1 nerve cell and the beginning of another nerve cell.

dopamine Type of neurotransmitter in the central nervous system that leads to feelings of euphoria, among other functions; also used to form norepinephrine, another neurotransmitter.

norepinephrine Neurotransmitter released from nerve endings; also a hormone produced by the adrenal gland in times of stress.

acetylcholine Neurotransmitter released from nerve endings.

serotonin Neurotransmitter, synthesized from the amino acid tryptophan, that affects mood (sense of calmness), behavior, and appetite and induces sleep.

adrenergic Relating to the actions of epinephrine and norepinephrine.

- Neurotransmitter
- Synaptic vesicle
- Presynaptic membrane of a neuron
- Synapse
- Postsynaptic membrane of another neuron or nearby cell
- Receptor

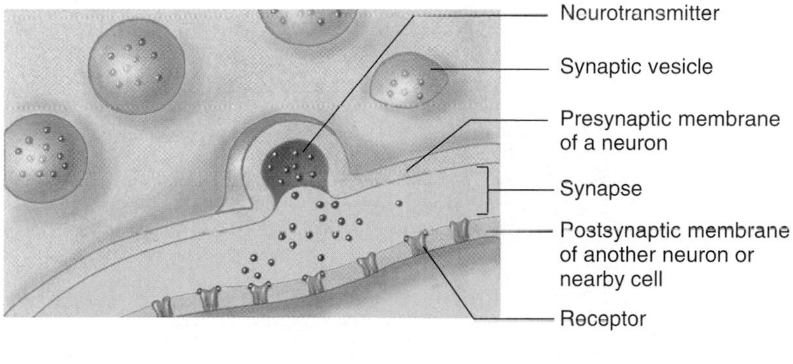

Figure A-12 Transmission of a message from 1 neuron to another neuron or another cell relies on neurotransmitters. Vesicles containing neurotransmitters fuse with the membrane of the neuron, and the neurotransmitter is released into the synapse. The neurotransmitter then binds to the receptors on the nearby neuron (or cell). In this way, the message is sent from 1 neuron to another, or to the cell that ultimately performs the action directed by the message.

epinephrine Hormone produced by the adrenal gland in times of stress. It may also have neurotransmitter functions, such as in the brain.

cholinergic Relating to the actions of acetylcholine.

▶ The most important nutrient for continued efficient brain function is carbohydrate in the form of glucose. Should the diet fail to deliver enough carbohydrate that can form glucose, the body will synthesize it in sufficient amounts to provide for the needs of the brain. Alternately, the brain will use an alternative fuel called ketone bodies, but this is not healthy for the body over the long term (see Chapter 9).

Calcium allows the release of neurotransmitters from the axon of a neuron. As we have seen, the neurotransmitter carries the signal to the next neuron as it jumps the synapse. Fortunately, a calcium-deficient diet will never have a major effect on nerve transmission; the body can always find enough calcium to keep the nervous system functioning. There are, however, rare instances when a deficiency of calcium causes tetany. (More about tetany appears in Chapter 14.)

Other nutrients required for the nervous system are various amino acids. One amino acid we obtain from dietary protein, tryptophan, is converted to serotonin by neurons. This neurotransmitter has a variety of behavioral effects. Varying the amount of dietary tryptophan controls the amount of serotonin produced by neurons. The amino acid tyrosine can be converted to dopamine and norepinephrine.

The GI tract has its own nervous system. The sight or smell of food, or one's emotions, can signal muscle cells and glands to prepare the way for food and turn on digestive processes (Chapter 4 has more details).

Endocrine System and Hormones

Endocrine glands secrete regulatory substances, hormones, into the blood for distribution to target tissues or organs. The endocrine gland that secretes a hormone is responding to the need to restore homeostasis. This section is not a complete exploration of all the body's hormones; it concentrates on those that affect nutrition (Fig. A-13).

Some hormones control metabolic functions, such as appetite, and the transport of substances through cell membranes. Others control growth, and still others are responsible for sex and reproduction. Of all these hormones, some are described as "local," in that they function in the immediate vicinity of their production. There are also

Figure A-13 **The major endocrine glands. These glands secrete a variety of hormones.**

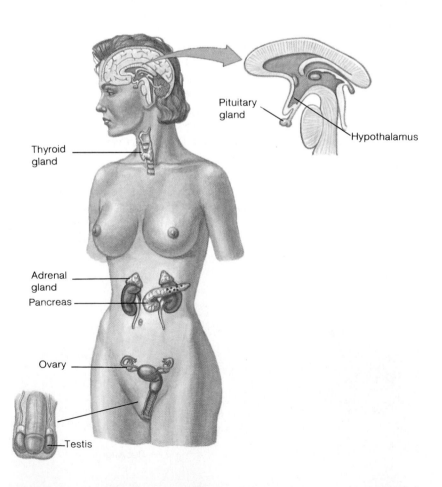

Pituitary gland

Hypothalamus

Thyroid gland

Adrenal gland

Pancreas

Ovary

Testis

many interrelationships between hormones and the nervous system. For example, the adrenal gland and the pituitary gland respond to neural stimuli.

Some hormones from the pituitary gland control the secretion of other endocrine glands. And, as mentioned in the previous section, a substance such as norepinephrine secreted as a neurotransmitter can act as a hormone.

Chemical Classification of Hormones

General hormones are classified according to chemical categories: **steroids, glycoproteins, polypeptides,** and **amines.**

Steroid hormones are lipid substances synthesized from cholesterol (Table A-2). The glycoproteins are long chains of amino acids (100 or more) bound to carbohydrate (Table A-3). Follicle-stimulating hormone (FSH), luteinizing hormone (LH), thyroid-stimulating hormone (TSH), and several other pituitary hormones are such hormones and are referred to as **tropic hormones** because they stimulate the secretion of another hormone and usually stimulate the growth of the associated gland. For example, TSH stimulates the production of the thyroid hormone. Another group of hormones are polypeptide chains made of fewer than 100 amino acids per chain (Table A-4). Amines are hormones synthesized from the amino acids tyrosine and tryptophan (Table A-5).

There are also special hormones that regulate the digestive tract. (These are discussed in Chapter 4.)

Interesting Features of Hormones

Steroid and thyroid hormones can be taken in pill form because they are not digested in the GI tract; thus, they can be absorbed into the body in their active state. All the other hormones are deactivated when taken by mouth because their biological activity is destroyed by digestive enzymes. That is why the hormone insulin must be taken by injection to bypass the digestive tract.

Some hormones must undergo chemical changes before they can function. For example, vitamin D synthesized in the skin and/or obtained from food is converted to an active hormone by the kidneys and liver.

steroid Group of hormones and related compounds that are derivatives of cholesterol.

glycoprotein Protein containing a carbohydrate group.

polypeptide Fifty to 2000 or more amino acids bonded together.

amine Can refer to hormone made of 1 or a few amino acids.

tropic hormone Hormone that stimulates the secretion of another secreting gland.

▶ In most cases, a single gland secretes a single hormone but, in a few cases, a gland secretes more than 1 hormone. In addition, sometimes a hormone is produced by more than 1 gland.

Table A-2 Steroid Hormones

Hormone	Gland	Target	Effect	Role in Nutrition
Testosterone	Testes, adrenal glands	Reproductive organs	Reproduction, secondary sexual development	Muscle growth
Estrogens, progesterone	Ovaries, adrenal glands	Reproductive organs	Reproduction, secondary sexual characteristics	Maintenance of bone
Cortisol	Adrenal glands	Liver	Glucocorticoid activity	Metabolism of protein, carbohydrate, fat
Aldosterone	Adrenal glands	Kidneys	Mineral-corticoid activity	Electrolyte balance

Table A-3 Glycoprotein Hormones

Hormone	Gland	Target	Effect	Role in Nutrition
FSH, LH, TSH	Pituitary gland	Variety of organs	Stimulation of target organ to produce its own hormone	None directly

Table A-4 Polypeptide Hormones

Hormone	Gland	Target	Effect	Role in Nutrition
Antidiuretic hormone	Pituitary gland	Kidneys	Water retention, vasoconstriction	Maintenance of normal blood volume
Prolactin	Pituitary gland	Mammary glands	Milk production; in males, indirect enhancement of testosterone secretions	Nourishment of newborn
Oxytocin	Pituitary gland	Uterus, mammary glands	Contraction of uterus, mammary secretions	Milk production
Insulin	Pancreas	Fat and muscle cells	Decreased blood glucose concentration	Storage of glucose as glycogen, increased fat storage, increased amino acid uptake by cells
Glucagon	Pancreas	Liver	Increased blood glucose concentration	Release of glucose from liver stores, increased fat mobilization
ACTH (adrenocorticotropic hormone)	Pituitary gland	Adrenal glands	Secretion of glucocorticoids	Secretion of adrenal cortical hormones
Growth hormone	Pituitary gland	Most cells	Promotion of amino acid uptake by cells	Promotion of protein synthesis and growth, increased fat utilization for energy
Parathyroid hormone	Parathyroid glands	Intestinal tract, kidneys	Increased blood calcium	Release of calcium from bone into blood
Calcitonin	Thyroid gland	Bone	Inhibition of breakdown of bone, stimulation of calcium excretion by kidneys	Reduced blood calcium concentration
Leptin	No gland, just adipose tissue	Hypothalamus	Targeting of satiety center	Decreased appetite

Table A-5 Amine Hormones

Hormone	Gland	Target	Effect	Role in Nutrition
Epinephrine, norepinephrine*	Adrenal glands	Heart, blood vessels, brain, lungs	Increased metabolic rate	Release of glucose into the blood, fat mobilization
Thyroid hormone	Thyroid gland	Most organs	Increased oxygen consumption, growth, brain development, development of CNS in fetus	Protein synthesis, increased metabolic rate
Melatonin	Pineal gland	Specific neurons	Maintenance of body (circadian) rhythms, sleep	Scavenging of atoms and molecules that are highly reactive and dangerous

*Norepinephrine also functions as a neurotransmitter, depending on location in the body. Epinephrine is suspected of doing the same, such as in the brain.

Neural and Endocrine Regulation

Whether a chemical is acting as a hormone or a neurotransmitter, the target cell must have a receptor protein to combine with it. This causes a change in the target cell (Chapter 4 provides a fuller discussion of this concept). This also means that there must be a mechanism to turn off the action. Hormones are subject to control by an "off" switch. For example, when the blood glucose concentration has been returned to normal by the action of the hormone insulin, insulin production is turned off. If it were not, the person would experience decreasing glucose concentrations until the concentration dropped so low that the person would go into shock and die.

Urinary System

The urinary system is composed of 2 kidneys located on the back of the abdominal wall, 1 on each side of the vertebral column (Fig. A-14). Each is connected to the urinary bladder by a **ureter.** The bladder is emptied by way of the **urethra.**

Each bean-shaped kidney has an outer section called the cortex and an inner section called the medulla. The medulla is composed of cone-shaped pyramid structures, which empty waste materials into a funnel-shaped tube ending in the ureter. Ureters carry urine from the kidneys to the bladder for temporary storage. Blood flows through the kidneys at a rate of about 120 ml/minute.

> **ureter** Tube that transports urine from the kidney to the urinary bladder.
>
> **urethra** Tube that transports urine from the urinary bladder to the outside of the body.

Kidney Functions

The kidneys regulate the composition of the blood (plasma) and the interstitial fluid, known together as the extracellular fluid. This regulation is accomplished by filtering the blood and forming urine, which is basically the filtrate. As a result of kidney action and

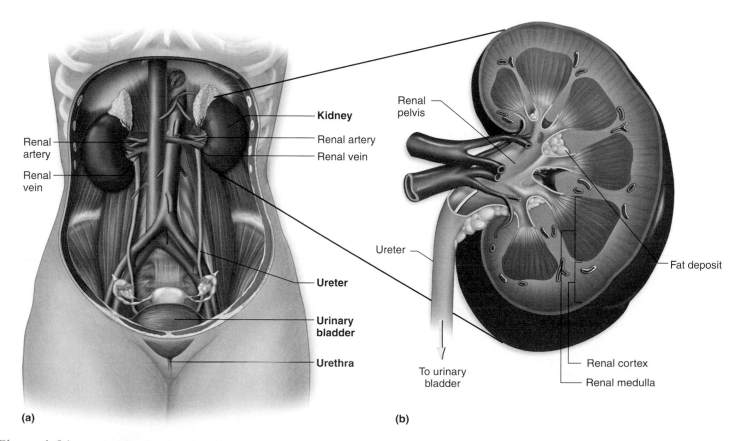

(a)

Renal artery
Renal vein

Kidney
Renal artery
Renal vein

Ureter

Urinary bladder

Urethra

(b)

Renal pelvis

Ureter

To urinary bladder

Fat deposit

Renal cortex

Renal medulla

Figure A-14 **Organs of the urinary system. (***a***)** The urinary system of the female. The male's urinary system is the same, except that the urethra extends through the penis. (***b***)** A cross section of the kidney. The kidneys are bean-shaped organs located on each side of the spinal column. They filter waste from the blood, which is then stored in the bladder as urine. The kidneys are connected to the urinary bladder by ureters. The outer section of the kidney is the cortex; the inner section is the medulla. The functional unit of the kidney, the nephron, loops through the cortex and medulla, and the fluid that flows through these tiny structures is separated, so that the waste is removed from the blood into collecting ducts and drains into the renal pelvis. Thus, the urine exits by way of the ureter to the bladder. The remaining fluid is returned to the circulatory system to maintain the normal composition of the blood.

▶ Together with the lungs, the kidneys maintain the pH of the blood.

erythropoietin Hormone, secreted mostly by the kidneys, that enhances red blood cell synthesis and stimulates red blood cell release from bone marrow.

nephron Functional unit of the kidney.

glomerulus Capillaries in the kidney that filter waste products from the blood.

the formation of urine, the volume of blood plasma is controlled, and blood pressure is maintained. The kidneys remove metabolic waste and foreign chemicals from the blood, and they maintain a certain concentration of electrolytes, such as Na^+, K^+, and HCO_3^- (bicarbonate) in the plasma. The kidneys constantly monitor the composition of the blood and produce hormones to maintain homeostasis. For example, the kidneys produce the hormone **erythropoietin,** which is responsible for the synthesis of red blood cells. The kidneys convert a form of vitamin D into its active hormone form. During times of fasting, the kidneys can produce glucose from amino acids.

Kidney Structure

Each kidney is enclosed in a fatty, fibrous sac that protects it from external physical damage. Examined microscopically, the functional unit of the kidney, the **nephron,** is disclosed. Nephrons extend through the renal cortex and the renal medulla. There are more than 1 million nephrons per kidney. A nephron consists of small tubules allied with small blood vessels. The tiny capillary filtration unit, the **glomerulus,** is held in a small capsule (Bowman's capsule). The glomerulus filters large amounts of fluid from the blood, removing the dissolved waste and excess fluid to form urine, which leaves by way of the tubules. The remaining fluid is returned to the blood.

This ingenious mechanism constantly adjusts the composition of the blood. In this process, the essential components are recovered and returned to general circulation, waste products and excess water are removed, and unneeded nutrients (ones in which storage compartments are full or there are no storage facilities) are flushed away by the urine.

Reproductive System

Reproduction is a fundamental property of all living things. We die, but our genes live on in our progeny. In humans, both ova and sperm, called gametes (sex cells), contain 23 chromosomes. The fertilized egg contains 46 chromosomes (23 from each parent) and is programmed to produce a new human. At conception, the instructions for the developing embryo are all present. Through the actions of the female reproductive organs, supported by hormonal secretions, a human is produced about 40 weeks after conception, if essential nutrients are present and no genetic defects are encountered. The most precarious time of pregnancy is during the first 13 weeks when a woman is least likely to know she is pregnant.

The male reproductive organs consist of the scrotum (containing the testes), penis, urethra, seminal vesicles, and prostate. The female reproductive organs consist of the ovaries, uterus, and vagina.

In addition to reproduction, the sex hormones stimulate bone growth and the closure of the epiphyseal plate, thus ending bone growth. Estrogens protect against bone loss. The sex hormone testosterone stimulates protein synthesis, such as muscle growth and bone growth.

Puberty, or the onset of adult sex life, takes place during early adolescence. **Menarche,** the onset of menstruation, occurs usually between the ages of 11 and 16 in females. In the male, sexual maturation occurs somewhat later and is initiated by hormonal secretions from the brain. (The female reproductive system is discussed in Chapter 16 in more detail.)

menarche Onset of menstruation. Menarche usually occurs around age 13, 2 or 3 years after the first signs of puberty appear.

Appendix B

CHEMISTRY: A TOOL FOR UNDERSTANDING NUTRITION

The study of human nutrition requires a basic awareness of and familiarity with general chemistry, organic chemistry, and biochemistry. This appendix provides only a review of key chemistry principles and fundamental concepts regarding atoms, molecules, chemical bonds, pH, organic compounds, and biochemical structures that may come up as you study nutrition. An understanding of basic chemistry makes the study of nutrition easier and more interesting. It helps connect nutrient characteristics with the structural and chemical attributes of the individual components of food (Table B-1).

▶ The physical and chemical properties of almost anything—whether atoms, molecules or organisms—are intimately related to its structure. A basic knowledge of chemical structures can help you visualize important fundamental concepts in nutrition.

Properties of Matter and Mass

All living and nonliving things are composed of matter. Matter exists in 3 states: solid, liquid, or gas. An example of a solid is ice, a liquid is water, and a gas is steam. Two characteristics of matter are it has mass and it occupies space (volume). Mass is related to the amount of force it takes to move an object—it takes less force to move a paper clip than a pencil; therefore, the clip has less mass. Volume is related to the amount of space an object occupies—a pint of water occupies less space than a gallon; therefore, a pint has a smaller volume. Both these properties depend on how much of the substance there is.

Another property of matter is density. Density is defined as the mass of an object divided by its volume:

$$\text{Density} = \frac{\text{Mass}}{\text{Volume}}$$

Density is independent of how much matter is available. The density of water in a lake is the same as in a cup. Density is commonly expressed in units of grams per cubic centimeter (g/cm^3).

You can use density to compare objects. Using the density of pure water as a comparison ($1.0 \ g/cm^3$), lean body tissue has a density of about $1.1 \ g/cm^3$. The density of body fat in comparison is about $0.9 \ g/cm^3$. Substances that are less dense than water are buoyant (they tend to float), whereas substances that are more dense than water sink. The next time you are in a swimming pool, note the density of men and women. Women tend to have more body fat, so they float; men are generally more muscular (have more lean tissue), so they tend to sink deeper in the water. This physical property is used to determine the amount of body fat stored in a person (see Chapter 10).

Physical and Chemical Properties of Substances

Every substance has a characteristic set of physical and chemical properties. Physical properties can be determined without altering the chemical composition of the substance. Ice melts at 1°C. Sugar melts at 186°C. Melting and boiling points are common examples of physical properties.

Table B-1 Periodic Table of the Elements

Main-Group Elements

Transitional Metals

Inner-Transitional Metals

1 H 1.00794

Atomic Number
Symbol
Atomic Mass (Atomic Weight)

Period	1 IA	2 IIA	3 IIIB	4 IVB	5 VB	6 VIB	7 VIIB	8	9 VIIIB	10	11 IB	12 IIB	13 IIIA	14 IVA	15 VA	16 VIA	17 VIIA	18 VIIIA
1	1 H 1.00794																	2 He 4.002602
2	3 Li 6.941	4 Be 9.012182											5 B 10.811	6 C 12.011	7 N 14.00674	8 O 15.9994	9 F 18.998403	10 Ne 20.1797
3	11 Na 22.989768	12 Mg 24.3050											13 Al 26.981539	14 Si 28.0855	15 P 30.973762	16 S 32.066	17 Cl 35.4527	18 Ar 39.948
4	19 K 39.0983	20 Ca 40.078	21 Sc 44.955910	22 Ti 47.88	23 V 50.9415	24 Cr 51.9961	25 Mn 54.93805	26 Fe 55.847	27 Co 58.93320	28 Ni 58.69	29 Cu 63.546	30 Zn 65.39	31 Ga 69.723	32 Ge 72.61	33 As 74.92159	34 Se 78.96	35 Br 79.904	36 Kr 83.80
5	37 Rb 85.4678	38 Sr 87.62	39 Y 88.90585	40 Zr 91.224	41 Nb 92.90638	42 Mo 95.94	43 Tc (98)	44 Ru 101.07	45 Rh 102.90550	46 Pd 106.42	47 Ag 107.8682	48 Cd 112.411	49 In 114.82	50 Sn 118.710	51 Sb 121.75	52 Te 127.60	53 I 126.90447	54 Xe 131.29
6	55 Cs 132.90543	56 Ba 137.327	57 La* 138.9055	72 Hf 178.49	73 Ta 180.9479	74 W 183.85	75 Re 186.207	76 Os 190.2	77 Ir 192.22	78 Pt 195.08	79 Au 196.96654	80 Hg 200.59	81 Tl 204.3833	82 Pb 207.2	83 Bi 208.98037	84 Po (209)	85 At (210)	86 Rn (222)
7	87 Fr (223)	88 Ra (226)	89 Ac** (227)	104 RF (261)	105 Db (262)	106 Sg (263)	107 Bh (262)	108 Hs (265)	109 Mt (267)	110 Uun (269)	111 Uuu (272)	112 Uub (277)	113 Uut	114 Uuq	115 Uup	116 Uuh	117 Uus	118 Uuo

*Lanthanides

58 Ce 140.115	59 Pr 140.90765	60 Nd 144.24	61 Pm (145)	62 Sm 150.36	63 Eu 151.965	64 Gd 157.25	65 Tb 158.92534	66 Dy 162.50	67 Ho 164.93032	68 Er 167.266	69 Tm 168.93421	70 Yb 173.04	71 Lu 174.967

**Actinides

90 Th 232.0381	91 Pa (231)	92 U 238.0289	93 Np (237)	94 Pu (244)	95 Am (243)	96 Cm (247)	97 Bk (247)	98 Cf (251)	99 Es (252)	100 Fm (257)	101 Md (258)	102 No (259)	103 Lr (262)

A-26

Table B-1 Periodic Table of the Elements
Concluded

Key to Abbreviations

Name	Symbol	Name	Symbol	Name	Symbol	Name	Symbol
Actinium	Ac	Erbium	Er	Mercury	Hg	Scandium	Sc
Aluminum	Al	Europium	Eu	Molybdenum	Mo	Seaborgium	Sg
Americium	Am	Fermium	Fm	Neodymium	Nd	Selenium	Se
Antimony	Sb	Fluorine	F	Neon	Ne	Silicon	Si
Argon	Ar	Francium	Fr	Neptunium	Np	Silver	Ag
Arsenic	As	Gadolinium	Gd	Nickel	Ni	Sodium	Na
Astatine	At	Gallium	Ga	Niobium	Nb	Strontium	Sr
Barium	Ba	Germanium	Ge	Nitrogen	N	Sulfur	S
Berkelium	Bk	Gold	Au	Nobelium	No	Tantalum	Ta
Beryllium	Be	Hafnium	Hf	Osmium	Os	Technetium	Tc
Bismuth	Bi	Hassium	Hs	Oxygen	O	Tellurium	Te
Bohrium	Bh	Helium	He	Palladium	Pd	Terbium	Tb
Boron	B	Holmium	Ho	Phosphorus	P	Thallium	Tl
Bromine	Br	Hydrogen	H	Platinum	Pt	Thorium	Th
Cadmium	Cd	Indium	In	Plutonium	Pu	Thulium	Tm
Calcium	Ca	Iodine	I	Polonium	Po	Tin	Sn
Californium	Cf	Iridium	Ir	Potassium	K	Titanium	Ti
Carbon	C	Iron	Fe	Praseodymium	Pr	Tungsten	W
Cerium	Ce	Krypton	Kr	Promethium	Pm	Uranium	U
Cesium	Cs	Lanthanum	La	Protactinium	Pa	Vanadium	V
Chlorine	Cl	Lawrencium	Lr	Radium	Ra	Xenon	Xe
Chromium	Cr	Lead	Pb	Radon	Rn	Ytterbium	Yb
Cobalt	Co	Lithium	Li	Rhenium	Re	Yttrium	Y
Copper	Cu	Lutetium	Lu	Rhodium	Rh	Zinc	Zn
Curium	Cm	Magnesium	Mg	Rubidium	Rb	Zirconium	Zr
Dubnium	Db	Manganese	Mn	Ruthenium	Ru		
Dysprosium	Dy	Meitnerium	Mt	Rutherfordium	Rf		
Einsteinium	Es	Mendelevium	Md	Samarium	Sm		

chemical reaction Interaction between 2 chemicals that changes both participants.

Chemical properties, such as whether the compound is an acid or a base, determine the changes that a substance undergoes in **chemical reactions.** Other substances affect the chemical properties of a substance. A chemical reaction is a process whereby the composition of 1 or more substances is changed. What actually takes place is affected by the chemical properties of the participants. For example, given the right conditions, exposing glucose to oxygen causes it to break down to carbon dioxide and water.

$$C_6H_{12}O_6 \quad + \quad 6O_2 \quad \rightarrow \quad 6CO_2 \quad + \quad 6H_2O$$

| Glucose | Oxygen | Carbon dioxide | Water |

Units

The SI units (*Système International d'Unités*) used for scientific measurements designate specific metric units. The units used most frequently in nutrition are mass (kilogram), length (meter), temperature, and amount of substance. Prefixes indicate decimal fractions or multiples of the various units. For example, *kilo* means 1×10^3, and 1 *milli* is 1×10^{-3}.

Celsius Centigrade measure of temperature. For conversion: (°Fahrenheit − 32) × 5/9 = °C (°Celsius × 9/5) + 32 = °F.

The temperature scale commonly used in scientific studies is the **Celsius** scale. On this scale, water freezes at 0°Celsius (32°Fahrenheit). Water boils at 100°C (212°F). Normal body temperature is 37.0°C (98.6°F). For English-metric conversions for length, weight, temperature, and volume (amount) see Appendix H.

Calories and Joules

Energy is measured in calories or joules. A calorie is the amount of energy required to raise the temperature of 1 gram of water 1 degree C. The SI unit of energy is the joule (J). A mass of 1 gram moving at a velocity of 1 meter per second possesses the energy equivalent of 1 J. A calorie or joule is not a large amount of energy, so kilocalories (kcal) and kilojoules (kJ) are widely used in nutrition chemistry, biology, and biochemistry. In terms of the joule, 1 kcal = 4.184 kJ.

Scientific Notation

▶ To change a number greater than 1 into scientific notation, move the decimal point to the left until the number is greater than 1 but less than 10. This number is the coefficient. The number of places that the decimal is moved becomes the exponent of 10. To change a number less than 1 into scientific notation, move the decimal point to the right until the number is greater than 1 but less than 10. This number is the coefficient. The number of places that the decimal is moved is again the exponent of 10, but this time a negative sign is placed in front of it.

In science, very large and very small numbers frequently must be used, but they are awkward because large numbers have a long string of trailing zeros, and small numbers have a long string of leading zeros. A more convenient way to express these numbers is to use the power of 10, or scientific notation.

In scientific notation, a number is expressed as a product of a coefficient multiplied by a power of 10. The coefficient is a number equal to or greater than 1 but less than 10. The power of 10 is the exponent. In other words:

$$a \times 10^b$$

where a is the coefficient and b is the exponent.

$$6.02217 \times 10^{23} = 602,217,000,000,000,000,000,000$$

$$2.99161 \times 10^{-23} = 0.0000000000000000000000299161$$

In the previous examples, the positive exponent for the number indicates that the number is very large, whereas the negative exponent indicates a very small number.

Atoms

atom Smallest combining unit of an element. An atom contains protons, neutrons, and electrons.

The smallest unit of matter that can undergo a chemical change is called an **atom.** An element is composed of atoms of only 1 kind. For example, the element carbon is composed of just carbon atoms. There are more than 100 different elements.

Atomic Structure

The center of an atom is, for the most part, a nucleus containing 2 (subatomic) particles: **protons,** which carry a positive charge, and **neutrons,** with no charge. Usually, the mass of the proton equals the mass of the neutron. Adding the number of protons and number of neutrons together yields the atomic mass of the atom. An atom of carbon containing 6 protons and 6 neutrons has an atomic mass of 12. The atomic mass of nitrogen is 14 and the atomic mass of oxygen is 16.

The atomic number is equal to the number of protons in the nucleus. What are the atomic numbers of hydrogen, carbon, nitrogen, and oxygen?

Surrounding the nucleus of the atom are negatively charged subatomic particles called **electrons.** The nucleus is actually surrounded by an electron cloud. Electrons have about 2000 times less mass than the mass of protons or neutrons. Thus, all the mass of an atom essentially is located within the nucleus. The structure of an atom can therefore be pictured as a very tiny, highly dense nuclear core surrounded by a cloud of electrons. The number of electrons in an atom equals the number of protons, so the net charge is 0.

Electrons surrounding the nucleus have a somewhat peculiar, non-intuitive (contrary to what would be expected) behavior. For instance, it's impossible to know precisely where any given electron is located at any given moment. It is only possible to define a volume of space where the electron is most likely to be found. This volume has a specific distribution of electron density in space and is called an orbital. An orbital is a volume of space. Each orbital has its own characteristic energy and shape.

Orbitals of similar energy are grouped together into energy levels. The energy levels are assigned coordinate numbers—1, 2, 3, etc.—that increase as one moves away from the nucleus. Energy level 1 contains only 1 orbital, an "s" orbital. This orbital can hold a maximum of 2 electrons. Energy level 2 contains an "s" orbital and a "p" orbital; the "s" orbital can contain up to 2 electrons, and the "p" orbital up to 6. Energy level 3 contains an "s" orbital, a "p" orbital, and a "d" orbital. As before, the "s" orbital and "p" orbital can hold up to 2 and 6 electrons, respectively, whereas the "d" orbital can contain as many as 10. Thus, each energy level can hold a maximum of 2, 8, or 18 electrons, depending on the number of orbitals, and any energy level can hold less than the maximum number of electrons.

Atoms tend to exist in the lowest possible energy state. Thus, electrons tend to occupy orbitals at low energy levels before filling orbitals at higher energy levels. The first energy level outside the nucleus has room for just 2 electrons. When that is full, the next energy level away from the nucleus is available for electrons, and there is room for 8 electrons. For example, hydrogen has 1 electron in energy level 1. Carbon has 2 electrons in energy level 1 and 4 in energy level 2. In energy level 3, there is room for 8 electrons. Sulfur, with an atomic number of 16, has 2 electrons in the first energy level, 8 in the second, and 6 in the third (Table B-2).

An atom tends to bond with other atoms that will fill its outermost energy level and produce a number of valence electrons equal to the noble gas that is the farthest to the right in its row in the periodic table (e.g., helium and argon). For instance, a hydrogen atom, with only a single electron, will react with other atoms that provide another electron and fill the energy level with 2 electrons, the same number of electrons as in the noble gas helium.

proton Part of an atom that is positively charged.

neutron Part of an atom that has no charge.

electron Part of an atom that is negatively charged. Electrons orbit the nucleus.

► Hydrogen has an atomic mass of 1 because it has 1 proton and no neutrons.

► Only the electrons in the outermost energy level (if it is incomplete) can participate in chemical reactions to form chemical bonds. The outermost electrons of an atom are known as its valence electrons.

Table B-2 Atoms Commonly Present in Organic Molecules

Atom	Symbol	Atomic Number	Atomic Mass	Energy Level 1	Energy Level 2	Energy Level 3	Number of Chemical Bonds to Attain Electron Stability
Hydrogen	H	1	1	1	0	0	1
Carbon	C	6	12	2	4	0	4
Nitrogen	N	7	14	2	5	0	3
Oxygen	O	8	16	2	6	0	2
Sulfur	S	16	32	2	8	6	2

Isotopes and Atomic Weight

isotope Alternate form of a chemical element. It differs from other atoms of the same element in the number of neutrons in its nucleus.

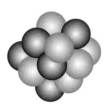

¹²Carbon
6 Protons
6 Neutrons
6 Electrons

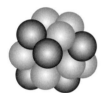

¹³Carbon
6 Protons
7 Neutrons
6 Electrons

¹⁴Carbon
6 Protons
8 Neutrons
6 Electrons

▶ *Dalton* is another term used to indicate atomic mass, such as for proteins, DNA, and RNA. One Dalton is equivalent to 1 atomic mass unit (amu).

All the atoms of an element have the same number of protons in the nucleus, but the number of neutrons in the nuclei of elements such as carbon, nitrogen, and oxygen may vary. All elements have such varieties, called **isotopes,** that differ from each other only in the number of neutrons and, consequently, atomic mass. Most hydrogen atoms have only 1 proton, but isotopic forms can have 1 or 2 neutrons. Some isotopes are radioactive, but most are not. Tritium, a radioactive isotope of hydrogen, has 1 proton and 2 neutrons. Carbon nuclei can contain 5, 6, 7, or 8 neutrons.

Isotopes are distinguished by adding the number of protons and neutrons together and writing the resultant sum as a superscript to the left of the symbol for the element. For example, a carbon nuclei with 6 protons and 6 neutrons is written as ^{12}C. The isotope containing 7 neutrons is labeled ^{13}C, and the isotope containing 8 neutrons is labeled ^{14}C. Note that, because all these atoms have 6 protons, they are all carbon atoms. However, because they possess different numbers of neutrons, they represent isotopes of carbon. All isotopes of an element behave the same way chemically.

Atomic weight takes into account that an element is a mixture of isotopes. If all carbon were ^{12}C, the atomic weight would be the same as its atomic mass, 12. But, because some carbon exists as ^{13}C and ^{14}C, the atomic weight is slightly higher, 12.011. The atomic weight is based on the relative abundance of the various isotopes.

Although the ordinary chemical behavior of different isotopes of the same element is virtually identical, the radiochemical behavior is sometimes different. Isotopes exhibit such differences in physical behavior because they decay (break down) to more stable isotopes by giving off nuclear particles of ionizing radiation. Certain unstable isotopes (radioisotopes) are in an obvious process of decay. Every element has at least 1 such radioisotope. These radioisotopes have a physical half-life, which is the time required for 50% of its atoms to decay to a more stable state. Isotopes such as ^{32}P (phosphorus) emit radiation that can be measured by instruments, such as Geiger counters and scintillation counters. The isotope ^{14}C decays more rapidly than other isotopes of carbon.

Other isotopes are not radioactive but can still be traced in body fluids or tissues using other types of instruments. Examples include ^{13}C and ^{15}N; these are called stable isotopes because they decay very slowly and do not emit radiation.

Isotope "markers," such as ^{32}P and ^{13}C, have a practical use because they can be used to trace nutrients as they follow various chemical pathways in the body. For example, researchers can "mark" a glucose molecule with a radioactive carbon atom (^{14}C). This marking allows the researchers to see where the carbons of glucose are distributed in the body, and it helps indicate what chemical transformations glucose undergoes when metabolized. Such studies have demonstrated that glucose can become part of the lipid stored in adipose cells and can form CO_2 (detected as $^{14}CO_2$) that is exhaled. Isotope techniques are widely used in nutrition research.

Atomic and Molar Mass

Atoms are very small. One ^{12}C atom has a mass of 1.993×10^{-23}g. The units used to quantify atomic mass are called atomic mass units (amu). The carbon amu is calculated by dividing the mass of a carbon atom by 1.6605×10^{-24}, which is essentially the mass of 1 proton or neutron. By performing this calculation on ^{12}C, you will find that the mass of a carbon atom is 12 amu. The amu for each element is listed in the bottom portion of each entry in the periodic table. Each amu is based on comparing the element's mass with that of ^{12}C.

You are familiar with counting units, such as the number of sticks in a package of chewing gum. In chemistry, the unit for counting atoms, ions (an electrically charged atom), and molecules (a combination of atoms) is the mole. A mole is defined as the amount of matter that contains as many objects as the number of atoms in 12 g of ^{12}C. The number of atoms in 12 g of ^{12}C is

$$12 \text{ g } ^{12}C \times \frac{1 \text{ atom}}{1.993 \times 10^{-23}\text{g } ^{12}C} = 6.023 \times 10^{23} \text{ atoms}$$

It is not the weight but the *number* of molecules that determines the physiological effect of a substance. Therefore, the number of "objects" in a mole of carbon (or any other substance) is 6.02×10^{23}, which is called Avogadro's number—for example,

$$1 \text{ mol } ^{12}C \text{ atoms} = 6.02 \times 10^{23} \text{ }^{12}C \text{ atoms}$$

$$1 \text{ mol of water molecules} = 6.02 \times 10^{23} \text{ H}_2\text{O molecules}$$

$$1 \text{ mol NO}_3^- \text{ ions} = 6.02 \times 10^{23} \text{ NO}_3^- \text{ ions}$$

A single ^{12}C atom has a mass of 12 amu, but a single ^{24}Mg is twice as massive, 24 amu. Because a mole always has the same number of particles, a mole of Mg is twice as massive as a mole of ^{12}C atoms. A mole of carbon weighs 12 g; a mole of Mg weighs 24 g. The same number that refers to the mass of a single atom of an element (in amu) also represents the mass (in g) of 1 mol of atoms of that element. For example, 1 ^{12}C atom weighs 12 amu. One mol ^{12}C weighs 12 g. One ^{24}Mg atom weighs 24 amu, and 1 mol ^{24}Mg weighs 24 g.

The mass in g of 1 mole of a substance is called its molar mass. The molar mass (in g) of any substance is always numerically equal to its formula weight (in amu). For example, 1 H_2O molecule weighs 18.0 amu, and 1 mol of H_2O weighs 18.0 g. One NaCl molecule weighs 58.5 amu, and 1 mol of NaCl weighs 58.5 g.

molecule Group of atoms chemically linked together—that is, tightly connected by attractive forces (see also *compound*).

bond Sharing of electrons, charges, or attractions linking 2 atoms.

compound Group of different types of atoms bonded together in definite proportion (see also *molecule*). Not all chemical compounds exist as molecules. Some compounds are made up of ions attracted to each other, such as Na^+Cl^- (table salt).

Molecules, Covalent Bonds, Hydrogen Bonds, and Ions and Ionic Compounds

Molecules

Molecules are formed through the interaction of the electrons in the outermost orbitals (valence electrons) of 2 or more electrons. When electrons are shared, chemical **bonds** are formed. The term **compound** refers to molecules composed of more than 1 element. Water is a compound. Each molecule (or compound) possesses its own properties, such as color, taste, and density.

Hydrogen can form just 1 chemical bond because it has room for just 1 electron in its orbital of 2 electrons, in turn yielding a noble gas electron configuration. Carbon can form 4 chemical bonds, nitrogen 3, and oxygen 2 (see Table B-3).

A molecular formula gives the elemental composition of a molecule or compound. This formula consists of the symbols of the atoms in the molecule plus a subscript denoting the number of each type of atom.

A structural formula shows how the atoms are arranged with respect to each other. As an extension, molecular and ball-and-stick models approximate the shape of the molecule (Fig. B-1).

When molecules combine with each other, atoms do not increase or decrease in number. Atoms present in starting materials must be present in the products. For example, compare the number of oxygen atoms in glucose and the oxygen itself with the number in the products of the reaction (18 vs. 18). This example also illustrates the process of conservation of mass.

$$C_6H_{12}O_6 + 6 \text{ O}_2 \rightarrow 6 \text{ CO}_2 + 6 \text{ H}_2\text{0}$$

Figure B-1 Examples of the molecular and structural formulas and the molecular models of ethanol. The space-filling model gives a more realistic feeling of the space occupied by the atoms. On the other hand, the ball-and-stick type shows the bonds and bond angles more clearly.

Figure B-2 Covalent bonds. In each of the 4 bonds, 1 electron of the carbon is shared with the electron of a hydrogen atom in a single, sausage-shaped molecular orbital encompassing the 2 nuclei. Methane is the simplest organic molecule. Even the largest organic molecules are held together by strong covalent bonds like these.

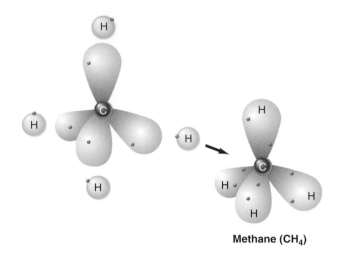

Methane (CH$_4$)

Covalent Bonds

covalent bond Union of 2 atoms formed by the sharing of electrons.

When atoms share their valence electrons, a **covalent bond** is formed (Fig. B-2). The electrons shared between atoms are bonding electrons; these represent the adhesive that holds the atoms together in molecular form.

When 2 identical atoms share electrons, such as in the formation of hydrogen gas (H$_2$) or oxygen gas (O$_2$), the covalent bond is very strong because the electrons are shared equally. This equal distribution between the atoms makes the molecule nonpolar. Consider the simple compound methane (CH$_4$). Hydrogen has 1 valence electron and its outermost (only) orbital can hold a maximum of 2 electrons. Carbon has 4 electrons in its outermost energy level, or valence shell, and that shell can hold a maximum of 8 electrons. Both carbon and hydrogen fill their valence shells to the maximum by sharing electrons with each other. Notice that each hydrogen in methane contains 2 electrons and that the carbon atom ends up with 8 electrons. A good way to look at this is that the hydrogen atoms share 1 pair of electrons, whereas the carbon atoms share 4 pairs of electrons (see Figure B-2).

Guidelines that govern the formation of covalent bonds are as follows:

1. The valence shell of each element must have room to accommodate additional electrons.
2. Second-row non-metallic elements of the periodic table (e.g., carbon, nitrogen, and oxygen) and hydrogen typically fill their outermost energy levels by sharing the necessary number of electrons with another element.
3. Third-row non-metals and those beyond this point in the periodic table (e.g., phosphorus and sulfur) frequently attain stability by giving up electrons in the outermost energy level rather than adding them. Phosphorus, for example, typically makes 5 bonds to attain stability instead of the 3 that are needed to have the electron configuration of the noble gas argon (18 electrons).

A single covalent bond forms when 2 atoms share 1 electron pair. A double covalent bond forms when 2 atoms share 2 electron pairs.

When electrons spend approximately equal time around each atom nucleus, the bond is called a nonpolar covalent bond. These are the strongest covalent bonds. If the 2 nuclei are not equally attractive to electrons, their atoms can form a polar covalent bond in which the electrons spend more time orbiting the more attractive nucleus. For example, when hydrogen bonds with oxygen, the electrons are more attracted to the oxygen nucleus and orbit that nucleus more than they do the hydrogen nucleus. Electrons carry a negative charge, which makes the oxygen region of the molecule slightly negative and the hydrogen region slightly positive. The Greek letter delta (δ) is used to symbolize a charge less than that of 1 electron or proton. A slightly negative region of a molecule is shown as δ^- and a slightly positive region is shown as δ^+. A molecule such as this is called a dipole because it has 2 charged ends.

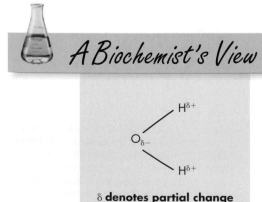

A Biochemist's View

$H^{\delta+}$

$O_{\delta-}$

$H^{\delta+}$

δ **denotes partial change**

When 2 different atoms form a covalent bond, the bonding electrons are never shared equally. Consider again the H–O bond in water. It is unreasonable to expect that the hydrogen nucleus (containing 1 proton) and the oxygen nucleus (containing 8 protons) have identical forces of attraction for the shared electron pair. In addition, other factors come into play, such as how many energy levels each atom has, how many electrons are in each, and the distance the shared electrons are from each nucleus. All these factors lead to an unequal sharing of electrons in a covalent bond between different atoms.

The ability of an atom in a molecule to attract electrons is called electronegativity. Elements toward the top right corner of the periodic table have the highest electronegativity, and those toward the bottom left have the lowest (electronegativity generally increases from left to right in a row of the periodic table, and it decreases going down a column; the difference in the electronegativities of bonded atoms can be used to determine the polarity of a bond). Metals have low electronegativity, whereas non-metals have relatively high electronegativity. Oxygen and nitrogen have the highest electronegativities of the elements typically found in compounds important to nutrition. The electronegativity values of atoms determine the type of chemical bond formed. If the electronegativity values are not very different, a covalent bond is formed. If the electronegativities of 2 bonding atoms differ greatly, electron transfer occurs to yield an ionic bond, as in Na^+Cl^- (see the section "Ions and Ionic Compounds").

Hydrogen Bonds

Water, and most other molecules containing an O—H or N—H bond, exhibit a particularly strong interaction called hydrogen bonding (Fig. B-3). In this case, the hydrogen atom of 1 molecule is attracted to a non-bonded electron pair (called a lone pair) of a highly electronegative atom on a neighboring molecule, such as oxygen. Water molecules are attracted to each other by hydrogen bonds. This attraction is responsible for many of the biologically important properties of water. Hydrogen bonds, such as those found in large proteins and DNA, help hold the molecule together. These molecules fold or twist into 3-dimensional shapes due in part to the action of hydrogen bonds. Hydrogen bonds are usually symbolized by a dotted line between the atoms: —C—O · · · H—N—. Hydrogen bonds are the weakest of all chemical bonds.

Ions and Ionic Compounds

Atoms that have an equal number of positively charged protons and negatively charged electrons are electrically neutral. Atoms or molecules that have positive or negative charges

▶ Water is a good example of a dipole compound. The oxygen atom pulls electrons from the 2 hydrogen atoms toward its side of the water molecule, so that the oxygen side is more negatively charged than the hydrogen side of the molecule. Water, the most abundant molecule in the body, is a good solvent because of the nature of its basic structure.

▶ Polar molecules are weakly attracted both to ions and to other polar molecules. The positive end of the molecule can align itself with an anion or with the negative end of another molecule. These attractive forces, called, respectively, ion-dipole and dipole-dipole forces, are much weaker than covalent bonds individually but, when there are many of them, they make a significant contribution to the total energy of a collection of molecules. Water, for instance, has a much higher boiling point than expected because the molecules are held together by such forces.

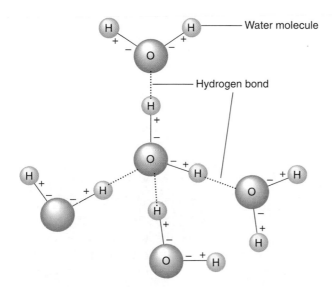

Figure B-3 Hydrogen bonds between water molecules. The oxygen atoms of water molecules are weakly joined together by the attraction of the electronegative oxygen for the positively charged hydrogen. These weak bonds are called hydrogen bonds.

ionic bond Union between 2 atoms formed by an attraction of a positive ion to a negative ion, as seen in table salt (Na^+Cl^-).

▶ Water molecules that surround ions attract other water molecules to form hydration spheres around each ion. This mechanism makes ions and numerous molecules soluble in water.

are called ions. **Ionic bonds** result when 1 or more valence electrons from 1 atom are completely transferred to another atom or molecule. Elements that have 1 to 3 valence electrons have a tendency to give up electrons, and those with 4 to 7 valence electrons have a tendency to accept electrons. The electrons are not shared. In both cases, the elements are giving up or taking on electrons to achieve the electron configuration of the closest noble gas. Consider sodium chloride. One atom loses electrons, so its number of electrons becomes smaller than its number of protons; thus, it becomes positively charged as Na^+ in sodium chloride. Now, sodium has the same number of electrons as neon. The other atom gains electrons, so its number of electrons is greater than its number of protons; it becomes negatively charged as Cl^- in sodium chloride. Now, chloride has the same number of electrons as argon.

Positively charged ions are called cations; they move toward the negative pole in an electric field. An atom with more electrons than protons is negatively charged and is known as an anion; it moves to the positive pole. NaCl is an example of an ionic compound. Note the name change that occurs when an element gains an electron to become a negative ion; the suffix becomes –*ide*.

These charged atoms, where electron(s) have been added or removed, are collectively known as ions. Sodium (Na^+), potassium (K^+), and calcium (Ca^{2+}) are found in the body as cations. Chloride (Cl^-) is a common anion in the body. See Table B-3 for a more complete list of common ions found in the body.

Ionic bonds are weaker than polar covalent bonds. Ionic compounds easily separate when dissolved in water. Table salt (NaCl) is obvious when poured out of the salt shaker, but when the salt is stirred into a cup of water it disappears. It *dissociates*. The polar water's negative side (oxygen) is attracted to the Na^+, and the positive side (hydrogen) is attracted to Cl^-.

Salts

Salts are substances composed of cations and anions. Table salt is NaCl. The Na^+ and Cl^- are attracted to each other by electrostatic force, and the resulting ionic compound is known chemically as sodium chloride. Salts are formed by the interaction of acids and bases

Table B-3 Important Ions in the Human Body

Common Ion	Symbol	Some Functions
Calcium	Ca^{2+}	Component of bones and teeth; necessary for blood clotting, muscle contraction, and nerve transmission
Sodium	Na^+	Helps maintain membrane potentials (electrical charge differences across a membrane) and water balance
Potassium	K^+	Helps maintain membrane potentials
Hydrogen	H^+	Helps maintain acid-base balance
Hydroxide	OH^-	Helps maintain acid-base balance
Chloride	Cl^-	Helps maintain acid-base balance
Bicarbonate	HCO_3^-	Helps maintain acid-base balance
Ammonium	NH_4^+	Helps maintain acid-base balance
Phosphate	PO_{43}^-	Component of bones and teeth; involved in energy exchange and acid-base balance
Iron	Fe^{2+}	Necessary for red blood cell formation and function
Magnesium	Mg^{2+}	Necessary for enzyme function
Iodide	I^-	Part of the thyroid hormones
Fluoride	F^-	Strengthens bones and teeth

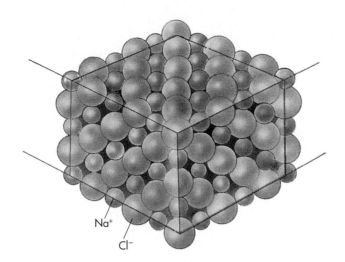

Figure B-4 Molecules of sodium chloride (table salt) in typical cube-shape formation.

in a neutralization reaction. Water also is formed in such a reaction. In this type of reaction, hydrogen ions of an acid are replaced by the positive ions of a base, and a salt forms. For example, when hydrochloric acid reacts with sodium hydroxide, table salt is produced:

HCl	+	NaOH	$\rightarrow$	NaCl	+	H_2O
Hydrochloric acid		Sodium hydroxide		Salt		Water
		(neutralization reaction)				

The formula for salts can be misleading. For example, NaCl suggests that table salt exists as a discrete entity containing 1 sodium ion and 1 chloride ion. An inspection of the chemical structure of table salt shows that it is actually a 3-dimensional stack of layers—much like a ream of paper with all the pages glued together (Fig. B-4).

▶ Salts separate to form positively and negatively charged ions when dissolved in water. Substances that dissolve in water and conduct electricity are called electrolytes. (A solute that produces ions in solution forms an electrolytic solution that conducts an electrical current.) Sodium (Na^+), potassium (K^+), calcium (Ca^{2+}), chloride (Cl^-), magnesium (Mg^{2+}), phosphate (PO_4^{3-}), and bicarbonate (HCO_3^-) are electrolytes commonly found in the body.

Acids, Bases, and the pH Scales

You have a pretty good idea of what acids and bases are. You know that lemon juice is an acid and drain cleaners are strong bases.

A solution that has a higher concentration of protons (H^+) is said to be acidic, and one that is lower is basic, or alkaline. An acid is defined as a substance that can ionize and release protons (H^+) into solution. It is a proton donor.

Any substance that releases protons (hydrogen ions) when in water is an acid. For example, hydrogen chloride (HCl) forms hydrogen and chloride ions (H^+ and Cl^-) in solution and therefore is an acid.

$$HCl \rightarrow H^+ + Cl^-$$

Figure B-5 lists several common acids and bases. A base is a negatively charged ion or a molecule that ionizes to produce an anion. This then can combine with a proton (H^+), removing it from solution. This base is a proton acceptor. Any substance that can accept hydrogen ions while in water is a base.

Many bases can function as proton acceptors by releasing hydroxide ions (OH^-) when dissolved in water. Most strong bases release OH^- into solution. The OH^- combines with H^+ to form water.

NaOH	$\rightarrow$	Na^+	+	OH^-
Sodium hydroxide		Sodium ion		Hydroxide ion

OH^-	+	H^+	$\rightarrow$	H_2O
Hydroxide ion		Hydrogen ion		Water

▶ Water molecules of 2 hydrogens and 1 oxygen are held together by polar covalent bonds. Although these are strong bonds, a *small* proportion of them break, releasing a hydrogen ion and a hydroxide ion. The hydrogen ion (a proton) is transferred to another oxygen in a water molecule, forming a *hydronium ion.* This means that a pair of water molecules can act as an acid and a base because water self-ionizes, forming hydronium ions and hydroxide ions:

$2H_2O$	$\longleftrightarrow$	H_3O^+	+	OH^-
Water		**Hydronium ion**		**Hydroxide ion**

For simplicity, ionized water will be represented by H^+ and OH^-.

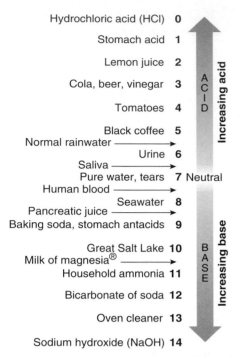

Figure B-5 **pH of various substances. Any pH value above 7 is basic, and any pH value below 7 is acidic.**

acidic pH pH less than 7. Lemon juice has an acidic pH.

alkaline pH pH greater than 7. Baking soda in water yields an alkaline pH.

pH

Acidity is expressed in terms of pH, a measure of the molarity (the ratio of solute per liter of solution) of H^+. Molarity is expressed by square brackets, so the molarity of H^+ is symbolized as $[H^+]$. pH is defined as the negative logarithm of the hydrogen ion molarity (concentration), or $pH = -log\,[H^+]$. The pH unit is the H^+ concentration of a solution. Pure water has a neutral pH because it contains equal amounts of hydrogen (hydronium) and hydroxyl ions. The pH scale runs from 0 to 14 (see Fig. B-5).

Because pH is a negative logarithmic scale, a solution with a pH of 4 has an **acidic pH** that is 10 times greater than that of a solution with a pH of 5, and it is 100 times more acidic than a solution with a pH of 6. These numbers may be confusing because they are inversely related to the hydrogen ion concentration: a solution with a high hydrogen ion concentration has a low pH number. A solution with a low hydrogen concentration has a high pH number. Acid solutions have a pH of less than 7. Basic, or **alkaline pH,** solutions have a pH greater than 7.

A slight disruption of pH can seriously disturb normal physiological functions, so it is important for the body to be able to control pH. Blood normally has a pH range from 7.35 to 7.45. Any deviations from this range can cause dizziness, fainting, coma, paralysis, or death.

Acids and bases are classified as strong or weak. Strong acids and strong bases dissociate completely when dissolved in water. Consequently, they release all their hydrogen ions or hydroxide ions when dissolved. In general, the more completely an acid or a base dissociates, the stronger it is. Hydrochloric acid, for example, is a strong acid because it completely dissociates in water.

Weak acids only partially dissociate in water. Consequently, they release only some of their acidic hydrogens. For example, when acetic acid (CH_3C—OH, the principal component of vinegar) dissolves in water, it dissociates only partially.

$$
\underset{\textbf{Acetic acid}}{CH_3\overset{\textstyle O}{\overset{||}{C}}-OH} \quad \longleftrightarrow \quad \underset{\textbf{Acetate ion}}{CH_3\overset{\textstyle O}{\overset{||}{C}}-O^-} \quad + \quad \underset{\textbf{Proton}}{H^+}
$$

The equilibrium lies far to the left, so that only a small fraction of the acetic acid in the vinegar is dissociated into acetate ions and protons.

Most weak bases release hydroxide into solution by reacting with the water itself. For example, ammonia (NH_3) reacts with water to form NH_4^+ and OH^-.

$$
\underset{\textbf{Ammonia}}{NH_3} \quad + \quad \underset{\textbf{Water}}{H_2O} \quad \longleftrightarrow \quad \underset{\textbf{Ammonium ion}}{NH_4^+} \quad + \quad \underset{\textbf{Hydroxide ion}}{OH^-}
$$

Buffers

Many of the biochemical reactions that occur in living tissues require tight control of pH. To prevent changes in the H^+ concentration in the body and to control the pH, a system of buffers is maintained. These buffers are ions and molecules that stabilize the pH of a solution. In the blood (plasma), the pH is maintained by the carbonic acid–bicarbonate buffer system. The acid is formed by the combination of water and carbon dioxide. Carbonic acid separates into bicarbonate ion (HCO_3^-) and the hydrogen ion (H^+).

$$
\underset{\textbf{Biocarbonate}}{HCO_3^-} \quad + \quad \underset{\textbf{Hydrogen ion}}{H^+} \quad \longleftrightarrow \quad \underset{\textbf{Carbonic acid}}{H_2CO_3} \quad \longleftrightarrow \quad \underset{\textbf{Water}}{H_2O} \quad + \quad \underset{\textbf{Carbon dioxide}}{CO_2}
$$

The reaction can go either way. The direction depends on the concentration of ions on either side of the arrows. For example, if an acid were released into the blood plasma (more H^+ in solution), the reaction would be driven to the right. The carbon dioxide produced could then be exhaled via the lungs. Acids that are present in the plasma come from cellular activities, but despite the increase in H^+ ions by these activities, the blood plasma pH hardly changes; it is essentially constant. The buffer, bicarbonate, accomplishes this. It is constantly formed to maintain normal pH.

Free Radicals

You are aware that atoms tend to share electron pairs when forming chemical bonds, and they tend to share enough electrons to completely fill the valence shell to form a noble gas configuration. A consequence is that atoms or elements are rarely found with unpaired electrons. When a molecule with an extra electron does arise, however, it is called a **free radical**. An example is the superoxide anion. Oxygen is composed of 2 oxygen atoms (O_2); if an electron is added, it becomes superoxide, or $O_2^{\bullet -}$. The dot signifies an unpaired electron.

Superoxide and other free radicals are reactive, primarily because they contain an unpaired electron. Free radicals seek an electron by attacking and removing electrons from other compounds, such as at the location where hydrogens are attached to carbon. This not only damages the other molecule but also transforms it into a free radical.

$$R^{\bullet} + {-}CH_2 \rightarrow RH^+{-}CH^{-\bullet}$$

Free radicals also are formed when a covalent bond breaks and each atom or molecule fragment recovers the electron originally used to make the bond. In this case, energy—usually in the form of sunlight, ultraviolet radiation, or heat—is used to break the bond.

$$A{-}B + energy \rightarrow A^{\bullet} + B^{\bullet}$$

Because free radicals are reactive, they can generate thousands of other free radicals within minutes in a chain-reaction process. The reactivity of free radicals sometimes produces detrimental effects in living systems. For instance, the development of cardiovascular disease and some types of cancer, such as skin and lung cancer, is probably promoted by free radicals. However, some normal physiological functions in the body involve free radical formation; for example, various white blood cells use free radicals to kill invading bacteria.

The body has a number of mechanisms, such as antioxidants, for neutralizing free radicals. Antioxidants are substances that react with and neutralize free radical forms of oxygen and nitrogen. The enzyme superoxide dismutase (SOD) converts superoxide into oxygen and hydrogen peroxide. One form of SOD contains the minerals copper and zinc, whereas another form contains manganese. Other antioxidants obtained from the diet are vitamin E and various phytochemicals.

Some substances are used extensively in the food industry to trap free radicals or prevent their formation. This use allows for increased food storage time by decreasing chemical breakdown. These substances are part of a class of food additives called preservatives (see Chapter 3). Vitamin E added to cooking oils protects C—C bonds by trapping free radicals.

Organic Chemistry

Organic compounds contain carbon in combination with other elements, such as hydrogen, oxygen, and nitrogen. Carbon compounds are associated with living things, but why carbon? It is because carbon forms very stable covalent bonds, such as single, double, and even triple bonds. Carbon also forms these bonds with many other atoms. Carbon atoms can even form rings and chains by bonding to other carbons. Variation in

▶ The kidneys play a buffering role in the body by absorbing or releasing H^+ or HCO_3^-, depending on the acid-base balance in the person. In fact, much of the excess acid leaves the body via the urine (urine has an acid pH). Thus, the kidneys and lungs keep this buffering system functioning and, in turn, are key to acid-base balance in the body.

free radical Short-lived form of a compound that has an unpaired electron, causing it to seek an electron from another compound. Free radicals are strong oxidizing agents and can be very destructive to electron-dense cell components, such as the DNA and cell membranes.

organic compound Substance that contains carbon atoms bonded to hydrogen atoms in the chemical structure.

Glucose

Butyric acid

the length of the chains, and their atomic configurations, allows the formation of a wide variety of molecules. Organic molecules generally also contain hydrogen.

Cyclic and Chain Compounds

Cyclic organic compounds are common forms of hydrocarbons. Note the diagram of butyric acid (a chain) in the margin and compare that with the structure of glucose, which is a ring. Even though the 2 compounds are only carbon, oxygen, and hydrogen, their structures each confer a very different property. Some ring structures are referred to as **aromatic compounds.**

Hydrocarbons as chains or rings provide the backbone of many groups of compounds that make up important organic nutrients. Other groups are attached to these backbones. They usually contain atoms of oxygen, nitrogen, phosphorus, and sulfur. The functional or reactive groups provide the unique chemical properties of organic molecules. Classes of organic molecules are known by their functional groups.

A Closer Look at Functional Groups

Several important organic compounds contain a functional group called a carbonyl group ($C = O$). The **carbonyl group** is the parent compound for ketones, aldehydes, and many related groups. Table B-4 has a list of all these compounds that are important to nutrition.

Ketones are organic compounds in which the carbonyl group occurs in the interior of a carbon chain and is therefore flanked by carbon atoms. Body fat that is breaking down at a rapid rate produces ketones ($C—\overset{\overset{\textstyle O}{\|}}{C}—C$), some of which are removed from the body by way of the urine (see Chapter 9).

Aldehydes ($—\overset{\overset{\textstyle O}{\|}}{C}—H$) are organic compounds that contain a carbonyl group to which at least 1 hydrogen atom is attached. This active group is found in an important form of vitamin A. As an aldehyde, it plays a central role in vision.

Many of the most common substances in both foods and the body contain carboxylic acids. A **carboxylic acid** ($—\overset{\overset{\textstyle O}{\|}}{C}—OH$) contains the carbonyl group with an OH group attached. These acids are widely distributed in tissues and natural products. Vinegar contains acetic acid. Citrus fruits contain citric acid, and vitamin C is ascorbic acid.

The **carboxyl group** is an acid because it can donate a H^+ (proton) to a solution. A very common acid formed in muscle cells is lactic acid. When lactic acid ionizes, it releases the H^+ and becomes lactate. Because both forms of the acid (ionized and non-ionized) are in solution, the proportion depends on the pH of the solution.

An **alcohol** has the carbon-oxygen bond, but the O is also bonded to a single hydrogen. This leaves only a single bond between the carbon and oxygen, forming an —OH or hydroxide group (ROH).

An **ester** ($R—\overset{\overset{\textstyle O}{\|}}{C}—O—C$) is an organic compound that has an O—C group attached to a carbonyl group. An ester is the product of a reaction between a carboxylic acid and an alcohol. The formation of lipids called triglycerides involves the formation of ester bonds.

The carbonyl portion of a compound such as an ester is called an **acyl group.** Thus, removal of the hydroxyl group (OH) from an organic acid forms an acyl group.

Two sulfur atoms (S—S), each attached to a carbon, produce a **disulfide group.** This group is important to the structural characteristics of certain proteins.

A single carbon with an **amine** (also called **amino**) **group** attached ($—NH_2$) is a component of all amino acids.

Table B-4 Typical Chemical Groups Found in Nutrients

Functional Group	Name	Typically Found In	Example
—OH	Hydroxide	Alcohols	CH_3—OH
—C=O (with H below)	Aldehyde	Sugars	CH_3C=O (with H below)
C—C=O (with C below)	Ketone	Ketones	CH_3C=O (with CH_3 below)
—C=O (with OH below)	Carboxyl	Acids	CH_3C=O (with OH below)
—S—S—	Disulfide	Proteins	—CH_2—S—S—CH_2—
—C=O	Carbonyl	Aldehydes, ketones, carboxylic acids, amides	$(CH_3)_2C$=O
—C—NH_2	Amine	Proteins	CH_3—NH_2
—C=O (with NH_2 below)	Amide	Vitamins	—CH_2C=O (with NH_2 below)
$^-$O—P=O (with O— above and O— below)	Phosphate	High-energy compounds	—CH_2—O—P=O (with O— above and O—CH_2- below)
	Ester		
—O—C—CH_2- (with O double bond above)	Acyl	Triglycerides	

Isomerism

Molecules that have identical chemical formulas but different structures are called **isomers.** A simple example is 2 compounds with the formula C_2H_6O.

isomers Different chemical structures for compounds that share a chemical formula.

$$CH_3CH_2OH \qquad CH_3OCH_3$$
Ethanol   **Methyl ether**

Both these compounds can be harmful. However, there are intake levels at which ethanol produces no toxic symptoms (i.e., the amount in a small glass of wine) but at which methyl ether would cause very toxic effects. This fact illustrates an important point about isomers: because they have different structures, they can have different *chemical* properties.

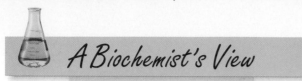

A Biochemist's View

$$CH_3 - CH_2 - CH_2 - CH_2 - CH_3$$

Pentane

$$CH_3 - CH_2 - \overset{\displaystyle |}{\underset{\displaystyle |}{CH}} - CH_3$$
$$CH_3$$

Neopentane

$$CH_3 - \overset{\displaystyle CH_3}{\underset{\displaystyle CH_3}{\overset{|}{\underset{|}{C}}}} - CH_3$$

Isopentane

Isomers of pentane.

---

cis configuration Form seen in compounds with double bonds, such as fatty acids, in which the hydrogens on both ends of the double bond lie on the same side of the plane of that bond.

trans configuration Compound in which the hydrogens lie opposite each other across a carbon-carbon double bond.

▶ *Trans* isomers of fatty acids are associated with an increased risk of cardiovascular disease (see Chapter 6).

The difference in properties between 2 isomers can be great (as in the preceding example) or very subtle, but the differences are detectable. There are different types of isomerism, but only 2 of the common types will be briefly reviewed in this section: structural isomers and stereoisomers.

Structural Isomers

Isomers in which the number and kinds of bonds differ are called **structural isomers**. Molecules containing chains of carbon atoms typically have many structural isomers. Any variation in the way the chain is branched gives rise to a new isomer. For example, pentane (C_5H_{12}) has 3 isomers, as shown in the margin.

Stereoisomers

Stereoisomers have the same number and types of chemical bonds but with different spatial arrangements (different configurations in space). Molecules containing double bonds illustrate stereoisomers. Because there is no freedom to rotate around a C—C bond, molecules containing such bonds frequently exhibit stereoisomerism. For example, hydrogens or various chemical compounds can be located on the same side of the bond (*cis* configuration) or on opposite sides of the double bond (*trans* configuration).

Consider oleic acid and its isomer elaidic acid (Fig. B-6*a*). Oleic acid is a *cis* isomer, or the form found naturally in food. With food-processing technology, such as hydrogenation, some *cis* bonds of fatty acids are converted to *trans* bonds. When vegetable oils are converted to vegetable fats, such as in margarine or shortening, some of the *trans* isomers are formed. The *trans* isomer elaidic acid is not the natural form. Isomers of these types (i.e., *cis* and *trans*) are called geometric isomers.

Describing each stereoisomerism depends on which way the functional groups are arranged with respect to each other. If there are 2 isomers, *D* stands for dextro or right-handed, and *L* stands for levo or left-handed, such as alanine in D-alanine and L-alanine (Fig. B-6*b*). Stereoisomers that can't be superimposed on their mirror images are called optical isomers. Optical isomers can be identified from each other by their reaction to polarized light. One solution of an isomer that rotates the plane of polarized light to the right is dextrorotary. And the solution of its optical isomer rotates the plane of light to the left and, so, is levorotary.

The difference between 2 stereoisomers is "fit." This difference is important because the molecule has to fit an enzyme to make the chemical reaction proceed. For example, human enzymes use only L-amino acids (building blocks of protein) and D-sugars to build compounds. D-amino acids and L-sugars just won't function as such in the body. It is rather like trying to wear a left-hand glove on the right hand and do anything that requires manual skill.

In living organisms, many molecules are chiral. A carbon atom with 4 different atoms or groups of atoms attached is described as being **chiral** (also called asymmetric). A molecule with 1 chiral carbon can have 2 stereoisomers, such as alanine (see Fig. B-6*b*). When 2 or more (n) chiral carbons are present, there can be 2^n stereoisomers. Some stereoisomers are mirror images of each other; others are not.

$$CH_3 - CH_2 - \overset{\displaystyle OH}{\underset{\displaystyle H}{\overset{|}{\underset{|}{C}}}} - CH_3 \qquad \text{Chiral carbon}$$

$$CH_3 - \overset{\displaystyle OH}{\underset{\displaystyle H}{\overset{|}{\underset{|}{C}}}} - CH_3 \qquad \text{Achiral carbon}$$

When compounds have more than 1 chiral center, the "RS" system of naming is used, rather than the D and L system. Every chiral carbon is designated either *R* or *S*, based on specific rules.

This RS terminology is important to understanding vitamin E chemistry. It is now known that vitamin E as alpha-tocopherol has 3 chiral centers and, so, has 8 different stereoisomers ($2^3 = 8$). All 3 are found in synthetic preparations. The 3 chiral centers are identified as 2, 4, and 8 as related to the position on the tail of the molecule (see Chapter 12). The RRR isomer (i.e., R form at all of the 3 chiral centers on the tail) is the natural form. A

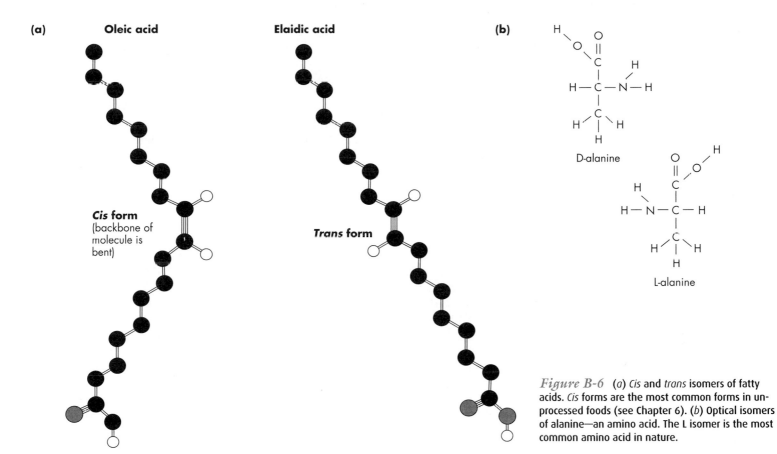

(a) Oleic acid Elaidic acid

Cis form
(backbone of
molecule is
bent)

Trans form

(b)

D-alanine

L-alanine

Figure B-6 (*a*) *Cis* and *trans* isomers of fatty acids. *Cis* forms are the most common forms in unprocessed foods (see Chapter 6). (*b*) Optical isomers of alanine—an amino acid. The L isomer is the most common amino acid in nature.

transfer protein in the liver only recognizes the R form of the chiral center at the 2 position. Of all the 8 combinations of R and S in the tail of synthetic vitamin E, the only biologically active ones are RRR, RSR, RSS, RRS because they all have the R form in the 2 position.

Biochemistry

The study of the chemistry or molecular basis of life and the reactions, structures, and composition of living materials is known as biochemistry. Biochemical reactions are possible because of enzymes. Living organisms convert the energy they extract from food into energy for growth, maintenance, and reproduction. Energy can be stored for future use. The energy in the food is converted and used in the form of chemical energy contained in adenosine triphosphate (ATP). The fact that living organisms can self-replicate depends on deoxyribonucleic acid (DNA) and the genetic code. All forms of life store and transmit genetic information in the form of DNA.

Approximately 98.5% of the body's weight is composed of the elements oxygen, carbon, hydrogen, nitrogen, calcium, and phosphorus. Elements such as iron, zinc, and copper are present in trace amounts in the body, but that doesn't mean they are unimportant. For instance, iron combines with a blood protein to form hemoglobin, an oxygen carrier. Hemoglobin transports oxygen from the lungs to the tissues and assists in returning carbon dioxide from the tissues to the lungs for removal.

Water is the most abundant chemical in the body, making up to about 70% of human tissue. Other important classes of compounds in the body are the proteins, carbohydrates, lipids, and nucleic acids.

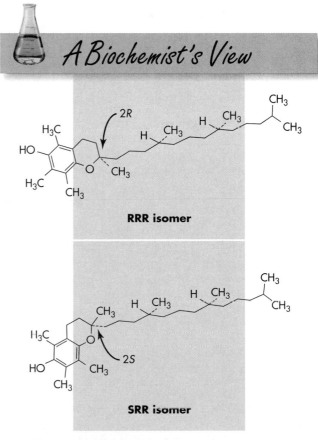

A Biochemist's View

RRR isomer

SRR isomer

RRR and SRR isomers of vitamin E. Of the 2, only the RRR isomer contributes to vitamin E needs.

Biochemical Reactions

All the biochemical reactions that occur in the body are described as **metabolism**. The intermediate compounds in metabolism are termed metabolites. Metabolic reactions that build (synthesize) complex molecules are described as **anabolic**. An example is the synthesis of protein from amino acids. The reactions that break down (degrade) larger molecules into smaller ones are described as **catabolic**. An example is starch breaking down to glucose molecules.

Carbohydrates

▶ Di- and *poly*saccharides are assembled by a condensation reaction. Water is a by-product of the reaction. In contrast, **hydrolysis**, or the splitting by the addition of water, digests di- and polysaccharides to smaller sugar units (for details, see the section "Important Chemical Reactions Related to the Study of Nutrition").

Carbohydrates are aldehydes with hydroxyl groups and ketones, containing carbon, hydrogen, and oxygen with the general formula CH_2O. (There are twice as many hydrogen atoms as carbon and oxygen atoms.) The suffix -*ose* indicates a sugar. *Hexose* refers to a 6-carbon monosaccharide. There are 3 structural isomers of hexose: galactose, glucose, and fructose. All have the same formula, $C_6H_{12}O_6$, but the arrangements of their individual atoms differ slightly.

The simplest carbohydrates are **monosaccharides**. When 2 monosaccharides are chemically bonded, they form a **disaccharide**, or double sugar. The table sugar sucrose is an example of a disaccharide, formed from glucose and fructose.

Polysaccharides are many monosaccharides joined by covalent bonds. Plant starch and cellulose are polysaccharides. Some starches have thousands of glucose subunits. In animals, carbohydrate is stored as an animal starch called glycogen, found in liver and muscle tissue.

Lipids

Lipids are a class of nonpolar compounds that are grouped according to solubility in organic solvents. They don't readily dissolve in water because most are nonpolar or hydrophobic.

Simple lipids include fatty acids and steroids. The lipid cholesterol serves as the precursor (parent) for the steroid hormones, such as testosterone, estrogen, and progesterone. Complex lipids include triglycerides (often referred to as *triacylglycerols*), which are esters of glycerol and fatty acids. Phospholipids are composed of glycerol, phosphoric acid, and long chain fatty acids; sphingolipids are composed of sphingosine, phosphoric acid, long chain fatty acids, and choline; and glycosphingolipids are composed of sphingosine, fatty acids, and carbohydrates.

▶ Prostaglandins are a special type of fatty acid produced by almost all organs in the body; they have specific regulatory functions. They are all derived from certain dietary (essential) fatty acids (see Chapter 6 and Appendix A).

Triglycerides represent fuel found in food and stored in adipose tissues. Phospholipids are part polar and part nonpolar, which allows them to interact with water and function as emulsifiers. Sphingophospholipids make up the material surrounding nerves. Glycosphingolipids are structural material for brain and nerve tissue. These complex lipids can be hydrolyzed to yield fatty acids.

Proteins

Proteins are polymers of amino acids. Twenty common amino acids are incorporated into the great variety of body proteins. Although the amino acids contain an amine (amino)

$$\overset{\displaystyle O}{\overset{\displaystyle \|}{}}$$

group (NH_2) and a carboxylic acid group ($—C—OH$), each has a distinctive structure (Fig. B-7). Proteins typically contain many atoms, such as carbon, nitrogen, sulfur, hydrogen, and oxygen.

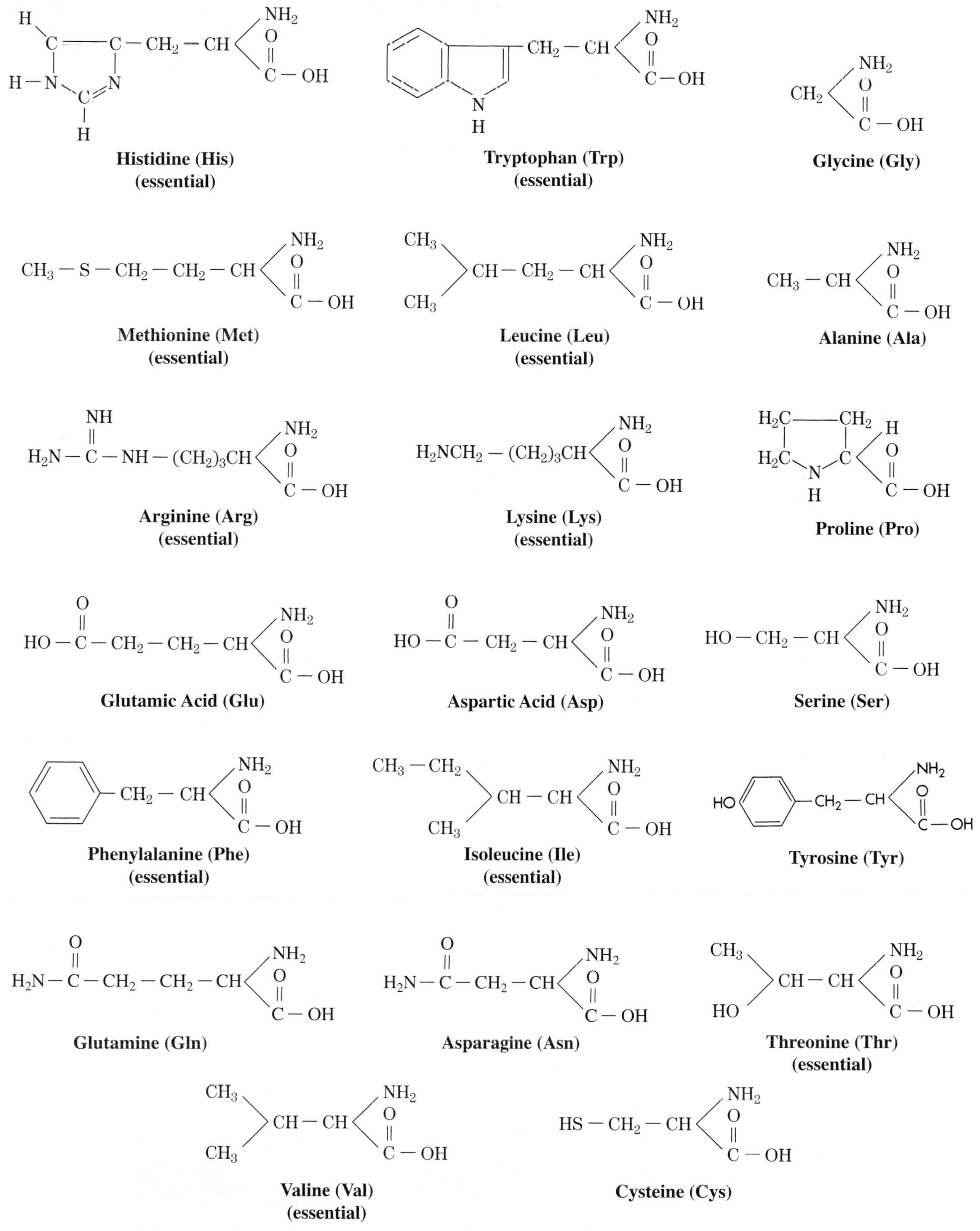

Histidine (His)
(essential)

Tryptophan (Trp)
(essential)

Glycine (Gly)

Methionine (Met)
(essential)

Leucine (Leu)
(essential)

Alanine (Ala)

Arginine (Arg)
(essential)

Lysine (Lys)
(essential)

Proline (Pro)

Glutamic Acid (Glu)

Aspartic Acid (Asp)

Serine (Ser)

Phenylalanine (Phe)
(essential)

Isoleucine (Ile)
(essential)

Tyrosine (Tyr)

Glutamine (Gln)

Asparagine (Asn)

Threonine (Thr)
(essential)

Valine (Val)
(essential)

Cysteine (Cys)

Figure B-7 The 20 common amino acids in foods.

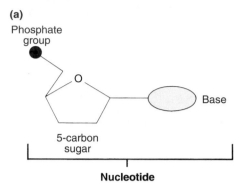

(a)

Phosphate group

O

Base

5-carbon sugar

Nucleotide

(b)

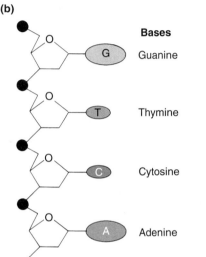

Bases

G Guanine

T Thymine

C Cytosine

A Adenine

Figure B-8 (*a*) General structure of a nucleotide. (*b*) A polymer of nucleotides, or polynucleotide, is formed by sugar-phosphate bonds between nucleotides.

The genetic information in the DNA in a cell's nucleus is the code book for constructing a protein. The sequence of amino acids in a protein follows the DNA code for synthesizing the protein. This protein can be made over and over again because of the code carried in the genes.

Nucleic Acids (DNA and RNA)

Nucleic acids include DNA (deoxyribonucleic acid), RNA (ribonucleic acid), and the subunits from which they are formed, called nucleotides. A nucleotide is made of 3 components: a 5-carbon pentose sugar, a phosphate group, and a nitrogenous base (Fig. B-8). There are 2 kinds of nitrogenous base: purines (double ring) and pyrimidines (single ring).

The sugar contained in RNA is ribose. The pyrimidine bases in ribonucleic acids are uracil and cytosine, and the purine bases are guanine and adenine. RNA is a single polynucleotide strand, not a double strand like DNA.

DNA in the nucleus of the cell is the basis of the genetic code. The sugar in DNA deoxyribose can be covalently bonded to the purine bases adenine and guanine and to the pyrimidine bases cytosine and thymine (Fig. B-9). These 4 types of nucleotides can produce the long chain that makes up a single strand of DNA. The DNA is a 2-stranded sugar phosphate chain that twists around in such a way to form a helix. The bases project into the center of the helix, forming a staircase structure. The 2 strands are held together by hydrogen bonds (Fig. B-10).

DNA always contains an equal number of purine and pyrimidine bases. And there is a relationship called complementary base pairing—adenine pairs only with thymine, and guanine pairs only with cytosine. (In RNA, adenine pairs with uracil.)

Although there are only 4 bases, the number of sequences of bases is endless. The total human genome consists of billions of base pairs, making up about 35,000 genes. The

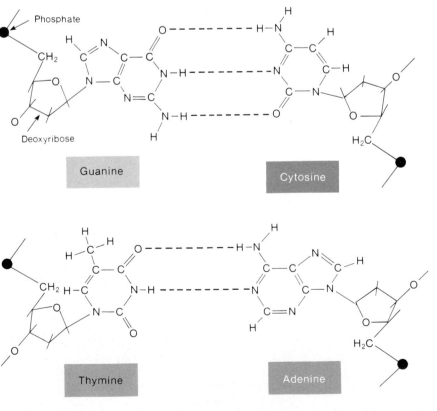

Phosphate

CH_2

Deoxyribose

Guanine

Cytosine

H_2C

Thymine

Adenine

H_2C

Figure B-9 The 4 nitrogenous bases in deoxyribonucleic acid (DNA). Hydrogen bonds can form between guanine and cytosine and between thymine and adenine.

applications of this knowledge can lead to genetic screening for breast cancer and, in the future, are likely to help produce drugs to treat obesity and inborn errors of metabolism.

During replication, the helix uncoils and separates, so that each chain or strand serves as a template for the synthesis of its complementary chain. This step is important for cell division. Each daughter cell receives DNA containing 1 strand of the original molecule and 1 new strand.

RNA, another nucleic acid, takes its instructions from DNA. There are 3 types of RNA: ribosomal RNA, transfer RNA, and messenger RNA. Ribosomal RNA forms part of the structure of ribosomes in the cell; this is where proteins are synthesized. Messenger RNA contains the code for the synthesis of a specific protein transcribed from DNA. Transfer RNA decodes the genetic message in RNA and assembles the amino acids for the protein assembly line (see Chapter 7 for details). The process is called **translation**.

Important Chemical Reactions Related to the Study of Nutrition

One of the most important properties of chemical compounds is the type of reactions they undergo. Chemical reactions are responsible for vision, thinking, movement, and everything else that occurs in the human body.

In a chemical reaction, a compound or set of compounds (the reactants) is converted into another compound or set of compounds (the products), accompanied by the absorption or release of energy, which is typically heat in biological processes. In effect, the reactants reshuffle their atoms to form products. Clearly, then, no atoms lose their identity during a chemical reaction, and no atoms are gained, lost, or converted to another kind of atom during the course of chemical activity.

Chemists have grouped reactions according to their similarities in chemical behavior. Some of these reactions are performed over and over within each cell. Following is a brief overview of some important reaction types.

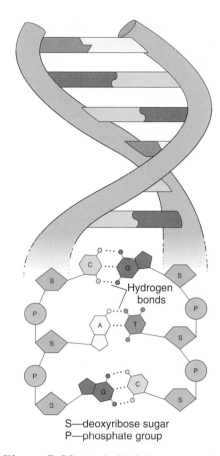

S—deoxyribose sugar
P—phosphate group

Figure B-10 The double-helix structure of DNA. The 2 strands are held together by hydrogen bonds between complementary bases in each strand.

Condensation Reactions

A **condensation reaction** occurs when 2 molecules join together to form a larger molecule and water is released. The 2-reactant molecules typically contain hydroxyl groups, meaning that there are 2 OH groups. A simple example is the condensation of glucose and galactose to make lactose and water.

$$C_6H_{12}O_6 \quad + \quad C_6H_{12}O_6 \quad \rightarrow \quad C_{12}H_{22}O_{11} \quad + \quad H_2O$$

Glucose   Galactose   Lactose   Water

One –OH group on the single sugar gains a proton and forms a water molecule. The OH group on the other single sugar loses a proton and forms a bond with the other molecule—in exactly the same place that the water molecule leaves. Note that this is an overall description of what happens, not how it happens. In addition, although it is typical for both molecules to contain an –OH group in a condensation reaction, it is not a requirement for the reaction. A condensation reaction can occur in which only 1 of the reactants contains an –OH group.

Hydrolysis Reactions

Hydrolysis reactions are reactions that occur when water is added to a compound. In biological systems, hydrolysis reactions are very frequently the reverse of condensation

▶ Many important compounds in cells are formed through condensation reactions, and the breakdown of many compounds into smaller fragments occurs via hydrolysis reactions.

▶ In organic chemistry, oxidation is the loss of hydrogen (or gain of oxygen).

▶ In organic chemistry, reduction is the gain of hydrogen (or loss of oxygen).

reactions. That is, water is added to a large molecule, which results in the formation of 2 smaller molecules. This can be illustrated by the hydrolysis of lactose.

$$C_{12}H_{22}O_{11} \quad + \quad H_2O \quad \rightarrow \quad C_6H_{12}O_6 \quad + \quad C_6H_{12}O_6$$

| Lactose | Water | Glucose | Galactose |

Oxidation-Reduction Reactions

Oxidation-reduction (redox) reactions are important in nutrition science because they release energy from food during oxidation and synthesize carbohydrates, fatty acids, and other organic compounds during reduction. Redox reactions follow 3 rules:

1. No oxidation reaction takes place without something being reduced at the same time, and no reduction takes place without something being oxidized.
2. Oxidation is the loss of electrons.
3. Reduction is the gain in electrons.

A simple redox reaction involving iron is as follows:

$$Fe^{3+} + e- \longleftrightarrow Fe^{2+}$$

A biochemical redox reaction involving the coenzyme form of riboflavin occurs as follows:

$$\overset{+2H}{\underset{-2H}{FAD \longleftrightarrow FADH_2}}$$

(Chapters 9, 10, and 12 provide more information about coenzymes, cofactors, and oxidation-reduction reactions.)

catalyst Compound that speeds reaction rates but is not altered by the reaction.

Energy and Enzymatic Reactions

Enzymes are large proteins with varying amino acid composition that behave as organic **catalysts.** They are highly specific. Enzymes help a reaction proceed by lowering the "energy of activation," so that the reaction can go faster (Fig. B-11). Enzymes lower this energy barrier between the reactants and the products. Some of the enzyme reactions that occur in the cell require coenzymes (vitamins) at the active site to make the reaction go, whereas many others don't. Fortunately, an enzyme isn't consumed by the reaction, so it can be used over and over.

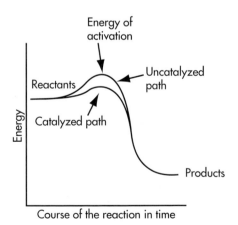

Figure B-11 Enzymes and other catalysts accelerate chemical reactions by reducing the energy barrier to the reactions. Reactant molecules free in solution can react only if they meet in just the right orientation and with enough energy. An enzyme holds its substrate molecules in the right orientation to react and exerts forces on them that cause chemical bonds to break and form. In this way, an enzyme lowers the energy barrier that substrates must pass and, so, increases their reaction rates.

Common Chemical Structures

Most compounds in the body are composed of carbon, hydrogen, and oxygen, with carbon often being the predominant atom. Some commonly encountered combinations of atoms, called functional groups, have been given specific names because they appear in many molecules. You need to be familiar with them, for they are the most important features in many nutrients. The important ones were listed in Table B-5.

The Drawing of Chemical Structures

Chemists have developed a shorthand notation for writing chemical formulas, called **skeletal structures.** In skeletal structures, neither carbon atoms nor the hydrogens bonded to the carbon atoms are expressly shown. What are shown are the bonds between the carbon atoms and the position of all atoms other than carbon and hydrogen. Keep in mind that there are carbon atoms at the apices (corners) of every angle in the structure (with the appropriate number of hydrogens attached to the carbon) and at the terminal end of the sticks. By way of illustration, look at a skeletal structure of propane ($CH_3CH_2CH_3$).

The advantage of using skeletal structures is that they allow for a clear representation of complex molecules without cluttering up the picture. **They are handy when large structures, such as fatty acids, have to be represented.** This notation is used throughout the text.

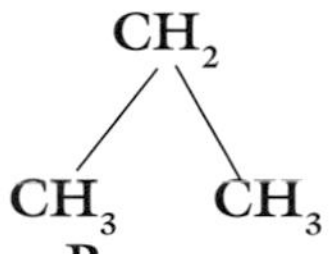

CH_2

CH_3 CH_3
Propane

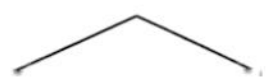

Skeletal structure
of propane

Appendix C

DETAILED DEPICTIONS OF GLYCOLYSIS, CITRIC ACID CYCLE, ELECTRON TRANSPORT CHAIN, CLASSES OF EICOSANOIDS, AND HOMOCYSTEINE METABOLISM

The following illustrations are provided to help you better visualize the changes in chemical structures throughout the metabolic processes described. These figures reflect greater scientific detail than the more simplified versions in Chapters 6, 9, and 13.

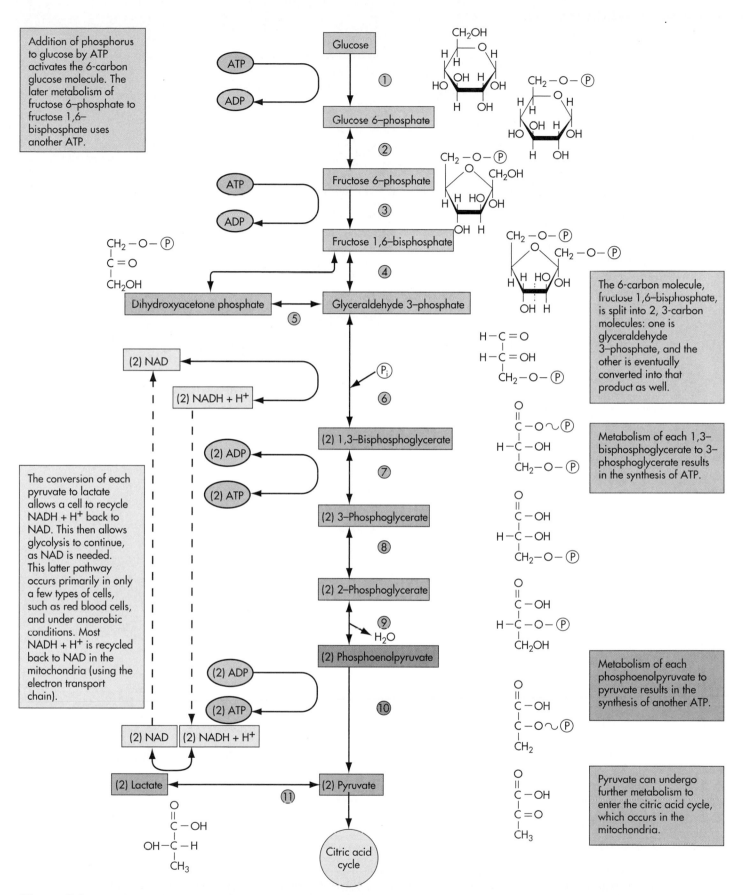

Figure C-1 Detailed depiction of the individual chemical reactions that constitute glycolysis—glucose to pyruvate. Glycolysis takes place in the cytosol of the cell. The enzymes in the cytosol that participate at the following steps are (1) hexokinase, (2) phosphohexose isomerase, (3) phosphofructokinase, (4) aldolase, (5) phosphotriose isomerase, (6) glyceraldehyde-3-phosphate dehydrogenase, (7) phosphoglycerate kinase, (8) phosphoglycerate mutase, (9) enolase, and (10) pyruvate kinase. Sometimes (11) lactate dehydrogenase is used to recycle NADH + H⁺ back to NAD (anaerobic glycolysis). P_i represents a phosphate group.

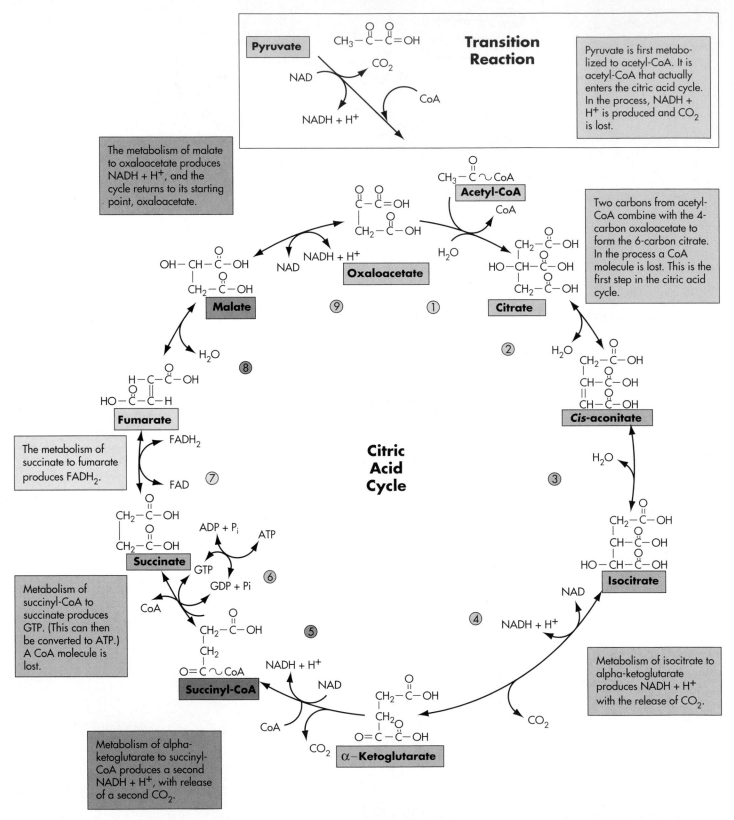

Figure C-2 Detailed depiction of conversion of pyruvate to acetyl-CoA in the transition reaction and the individual chemical reactions of the citric acid cycle. Conversion of pyruvate to acetyl-CoA uses an enzyme complex that includes pyruvate dehydrogenase. The enzymes used in the citric acid cycle at the following steps are (1) citrate synthase, (2) aconitase, (3) aconitase, (4) isocitrate dehydrogenase, (5) alpha-ketoglutarate dehydrogenase, (6) succinate thiokinase, (7) succinate dehydrogenase, (8) fumarase, and (9) malate dehydrogenase. *CoA* stands for coenzyme A, which is made from the vitamin pantothenic acid (see Chapter 12 for the chemical structure). Note that the CO_2 molecules lost during 1 turn of the citric acid cycle are not those from the carbons donated by acetyl-CoA. Instead, the carbons are broken off the portion of the citrate molecule derived from oxaloacetate.

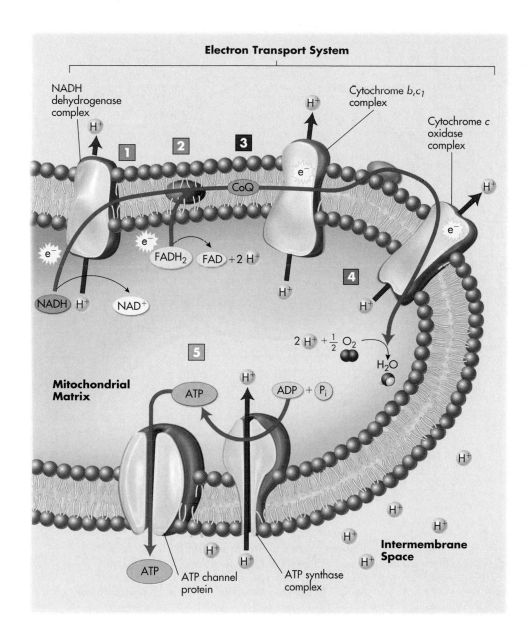

Electron Transport System

Figure C-3 Organization of the electron transport chain. As electrons move from 1 molecular complex to the other, hydrogen ions (H^+) are pumped from the mitochondrial matrix into the intermembrane space (Steps 1–4). (Each mitochondrion has an inner and an outer membrane.) As hydrogen ions flow down a concentration gradient from the intermembrane space into the mitochondrial matrix, ATP is synthesized by the enzyme ATP synthase (Step 5). ATP leaves the mitochondrial matrix by way of a channel protein.

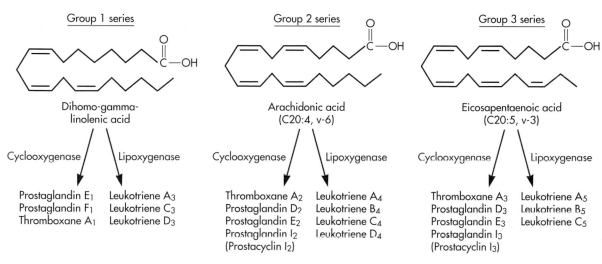

Group 1 series		Group 2 series		Group 3 series	
Dihomo-gamma-linolenic acid		Arachidonic acid (C20:4, v-6)		Eicosapentaenoic acid (C20:5, v-3)	
Cyclooxygenase	Lipoxygenase	Cyclooxygenase	Lipoxygenase	Cyclooxygenase	Lipoxygenase
Prostaglandin E_1	Leukotriene A_3	Thromboxane A_2	Leukotriene A_4	Thromboxane A_3	Leukotriene A_5
Prostaglandin F_1	Leukotriene C_3	Prostaglandin D_2	Leukotriene B_4	Prostaglandin D_3	Leukotriene B_5
Thromboxane A_1	Leukotriene D_3	Prostaglandin E_2	Leukotriene C_4	Prostaglandin E_3	Leukotriene C_5
		Prostaglandin I_2 (Prostacyclin I_2)	Leukotriene D_4	Prostaglandin I_3 (Prostacyclin I_3)	

Figure C-4 Examples of eicosanoids from the 3 major groups. The parent fatty acid produces profound difference in how eicosanoids across the 3 groups act in the body (e.g., thromboxane A_1 vs. A_2 vs. A_3).

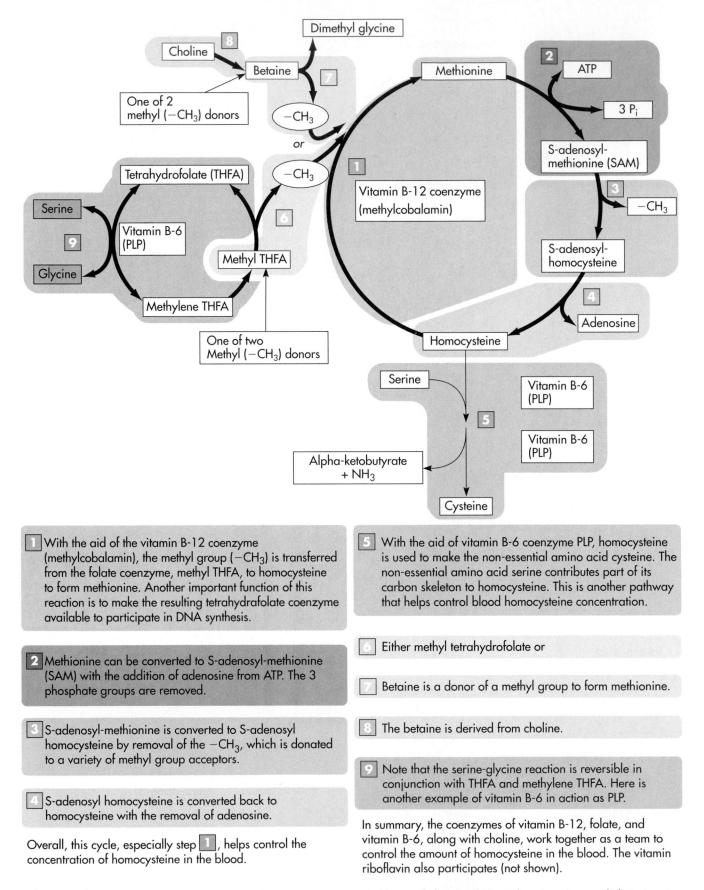

1. With the aid of the vitamin B-12 coenzyme (methylcobalamin), the methyl group (−CH₃) is transferred from the folate coenzyme, methyl THFA, to homocysteine to form methionine. Another important function of this reaction is to make the resulting tetrahydrafolate coenzyme available to participate in DNA synthesis.

2. Methionine can be converted to S-adenosyl-methionine (SAM) with the addition of adenosine from ATP. The 3 phosphate groups are removed.

3. S-adenosyl-methionine is converted to S-adenosyl homocysteine by removal of the −CH₃, which is donated to a variety of methyl group acceptors.

4. S-adenosyl homocysteine is converted back to homocysteine with the removal of adenosine.

Overall, this cycle, especially step 1, helps control the concentration of homocysteine in the blood.

5. With the aid of vitamin B-6 coenzyme PLP, homocysteine is used to make the non-essential amino acid cysteine. The non-essential amino acid serine contributes part of its carbon skeleton to homocysteine. This is another pathway that helps control blood homocysteine concentration.

6. Either methyl tetrahydrofolate or

7. Betaine is a donor of a methyl group to form methionine.

8. The betaine is derived from choline.

9. Note that the serine-glycine reaction is reversible in conjunction with THFA and methylene THFA. Here is another example of vitamin B-6 in action as PLP.

In summary, the coenzymes of vitamin B-12, folate, and vitamin B-6, along with choline, work together as a team to control the amount of homocysteine in the blood. The vitamin riboflavin also participates (not shown).

Figure C-5 Detailed diagram of folate, vitamin B-12, vitamin B-6, and choline metabolism in relation to homocysteine metabolism. Step 9 (serine → glycine) is the major source of methyl groups for this overall pathway.

Appendix D

DIETARY ADVICE FOR CANADIANS

The information in this appendix includes advice on dietary patterns as well as regulations that apply to food labeling. Previous **Recommended Nutrient Intakes (RNIs)** for nutrients have been replaced by the Dietary Reference Intakes (DRIs) that apply to Canadian and U.S. citizens. These are listed on the back inside cover. Both Canadian and American scientists worked on the various DRI committees, creating a set of harmonized DRIs for both countries.

> **Recommended Nutrient Intake (RNI)** Canadian version of RDA published in 1990.

Summary of the Nutrition Recommendations for Canadians

The latest Nutrition Recommendations of the Scientific Review Committee of the Office of Nutrition Policy and Promotion suggest that the Canadian diet should supply

- Essential nutrients in the amounts specified in the updated RNIs
- Sufficient energy to maintain a healthy weight when balanced with physical activity (energy intakes for adults should not be lower than 1800 kilocalories in order to meet RNIs)
- No more than 30% of energy as fat and no more than 10% of energy as saturated fat
- At least 55% energy as carbohydrates
- Less sodium than is now used
- No more than 5% of energy as alcohol, or 2 drinks per day (whichever is less), with no alcohol during pregnancy
- No more caffeine than the equivalent of 4 regular cups of coffee per day
- Water containing no less than 1 mg/liter of fluoride

> ► Resources for Canadians are Health Canada (**www. hc-sc.gc.ca**), Dietitians of Canada (**www.dietitians.ca**), and the National Institute of Nutrition (**www. nin.ca**).

In essence, suggested actions toward healthful eating as listed in Canada's Guidelines for Healthy Eating include the following:

- Enjoy a variety of foods.
- Emphasize cereals, breads, other grain products, vegetables, and fruit.
- Choose lower-fat dairy products, leaner meats, and foods prepared with little or no fat.
- Achieve and maintain a healthful body weight by enjoying regular physical activity and healthy eating.
- Limit salt, alcohol, and caffeine.

Canada's Food Guide is a guide to help Canadians make wise food choices (Fig. D-1). The rainbow side of the Food Guide places foods into 4 groups: vegetables and fruit; grain products; milk products; and meat and meat alternatives. The rainbow includes information about the types of foods to choose from each food group for healthy eating. *Canada's Food Guide* also provides recommended servings per day, dietary advice for different age groups, and physical activity recommendations.

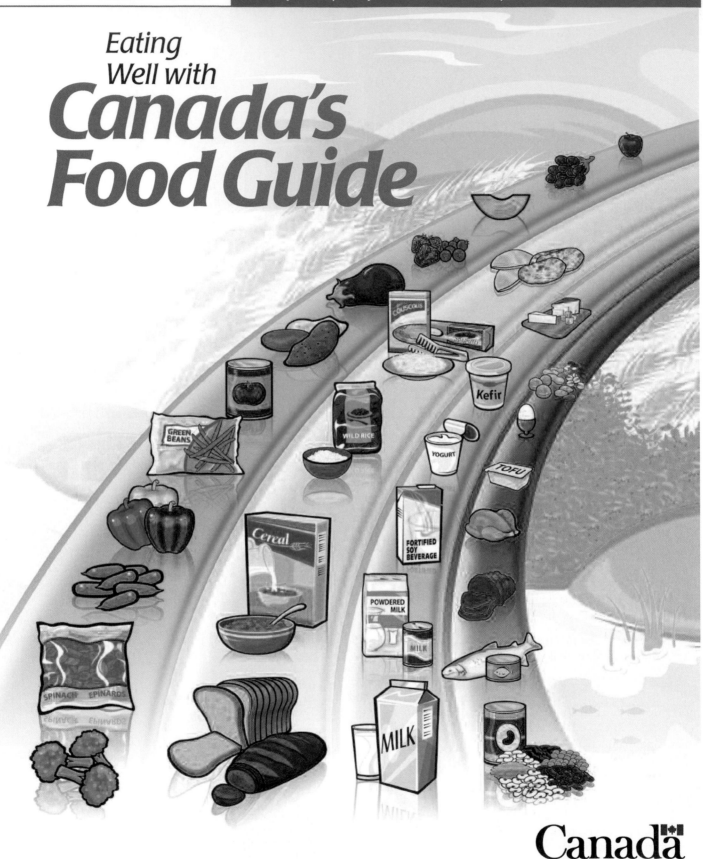

Figure D-1 Canada's Food Guide.

Recommended Number of *Food Guide Servings* per Day

	Children			Teens		Adults			
Age in Years	2-3	4-8	9-13	14-18		19-50		51+	
Sex	Girls and Boys			Females	Males	Females	Males	Females	Males
Vegetables and Fruit	4	5	6	7	8	7-8	8-10	7	7
Grain Products	3	4	6	6	7	6-7	8	6	7
Milk and Alternatives	2	2	3-4	3-4	3-4	2	2	3	3
Meat and Alternatives	1	1	1-2	2	3	2	3	2	3

The chart above shows how many Food Guide Servings you need from each of the four food groups every day.

Having the amount and type of food recommended and following the tips in *Canada's Food Guide* will help:

- Meet your needs for vitamins, minerals and other nutrients.
- Reduce your risk of obesity, type 2 diabetes, heart disease, certain types of cancer and osteoporosis.
- Contribute to your overall health and vitality.

What is One Food Guide Serving?
Look at the examples below.

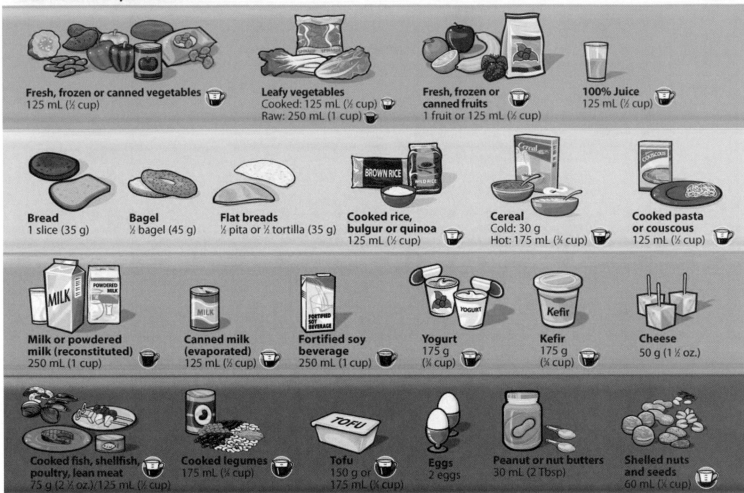

Fresh, frozen or canned vegetables
125 mL (½ cup)

Leafy vegetables
Cooked: 125 mL (½ cup)
Raw: 250 mL (1 cup)

Fresh, frozen or canned fruits
1 fruit or 125 mL (½ cup)

100% Juice
125 mL (½ cup)

Bread
1 slice (35 g)

Bagel
½ bagel (45 g)

Flat breads
½ pita or ½ tortilla (35 g)

Cooked rice, bulgur or quinoa
125 mL (½ cup)

Cereal
Cold: 30 g
Hot: 175 mL (¾ cup)

Cooked pasta or couscous
125 mL (½ cup)

Milk or powdered milk (reconstituted)
250 mL (1 cup)

Canned milk (evaporated)
125 mL (½ cup)

Fortified soy beverage
250 mL (1 cup)

Yogurt
175 g
(¾ cup)

Kefir
175 g
(¾ cup)

Cheese
50 g (1 ½ oz.)

Cooked fish, shellfish, poultry, lean meat
75 g (2 ½ oz.)/125 mL (½ cup)

Cooked legumes
175 mL (¾ cup)

Tofu
150 g or
175 mL (¾ cup)

Eggs
2 eggs

Peanut or nut butters
30 mL (2 Tbsp)

Shelled nuts and seeds
60 mL (¼ cup)

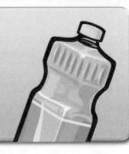

Oils and Fats
- Include a small amount – 30 to 45 mL (2 to 3 Tbsp) – of unsaturated fat each day. This includes oil used for cooking, salad dressings, margarine and mayonnaise.
- Use vegetable oils such as canola, olive and soybean.
- Choose soft margarines that are low in saturated and trans fats.
- Limit butter, hard margarine, lard and shortening.

Make each Food Guide Serving count...
wherever you are – at home, at school, at work or when eating out!

▸ **Eat at least one dark green and one orange vegetable each day.**
- Go for dark green vegetables such as broccoli, romaine lettuce and spinach.
- Go for orange vegetables such as carrots, sweet potatoes and winter squash.

▸ **Choose vegetables and fruit prepared with little or no added fat, sugar or salt.**
- Enjoy vegetables steamed, baked or stir-fried instead of deep-fried.

▸ **Have vegetables and fruit more often than juice.**

▸ **Make at least half of your grain products whole grain each day.**
- Eat a variety of whole grains such as barley, brown rice, oats, quinoa and wild rice.
- Enjoy whole grain breads, oatmeal or whole wheat pasta.

▸ **Choose grain products that are lower in fat, sugar or salt.**
- Compare the Nutrition Facts table on labels to make wise choices.
- Enjoy the true taste of grain products. When adding sauces or spreads, use small amounts.

▸ **Drink skim, 1%, or 2% milk each day.**
- Have 500 mL (2 cups) of milk every day for adequate vitamin D.
- Drink fortified soy beverages if you do not drink milk.

▸ **Select lower fat milk alternatives.**
- Compare the Nutrition Facts table on yogurts or cheeses to make wise choices.

▸ **Have meat alternatives such as beans, lentils and tofu often.**

▸ **Eat at least two Food Guide Servings of fish each week.***
- Choose fish such as char, herring, mackerel, salmon, sardines and trout.

▸ **Select lean meat and alternatives prepared with little or no added fat or salt.**
- Trim the visible fat from meats. Remove the skin on poultry.
- Use cooking methods such as roasting, baking or poaching that require little or no added fat.
- If you eat luncheon meats, sausages or prepackaged meats, choose those lower in salt (sodium) and fat.

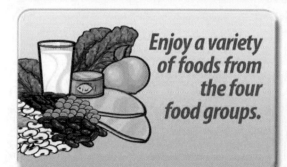

Enjoy a variety of foods from the four food groups.

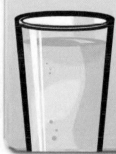

Satisfy your thirst with water!

Drink water regularly. It's a calorie-free way to quench your thirst. Drink more water in hot weather or when you are very active.

* Health Canada provides advice for limiting exposure to mercury from certain types of fish. Refer to www.healthcanada.gc.ca for the latest information.

Advice for different ages and stages...

Children

Following *Canada's Food Guide* helps children grow and thrive.

Young children have small appetites and need calories for growth and development.

- Serve small nutritious meals and snacks each day.
- Do not restrict nutritious foods because of their fat content. Offer a variety of foods from the four food groups.
- Most of all... be a good role model.

Women of childbearing age

All women who could become pregnant and those who are pregnant or breastfeeding need a multivitamin containing **folic acid** every day. Pregnant women need to ensure that their multivitamin also contains **iron**. A health care professional can help you find the multivitamin that's right for you.

Pregnant and breastfeeding women need more calories. Include an extra 2 to 3 Food Guide Servings each day.

Here are two examples:
- Have fruit and yogurt for a snack, or
- Have an extra slice of toast at breakfast and an extra glass of milk at supper.

Men and women over 50

The need for **vitamin D** increases after the age of 50.

In addition to following *Canada's Food Guide*, everyone over the age of 50 should take a daily vitamin D supplement of 10 µg (400 IU).

How do I count Food Guide Servings in a meal?

Here is an example:

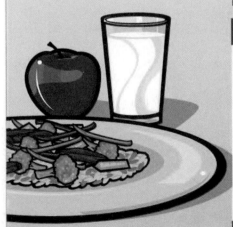

Vegetable and beef stir-fry with rice, a glass of milk and an apple for dessert		
250 mL (1 cup) mixed broccoli, carrot and sweet red pepper	=	2 **Vegetables and Fruit** Food Guide Servings
75 g (2 ½ oz.) lean beef	=	1 **Meat and Alternatives** Food Guide Serving
250 mL (1 cup) brown rice	=	2 **Grain Products** Food Guide Servings
5 mL (1 tsp) canola oil	=	part of your **Oils and Fats** intake for the day
250 mL (1 cup) 1% milk	=	1 **Milk and Alternatives** Food Guide Serving
1 apple	=	1 **Vegetables and Fruit** Food Guide Serving

Eat well and be active today and every day!

The benefits of eating well and being active include:

- Better overall health.
- Feeling and looking better.
- Lower risk of disease.
- More energy.
- A healthy body weight.
- Stronger muscles and bones.

Be active

To be active every day is a step towards better health and a healthy body weight.

Canada's Physical Activity Guide recommends building 30 to 60 minutes of moderate physical activity into daily life for adults and at least 90 minutes a day for children and youth. You don't have to do it all at once. Add it up in periods of at least 10 minutes at a time for adults and five minutes at a time for children and youth.

Start slowly and build up.

Eat well

Another important step towards better health and a healthy body weight is to follow *Canada's Food Guide* by:

- Eating the recommended amount and type of food each day.
- Limiting foods and beverages high in calories, fat, sugar or salt (sodium) such as cakes and pastries, chocolate and candies, cookies and granola bars, doughnuts and muffins, ice cream and frozen desserts, french fries, potato chips, nachos and other salty snacks, alcohol, fruit flavoured drinks, soft drinks, sports and energy drinks, and sweetened hot or cold drinks.

Read the label

- Compare the Nutrition Facts table on food labels to choose products that contain less fat, saturated fat, trans fat, sugar and sodium.
- Keep in mind that the calories and nutrients listed are for the amount of food found at the top of the Nutrition Facts table.

Nutrition Facts

Per 0 mL (0 g)

Amount	% Daily Value
Calories 0	
Fat 0 g	0 %
Saturates 0 g	0 %
+ Trans 0 g	
Cholesterol 0 mg	
Sodium 0 mg	0 %
Carbohydrate 0 g	0 %
Fibre 0 g	0 %
Sugars 0 g	
Protein 0 g	

Vitamin A	0 %	Vitamin C	0 %
Calcium	0 %	Iron	0 %

Limit trans fat

When a Nutrition Facts table is not available, ask for nutrition information to choose foods lower in trans and saturated fats.

Take a step today...

✓ Have breakfast every day. It may help control your hunger later in the day.

✓ Walk wherever you can – get off the bus early, use the stairs.

✓ Benefit from eating vegetables and fruit at all meals and as snacks.

✓ Spend less time being inactive such as watching TV or playing computer games.

✓ Request nutrition information about menu items when eating out to help you make healthier choices.

✓ Enjoy eating with family and friends!

✓ Take time to eat and savour every bite!

For more information, interactive tools, or additional copies visit Canada's Food Guide on-line at:
www.healthcanada.gc.ca/foodguide

or contact:

Publications
Health Canada
Ottawa, Ontario K1A 0K9
E-Mail: publications@hc-sc.gc.ca
Tel.: 1-866-225-0709
Fax: (613) 941-5366
TTY: 1-800-267-1245

Également disponible en français sous le titre :
Bien manger avec le Guide alimentaire canadien

This publication can be made available on request on diskette, large print, audio-cassette and braille.

Recommended Daily Intakes and Reference Standards

Following are the **Recommended Daily Intakes** and **Reference Standards** used on Nutrition Labels for persons 2 years of age and older.[*][†][‡]

Dietary Constituent	Amount	Dietary Constituent	Amount
Fat	**65 g**	Folacin	220 µg
Sum of saturated fatty	Vitamin B_{12}	2 µg	
acids and *trans* fatty acids	**20 g**	Pantothenic acid or	
Cholesterol	**300 mg**	pantothenate	7 mg
Carbohydrate	**300 g**	Vitamin K	**80 mg**
Fibre	**25 g**	Biotin	**30 µg**
Sodium	**2400 mg**	Calcium	1100 mg
Chloride	**3400 µg**	Phosphorus	1100 mg
Potassium	**3500 mg**	Magnesium	250 mg
Vitamin A	1000 RE	Iron	14 mg
Vitamin D	5 µg	Zinc	9 mg
Vitamin E	10 mg	Iodide	160 µg
Vitamin C	60 mg	Selenium	**50 µg**
Thiamin, or vitamin B_1	1.3 mg	Copper	**2 mg**
Riboflavin or vitamin B_2	1.6 mg	Manganese	**2 mg**
Niacin	23 NE	Chromium	**120 µg**
Vitamin B_6	1.8 mg	Molybdenum	**75 µg**

[*]RE = retinol equivalents
[†]NE = niacin equivalents
[‡]Together, these constitute the Daily Values used on the new Canadian Nutrition Label. Reference Standards are bolded.

Approved Nutrient Content Claims for Food Labels

The following is a sample of approved nutrient content claims for food labels.

Energy

- *Free of energy:* The food provides less than 5 Calories or 21 kilojoules per reference amount and serving of stated size.
- *Low in energy:* The food provides 40 Calories or 167 kilojoules or less per reference amount and serving of stated size.
- *Reduced in energy:* The food is processed, formulated, reformulated, or otherwise modified so that it provides at least 25% less energy per reference amount of a similar food.
- *Lower in energy:* The food provides at least 25% less energy per reference amount of a similar food.
- *Source of energy:* The food provides at least 100 Calories or 420 kilojoules per reference amount and serving of stated size.
- *More energy:* The food provides at least 25% more energy, totalling at least 100 more Calories or 420 more kilojoules per reference amount of a similar food.

Protein

- *Low in protein:* The food contains no more than 1 g of protein per 100 g of the food.
- *Source of protein:* The food has a protein rating of 20 or more, as determined by official method FO-1, *Determination of Protein Rating,* October 15, 1981, (*a*) per reasonable daily intake; or (*b*) per 30 g combined with 125 mL of milk, if the food is a breakfast cereal.
- *Excellent source of protein:* The food has a protein rating of 40 or more, as determined by official method FO-1, *Determination of Protein Rating,* October 15, 1981, (*a*) per

reasonable daily intake; or (*b*) per 30 g combined with 125 mL of milk, if the food is a breakfast cereal.

- *More protein:* The food (*a*) has a protein rating of 20 or more, as determined by official method FO-1, *Determination of Protein Rating,* October 15, 1981, (i) per reasonable daily intake, or (ii) per 30 g combined with 125 mL of milk, if the food is a breakfast cereal; and (*b*) contains at least 25% more protein, totalling at least 7 g more, per reasonable daily intake compared to the reference food of the same food group or the similar reference food.

Fat

- *Free of fat:* The food contains less than 0.5 g of fat per reference amount and serving of stated size.
- *Low in fat:* The food contains 3 g or less of fat per reference amount and serving of stated size and, if the reference amount is 30 g or 30 mL or less, per 50 g.
- *Reduced in fat:* The food is processed, formulated, reformulated, or otherwise modified so that it contains at least 25% less fat than the reference amount of a similar food.
- *Lower in fat:* The food contains at least 25% less fat per reference amount of the food, than the reference amount of the reference food of the same food group.
- *100% fat-free:* The food (*a*) contains less than 0.5 g of fat per 100 g; (*b*) contains no added fat.
- *No added fat:* (1) The food contains no added fats or oils set out in Division 9, or added butter or ghee, or ingredients that contain added fats or oils, or butter or ghee.
- *Free of saturated fatty acids:* The food contains less than 0.2 g saturated fatty acids and less than 0.2 g *trans* fatty acids per reference amount and serving of stated size.
- *Low in saturated fatty acids:* (1) The food contains 2 g or less of saturated fatty acids and *trans* fatty acids combined per reference amount and serving of stated size. (2) The food provides 15% or less energy from the sum of saturated fatty acids and *trans* fatty acids.
- *Reduced in saturated fatty acids:* The food is processed, formulated, reformulated, or otherwise modified, without increasing the content of *trans* fatty acids, so that it contains at least 25% less saturated fatty acids per reference amount of the food than the reference amount of the similar reference food.
- *Lower in saturated fatty acids:* The food contains at least 25% less saturated fatty acids and the content of *trans* fatty acids is not higher per reference amount of the food, than the reference amount of the reference food of the same food group.
- *Free of* trans *fatty acids:* The food contains less than 0.2 g of *trans* fatty acids per reference amount and serving of stated size.
- *Reduced in* trans *fatty acids:* The food is processed, formulated, reformulated, or otherwise modified, without increasing the content of saturated fatty acids, so that it contains at least 25% less *trans* fatty acids per reference amount of the food than the reference amount of the similar reference food.
- *Lower in* trans *fatty acids:* The food contains at least 25% less *trans* fatty acids and the content of saturated fatty acids is not higher per reference amount of the food compared to the reference amount of a similar food.
- *Source of omega-3 polyunsaturated fatty acids:* The food contains 0.3 g or more of omega-3 polyunsaturated fatty acids per reference amount and serving of stated size.
- *Source of omega-6 polyunsaturated fatty acids:* The food contains 2 g or more of omega-6 polyunsaturated fatty acids per reference amount and serving of stated size.

Cholesterol

- *Free of cholesterol:* The food contains less than 2 mg of cholesterol per reference amount and serving of stated size.
- *Low in cholesterol:* The food contains 20 mg or less of cholesterol per reference amount and serving of stated size (if the reference amount is 30 g or 30 mL or less, per 50 g.)

- *Reduced in cholesterol:* The food is processed, formulated, reformulated, or otherwise modified so that it contains at least 25% less cholesterol per reference amount of a similar food.
- *Lower in cholesterol:* The food contains at least 25% less cholesterol per reference amount of a similar food.

Sodium or Salt

- *Free of sodium or salt:* The food contains less than 5 mg of sodium per reference amount and serving of stated size.
- *Low in sodium or salt:* The food contains 140 mg or less of sodium per reference amount and serving of stated size.
- *Reduced in sodium or salt:* (1) The food is processed, formulated, reformulated, or otherwise modified so that it contains at least 25% less sodium per reference amount of a similar food.
- *Lower in sodium or salt:* The food contains at least 25% less sodium per reference amount of the food.
- *No added sodium or salt:* The food contains no added salt, other sodium salts, or ingredients that contain sodium that functionally substitute for added salt.
- *Lightly salted:* The food contains at least 50% less added sodium than the sodium added to a similar reference food.

Sugars

- *Free of sugars:* The food contains less than 0.5 mg of sugars per reference amount and serving of stated size.
- *Reduced in sugars:* The food is processed, formulated, reformulated, or otherwise modified so that it contains at least 25% less sugars, totalling at least 5 g less per reference amount of the food.
- *Lower in sugars:* The food contains at least 25% less sugars, totalling at least 5 g less per reference amount of the food.
- *No added sugars:* (1) The food contains no added sugars, no ingredients containing added sugars, or ingredients that contain sugars that functionally substitute for added sugars.

Fibre

- *Source of fibre:* (1) The food contains 2 g or more (*a*) of fibre per reference amount and serving of stated size, if no fibre or fibre source is identified in the statement or claim; or (*b*) of each identified fibre or fibre from an identified fibre source per reference amount and serving of stated size, if a fibre or fibre source is identified in the statement or claim.
- *High source of fibre:* The food contains 4 g or more (*a*) of fibre per reference amount and serving of stated size, if no fibre or fibre source is identified in the statement or claim; or (*b*) of each identified fibre or fibre from an identified fibre source per reference amount and serving of stated size, if a fibre or fibre source is identified in the statement or claim.
- *Very high source of fibre:* The food contains 6 g or more (*a*) of fibre per reference amount and serving of stated size, if no fibre or fibre source is identified in the statement or claim; or (*b*) of each identified fibre or fibre from an identified fibre source per reference amount and serving of stated size, if a fibre or fibre source is identified in the statement or claim.
- *More fibre:* The food contains at least 25% more fibre, totalling at least 1 g more, if no fibre or fibre source is identified in the statement or claim, or at least 25% more of an identified fibre or fibre from an identified fibre source, totalling at least 1 g more, if a fibre or fibre source is identified in the statement or claim compared to reference amount of a similar food.

Light and Lean

- *Light in energy or fat:* The food meets the conditions set out for the subject "reduced in energy" or "reduced in fat."
- *Lean:* The food (*a*) is meat or poultry that has not been ground, a marine or fresh water animal, or a product of any of these; and (*b*) contains 10% or less fat.
- *Extra lean:* The food (*a*) is meat or poultry that has not been ground, a marine or fresh water animal, or a product of any of these; and (*b*) contains 7.5% or less fat.

Approved Health Claims for Nutrition Labels

If a manufacturer follows specific guidelines addressing both the nutrients noted in the claim as well as guidelines pertaining to other nutrients in a food, the following health claims can be made.

- A healthy diet containing foods high in potassium and low in sodium may reduce the risk of high blood pressure, a risk factor for stroke and heart disease.
- A healthy diet with adequate calcium and vitamin D, and regular physical activity, helps achieve strong bones and may reduce the risk of osteoporosis.
- A healthy diet low in saturated and *trans* fats may reduce the risk of heart disease.
- A healthy diet rich in a variety of vegetables and fruit may help reduce the risk of some types of cancer.
- Foods very low in starch and fermentable sugars can make the following health claims:
  - Won't cause cavities
  - Does not promote tooth decay
  - Does not promote dental caries
  - Is non-carciogenic

Appendix E

THE EXCHANGE SYSTEM AND LISTS: A HELPFUL MENU PLANNING TOOL

Exchange System System for classifying foods into numerous lists based on the foods' macronutrient composition and establishing serving sizes, so that 1 serving of each food on a list contains the same amount of carbohydrate, protein, fat, and energy content.

exchange Serving size of a food on a specific exchange list.

The **Exchange System** is a valuable tool for roughly estimating the energy, protein, carbohydrate, and fat content of a food or meal. This tool organizes many details of the nutrient composition of foods into a manageable framework. By using the Exchange System, you can plan daily menus to fall roughly within specific percentages of macronutrients without having to look up or memorize the nutrient values of numerous foods, so the time you spend now becoming familiar with the Exchange System will pay dividends in the future.

In the Exchange System, individual foods are placed into 3 broad groups: carbohydrate, meat and meat substitutes, and fat. Within these groups are lists of foods of similar macronutrient composition: various types of milk, fruits, vegetables, starch, other carbohydrates, meat and meat substitutes, and fat. These lists are designed so that, when the correct serving size is used, each food on a list provides about the same amount of carbohydrate, protein, fat, and energy. This equality allows the exchange of foods on each list, hence the term *Exchange System*.

The Exchange System was originally developed for planning diabetic diets. Diabetes is easier to control if the person's diet has about the same composition day after day. If a certain number of **exchanges** from each of the various lists is eaten each day, that regularity is easier to achieve. However, because the Exchange System provides a quick way to estimate the energy, carbohydrate, protein, and fat content in any food or meal, it is a valuable menu planning tool.

Becoming Familiar with the Exchange System

To use the Exchange System, you must know which foods are on each list and the serving sizes for each food. Table E-1 gives the serving sizes for foods on each exchange list as well as the carbohydrate, protein, fat, and energy content per exchange. Note that the meat and milk lists are divided into subclasses, which vary in fat content and, hence, in the amount of energy they provide. Foods on the meat and fat lists contain essentially no carbohydrate; those on the fruit and fat lists lack appreciable amounts of protein; and those on the vegetable, fruit, and other carbohydrates lists contain essentially no fat. You need to study Table E-1 and Figure E-1 to become familiar with the exchange lists, the sizes of the exchanges (that is, serving sizes) on each list, and the amounts of carbohydrate, protein, fat, and energy per exchange.

Before you can turn a group of exchanges into a daily meal plan, you must be aware of which foods are on each exchange list (see Fig. E-1). The entire U.S. Exchange System is presented in this appendix, which you should consult frequently while exploring the system to discover its various peculiarities. For example, the starch list includes not only bread, dry cereal, cooked cereal, rice, and pasta but also baked beans, corn on the cob, and potatoes. These foods are not identical to those composing the grain group in MyPyramid.

Table E-1 Nutrient Composition of Exchange System Lists (2003 Edition)

Groups/Lists	Household Measures*	Carbohydrate (g)	Protein (g)	Fat (g)	Energy (kcal)
Carbohydrate Group					
Starch	1 slice, ¾ cup raw, or ½ cup cooked	15	3	1 or less†	80
Fruit	1 small/medium piece	15	—	—	60
Milk	1 cup				
Fat-free/very low fat		12	8	0–3†	90
Reduced-fat		12	8	5	120
Whole		12	8	8	150
Other carbohydrates	Varies	15	Varies	Varies	Varies
Nonstarchy vegetables	1 cup raw or ½ cup cooked	5	2	—	25
Meat and Meat Substitutes Group	**1 oz**				
Very lean		—	7	0–1	35
Lean		—	7	3	55
Medium-fat		—	7	5	75
High-fat		—	7	8	100
Fat Group	**1 tsp**	—	—	**5**	**45**

Reproduction of the exchange lists in whole or in part, without permission of The American Dietetic Association or the American Diabetes Association, Inc. is a violation of federal law. This material has been modified from *Exchange Lists for Meal Planning,* which is the basis of a meal planning system designed by a committee of the American Diabetes Association and The American Dietetic Association. While designed primarily for people with diabetes and others who must follow special diets, the exchange lists are based on principles of good nutrition that apply to everyone. Copyright © 2003 by the American Diabetes Association and the American Dietetic Association.

*Just an estimate; see exchange lists for actual amounts.

†Calculated as 1 g for purposes of energy contribution.

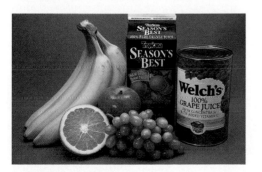

Starch exchange choices

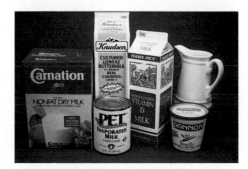

Meat and meat substitute exchange choices

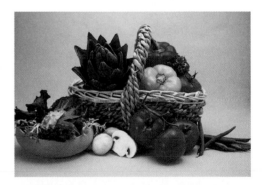

Vegetable exchange choices

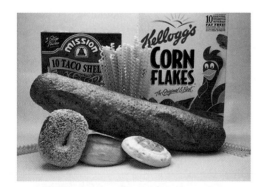

Fruit exchange choices

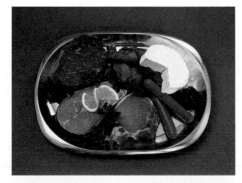

Milk exchange choices

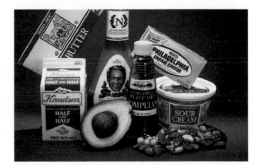

Fat exchange choices

Figure E-1 Foods arranged according to the Exchange System lists.

The Exchange System is not concerned with the origin of a food, whether animal or vegetable. It is primarily concerned with the macronutrients carbohydrate, protein, and fat in each food on a specific list. For example, the carbohydrate composition of potatoes resembles that of bread more than that of broccoli, although potatoes are vegetables. In addition, several foods on the meat and meat substitutes list are not meats. The list of other carbohydrates includes jam, angel food cake, fat-free frozen yogurt, and foods, such as frosted cake, that count as both other carbohydrate exchanges and fat exchanges. Bacon appears in the fat list rather than the high-fat meat category.

Free foods (essentially calorie-free) include bouillon, diet soda, coffee, tea, dill pickles, and vinegar, as well as herbs and spices. Most vegetables, such as cabbage, celery, mushrooms, lettuce, and zucchini, also can be considered free foods; their minimal energy contribution need not count in the calculations when they are eaten in moderation (1 to 2 servings per meal or snack).

Using the Exchange System to Develop Daily Menus

Use the Exchange System to plan a 1-day menu. Target an energy content of 2000 kcal, with 55% derived from carbohydrates (1100 kcal), 15% from protein (300 kcal), and 30% from fat (600 kcal). These specifications can be translated into 2 low-fat milk exchanges, 3 vegetable exchanges, 5 fruit exchanges, 11 starch exchanges, 4 lean meat exchanges, and 6 fat exchanges (Table E-2). Note that this example is only 1 of many possible combinations; the Exchange System offers great flexibility.

Table E-3 arbitrarily separates these exchanges into breakfast, lunch, dinner, and a snack. Breakfast includes 1 reduced-fat milk exchange, 2 fruit exchanges, 2 starch exchanges, and 1 fat exchange. This total corresponds to ¾ cup of a ready-to-eat breakfast cereal, 1 cup of reduced-fat milk, 1 slice of bread with 1 tsp margarine, and 1 cup of orange juice.

Lunch consists of 2 fat exchanges, 4 starch exchanges, 1 vegetable exchange, 1 reduced-fat milk exchange, and 2 fruit exchanges. This total translates into 1 slice of bacon with 1 teaspoon of mayonnaise on 2 slices of bread, with tomato—in other words, a bacon and tomato sandwich. You also can add lettuce to the sandwich. Lettuce can be considered a free vegetable choice. Add to this meal a 9-inch banana (1 exchange = 1 small banana), 1 cup of reduced-fat milk, and 6 graham crackers (2½ inches by 2½ inches). Later, add a snack of ¾ oz of pretzels for another starch exchange.

Table E-2 Possible Exchange Patterns That Yield 55% of Energy as Carbohydrate, 30% as Fat, and 15% as Protein for Energy Intakes Greater Than 2000 kcal

kcal/Day Exchange List	1200*	1600*	2000	2400	2800	3200	3600
Milk (reduced-fat)	2	2	2	2	2	2	2
Vegetable	3	3	3	4	4	4	4
Fruit	3	4	5	6	8	9	9
Starch	5	8	11	13	15	18	21
Meat (lean)	4	4	4	5	6	7	8
Fat	2	4	6	8	10	11	13

This is just 1 set of options. More meat could be included if less milk were used, for example.

*Energy intakes of 1200 and 1600 kcal contain 20% of energy as protein and 50% energy as carbohydrate to allow for greater flexibility in diet planning.

Table E-3 Sample 1-Day 2000-kcal Menu Based on the Exchange System Plan*

Breakfast

1 reduced-fat milk exchange	1 cup reduced-fat milk (some on cereal)
2 fruit exchanges	1 cup orange juice
2 starch exchanges	¾ cup ready-to-eat breakfast cereal, 1 piece whole-wheat toast
1 fat exchange	1 tsp soft margarine on toast

Lunch

4 starch exchanges	2 slices whole-wheat bread, 6 graham crackers (2½ inches by 2½ inches)
2 fat exchanges	1 slice bacon, 1 tsp mayonnaise
1 vegetable exchange	1 sliced tomato
2 fruit exchanges	1 banana (9 inches)
1 reduced-fat milk exchange	1 cup reduced-fat milk

Snack

1 starch exchange	¾ oz pretzels

Dinner

4 lean meat exchanges	4 oz lean steak (well trimmed)
2 starch exchanges	1 medium baked potato
1 fat exchange	1 tsp soft margarine
2 vegetable exchanges	1 cup cooked broccoli
1 fruit exchange	1 kiwi fruit
	Coffee (if desired)

Snack

2 starch exchanges	1 bagel
2 fat exchanges	2 tbsp regular cream cheese

*The target plan was a 2000-kcal energy intake, with 55% from carbohydrate, 15% from protein, and 30% from fat. Computer analysis indicates that this menu yielded 2040 kcal, with 53% from carbohydrate, 16% from protein, and 31% from fat—in close agreement with the targeted goals.

Dinner consists of 4 lean meat exchanges, 1 fruit exchange, 2 vegetable exchanges, 1 fat exchange, and 2 starch exchanges. This total corresponds to a 4-oz broiled steak (meat only, no bone), 1 medium baked potato (1 exchange = 1 small baked potato) with 1 tsp of margarine, 1 cup of broccoli, and 1 kiwi fruit. Coffee (if desired) is not counted, because it contains no appreciable energy.

Finally, you can have a snack containing 2 starch exchanges and 2 fat exchanges. This total translates into 1 bagel with 2 tbsp of regular cream cheese.

This 1-day menu is only 1 of many that are possible with the exchange lists. Apple juice could replace the orange juice; 2 apples could be exchanged for the banana. The choices are endless. Notice that an exchange diet is much easier to plan if you use individual foods, as was done here; however, the Exchange System tables list some combination foods to help you. Using combination foods, such as pizza or lasagna, however, makes it more difficult to calculate the number of exchanges in a serving. For instance, lasagna typically has meat exchanges, vegetable exchanges, and starch exchanges. With practice, you will be able to tackle such complex foods (Fig. E-2). For now, using individual foods makes learning the Exchange System much easier. Finally, you might want to prove to yourself that the food choices listed in Table E-3 really meet the exchange plan. This demonstration will give you practice turning exchanges into actual food servings.

Figure E-2 Record the Exchange System pattern you have chosen in the left column. Then distribute the exchanges throughout the day, noting the food to be used and the serving size.

Exchange List	Total Exchanges to Be Consumed Daily	Exchanges Consumed at Each Meal		
		Breakfast	Lunch	Dinner
MILK				
VEGETABLE				
FRUIT				
STARCH				
MEAT AND SUBSTITUTES				
FAT				

Exchange System Lists*

Milk Exchange List

Fat-Free and Low-Fat Milk

(12 g carbohydrate, 8 g protein, 0–3 g fat, 90 kcal)

1 cup	fat-free, ½%, and 1% milk and buttermilk
⅓ cup	powdered (fat-free dry, before adding liquid)
½ cup	canned, evaporated fat-free milk
1 cup	buttermilk made from fat-free or low-fat milk
1 cup	soy milk (low-fat or fat-free)
⅔ cup (6 oz)	yogurt made from fat-free milk (plain, unflavored)
⅔ cup (6 oz)	yogurt, fat-free, flavored, sweetened with non-nutritive sweetener and fructose

*The exchange lists are the basis of a meal planning system designed by a committee of the American Diabetes Association and the American Dietetic Association. While designed primarily for people with diabetes and others who must follow special diets, the exchange lists are based on principles of good nutrition that apply to everyone. Copyright © 2003 by the American Diabetes Association and the American Dietetic Association.

Reduced-Fat Milk

(12 g carbohydrate, 8 g protein, 5 g fat, 120 kcal)

1 cup	2% milk
1 cup	soy milk
¾ cup	yogurt plain, low-fat (added milk solids)
1 cup	sweet acidophilus milk

Whole Milk

(12 g carbohydrate, 8 g protein, 8 g fat, 150 kcal)

1 cup	whole milk
½ cup	evaporated whole milk
1 cup	goat's milk
1 cup	kefir
1 cup	yogurt, plain (made from whole milk)

Non-Starchy Vegetable Exchange List

(5 g carbohydrate, 2 g protein, 0 g fat, 25 kcal)
1 vegetable exchange equals:

½ cup cooked vegetables or vegetable juice
1 cup raw vegetables

artichoke	carrots	mixed vegetables (without	sauerkraut
artichoke hearts	cauliflower	corn, peas, or pasta)	spinach
asparagus	celery	mushrooms	squash (summer)
beans (green, wax, Italian)	cucumber	okra	tomato (fresh, canned, sauce)
bean sprouts	eggplant	onions	tomato/vegetable juice
beets	green onions or scallions	pea pods	turnips
broccoli	greens (e.g., collard)	peppers (all varieties)	water chestnuts
Brussels sprouts	kohlrabi	radishes	watercress
cabbage	leeks	salad greens (all varieties)	zucchini

Fruit Exchange List

Fruit

(15 g carbohydrate, 0 g protein, 0 g fat, 60 kcal)
1 fruit exchange equals:

1 (4 oz)	apple, unpeeled (small)	4 (5½ oz)	apricots, fresh
4 rings	apple, dried	8 halves	apricots, dried
½ cup	applesauce (unsweetened)	½ cup	apricots, canned

1 (4 oz)	banana (small)	1 (5 oz)	nectarine (small)
¾ cup	blackberries	1 (6½ oz)	orange (small)
¾ cup	blueberries	½ (8 oz)	papaya (or 1 cup cubes)
⅓ melon (11 oz)	cantaloupe (small)	1 (4 oz)	peach, fresh (medium)
1 cup cubes	cantaloupe	½ cup	peaches, canned
12 (3 oz)	cherries	½ (4 oz)	pear, fresh
½ cup	cherries, canned	½ cup	pear, canned
3	dates	¾ cup	pineapple, fresh
2 (3½ oz)	figs, fresh (large)	½ cup	pineapple, canned
1½	figs, dried	2 (5 oz)	plums (small)
½ cup	fruit cocktail	½ cup	plums, canned
½ (11 oz)	grapefruit (large)	3	plums, dried (prunes)
¾ cup	grapefruit sections, canned	2 tbsp	raisins
17 (3 oz)	grapes (small)	1 cup	raspberries
1 slice (10 oz)	honeydew melon (or 1 cup cubes)	1¼ cups	strawberries (raw, whole)
1 (3½ oz)	kiwi	2 (8 oz)	tangerines (small)
¾ cup	mandarin orange sections	1 slice (13½ oz)	watermelon (or 1¼ cups cubes)
½ (5½ oz)	mango (or ½ cup)		

Fruit Juice

½ cup	apple juice/cider	½ cup	grapefruit juice
⅓ cup	cranberry juice cocktail	½ cup	orange juice
1 cup	cranberry juice cocktail, reduced-calorie	½ cup	pineapple juice
⅓ cup	fruit juice blends, 100% juice	⅓ cup	prune juice
⅓ cup	grape juice		

Starch Exchange List

(15 g carbohydrate, 3 g protein, 0–1 g fat, 80 kcal)
1 starch exchange equals:

Bread

¼ (1 oz)	bagel	½	pita, 6 inches across
2 slices (1½ oz)	bread, reduced-calorie	1 slice (1 oz)	raisin bread, unfrosted
1 slice (1 oz)	bread, white, whole-wheat, pumpernickel, or rye	1 (1 oz)	roll, plain (small)
4 (⅔ oz)	bread sticks, crisp, 4-inch × ½-inch	1	tortilla, corn, 6 inches across
½	English muffin	1	tortilla, flour, 6 inches across
½ (1 oz)	hot dog or hamburger bun	⅓	tortilla, flour, 10 inches across
¼	naan, 8-inch × 2 inch	1	waffle, 4 inches square or across, reduced-fat
1	pancake, 4 inches across × ¼ inch thick		

Cereals and Grains

½ cup	bran cereal	½ cup	kasha
½ cup	bulgur	⅓ cup	millet
½ cup	cereal, cooked	¼ cup	muesli
¾ cup	cereal, unsweetened, ready-to-eat	½ cup	oats
3 tbsp	cornmeal (dry)	⅓ cup	pasta
⅓ cup	couscous	1½ cups	puffed cereal
3 tbsp	flour (dry)	⅓ cup	rice, white or brown
¼ cup	granola, low-fat	½ cup	Shredded Wheat
¼ cup	Grape-Nuts	½ cup	sugar-frosted cereal
½ cup	grits	3 tbsp	wheat germ

Starchy Vegetables

⅓ cup	baked beans	½ cup or	potato, boiled
½ cup	corn	½ medium (3 oz)	
½ (5 oz)	corn on the cob (large)	¼ large (3 oz)	potato, baked with skin
1 cup	mixed vegetables with corn, peas, or pasta	½ cup	potato, mashed
½ cup	peas, green	1 cup	squash, winter (acorn, butternut, pumpkin)
½ cup	plantain	½ cup	yam, sweet potato, plain

Crackers and Snacks

8	animal crackers	¾ oz	pretzels
3	graham crackers, 2½-inch square	2	rice cakes, 4 inches across
¾ oz	matzoh	6	saltine-type crackers
4 slices	melba toast	15–20 (¾ oz)	snack chips, fat-free (tortilla, potato)
24	oyster crackers	2–5 (¾ oz)	whole-wheat crackers, no fat added
3 cups	popcorn (popped, no fat added or low-fat microwave)		

Dried Beans, Peas, and Lentils

(counts as 1 starch exchange plus 1 very lean meat exchange)

½ cup	beans and peas (garbanzo, pinto, kidney, white, split, black-eyed)	½ cup	lentils
		3 tbsp	miso
⅔ cup	lima beans		

Starchy Foods Prepared with Fat

(counts as 1 starch exchange plus 1 fat exchange)

1	biscuit, 2½ inches across	⅓ (1 oz)	muffin, 5 oz
½ cup	chow mein noodles	3 cups	popcorn, microwaved
1 (2 oz)	corn bread, 2-inch cube	3	sandwich crackers, cheese or peanut butter filling
6	crackers, round butter type		
1 cup	croutons	9–13 (¾ oz)	snack chips (potato, tortilla)
1 cup (2 oz)	french-fried potatoes (oven-baked) (see also the fast-foods list)	⅓ cup	stuffing, bread (prepared)
		2	taco shell, 6 inches across
¼ cup	granola	1	waffle, 4-inch square or across
⅕ cup	hummus	4–6 (1 oz)	whole-wheat crackers, fat added

Sweets, Desserts, and Other Carbohydrates Exchange List

One exchange equals 15 g carbohydrate, or 1 starch, or 1 fruit, or 1 milk.

Exchanges per Serving

1/12 th cake (about 2 oz)	angel food cake, unfrosted	2 carbohydrates
2-inch square (about 1 oz)	brownie, unfrosted (small)	1 carbohydrate, 1 fat
2-inch square (about 1 oz)	cake, unfrosted	1 carbohydrate, 1 fat
2-inch square (about 2 oz)	cake, frosted	2 carbohydrates, 1 fat
2	cookies, fat-free (small)	1 carbohydrate
2 (about ⅔ oz)	cookies or sandwich cookies with creme filling (small)	1 carbohydrate, 1 fat
¼ cup	cranberry sauce, jellied	1½ carbohydrates
1 (about 2 oz)	cupcake, frosted (small)	2 carbohydrates, 1 fat
1 (1½ oz)	doughnut, plain cake (medium)	1½ carbohydrates, 2 fats
3¾ inches across (2 oz)	doughnuts, glazed	2 carbohydrates, 2 fats
1 bar (1⅓ oz)	energy, sport or breakfast bar	2 carbohydrates, 1 fat
1 bar (2 oz)	energy, sport or breakfast bar	3 carbohydrates, 1 fat
½ cup (3½ oz)	fruit cobbler	3 carbohydrates, 1 fat
1 bar (3 oz)	fruit juice bars, frozen, 100% juice	1 carbohydrate

1 roll (¾ oz)	fruit snacks, chewy (puréed fruit concentrate)	1 carbohydrate
1 tbsp	honey	1 carbohydrate
1 tbsp	sugar	1 carbohydrate
1½ tbsp	fruit spread, 100% fruit	1 carbohydrate
½ cup	gelatin, regular	1 carbohydrate
3	gingersnaps	1 carbohydrate
1 bar (1 oz)	granola or snack bar (regular and low-fat)	1½ carbohydrates
½ cup	ice cream, low-fat	1½ carbohydrates
½ cup	ice cream	1 carbohydrate, 2 fats
½ cup	ice cream, light	1 carbohydrate, 1 fat
½ cup	ice cream, fat-free, no sugar added	1 carbohydrate
1 tbsp	jam or jelly, regular	1 carbohydrate
1 cup	milk, chocolate, whole	2 carbohydrates, 1 fat
⅙ pie	pie, fruit, 2 crusts (8 inches across)	3 carbohydrates, 2 fats
⅛ pie	pie, pumpkin or custard (8 inches across)	2 carbohydrates, 2 fats
½ cup	pudding, regular (made with reduced-fat milk)	2 carbohydrates
½ cup	pudding, sugar-free (made with fat-free milk)	1 carbohydrate
1 can (10–11 oz)	reduced-calorie meal replacement (shake)	1½ carbohydrates, 0–1 fat
1 cup	rice milk, low-fat or fat-free, plain	1 carbohydrate
1 cup	rice milk, low-fat, flavored	1½ carbohydrates
¼ cup	salad dressing, fat-free	1 carbohydrate
½ cup	sherbet, sorbet	2 carbohydrates
½ cup	spaghetti or pasta sauce, canned	1 carbohydrate, 1 fat
1 cup (8 oz)	sports drinks	1 carbohydrate
1 tbsp	sugar	1 carbohydrate
1 (2½ oz)	sweet roll or Danish	2½ carbohydrates, 2 fats
2 tbsp	syrup, light	1 carbohydrate
1 tbsp	syrup, regular	1 carbohydrate
5	vanilla wafers	1 carbohydrate, 1 fat
⅓ cup	yogurt, frozen, fat-free	1 carbohydrate
1 cup	yogurt, low-fat with fruit	3 carbohydrates, 0–1 fat

Meat and Meat Substitutes Exchange List

Very Lean Meat and Substitutes List

(0 g carbohydrate, 7 g protein, 0–1 g fat, and 35 kcal)
1 very lean meat exchange equals:

Poultry

1 oz   chicken or turkey (white meat, no skin), Cornish hen (no skin)

Fish

1 oz   fresh or frozen cod, flounder, haddock, halibut, trout; tuna, fresh or canned in water

Shellfish

1 oz   clams, crab, lobster, scallops, shrimp, imitation shellfish

Game

1 oz   duck or pheasant (no skin), venison, buffalo, ostrich

Cheese with 1 g or less fat per oz

¼ cup   fat-free or low-fat cottage cheese
1 oz   fat-free cheese

Other

1 oz   processed sandwich meats with 1 g or less fat per oz, such as deli thin, shaved meats, chipped beef, turkey, ham
2   egg whites
¼ cup   egg substitute, plain
1 oz   hot dogs with 1 g or less fat per oz
1 oz   kidney (high in cholesterol)
1 oz   sausage with 1 g or less fat per oz

Counts as 1 very lean meat and 1 starch exchange:

½ cup   dried beans, peas, lentils (cooked)

Lean Meat and Substitutes List

(0 g carbohydrate, 7 g protein, 3 g fat, and 55 kcal)
1 lean meat exchange equals:

	Beef
1 oz	USDA Select or Choice grades of lean beef trimmed of fat, such as round, sirloin, and flank steak; tenderloin; roast (rib, chuck, rump); steak (T-bone, porterhouse, cubed), ground round
	Pork
1 oz	lean pork, such as fresh ham; canned, cured, or boiled ham; Canadian bacon; tenderloin, center loin chop
	Lamb
1 oz	roast, chop, leg
	Veal
1 oz	lean chop, roast
	Poultry
1 oz	chicken, turkey (dark meat, no skin), chicken white meat (with skin), domestic duck or goose (well drained of fat, no skin)

	Fish
1 oz	herring (uncreamed or smoked)
6	oysters (medium)
1 oz	salmon (fresh or canned), catfish
2	sardines (canned, medium)
1 oz	tuna (canned in oil, drained)
	Game
1 oz	goose (no skin), rabbit
	Cheese
¼ cup	4.5%–fat cottage cheese
2 tbsp	grated Parmesan
1 oz	cheeses with 3 g or less fat per oz
	Other
1½ oz	hot dogs with 3 g or less fat per oz
1 oz	processed sandwich meat with 3 g or less fat per oz, such as turkey pastrami or kielbasa
1 oz	liver, heart (high in cholesterol)

Medium-Fat Meat and Substitutes List

(0 g carbohydrate, 7 g protein, 5 g fat, and 75 kcal)
1 medium-fat meat exchange equals:

	Beef
1 oz	most beef products (ground beef, meatloaf, corned beef, short ribs, prime grades of meat trimmed of fat, such as prime rib)
	Pork
1 oz	top loin, chop, Boston butt, cutlet
	Lamb
1 oz	rib roast, ground
	Veal
1 oz	cutlet (ground or cubed, unbreaded)
	Poultry
1 oz	chicken dark meat (with skin), ground turkey or ground chicken, fried chicken (with skin)

	Fish
1 oz	any fried fish product
	Cheese (with 5 g or less fat per oz)
1 oz	feta
1 oz	mozzarella
¼ cup (2 oz)	ricotta
	Other
1	egg (high in cholesterol, limit to 3 per week)
1 oz	sausage with 5 g or less fat per oz
¼ cup	tempeh
4 oz (½ cup)	tofu

High-Fat Meat and Substitutes List

(0 g carbohydrate, 7 g protein, 8 g fat, and 100 kcal)
1 high-fat meat exchange equals:

	Pork
1 oz	spareribs, ground pork, pork sausage
	Cheese
1 oz	all regular cheeses, such as American, cheddar, Monterey Jack, Swiss
	Other
1 oz	processed sandwich meats with 8 g or less fat per oz, such as bologna, pimento loaf, salami

1 oz	sausage, such as bratwurst, Italian, knockwurst, Polish, smoked
1	hot dog (turkey or chicken) (10 per pound)
3 slices	bacon (20 slices per pound)

Counts as 1 high-fat meat plus 1 fat exchange:

1	hot dog (beef, pork, or combination) (10 per pound)

Fat Exchange List

Monounsaturated Fats List

(5 g fat and 45 kcal)
1 exchange equals:

2 tbsp (1 oz)	avocado (medium)	6 nuts	almonds, cashews
1 tsp	oil (canola, olive, peanut)	6 nuts	mixed (50% peanuts)
	olives:	10 nuts	peanuts
8	ripe, black (large)	4 halves	pecans
10	green, stuffed (large)	½ tbsp	peanut butter, smooth or crunchy
		1 tbsp	sesame seeds
		2 tsp	tahini or sesame paste

Polyunsaturated Fats List

(5 g fat and 45 kcal)
1 exchange equals:

	margarine:		salad dressing:
1 tsp	stick, tub, or squeeze	1 tbsp	regular
1 tbsp	lower-fat (30 to 50% vegetable oil)	2 tbsp	reduced-fat
	mayonnaise:		Miracle Whip Salad Dressing:
1 tsp	regular	2 tsp	regular
1 tbsp	reduced-fat	1 tbsp	reduced-fat
4 halves	English walnuts	1 tbsp	seeds: pumpkin, sunflower
1 tsp	oil (corn, safflower, soybean)		

Saturated Fats List

(5 g fat and 45 kcal)
1 exchange equals:

1 slice	bacon, cooked (20 slices per pound)		butter:
1 tsp	bacon, grease	1 tsp	stick
2 tbsp (½ oz)	chitterlings, boiled	2 tsp	whipped
	cream cheese:	1 tbsp	reduced-fat
1 tbsp (½ oz)	regular		sour cream:
2 tbsp (1 oz)	reduced-fat	2 tbsp	regular
1 tsp	shortening or lard	3 tbsp	reduced-fat

Free Foods List

A *free food* is any food or drink that contains less than 20 kcal or less than 5 g of carbohydrate per serving. Foods with a serving size listed should be limited to 3 servings per day. Foods listed without a serving size can be eaten as often as you like.

Fat-Free or Reduced-Fat Foods

1 tbsp (½ oz)	cream cheese, fat-free	1 tbsp	salad dressing, fat-free
1 tbsp	creamers, nondairy, liquid		nonstick cooking spray
2 tsp	creamers, nondairy, powdered	1 tbsp	salad dressing, fat-free or low-fat, Italian
1 tbsp	mayonnaise, fat-free	2 tbsp	salad dressing, fat-free, Italian
1 tsp	mayonnaise, reduced-fat	1 tbsp	sour cream, fat-free, reduced-fat
4 tbsp	margarine, fat-free	1 tbsp	whipped topping, regular
1 tsp	margarine, reduced-fat	2 tbsp	whipped topping, light or fat-free
1 tbsp	Miracle Whip, fat-free		
1 tsp	Miracle Whip, reduced-fat nonstick cooking spray		

Sugar-Free Foods

1 candy	candy, hard, sugar-free	2 tsp	jam or jelly, light
	gelatin dessert, sugar-free		sugar substitutes*
	gelatin, unflavored	2 tbsp	syrup, sugar-free
	gum, sugar-free		

*Sugar substitutes, alternatives, or replacements that are approved by the Food and Drug Administration (FDA) are safe to use.

Drinks

	bouillon, broth, consommé		coffee
	bouillon or broth, low-sodium		diet soft drinks, sugar-free
	carbonated or mineral water		drink mixes, sugar-free
	club soda		tea
1 tbsp	cocoa powder, unsweetened		tonic water, sugar-free

Condiments

1 tbsp	catsup	2 slices	pickles, sweet (bread and butter)
	horseradish	¾ oz	pickles, sweet (gherkin)
	lemon juice	¼ cup	salsa
	lime juice	1 tbsp	soy sauce, regular or light
	mustard	1 tbsp	taco sauce
1 tbsp	pickle relish		vinegar
1½	pickles, dill (medium)	2 tbsp	yogurt

Seasonings

flavoring extracts	spices
garlic	Tabasco or hot pepper sauce
herbs, fresh or dried	wine, used in cooking
pimento	Worcestershire sauce

Combination Foods List

	Entrées	**Exchanges per Serving**
1 cup (8 oz)	tuna noodle casserole, lasagna, spaghetti with meatballs, chili with beans, macaroni and cheese	2 carbohydrates, 2 medium-fat meats
2 cups (16 oz)	chow mein (without noodles or rice)	1 carbohydrate, 2 lean meats
½ cup (3½ oz)	tuna or chicken salad	½ carbohydrate, 2 lean meats, 1 fat
	Frozen Entrées and Meals	
generally 14–17 oz	dinner-type meal	3 carbohydrates, 3 medium-fat meats, 3 fats
3 oz	meatless burger, soy-based	½ carbohydrate, 2 lean meats
3 oz	meatless burger, vegetable and starch-based	1 carbohydrate, 1 lean meat
¼ of 12-inch (6 oz)	pizza, cheese, thin crust	2 carbohydrates, 2 medium-fat meats, 1 fat
¼ of 12-inch (6 oz)	pizza, meat topping, thin crust	2 carbohydrates, 2 medium-fat meats, 2 fats
1 (7 oz)	pot pie	2½ carbohydrates, 1 medium-fat meat, 3 fats
8–11 oz	entrée or meal with less than 340 kcal	2–3 carbohydrates, 1–2 lean meats
	Soups	
1 cup	bean	1 carbohydrate, 1 very lean meat
1 cup (8 oz)	cream (made with water)	1 carbohydrate, 1 fat
6 oz prepared	instant	1 carbohydrate
8 oz prepared	instant with beans/lentils	2½ carbohydrates, 1 very lean meat
½ cup (4 oz)	split pea (made with water)	1 carbohydrate
1 cup (8 oz)	tomato (made with water)	1 carbohydrate
1 cup (8 oz)	vegetable beef, chicken noodle, or other broth-type	1 carbohydrate

Fast-Foods

		Exchanges per Serving
1 (5–7 oz)	burritos with beef	3 carbohydrates, 1 medium-fat meat, 1 fat
6	chicken nuggets	1 carbohydrate, 2 medium-fat meats, 1 fat
1 each	chicken breast and wing, breaded and fried	1 carbohydrate, 4 medium-fat meats, 2 fats
1	chicken sandwich, grilled	2 carbohydrates, 3 very lean meats
6 (5 oz)	chicken wings, hot	1 carbohydrate, 3 medium-fat meats, 4 fats
1	fish sandwich/tartar sauce	3 carbohydrates, 1 medium-fat meat, 3 fats
1 medium serving (5 oz)	french fries	4 carbohydrates, 4 fats
1	hamburger (regular)	2 carbohydrates, 2 medium-fat meats
1	hamburger (large)	2 carbohydrates, 3 medium-fat meats, 1 fat
1	hot dog with bun	1 carbohydrate, 1 high-fat meat, 1 fat
1	individual pan pizza	5 carbohydrates, 3 medium-fat meats, 3 fats
¼ 12-inch (about 6 oz)	pizza, cheese, thin crust	2½ carbohydrates, 2 medium-fat meats
¼ 12-inch (about 6 oz)	pizza, meat, thin crust	2½ carbohydrates, 2 medium-fat meats, 1 fat
1 (5 oz)	soft serve cone (small)	2½ carbohydrates, 1 fat
1 sub (6 inches)	submarine sandwich	3 carbohydrates, 1 vegetable, 2 medium-fat meats, 1 fat
1 (3–3½ oz)	taco, hard or soft shell	1 carbohydrate, 1 medium-fat meat, 1 fat

Appendix F

FATTY ACIDS, INCLUDING OMEGA-3 FATTY ACIDS, IN FOODS

Chain Length, Number, and Site of Double Bonds for Common Fatty Acids	
Common Name of Fatty Acid	Number of Carbon Atoms and Number and Site of Double Bond(s), Counting from Methyl End ($-CH_3$) If Appropriate
Saturated Fatty Acids (No Double Bonds)	
Formic	1
Acetic	2
Propionic	3
Butyric	4
Valeric	5
Caproic	6
Caprylic	8
Capric	10
Lauric	12
Myristic	14
Palmitic	16
Stearic	18
Unsaturated Fatty Acids	
Oleic	18:1 (9-10) ω-9
Linoleic	18:2 (6-7, 9-10) ω-6
Alpha-linolenic	18:3 (3-4, 6-7, 9-10) ω-3
Arachidonic	20:4 (6-7, 9-10, 12-13, 15-16) ω-6
Eicosapentaenoic	20:5 (3-4, 6-7, 9-10, 12-13, 15-16) ω-3
Docosahexaenoic	22:6 (3-4, 6-7, 9-10, 12-13, 15-16, 18-19) ω-3

Fatty Acid Composition of Selected Foods*

Food Item	Fatty Acid[†]									
	Saturated					Unsaturated				
	< C12:0	C12:0	14:0	C16:0	C18:0	C18:1 ω-9	C18:2 ω-6	C18:3 ω-3	C20:5 ω-3	C22:6 ω-3
		Lauric Acid	Myristic Acid	Palmitic Acid	Stearic Acid	Oleic Acid	Linoleic Acid	Alpha-Linolenic Acid	EPA[‡]	DHA[‡]
Fats and Oils										
Beef tallow	0.0	0.90	3.70	24.9	18.9	36.0	3.1	0.60	0.00	0.00
Butter	8.9	2.6	7.4	21.7	10.0	20.0	2.2	0.3	0.0	0.0
Cocoa butter	0.0	0.0	0.10	25.4	33.2	32.6	2.8	0.10	0.0	0.0
Corn oil	0.0	0.0	0.02	10.6	1.8	27.3	53.2	1.2	0.0	0.0
Cottonseed oil	0.0	0.0	0.80	22.7	2.3	17.0	51.5	0.20	0.0	0.0
Lard	0.1	0.20	1.30	23.8	15.5	41.2	10.2	1.0	0.0	0.0
Olive oil	0.0	0.0	0.0	11.3	2.0	71.3	9.8	0.8	0.0	0.0
Palm kernel oil	7.2	47.00	16.40	8.1	2.8	11.4	1.6	0.0	0.0	0.0
Palm oil	0.0	0.10	1.00	43.5	4.3	36.6	9.1	0.20	0.0	0.0
Safflower oil, high oleic	—	—	—	4.3	1.9	74.6	14.4	0.0	0.0	0.0
Shortenings	0.0	0.0	0.1	12.5	11.4	41.0	23.7	1.9	0.0	0.0
Margarine, stick	0.0	0.0	0.05	8.4	6.2	38.7	21.5	2.0	0.0	0.0
Margarine, tub	0.04	0.4	0.2	7.1	5.8	30.3	21.0	4.7	0.0	0.0
Canola oil	0.0	0.0	0.0	4.3	2.1	61.7	18.6	9.1	0.0	0.0
Soybean oil	0.0	0.0	0.04	10.7	4.0	22.6	50.1	6.5	0.0	0.0
Coconut oil	14.1	44.6	16.8	8.2	2.8	5.8	1.8	0.0	0.0	0.0
Peanut oil	0.0	0.0	0.10	9.5	2.8	44.8	32.0	0.0	0.0	0.0
Cod liver oil	—	—	3.6	10.6	2.8	20.6	0.9	0.9	6.9	11.0
Menhaden oil	—	—	8.0	15.1	3.8	14.5	2.2	1.5	13.1	8.6
Meat, Fish, and Poultry										
Beef, lean only, cooked	0.01	0.01	0.3	2.0	1.1	3.4	0.2	0.03	0.0	0.0
Chicken, white meat, cooked	0.0	0.01	0.03	0.7	0.3	1.0	0.6	0.03	0.01	0.02
Salmon, coho, wild, cooked	0.0	0.0	0.15	0.7	0.2	0.9	0.06	0.06	0.40	0.7
Tuna, light, canned in water	0.0	0.0	0.02	0.2	0.06	0.09	0.0	0.0	0.05	0.22
Nuts and Seeds										
Walnuts, English	0.0	0.0	0.0	4.4	1.7	8.8	38	9	0.0	0.0
Flaxseeds	0.0	0.0	0.0	2.2	1.3	7.4	5.9	22.8	0.0	0.0

From USDA Nutrient Database for Standard Reference, Release 20.

*Only major fatty acids are presented.

[†]All values represent grams per 100 g edible portion.

[‡]EPA eicosapentaenoic acid
DHA docosahexaenoic acid } fish oil fatty acids

Appendix G

METROPOLITAN LIFE INSURANCE COMPANY HEIGHT-WEIGHT TABLE AND DETERMINATION OF FRAME SIZE

1983 Metropolitan Life Insurance Company Height-Weight Table*†

Women					Men				
Height		Frame			Height		Frame		
Ft.	In.	Small	Medium	Large	Ft.	In.	Small	Medium	Large
4	10	102–111	109–121	118–131	5	2	128–134	131–141	138–150
4	11	103–113	111–123	120–134	5	3	130–136	133–143	140–153
5	0	104–115	113–126	122–137	5	4	132–138	135–145	142–156
5	1	106–118	115–129	125–140	5	5	134–140	137–148	144–160
5	2	108–121	118–132	128–143	5	6	136–142	139–151	146–164
5	3	111–124	121–135	131–147	5	7	138–145	142–154	149–168
5	4	114–127	124–138	134–151	5	8	140–148	145–157	152–172
5	5	117–130	127–141	137–155	5	9	142–151	148–160	155–176
5	6	120–133	130–144	140–159	5	10	144–154	151–163	158–180
5	7	123–136	133–147	143–163	5	11	146–157	154–166	161–184
5	8	126–139	136–150	146–167	6	0	149–160	157–170	164–188
5	9	129–142	139–153	149–170	6	1	152–164	160–174	168–192
5	10	132–145	142–156	152–173	6	2	155–168	164–178	172–197
5	11	135–148	145–159	155–176	6	3	158–172	167–182	176–202
6	0	138–151	148–162	158–179	6	4	162–176	171 187	181 207

*Based on a weight-height mortality study conducted by the Society of Actuaries and the Association of Life Insurance Medical Directors of America, Metropolitan Life Insurance Medical Directors of America, Metropolitan Life Insurance Company, 1983 (latest revision).

†Weights at ages 25 to 59 based on lowest mortality. Height includes 1-in. heel. Weight for women includes 3 lb for indoor clothing. Weight for men includes 5 lb for indoor clothing.

Reprinted courtesy of Metropolitan Life Insurance Company, *Statistical Bulletin*.

Permission granted courtesy of Metropolitan Life Insurance Company, *Statistical Bulletin*.

Using the Metropolitan Life Insurance Table to Estimate Healthy Weight

The Metropolitan Life Insurance table was a common method for estimating healthy weight (body mass index is more commonly used now). The table lists for any height the weight that is associated with a maximum life span. The table does not tell the healthiest weight for a living person; it simply lists the weight associated with longevity.

Criticisms of this table stem from the inclusion of some people and the exclusion of others. For example, only policyholders of life insurance are included. In addition, smokers are included, but anyone over the age of 60 is excluded. Weight is measured only at the time of purchase of insurance, and there is no follow-up. All these factors contribute to the fact that this table should be used only as a rough screening tool; not meeting the exact recommendations should not be cause for alarm.

To diagnose overweight or obesity using the table, calculate the percentage of the Metropolitan Life Insurance table weight. Use the midpoint of a weight range for a specific height.

$$\frac{(\text{Current wt.} - \text{wt. from table})}{\text{Weight from table}} \times 100$$

Example:

$$\frac{140 - 120}{120} \times 100 = 17\% \text{ over standard}$$

Overweight can be defined as weighing at least 10% more than the weight listed on the table. Obesity weighs in at 20% more than that listed on the table. Moreover, this measure of obesity comes in degrees. Whereas mild obesity carries little health risk, severe obesity raises overall health risk 12-fold.

Degrees of Obesity

% over Healthy Body Weight	Form of Obesity
20–40%	Mild
41–99%	Moderate
100%+	Severe

Determining Frame Size

Method 1

Height is recorded without shoes. Wrist circumference is measured just beyond the bony (styloid) process at the wrist joint on the right arm, using a tape measure. The following formula is used:

$$r = \frac{\text{Height } (cm)}{\text{Wrist circumference (cm)}}$$

Frame size can be determined as follows:[†]

Males	Females
$r > 10.4$ small	$r > 11$ small
$r = 9.6–10.4$ medium	$r = 10.1–11$ medium
$r < 9.6$ large	$r < 10.1$ large

[†]From Grant JP: *Handbook of total parenteral nutrition.* Philadelphia: WB Saunders; 1980.

Method 2

The patient's right arm is extended forward, perpendicular to the body, with the arm bent so the angle at the elbow forms 90 degrees, with the fingers pointing up and the palm turned away from the body. The greatest breadth across the elbow joint is measured with a sliding caliper along the axis of the upper arm, on the 2 prominent bones on either side of the elbow. This measurement is recorded as the elbow breadth. The following table gives elbow breadth measurements for medium-framed men and women of various heights. Measurements lower than those listed indicate a small frame size; higher measurements indicate a large frame size.

Men		Women	
Height in 1″ Heels	Elbow Breadth	Height in 1″ Heels	Elbow Breadth
5′2″–5′3″	2½–2⅞″	4′10″–4′11″	2¼–2½″
5′4″–5′7″	2⅝–2⅞″	5′0″–5′3″	2¼–2½″
5′8″–5′11″	2¾–3″	5′4″–5′7″	2⅜–2⅝″
6′0″–6′3″	2¾–3¼″	5′8″–5′11″	2⅜–2⅝″
6′4″ and over	2⅞–3¾″	6′0″ and over	2½–2¾″

Appendix H

ENGLISH-METRIC CONVERSIONS AND NUTRITION CALCULATIONS

English-Metric Conversions

Length

English (USA)	Metric
inch (in.)	= 2.54 cm, 25.4 mm
foot (ft)	= 0.30 m, 30.48 cm
yard (yd)	= 0.91 m, 91.4 cm
mile (statute) (5280 ft)	= 1.61 km, 1609 m
mile (nautical) (6077 ft, 1.15 statute mi)	= 1.85 km, 1850 m

Metric	English (USA)
millimeter (mm)	= 0.039 in. (thickness of a dime)
centimeter (cm)	= 0.39 in.
meter (m)	= 3.28 ft, 39.37 in.
kilometer (km)	= 0.62 mi, 1091 yd, 3273 ft

Weight

English (USA)	Metric
grain	= 64.80 mg
ounce (oz)	= 28.35 g
pound (lb)	= 453.60 g, 0.45 kg
ton (short—2000 lb)	= 0.91 metric ton (907 kg)

Metric	English (USA)
milligram (mg)	= 0.002 grain (0.000035 oz)
gram (g)	= 0.04 oz (1/28 oz)
kilogram (kg)	= 35.27 oz, 2.20 lb
metric ton (1000 kg)	= 1.10 tons

Volume

English (USA)	Metric
cubic inch	= 16.39 cc
cubic foot	= 0.03 m^3
cubic yard	= 0.765 m^3
teaspoon (tsp)	= 5 ml
tablespoon (tbsp)	= 15 ml
fluid ounce	= 0.03 liter (30 ml)*
cup (c)	= 237 ml
pint (pt)	= 0.47 liter
quart (qt)	= 0.95 liter
gallon (gal)	= 3.79 liters

Metric	English (USA)
milliliter (ml)	= 0.03 oz
liter (L)	= 2.12 pt
liter	= 1.06 qt
liter	= 0.27 gal

Metric and Other Common Units

Unit/Abbreviation	Other Equivalent Measure
milligram/mg	$^1/_{1000}$ of a gram
microgram/μg	$^1/_{1,000,000}$ of a gram
deciliter/dl	$^1/_{10}$ of a liter (about ½ cup)
milliliter/ml	$^1/_{1000}$ of a liter (5 ml is about 1 tsp)
International Unit/IU	Crude measure of vitamin activity generally based on growth rate seen in animals

1 liter ÷ 1000 = 1 milliliter or 1 cubic centimeter (10^{-3} liter)
1 liter ÷ 1,000,000 = 1 microliter (10^{-6} liter)
*Note: 1 ml = 1 cc

Fahrenheit-Celsius Conversion Scale

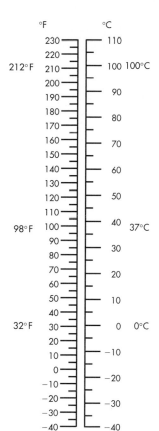

To convert temperature scales:
Fahrenheit to Celsius: $°C = (°F - 32) \times 5/9$
Celsius to Fahrenheit: $°F = 9/5 (°C) + 32$

Household Units

3 teaspoons	= 1 tablespoon
4 tablespoons	– ¼ cup
5⅓ tablespoons	= ⅓ cup
8 tablespoons	= ½ cup
10⅔ tablespoons	= ⅔ cup
16 tablespoons	= 1 cup
1 tablespoon	= ½ fluid ounce
1 cup	= 8 fluid ounces
1 cup	= ½ pint
2 cups	= 1 pint
4 cups	= 1 quart
2 pints	= 1 quart
4 quarts	= 1 gallon

Nutrition Calculations

Conversions are mathematical techniques for expressing the same quantity in different measurements. This section will walk you step by step through a few basic conversions that are important to understand when studying human nutrition.

Example 1: Converting Pounds to Kilograms. Begin with 2.2 pounds and 1 kilogram; they are equivalent. Each represents the same weight but is expressed in different units. The following is the conversion factor to change pounds to kilograms and kilograms to pounds.

$$\frac{2.2 \text{ lb}}{1 \text{ kg}} \quad \text{or} \quad \frac{1 \text{ kg}}{2.2 \text{ lb}}$$

Because these factors equal 1, they can be multiplied by a number without changing the measurement value. This allows the units to be changed.

Convert the weight of 150 lb to kg.

Step 1: Choose the conversion factor in which the unit you are seeking is on top.

$$\frac{1 \text{ kg}}{2.2 \text{ lb}}$$

Step 2: Multiply 150 pounds by the factor

$$150 \text{ lb} \times \frac{1 \text{ kg}}{2.2 \text{ lb}} = \frac{150 \text{ kg}}{2.2} = 59 \text{ kg}$$

Example 2: Converting Cups to Milliliters. Convert ½ cup to an approximate number of milliliters for use in a recipe.

Step 1: The conversion factor is

$$\frac{1 \text{ cup}}{240 \text{ ml}} \quad \text{or} \quad \frac{240 \text{ ml}}{1 \text{ cup}}$$

Step 2: Multiply ½ cup by the conversion factor.

$$\frac{1}{2} \text{ cup} \times \frac{240 \text{ ml}}{1 \text{ cup}} = 120 \text{ ml}$$

Example 3: Calculating Percent of Calories Supplied by Carbohydrate, Fat, Protein, and Alcohol. Suppose that for 1 day in your diet you consumed 290 g of carbohydrate, 60 g of fat, 70 g of protein, and 15 g of alcohol. Calculate the energy intake for the day, as well as the percentage of carbohydrate, fat, protein, and alcohol in the day's diet.

Step 1: Calculate the total energy intake. Begin by multiplying the grams of carbohydrate, fat, protein, and alcohol by the number of kcal that each gram yields.

$$\text{Carbohydrate: } 290 \text{ g} \times \frac{4 \text{ kcal}}{\text{g}} = 1160 \text{ kcal}$$

$$\text{Fat: } 60 \text{ g} \times \frac{9 \text{ kcal}}{\text{g}} = 540 \text{ kcal}$$

$$\text{Protein: } 70 \text{ g} \times \frac{4 \text{ kcal}}{\text{g}} = 280 \text{ kcal}$$

$$\text{Alcohol: } 15 \text{ g} \times \frac{7 \text{ kcal}}{\text{g}} = 105 \text{ kcal}$$

Step 2: Add all the values together for total energy intake.

$$1160 + 540 + 280 + 105 = 2085 \text{ total kcal}$$

Step 3: Calculate the percentage of total carbohydrate by multiplying the kcal from carbohydrate by the total energy intake.

$$\frac{1160 \text{ kcal from carbohydrate}}{2085 \text{ total kcal}} = 56\% \text{ carbohydrate}$$

Step 4: Calculate the percentage of total fat by multiplying the grams of fat by the energy yield and total energy factor.

$$\frac{540 \text{ kcal from fat}}{2085 \text{ total kcal}} = 26\% \text{ fat}$$

Step 5: Calculate the percentage of total protein by multiplying the grams of protein by the energy yield and total energy factor.

$$\frac{280 \text{ kcal from protein}}{2085 \text{ total kcal}} = 13\% \text{ protein}$$

Step 6: Calculate the percentage of total alcohol by multiplying the grams of alcohol by the energy yield and total energy factor.

$$\frac{105 \text{ kcal from alcohol}}{2085 \text{ total kcal}} = 5\% \text{ alcohol}$$

Example 4: Converting Amount of a Nutrient in a Quantity of Food to Another Quantity. How many grams of saturated fat are contained in a 3-oz hamburger? A 5-oz hamburger contains 8.5 g of saturated fat.

Step 1: The conversion factor for grams of saturated fat is

$$\frac{8.5 \text{ g saturated fat}}{5\text{-oz hamburger}}$$

Step 2: Multiply 3-oz hamburger by the conversion factor.

$$3 = \text{oz hamburger} \times \frac{8.5 \text{ g saturated fat}}{5\text{-oz hamburger}} = \frac{3 \times 8.5 \text{ g}}{5} = \frac{25.5}{5}$$

Example 5: Converting Sodium to Salt. The conversion factor to change milligrams of sodium to milligrams of salt, and milligrams of salt to milligrams of sodium, is

$$\frac{1000 \text{ mg sodium}}{2500 \text{ mg salt}} \quad \text{or} \quad \frac{2500 \text{ mg salt}}{1000 \text{ mg sodium}}$$

A frozen pepperoni pizza contains 2200 mg of salt. How much sodium is in the pizza?

Step 1: Choose the conversion factor with the unit you are seeking on top.

$$\frac{1000 \text{ mg sodium}}{2500 \text{ mg salt}}$$

Step 2: Multiply 2200 mg of salt by the conversion factor.

$$2200 \text{ mg salt} \times \frac{1000 \text{ mg sodium}}{2500 \text{ mg salt}} = 880 \text{ mg of sodium}$$

Example 6: Converting Folate to Dietary Folate Equivalents. To convert micrograms of synthetic folate in supplements and enriched foods to Dietary Folate Equivalents (micrograms DFE), use this conversion factor:

$$\frac{1 \text{ μg synthetic folic acid}}{1.7 \text{ μg DFE}} \quad \text{or} \quad \frac{1.7 \text{ μg DFE}}{1 \text{ μg synthetic folic acid}}$$

If a ready-to-eat breakfast cereal contains 200 μg of synthetic folic acid, how many μg of folate in the product are in DFE units?

Step 1: Choose the conversion factor with the unit you are seeking on top.

$$\frac{1.7 \text{ μg DFE}}{1 \text{ μg synthetic folic acid}}$$

Step 2: Multiply 200 μg of synthetic folic acid by the conversion factor.

$$200 \text{ μg synthetic folic acid} \times \frac{1.7 \text{ ug DFE}}{1 \text{ μg synthetic folic acid}}$$

For naturally occurring folate, assign each microgram of food folate a value of 1 microgram DFE:

$$\frac{1 \text{ μg food folate}}{1 \text{ μg DFE}} \quad \text{or} \quad \frac{1 \text{ μg DFE}}{1 \text{ μg synthetic folic acid}}$$

An orange has 50 μg of food folate. How many μg of folate in DFE does the orange contain?

Step 1: Choose the conversion factor with the unit you are seeking on top.

$$\frac{1 \text{ μg DFE}}{1 \text{ μg food folate}}$$

Step 2: Multiply 50 μg of food folate by the conversion factor.

$$50 \text{ μg food folate} \times \frac{1 \text{ μg DFE}}{1 \text{ μg food folate}} = 50 \text{ μg DFE}$$

Appendix I

CAFFEINE CONTENT OF BEVERAGES, FOODS, AND OVER-THE-COUNTER DRUGS*

Beverage or Food	Serving Size	Caffeine (mg)
Coffee Drinks		
Brewed, generic	8 oz	95
Brewed, Starbucks	12 oz	248
Brewed, decaffeinated	8 oz	2
Espresso	1 oz	63–75
Caffé latté	12 oz	75–233
Starbucks® frappuccino blended coffee beverage, average	9.5 oz	115
Instant coffee	8 oz	69
Tea		
Brewed, black	8 oz	47
Brewed, green	8 oz	
Brewed, herbal	8 oz	0
Starbucks® Tazo Chai Tea Latté	16 oz	100
Bottled iced teas	16 oz	10–76
Soda†		
FDA limit	12 oz	72
Jolt Cola	12 oz	72
Mountain Dew®, MDX	12 oz	72
Citrus-type (e.g., Mountain Dew®, Mello Yello®)	12 oz	50–74
Cola-type	12 oz	34–57
Pepper-type	12 oz	37–41
Miscellaneous: Barq's Root Beer® A & W® cream soda, Sunkist®, Big Red	12 oz	22–42
Energy Drinks		
AMP Tall Boy® energy drink	16 oz	143
Enviga®	12 oz	100
Full Throttle®	16 oz	144
Monster Energy®	16 oz	160
Red Bull®	8.3 oz	80
Rockstar®	16 oz	160–240

(continued)

Beverage or Food	Serving Size	Caffeine (mg)
Energy Drinks, *continued*		
SoBe® Adrenaline Rush	16 oz	152
SoBe® No Fear	16 oz	174
Chocolate and Candies		
Coffee ice cream	½ cup	24–42
Hershey's® milk chocolate	1.45 oz	8
Hershey's® special dark chocolate	1.45 oz	18–27
Hot chocolate from mix	8 oz	3–13
Over-the-Counter Drugs		
Anacin® (maximum strength)	2 tablets	64
Excedrin® (extra strength)	2 tablets	130
NoDoz® (maximum strength)	1 tablet	200
Vivarin®	1 tablet	200

*Each of the following ingredients listed on food, supplement, or drug labels contributes to caffeine: caffeine; coffee or coffee beans; cocoa or cacao, Theobroma cacao; guarana or paullinia cupana; kola nuts or cola seeds, cola nitida; green tea, black tea, or Camellia Sinesis, Thea Sinesis, Camellia; yerba mate or Mate, Ilex paraguariensis.

†Caffeine levels can vary considerably from brand to brand. Many soft drinks contain no caffeine.

Sources: USDA National Nutrient Database for Standard Reference 20; *Caffeine content of food & drugs*, Center for Science in the Public Interest; 2007. www.cspinet.org/new/cafchart.htm; How much caffeine is in your daily habit? MayoClinic.com; 2007. www.mayoclinic.com/caffeine; Chou K-H, Bell LN. Caffeine content of prepackaged national-brand and private-label carbonated beverages. *J Food Sci.* 2007;72:C337. Dietary Supplement Ingredient Database, Agricultural Research Service, United States Department of Agriculture.

Appendix J

ESTIMATED AVERAGE REQUIREMENTS (EARs) FOR NUTRIENTS

Estimated Average Energy Requirements Set by the Food and Nutrition Board, Institute of Medicine, National Academies

Life Stage Group	CHO (g/d)	PROT (g/kg/d)	Vitamin A (µg/d)	Vitamin C (mg/d)	Vitamin E (mg/d)	Thiamin (mg/d)	Riboflavin (mg/d)	Niacin (mg/d)	Vitamin B-6 (mg/d)
Children									
1–3 y	100	0.88	210	13	5	.4	.4	5	.4
4–8 y	100	0.76	275	22	6	.5	.5	6	.5
Males									
9–13 y	100	0.76	445	39	9	.7	.8	9	.8
14–18 y	100	0.73	630	63	12	1.0	1.1	12	1.1
19–30 y	100	0.66	625	75	12	1.0	1.1	12	1.1
31–50 y	100	0.66	625	75	12	1.0	1.1	12	1.1
51–70 y	100	0.66	625	75	12	1.0	1.1	12	1.4
> 70 y	100	0.66	625	75	12	1.0	1.1	12	1.4
Females									
9–13 y	100	0.76	420	39	9	.7	.8	9	.8
14–18 y	100	0.71	485	56	12	.9	.9	11	1.0
19–30 y	100	0.66	500	60	12	.9	.9	11	1.1
31–50 y	100	0.66	500	60	12	.9	.9	11	1.1
51–70 y	100	0.66	500	60	12	.9	.9	11	1.3
> 70 y	100	0.66	500	60	12	.9	.9	11	1.3
Pregnancy									
≤ 18 y	135	0.88	530	66	12	1.2	1.2	14	1.6
19–30 y	135	0.88	550	70	12	1.2	1.2	14	1.6
31–50 y	135	0.88	550	70	12	1.2	1.2	14	1.6
Lactation									
≤ 18 y	160	1.05	880	96	16	1.2	1.3	13	1.7
19–30 y	160	1.05	900	100	16	1.2	1.3	13	1.7
31–50 y	160	1.05	900	100	16	1.2	1.3	13	1.7

This information taken from the various DRI reports (see www.nap.edu).

Folate (µg/d)	Vitamin B-12 (µg/d)	Copper (µg/d)	Iodine (µg/d)	Iron (mg/d)	Magnesium (mg/d)	Molybdenum (µg/d)	Phosphorus (mg/d)	Selenium (µg/d)	Zinc (mg/d)
120	.7	260	65	3.0	65	13	380	17	2.2
160	1.0	340	65	4.1	110	17	405	23	4
250	1.5	540	73	5.9	200	26	1055	35	7
330	2.0	685	95	7.7	340	33	1055	45	8.5
320	2.0	700	95	6	330	34	580	45	9.4
320	2.0	700	95	6	350	34	580	45	9.4
320	2.0	700	95	6	350	34	580	45	9.4
320	2.0	700	95	6	350	34	580	45	9.4
250	1.5	540	73	5.7	200	26	1055	35	7
330	2.0	685	95	7.9	300	33	1055	45	7.5
320	2.0	700	95	8.1	255	34	580	45	6.8
320	2.0	700	95	8.1	265	34	580	45	6.8
320	2.0	700	95	5	265	34	580	45	6.8
320	2.0	700	95	5	265	34	580	45	6.8
520	2.2	785	160	23	355	40	1055	49	10.5
520	2.2	800	160	22	290	40	580	49	9.5
520	2.2	800	160	22	300	40	580	49	9.5
450	2.4	985	209	7	300	50	1055	59	11.6
450	2.4	1000	209	6.5	255	50	580	59	10.4
450	2.4	1000	209	6.5	265	50	580	59	10.4

Appendix K

CDC GROWTH CHARTS

Birth to 36 months: Boys
Length-for-age and Weight-for-age percentiles

NAME _____

RECORD # _____

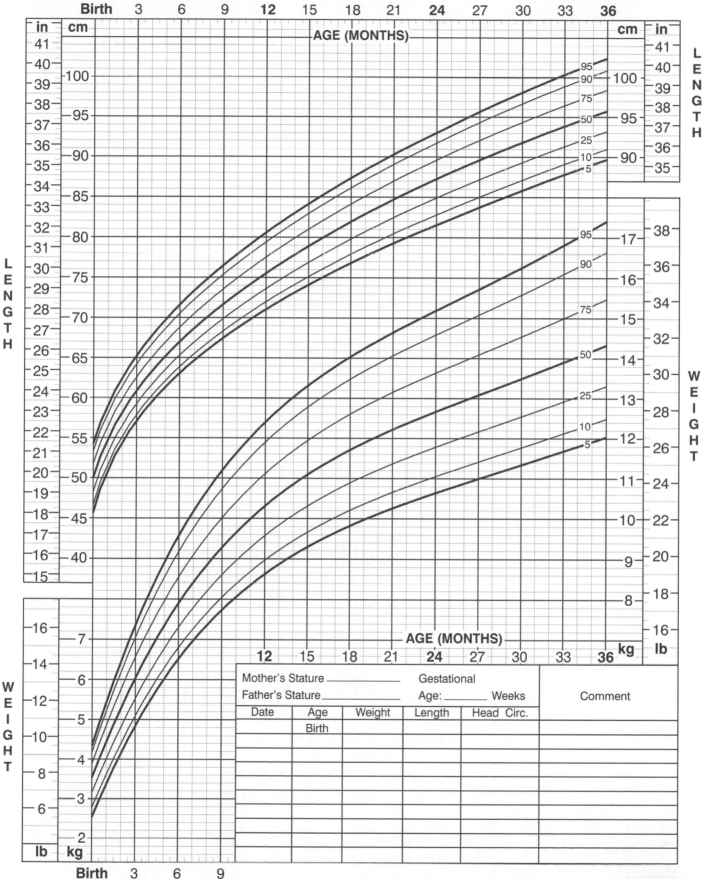

AGE (MONTHS)

Mother's Stature _____ Gestational
Father's Stature _____ Age: _____ Weeks

Comment

Date	Age	Weight	Length	Head Circ.
Birth				

Published May 30, 2000 (modified 4/20/01).
SOURCE: Developed by the National Center for Health Statistics in collaboration with
the National Center for Chronic Disease Prevention and Health Promotion (2000).
http://www.cdc.gov/growthcharts

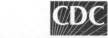

SAFER · HEALTHIER · PEOPLE™

Birth to 36 months: Boys
Head circumference-for-age and
Weight-for-length percentiles

NAME _____

RECORD # _____

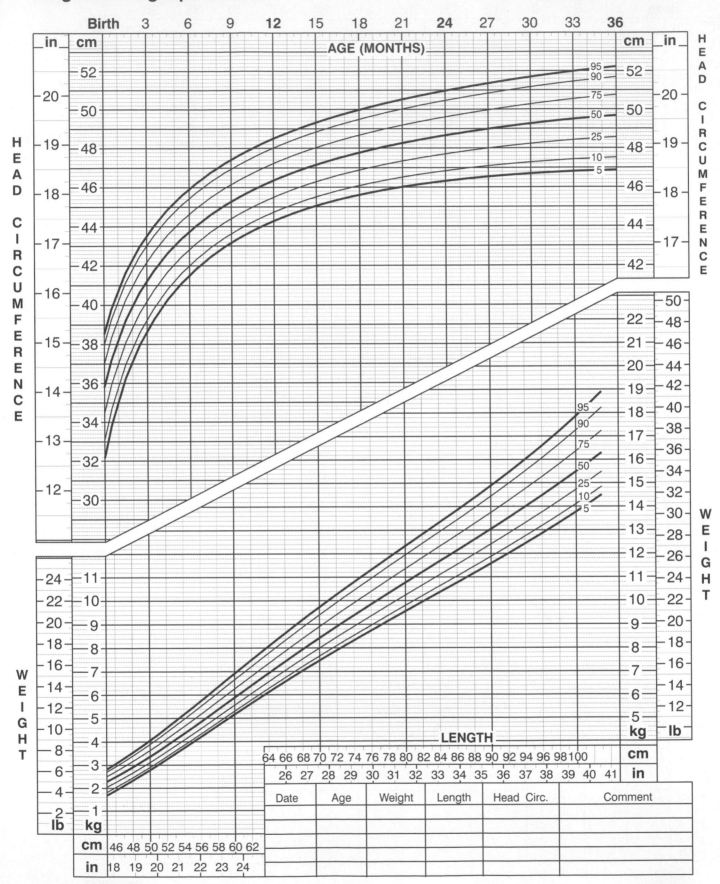

Date	Age	Weight	Length	Head Circ.	Comment

Published May 30, 2000 (modified 10/16/00).
SOURCE: Developed by the National Center for Health Statistics in collaboration with
the National Center for Chronic Disease Prevention and Health Promotion (2000).
http://www.cdc.gov/growthcharts

CDC

SAFER · HEALTHIER · PEOPLE™

Birth to 36 months: Girls
Length-for-age and Weight-for-age percentiles

NAME _____

RECORD # _____

AGE (MONTHS)

Birth 3 6 9 12 15 18 21 24 27 30 33 36

Length percentile curves: 95, 90, 75, 50, 25, 10, 5

Weight percentile curves: 95, 90, 75, 50, 25, 10, 5

LENGTH (in / cm): 41, 40, 39, 38, 37, 36, 35, 34, 33, 32, 31, 30, 29, 28, 27, 26, 25, 24, 23, 22, 21, 20, 19, 18, 17, 16, 15 / 100, 95, 90, 85, 80, 75, 70, 65, 60, 55, 50, 45, 40

WEIGHT (in / cm): 38, 36, 34, 32, 30, 28, 26, 24, 22, 20, 18 / 17, 16, 15, 14, 13, 12, 11, 10, 9, 8

AGE (MONTHS)

12 15 18 21 24 27 30 33 36 kg lb

Mother's Stature _____		Gestational		
Father's Stature _____		Age: _____ Weeks		Comment
Date	Age	Weight	Length	Head Circ.	
	Birth				

WEIGHT (lb / kg): 16, 14, 12, 10, 8, 6 / 7, 6, 5, 4, 3, 2

Birth 3 6 9

Published May 30, 2000 (modified 4/20/01).
SOURCE: Developed by the National Center for Health Statistics in collaboration with
the National Center for Chronic Disease Prevention and Health Promotion (2000).
http://www.cdc.gov/growthcharts

SAFER · HEALTHIER · PEOPLE™

Birth to 36 months: Girls
Head circumference-for-age and
Weight-for-length percentiles

NAME _____

RECORD # _____

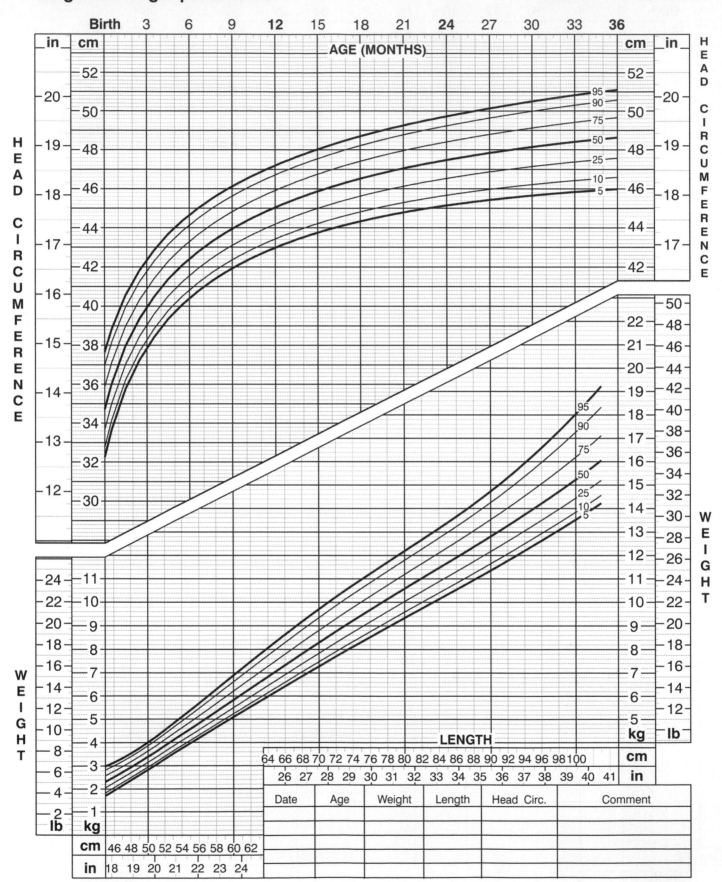

Published May 30, 2000 (modified 10/16/00).
SOURCE: Developed by the National Center for Health Statistics in collaboration with
the National Center for Chronic Disease Prevention and Health Promotion (2000).
http://www.cdc.gov/growthcharts

CDC
SAFER · HEALTHIER · PEOPLE™

2 to 20 years: Boys
Stature-for-age and Weight-for-age percentiles

NAME _____

RECORD # _____

Mother's Stature _____		Father's Stature _____		
Date	Age	Weight	Stature	BMI*

*To Calculate BMI: Weight (kg) ÷ Stature (cm) ÷ Stature (cm) x 10,000
or Weight (lb) ÷ Stature (in) ÷ Stature (in) x 703

AGE (YEARS)

12 13 14 15 16 17 18 19 20

STATURE

in   cm   3   4   5   6   7   8   9   10 11

cm   in

190 — 74
185
180 — 72
175 — 70
170 — 68
66

95
90
75
50
25
10
5

WEIGHT

95
90
75
50
25
10
5

lb   kg

AGE (YEARS)

2 3 4 5 6 7 8 9 10 11 12 13 14 15 16 17 18 19 20

Published May 30, 2000 (modified 11/21/00).
SOURCE: Developed by the National Center for Health Statistics in collaboration with
the National Center for Chronic Disease Prevention and Health Promotion (2000).
http://www.cdc.gov/growthcharts

SAFER · HEALTHIER · PEOPLE™

2 to 20 years: Boys
Body mass index-for-age percentiles

NAME _____

RECORD # _____

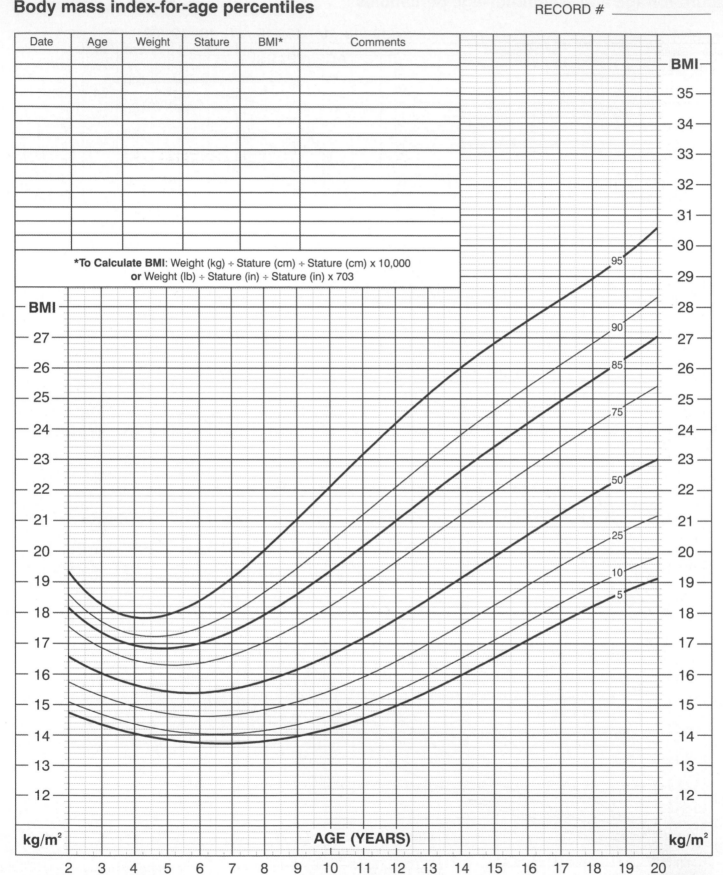

Date	Age	Weight	Stature	BMI*	Comments

*To Calculate BMI: Weight (kg) ÷ Stature (cm) ÷ Stature (cm) x 10,000
or Weight (lb) ÷ Stature (in) ÷ Stature (in) x 703

AGE (YEARS)

kg/m²

BMI

SOURCE: Developed by the National Center for Health Statistics in collaboration with
the National Center for Chronic Disease Prevention and Health Promotion (2000).
http://www.cdc.gov/growthcharts

CDC

SAFER • HEALTHIER • PEOPLE™

2 to 20 years: Girls
Stature-for-age and Weight-for-age percentiles

NAME _____

RECORD # _____

Mother's Stature _____		Father's Stature _____		
Date	Age	Weight	Stature	BMI*

*To Calculate BMI: Weight (kg) ÷ Stature (cm) ÷ Stature (cm) x 10,000
or Weight (lb) ÷ Stature (in) ÷ Stature (in) x 703

AGE (YEARS)

12 13 14 15 16 17 18 19 20

STATURE

in cm   3 4 5 6 7 8 9 10 11

STATURE

WEIGHT

WEIGHT

lb kg

AGE (YEARS)

2 3 4 5 6 7 8 9 10 11 12 13 14 15 16 17 18 19 20

kg lb

Percentile curves labeled: 95, 90, 75, 50, 25, 10, 5

Published May 30, 2000 (modified 11/21/00).
SOURCE: Developed by the National Center for Health Statistics in collaboration with
the National Center for Chronic Disease Prevention and Health Promotion (2000).
http://www.cdc.gov/growthcharts

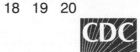

SAFER • HEALTHIER • PEOPLE™

2 to 20 years: Girls
Body mass index-for-age percentiles

NAME _____

RECORD # _____

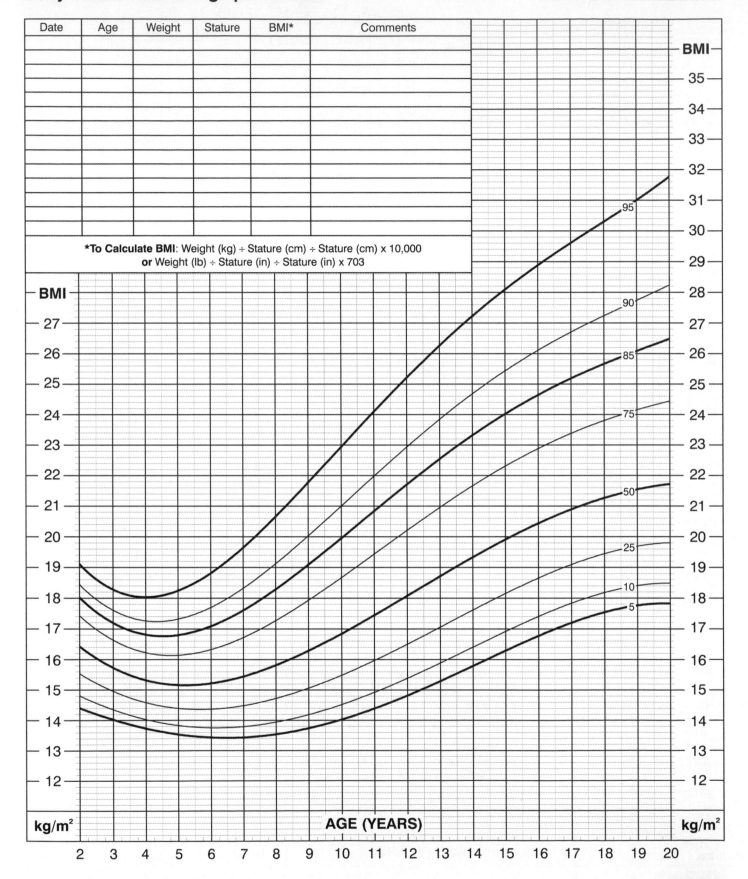

Date	Age	Weight	Stature	BMI*	Comments

*To Calculate BMI: Weight (kg) ÷ Stature (cm) ÷ Stature (cm) x 10,000
or Weight (lb) ÷ Stature (in) ÷ Stature (in) x 703

AGE (YEARS)

kg/m²

Published May 30, 2000 (modified 10/16/00).
SOURCE: Developed by the National Center for Health Statistics in collaboration with
the National Center for Chronic Disease Prevention and Health Promotion (2000).
http://www.cdc.gov/growthcharts

CDC

SAFER · HEALTHIER · PEOPLE™

Appendix L

SOURCES OF NUTRITION INFORMATION

Consider the following reliable sources of food and nutrition information:

Journals That Regularly Cover Nutrition Topics

American Family Physician*
American Journal of Clinical Nutrition
American Journal of Epidemiology
American Journal of Medicine
American Journal of Nursing
American Journal of Obstetrics and
    Gynecology
American Journal of Physiology
American Journal of Public Health
American Scientist
Annals of Internal Medicine
Annual Reviews of Medicine
Annual Reviews of Nutrition
Archives of Disease in Childhood
Archives of Internal Medicine
BMJ (British Medical Journal)
British Journal of Nutrition
Cancer
Cancer Research
Circulation
Diabetes

Diabetes Care
Disease-a-Month
FASEB Journal
FDA Consumer*
Food Chemical Toxicology
Food Engineering
Gastroenterology
Geriatrics
Gut
Human Nutrition: Applied Nutrition
Human Nutrition: Clinical Nutrition
JAMA (Journal of the American Medical
    Association)
JNCI (Journal of the National Cancer
    Institute)
Journal of the American College of
    Nutrition*
Journal of the American Dietetic
    Association*
Journal of the American Geriatric Society
Journal of Applied Physiology
Journal of the Canadian Dietetic
    Association*

Journal of Clinical Investigation
Journal of Food Service
Journal of Food Technology
Journal of Nutrition
Journal of Nutritional Education*
Journal of Nutrition for the Elderly
Journal of Pediatrics
Lancet
Mayo Clinic Proceedings
Medicine & Science in Sports and Exercise
Nature
The New England Journal of Medicine
Nutrition
Nutrition Reviews
Nutrition Today*
Pediatrics
The Physician and Sports Medicine
Postgraduate Medicine*
Proceedings of the Nutrition Society
Science
Science News*
Scientific American*

The majority of these journals are available in college and university libraries. As indicated, a few journals will be filed under their abbreviations rather than the first word in their full name. A reference librarian can help you locate any of these sources. The journals with an asterisk (*) are those you may find especially interesting and useful because of the number of nutrition articles presented each month or the less technical nature of the presentation.

Textbooks and Other Sources for Advanced Study of Nutrition Topics

Groff JL, Smith JL, Gropper SS. *Advanced human nutrition and metabolism.* 4th ed. Belmont, CA: Wadsworth; 2005.

International Life Sciences Institute. *Present knowledge in nutrition.* 9th ed. Washington DC: Nutrition Foundation; 2006.

Mahan LK, Escott-Stump S. *Krause's food, nutrition, and diet therapy.* 12th ed. Philadelphia: WB Saunders; 2007.

Murray RK and others. *Harper's biochemistry.* 27th ed. New York: McGraw-Hill; 2007.

Schils ME and others. *Modern nutrition in health and disease.* 10th ed. Philadelphia: Lippincott Williams & Wilkins; 2006.

Stipanuk MH. *Biochemical and physiological aspects of human nutrition.* 2nd ed. Philadelphia: WB Saunders; 2006.

Newsletters That Cover Nutrition Issues on a Regular Basis

American Institute for Cancer Research Newsletter
www.aicr.org

Consumer Health Digest
www.quackwatch.com

Dairy Council Digest
www.nationaldairycouncil.org

Environmental Nutrition
www.environmentalnutrition.com

Harvard Health Letter
www.hms.harvard.edu/news/index.html

Mayo Clinic Health Letter
www.mayohealth.org

National Council Against Health Fraud Newsletter (NCAHF)
www.ncahf.org

Nutrition Action Healthletter
www.cspinet.org

Nutrition Close-Up
www.enc-online.org

Tufts University Health & Nutrition Letter
www.healthletter.tufts.edu

University of California at Berkeley Wellness Letter
www.wellnessletter.com

Professional Organizations with a Commitment to Nutrition Issues

American Academy of Pediatrics
www.aap.org

American Cancer Society
www.cancer.org

American College of Sports Medicine
www.acsm.org

American Dental Association
www.ada.org

American Diabetes Association
www.diabetes.org

American Dietetic Association
www.eatright.org

American Geriatrics Society
www.americangeriatrics.org

American Heart Association
www.americanheart.org

American Medical Association
www.ama-assn.org

American Public Health Association
www.apha.org

American Society for Clinical Nutrition
www.faseb.org/ajcn

American Society for Nutrition
www.nutrition.org

Canadian Council of Food & Nutrition
www.ccfn.ca

Canadian Diabetes Association
www.diabetes.ca

Canadian Dietetic Association
www.dietitians.ca

Canadian Society for Nutritional Sciences
www.nutritionalsciences.ca

Environmental Working Group
www.ewg.org

Food and Nutrition Board
www.nas.edu

Institute of Food Technologies
www.ift.org

National Council on the Aging
www.ncoa.org

National Osteoporosis Foundation
www.nof.org

Society for Nutrition Education
www.sne.org

Professional or Lay Organizations Concerned with Nutrition Issues

Bread for the World Institute
www.bread.org

Children's Foundation
www.childrenfoundation.com

Food Research and Action Center
www.frac.org

Institute for Food and Development Policy
www.foodfirst.org

La Leche League International, Inc.
www.lalecheleague.org

March of Dimes Birth Defects Foundation
www.marchofdimes.com

National Council Against Health Fraud, Inc.
www.ncahf.org

National WIC Association
www.nwica.org

Overeaters Anonymous
www.oa.org

Oxfam America
www.oxfamamerica.org

Local Resources for Advice on Nutrition Issues

Registered dietitians (R.D.s or in Canada also RDNs) in health-care, city, county, or state agencies, as well as in private practice

Cooperative extension agents in county extension offices and specialists at land-grant universities

Nutrition faculty affiliated with departments of food and nutrition, human ecology, family and consumer sciences, and dietetics

Government Agencies Concerned with Nutrition Issues or That Distribute Nutrition Information

United States
Centers for Disease Control and Prevention
www.cdc.org

Consumer Information Center
www.pueblo.gsa.gov

Food and Drug Administration (FDA)
www.fda.gov

Food and Nutrition Information and Education Resources Center
www.fnic.nal.usda.gov

Human Nutrition Research Division Agricultural Research Center
www.ars.usda.gov

National Center for Health Statistics
www.cdc.gov/nchs

National Heart, Lung, and Blood Institute
www.nhlbi.nih.gov

National Institute on Aging
www.nia.nih.gov

National Cancer Institute
www.nci.nih.gov

USDA, Center for Nutrition Policy and Promotion
MyPyramid
www.mypyramid.gov

USDA, Food Safety & Inspection Service
www.fsis.usda.gov

U.S. Government Printing Office
www.gpo.gov

Canada
Canadian Food Inspection Agency
www.inspection.gc.ca

Health and Welfare Canada
www.hc-sc.gc.ca

Nutrition Programs
www.hc-sc.gc.ca

United Nations
Food and Agriculture Organization (FAO)
www.fao.org

World Health Organization (WHO)
www.who.org

Appendix M

DIETARY INTAKE AND ENERGY EXPENDITURE ASSESSMENT

Although it may seem overwhelming at first, it is actually very easy to track the foods you eat. One tip is to record foods and beverages consumed as soon as possible after the actual time of consumption.

I. Fill in the food record form that follows. This appendix contains a blank copy (see the completed example in Table M-1). Then, to estimate the nutrient values of the foods you are eating, consult food labels and a nutrient database. If these resources do not have the serving size you need, adjust the value (see Appendix H). If you drink ½ cup of orange juice, for example, but a table has values only for 1 cup, halve all values before you record them. Then, consider grouping all servings of the same food to save time; if you drink a cup of 1% milk 3 times throughout the day, enter milk consumption only once as 3 cups. As you record your intake for use on the nutrient analysis form that follows, consider the following tips:

- Measure and record the amounts of foods eaten in portion sizes of cups, teaspoons, tablespoons, ounces, slices, or inches (or convert metric units to these units).
- Record brand names of all food products.
- Measure and record all those little extras, such as gravies, salad dressings, taco sauces, pickles, jelly, sugar, catsup, and margarine.
- For beverages
  —List the type of milk, such as whole, fat-free, 1%, evaporated, or chocolate.
  —Indicate whether fruit juice is fresh, frozen, or canned.
  —Indicate type for other beverages, such as fruit drink, fruit-flavored drink, and hot chocolate made with water or milk.
- For fruits
  —Indicate whether fresh, frozen, dried, or canned and whether processed in water, light syrup, or heavy syrup.
  —If whole, record number eaten and size with approximate measurements (such as 1 apple—3 in. in diameter).
- For vegetables
  —Indicate whether fresh, frozen, dried, or canned.
  —Record as portion of cup, teaspoon, or tablespoon, or as pieces (such as carrot sticks—4 in. long, ½ in. thick).
  —Record, preparation method.
- For cereals
  —Record cooked cereals in portions of tablespoon or cup (a level measurement after cooking).
  —Record dry cereal in level portions of tablespoon or cup.
  —If margarine, milk, sugar, fruit, or another ingredient is added, measure and record amount and type.
- For breads
  —Indicate whether whole-wheat, rye, white, and so on.
  —Measure and record number and size of portion (biscuit—2 in. across, 1 in. thick; slice of homemade rye bread—3 in. by 4 in., ¼ in. thick).
  —Sandwiches: list *all* ingredients (lettuce, mayonnaise, tomato, and so on).

Table M-1 Food Record Example

Time	Minutes Spent Eating	M or S*	H† (0–3)	Activity While Eating	Place of Eating	Food Eaten and Amount	Others Present	Reason for Choosing Food
7:10 A.M.	15	M	2	Standing, fixing lunch	Kitchen	Orange juice, 1 cup Crispix®, 1 cup Fat-free milk, ½ cup Sugar, 2 tsp Black coffee	———	Health Habit Health Taste Habit
10:00 A.M.	4	S	1	Sitting, taking notes	Classroom	Diet cola, 12 oz	Class	Weight control
12:15 P.M.	40	M	2	Sitting, talking	Student center	Chicken sandwich with lettuce and mayonnaise (3 oz chicken, 2 slices bread, 2 tsp mayonnaise) Pear, 1 medium 1% milk, 1 cup	Friends	Taste Health Health
2:30 P.M.	10	S	1	Sitting, studying	Library	Regular cola, 12 oz	Friend	Hunger
6:30 P.M.	35	M	3	Sitting, talking	Kitchen	Pork chop, 1 Baked potato, 1 Margarine, 2 tbsp Lettuce and tomato salad, 1½ cups Ranch dressing, 2 tbsp Peas, ½ cup Whole milk, 1 cup Cherry pie, 1 small piece Ice tea, 12 oz	Boyfriend	Convenience Health Taste Health Taste Health Habit Taste Health
9:10 P.M.	10	S	2	Sitting, studying	Living room	Apple, 1 Mineral water, 12 oz	———	Weight control Weight control

*M or S: Meal or snack
†H: Degree of hunger (0 = none; 3 = maximum)

- For meat, fish, poultry, and cheese
  - —Give size (length, width, thickness) in inches or weight in ounces after cooking for meat, fish, and poultry (e.g., cooked hamburger patty—3 in. across, ½ in. thick).
  - —Give size (length, width, thickness) in inches or weight in ounces for cheese.
  - —Record measurements only for the cooked, edible part—without bone or fat that is left on the plate.
  - —Describe how meat, poultry, or fish was prepared.
- For eggs
  - —Record as soft or hard-cooked, fried, scrambled, poached, or omelet.
  - —If milk, butter, or other ingredients are used, specify kinds and amount.
- For desserts
  - —List commercial brand or "homemade" or "bakery" under brand.
  - —Specify kind and size of purchased candies, cookies, and cakes.
  - —Measure and record portion size of cakes, pies, and cookies by specifying thickness, diameter, and width or length, depending on the item.

II. Now complete the nutrient analysis form as shown, using your food record. A blank copy of this form is printed in this appendix for your use. See the example in Table M-2.

Table M-2 Nutrient Analysis Example

Name	Quantity	kcal	Protein (g)	Carbohydrates (g)	Fiber (g)	Total Fat (g)	Monounsaturated Fat (g)	Polyunsaturated Fat (g)	Saturated Fat (g)	Cholesterol (g)	Calcium (mg)	Iron (mg)
Egg bagel, 4-inch	1	180	7.45	34.7	0.748	1.00	0.286	0.400	0.171	44.0	20.0	2.10
Jelly	1 tbsp	49.0	0.018	12.7	——	0.018	0.005	0.005	0.005	——	2.00	0.120
Orange juice, prepared fresh or frozen	1½ cups	165	2.52	40.2	1.49	0.210	0.037	0.045	0.025	——	33.0	0.411
Cheeseburger, McDonald's®	2	636	30.2	57.0	0.460	32.0	12.2	2.18	13.3	80.0	338	5.68
French fries, McDonald's®	1 order	220	3.00	26.1	4.19	11.5	4.37	0.570	4.61	8.57	9.10	0.605
Cola beverage, regular	1½ cups	151	——	38.5	——	——	——	——	——	——	9.00	0.120
Pork loin chop, broiled, lean	4 oz	261	36.2	——	——	11.9	5.35	1.43	4.09	112	5.67	1.04
Baked potato with skin	1	220	4.65	51.0	3.90	0.200	0.004	0.087	0.052	——	20.0	2.75
Peas, frozen, cooked	½ cup	63.0	4.12	11.4	3.61	0.220	0.019	0.103	0.039	——	19.0	1.25
Margarine, regular or soft, 80% fat	20 g	143	0.160	0.100	——	16.1	5.70	6.92	2.76	——	5.29	——
Iceberg lettuce, chopped	2 cups	14.6	1.13	2.34	1.68	0.212	0.008	0.112	0.028	——	21.2	0.560
French dressing	2 oz	300	0.318	3.63	0.431	32.0	14.2	12.4	4.94	——	7.10	0.227
Reduced-fat milk	1 cup	121	8.12	11.7	——	4.78	1.35	0.170	2.92	22.0	297	0.120
Graham crackers	2	60.0	1.04	10.8	1.40	1.46	0.600	0.400	0.400	——	6.00	0.367
Totals		2584	99.0	300	17.9	112	44.1	24.8	33.4	266	792	15.4
RDA or related nutrient standard*		2900	58	130	38						1000	8
% of nutrient needs		89	170	230	47						79	193

Abbreviations: g = grams, mg = milligrams, µg = micrograms

*Values from inside cover. The values listed are for a male age 19 years. Note that number of kcal is just a rough estimate. It is better to base energy needs on actual energy output.

†In RAE units. Table values generally are in RE units today because the food values have not been updated to reflect the latest vitamin A standards. RAE equal RE for foods with preformed vitamin A, such as for the pork chop, but RAE are only about half the RE listed for foods with provitamin A carotenoids, such as for the peas (see Chapter 12 for details).

‡Amounts refer to actual folate content rather than dietary folate equivalents (DFEs). This difference is important to consider if the food contains added synthetic folic acid as part of enrichment or fortification. Any such folic acid is absorbed about twice as much as the folate present naturally in foods. Thus, the total contribution of folate in the food in comparison with human needs will be greater than if all the folate were naturally in the food product. Nutrient analysis tables have yet to be updated to reflect the dietary folate equivalents of products (see Chapter 13 for more details).

Magnesium (mg)	Phosphorus (mg)	Potassium (mg)	Sodium (mg)	Zinc (mg)	Vitamin A (RE)	Vitamin C (mg)	Vitamin E (mg)	Thiamin (mg)	Riboflavin (mg)	Niacin (mg)	Vitamin B-6 (mg)	Folate (μg)	Vitamin B-12 (μg)
18.0	61.0	65.0	300	0.612	7.00	——	1.80	2.58	0.197	2.40	0.030	16.3	0.065
0.72	1.00	16.0	4.00	——	0.200	0.710	0.016	0.002	0.005	0.036	0.005	2.00	——
36.0	60.0	711	3.00	0.192	28.5	145	0.714	0.300	0.060	0.750	0.165	163	
45.8	410	314	1460	5.20	134	4.10	0.560	0.600	0.480	8.66	0.230	42.0	1.82
26.7	101	564	109	0.320	5.00	12.5	0.203	0.122	0.020	2.26	0.218	19.0	0.027
3.00	46.0	4.00	15.0	0.049	——	——	——	——	——	——	——	——	——
34.0	277	476	88.2	2.54	3.15	0.454	0.405	1.30	0.350	6.28	0.535	6.77	0.839
55.0	115	844	16.0	0.650	——	26.1	0.100	0.216	0.067	3.32	0.701	22.2	——
23.0	72.0	134	70.0	0.750	53.4	7.90	0.400	0.226	0.140	1.18	0.090	46.9	——
0.467	4.06	7.54	216	0.041	199	0.028	2.19	0.002	0.006	0.004	0.002	0.211	0.017
10.1	22.4	177	10.1	0.246	37.0	4.36	0.120	0.052	0.034	0.210	0.044	62.8	——
5.81	3.63	7.03	666	0.045	0.023	——	15.9	——	——	——	0.006	——	——
33.0	232	377	122	0.963	140	2.32	0.080	0.095	0.403	0.210	0.105	12.0	0.89
6.00	20.0	36.0	86.0	0.113	——	——	——	0.020	0.030	0.600	0.011	1.80	——
298	1425	3732	3165	11.7	607	204	22.5	5.52	1.79	25.9	2.14	395	3.65
400	700	4700	1500	11	900[†]	90	15	1.2	1.3	16	1.3	400[‡]	2.4
75	204	80	210	106	67	226	150	450	138	162	160	99	152

Time	Minutes Spent Eating	M or S*	H† (0–3)	Activity While Eating	Place of Eating	Food Eaten and Amount	Others Present	Reason for Choosing Food

*M or S: Meal or snack
†H: Degree of hunger (0 = none; 3 = maximum)

III. Complete the following table to summarize dietary intake.

Percent of kcal from Protein, Fat, Carbohydrate, and Alcohol

Intake

Protein (P):	____ g/day × 4 kcal/g	=	(P) ____ kcal/day
Fat (F):	____ g/day × 9 kcal/g	=	(F) ____ kcal/day
Carbohydrate (C):	____ g/day × 4 kcal/g	=	(C) ____ kcal/day
Alcohol (A):		=	(A) ____ kcal/day
	Total kcal (T)/day	=	(T) ____ kcal/day

Percent of kcal from protein:

$\frac{(P)}{(T)}$ × 100 = ____%

Percent of kcal from fat:

$\frac{(F)}{(T)}$ × 100 = ____%

Percent of kcal from carbohydrate:

$\frac{(C)}{(T)}$ × 100 = ____%

Percent of kcal from alcohol:

$\frac{(A)}{(T)}$ × 100 = ____%

NOTE: The 4 percentages can total slightly more or less than 100% due to rounding. To calculate kcal provided by alcohol, subtract kcal from carbohydrate, fat, and protein from total kcal. The remaining kcal are from alcohol.

Nutrient Analysis Form

Name	Quantity	kcal	Protein (g)	Carbohydrates (g)	Fiber (g)	Total Fat (g)	Monounsaturated Fat (g)	Polyunsaturated Fat (g)	Saturated Fat (g)	Cholesterol (g)	Calcium (mg)	Iron (mg)
Totals												
RDA or related nutrient standard*												
% of nutrient needs												

*Values from inside cover. Note that number of kcals is just a rough estimate. It is better to base energy neeeds on actual energy input.
†Use RAE values, even though food table is based on RE units.
‡Use DFE values, even though the food is based on total folate content, irrespective of natural or synthetic sourcs.
**See Chapter 2.

Note that a food such as toast with soft margarine contributes to 2 categories—the grain group and the oils group. You can expect that many food choices will contribute to more than 1 group.

Magnesium (mg)	Phosphorus (mg)	Potassium (mg)	Sodium (mg)	Zinc (mg)	Vitamin A (RE)	Vitamin C (mg)	Vitamin E (mg)	Thiamin (mg)	Riboflavin (mg)	Niacin (mg)	Vitamin B-6 (mg)	Folate (µg)	Vitamin B-12 (µg)

IV. Evaluation. Are there weaknesses suggested in your nutrient intake that correspond to missing servings in MyPyramid? Consider replacing the missing servings to improve your nutrient intake.

V. For the same day you keep your food record, also keep a 24-hour record of your activities. Include sleeping, sitting, and walking, as well as the obvious forms of exercise. Calculate your energy expenditure for these activities using Table 10-5 in Chapter 10 or the software available with this book. Try to substitute a similar activity if your particular activity is not listed. Calculate the total kcal you used for the day. Following is an example of an activity record and a blank form for your use.

Weight (kg)*: 70 kg

Activity	Time (Minutes): Convert to Hours	Energy Cost Column 1 kcal/kg/hr (from Table 10-5)	Column 2 (Column 1 × Time)	Column 3 (Column 2 × Weight in kg)
Brisk walking	(60 min) 1 hr	4.4	(× 1) = 4.4	(× 70) = 308

*lb/2.2

Weight (kg)*:

Activity	Time (Minutes): Convert to Hours	Energy Cost Column 1 kcal/kg/hr (from Table 10-5)	Column 2 (Column 1 × Time)	Column 3 (Column 2 × Weight in kg)

Total kcal used (add all items listed in column 3)

*lb/2.2

A

absorption Process by which nutrient molecules are absorbed by the GI tract and enter the bloodstream.

absorptive cells Class of cells, also called *enterocytes*, that cover the surface of the villi (fingerlike projections in the small intestine) and participate in nutrient absorption.

Acceptable Daily Intake (ADI) Amount of a food additive considered safe for daily consumption over one's lifetime.

Acceptable Macronutrient Distribution Range (AMDR) Range of intake for a specific macronutrient that is associated with a reduced risk of chronic diseases while providing for recommended intakes of essential nutrients. AMDR are set for carbohydrate, protein, and fat (various forms). Each is intended to provide guidance in dietary planning.

acesulfame K (ay-SUL-fame) Alternative sweetener that yields no energy to the body; 200 times sweeter than sucrose.

acetic acid (a-SEE-tic) Two-carbon fatty acid used in the synthesis of lipids.

$$CH_3-\overset{\overset{\displaystyle O}{\|}}{C}-OH$$

acetylcholine (a-SEE-tul-coal-ene) Neurotransmitter, formed from choline, that is associated with attention, learning, memory, muscle control, and other functions.

acetyl-CoA (acetyl coenzyme A) (a-SEE-tul) An important metabolic intermediate formed by the breakdown of glucose, fatty acids, and some amino acids. Its synthesis requires coenzyme A derived from panthothenic acid and acetic acid.

achlorhydria (ay-clor-HIGH-dre-ah) Decrease in stomach acid primarily due to age-associated loss of acid-producing gastric cells.

acidic pH pH less than 7; for example, lemon juice has an acidic pH.

acquired immunodeficiency syndrome (AIDS) Disorder in which a virus (human immunodeficiency virus [HIV]) infects specific types of immune system cells. This leaves the person with reduced immune function and, in turn, defenseless against numerous infectious agents.

acrodermatitis enteropathica (Ak-roh-der-MAH-tight-tis INN-teer-oh-PATH-ih-cah) Rare inherited childhood disorder that results in the inability to absorb adequate amounts of zinc from the diet. Symptoms include skin lesions, hair loss, and diarrhea. If untreated, the condition can result in death during infancy or early childhood. Management of this condition is with zinc supplements.

actin (AK-tin) Protein in muscle fiber that, together with myosin, is responsible for contraction.

active absorption Absorption using a carrier and expending ATP energy. In this way, the absorptive cell can absorb nutrients, such as glucose, against a concentration gradient.

acute alcohol intoxication Temporary deterioration in mental and physical function, arising from drinking alcoholic beverages too rapidly. An intoxicated person may be confused, disoriented, lack coordination, and have increasing lethargy. Coma and death can occur.

acyl carrier protein Protein, formed from the vitamin pantothenic acid, that attaches to fatty acids and shuttles them through the metabolic pathway that increases their chain length.

acyl group Carbonyl portion of a compound, such as an ester.

adenine Nitrogenous base that forms part of the structure of DNA and RNA; a purine.

adenosine diphosphate (ADP) (ah-DEN-o-scene di-FOS-fate) Breakdown product of ATP. ADP is synthesized into ATP using energy from foods and a phosphate group (abbreviated P_i).

adenosine monophosphate (AMP) (ah-DEN-o-scene mono-FOS-fate) Breakdown product of ADP when a phosphate group is removed. AMP is produced when ATP is in short supply.

adenosine triphosphate (ATP) (ah-DEN-o-scene tri-FOS-fate) Main energy currency for cells. ATP energy is used to promote ion pumping, enzyme activity, and muscular contraction.

Adequate Intake (AI) Recommendation for nutrient intake when not enough information is available to establish an RDA. AIs are based on observed or experimentally determined estimates of the average nutrient intake that appears to maintain a defined nutritional state (e.g., bone health) in a specific population. It is used when no RDA can be set.

adipose tissue (ad-i-POSE) Group of fat-storing cells.

ad libitum (ad-LIB-itum) At one's desire or pleasure.

ADP See *adenosine diphosphate*.

adrenergic (ADD-ren-er-gic) Relating to the actions of epinephrine and norepinephrine.

aerobic (air-ROW-bic) Requiring oxygen.

aerobic exercise Physical activity that uses large muscles groups and aerobic respiration.

aflatoxin Mycotoxin found in peanuts, corn, tree nuts, and oilseeds that can cause liver cancer.

aging Time-dependent physical and physiological changes in body structure and function that occur normally and progressively throughout adulthood as humans mature and become older.

air displacement Method for estimating body composition based on the volume of space taken up by a body inside a small chamber.

alcohol Compound with a carbon-oxygen bond with the oxygen also bonded to a single hydrogen; also the type of alcohol consumed, ethyl alcohol or ethanol (CH_3CH_2OH).

alcohol abuse Alcohol consumption that results in severe physical, psychological, or social problems.

alcohol dehydrogenase (dee-high-DRO-jen-ase) Enzyme used in alcohol (ethanol) metabolism; the major enzyme used in the liver when alcohol is in low concentration.

alcohol dependence A chronic disease that includes the following symptoms: craving, loss of control, withdrawal symptoms, tolerance, and unsuccessful attempts to cut down on use.

aldehyde (AL-dah-hide) Organic compound that contains a carbonyl group to which at least 1 hydrogen atom is attached; found in 1 form of vitamin A.

$$\overset{\displaystyle \overset{\textstyle O}{\|}}{-C-H}$$

aldosterone (al-DOS-ter-own) Hormone produced in the adrenal glands that acts on the kidneys, causing them to retain sodium and, therefore, water.

alkaline pH pH greater than 7. Baking soda in water yields an alkaline pH.

allergen A substance (e.g., a protein in food) that induces a hypersensitive response, with excess production of certain immune system antibodies. Subsequent exposure to the same protein leads to allergic symptoms.

allergy Hypersensitive immune response that occurs when immune bodies produced by us react with a protein we sense as foreign (an antigen).

alpha (α) bond Type of chemical bond that can be broken by human intestinal enzymes in digestion; drawn as $C-O-C$.

alpha-linolenic acid (AL-fah-lin-oh-LE-nik) Essential omega-3 fatty acid with 18 carbons and 3 double bonds (C18:3, omega-3).

alpha-tocopherol (to-ca-FUR-all) Most potent form of vitamin E for antioxidant function in humans.

alveoli (al-VE-o-lye), alveolus Basic functional units of the lungs where respiratory gases are exchanged.

Alzheimer's disease Irreversible, abnormal, progressive deterioration of the brain that causes victims to steadily lose the ability to remember, reason, and comprehend.

amenorrhea (A-men-or-ee-a) Absence of 3 or more consecutive menstrual cycles; absence of menses in a female.

amine A nitrogen-containing chemical compound derived from ammonia. Examples include tyramine and histamine.

amino acid (ah-MEE-noh) Building block for proteins, containing a central carbon atom, an amino group (NH_2), a carboxylic acid group (COOH) and a side group.

amino group Nitrogen-containing chemical group ($-NH_2$); attached to a single carbon in all amino acids.

amniotic fluid (am-nee-OTT-ik) Fluid contained in a sac within the uterus. This fluid surrounds and protects the fetus during development.

AMP See *adenosine monophosphate.*

amphetamine (am-FET-ah-mean) Group of medications that stimulate the central nervous system and have other effects in the body. Abuse is linked to physical and psychological dependence.

amylase (AM-uh-lace) Starch-digesting enzyme from the salivary glands or pancreas.

amylopectin (AM-uh-low-pek-tin) Digestible branched-chain type of starch composed of multiple glucose units.

amylose (AM-uh-los) Digestible straight-chain type of starch made of multiple glucose units.

anabolic/anabolism (an-AH-bol-iz-um) Pathways that use small, simple compounds to build larger, more complex compounds.

anabolic steroids Hormones that increase strength and muscle mass; known to have severe and sometimes deadly side effects. The use of anabolic steroids is illegal.

anaerobic (AN-ah-ROW-bic) Not requiring oxygen.

anaerobic exercise Physical activity such as sprinting that uses anaerobic respiration.

analog (AN-a-log) Chemical compound that differs slightly from another naturally occurring compound. Analogs generally contain extra or altered chemical groups and may have similar or opposite metabolic effects compared with the native compound; also spelled *analogue.*

anal sphincters Group of 2 sphincters (inner and outer) that help control expulsion of feces from the body.

anaphylactic shock (an-ah-fih-LAK-tic) Severe allergic response that results in lowered blood pressure and respiratory and gastrointestinal distress. This reaction can be fatal.

androgenic (AN-dro-jenic) Hormones that stimulate development in male sex organs—for example, testosterone.

android obesity (AN-droyd) Type of obesity in which fat is stored primarily in the abdominal area; defined as a waist circumference greater than 40 inches (102 centimeters) in men and greater than 35 inches (89 centimeters) in women; closely associated with a high risk of cardiovascular disease, hypertension, and type 2 diabetes.

anemia (ah-NEM-ee-a) Decreased oxygen-carrying capacity of the blood. This can be caused by many factors, such as iron deficiency or blood loss.

anencephaly (an-en-SEF-ah-lee) Fatal birth defect in which parts of the brain and skull are missing.

anergy (AN-er-jee) Lack of an immune response to foreign compounds entering the body.

angiotensin I (an-jee-oh-TEN-sin) Intermediary compound produced during the body's attempt to conserve water and sodium. It is converted in the lungs to angiotensin II.

angiotensin II Compound, produced from angiotensin I, that increases blood vessel constriction and triggers production of the hormone aldosterone.

angiotensinogen Blood protein, synthesized in the liver, that forms angiotensin I.

angular cheilitis (kee-LIE-tis) Deep cracks at the corners of the mouth; may result from a B-vitamin deficiency.

animal model Study of a disease in laboratory animals that duplicates human disease. This can be used to understand more about human disease.

anion Negatively charged ion.

anorexia nervosa (an-oh-REX-ee-uh ner-VOH-sah) Eating disorder characterized by a psychological loss or denial of appetite is followed by self-starvation; related in part to a distorted body image and to various social pressures commonly associated with puberty.

anthropometric assessment (an-throw-PO-met-rick) Pertaining to the measurement of body weight and the lengths, circumferences, and thicknesses of parts of the body.

antibody (AN-tih-bod-ee) Blood protein that inactivates foreign proteins found in the body; helps prevent and control infections.

antibody-mediated immunity Specific immunity provided by B lymphocytes; also known as humoral immunity.

antidiuretic hormone (an-tie-dye-u-RET-ik) Hormone, secreted by the pituitary gland, that acts on the kidney to cause a decrease in water excretion; also called arginine vasopressin.

antigen (AN-ti-jen) Foreign substance, generally large in size, that is capable of inducing a specific immune response. Often binds with an antibody.

antioxidant (an-tie-OX-ih-dant) Compound that stops the damaging effects of reactive substances seeking an electron (i.e., oxidizing agent). This compound prevents the breakdown of substances in food or the body, particularly lipids. An antioxidant is able to donate electrons to electron-seeking compounds, which helps prevent the breakdown of unsaturated fatty acids and other cell (and food) components by oxidizing agents. Some compounds have antioxidant capabilities (i.e., stop oxidation) but are not electron donors per se.

anus (A-nus) Last portion of the GI tract; serves as an outlet for that organ through which feces are expelled.

aorta (a-ORT-ah) Major blood vessel of the body, leaving from the left ventricle of the heart.

apoenzyme (ape-oh-EN-zime) Inactive enzyme without its cofactor.

apoferritin (ape-oh-FERR-ih-tin) Protein in the intestinal cell and liver that binds with the ferric form of iron (Fe^3) to form ferritin.

apolipoprotein (ape-oh-LIP-oh-pro-teen) Protein attached to the surface of a lipoprotein or embedded in its outer shell. Apolipoproteins can help enzymes function, act as lipid-transfer proteins, or assist in the binding of a lipoprotein to a cell-surface receptor.

apoptosis (ah-pop-TOE-sis) Process that occurs over time in which enzymes in a cell set off a series of events that disable numerous cell functions, eventually leading to cell death.

appetite Primarily psychological (external) influences that encourage us to find and eat food, often in the absence of obvious hunger.

arachidonic acid (ar-a-kih-DON-ik) Omega-6 fatty acid with 20 carbon atoms and 4 carbon-carbon double bonds (C20:4, omega-6); a precursor to some eicosanoids.

areola (ah-REE-oh-lah) Circular, dark area of skin surrounding the nipple of the breast.

ariboflavinosis (ah-rih-bo-flay-vih-NOH-sis) Condition resulting from a lack of riboflavin; *a* means "without," and *osis* means "a condition of."

aromatherapy Use of the vapors of essential oils extracted from flowers, leaves, stalks, fruits, and roots for therapeutic purposes.

arrhythmias (ah-RITH-me-ahs) Abnormal heart rhythms that may be too slow, too early, too rapid, or irregular.

arteriole (ar-TEAR-e-ol) Tiny artery branch that ends in capillaries.

arteriosclerosis (ar-TEAR-e-o-scle-ROH-sis) A chronic disease characterized by abnormal thickening and hardening of the arterial walls resulting in a lack of elasticity.

artery Blood vessel that carries blood away from the heart.

arthritis Inflammation at a point where bones join together. The disease has many possible causes.

ascending colon First part of the large intestine, between the ileocecal valve and the transverse colon.

ascites (a-SITE-ease) Fluid produced by the liver, accumulating in the abdomen, that is a sign of liver failure associated with cirrhosis.

ascorbic acid Water-soluble vitamin; also known as vitamin C.

aseptic processing (ah-SEP-tik) Method by which a food and a container are separately and simultaneously sterilized, allowing manufacturers to produce boxes of milk and other foods that can be stored at room temperature.

aspartame (AH-spar-tame) Alternative sweetener made of 2 amino acids and methanol; about 200 times sweeter than sucrose.

ataxia (a-TAX-ee-a) Inability to coordinate muscle activity during voluntary movement; incoordination.

atherosclerosis (ath-e-roh-scle-ROH-sis) Buildup of fatty material (plaque) in the arteries, including those surrounding the heart.

atom Smallest combining unit of an element. An atom contains protons, neutrons, and electrons.

ATP See *adenosine triphosphate*.

atria (A-tree-a) Plural of atrium. Two upper chambers of the heart that receive venous blood.

atrophic gastritis (A-troh-fik) Chronic inflammation of the stomach, in which the stomach glands and lining atrophy.

atrophy (AT-row-fee) Wasting away of tissue or organs.

autodigestion Literally, "self-digestion." The stomach limits autodigestion by covering itself with a thick layer of mucus and producing enzymes and acid only when needed for digestion of foodstuff.

autoimmune Immune reactions against normal body cells; self against self.

avidin (AV-ih-din) Protein, found in raw egg whites, that can bind biotin and inhibit its absorption. Cooking destroys avidin.

axon (Ay-on) Part of a nerve cell that conducts impulses away from the main body of the cell.

B

bacteria Single-cell microorganisms; some produce poisonous substances that cause illness in humans. They contain only 1 chromosome and lack many of the organelles found in human cells. Some can live without oxygen and survive harsh conditions by means of spore formation.

basal metabolic rate (BMR) Rate of energy use (e.g., kcal/min) by the body when at rest, fasting, and awake in a warm, quiet environment.

basal metabolism Minimal amount of energy the body uses to support itself in a fasting state when resting, fasting, and awake in a warm, quiet environment. It amounts to roughly 1 kcal per kilogram per hour for men and 0.9 kcal per kilogram per hour for women.

benign Non-cancerous; describes tumors that do not spread.

beriberi (BEAR-ee-BEAR-ee) Thiamin deficiency disorder characterized by muscle weakness, loss of appetite, nerve degeneration, and sometimes edema.

beta (β) bond Type of chemical bond that cannot be broken by human intestinal enzymes during digestion when it is part of a long chain of glucose molecules (e.g., cellulose); drawn as $C \frown O \cup C$.

betaine (bee-TAINE) Product of choline metabolism and a methyl ($-CH_3$) donor in methionine metabolism.

beta-oxidation Breakdown of a fatty acid into numerous acetyl-CoA molecules; also known as fatty acid oxidation.

BHA Butylated hydroxyanisole, a synthetic antioxidant added to food.

BHT Butylated hydroxytoluene, a synthetic antioxidant added to food.

bile Liver secretion that is stored in the gallbladder and released through the common bile duct into the duodenum. It is essential for the digestion and absorption of fat.

bile acids Emulsifiers synthesized by the liver and released by the gallbladder during digestion.

bilirubin (bi-li-RUBE-in) Bile pigment derived from hemoglobin during the destruction of red blood cells; excreted by the liver into the gallbladder. Excess in the blood causes skin and eyes to become yellow (jaundiced).

binge drinking Consumption of 5 or more drinks by men or 4 or more drinks by women at a single occasion.

binge-eating disorder Eating disorder characterized by recurrent binge eating and feelings of loss of control over eating that have lasted at least 6 months. Binge episodes can be triggered by frustration, anger, depression, anxiety, permission to eat forbidden foods, and excessive hunger.

bioavailability Degree to which the amount of an ingested nutrient is absorbed and is available to the body.

biochemical assessment Assessment focusing on biochemical functions (e.g., concentrations of nutrient by-products or enzyme activities in the blood or urine) related to a nutrient's function.

biochemical lesion Indication of reduced biochemical function (e.g., low concentrations of nutrient by-products or enzyme activities in the blood or urine) resulting from a nutritional deficiency.

biocytin (By-oh-si-tin) Protein-bound form of the vitamin biotin.

bioelectrical impedance Method to estimate total body fat that uses a low-energy electrical current. The more fat storage a person has, the more impedance (resistance) to electrical flow will be exhibited.

biological pest management Way to control agricultural pests by using natural predators, parasites, or pathogens.

biological value (BV) Measure of how efficiently food protein, once absorbed from the gastrointestinal tract, can be turned into body tissues.

biopharming Use of genetically engineered crops and livestock animals to produce pharmaceutical agents.

biotechnology Collection of processes that involve the use of biological systems for altering and, ideally, improving the characteristics of plants, animals, and other forms of life.

biotin (BY-oh-tin) Water-soluble vitamin that, in coenzyme form, participates in reactions where carbon dioxide is added to a compound. It is an essential cofactor for enzymes involved in energy and amino acid metabolism and in fatty acid synthesis. Peanuts, liver, and egg are rich sources. It also can be synthesized by intestinal bacteria.

bisphosphonates (bis-FOS-foh-nates) Medications composed primarily of carbon and phosphorus, that bind to bone mineral and in turn reduce bone breakdown.

bleaching process Process by which light depletes the rhodopsin concentration in the eye. This fall in rhodopsin concentration allows the eye to become adapted to bright light.

blind study Experiment in which the participants, the researchers, or both are unaware of each participant's assignment (test or placebo) or the outcome of the study until it is completed. See also *double-blind study*.

blood doping Technique by which an athlete's red blood cell count is increased. Blood is taken from the athlete, the red blood cells are concentrated, and then later they are reinjected into the athlete. Alternately, a hormone may be injected to increase red blood cell synthesis (erythropoetin [Epogen®]).

B lymphocyte (LIM-fo-site) Type of white blood cell that recognizes antigens (e.g., bacteria) present in extracellular sites in the body and is responsible for antibody-mediated immunity. B lymphocytes originate and mature in the bone marrow and are released into the blood and lymph.

body mass index (BMI) Weight (in kilograms) divided by height (in meters) squared. A normal value is 18.5 to 24.9. A value of 25 or greater indicates a risk for body weight–related health disorders, such as type 2 diabetes and cardiovascular disease, especially when it is 30 or greater. One BMI unit equals 6 to 7 lb.

bolus (BOWL-us) Mass of food that is swallowed.

bomb calorimeter (kal-oh-RIM-eh-ter) Instrument used to determine the energy content of a food.

bond Link between 2 atoms by the sharing of electrons, charges, or attractions.

bone mass Total mineral substance (e.g., calcium or phosphorus) in a cross section of bone, generally expressed as grams per centimeter of length.

bone mineral density Total mineral content of bone at a specific bone site divided by the width of the bone at that site, generally expressed as grams per cubic centimeter. Bone mineral density tests are used to diagnose osteopenia and osteoporosis.

bone remodeling Process by which bone is first resorbed by osteoclasts and then re-formed by osteoblasts. This process allows the body to form bone where needed, such as in areas of high mechanical stress.

bonking State of exercise when the muscles and liver have run out of glycogen, characterized by extreme fatigue, confusion, anxiety, and sweating; sometimes referred to as "hitting the wall."

botulism Foodborne illness caused by the bacterium *Clostridium botulinum*.

bran Outer layer of grains, such as wheat; rich source of dietary fiber.

branched-chain amino acids Amino acids that contain branched methyl groups in their side chains; the essential amino acids valine, leucine and isoleucine.

bronchial tree (BRON-key-al) Bronchi and the branches that stem out to bronchioles.

bronchioles Smallest division of the bronchi.

brown adipose tissue (ADD-ih-pose) Specialized form of adipose tissue that produces large amounts of heat by metabolizing energy-yielding nutrients without synthesizing much useful energy for the body. The unused energy is released as heat.

brush border Densely packed microvilli on the intestinal epithelial cells.

buffer Compound that helps maintain acid-base balance within a narrow range.

bulimia nervosa (boo-LEEM-ee-uh) Eating disorder characterized by eating large quantities of food at one time (binge eating) and purging it from the body by vomiting or by misusing laxatives, diuretics, or enemas. Alternate means to counteract the excess energy intake are fasting and excessive exercise.

B-vitamins Group of several water-soluble vitamins that includes thiamin, riboflavin, niacin, pantothenic acid, biotin, vitamin B-6, vitamin B-12, and folate. All B-vitamins function as coenzymes.

C

cachexia (ka-KEX-ee-a) Widespread wasting of the body due to undernutrition and usually associated with chronic disease.

calcitonin (kal-sih-TONE-in) Thyroid gland hormone that inhibits bone resorption and lowers blood calcium.

calcitriol (kal-sih-TRIH-ol) Name sometimes given to the active hormone form of vitamin D [1,25(OH)2 vitamin D].

calcium Major mineral component of bones and teeth. Calcium also aids in nerve impulse transmission, blood clotting, muscle contractions, and other cell functions. Milk and milk products, leafy vegetables, and tofu are good sources.

calmodulin (kal-MOD-ju-lyn) Cell protein that binds calcium ions. The resulting calmodulin-Ca2+ complex influences the activity of some enzymes in the cell.

calorie See *kilocalorie*.

***Campylobacter jejuni* (kam-PILE-o-bak-ter je-JUNE-ee)** Bacterium that produces a toxin that destroys the mucosal surfaces of the small and large intestines. *Campylobacter* is a leading cause of bacterial foodborne illness. The chief food sources are raw poultry and meat and unpasteurized milk. It is easily destroyed by cooking.

cancer Condition characterized by uncontrolled growth of abnormal body cells.

cancer initiation Stage in the process of cancer development that begins with the exposure of a cell to a carcinogen and that results in alterations in DNA. These alterations may cause the cell to no longer respond to normal physiological controls.

cancer progression Final stage in the cancer process, during which the cancer cells proliferate, invade surrounding tissue, and metastasize to other sites.

cancer promotion Stage in the cancer process during which cell division increases, in turn decreasing the time available for repair enzymes to act on altered DNA and encouraging cells with altered DNA to develop and grow.

capillary (KAP-ill-air-ee) Microscopic blood vessel that connects an arteriole and a venule; the functional unit of the circulatory system.

capillary bed Minute vessels 1 cell thick that create a junction between arterial and venous circulation. Gas and nutrient exchange occurs here between body cells and the bloodstream.

carbohydrate (kar-bow-HIGH-drate) Compound containing carbon, hydrogen, and oxygen atoms; most are known as sugars, starches, and fibers; supplies 4 kcal/gram.

carbohydrate counting Diet method that assigns points (1 point = 15 g of carbohydrate) to each meal and snack.

carbohydrate loading Process in which a very high carbohydrate intake is consumed for 6 days before an athletic event while tapering exercise duration in an attempt to increase muscle glycogen stores; sometimes referred to as glycogen loading.

carbon skeleton Remains of an amino acid after the amino group (—NH_2) has been removed.

carbonyl group (KAR-bow-neel) Parent compound for ketones, aldehydes, and many related groups; (C=O).

carboxyl group (KAR-BOX-ill) The COOH group in an organic acid.

carboxylic acid (KAR-BOX-ih-lik) Organic molecule with the carboxyl group. Examples include acetic acid and citric acid.

$$\overset{\displaystyle O}{\underset{\displaystyle (-C-OH)}{\|}}$$

carcinogenic (Kar-sin-oh-JEN-ik) Having the potential to cause cancer.

carcinoma (Kar-sih-NOH-mah) Invasive malignant tumor derived from epithelial tissues that cover external and internal areas of the body.

cardiac muscle Muscle that makes up the walls of the heart; produces rhythmic, involuntary contractions.

cardiac output Amount of blood pumped by the heart.

cardiomyopathy (Kar-dee-oh-my-OP-ah-thee) A disease in which the heart muscle is damaged and cannot pump blood efficiently.

cardiovascular (heart) disease Disease of the heart and circulatory system, characterized by the deposition of fatty material in the blood vessels (hardening of the arteries), which can lead to organ damage and death; also termed *coronary heart disease (CHD)* because the vessels of the heart are the primary sites of the disease.

cardiovascular system Body system consisting of the heart, blood vessels, and blood. This system transports nutrients, waste products, gases, and hormones throughout the body and plays an important role in immune responses and body temperature regulation.

cariogenic (CARE-ee-oh-jen-ik) Literally "caries producing;" a substance, often carbohydrate-rich (e.g., caramel), that promotes dental caries.

carnitine (CAR-nih-teen) Compound used to shuttle fatty acids from the cytosol of the cell into mitochondria.

carotenoids (kah-ROT-en-oyds) Pigmented materials in fruits and vegetables that range in color from yellow to orange to red (e.g., beta-carotene); 3 types yield vitamin A activity in humans and thus are called provitamin A. Many have antioxidant properties.

carpal tunnel syndrome (CAR-pull) Disease in which nerves that travel to the wrist are pinched as they pass through a narrow opening in a bone in the wrist.

cartilage Connective tissue, usually part of the skeleton, composed of cells in a flexible network.

case-control study Study in which individuals who have the condition in question, such as lung cancer, are compared with individuals who do not have the condition.

casein (KAY-seen) Protein, found in milk, that forms curds when exposed to acid and is difficult for infants to digest.

catabolic/catabolism (cat-ah-BOL-ik) Pathways that breakdown large compounds into smaller compounds. Energey is usually released.

catalase Enzyme that breaks down hydrogen peroxide (H_2O_2) to water.

catalase pathway Alternative enzyme pathway to alcohol metabolism. Alcohol is broken down in conjunction with the breakdown of hydrogen peroxide (H_2O_2) by this enzyme.

catalyst (CAT-ul-ist) Compound that speeds reaction rates but is not altered by the reaction.

cation Positively charged ion.

cecum (SEE-come) First portion of the large intestine, which connects to the ileum.

celiac disease (SEE-lee-ak) Immunological or allergic reaction to the protein gluten in certain grains, such as wheat and rye. The effect is to destroy the intestinal enterocytes, resulting in a much reduced surface area due to flattening of the villi. Elimination of wheat, rye, and certain other grains from the diet restores the intestinal surface.

cell Minute structure; the living basis of plant and animal organization. In animals, the cell is bounded by a cell membrane. Cells contain both genetic material and systems for synthesizing energy-yielding compounds. Cells have the ability to take up compounds from and excrete compounds into their surroundings.

cell differentiation Process of transforming an unspecialized cell into a specialized cell.

cell-mediated immunity Process in which T lymphocytes come in contact with invading cells in order to destroy them.

cell nucleus Organelle bound by its own double membrane and containing chromosomes that hold the genetic information for cell protein synthesis.

cellular respiration See *respiration*.

cellulose (SELL-you-lows) Straight-chain polysaccharide of glucose molecules that is indigestible because of the presence of beta bonds; part of insoluble fiber.

Celsius (SEL-see-us) Centigrade measure of temperature; for conversion: (degrees in Fahrenheit − 32) × 5/9 = °C; degrees in Celsius × 9/5) + 32 = °F.)

central nervous system (CNS) Brain and spinal cord portions of the nervous system.

cerebrovascular accident (CVA) (se-REE-bro-VAS-cue-lar) Death of part of the brain tissue due typically to a blood clot; also called *stroke* or brain attack.

ceruloplasmin (se-RUE-low-PLAS-min) Blue, copper-containing protein in the blood that can remove an electron from Fe^{2+} (ferrous form) to yield Fe^{3+} (ferric form). The Fe^{3+} form can bind with iron transport and storage proteins, such as transferrin.

chain-breaking Breaking the link between 2 or more behaviors that encourage overeating, such as snacking while watching television.

chelates (KEY-lates) Complexes formed between metal ions and substances with polar groups, such as proteins. The polar groups form 2 or more attachments with the metal ions, forming a ringed structure. The metal ion is then firmly bound and sequestered.

chelation (key-LAY-shun) Use of medicinal compounds, such as ethylene-diamine-tetra-acetic acid (EDTA), to bind metals and other constituents in the blood.

chemical reaction Interaction between 2 or more chemicals that changes the participants.

chemical score Ratio comparing the essential amino acid content of the protein in a food with the essential amino acid content in a reference protein. The lowest amino acid ratio calculated for any essential amino acid is the chemical score.

chief cell Gastric gland cell that secretes pepsinogen, precursor of pepsin.

Child and Adult Care Food Program U.S. government program that provides nutritious meals and snacks to low-income children enrolled in child-care centers or residing in emergency shelters, as well as adults who are functionally impaired or age 60 and older in non-residential adult day-care centers.

chiral (KI-rell) Carbon atom with 4 different atoms or groups of atoms attached.

chloride Major negative ion of extracellular fluid; aids in nerve impulse transmission and fluid balance in conjunction with sodium and potassium. It contributes to the function of white blood cells, aids in the transport of carbon dioxide from cells to the lungs, and is a component of hydrochloric acid production in the stomach. Salt supplies most of the chloride in the diet.

cholecystokinin (CCK) (ko-la-sis-toe-KY-nin) Hormone that stimulates enzyme release from the pancreas and bile release from the gallbladder.

cholera (KOL-er-a) See *Vibrio cholerae*.

cholesterol (ko-LES-te-rol) Waxy lipid found in all body cells. It has a structure containing multiple chemical rings. It is an important component of cell membranes and serves as a precursor to many important biological compounds. Dietary cholesterol is cholesterol found only in foods that contain animal products.

choline (COAL-ene) Water-soluble vitamin-like compound that functions as a precursor for acetylcholine, a neurotransmitter associated with attention, learning and memory, muscle control, and many other functions. Protein foods, especially eggs, are rich in choline.

cholinergic (coal-in-NER-jic) Relating to the actions of acetylcholine.

chromium Trace mineral that enhances the action of insulin. Egg yolks, whole grains, pork, nuts, and mushrooms are good sources.

chromosome Complex of DNA and protein containing the genetic material of a cell's nucleus. There are 46 chromosomes in the nucleus of each cell except in germ cells.

chronic (KRON-ik) Long-standing, developing over time. When referring to disease, this term indicates that the disease tends to progress slowly; an example is cardiovascular disease.

chylomicron (kye-lo-MY-kron) Lipoprotein made of dietary fats that are surrounded by a shell of cholesterol, phospholipids, and protein. Chylomicrons are formed in the absorptive cells (enterocytes) in the small intestine after fat absorption and travel through the lymphatic system to the bloodstream.

chyme (KIME) Liquid mixture of stomach secretions and partially digested food.

ciguatera toxin (see-gwah-TER-ah) Seafood toxin that causes gastrointestinal, neuromuscular, and respiratory symptoms. It is most common in large fish from tropical waters.

circular folds Numerous folds of the mucous membrane of the small intestine.

cirrhosis (see-ROH-sis) Loss of functioning liver cells, which are replaced by nonfunctioning connective tissue. Any substance that poisons liver cells can lead to cirrhosis. The most common cause is chronic, excessive alcohol intake. Exposure to certain industrial chemicals also can lead to cirrhosis.

***cis* configuration (SIS)** Form seen in compounds with double bonds, such as fatty acids, in which the hydrogens on both ends of the double bond lie on the same side of the plane of that bond in the cell mitochondria.

citric acid cycle Pathway that breaks down acetyl-CoA, yielding carbon dioxide, $FADH_2$, NADH+ H^+, and GTP. The pathway also can be used to synthesize compounds; also known as the tricarboxylic acid cycle (TCA cycle) and the Krebs cycle.

clinical assessment Physical evidence of diet-related disease. This type of assessment focuses on the general appearance of skin, eyes, and tongue; evidence of rapid hair loss; loss of sense of touch; and loss of ability to cough and walk.

clinical lesion Sign seen on physical examination or a symptom perceived by the patient resulting from a nutritional deficiency.

clinical symptoms Changes in health status noted by the individual (e.g., stomach pain) or clinician during physical examination (the latter is technically called a clinical sign).

cloning Creating genetically identical animals by non-sexual reproduction.

***Clostridium botulinum* (closs-TRID-ee-um bot-u-LYE-num)** Bacterium in soil and possibly in food in the form of bacteria or spores. This bacterium multiplies in the absence of air and produces a deadly toxin. *C. botulinum* thrives primarily in canned food, especially incorrectly home-canned, low-acid foods, such as string beans, corn, mushrooms, beets, asparagus, and garlic.

***Clostridium perfringens* (per-FRING-ens)** Toxin-producing bacterium living throughout the environment, especially in soil, the intestinal tract of humans and animals, and sewage. It is often referred to as the "cafeteria germ" because most outbreaks of foodborne illness caused by it are associated with the food service industry or with events where large quantities of food are prepared and served. *Clostridium* thrives in an oxygen-free environment and forms heat-resistant spores.

coagulation Blood clot formation.

cobalamin (Koh-BAL-ah-meen) Vitamin B-12, a water-soluble vitamin.

codon (KOH-don) A specific sequence of 3 nucleotide units within DNA that codes particular amino acids needed for protein synthesis.

coenzyme Compound that combines with an inactive protein, called an apoenzyme, to form a catalytically active enzyme, called a holoenzyme. In this manner, coenzymes aid in enzyme function.

cofactor Organic or inorganic substance that binds to a specific region on an enzyme and is necessary for the enzyme's activity.

cognitive behavior therapy Psychological therapy in which a person's assumptions about dieting, body weight, and related issues are challenged. New ways of thinking are explored and then practiced by the person. In this way, the person can learn new ways to control disordered eating behaviors and related life stress.

cognitive restructuring Changing one's frame of mind regarding eating—for example, instead of using a difficult day as an excuse to overeat, substituting other pleasures or rewards, such as a relaxing walk with a friend.

cohort study Research that follows a healthy population over time, looking for indicators of the development of disease.

colic (KOL-ik) Sharp abdominal pain that generally occurs in otherwise healthy infants and is associated with periodic spells of inconsolable crying.

colipase (co-LIE-pace) Protein, secreted by the pancreas, that changes the shape of pancreatic lipase, facilitating its action.

colitis (koh-LIE-tis) Inflammation of part of the large intestine (the colon). There are many possible causes of colitis.

collagen (KOL-ah-jen) Major protein of the material that holds together the various structures of the body.

colostrum (ko-LAHS-trum) First fluid secreted by the breast during late pregnancy and the first few days after birth. This thick fluid is rich in immune factors and protein.

Commodity Foods Program U.S. government program that distributes, free of charge, surplus agricultural products (e.g., cheese, peanut butter, canned foods), produced by U.S. farmers, to low-income households.

comorbid Disease process that accompanies another disease. For example, if hypertension develops as obesity is established, hypertension is said to be a comorbid condition accompanying the obesity.

complement Series of blood proteins that participate in a complex reaction cascade following stimulation by an antigen-antibody complex on the surface of a bacterial cell. Various activated complement proteins can enhance phagocytosis, contribute to inflammation, and destroy bacteria.

Complementary and Alternative Medicine (CAM) Medical or health-care system, practice, or product not presently part of conventional medicine; also called complementary care and integrative medicine.

complementary proteins Two food protein sources that make up for each other's inadequate supply of specific essential amino acids. Together, they yield a sufficient amount of all 9 and, so, provide high-quality (complete) protein for the diet.

complete proteins Proteins that contain ample amounts of all 9 essential amino acids.

complex carbohydrate Carbohydrate composed of many monosaccharide molecules. Examples include glycogen, starch, and fiber.

compound Group of different types of atoms bonded together in definite proportion (see also *molecule*). Not all chemical compounds exist as molecules. Some compounds are made up of ions attracted to each other, such as Na^+Cl^- (table salt).

compression of morbidity Delay of the onset of disabilities caused by chronic disease.

concentration gradient Gradation in concentration that occurs between 2 regions having different concentrations.

conceptus (kon-SEP-tus) Developmental stage derived from the fertilized ovum (zygote) until birth. The conceptus includes the extra-embryonic membranes, as well as the embryo or fetus.

condensation reaction Chemical reaction in which a bond is formed between 2 molecules by the elimination of a small molecule, such as water.

cones Sensory elements in the retina of the eye responsible for visual processes that occur under bright light, translating objects into color images.

congenital (con-JEN-i-tal) Literally, "present at birth." A congenital abnormality is a defect that has been present since birth. These defects may be inherited from the parents, may occur as a result of damage or infection while in the uterus, or may occur at the time of birth.

congestive heart failure Condition resulting from severely weakened heart muscle, resulting in ineffective pumping of blood. This leads to fluid retention, especially in the lungs. Symptoms include fatigue, difficulty breathing, and leg and ankle swelling.

conjugase (KON-ju-gase) Enzyme systems in the intestine that enhance folate absorption; they remove glutamate molecules from polyglutamate forms of folate.

conjunctiva (kon-junk-TEA-vah) Mucous membrane covering the front surface of the eye and the lining of the eyelids.

connective tissue Cells and their protein products that hold different structures in the body together. Some structures are made up of connective tissue—notably; tendons and cartilage. Connective tissue also forms part of bone and the non-muscular structures of arteries and veins.

constipation Condition characterized by infrequent and often painful bowel movements.

contingency management Forming a plan of action to respond to a situation in which overeating is likely, such as when snacks are within arm's reach at a party.

control group Participants in an experiment who are not given the treatment being tested.

copper Trace mineral that aids in iron metabolism, functions in antioxidant enzyme systems and with enzymes involved in connective tissue metabolism, and used in hormone synthesis. Liver, cocoa, beans, nuts, and whole grains are good sources.

cortical bone (KORT-ih-kal) Dense, compact bone that constitutes the outer surface and shafts of bone; also called compact bone. Cortical bone makes up 75 to 80% of total bone mass.

corticosteroid (kor-ti-ko-STARE-oyd) Steroid produced by the adrenal gland (e.g., cortisol).

cortisol (KORT-ih-sol) Hormone made by the adrenal glands that, among other functions, stimulates the production of glucose from amino acids and increases the desire to eat.

covalent bond (ko-VAY-lent) Union of 2 atoms formed by the sharing of electrons.

creatine (CREE-a-tin) Organic molecule in muscle cells that serves as a part of the high-energy compound creatine phosphate (or phosphocreatine).

creatinine (cree-A-tin-in) Nitrogenous waste product of the compound creatine found in muscles.

cretinism (KREET-in-ism) Stunting of body growth and mental development during fetal and later development that results from inadequate maternal intake of iodine during pregnancy.

critical period Finite period during pregnancy when cells for a particular tissue or organ can develop.

Crohn's disease Inflammatory disease of the gastrointestinal tract, generally more pronounced in the terminal ileum, that limits the absorptive capacity of the small intestine. Family history is a major risk factor.

crude fiber Outdated term for what remains of fiber after extended acid and alkaline treatment. Crude fiber consists primarily of cellulose and lignins.

cryptosporidiosis (krip-toe-spore-id-ee-O-sis) Intestinal disease, characterized by diarrhea, that originates from a protozoan parasite of the genus *Cryptosporidium*.

Cushing's disease Endocrine disorder characterized by elevated blood levels of the hormone cortisol. High cortisol levels can lead to the breakdown of body proteins, such as those in the skin and muscle.

cyclamate (sigh-cla-MATE) Alternative sweetener that yields no energy to the body; 30 times sweeter than sucrose. Not a legal food additive in the U.S.

cyclooxygenase (sigh-clo-OXY-jen-ase) (COX) Enzyme used to synthesize prostaglandins, thromboxanes, and other eicosanoids.

cystic fibrosis (SIS-tik figh-BRO-sis) Inherited disease that can cause overproduction of mucus. Mucus can block the pancreatic duct, decreasing enzyme output.

cytochrome (SITE-o-krome) Electron-transfer compound that participates in the electron transport chain.

cytochrome P450 Set of enzymes in cells, especially in the liver, that act on compounds foreign to the body. This action aids in their excretion but also creates short-lived, highly reactive forms.

cytokine (SITE-o-kine) Protein, secreted by a cell, that regulates the activity of neighboring cells.

cytoplasm (SITE-o-plas-um) Fluid and organelles (except the nucleus) in a cell.

cytosine (SIH-toe-zeen) Nitrogenous base that forms part of the structure of DNA and RNA; a pyrimidine.

cytosol (SHI-tae-sall) Water-based phase of the cytoplasm; excludes organelles, such as mitochondria.

cytotoxic T cell (cite o TOX-ik) Type of T cell that interacts with an infected host cell through special receptor sites on the T cell surface.

cytotoxic test Unreliable test to diagnose food allergies; it involves mixing white blood cells with food proteins.

D

Daily Reference Values (DRVs) Nutrient-intake standards established for protein, carbohydrate, and some dietary components lacking an RDA or a related nutrient standard, such as total fat intake. The DRVs for sodium and potassium are constant; those for the other nutrients increase as energy intake increases. The DRVs constitute part of the Daily Values used in food labeling.

Daily Values Standard nutrient-intake values developed by the FDA and used as a reference for expressing nutrient content on nutrition labels. The Daily Values include 2 types of standards—RDIs and DRVs.

danger zone Temperature range of 41°F to 135°F, which supports the growth of pathogenic bacteria.

dark adaptation Process by which the rhodopsin concentration in the eye increases in dark conditions, allowing improved vision in the dark.

deamination (dee-am-ih-NA-shun) Removal of an amino group from an amino acid.

decarboxylation (dee-car-box-ih-LAY-shun) Removal of 1 molecule of carbon dioxide from a compound.

decubitus ulcer (dee-CUBE-ih-tus) Chronic ulcer (also called bedsore) that appears in pressure areas of the skin over a body prominence. These sores develop when people are confined to bed or otherwise immobilized.

defecation Expulsion of feces from the rectum.

dehydroascorbic acid (DEE-hy-dro-ah-scor-bik) Oxidized form of ascorbic acid (vitamin C).

Delaney Clause Clause in the 1958 Food Additives Amendment of the Pure Food and Drug Act in the United States that prevents the intentional (direct) addition to foods of a compound that has been shown to cause cancer in laboratory animals or humans.

dementia (de-MEN-sha) General, persistent loss of or decrease in mental function.

denaturation (dee-NAY-ture-a-shun) Alteration of a protein's 3-dimensional structure, usually because of treatment by heat, enzymes, acid or alkaline solutions, or agitation.

dendrite (DEN-drite) Relatively short, highly branched nerve cell process that carries electrical activity to the main body of the nerve cell.

dental caries (KARE-ees) Erosions in the surface of a tooth caused by acids made by bacteria as they metabolize sugars.

deoxyribonucleic acid (DNA) (DEE-awks-ee-ry-boh-noo-KLAY-ik) Site of hereditary information in cells. DNA directs the synthesis of cell proteins.

depolarization Reversal of membrane potential, which triggers generation of the nerve impulse in nerve cells.

dermatitis (dur-ma-TIE-tis) Inflammation of the skin.

dermis (DUR-miss) Second, or deep, layer of the skin under the epidermis.

descending colon Part of the large intestine between the transverse colon and the sigmoid colon.

desirable nutritional status State in which body tissues have enough of a nutrient to support normal functions and build and maintain surplus stores.

DEXA See *dual energy X-ray absorptiometry.*

dextrin Partial breakdown product of starch that contains few to many glucose molecules. These appear when starch is being digested into many units of maltose by salivary and pancreatic amylase.

diabetes (DYE-uh-BEET-eez) Disease characterized by high blood glucose, resulting from either insufficient or no release of the hormone insulin by the pancreas or the general inability of insulin to act on certain body cells, such as muscle cells. The 2 major forms are type 1 (requires daily insulin therapy) and type 2 (may or may not require insulin therapy).

diarrhea Loose, watery stools occurring more than 3 times per day.

diastolic blood pressure (dye-ah-STOL-ik) Pressure in the arterial blood vessels when the heart is between beats.

dietary assessment Assessment that focuses on one's typical food choices, relying mostly on the recounting of one's usual intake or a record of one's intake of the previous day.

dietary fiber Fiber in food.

Dietary Guidelines for Americans General goals for nutrient intakes and diet composition set by the USDA and the U.S. Department of Health and Human Services.

Dietary Reference Intakes (DRIs) Latest nutrient recommendations made by the Food and Nutrition Board, a part of the Institute of Medicine, and the National Academy of Science. These include Estimated Average Requirements (EARs), Recommended Dietary Allowances (RDAs), Adequate Intakes (AIs), Tolerable Upper Intake Levels (Upper Levels, or ULs), and Estimated Energy Requirements (EERs).

dietitian See *registered dietitian.*

diffusion Net movement of molecules or ions from regions of higher concentration to regions of lower concentration.

digestibility (dye-JES-tih-bil-i-tee) Proportion of food substances eaten that can be broken down into individual nutrients in the intestinal tract for absorption into the body.

digestion Process by which large ingested molecules are mechanically and chemically broken down to produce smaller molecules that can be absorbed across the wall of the GI tract.

digestive system Body system consisting of the gastrointestinal tract and accessory structures, such as the liver, gallbladder, and pancreas. This system performs the mechanical and chemical processes of digestion, absorption of nutrients, and formation and elimination of feces.

diglyceride (dye-GLISS-er-ide) Breakdown product of a triglyceride; consists of 2 fatty acids bonded to a glycerol backbone.

dihomo-gamma-linolenic acid (dye-homo-gama-linoh-lenik) Omega-6 fatty acid with 20 carbons and 3 double bonds; the precursor to some eicosanoids.

direct calorimetry (kal-oh-RIM-eh-tree) Method of determining a body's energy use by measuring heat that is released from the body, usually using an insulated chamber.

disaccharide (dye-SACK-uh-ride) Class of sugars formed by the chemical bonding of 2 monosaccharides.

discretionary calories Amount of energy theoretically allowed in a diet after a person has met overall nutrition needs. This generally small amount of energy gives individuals the flexibility to consume some foods and beverages that contain alcohol, added sugars, or added fats (e.g., many snack foods).

disordered eating Abnormal change in eating pattern that occurs in relation to a stressful event, an illness, or a desire to modify one's diet for a variety of health and personal appearance reasons.

distillation (di-stah-lay-shun) Physical method used to separate liquids based on their boiling points.

disulfide group (dye-sul-fide) Two sulfur atoms (S-S), each attached to a carbon; important structural characteristic of some proteins.

diuretic (dye-u-RET-ik) Substance that, when ingested, increases the flow of urine.

diverticula (DYE-ver-TIK-you-luh) Pouches that protrude through the exterior wall of the large intestine.

diverticulitis (DYE-ver-tik-you-LITE-us) Inflammation of the diverticula caused by acids produced by bacterial metabolism inside the diverticula.

diverticulosis (DYE-ver-tik-you-LOW-sus) Condition of having many diverticula in the large intestine.

DNA See *deoxyribonucleic acid.*

DNA transcription Formation of messenger RNA (mRNA) from a portion of DNA.

docosahexaenoic acid (DHA) (DOE-co-sa-hex-ee-noik) Omega-3 fatty acid with 22 carbons and 6 carbon-carbon double bonds (C22:6, omega-3). It is present in large amounts in fatty fish and is slowly synthesized in the body from alpha-linolenic acid. DHA is concentrated in the retina and brain.

dopamine (DOE-pah-mean) Type of neurotransmitter in the central nervous system that leads to feelings of euphoria, among other functions; also used to form norepinephrine, another neurotransmitter.

double-blind study Experiment in which neither the participants nor the researchers are aware of each participant's assignment (test or placebo) or the outcome of the study until it is completed. An independent third party holds the code and the data until the study has been completed.

dual energy X-ray absorptiometry (DEXA) Highly accurate method of measuring body composition and bone mass and density using multiple low-energy X rays.

dual energy X-ray absorptiometry (DEXA) bone scan Method to measure bone density that uses small amounts of X-ray radiation. A bone's ability to block the path of the radiation is used as a measure of bone density at that bone site.

duodenum (doo-oh-DEE-num, or doo-ODD-num) First portion of the small intestine; leads from the pyloric sphincter to the jejunum.

duration Length of time (e.g., duration of an exercise session).

dyslipidemia (DIS-lip-ah-DEEM-E-ah) State in which various blood lipids, such as LDL or triglycerides, are greatly elevated or, in the case of HDL, are very low.

E

early childhood caries Tooth decay that results from formula or juice (and even human milk) bathing the teeth as the child sleeps with a bottle in his or her mouth. Upper teeth are affected mostly because the lower teeth are protected by the tongue; formerly called *nursing bottle syndrome* and *baby bottle tooth decay*.

eating disorder Severe alterations in eating patterns linked to physiological changes. The alterations are associated with food restricting, binge eating, purging, and fluctuations in weight. They also involve a number of emotional and cognitive changes that affect the way a person perceives and experiences his or her body.

eclampsia (ee-KLAMP-see-ah) See *pregnancy-induced hypertension*.

E. coli See *Escherichia coli*.

ecosystem (ek-OH-sis-tum) "Community" in nature that includes plants, animals, and the environment.

edamame (ed-a-MOM-ee) Fresh green soybeans.

edema (uh-DEE-muh) Buildup of excess fluid in extracellular spaces.

EFNEP See *Expanded Food and Nutrition Education Program*.

eicosanoids (eye-KOH-san-oyds) Hormone-like compounds synthesized from polyunsaturated fatty acids, such as arachidonic acid. Within this class of compounds are prostacyclins, prostaglandins, thromboxanes, and leukotrienes.

eicosapentaenoic acid (EPA) (eye-KOH-sah-pen-tahee-NO-ik) Omega-3 fatty acid with 20 carbons and 5 carbon-carbon double bonds (C20:5, omega-3). It is present in large amounts in fatty fish and slowly synthesized in the body from alpha-linolenic acid. EPA is a precursor to some eicosanoids.

Elderly Nutrition Program U.S. government program that provides nutrition services through the Congregate Meal Program and Home Delivered Meal Program (often referred to as Meals on Wheels) to anyone age 60 and older.

electrolytes (ih-LEK-tro-lites) Compounds that separate into ions in water and, in turn, are able to conduct an electrical current. These include sodium, chloride, and potassium.

electron Part of an atom that is negatively charged. Electrons orbit the nucleus.

electron transport chain Series of reactions using oxygen to convert NADH+H$^+$ and FADH$_2$ molecules to free NAD$^+$ and FAD molecules with the donation of electrons and hydrogen ions to oxygen, yielding water and ATP.

element Substance that cannot be separated into simpler substances by chemical processes. Common elements in nutrition include carbon, oxygen, hydrogen, nitrogen, calcium, phosphorus, and iron.

elimination diet Restrictive diet that systematically tests foods that may cause an allergic response by first eliminating them for 1 to 2 weeks and then adding them back, 1 at a time.

embryo (EM-bree-oh) In humans, the developing in utero offspring from about the beginning of the third week to the end of the eighth week after conception.

emulsifier (ee-MULL-sih-fire) Compound that can suspend fat in water by isolating individual fat droplets using a shell of water molecules or other substances to prevent the fat from coalescing.

endemic (en-DEM-ik) Habitual presence within a given geographic area (e.g., an endemic disease).

endocrine cells Cells throughout the gastrointestinal tract that contain regulatory peptides and/or biogenic amines.

endocrine gland (EN-doh-krin) Hormone-producing gland.

endocrine system Body system consisting of the various glands and the hormones these glands secrete. This system has major regulatory functions in the body, such as in reproduction and cell metabolism.

endocytosis (phagocytosis/pinocytosis) Active absorption in which the absorptive cell forms an indentation in its membrane, and then particles (phagocytosis) or fluids (pinocytosis) entering the indentation are engulfed by the cell.

endometrium (en-doh-ME-tree-um) Membrane that lines the inside of the uterus. It increases in thickness during the menstrual cycle until ovulation occurs. The surface layers are shed during menstruation if conception does not take place.

endoplasmic reticulum (ER) (en-doh-PLAZ-mik re-TIK-u-lum) Organelle in the cytoplasm composed of a network of canals running through the cytoplasm. Rough ER contains ribosomes. Smooth ER contains no ribosomes.

endorphins (en-DOR-fins) Natural body tranquilizers that may be involved in the feeding response and function in pain reduction.

endosperm Starch interior of a cereal grain.

endothelial cells (en-doh-THEE-lee-al) Flat cells lining the blood and lymphatic vessels and the chambers of the heart.

enema (EN-ah-mah) Injection of liquid through the rectum to cause the elimination of fecal matter.

energy balance State in which energy intake, in the form of food and beverages, matches energy expended, primarily through basal metabolism and physical activity.

energy density Comparison of the energy content of a food with the weight of the food. An energy-dense food is high in energy but weighs very little (e.g., many fried foods), whereas a food low in energy density (e.g., an orange) weighs a lot but is low in energy content.

energy equilibrium See *equilibrium*.

enriched Term generally meaning that the vitamins thiamin, niacin, riboflavin, and folate and the mineral iron have been added to a grain product to improve its nutritional quality.

enterocytes (en-TER-oh-sites) Epithelial cells, which are highly specialized for digestion and absorption, that line the intestinal villi.

enterohepatic circulation (EN-ter-oh-heh-PAT-ik) Continual recycling of compounds between the small intestine and the liver; bile acids are an example of a recycled compound.

environmental assessment Assessment that focuses on one's education and economic background and other factors that affect one's ability to purchase, transport, and cook food and follow instructions given by health-care providers.

enzyme (EN-zime) Compound that speeds the rate of a chemical process but is not altered by the process. Almost all enzymes are proteins (some are made of nucleic acids).

epidemiology (ep-uh-dee-me-OLL-uh-gee) Distribution and determinants of diseases in human populations.

epidermis (ep-ih-DUR-miss) Outermost layer of the skin; composed of epithelial layers.

epigenetic carcinogens (promoters) (ep-ih-je-NET-ik car-SIN-oh-jens) Compounds that increase cell division and thereby increase the chance that a cell with altered DNA will develop into cancer.

epiglottis (ep-ih-GLOT-iss) Flap that folds down over the trachea during swallowing.

epinephrine (ep-ih-NEF-rin) Hormone produced by the adrenal gland in times of stress. It also may have neurotransmitter functions, such as in the brain.

epiphyseal line (ep-ih-FEES-ee-al) Line that replaces the epiphyseal plate when bone growth is complete.

epiphyseal plate Cartilage-like layer in the long bone sometimes referred to as the growth plate. It functions in linear growth. During childhood, the cartilage cells multiply and absorb calcium to develop into bone.

epiphyses (e-PIF-ih-seas) Ends of long bones.

epithelial tissue (ep-ih-THEE-lee-ul) Surface cells that line the outside of the body and all passageways within it.

epithelium (ep-ih-THEE-lee-um) Covering of internal and external surfaces of the body, including the lining of vessels and other small cavities. It consists of epithelial cells joined by a small amount of cementing material.

equilibrium (ee-kwih-LIB-ree-um) In nutrition, a state in which nutrient intake equals nutrient losses. Thus, the body maintains a stable condition, such as energy equilibrium.

ergogenic (ur-go-JEN-ic) Work-producing. An ergogenic aid is a mechanical, nutritional, psychological, pharmacological, or physiological substance or treatment that is intended to directly improve exercise performance.

erythrocyte (eh-RITH-row-site) Mature red blood cell. It has no nucleus and a life span of about 120 days. It contains hemoglobin, which transports oxygen and carbon dioxide.

erythropoietin (eh-REE-throw-POY-eh-tin) Hormone, secreted mostly by the kidneys, that enhances red blood cell synthesis and stimulates red blood cell release from bone marrow.

Escherichia coli Bacterium commonly found in the intestinal tract of humans and animals (commonly called *E. coli*). The especially virulent strains 0157:H7 and 0111:H8 have been found in undercooked beef, especially ground beef. Foods implicated in *E. coli* infection include unpasteurized milk, unpasteurized fresh apple cider, salad greens, cantaloupe, dry-cured salami, and many types of sprouts. Cooking destroys *E. coli*.

esophagus (eh-SOF-ah-gus) Tube in the GI tract that connects the pharynx with the stomach.

essential amino acids Amino acids that cannot be synthesized by humans in sufficient amounts or at all and therefore must be included in the diet. There are 9 essential amino acids. They also are called *indispensable amino acids*.

essential fatty acids Fatty acids that must be supplied by the diet to maintain health. Currently, only linoleic acid and alpha-linolenic acid are classified as essential.

essential nutrient In nutritional terms, a substance that, when left out of a diet, leads to signs of poor health. The body either can't produce this nutrient or can't produce enough of it to meet its needs. Then, if added back to a diet before permanent damage occurs, the affected aspects of health are restored.

ester (ES-ter) Organic compound that has an O=C group attached to a carbonyl group; product of a reaction between a carboxylic acid and an alcohol; formation of triglycerides involves forming ester bonds.

esterification (e-ster-ih-fih-KAY-shun) Process of attaching fatty acids to a glycerol molecule, creating an ester bond and releasing water. Removing a fatty acid is called deesterification; reattaching a fatty acid is called reesterification.

Estimated Average Requirement (EAR) Amount of nutrient intake that is estimated to meet the needs of 50% of the individuals in a specific age and gender group.

Estimated Energy Requirement (EER) An estimate of the amount of energy intake that will meet the energy needs of an average person within specific gender, age, and other considerations.

ethanol Chemical term for the form of alcohol found in alcoholic beverages.

eustachian tubes (you-STAY-shun) Thin tubes connected to the middle ear that open into the throat.

exchange Serving size of a food on a specific exchange list.

Exchange System System for classifying foods into numerous lists based on the foods' macronutrient composition and establishing serving sizes, so that 1 serving of each food on a list contains the same amount of carbohydrate, protein, fat, and calories.

exercise Physical activity done with the intent of providing a health benefit, such as improved muscle tone or stamina.

exocrine gland (EK-so-krin) Cluster of epithelial cells specialized for secretion. They have ducts that lead to an epithelial surface.

exocytosis (ek-so-sigh-TOE-sis) Process of cellular secretion in which the secretory products are contained within a membrane-enclosed vesicle. The vesicle fuses with the cell membrane and is open to the extracellular environment.

Expanded Food and Nutrition Education Program (EFNEP) U.S. government program that provides nutrition education for families with limited resources.

experiment Test made to examine the validity of a hypothesis.

extracellular Outside cells.

extracellular fluid (ECF) Fluid present outside the cells. It includes intravascular and interstitial fluids and represents one-third of all body fluid.

extrusion reflex Reflex present in first few months of life that helps a baby express milk from a nipple, but it also causes an infant to push objects placed on the tip of the tongue, such as a spoon or food, out of the mouth; also called tongue-thrusting.

F

facilitated diffusion Absorption in which a carrier shuttles substances into the absorptive cell but no energy is expended. Absorption is driven by a concentration gradient that is higher in the intestinal contents than in the absorptive cell.

failure to thrive Inadequate gains in height and weight in infancy, often due to an inadequate food intake.

famine Extreme shortage of food that leads to massive starvation in a population; often associated with crop failures, war, and political unrest.

fasting blood sugar (FBS) Measurement of blood glucose levels after a period of 8 hours or more without food or beverages.

fasting hypoglycemia (HIGH-po-gligh-SEE-meah) Low blood glucose that follows after about a day of fasting.

fat Substance that dissolves in organic solvents, such as benzene and ether. Fats are mostly composed of carbon and hydrogen, with relatively small amounts of oxygen and other elements. Dietary fat supplies 9 kcal/gram.

fat-soluble vitamins Vitamins that dissolve in fat and such substances as ether and benzene, but not readily in water; vitamins A, D, E, and K.

fatty acid Chain of carbons chemically bonded together and surrounded by hydrogen molecules. These hydrocarbons are found in lipids and contain a carboxyl (acid

$$\overset{\text{O}}{\underset{\|}{}}$$

group ($-C-OH$) at 1 end and a methyl group ($-CH_3$) at the other.

fatty acid oxidation Breakdown of fatty acids into compounds that enter the citric acid cycle.

favorable pregnancy outcome In humans, a full-term gestation period (longer than 37 weeks) that results in a live, healthy infant weighing more than 5.5 pounds.

feces (FEE-seas) Substances discharged from the bowel during defecation, including undigested food residue, dead GI tract cells, mucus, bacteria, and other waste material.

feeding center Group of cells in the hypothalamus that, when stimulated, causes hunger.

female athlete triad Condition characterized by low energy availability, menstrual disorders, and low bone mineral density.

fermentation Metabolism, without the use of oxygen, of carbohydrates to alcohols, acids, and carbon dioxide.

ferritin (FER-ih-tin) Iron-binding protein in the intestinal mucosa that binds iron and prevents it from entering the bloodstream; also the primary storage form of iron in liver and other tissues.

fetal alcohol effect (FAE) (FEET-al) Hyperactivity, attention deficit disorder, poor judgment, sleep disorders, and delayed learning as a result of prenatal exposure to alcohol.

fetal alcohol syndrome (FAS) Group of irreversible physical and mental abnormalities in an infant that results from the mother's consuming alcohol during pregnancy.

fetus (FEET-us) In humans, developing offspring from about the beginning of the ninth week after conception until birth.

fiber Substance in plant foods that is not broken down by the digestive processes of the stomach or small intestine. Fiber adds bulk to feces. Fiber naturally found in foods is called dietary fiber.

flatulence (FLAT-u-lens) Intestinal gas.

flatus (FLA-tus) Gas generated in the intestinal tract that may be passed through the anus.

flavin Group of compounds that contains riboflavin or a related compound.

flavin adenine dinucleotide (FAD) Coenzyme that readily accepts and donates electrons and hydrogen ions; formed from the vitamin riboflavin.

flavin mononucleotide (FMN) Coenzyme, formed from the vitamin riboflavin, that participates in oxidation reduction reactions.

flexibility exercise Ability to move a joint through its full range of motion.

fluoride Trace mineral that increases the resistance of tooth enamel to dental caries. Typical sources are fluoridated water and toothpaste.

fluoroapatite (fleur-oh-APP-uh-tite) Fluoride-containing, acid-resistant, crystalline substance produced during bone and tooth development. Its presence in teeth helps prevent dental caries.

folate Water-soluble vitamin that shares a close relationship with vitamin B-12. In its coenzyme form, folate is necessary for the synthesis of DNA and in the metabolism of various amino acids and their derivatives, such as homocysteine. It also functions in the formation of neurotransmitters in the brain. A maternal deficiency of folate can lead to neural tube defects in the very early development of the fetus. Asparagus, spinach, fortified grain products, and legumes are good sources.

folic acid Form of folate found in supplements and fortified foods.

folk medicine Medical treatment based on the beliefs, traditions, or customs of a particular society or ethnic/cultural group.

follicular hyperkeratosis (fo-LICK-you-lar high-per-ker-ah-TOE-sis) Condition in which keratin, a protein, accumulates around hair follicles.

food additive Substance added to foods to produce a desired effect, such as preservation or nutritional fortification. Over 3000 food additives are regulated by the FDA.

foodborne illness Sickness caused by the ingestion of food containing pathogenic microorganisms and/or their toxins.

food diary Written record of sequential food intake for a period of time. Details associated with the food intake are often recorded as well.

food insecure Condition in which the quality, variety, and/or desirability of the diet is reduced and there is difficulty at times providing enough food for everyone in the household.

food intolerance Adverse reaction to food that does not involve an allergic reaction.

food secure Condition in which food needs are met all of the time.

food sensitivity Mild reaction to a substance in a food; might be expressed as light itching or redness of the skin.

Food Stamp Program U.S. government program that provides nutrition education and foods for those with limited financial resources.

fore milk First breast milk delivered in a breastfeeding session.

fortified Term generally meaning that vitamins, minerals, or both have been added to a food product in excess of what was originally found in the product.

fraternal twins Offspring that develop from 2 separate ova and sperm and therefore have separate genetic identities but develop simultaneously in the mother.

free fatty acid Fatty acid that is not attached to a glycerol molecule.

free radical Short-lived form of a compound that has an unpaired electron, causing it to seek an electron from another compound. Free radicals are strong oxidizing agents and can be very destructive to electron-dense cell components, such as DNA and cell membranes.

free water Water not bound to the compounds in a food. This water is available for microbial use.

frequency In terms of exercise, number of activity sessions performed per week.

fructans (FROOK-tans) Polysaccharides composed of fructose units.

fructose (FROOK-tose) Monosaccharide with 6 carbons that forms a 5-membered or 6-membered ring with oxygen in the ring; found in fruits and honey.

fruitarian (froot-AIR-ee-un) Person who eats primarily fruits, nuts, honey, and vegetable oils.

functional fiber Fiber added to foods that has shown to provide health benefits.

functional foods Foods that provide health benefits beyond those supplied by the traditional nutrients they contain. For example, a tomato contains the phytochemical lycopene, so it can be called a functional food.

fungi Simple parasitic life forms, including molds, mildews, yeasts, and mushrooms. They live on dead or decaying organic matter. Fungi can grow as single cells, such as yeast, or as multicellular colonies, as seen with molds.

G

galactose (gah-LAK-tos) Six-carbon monosaccharide that forms a 6-membered ring with oxygen in the ring; an isomer of glucose.

galactosemia (gah-LAK-toh-SEE-mee-ah) Rare genetic disease characterized by the buildup of the single sugar galactose in the bloodstream, resulting from the liver's inability to metabolize it. If present at birth and left untreated, this disease can cause severe mental retardation and cataracts in the infant.

gallbladder Organ attached to the underside of the liver and in which bile is stored and secreted.

gamma-aminobutyric acid (GABA) (ah-MEE-noh-bu-tir-ik) Inhibitory neurotransmitter synthesized from the amino acid glutamic acid.

gastric inhibitory peptide (GIP) (GAS-trik in-HIB-ih-tor-ee PEP-tide) Hormone that slows gastric motility and stimulates insulin release from the pancreas.

gastrin (GAS-trin) Hormone that stimulates enzyme and acid secretion by the stomach.

gastroesophageal reflux disease (GERD) (gas-troh-eh-SOF-ah-jee-al) Disease that results from stomach acid backing up into the esophagus. The acid irritates the lining of the esophagus, causing pain.

gastrointestinal distension (gas-troh-in-TEST-in-al) Expansion of the wall of the stomach or intestines due to pressure caused by the presence of gases, food, drink, or other factors. This expansion contributes to a feeling of satiety brought on by food intake.

gastrointestinal (GI) tract Comprises the main sites in the body used in digestion and absorption of nutrients. The GI tract consists of the mouth, esophagus, stomach, small intestine, large intestine, rectum, and anus.

gastroplasty (GAS-troh-plas-tee) Surgery performed on the stomach to limit its volume to approximately 30 milliliters.

gene expression (JEAN) Activation of a specific site on DNA, which results in either the activation or the inhibition of the gene.

generally recognized as safe (GRAS) List of food additives that in 1958 were considered safe for consumption. Manufacturers were allowed to continue to use these additives, without special clearance, when needed for food products. The FDA bears responsibility for proving they are not safe; it can remove unsafe products from the list.

genes (JEANS) Hereditary material on chromosomes that makes up DNA. Genes provide the blueprint for the production of cell proteins. The nucleus of the cell contains about 30,000 genes.

genetically modified organism (GMO) Organism created by genetic engineering.

genetic engineering Manipulation of the genetic makeup of any organism with recombinant DNA technology.

genotoxic carcinogen (initiator) (JEE-no-TOK-sik car-SIN-oh-jen) Compound that directly alters DNA or is converted in cells to metabolites that alter DNA, thereby providing the potential for cancer to develop.

germ Vitamin- and lipid-rich core of the whole grain.

gestation (jes-TAY-shun) Period of intrauterine development of offspring, from conception to birth. In humans, gestation lasts for about 40 weeks after the woman's last menstrual period.

gestational diabetes (jes-TAY-shun-al) High blood glucose concentration that develops during pregnancy and returns to normal after birth.

ghrelin (GREL-in) Hormone, made by the stomach, that increases food intake.

glomerulus (glo-MER-you-lus) Capillaries in the kidney that filter the blood.

glossitis (glah-SI-tis) Inflammation of the tongue. It becomes red, smooth, shiny, and sore.

glucagon (GLOO-kuh-gon) Hormone, made by the pancreas, that stimulates the breakdown of glycogen in the liver into glucose. This breakdown increases blood glucose.

glucogenic amino acid (gloo-ko-JEN-ik) Amino acid that can be converted into glucose via gluconeogenesis.

gluconeogenesis (gloo-ko-nee-oh-JEN-uh-sis) Production of new glucose by metabolic pathways in the cell. Amino acids derived from protein usually provide the carbons for this glucose.

glucose (GLOO-kos) Monosaccharide with 6 carbons; also called *dextrose;* a primary source of energy in the body; found in table sugar (sucrose) bound to fructose.

glucose polymer (PAH-lah-mer) Carbohydrate, used in some sports drinks, that consists of a few glucose molecules bonded together.

glutamine (GLOO-tah-meen) Amino acid that enhances the immune system during trauma and illness.

glutathione (gloo-tah-THIGH-on) Reducing agent; can remove toxic peroxides that form in the cell during aerobic respiration.

glutathione peroxidase (gloo-tah-THIGH-on per-OX-ih-dase) Selenium-containing enzyme that can destroy peroxides; acts in conjunction with vitamin E to reduce free radical damage to cells.

glycemic index (GI) (gli-SEA-mik) Ratio of the blood glucose response to a given food, compared with a standard (typically, glucose or white bread).

glycemic load (GL) Amount of carbohydrate in a food multiplied by the glycemic index of that carbohydrate. The result is then divided by 100.

glycerol (GLIS-er-ol) 3-carbon alcohol that provides the backbone of triglycerides.

glycocalyx (gli-ko-KAL-iks) Projections of proteins on the microvilli. They contain enzymes to digest protein and carbohydrate.

glycogen (GLI-ko-jen) Carbohydrate made of multiple units of glucose with a highly branched structure; sometimes known as *animal starch;* the storage form of glucose in humans; is synthesized (and stored) in the liver and muscles.

glycogen storage disease Genetic defect that does not allow glycogen to be stored in the muscles or liver.

glycolipid (gli-ko-LIP-id) Lipid (fat) containing a carbohydrate group.

glycolysis (gli-KOL-ih-sis) Metabolic pathway that converts glucose into 2 molecules of pyruvic acid, with the net gain of 2 ATP and 2 NADH+2H$^+$.

glycoprotein (gli-ko-PRO-teen) Protein containing a carbohydrate group.

glycosylation (gli-COS-ih-lay-shun) Process by which glucose attaches to (glycates) other compounds, such as proteins.

goiter (GOY-ter) Enlargement of the thyroid gland; can be caused by a lack of iodide in the diet.

goitrogens (GOY-troh-jens) Substances in food and water that interfere with thyroid gland metabolism and thus may cause goiter if consumed in large amounts.

Golgi complex (GOAL-jee) Cell organelle near the nucleus; processes newly synthesized protein for secretion or distribution to other organelles.

gout (gowt) Joint inflammation caused by accumulation of uric acid. Obesity is a risk factor for developing gout.

green revolution Increases in crop yields accompanying the introduction of new agricultural technologies in less developed countries, beginning in the 1960s. The key technologies were high-yielding, disease-resistant strains of rice, wheat, and corn; greater use of fertilizer and water; and improved cultivation practices.

growth hormone Pituitary hormone that stimulates body growth and the release of fat from storage, as well as other effects.

guanine (GWAH-heen) Nitrogenous base that forms part of the structure of DNA and RNA; a purine.

gum Soluble fiber consisting of chains of galactose and other monosaccharides; characteristically found in exudates from plant stems.

gynecoid obesity (GI-nih-coyd) Excess fat storage located primarily in the buttocks and thigh area.

H

H$_2$ blocker Medication, such as cimetidine (Tagamet®), that blocks the increase of stomach acid production caused by histamine.

Harris-Benedict equation Equation that predicts resting metabolic rate based on a person's weight, height, and age.

health claim Claim that describes a well-researched and documented relationship between a disease and a nutrient, food, or food constituent. See also *preliminary health claim.*

heart attack Rapid fall in heart function caused by obstructed blood flow through the heart's blood vessels. Often, part of the heart dies in the process. It is technically called a myocardial infarction.

heartburn Pain caused by stomach acid backing up into the esophagus and irritating the tissue in that organ.

heart disease See *cardiovascular disease.*

heat cramps Frequent complication of heat exhaustion. They usually occur in individuals who have experienced large sweat losses from exercising for several hours in a hot climate and have consumed a large volume of water. The cramps occur in skeletal muscles and consist of contractions for 1 to 3 minutes at a time.

heat exhaustion First stage of heat-related illness that occurs because of depletion of blood volume from fluid loss by the body. This depletion increases body temperature and can lead to headaches, dizziness, muscle weakness, and visual disturbances, among other effects.

heatstroke Condition in which the internal body temperature reaches 104°F. Sweating generally ceases if left untreated, and blood circulation is greatly reduced. Nervous system damage may ensue, and death is likely. Often, the skin of individuals who suffer heatstroke is hot and dry.

helminth (HEL-menth) Parasitic worm that can contaminate food, water, feces, animals, and other substances.

helper T cell Type of T cell that interacts with macrophages and secretes substances to signal an invading pathogen; stimulates B lymphocytes to proliferate.

hematocrit (hee-MAT-oh-krit) Percentage of total blood volume occupied by red blood cells.

hematopoiesis (hee-mat-oh-po-EE-sis) Production of blood cells.

heme Iron-containing structure found in hemoglobin and myoglobin.

heme iron (HEEM) Iron provided from animal tissues primarily as a component of hemoglobin and myoglobin. Approximately 40% of the iron in meat is heme iron; it is readily absorbed.

hemicellulose (hem-ih-SELL-you-los) Mostly insoluble fiber containing galactose, glucose, and other monosaccharides bonded together.

hemochromatosis (heem-oh-krom-ah-TOE-sis) Disorder of iron metabolism characterized by increased absorption of iron, saturation of iron-binding proteins, and deposition of hemosiderin in the liver tissue.

hemoglobin (HEEM-oh-glow-bin) Iron-containing protein in red blood cells that transports oxygen to the body tissues and some carbon dioxide away from the tissues. It also is responsible for the red color of blood.

hemolysis (hee-MOL-ih-sis) Destruction of red blood cells caused by the breakdown of the red blood cell membranes. This causes the cell contents to leak into the fluid portion (plasma) of the blood.

hemolytic anemia (hee-moe-LIT-ik) Disorder that causes red blood cells to break down faster than they can be replaced.

hemorrhage (hem-OR-ij) Escape of blood from blood vessels, causing bleeding.

hemorrhagic stroke (hem-oh-RAJ-ik) Damage to part of the brain resulting from rupture of a blood vessel and subsequent bleeding within or over the internal surface of the brain.

hemorrhoid (HEM-or-oid) Pronounced swelling in a large vein, particularly a vein in the anal region.

hemosiderin (heem-oh-SID-er-in) Insoluble iron-protein compound in the liver. Hemosiderin stores iron when the amount of iron in the body exceeds the storage capacity of ferritin.

hepatic portal system (vein) (he-PAT-ik) Vein in the GI tract that conveys blood from capillaries in the intestines and portions of the stomach to capillaries in the liver; also called the portal vein.

hepatic vein (he-PAT-ik) Vein that drains the liver.

hepatitis A (hep-ah-TIE-tis) Virus found in the human intestinal tract and feces; causes inflammation and loss of function of the liver. It can contaminate many foods, especially shellfish and raw foods, and can endure significant heat, cold, and drying.

herbicide (ERB-ih-side) Compound that reduces the growth and reproduction of plants.

hexose (HEK-sos) Carbohydrate containing 6 carbons.

hiatal hernia (high-AY-tal HUR-nee-ah) Protrusion of part of the stomach through the diaphragm. It is often associated with gastroesophageal reflux disease.

high-density lipoprotein (HDL) Lipoprotein that picks up cholesterol from cells and transfers it in the bloodstream to the liver. A low blood HDL value increases the risk of cardiovascular disease.

high-fructose corn syrup Corn syrup that has been manufactured to contain between 42 and 90% fructose.

high-quality (complete) proteins Dietary proteins that contain ample amounts of all 9 essential amino acids.

hind milk (HYND) Milk secreted at the end of a breastfeeding session. It is higher in fat than fore milk.

histamine (HISS-tuh-meen) Breakdown product of the amino acid histidine; stimulates acid secretion by the stomach and has other effects on the body, such as contraction of smooth muscles, increased nasal secretions, relaxation of blood vessels, and changes in constriction of airways.

holoenzyme Active enzyme complex composed of the apoenzyme and the cofactor.

homeostasis (home-ee-oh-STAY-sis) Series of adjustments that prevent change in the internal environment in the body.

homocysteine (homo-SIS-teen) Amino acid not used in protein synthesis. Instead, it arises during metabolism of the amino acid methionine. Homocysteine likely is toxic to many cells, such as those lining the blood vessels.

hormone Compound with a specific site of synthesis that, when secreted into the bloodstream, controls the function of cells in its target organ or organs. Hormones can be amino acidlike (epinephrine), proteinlike (insulin), or fatlike (estrogen).

hormone-sensitive lipase Hormone that is responsible for breaking down stored triglycerides in fat cells into free fatty acids and glycerol.

hospice care (HAHS-pis) Supportive care that emphasizes comfort and dignity in death.

human immunodeficiency virus (HIV) Virus that leads to acquired immunodeficiency syndrome (AIDS).

hunger Primarily physiological (internal) drive for food.

hydrogenation (high-dro-jen-AY-shun) Addition of hydrogen to a carbon-carbon double bond, producing a single carbon-carbon bond with 2 hydrogens attached to each carbon. Because hydrogenation of unsaturated fatty acids in a vegetable oil increases its hardness, this process is used to convert liquid oils into more solid fats, which are used in making margarine and shortening. *Trans* fatty acids are a by-product of the hydrogenation of vegetable oils.

hydrogen peroxide (pur-OX-ide) Chemically, H_2O_2.

hydrolysis (high-DROL-ih-sis) Chemical reaction in which a compound is broken down by the addition of water. One product receives a hydrogen ion (H^+), whereas the other product receives a hydroxyl ion (—OH). Hydrolytic enzymes break down compounds using water in this manner.

hydrolysis reaction Chemical reaction in which a bond between 2 molecules is broken by the inclusion of a water molecule. The water donates a hydrogen to 1 reactant and a hydroxyl (—OH) group to the other reactant.

hydrophilic (high-dro-FILL-ik) Literally, "water-loving;" attracts water.

hydrophobic (high-dro-FO-bik) Literally, "water-fearing;" repels water.

hydroxyapatite (high-drox-ee-APP-uh-tite) Compound composed primarily of calcium and phosphate; is deposited in bone protein matrix to give bone strength and rigidity ($Ca_{10}[PO_4]6OH_2$).

hyperactivity Inattention, irritability, and excessively active behavior in children; technically referred to as *attention deficit hyperactive disorder.*

hypercalcemia (high-per-kal-SEE-mee-ah) High concentration of calcium in the bloodstream. This condition can lead to loss of appetite, calcium deposits in organs, and other health problems.

hypercarotenemia (high-per-car-oh-teh-NEEM-ee-ah) Elevated amounts of carotenoids in the bloodstream, usually caused by consuming a diet high in carrots or squash or by taking beta-carotene supplements.

hyperemesis gravidarum (high-per-EM-eh-sis gra-va-DAR-um) Severe nausea and vomiting experienced during pregnancy that continues beyond 14 weeks of gestation.

hyperglycemia (HIGH-per-gligh-SEE-me-uh) High blood glucose, above 125 mg/100 ml (dl) of blood.

hypergymnasia (high-per-jim-NAY-zee-ah) Exercising more than is required for good physical fitness or maximum performance in a sport; excessive exercise.

hyperkalemia (high-per-kah-LEE-mee-ah) High potassium levels in the blood.

hypernatremia (high-per-nay-TREE-mee-ah) High sodium levels in the blood.

hyperlipidemia (high-per-lip-ih-DEE-me-ah) Presence of an abnormally large amount of lipids in the circulating blood.

hyperparathyroidism (high-per-pair-ah THY-royd-iz-um) Overproduction of parathyroid hormone by the parathyroid glands, usually caused by a tumor. In most cases, there are no symptoms except hypercalcemia. In severe cases, weakness, confusion, nausea, and bone pain occur.

hyperplasia (high-per-PLAY-zee-uh) Increase in cell number.

hypertension (high-per-TEN-shun) Persistently elevated blood pressure. Obesity, inactivity, alcohol intake, and excess salt intake all can contribute to the problem.

hyperthyroidism Condition characterized by high blood levels of thyroid hormone.

hypertriglyceridemia (high-PURR-tri-GLISS-uh-ride-ee-me-ah) Condition in which there are excess triglycerides in the blood.

hypertrophy (high-PURR-tro-fee) Increased tissue or organ size.

hypervitaminosis A (HIGH-per-vi-tah-mi-NO-sis) Condition resulting from intake of excessive amounts of vitamin A.

hypocalcemia (HIGH-po-kal-SEE-me-ah) Low blood calcium, typically arising from inadequate parathyroid hormone release or action.

hypochromic (high-po-KROM-ik) Pale; red blood cells lacking sufficient hemoglobin. Hypochromic cells have a reduced oxygen-carrying ability.

hypoglycemia (HIGH-po-gligh-SEE-me-uh) Low blood glucose, below 50 mg/100 ml (dl) of blood.

hypokalemia (high-po-kah-LEE-me-ah) Low postassium levels in the blood.

hyponatremia (high-po-nay-TREE-me-ah) Low sodium levels in the blood.

hypothalamus (high-po-THALL-uh-mus) Region at the base of the brain; contains cells that play a role in the regulation of hunger, respiration, body temperature, and other body functions.

hypothesis (high-POTH-eh-sis) Tentative explanation by scientists to explain a phenomenon.

hysterectomy (hiss-te-RECK-toe-mee) Surgical removal of the uterus.

I

identical twins Two offspring that develop from a single ovum and sperm and, consequently, have the same genetic makeup.

ileocecal valve (ill-ee-oh-SEE-kal) Ring of smooth muscle between the ileum of the small intestine and the colon; also known as the ileocecal sphincter.

ileum (ILL-ee-um) Terminal portion of the small intestine.

immune system Body system consisting of white blood cells, lymph glands, lymphocytes, antibodies, and other body tissues and cells. The immune system defends against foreign invaders.

immunoglobulins (em-you-no-GLOB-you-lins) Proteins (also called antibodies) in the blood that are responsible for identifying and neutralizing antigens, as well as pathogens that bind specifically to antigens.

incidence Number of new cases of a disease in a defined population over a specific period of time, such as 1 year.

incidental food additives Additives that appear in food products indirectly, from environmental contamination of food ingredients or during the manufacturing process.

incomplete (lower-quality) protein Food protein that lacks enough of 1 or more of the essential amino acids to support human protein needs.

indirect calorimetry (kal-oh-RIM-eh-tree) Method to measure energy use by the body by measuring oxygen uptake. Formulas are used to convert this gas exchange value into energy use.

infancy Earliest stage of childhood—from birth to 1 year of age.

infectious disease (in-FEK-shus) Disease caused by an invasion of the body by microorganisms, such as bacteria, fungi, or viruses.

infrastructure Basic framework of a system or an organization. For a society, this includes roads, bridges, telephones, and other basic technologies.

inorganic (in-or-GAN-ik) Substance lacking carbon atoms bonded to hydrogen atoms in the chemical structure.

insensible water losses Water losses not readily perceived, such as water lost with each breath.

insoluble fibers Fibers that mostly do not dissolve in water and are not metabolized by bacteria in the large intestine. These include cellulose, some hemicelluloses, and lignins; more formally called *nonfermentable fibers*.

insulin (IN-su-lynn) Hormone produced by beta cells of the pancreas. Among other processes, insulin increases the synthesis of glycogen in the liver and the movement of glucose from the bloodstream into muscle and adipose cells.

integumentary system (in-teg-you-MEN-tah-ree) Having to do with the skin, hair, glands, and nails.

intensity In terms of exercise, the amount of effort expended or how difficult the activity is to perform.

intentional food additive Additive knowingly (directly) incorporated into food products by manufacturers.

interferon (in-ter-FEAR-on) Protein released by virus-infected cells that bind to other cells, stimulating the synthesis of antiviral proteins, which in turn inhibit viral multiplication.

intermediate Chemical compound formed in 1 of many steps in a metabolic pathway.

international unit (IU) Crude measure of vitamin activity, often based on the growth rate of animals. Today, IUs have generally been replaced by precise measurements of actual quantities, such as milligrams or micrograms.

interstitial fluid (in-ter-STISH-al) Fluid between cells.

interstitial spaces Spaces between cells.

intracellular fluid (in-tra-SELL-you-lar) Fluid contained within a cell; represents about two-thirds of all body fluid.

intravascular fluid (in-tra-VAS-kyu-lar) Fluid within the bloodstream (i.e., in the arteries, veins, capillaries, and lymphatic vessels); represents about 25% of all body fluids.

intrinsic factor (in-TRIN-zik) Substance produced by parietal cells of the stomach; enhances vitamin B-12 absorption.

inulin (IN-u-lin) Type of soluble fiber made up mainly of fructose molecules; found in foods such as onion and chicory; acts as a prebiotic.

in utero (in-YOU-ter-oh) "In the uterus," or during pregnancy.

in vitro (in-VEE-troh) Literally, "in glass," such as in a test tube (e.g., experiments performed outside the body).

in vivo (in-VEE-vo) Within the living body.

iodine Trace mineral that is a component of thyroid hormones. A deficiency can result in goiter. Iodized salt, saltwater fish, and iodine-fortified foods are good sources.

ion (EYE-on) Atom with an unequal number of electrons and protons. Negative ions have more electrons than protons; positive ions have more protons than electrons.

ionic bond (eye-ON-ik) Union between 2 atoms formed by an attraction of a positive ion to a negative ion, as in table salt (Na^+Cl^-).

iron Trace mineral that functions as a component of hemoglobin and other key compounds used in respiration; also important in immune function and cognitive development. Meats, seafood, molasses, and fortified foods are good sources.

irradiation (ir-RAY-dee-AY-shun) Process in which radiation energy is applied to foods, creating compounds (free radicals) within the food that destroy microorganisms that can lead to food spoilage. This process does not make the food radioactive.

irritable bowel syndrome Bowel disease characterized by diarrhea, constipation, abdominal pain, and distension; believed to be caused by abnormal function of the muscles and nerves of the gastrointestinal tract. It is more common in women than men.

ischemia (ih-SKEE-mee-ah) Lack of blood flow due to mechanical obstruction of the blood supply, mainly from arterial narrowing.

ischemic stroke (ih-SKEE-mik) Stroke caused by the absence of blood flow to a part of the brain.

isomers (EYE-so-merz) Different chemical structures for compounds that share the same chemical formula.

isotope (EYE-so-towp) Alternate form of a chemical element. It differs from other atoms of the same element in the number of neutrons in its nucleus.

J

jaundice (JOHN-diss) Yellowish staining of skin, sclerae of the eyes, and other tissues by bile pigments that build up in the blood.

jejunum (je-JOO-num) Middle section of the small intestine. (The first 12 inches is the duodenum.)

K

ketogenic amino acid (kee-toe-JEN-ik) Amino acid that can be converted to acetyl-CoA and can form ketones

ketone (kee-tone) Produced in the liver during the breakdown of fat when carbohydrate intake is very low.

ketone bodies (KEE-tone) Incomplete breakdown products of fat, containing 3 or 4 carbons. Most contain a chemical group called a ketone, hence the name. An example is aceto acetic acid.

ketosis (kee-TOE-sis) Condition of having a high concentration of ketone bodies and related breakdown products in the blood stream and tissues.

kidney nephron (NEF-ron) Functional unit of kidney cells that filters the blood for reabsorption of compounds and elimination of waste.

kilocalorie (kill-oh-KAL-oh-ree) (kcal) Heat energy needed to raise the temperature of 1000 grams (1 L) of water 1 degree Celsius; also written as *Calories*.

kilojoule (KIL-oh-jool) (kJ) Measure of work. A mass of 1 kilogram moving at a velocity of 1 m/sec possesses the energy of 1 Kj; 1 kcal equals 4.18 kJ.

kwashiorkor (kwash-ee-OR-core) Disease occurring primarily in young children who have an existing disease and who consume a marginal amount of energy and considerably insufficient amounts of protein in relation to needs. Characterized by edema, poor growth, weakness, and an increased susceptibility to further illness and infection.

kyphosis (ky-FOH-sis) Abnormal convex curvature of the spine, resulting in a bulge at the upper back; often caused by osteoporosis of the spine.

L

lactase Enzyme made by absorptive cells of the small intestine; digests lactose to glucose and galactose.

lactate (LAK-tate) Three-carbon acid formed during anaerobic cell respiration; a partial breakdown product of glucose; also called lactic acid.

lactation Period of milk secretion following pregnancy; typically called breastfeeding.

lacteal (LACK-tee-al) Small lymphatic duct within a villus of the small intestine.

***Lactobacillus bifidus* factor (lak-toe-bah-SIL-us BIFF-id-us)** Protective factor secreted in colostrum; encourages growth of beneficial bacteria in a newborn's intestines.

lacto-ovo-pesco vegetarian (lak-toe-o-vo-pes-co vej-eh-TEAR-ree-an) Person who consumes only plant products, dairy products, eggs, and fish.

lacto-ovo vegetarian (lak-toe-o-vo vej-eh-TEAR-ree-an) Person who consumes plant products, dairy products, and eggs.

lactose (LAK-tose) Glucose bonded to galactose.

lactose intolerance Condition caused by a lack of the enzyme that digests lactose (lactase); symptoms include abdominal gas, bloating, and diarrhea.

lacto-vegetarian (lak-toe-vej-eh-TEAR-ree-an) Person who consumes plant products and dairy products.

lanugo (lah-NEW-go) Downlike hair that appears after a person has lost much body fat through semi-starvation. The hair stands erect and traps air, acting as insulation for the body to compensate for the relative lack of body fat, which usually functions as insulation.

larva (LAR-vah) Early developmental stage in the life history of some organisms, such as parasites.

larynx (LAYR-ingks) Structure located between the pharynx and trachea; contains the vocal cords.

laxative Medication or other substance used to relieve constipation.

lean body mass Body weight after subtracting the weight of body fat. Lean body mass includes organs such as the brain, muscles, and liver, as well as blood and other body fluids.

leavened bread (LEV-end) Bread prepared using a leavening agent, such as yeast or baking powder. Leavening agents create gas, which causes bread dough to rise. Flat breads, such as pita bread, do not contain leavening.

lecithin (LESS-uh-thin) Group of phospholipids containing 2 fatty acids, a phosphate group, and a choline molecule. Lecithins differ based on the types of fatty acids found on each lecithin molecule.

leptin (LEP-tin) Hormone (167 amino acids) made by adipose tissue that influences long-term regulation of fat mass. Leptin also influences reproductive functions, as well as other body processes, such as insulin release.

let-down reflex Reflex stimulated by infant suckling; causes the release (ejection) of milk from milk ducts in the mother's breasts; also called *milk ejection reflex*.

leukemia (loo-KEY-mee-ah) Malignant neoplasm of blood-forming tissues, the bone marrow.

leukocyte (LOO-ko-site) White blood cell.

leukotriene (LT) (loo-ko-TRY-een) Eicosanoid involved in inflammatory or hypersensitivity reactions, such as asthma.

life expectancy Average length of life for a given group of people (usually determined by the year of birth).

life span Oldest age a person can reach.

lignan (LIG-nan) Phytochemical class that acts as a phytoestrogen in the body. Food sources are whole grains and flaxseeds.

lignin (LIG-nin) Insoluble fiber made of a multi-ringed alcohol (non-carbohydrate) structure.

limiting amino acid Essential amino acid in the lowest concentration in a food or diet relative to body needs.

linoleic acid (lin-oh-LEE-ik) Essential omega-6 fatty acid with 18 carbon and 2 double bonds (C18:2, omega-6).

lipase (LYE-pace) Fat-digesting enzyme; produced by the stomach, salivary glands, and pancreas.

lipid Group of organic compounds that includes oils and fats; triglycerides, phospholipids, and sterols. All these compounds contain carbon, hydrogen, and oxygen. None dissolve in water but do dissolve in organic solvents, such as chloroform, benzene, and ether.

lipid peroxidation (per-OX-ih-day-shun) Process initiated by an environmental component that induces the formation of an organic free radical, R·. In the formation of a fatty acid of this type, first a carbon-carbon double bond is broken. The resulting breakdown products react with oxygen to form peroxides (a) or free radicals (b):

a.
$$\begin{array}{ccc} H & H \\ | & | \\ -C-C-O-O-H \\ | & | \\ H & H \end{array}$$

b.
$$\begin{array}{ccc} H & H \\ | & | \\ -C-C-O-O^{\bullet} \\ | & | \\ H & H \end{array}$$

lipogenesis (lye-poh-JEN-eh-sis) Building of fatty acids using derivatives of acetyl-CoA.

lipogenic (lye-poh-JEN-ik) Creation of lipid. The liver is the major organ with lipogenic potential in the human body.

lipolysis (lye-POL-ih-sis) Breakdown of triglycerides to glycerol and fatty acids.

lipoprotein (ly-poh-PRO-teen) Compound, found in the bloodstream, containing a core of lipids with a shell composed of protein, phospholipid, and cholesterol.

lipoprotein lipase (lye-poh-PRO-teen LYE-pace) Enzyme attached to the outside of endothelial cells that line the capillaries in the blood vessels. It breaks down triglycerides into free fatty acids and glycerol.

lipoxin (LX) (lih-POX-in) Eicosanoid made by white blood cells that is involved in the immune system and allergic response.

lipoxygenase (lih-POX-ih-jen-ace) Enzyme used to synthesize leukotrienes and some other types of eicosanoids.

Listeria monocytogenes (lis-TEER-i-a mono-sy-TODGE-en-ees) Bacterium widely distributed in the environment, often entering food from contamination with animal or human feces. Soft cheeses made with unpasteurized milk and unpasteurized milk itself are most often implicated. *Listeria* is very hardy, resisting heat, salt, cold, nitrate, and acidity much better than

any other bacterium. Thorough cooking and pasteurization destroy *Listeria*.

liter (L) (LEE-ter) Measure of volume in the metric system. One liter equals 0.96 quart.

liver Organ located in the abdominal cavity below the diaphragm; performs many vital functions that maintain balance in blood composition.

lobules (LOB-you-elz) Saclike structures in the breast that store milk.

long chain fatty acids Fatty acids that contain 12 or more carbons.

low birth weight (LBW) Infant weight of less than 5.5 pounds (2.5 kilograms) at birth; most commonly results from preterm birth.

low-density lipoprotein (LDL) (lye-po-PRO-teen) Lipoprotein in the blood containing primarily cholesterol; elevated LDL cholesterol is strongly linked to cardiovascular disease risk.

lower esophageal sphincter (e-sof-ah-GEE-al SFINK-ter) Circular muscle that constricts the opening of the esophagus to the stomach.

lower-quality (incomplete) proteins Dietary proteins that are low in or lack 1 or more essential amino acids.

lumen (LOO-men) Inside of a tube, such as the inside cavity of the GI tract.

lymph (LIMF) Clear, plasmalike fluid that flows through lymphatic vessels.

lymphatic system (lim-FAT-ick) System of vessels that can accept fluid surrounding cells and large particles, such as products of fat absorption. Lymph fluid eventually passes into the bloodstream via the lymphatic system.

lymphatic vessel (lim-FAT-ick) Vessel that carries lymph.

lymph duct Large lymphatic vessel that empties lymph into the circulatory system.

lymph node Small structure located along the course of the lymphatic vessels.

lymphocyte (LIM-fo-site) Class of white blood cells involved in the immune system, generally comprising about 25% of all white blood cells. There are several types of lymphocytes with diverse functions, including antibody production, allergic reactions, graft rejections, tumor control, and regulation of the immune system.

lymphoma (lim-FO-ma) Malignant tumor arising from lymph nodes or other lymphatic tissues.

lysosome (LYE-so-som) Cell organelle that contains digestive enzymes for use inside the cell for turnover of cell parts.

lysozyme (LYE-so-zime) Set of enzyme substances produced by a variety of cells; can destroy bacteria by rupturing cell membranes.

M

macrocyte (MACK-ro-site) Literally, "large cell," such as a large red blood cell.

macrocytic anemia (mack-ro-SIT-ik ah-NEM-ee-a) Anemia characterized by the presence of abnormally large red blood cells in the bloodstream.

macronutrient Nutrient needed in gram quantities in the diet. Fat, protein, and carbohydrates are macronutrients.

macrophage (MACK-ro-faj) Large, mononuclear, phagocytic cell derived from a monocyte in the blood and found in body tissues. Besides functioning as phagocytes, macrophages secrete numerous cytokines and act as antigen-presenting cells.

macular degeneration (MAK-u-lar) Chronic eye disease that occurs when tissue in the macula (the part of the retina responsible for central vision) deteriorates. It causes a blind spot or blurred vision in the center of the visual field.

magnesium (mag-NEE-zee-um) Major mineral essential to many biochemical and physiological processes, including calcium metabolism, active ATP formation, enzyme function, DNA and RNA synthesis, nerve and heart function, and insulin function. Spinach, squash, and wheat bran are good sources.

major mineral Mineral vital to health; required in the diet in amounts greater than 100 mg/day; also called a *macromineral*.

malignant (ma-LIG-nant) In reference to a tumor, the property of spreading locally and to distant sites.

malnutrition Can refer to either undernutrition or overnutrition. Eventually contributes to failing health.

malonyl-CoA (MAL-o-kneel) Building block in fatty acid synthesis.

maltase (MALL-tace) Enzyme made by absorptive cells of the small intestine; digests maltose to 2 glucoses.

maltose (MALL-tos) Disaccharide made of 2 glucose molecules.

manganese Trace mineral that functions as a cofactor of some enzymes, such as those involved in carbohydrate metabolism and antioxidant protection. Nuts, oats, beans, and tea are good sources.

mannitol (MAN-ih-tahl) Alcohol derivative of fructose.

marasmus (ma-RAZ-mus) Disease resulting from a severe deficit of protein and energy; classed as protein-energy malnutrition; results in an extreme loss of fat stores, muscle mass, and strength. Death from infections is common.

mass movement Peristaltic wave that simultaneously coordinates contraction over a large area of the large intestine. Mass movements propel material from 1 portion of the large intestine to another and from the large intestine to the rectum.

mast cell Tissue cell that releases histamine and other chemicals involved in inflammation.

meconium (me-KO-nee-um) First thick, mucouslike stool passed by an infant after birth.

medium chain fatty acid Fatty acid that contains 6 to 10 carbons.

Mediterranean Diet Dietary pattern that includes large amounts of fruits, vegetables, and olive oil; associated with a low incidence of coronary heart disease.

megadose Intake of a nutrient far beyond human needs.

megaloblast (MEG-ah-low-blast) Large, nucleated, immature red blood cell in the bone marrow that results from the inability of a precursor cell to divide when it normally should.

megaloblastic anemia (MEG-ah-low-BLAST-ik) Form of anemia characterized by large, nucleated, immature red blood cells that result from the inability of precursor cells to divide normally.

memory cells B lymphocytes that remain after an infection and provide long-lasting or permanent immunity.

menaquinone (men-ah-KWIH-nohn) Form of vitamin K found in fish oils and meats; also is synthesized by bacteria in the human intestine.

menarche (men-AR-kee) Onset of menstruation. Menarche usually occurs around age 13, 2 or 3 years after the first signs of puberty start to appear.

menopause (MEN-oh-pawz) Cessation of menses in women, usually beginning at about age 50.

meta-analysis Summary of several scientific studies grouped together.

metabolic equivalent (MET) Exercise intensity that is relative to a person's metabolic rate.

Metabolic Syndrome Condition characterized by poor blood glucose regulation, hypertension, increased blood lipids, and abdominal obesity; usually accompanied by lack of physical activity; previously called *Syndrome X.*

metabolism (meh-TAB-oh-liz-m) Chemical processes in the body that provide energy in useful forms and sustain vital activities.

metabolites Intermediate compounds in metabolism.

metalloenzyme (meh-tal-oh-EN-zyme) Enzyme that contains 1 or more metal ions that are required for enzymatic activity.

metallothionein (meh-TAL-oh-THIGH-oh-neen) Protein that binds and regulates the release of zinc and copper in intestinal and liver cells.

metastasize (ma TAS tah size) Spread of disease from 1 part of the body to another, even to parts of the body that are remote from the site of the original tumor. Cancer cells can spread via blood vessels, the lymphatic system, or direct growth of the tumor.

meter (mee-ter) Measure of length in the metric system; 1 meter equals 39.4 inches.

micelles (my-SELLS) Water-soluble, spherical structures formed by lecithin and bile acids in which the hydrophobic parts of the molecules face inward and the hydrophilic parts face outward. Lipids enclosed within micelles do not separate out into an oily layer, as they normally do when mixed with water.

microcytic (my-kro-SIT-ik) Literally, "small cell" (e.g., red blood cells that are smaller than normal.

microcytic hypochromic anemia (high-po-KROME-ik) Anemia characterized by small, pale red blood cells that lack sufficient hemoglobin and thus have reduced oxygen-carrying ability. It is often caused by an iron deficiency.

microfractures Small fractures, undetectable by X rays or other bone scans, that may develop constantly in bones.

micronutrient Nutrient needed in milligram or microgram quantities in a diet. Vitamins and minerals are micronutrients.

microsomal ethanol oxidizing system (my-kro-SO-mol) Alternative pathway for alcohol metabolism when alcohol is in high concentration in the liver; uses rather than yields energy for the body.

microvilli (my-kro-VIL-eye) Microscopic, hairlike projections of cell membranes of certain epithelial cells.

migrant study Research that examines the health of people who move from 1 country to another.

mineral Element used in the body to promote chemical reactions and to form body structures.

miscarriage Non-elective termination of pregnancy that occurs before the fetus can survive; typically called *spontaneous abortion.*

mitochondria (my-toe-KON-dree-ah) Main sites of energy production in a cell. They also contain the pathway for oxidizing fat for fuel, among other metabolic pathways.

mode Type, as in the type of exercise that is performed.

modified food starch Product consisting of chemically linked starch molecules; is more stable than normal, unmodified starches.

mold Type of fungus that grows best in warm, dark, moist environments. Some molds produce toxins (mycotoxins) that cause illness when ingested by humans.

molecule Group of atoms chemically linked together—that is, tightly connected by attractive forces (see also *compound*).

molybdenum (mo-LIB-den-um) Trace mineral that aids in the action of some enzymes in the body. Beans, whole grains, and nuts are good sources.

monoamine (MON-oh-ah-MEAN) Molecule containing one amide group.

monoglyceride (mon-oh-GLIS-er-ide) Breakdown product of a triglyceride consisting of 1 fatty acid bonded to a glycerol backbone.

monosaccharide (mon-oh-SACK-uh-ride) Simple sugar, such as glucose, that is not broken down further during digestion.

monounsaturated fatty acid (MUFA) (mon-oh-un-SAT-urated) Fatty acid containing 1 carbon-carbon double bond.

morbidity Disease condition or state; amount of illness present in a population

mortality Death rate of a population.

motility Ability to move spontaneously; also movement of food through the GI tract.

mottling (MOT-ling) Discoloration or marking of the surface of teeth from exposure to excessive amounts of fluoride (also called *enamel fluorosis*).

mRNA translation Synthesis of polypeptide chains at the ribosome according to information contained in strands of messenger RNA (mRNA).

mucilage (MYOO-sih-laj) Soluble fiber consisting of chains of galactose and other monosaccharides; characteristically found in seaweed.

mucopolysaccharide (MYOO-ko-POL-ee-SAK-ah-ride) Substance containing protein and carbohydrate parts; found in bone and other organs.

mucosa (MYOO-co-sa) Mucous membrane consisting of cells and supporting connective tissue. Mucosa lines cavities that open to the outside of the body, such as the stomach and intestine, and generally contains glands that secrete mucus.

mucous membranes (MYOO-cuss) Membranes that line passageways open to the exterior environment; also called mucosae.

mucus (MYOO-cuss) Thick fluid, secreted by glands throughout the body, that lubricates and protects cells; contains a compound that has both a carbohydrate and a protein nature.

muscle Body tissue made of groups of muscle fibers that contract to allow movement. There are 3 muscle types: smooth, striated, and cardiac.

muscle fiber One muscle cell; an elongated cell, with contractile properties, that forms the muscles of the body.

muscle tissue Type of tissue adapted for contraction.

muscular system System consisting of smooth, cardiac, and skeletal muscle. This system produces body movement, maintains posture, and produces body heat.

mutagen (MYOO-tah-jen) Agent that promotes a mutation (e.g., radioactive substances, X rays, or certain chemicals).

mutagenicity Agent that can induce or increase the frequency of mutation in an organism.

mutase (MYOO-tace) Enzyme that rearranges the functional groups on a molecule.

mutation (myoo-TAY-shun) Change in the chemistry of a gene; change is perpetuated in subsequent divisions of the cell in which it occurred; a change in the sequence of the DNA.

mycotoxin (MY-ko-tok-sin) Toxic compound produced by molds, such as aflatoxin B-1, found on moldy grains.

myelin sheath (MY-eh-lyn) Combined lipid and protein structure (lipoprotein) that covers nerve fibers.

myocardial depression Decreased activity of the heart muscle.

myocardial infarction (MY-oh-CARD-ee-ahl in-FARK-shun) Death of part of the heart muscle.

myofibril (my-oh-FIB-ril) Bundle of contractile fibers within a muscle cell.

myoglobin (my-oh-GLOW-bin) Iron-containing protein that controls the rate of diffusion of oxygen (O_2) from red blood cells to muscle cells.

myosin (MY-oh-sin) Thick filament protein that connects with actin to cause a muscle contraction.

N

narcotic Agent that reduces sensations or consciousness.

natural food Food that has undergone minimal processing and does not contain food additives.

natural toxins Naturally occurring toxins in foods, especially plants. They rarely cause disease in humans.

negative energy balance State in which energy intake is less than energy expended, resulting in weight loss.

negative nitrogen balance State in which nitrogen losses from the body exceed intake, as in starvation.

neoplasm (NEE-oh-plaz-em) New and abnormal growth of tissues, which may be benign or cancerous.

neotame General-purpose non-nutritive sweetener that is approximately 7000 to 13,000 times sweeter than table sugar. It has a chemical structure similar to aspartame's. Neotame is heat stable and can be used as a tabletop sweetener, as well as in cooking applications. It is not broken down to its amino acid components in the body after consumption.

nephron (NEF-ron) Functional unit of the kidneys.

nephrotic syndrome (NEF-rot-ick) Type of kidney disease that results from damage to the kidney, often caused by another disease, such as diabetes. Symptoms include protein loss and fluid retention, high blood cholesterol.

nerve Bundle of nerve cells outside the central nervous system.

nervous system Body system consisting of the brain, spinal cord, nerves, and sensory receptors. This system detects sensations and controls physiological and intellectual functions and movement.

nervous tissue Tissue composed of highly branched, elongated cells that transport nerve impulses from 1 part of the body to another.

neural tube defect Defect in the formation of the neural tube occurring during early fetal development. This type of defect results in various nervous system disorders, such as spina bifida. A very severe form is anencephaly. Folate deficiency in a pregnant woman increases the risk that the fetus will develop this disorder.

neuroendocrine (NEW-row-EN-do-krin) Linked to the combined action of the endocrine glands and the nervous system. Examples include substances released from glands in response to nerve stimulation.

neuroglia (NEW-row-GLEE-ah) (glial cells) Specialized support cells of the central nervous system.

neuromuscular junction (NEW-row-MUS-kyo-lar) Chemical synapse between a motor neuron and a muscle fiber.

neuron (NEW-ron) Structural and functional unit of the nervous system, consisting of cell body, dendrites, and axon.

neuropeptide Y (NEW-row-PEP-tide) Small protein (36 amino acids) that increases food intake and reduces energy expenditure when injected into the brains of experimental animals.

neurotransmitter (NEW-row-TRANS-mit-er) Compound made by a nerve cell that allows for communication between it and other cells.

neutron (NEW-tron) Part of an atom that has no charge.

neutrophil (NEW-tro-fil) Type of phagocytic white blood cell, normally constituting about 60 to 70% of the white blood cell count; forms highly toxic compounds, which destroy bacteria.

neutrophil/activation Type of white blood cell being prepared for immune response.

niacin Water-soluble vitamin that, in coenzyme form, participates in numerous oxidation-reduction reactions in cellular metabolic pathways, especially those used to produce ATP. Tuna, chicken, beef, peanuts, and salmon are good sources.

nicotinamide (nick-ah-TIN-ah-mide) One of the 2 forms of the vitamin niacin.

nicotinamide adenine dinucleotide (NAD) (nick-ah-TIN-ah-mide- AD-ah-neen di-NEW-klee-a-tide) Coenzyme that readily accepts and donates electrons and hydrogen ions; formed from the vitamin niacin.

nicotinamide adenine dinucleotide phosphate (NADP) Coenzyme that readily accepts and donates electrons and hydrogen ions; formed from the vitamin niacin.

nicotinic acid (nick-ah-TIN-ick) One of the 2 forms of the vitamin niacin. Physicians sometimes prescribe it to lower LDL cholesterol and increase HDL cholesterol levels.

night blindness Vitamin A deficiency condition in which the retina in the eye cannot adjust to low amounts of light.

nitrate (NIE-trate) Nitrogen-containing compound used to cure meats. Its use contributes a pink color to meats and confers some resistance to bacterial growth.

nitrosamine (ni-TROH-sa-mean) Carcinogen formed from nitrates and breakdown products of amino acids; can lead to stomach cancer.

non-essential amino acids Amino acids that can be synthesized by a healthy body in sufficient amounts. There are 11 non-essential amino acids. These are also called *dispensable amino acids.*

non-heme iron (non-HEEM) Iron provided from plant sources and elemental iron components of animal tissues. Non-heme iron is less efficiently absorbed than heme iron, and absorption is more closely dependent on body needs.

non-polar Neutral compound, no positive or negative poles present.

non-specific immunity Defenses that stop the invasion of pathogens; requires no previous encounter with a pathogen.

nonsteroidal anti-inflammatory drugs (NSAIDs) Medication used to reduce inflammation; include aspirin, ibuprofen, and naproxen.

no-observable-effect level (NOEL) Highest dose of an additive that produces no deleterious health effects in animals.

norepinephrine (nor-ep-ih-NEF-rin) Neurotransmitter released from nerve endings; also a hormone produced by the adrenal gland in times of stress.

norovirus (NOR-oh-VIE-rus) Virus in the human intestinal tract and feces. It contaminates food via direct hand-to-food contact, when sewage is used to enrich garden/farm soil, or when shellfish are harvested from waters contaminated by sewage. Cooking destroys the virus. Shellfish and salads are the foods most often implicated. Noroviruses cause more cases of foodborne illness than any other microorganism. They can survive chlorination, and a relatively small amount can cause illness.

nuclear receptor (NEW-klee-er) Site on the DNA in a cell where compounds (e.g., hormones) bind. Cells that contain DNA receptors for a specific compound are affected by that compound.

nucleolus (NEW-klee-o-less) Center for production of ribosomes within the cell nucleus.

nucleus (NEW-klee-us) In chemistry, the core of an atom; contains protons and neutrons.

nutrient Chemical substance in food that contributes to health. Nutrients nourish us by providing energy, materials for building body parts, and factors to regulate necessary chemical processes in the body.

nutrient content claim Claim that describes the nutrients in a food, such as "low in fat" and "calorie free."

nutrient density Ratio derived by dividing a food's contribution to nutrient needs by its contribution to energy needs. When its contribution to nutrient needs exceeds its energy contribution, the food is considered to have a favorable nutrient density.

nutrient receptors Proposed sites in the small intestine that contribute signals to the brain, which in turn elicit a feeling of satiety. These receptors are stimulated by nutrient exposure in the lumen of the small intestine.

nutrient requirement Amount of a nutrient required to maintain health. This varies between individuals.

nutrition Science of food; the nutrients and the substances therein; their action, interaction, and balance in relation to health and disease; and the process by which the organism (i.e., body) ingests, digests, absorbs, transports, utilizes, and excretes food substances.

nutritional status Nutritional health of a person as determined by anthropometric measures (e.g., height, weight, circumferences), biochemical measurements of nutrients or their by-products in blood and urine, a clinical (physical) examination, a dietary analysis, and an economic evaluation.

nutritionist Person who advises about nutrition and/or works in the field of food and nutrition. In many states in the United States, a person does not need formal training to use this title. Some states reserve this title for registered dietitians.

nutrition label Label containing "Nutrition Facts;" must be included on most foods. It depicts nutrient content in comparison with the Daily Values set by the FDA. Canada has a separate set of nutrition labels.

O

obesity (oh-BEES-ih-tee) Condition characterized by excess body weight and/or body fat; typically defined in clinical settings as a body mass index (BMI) of 30 or above, but this cutoff is not always appropriate.

Older Americans Act U.S. government legislation administered by Administration on Aging designed to help adults ages 60 years and older remain living independently in their homes and communities; community-based nutrition, health, and supportive services may include adult day care, senior center activities, transportation, information and counseling services, and health and physical activity programs. In-home care can include health and personal care, home maintenance assistance, and caregiver support services.

oleic acid (oh-LAY-ik) Omega-9 fatty acid with 18 carbons and 1 double bond (C18:1, omega-9).

olfactory (ol-FAK-toe-ree) Related to the sense of smell.

olfactory cells Cells in the nasal region that discriminate among numerous chemical molecules and transmit that information to the brain. This information represents a component of flavor.

oligosaccharide (ol-ih-go-SAK-ah-ride) Carbohydrate containing 3 to 10 single sugar units.

omega-3 (n-3) fatty acid Unsaturated fatty acid with the first double bond on the third carbon from the methyl end (—CH3).

omega-6 (n-6) fatty acid Unsaturated fatty acid with the first double bond on the sixth carbon from the methyl end (—CH3).

omnivore (AHM-nih-voor) Person who consumes foods from both plant and animal sources.

oncogene (AHN-ko-jeen) Protooncogene out of control.

oncotic force (ahn-KAH-tik) Osmotic potential exerted by blood proteins in the bloodstream.

opportunistic infection Infection that arises primarily in people who are already ill because of another disease.

opsin (AHP-sin) Protein in the rods of the retina in the eye that binds to ll-*cis*-retinal to form the visual pigment rhodopsin.

organ Group of tissues designed to perform a specific function—for example, the heart. It contains muscle tissue, nerve tissue, and so on.

organelle (OAR-gan-ell) Compartment, particle, or filament that performs specialized functions within a cell.

organic Substance that contains carbon atoms bonded to hydrogen atoms in the chemical structure.

organic food Food grown with farming practices such as biological pest management, composting, manure application, and crop rotation and without the use of synthetic pesticides, fertilizers, antibiotics, sewage sludge, genetic engineering, irradiation, and hormones.

organism Living thing (e.g., the human body is an organism consisting of many organs, which act in a coordinated manner to support life).

organ system Collection of organs that work together to perform an overall function.

osmolality (oz-mo-LAL-ih-tee) Measure of the total concentration of a solution; number of particles of solute per kilogram of solvent.

osmosis (oz-MO-sis) Passage of a solvent, such as water, through a semipermeable membrane from a less concentrated compartment to a more concentrated compartment.

osmotic pressure (oz-MAH-tick) Exerted pressure needed to keep particles in a solution from drawing liquid toward them across a semipermeable membrane.

osteoblast (OS-tee-oh-blast) Cell in bone; secretes mineral and bone matrix.

osteocalcin (OS-tee-oh-KAL-sin) Protein produced in bone that is thought to bind calcium. Synthesis of osteocalcin is aided by vitamin K.

osteoclast (OS-tee-oh-klast) Bone cell that arises from a type of white blood cell; secretes substances that lead to bone erosion. This erosion can set the stage for subsequent bone mineralization.

osteocytes (OS-tee-oh-sites) Bone cell formed from osteoblasts that have become embedded within bone matrix.

osteomalacia (OS-tee-oh-mal-AY-shuh) Weakening of bones that occurs in adults as a result of poor bone mineralization linked to inadequate vitamin D status.

osteopenia (os-tee-oh-PEE-nee-ah) Decreased bone mass caused by cancer, hyperthyroidism, or other health conditions.

osteoporosis (os-tee-oh-po-ROH-sis) Decreased bone mass leading to risk of bone fractures. This bone loss is related to the effects of aging, genetic background, poor diet, and hormonal changes occurring in postmenopausal women.

ostomy (OS-toe-me) Surgically created opening in the intestinal tract. The end point usually opens from the abdominal cavity rather than the anus (e.g., a colostomy).

overnutrition State in which nutritional intake greatly exceeds the body's needs.

overweight Body weight that is greater than an acceptable standard for a given height. Excess weight is usually due to excess body fat; however, in very muscular individuals, higher weight may be due to muscle.

ovum (OH-vum) Egg cell from which a fetus eventually develops if the egg is fertilized by a sperm cell.

oxalic acid (ox-al-ick) (oxalate) (ox-ah-late) Organic acid in spinach, rhubarb, and other leafy green vegetables; can depress the absorption of certain minerals, such as calcium, present in food.

oxidation (ox-ih-DAY-shun) Loss of an electron by an atom or a molecule; in metabolism, often associated with a gain of oxygen or a loss of hydrogen. Oxidation (loss of an electron) and reduction (gain of an electron) take place simultaneously in metabolism because an electron that is lost by 1 atom is accepted by another.

oxidative phosphorylation Process by which energy derived from the oxidation of NADH + H$^+$ and FADH$_2$ is transferred to ADP + P$_i$ to form ATP.

oxidative stress Damage to lipids, proteins, and DNA produced by excessive production of free radicals.

oxidize (OX-ih-dize) Loss of an electron or gain of an oxygen in a chemical substance. This change typically alters the shape and/or function of the substance. An oxidizing agent is a substance capable of capturing an electron from another source. That source is then "oxidized" when it loses the electron.

oxidized LDL LDL (low density lipoprotein) that has been damaged by free radicals. This type of damage is seen in both the lipids and the proteins that make up LDL.

oxidizing agent Substance capable of capturing an electron from another compound. A compound is "oxidized" when it loses an electron.

oxygenase (OK-si-jen-ace) Enzyme that incorporates oxygen directly into a molecule.

oxytocin (ok-si-TO-sin) Hormone secreted by the pituitary gland. It causes contraction of the musclelike cells surrounding the ducts of the breasts and the smooth muscle of the uterus.

P

p53 gene Tumor suppressor gene that can prevent inappropriate cell division.

palatable (PAL-it-ah-bull) Pleasing to taste.

pancreas (PAN-kree-us) Endocrine organ, located near the stomach, that secretes digestive enzymes into the small intestine and produces hormones—notably, insulin.

pantothenic acid Water-soluble vitamin that functions as a component of coenzyme A (CoA), which itself plays a pivotal role in energy metabolism and fatty acid synthesis. Most foods are sources.

para-aminobenzoic acid (ah-MEE-noh-ben-ZOH-ick) Compound that is a part of the B-vitamin folate.

parasite Organism that lives in or on another organism and derives nourishment from it.

parasthesia (par-a-STEE-zya) Abnormal spontaneous sensation, such as burning, prickling, and numbness.

parathyroid hormone (PTH) Hormone made by the parathyroid glands; increases synthesis of the vitamin D hormone and aids calcium release from bone and calcium uptake by the kidneys, among other functions.

parietal cell (PAH-rye-ah-tahl) Gastric gland cell that secretes hydrochloric acid and intrinsic factor.

passive diffusion Absorption that requires permeability of the substance through the wall of the small intestine and a concentration gradient higher in the intestinal contents than in the absorptive cell.

pasteurizing (PAS-tur-eye-zing) Heating food products to kill pathogenic microorganisms and reduce the total number of bacteria.

pathogen Disease-causing microorganism.

pathway Metabolic progression of individual steps from starting materials to ending products, such as $C_6H_{12}O_6$ (glucose) + O_2 eventually yielding CO_2 + H_2O.

pectin (PEK-tin) Soluble fiber containing chains of various monosaccharides; characteristically found between plant cell walls.

peer-reviewed journal Journal that publishes research only after 2 or 3 scientists who were not part of the study agree the study was well conducted and the results are fairly represented. Thus, the research has been approved by peers of the research team.

pellagra (peh-LAHG-rah) Disease characterized by inflammation of the skin, diarrhea, and eventual mental incapacity; results from an insufficient amount of the vitamin niacin in the diet.

pepsin (PEP-sin) Protein-digesting enzyme produced by the stomach.

pepsinogen (PEP-sin-oh-jin) Inactive protein precursor to pepsin.

peptic ulcer Hole in the lining of the stomach or duodenum.

peptide Amino acids (usually 2 to 4) chemically bonded together.

peptide bond Chemical bond formed between amino acids in a protein.

percentile Classification of a measurement of a unit into divisions of 100 units.

peripheral nervous system (PNS) (peh-RIF-er-al) System of nerves that lie outside the brain and spinal cord.

peripheral neuropathy (peh-RIF-er-al new-ROP-ah-thee) Impaired sensory, motor, and reflex actions affecting arms and legs and causing calf muscle tenderness and difficulty in rising from a squatting position.

peristalsis (per-ih-STALL-sis) Coordinated muscular contraction that propels food down the GI tract.

pernicious anemia (per-NISH-us) Anemia that results from the inability to absorb sufficient vitamin B-12; is associated with nerve degeneration, which can result in eventual paralysis and death.

peroxisome (per-OK-si-som) Cell organelle that uses oxygen to remove hydrogens from compounds. This produces hydrogen peroxide (H_2O_2), which breaks down into O_2 and H_2O.

peroxyl radical (per-OK-syl) Peroxide compound containing a free radical; designated ROO•, where R is a carbon-hydrogen chain broken off a fatty acid and the dot is an unpaired electron.

pesticide Agent that can destroy bacteria, fungi, insects, rodents, or other pests.

pH Measure of relative acidity or alkalinity of a solution. The pH scale is 0 to 14. A pH below 7 is acidic; a pH above 7 is alkaline.

phagocytic cells (fag-oh-SIT-ick) Cells that engulf substances; include neutrophils and macrophages.

phagocytosis (FAG-oh-sigh-TOW-sis) Form of active absorption in which the absorptive cell forms an indentation, and particles or fluids entering the indentation are then engulfed by the cell.

pharynx (FAIR-ingks) Organ of the digestive tract and respiratory tract located at the back of the oral and nasal cavities.

phenobarbital (fee-noe-BAR-bit-ahl) Medication used to treat seizure disorders.

phenylalanine (fen-ihl-AL-ah-neen) Essential (indispensable) amino acid.

phenylketonuria (PKU) (fen-ihl-kee-toh-NEW-ree-ah) Disease caused by a defect in the liver's ability to metabolize the amino acid phenylalanine into the amino acid tyrosine; untreated, toxic by-products of phenylalanine build up in the body and lead to mental retardation.

phosphocreatine (PCr) (fos-fo-CREE-a-tin) High-energy compound that can be used to re-form ATP from ADP.

phospholipase (fos-fo-LY-pase) Enzyme that splits a fatty acid from a cell membrane phospholipid.

phospholipid Class of fat-related substances that contain phosphorus, fatty acids, and a nitrogen-containing base. Phospholipids are an essential part of every cell.

phosphorus Major ion of intracellular fluid. It contributes to acid-base balance, bone and tooth strength, and various metabolic processes. Milk, milk products, and nuts are good sources.

photoisomerization (foto-eye-SOM-er-eye-zay-shun) Molecular isomerization of a compound by the energy of light.

photon (FO-ton) Unit of light intensity at the retina having the brightness of 1 candle.

photosynthesis (fo-to-SIN-tha-sis) Process by which plants use energy from the sun to produce energy-yielding compounds, such as glucose.

phylloquinone (fil-oh-KWIN-own) Form of vitamin K that comes from plants; also called *vitamin K1*.

physical activity Body movement caused by muscular contraction, resulting in the expenditure of energy.

physiological anemia Normal increase in blood volume in pregnancy that dilutes the concentration of red blood cells, resulting in anemia; also called *hemodilution*.

physiological fuel value Calories supplied by each macronutrient; equal to 4, 9, 4, and 7 kcal/g for carbohydrate, fat, protein, and alcohol, respectively.

phytic acid (phytate) (FY-tick, FY-tate) Constituent of plant fibers that binds positive ions to its multiple phosphate groups and decreases their bioavailability.

phytobezoar (fy-tow-BEE-zor) Pellet of fiber characteristically found in the stomach.

phytochemical (fie-toe-KEM-i-kahl) Chemical in plants. Some phytochemicals may contribute to a reduced risk of cancer or cardiovascular disease in people who consume them regularly.

pica (PIE-kah) Practice of eating non-food items, such as dirt, laundry starch, or clay.

pinocytosis (pee-no-sigh-TOE-sis) Formation of a vesicle that brings molecules into a cell; also called *cell drinking*.

placebo (plah-SEE-bo) Fake treatment (e.g., a sham medicine, supplement, or procedure) that seems like the experimental treatment; used to disguise whether a study participant is in the experimental or control group.

placebo effect Effect that occurs in research when control group participants experience changes that cannot be explained by the action of the placebo they have received.

placenta (plah-SEN-tah) Organ that forms in the uterus in pregnant women. Through this organ, oxygen and nutrients from the mother's blood are transferred to the fetus and fetal wastes are removed. The placenta also releases hormones that maintain the state of pregnancy.

plaque (PLACK) Cholesterol-rich substance deposited in the blood vessels; contains white blood cells, smooth muscle cells, connective tissue (collagen), cholesterol and other lipids, and eventually calcium.

plasma Fluid, non-cellular portion of the circulating blood. This includes the blood serum plus all blood-clotting factors. In contrast, serum is the fluid that results after the blood is first allowed to clot before being centrifuged; does not contain the blood-clotting factors.

plasma cells B lymphocytes that produce about 2000 antibodies per second.

polar Compound with distinct positive and negative charges (poles) on it. These charges act as poles on a magnet.

polyglutamate form of folate (POL-ee-GLOO-tah-mate) Folate with more than 1 glutamate molecule attached.

polyneuropathy (POL-ee-nyoo-ROP-ah-thee) Disease process involving a number of peripheral nerves.

polypeptide (POL-ee-PEP-tide) Ten or more amino acids bonded together.

polyphenol Group of compounds containing at least 2 ring structures each with at least 1 hydroxyl group (—OH) attached. Polyphenols occur naturally in tea, dark chocolate, and wine and can lower the bioavailability of minerals, especially iron and calcium.

polysaccharide (POL-ee-SACK-uh-ride) Large carbohydrate containing from 10 to 1000 or more monosaccharide units; also known as *complex carbohydrate*.

polyunsaturated fatty acid (PUFA) Fatty acid containing 2 or more carbon-carbon double bonds.

pool Amount of a nutrient within the body that can be easily mobilized when needed.

portal system Veins in the GI tract that convey blood from capillaries in the intestines and portions of the stomach to the liver.

portal vein Large vein leaving from the intestine and stomach and connecting to the liver.

positive energy balance State in which energy intake is greater than energy expended, generally resulting in weight gain.

positive nitrogen balance State in which nitrogen intake exceeds related losses. This state causes a net gain of nitrogen in the body, such as when tissue protein is gained during growth.

potassium Major positive ion in intracellular fluid. It performs many of the same functions as sodium, such as fluid balance and nerve impulse transmission. Potassium also influences the contractility of smooth, skeletal, and cardiac muscle. Spinach, squash, and bananas are good sources.

poverty guidelines Federal poverty level; income level calculated each year by the U.S. Census Bureau. Guidelines are used to determine eligibility for many federal food and assistance programs.

power stroke Movement of the thick filament alongside the thin filament in a muscle cell, causing muscle contraction.

prebiotic Substance that stimulates bacterial growth in the large intestines.

precursor Compound that comes before; a precedent.

preeclampsia (pre-ee-KLAMP-see-ah) Part of the disease called pregnancy-induced hypertension. This serious disorder can include high blood pressure, kidney failure, convulsions, and even death of the mother and fetus. Mild cases are known as preeclampsia; more severe cases are called eclampsia or, formerly, toxemia.

pregnancy-induced hypertension Serious disorder that can include high blood pressure, kidney failure, convulsions, and even death of the mother and fetus. Although its exact cause is not known, an adequate diet (especially adequate calcium intake) and prenatal care may prevent this disorder or limit its severity. Mild cases are known as preeclampsia; more severe cases are called eclampsia (formerly called toxemia).

preliminary health claim Claim made about foods that is based on incomplete scientific evidence.

premenstrual syndrome (PMS) Disorder occurring in some women a few days before a menstrual period begins; characterized by depression, anxiety, headache, bloating, and mood swings. Severe cases are currently termed premenstrual dysphoric disorder (PDD).

preservatives Compounds that extend the shelf life of foods by inhibiting microbial growth or minimizing the destructive effect of oxygen and metals.

preterm Born before 37 weeks of gestation; such an infant also also referred to as premature.

prevalence The proportion of people in a population at a specific time who have a certain disease, such as obesity or cancer.

previtamin D3 Precursor of 1 form of vitamin D, produced as a result of sunlight opening a ring on 7-dehydrocholesterol in the skin.

primary disease Disease process that is not simply caused by another disease process.

primary prevention Attempt to prevent a disease from developing—for example, following a diet low in saturated fat and cholesterol in an attempt to prevent cardiovascular disease.

primary structure of a protein Order of amino acids in the protein molecule.

prions (PRE-onz) Proteins involved in maintaining nerve cell function. Prions can become infectious and lead to diseases, such as bovine spongiform encephalopathy, also known as mad cow disease.

prior sanctioned substances Food additives in use prior to 1958 that have been approved by the FDA or the USDA.

probiotic (PRO-bye-ah-tic) Product that contains specific types of bacteria. Use is intended to colonize the large intestine with the specific bacteria in the product. An example is yogurt.

progestin (pro-JES-tin) Hormone, including progesterone, that is necessary for maintaining pregnancy and lactation.

prognosis (prog-NO-sis) Forecast of the course and end of a disease.

progression Increase in exercise frequency, duration, and intensity over time.

prohormone Precursor of a hormone.

prolactin (pro-LACK-tin) Hormone secreted by a mother's pituitary gland that stimulates the synthesis of milk in the breast.

prospective Type of research that follows individuals during a current course of treatment, in contrast with retrospective research, which examines the past habits of individuals.

prostacyclin (PGI) (prost-ah-SIGH-klin) Eicosanoid made by the blood vessel walls; a potent inhibitor of blood clotting.

prostaglandin (PG) (pros-tah-GLAN-din) Potent eicosanoid compound, made of polyunsaturated fatty acids, that produces diverse effects in the body.

prostanoids (PROS-ta-noidz) Group of prostaglandins, prostacyclins, and thromboxanes produced from 20 carbon (C:20)

fatty acids; not as inclusive a term as *eicosanoids* because leukotrienes and lipoxins are not included.

prostate gland (PROS-tait) Solid, chestnut-shaped organ surrounding the first part of the urinary tract in males. The prostate gland secretes substances into the semen.

protease (PRO-tea-ace) Protein-digesting enzyme.

protein Food and body components made of amino acids. Proteins contain carbon, hydrogen, oxygen, nitrogen, and sometimes other atoms in a specific configuration. Proteins contain the form of nitrogen most easily used by the human body. Protein supplies 4 kcal/gram.

protein digestibility corrected amino acid score (PDCAAS) Chemical score of a food multiplied by its digestibility.

protein-efficiency ratio (PER) Measure of protein quality in a food, determined by the ability of a protein to support the growth of a young animal.

protein-energy malnutrition (PEM) Condition resulting from regularly consuming insufficient amounts of energy and protein; results in body wasting, primarily of lean tissue, and an increased susceptibility to infections.

protein quality Measure of the ability of a food protein to support body growth and maintenance.

protein turnover Process by which a cell breaks down existing proteins and then synthesizes new proteins.

prothrombin (pro-THROM-bin) Protein that participates in the formation of blood clots. Conversion of its precursor protein to the active blood-clotting factor in the liver requires vitamin K.

proton (PRO-ton) Part of an atom that is positively charged.

proton pump inhibitor Medication that inhibits the ability of gastric cells to secrete hydrogen ions (e.g., esomeprazole [Nexium®], lansoprazole [Prevacid®], and omeprazole [Prilosec®]).

protooncogenes (pro-toe-ON-ko-jeans) Genes that cause a resting cell to divide.

protozoa (pro-tah-ZOE-ah) One-celled animals that are more complex than bacteria. Disease-causing protozoa can be spread through food and water.

provitamin Substance that can be made into a vitamin.

psoriasis (sah-RIE-ah-sis) Immune system disorder that causes a chronic inflammatory skin condition (painful patches of red, scaly skin).

psyllium (SIL-ee-um) Mostly soluble type of dietary fiber found in the seeds of the

plantago plant (native to India and Mediterranean countries).

pteridine (TER-ih-deen) Bi-cyclic compound that makes up part of the structure of folate.

puberty Period when a child physically matures into an adult capable of reproduction. Puberty is initiated by the secretion of sex hormones: primarily estrogen in females and testosterone in males.

pulmonary circulation (pulmonary circuit) System of blood vessels from the right ventricle of the heart to the lungs and back to the left atrium of the heart.

purine (PURE-een) Double-ringed compound that forms the nitrogenous bases adenine and guanine found in DNA and RNA.

pyloric sphincter (pi-LOR-ik SFINK-ter) Ring of smooth muscle between the stomach and the duodenum.

pyridoxal (pir-ih-DOX-ahl) One of the 3 forms of vitamin B-6.

pyridoxamine (pir-i-DOX-ah-meen) One of the 3 forms of vitamin B-6.

pyridoxine (pir-i-DOX-een) One of the 3 forms of vitamin B-6.

pyrimidine (pie-RIM-i-deen) Six-membered ring compound that forms the nitrogenous bases thymine and cytosine found in DNA and RNA.

pyruvate (pie-ROO-vate) Three-carbon compound formed during glucose metabolism; also called *pyruvic acid*.

R

racemase (RAS-ih-mace) Group of enzymes that catalyzes reactions involving structural rearrangement of a molecule (e.g., conversion of D-alanine isomer to L-alanine isomer).

radiation Energy that is emitted from a center in all directions. Various forms of radiation energy include X rays and ultraviolet rays from the sun.

raffinose (RAF-ih-nos) Indigestible oligosaccharide made of 3 monosaccharides (galactose-glucose-fructose).

rancid (RAN-sid) Containing products of decomposed fatty acids; yield unpleasant flavors and odors.

rating of perceived exertion (RPE) Scale that defines the difficulty level of any activity; can be used to determine intensity.

reactive hypoglycemia (HIGH-po-gligh-SEE-mee-uh) Low blood glucose that may follow a meal high in simple sugars, with corresponding symptoms of irritability, headache, nervousness, sweating, and confusion; actually called postprandial hypoglycemia.

reactive oxygen species (ROS) Several oxygen derivatives produced during the formation of ATP; formed constantly in the human body and shown to kill bacteria and inactivate proteins; also are implicated in a number of diseases and inflammatory processes.

receptive framework for learning Process by which a person opens up to learning more about a problem. It usually involves seeking more information about the issue from books and people. In the case of seeking behavior changes, it involves examining background experience to evaluate whether a behavior change is feasible.

receptor (ri-SEP-ter) Site in a cell where compounds (e.g., hormones) bind. Cells that contain receptors for a specific compound are partially controlled by that compound.

receptor pathway for cholesterol uptake Process by which LDL is bound by cell receptors and incorporated into the cell.

recombinant DNA (re-KOM-bih-nant) Molecule composed of the DNA from 2 different species spliced together, such as a combination of bacterial and human DNA used to produce unique bacteria that can synthesize human proteins.

recombinant DNA technology Test tube technology that rearranges DNA sequences in an organism by cutting the DNA, adding or deleting a DNA sequence, and rejoining DNA molecules with a series of enzymes.

Recommended Dietary Allowances (RDAs) Recommended intakes of nutrients that are sufficient to meet the needs of almost all individuals (97%) of similar age and gender; established by the Food and Nutrition Board of the Institute of Medicine, National Academy of Sciences.

Recommended Nutrient Intake (RNI) Canadian version of RDA, published in 1990.

rectum Terminal portion of the large intestine.

redox agents (RE-doks) Chemicals that can readily undergo both oxidation (loss of an electron) and reduction (gain of an electron).

reducing agent Compound capable of donating electrons (also hydrogen ions) to another compound.

reduction In chemical terms, the gain of an electron by an atom; takes place simultaneously with oxidation (loss of an electron by an atom) in metabolism because an electron that is lost by 1 atom is accepted by another. In metabolism, reduction often is associated with the gain of hydrogen.

Reference Daily Intakes (RDIs) Nutrient-intake standards set by the FDA based on the 1968 RDAs for various vitamins and minerals. RDIs have been set for 4 categories of people: infants, toddlers, people over 4 years of age, and pregnant or lactating women. Generally, the highest RDA value out of all categories is used as the RDI. The RDIs constitute part of the Daily Values used in food labeling.

registered dietitian (R.D.) Person who has completed a baccalaureate degree program approved by the American Dietetic Association, performed at least 900 hours of supervised professional practice, and passed a registration examination.

reinforcement Reaction by others in response to a person's behavior. Positive reinforcement entails encouragement; negative reinforcement entails criticism or penalty.

relapse prevention Series of strategies used to help prevent and cope with weight-control lapses, such as recognizing high-risk situations and deciding beforehand on appropriate responses.

remodeling Constant building and breakdown of bone throughout life.

renin (REN-in) Enzyme formed in the kidneys and released in response to low blood pressure. It acts on a blood protein called angiotensinogen to produce angiotensin I.

reproductive system Body system, consisting of the gonads, accessory structures, and genitals of males and females, that performs the process of reproduction and influences sexual functions and behaviors.

reserve capacity Extent to which an organ can preserve essentially normal function despite decreasing cell number or cell activity.

resistance exercise Physical activities that use muscular strength to move a weight or work against a resistant load.

resistant starch Starch, found in whole grains and some fruit, that resists the action of digestive enzymes.

resorption (ree-ZORP-shun) Loss of a substance by physiological or pathological means.

respiration Use of oxygen; in the human organism, the inhalation of oxygen and the exhalation of carbon dioxide; in cells, the oxidation (electron removal) of food molecules resulting in the eventual release of energy, CO_2, and water.

respiratory system Body system, consisting of the lungs and associated organs (e.g., the nose and various conducting tubes), that transports oxygen from outside air to the lungs and allows carbon dioxide to be expelled from the body. Oxygen and carbon dioxide are exchanged with the blood in the lungs. This system also regulates acid-base balance in the body.

resting metabolism Amount of energy the body uses when the person has not eaten in 4 hours and is resting (e.g., 15 to 30 minutes) and awake in a warm, quiet environment. It is approximately 6% higher than basal metabolism because of the less strict criteria for the test; often referred to as resting metabolic rate (RMR).

retina Light-sensitive layer at the back of the eye; contains the photoreceptors of the eye, called rods and cones.

retinoids (RET-ih-noydz) Biologically active forms of vitamin A, including retinol, retinal, and retinoic acid.

reverse transport of cholesterol Process by which cholesterol is picked up by HDL particles and transferred to the liver or to other lipoproteins that can dispose of it in the liver.

rhodopsin (row-DOP-sin) Photoreceptor in rod cells composed of 11-*cis*-retinal and opsin.

riboflavin (RYE-bo-fla-vin) Water-soluble vitamin that functions in coenzyme form in oxidation-reduction reactions, thereby playing a key role in energy metabolism. Milk and milk products, liver, mushrooms, and green leafy vegetables are rich sources of riboflavin.

ribonucleic acid (RNA) (RI-bow-new-CLAY-ik) Single-stranded nucleic acid involved in the transcription of genetic information and the translation of that information into protein structure.

ribose (RIGH-bos) Five-carbon sugar found in genetic material—specifically, RNA.

ribosomes (RI-bow-somz) Cytoplasmic particles that mediate the linking together of amino acids to form proteins; attached to endoplasmic reticulum as bound ribosomes or suspended in cytoplasm as free ribosomes.

rickets (RIK-its) Disease characterized by inadequate mineralization of the bones caused by poor calcium deposition during growth. This deficiency disease arises in infants and children with poor vitamin D status.

risk factor Term used frequently when discussing diseases and factors contributing to their development. Risk factors include inherited characteristics, lifestyle choices (e.g., smoking), and nutritional habits that affect the chances of developing a particular disease.

rods Sensory elements in the retina of the eye responsible for visual processes occurring in dim light, translating objects into black-and-white images, and detecting motion.

rough endoplasmic reticulum (EN-doe-PLAZ-mik re-TIK-you-lum) Portion of the endoplasmic reticulum that contains ribosomes; site of protein synthesis in a cell.

R-protein Protein produced by salivary glands that enhances absorption of vitamin B-12, possibly protecting the vitamin during its passage through the stomach.

RXR, RAR Abbreviations for retinoid X receptor and retinoic acid receptor. These 2 subfamilies of retinoid receptors in the nucleus interact with retinoic acid and bind with specific sites on DNA, allowing for gene expression.

S

saccharin (SACK-ah-rin) Alternative sweetener that yields no energy to the body; 300 times sweeter than sucrose.

S-adenosyl methione (SAM) (ES-ah-DEN-oh-sill-meh-THI-oh-neen) Compound formed from methionine; serves as a methyl donor in many biochemical reactions.

saliva (sah-LIGH-vah) Watery fluid, produced by the salivary glands in the mouth, that contains lubricants, enzymes, and other substances.

salivary amylase (SAL-ih-var-ee AM-ih-lace) Starch-digesting enzyme produced by salivary glands.

salmonella (sal-mo-NELL-a) Large class of bacteria, many strains of which are toxic, commonly found in animal and human feces. Salmonella can multiply in raw meats, poultry, eggs, fish, sprouts, unpasteurized milk, and foods made with these products. Cooking destroys salmonella.

salt Compound of sodium and chloride in a 40:60 ratio.

sarcoma (sar-KO-mah) Malignant tumor arising from connective tissues such as bone.

sarcomere (SAR-koe-mere) Portion of a muscle fiber that is considered the functional unit of a myofibril.

satiety (suh-TIE-uh-tee) State in which there is no longer a desire to eat; a feeling of satisfaction.

saturated fatty acid (SFA) Fatty acid containing no carbon-carbon double bonds.

scavenger pathway for cholesterol uptake Process by which LDL is taken up by scavenger cells embedded in the blood vessels.

schistosomiasis (shis-to-soh-MY-ah-sis) Diseases of liver, bladder, and GI tract caused by drinking water infested with a parasitic worm.

scurvy (SKER-vee) Deficiency disease that results after a few weeks to months of consuming a diet that lacks vitamin C. Pinpoint sites of bleeding on the skin are an early sign.

seborrheic dermatitis (seh-bor-REE-ik der-mah-TITE-is) Skin condition that results in scaly, flaky, itchy, and red skin; may result from a B-vitamin deficiency.

secondary deficiency Deficiency caused not by lack of the nutrient in question but by lack of a substance or process needed for that nutrient to function.

secondary disease Disease process that develops as a result of another disease.

secondary prevention Interventions to prevent further development of a disease so as to reduce the risk of further damage to health—for example, smoking cessation for a person who has already suffered a heart attack.

secretin (SEE-kreh-tin) Hormone that causes bicarbonate ion release from the pancreas.

secretory vesicles (see-KRE-tor-ee VES-ih-kels) Membrane-bound vesicles produced by the Golgi apparatus; contain proteins and other compounds to be secreted by the cell.

sedentary lifestyle Lifestyle that includes only the light physical activity associated with typical day-to-day life.

segmentation Contractions of the circular muscles in the intestines that lead to a dividing and mixing of the intestinal contents. This action aids digestion and absorption of nutrients.

selenium Trace mineral that functions as part of antioxidant enzyme systems and in thyroid hormone metabolism. Animal protein foods and whole grains are good sources.

self-monitoring Tracking behavior and conditions affecting that behavior; actions are usually recorded in a diary, along with location, time, and state of mind. This tool can help people understand more about their eating habits.

semiessential amino acids Amino acids that, when consumed, spare the need to use an essential amino acid for their synthesis. Tyrosine in the diet, for example, spares the need to use phenylalanine for tyrosine synthesis; also called *conditionally essential amino acids.*

Senior Farmers' Market Nutrition Program U.S. government program that provides low-income older adults with coupons that can be exchanged for fresh fruits, vegetables, and herbs at farmers' markets, roadside stands, and other community-support agriculture programs.

sensible water losses Water losses readily perceived, such as urine output and heavy perspiration.

sequestrants (see-KWES-trants) Compounds that bind free metal ions, thereby reducing the ability of ions to cause rancidity in foods containing fat.

serotonin (ser-oh-TONE-in) Neurotransmitter, synthesized from the amino acid tryptophan, that affects mood (sense of calmness), behavior, and appetite and induces sleep.

serum (SEER-um) Portion of the blood fluid remaining after the blood is allowed to clot and the red and white blood cells and other solid matter are removed by centrifugation.

set point Theory that humans have a genetically predetermined body weight which is closely regulated. It is not known what cells control this set point or how it actually functions in weight regulation.

sexually transmitted disease (STD) Contagious disease usually acquired by sexual intercourse or genital contact. Common examples include AIDS, gonorrhea, and syphilis; also called *venereal disease* and *sexually transmitted infection.*

shellfish poisoning Paralysis caused by eating shellfish contaminated with dinoflagellates (algae); also called *paralytic shellfish poisoning.*

short chain fatty acids Fatty acids that contain fewer than 6 carbon atoms.

sickle-cell disease (sickle-cell anemia) Genetic disease that creates red blood cells with incorrect primary structure in part of the hemoglobin protein chains. Malformed (sickle-shaped) red blood cells can lead to episodes of severe bone and joint pain, abdominal pain, headache, convulsions, paralysis, and even death.

sideroblastic anemia (si-der-oh-BLA-stik) Form of anemia characterized by red blood cells containing an internal ring of iron granules. This anemia may respond to vitamin B-6 treatment.

sigmoid colon (SIG-moyd) Part of the large intestine that connects the descending colon to the rectum.

sign Change in health status that is apparent on physical examination.

simple carbohydrate Carbohydrate composed of 1 or 2 sugars (e.g., glucose, fructose, galactose, sucrose, maltose, lactose).

simple sugar Monosaccharide or disaccharide in the diet.

skeletal fluorosis (flo-ROW-sis) Condition caused by a very high fluoride intake, characterized by bone pain and damage to skeletal structure.

skeletal muscle Muscle tissue responsible for voluntary body movements.

skeletal system Body system, consisting of the bones, associated cartilage, and joints, that supports the body, allows for body movement, produces blood cells, and stores minerals.

slough (SLUF) To shed or cast off.

small for gestational age (SGA) (jes-TAY-shun-al) Weighing less than the expected weight for length of gestation. This corresponds to less than 5.5 pounds (2.5 kilograms) in a full-term newborn. SGA infants are at increased risk of medical complications.

smooth endoplasmic reticulum (EN-doe-PLAZ-mik ri-TIK-you-lum) Portion of the endoplasmic reticulum that does not contain ribosomes. This is the site of lipid synthesis in a cell.

smooth muscle Muscle tissue under involuntary control; found in the GI tract, artery walls, respiratory passages, urinary tract, and reproductive tract.

sodium Major positive ion in extracellular fluid; essential for maintaining fluid balance and conducting nerve impulses. Salt added to foods during their production supplies most of the sodium in the diet.

sodium bicarbonate (SO-dee-um bi-KAR-bown-ait) Alkaline substance made basically of sodium and carbon dioxide ($NaHCO_3$).

soft palate (PAL-it) Fleshy posterior portion of the roof of the mouth.

solanine (sou-lah-neen) Toxin, produced in potatoes, that increases when potatoes are stored in a brightly lit environment; causes gastrointestinal and neurological symptoms.

soluble fibers (SOL-you-bull) Fibers that either dissolve or swell in water and are metabolized (fermented) by bacteria in the large intestine; include pectins, gums, and mucilages; more formally called *viscous fibers*.

solute Substance dissolved in a solution.

solvent Liquid substance that other substances dissolve in.

sorbitol (SOR-bih-tol) Alcohol derivative of glucose that yields about 3 kcal/g but is slowly absorbed from the small intestine; used in some sugarless gums and dietetic foods.

Special Supplemental Feeding Program for Women, Infants, and Children (WIC) U.S. government program that provides nutritious foods and nutrition education to low-income pregnant, postpartum, and breastfeeding women, as well as infants and children up to age 5 years who are at nutritional risk.

specific heat Amount of heat required to raise the temperature of any substance 1°C. Water has a high specific heat, meaning that a relatively large amount of heat is required to raise its temperature; therefore, it tends to resist large temperature fluctuations.

specific immunity Function of lymphocytes directed at specific antigens.

sphincter (SFINK-ter) Muscular valve that controls the flow of foodstuff in the GI tract.

sphincter of Oddi (ODD-ee) Ring of smooth muscle between the common bile duct and the upper part of the small intestine (duodenum); also called the *hepatopancreatic sphincter*.

spina bifida (SPY-nah BIF-ih-dah) Birth defect in which the backbone and spinal canal do not close.

spontaneous abortion Cessation of pregnancy and expulsion of the embryo or non-viable fetus prior to 20 weeks' gestation; result of natural causes, such as a genetic defect or developmental problem; also called *miscarriage*.

spore Dormant reproductive cell capable of turning into adult organisms without the help of another cell. Certain fungi and bacteria form spores.

sports anemia (ah-NEE-me-ah) Decrease in the blood's ability to carry oxygen, found in athletes, which may be caused by iron loss through perspiration and feces or increased blood volume.

stable isotope (EYE-so-tope) Specific, non-radioactive form of a chemical element; differs from atoms of other forms (isotopes) of the same element in the number of neutrons in its nucleus. *Stable* means that the isotope is not radioactive, in contrast to some other types of isotopes.

stachyose (STACK-ee-os) Indigestible oligosaccharide made of 4 monosaccharides (galactose-galactose-glucose-fructose).

***Staphylococcus aureus* (staf-i-lo-COCK-us OR-ee-us)** Bacterium found in nasal passages and in cuts on skin; produces a toxin when contaminated food is left for an extended time at danger zone temperature. Meats, poultry, fish, dairy, and egg products pose the greatest risk. *Staphylococcus aureus* can withstand prolonged cooking.

starch Carbohydrate made of multiple units of glucose attached together in a form the body can digest; also known as *complex carbohydrate*.

stem cell Unspecialized cells that can be transformed into specialized cells.

stenosis (ste-NO-sis) Narrowing, or stricture, of a duct or canal.

stereoisomers (stare-ee-oh-EYE-soh-mirz) Isomers with the same number and types of chemical bonds but with different spatial arrangements (different configurations in space).

steroid (STARE-oyd) Group of hormones and related compounds that are derivatives of cholesterol.

sterol (STARE-ol) Compound containing a multi-ring (steroid) structure and a hydroxyl group (—OH).

stimulus control Alteration of the environment to minimize the stimuli for eating—for example, removing foods from sight and storing them in kitchen cabinets.

stomatitis (stow-mah-TIE-tis) Inflammation and soreness of the mouth and throat.

stress fracture Fracture that occurs from repeated jarring of a bone. Common sites include bones of the foot.

striated muscle Muscles showing a striped pattern when viewed under a microscope. Stripes are due to the presence and specific organization of the contractile proteins actin and myosin.

stroke Loss of body function that results from a blood clot or another change in arteries in the brain that affects blood flow and leads to death of brain tissue; also called a *cerebrovascular accident*.

structural isomers (EYE-soh-mirz) Isomers in which the number and kinds of chemical bonds differ.

structure/function claim Claim that describes how a nutrient affects human body structure or function, such as "iron builds strong blood."

subclinical Present but not severe enough to produce signs and symptoms that can be detected or diagnosed (e.g., a subclinical disease or disorder).

submucosal layer (sub-myoo-KO-sal) Layer of blood and lymphatic vessels along with nerve fibers and connective tissue that stretch the whole length of the GI tract.

subsistence farmer Farmer who grows food only for the farm family rather than for sale.

successful aging Physical and physiological function decline that occurs only because one grows older, not because lifestyle choices, environmental exposures, and chronic disease have aggravated or sped up the rate of aging.

sucralose (SOO-kra-los) Alternative sweetener that has chlorines in place of 3 hydroxyl (—OH) groups on sucrose; 600 times sweeter than sucrose.

sucrase (SOO-krace) Enzyme made by the absorptive cells of the small intestine; digests sucrose to glucose and galactose.

sucrose (SOO-kros) Disaccharide composed of fructose bonded with glucose; also known as *table sugar*.

sugar Simple carbohydrate form with the chemical composition $(CH_2O)_n$. Most sugars form ringed structures when in solution; monosaccharides and disaccharides.

sulfur Major mineral primarily functioning in the body in non-ionic form as part of vitamins and amino acids. In ionic form, such as sulfate, it participates in the acid-base balance in the body. Protein-rich foods supply sulfur in the diet.

superoxide dismutase (soo-per-OX-ide DISS-myoo-tase) Enzyme that can quench (deactivate) a superoxide negative free radical (O_2^-); can contain manganese, copper, or zinc.

sustainable agriculture Agricultural system that provides a secure living for farm families; maintains the natural environment and resources; supports the rural community; and offers respect and fair treatment to all involved, from farm workers to consumers to the animals raised for food.

sympathetic nervous system Part of the nervous system that regulates involuntary vital functions, including the activity of the heart muscle, smooth muscle, and adrenal glands.

symptom Change in health status noted by the person with the problem, such as a stomach pain.

synapse (SIN-aps) Space between the end of 1 nerve cell and the beginning of another nerve cell.

system Collection of organs that work together to perform an overall function.

systemic circuit Part of the circulatory system concerned with the flow of blood from the heart's left ventricle to the body and back to the heart's right atrium.

systolic blood pressure (sis-TOL-lik) Pressure in the arterial blood vessels associated with the pumping of blood from the heart.

T

tagatose (TAG-uh-tose) Isomer of fructose that is poorly absorbed and, so, yields only 1.5 kcal/g to the body. Tagatose is 90% as sweet as sucrose.

taurine (TAH-reen) Non-essential sulfur-containing amino acid; has many vital functions and is included in some energy drinks.

telomerase (teh-LO-mer-ace) Enzyme that maintains length and completeness of chromosomes.

telomeres (TELL-oh-meers) Caps at the end of chromosomes.

tendon Dense connective tissue that attaches a muscle to a bone.

teratogenic (ter-A-toe-jen-ic) Tending to produce physical defects in a developing fetus (literally, "monster producing").

tertiary structure of a protein (TER-she-air-ee) Three-dimensional structure of a protein formed by interactions of amino acids placed far apart in the primary structure.

tetany (TET-ah-nee) Continuous, forceful muscle contraction without relaxation.

tetrahydrofolic acid (tet-rah-high-dro-FOE-lick) Central coenzyme formed from folic acid; participates in 1 carbon metabolism.

theory Explanation for a phenomenon that has numerous lines of evidence to support it.

thermic effect of food (TEF) Increase in metabolism that occurs during digestion, absorption, and metabolism of energy-yielding nutrients. TEF represents 5 to 10% of energy consumed.

thermogenesis (ther-mo-JEN-ih-sis) Ability of humans to regulate body temperature within narrow limits (thermoregulation); examples are fidgeting and shivering when cold. Other terms used to describe thermogenesis are *adaptive thermogenesis* and *non-exercise activity thermogenesis (NEAT)*.

thiamin (THIGH-a-min) Water-soluble B-vitamin that functions in coenzyme form to play a key role in energy metabolism. Pork is a good source of thiamin.

thiamin pyrophosphate (TPP) (pye-row-FOS-fate) Coenzyme form of thiamin.

thioredoxin (THIGH-o-re-dock-sin) Family of 3 selenium-dependent enzymes that have an antioxidant role and other roles in the body.

thrifty metabolism Metabolism that characteristically conserves more energy than normal, such that it increases risk of weight gain and obesity.

thromboxane (TX) (throm-BOK-sane) Eicosanoid made by blood platelets that is a stimulant of blood clotting.

thymine (THIGH-meen) Nitrogenous base that forms part of the structure of DNA and RNA; a pyrimidine.

thyroid hormone Hormone, produced by the thyroid gland, that increases the rate of overall metabolism in the body.

thyroid-stimulating hormone (TSH) Hormone that regulates the uptake of iodine by the thyroid gland and the release of thyroid hormone. TSH is secreted in response to a low concentration of circulating thyroid hormone (thyroxine).

tissue (TISH-you) Collection of cells adapted to perform a specific function.

T lymphocyte (tee LYMF-oh-site) Type of white blood cell that recognizes intracellular antigens (e.g., viral antigens in infected cells), fragments of which move to the cell surface. T lymphocytes originate in the bone marrow but must mature in the thymus gland.

tocopherols (tuh-KOFF-er-allz) Group of 4 structurally similar compounds that have vitamin E activity. The RRR ("d") isomer of alpha-tocopherol is the most active form.

tocotrienols (toe-co-TRY-en-olz) Group of 4 compounds with the same basic chemical structure as the tocopherols but containing slightly altered side chains. They exhibit much less vitamin E activity than the corresponding tocopherols.

Tolerable Upper Intake Level (UL) Maximum chronic daily intake of a nutrient that is unlikely to cause adverse health effects in almost all people in a population. This number applies to a chronic daily use.

total fiber Combination of dietary fiber and functional fiber in a food; also called *fiber*.

total parenteral nutrition Intravenous provision of all necessary nutrients, including the most basic forms of protein, carbohydrates, lipids, vitamins, minerals, and electrolytes. This solution is generally infused for 12 to 24 hours a day in a volume of about 2 to 3 L.

toxic Poisonous; caused by a poison.

toxicity Capacity of a substance to produce injury or illness at some dosage.

toxin Poisonous compound that can cause disease.

trabecular bone (trah-BEK-you-lar) Spongy, inner matrix of bone found primarily in the spine, pelvis, and ends of bones; also called *cancellous bone*. Trabecular bone makes up 20 to 25% of total bone mass.

trace mineral Mineral vital to health that is required in the diet in amounts less than 100 mg/day; also called *micromineral*.

trachea (TRAY-key-ah) Airway leading from the larynx to the bronchi.

transamination (trans-am-ih-NAY-shun) Transfer of an amino group from an amino acid to a carbon skeleton to form a new amino acid.

transcobalamin II (trans-koh-BAL-ah-meen) Blood protein that transports vitamin B-12.

trans **configuration** Compound that has hydrogens located opposite each other across a carbon-carbon double bond.

trans **fatty acids** Form of unsaturated fatty acids, usually a monounsaturated one when found in food, in which the hydrogens on both carbons forming that double bond lie on opposite sides of that bond (*trans* configuration). Margarine, shortenings, and deep fat–fried foods are rich sources.

transferrin (trans-FER-in) Blood protein that transports iron in the blood.

transgenic (trans-JEN-ik) Organism that contains genes originally present in another different organism.

transketolase (trans-KEY-toe-lace) Enzyme having TPP (thiamin pyrophosphate) as its functional component; converts glucose to various other sugars.

transverse colon Part of the large intestine between the ascending colon and descending colon.

Trichinella spiralis **(trik-i-NELL-a)** Parasitic nematode worm, found in wild game and pork, that causes the flulike disease trichinosis; easily destroyed by cooking. Modern sanitary feeding practices have drastically reduced *Trichinella* in commercial pork.

triglyceride (try-GLISS-uh-ride) Major form of lipid in the body and in food; composed of 3 fatty acids bonded to glycerol, an alcohol.

trimesters Three 13- to 14-week periods into which the normal pregnancy is somewhat arbitarily divided for purposes of discussion and analysis (the length of a normal pregnancy is about 40 weeks, measured from the first day of the woman's last menstrual period).

tropic hormone (TROW-pic) Hormone that stimulates the secretion of another secreting gland.

trypsin (TRIP-sin) Protein-digesting enzyme secreted by the pancreas to act in the small intestine.

tumor Mass of cells; may be cancerous (malignant) or non-cancerous (benign).

tumor suppressor genes Genes that prevent cells from dividing.

type 1 diabetes Form of diabetes in which the person is prone to ketosis and requires insulin therapy.

type 2 diabetes Most common form of diabetes in which ketosis is not commonly seen. Insulin therapy may be used but often is not required. This form of the disease is often associated with obesity.

U

ulcer (UL-sir) Erosion of the tissue lining, usually in the stomach (gastric ulcer) or the upper small intestine (duodenal ulcer). These are generally referred to as peptic ulcers.

umami (you-MA-mee) Brothy, meaty, savory flavor in some foods (e.g., mushrooms, Parmesan cheese). Monosodium glutamate enhances this flavor when added to foods.

undernutrition Failing health that results from a longstanding dietary intake that does not meet nutritional needs.

underwater weighing Method of estimating total body fat by weighing the individual on a standard scale and then weighing him or her again submerged in water. The difference between the 2 weights is used to estimate total body volume.

underweight Body mass index below 18.5.

unsaturated fatty acid Fatty acid with 1 or more carbon-carbon double bonds in its chemical structure.

upper-body obesity Type of obesity in which fat is stored primarily in the abdominal area; a waist circumference more than 40 inches (102 centimeters) in men and more than 35 inches (88 centimeters) in women; closely associated with a high risk of cardiovascular disease, hypertension, and type 2 diabetes.

uracil (YUR-ah-sil) Nitrogenous base that forms part of the structure of DNA and RNA; a pyrimidine.

urea (yoo-REE-ah) Nitrogenous waste product of protein metabolism; major source of nitrogen in the urine; chemically, NH_2—C—NH_2.

ureter (YOUR-ih-ter) Tube that transports urine from the kidney to the urinary bladder.

urethra (yoo-REE-thra) Tube that transports urine from the urinary bladder to the outside of the body.

urinary system Body system, consisting of the kidneys, urinary bladder, and the ducts that carry urine, that removes waste products from the circulatory system and regulates blood acid-base balance, overall chemical balance, and water balance in the body.

usual aging Age-related physical and physiological changes commonly thought to be a typical or expected part of aging.

V

vagus nerves (VAY-guss) Nerves arising from the brain that branch off to other organs and are essential for control of speech, swallowing, and gastrointestinal function.

vegan (VEE-gun) Person who eats only plant foods.

vegetarian Person who avoids eating animal products to a varying degree, ranging from consuming no animal products to simply not consuming mammals.

vein Blood vessel that conveys blood to the heart.

ventricles (VEN-tri-kelz) Two lower chambers of the heart, which contain blood to be pumped out of the heart.

venule (VEN-yool) Tiny vessel that carries blood from the capillary to a vein.

very-low-calorie diet (VLCD) Diet that contains 400 to 800 kcal per day, often in liquid form. Of this, 120 to 480 kcal are carbohydrate; the rest is mostly high-quality protein; also known as *protein-sparing modified fast (PSMF)*.

very-low-density lipoprotein (VLDL) Lipoprotein, created in the liver, that carries both cholesterol and lipids taken up from the bloodstream by the liver and those that are newly synthesized by the liver.

Vibrio cholerae Bacterium found in human and animal feces; causes the illness cholera; most often transmitted via contaminated drinking water.

villi (VIL-eye) Fingerlike protrusions into the small intestine that participate in digestion and absorption of food components.

virus Smallest known type of infectious agent (essentially, a piece of genetic material surrounded by a coat of protein), many of which cause disease in humans. Viruses reproduce with the aid of a living cellular host; do not metabolize, grow, or move by themselves.

visual cycle Chemical process in the eye that participates in vision. Forms of vitamin A participate in the process.

vitamin Compound needed in very small amounts in the diet to help regulate and support chemical reactions in the body.

vitamin A Fat-soluble vitamin that exists in retinoid and carotenoid forms and is crucial to vision in dim light, color vision, cell differentiation, growth, and immunity. Significant food sources are beef liver, sweet potato, spinach, and mangoes.

vitamin B-6 Group of water-soluble vitamins that, in coenzyme form, play a role in more than 100 enzymatic reactions in the body, almost all of which involve nitrogen-containing compounds. These reactions include amino acid metabolism, heme synthesis, and homocysteine metabolism. Salmon, potatoes, and bananas are good sources.

vitamin B-12 Water-soluble vitamin. In coenzyme form, it participates in folate metabolism and in the metabolism of fatty acids. Meats and shellfish are good sources; plants do not synthesize vitamin B-12.

vitamin C Water-soluble vitamin involved in many processes in the body, primarily as an electron donor; contributes to collagen synthesis, iron absorption, and immune function; likely has in vivo antioxidant capability; also known as *ascorbic acid*. Fruits and vegetables in general contain some vitamin C; citrus fruit, green vegetables, tomatoes, peppers, and potatoes are especially good sources.

vitamin D Fat-soluble vitamin crucial to maintenance of intracellular and extracellular calcium concentrations; exists in cholecalciferol and ergocalciferol forms. Vitamin D is abundant in fatty fish, such as herring, eel, salmon, and sardines, and, in North America, in fortified milk.

vitamin E Fat-soluble vitamin that functions in the body as an antioxidant, preventing the propagation of free radicals; exists as tocopherols or tocotrienols. Significant food sources are seeds, nuts, and plant oils.

vitamin K Fat-soluble vitamin that contributes to the liver's synthesis of blood-clotting factors and the synthesis of bone proteins; exists as phylloquinone or menaquinone. Green leafy vegetables, such as Brussels sprouts, kale, and lettuce, are excellent sources.

VO_{2max} Maximum volume of oxygen that can be consumed per unit of time.

W

water Universal solvent of life; chemically, H_2O. The body is composed of about 60% water. Water serves as a solvent for many chemical compounds, provides a medium in which many chemical reactions occur, and actively participates as a reactant or becomes a product in some reactions.

water-soluble vitamin Vitamin that dissolves in water; includes the B-vitamins and vitamin C.

wean (WEEN) To accustom an infant to a diet containing foods other than just breastmilk or infant formula.

weight cycling Successfully dieting to lose weight, regaining weight, and repeating the cycle.

Wernicke-Korsakoff syndrome (ver-NIK-ee KOR-sah-koff) Thiamin-deficiency disease caused by excessive alcohol consumption. Symptoms include eye problems, difficulty walking, and deranged mental functions.

whey (WAY) Protein, such as lactalbumin, found in great amounts in human milk; easy to digest.

white blood cell Formed element of the circulating blood system; also called *leukocyte*. Leukocyte types are lymphocytes, monocytes, neutrophils, basophils, and eosinophils. White blood cells are able to squeeze through intracellular spaces and migrate. Leukocytes phagocytize bacteria, fungi, and viruses, as well as detoxify proteins that may result from allergic reactions, cellular injury, and other immune system cells.

whole grains Grains containing the entire seed of the plant, including the bran, germ, and endosperm (starchy interior). Examples are whole wheat and brown rice.

WIC See *Special Supplemental Feeding Program for Women, Infants, and Children (WIC)*.

X

xanthine dehydrogenase (ZAN-thin de-HY-droj-ehn-ace) Enzyme containing molybdenum and iron; functions in the formation of uric acid and the mobilization of iron from liver ferritin stores.

xenobiotic (ZEE-no-bye-OT-ic) Compound that is foreign to the body; principal classes are drugs, chemical carcinogens, and environmental substances, such as pesticides.

xerophthalmia (zer-op-THAL-mee-uh) Condition marked by dryness of the cornea and eye membranes that results from vitamin A deficiency and can lead to blindness; specific cause is a lack of mucus production by the eye, which then leaves it more vulnerable to surface dirt and bacterial infections.

xylitol (ZY-lih-tol) Alcohol derivative of the 5-carbon monosaccharide xylose.

Y

***Yersinia enterocolitica* (yer-SIN-ee-ya)** Bacterium found throughout the environment; present in feces; can contaminate food and water; multiplies rapidly at room and refrigerator temperatures and is destroyed by thorough cooking.

yo-yo dieting See *weight cycling*.

Z

zinc Trace mineral required for many enzymes, including those that participate in antioxidant enzyme systems; stabilizes cell membranes and other body molecules. Seafood, meats, and whole grains are good sources.

zoochemical (zoh-uh-KEM-i-Kuhl) Compound in foods of animal origin that is physiologically active.

zygote (ZY-goat) Fertilized ovum; the cell resulting from the union of an egg cell (ovum) and a sperm until it divides.

zymogen (ZY-mow-gin) Inactive form of an enzyme that requires the removal of a minor part of the chemical structure for it to work. The zymogen is converted into an active enzyme at the appropriate time, such as when released into the stomach or small intestine.

Photo Credits

Chapter 1

Opener: Ed Carey/Cole Group/Getty Images RF; p. 5: The McGraw-Hill Companies, Inc./Jill Braaten, photographer; 1-2(left): © Stock Food/SuperStock; 1-2(right): Royalty Free/Corbis; p. 6: John A. Rizzo/Getty Images; 1-3: © PhotoDisc/Vol. 20; 1-4: © Comstock/PunchStock RF; p. 8: © Ingram Publishing/Alamy RF; p. 10(hamburger): Brand X; (cocktail): C Squared Studios/Getty Images RF; p. 11: © Creatas/PunchStock; 1-6: © BananaStock/PunchStock; p. 12(bottom): © Burke/Triolo Production/Getty Images RF; p. 13: © Eric Audras/Photoalto/PictureQuest RF; 1-7a: © Corbis/Vol. 76; 1-7b: © PhotoDisc/Vol. 29; 1-7c: © PhotoDisc Website; 1-7d: © Corbis/Vol. 130; 1-7e: Ryan McVay/Getty Images RF; p. 16(bottom): RF/Getty Images; p. 17: RF/Corbis; 1-9(fries): Brand X; (steak): Burke/Triolo Productions/Getty Images RF; (man & woman): RF/Getty Images; p. 18(bottom): © Digital Art/Corbis; p. 20: Rob Meinychuk/Getty Images RF; p. 21: Getty Images RF; p. 22: © Digital Vision/PunchStock RF; p. 24: G.K. & Vikki Hart/Getty Images RF; p. 29: © liquidlibrary/PictureQuest RF; p. 30: © E. Carey/Cole Group/Getty Images/RF

Chapter 2

Opener: Stockbyte/Getty Images RF; p. 36: © Digital Vision/Getty Images; p. 38: Royalty Free/Corbis; p. 40: © Stockdisc/PunchStock RF; p. 42(top): © PhotoDisc/Vol. 110; (bottom): © Royalty Free/Corbis; p. 44: © PhotoLink/Getty Images RF; p. 45: © The McGraw-Hill Companies, Inc./Jill Braaten, photographer; 46: The McGraw-Hill Companies, Inc./John Flournoy, photographer; p. 50: BananaStock/Jupiterimages RF; p. 51: USDA; p. 52(top): RF Getty Images; (middle): David Buffington/Getty Images RF; (bottom): © Bananastock; p. 53 (top): RF/Getty Images; (middle): © Photodisc/Getty Images RF; (bottom): © Comstock/Corbis RF; p. 54 (top): RF Getty Images; (middle): RF/Corbis; (bottom): Royalty Free/Corbis; p. 56(top): © Digital Vision/PunchStock RF; (bottom): RF/Corbis; p. 57: BananaStock/Jupiterimages RF; p. 60: Ryan McVay/Getty Images RF; p. 61: © Corbis/Vol. 192; Table 2-8(milk): © Ingram Publishing/Alamy; (meat): © Ingram Publishing/Alamy RF; (fruit): © Stockdisc/PunchStock RF; (vegetables): © Stockdisc/PunchStock RF; (grains): Jules Frazier/Getty Images RF; (oils): C Squared Studios/Getty Images RF; Fig 2-9(golf): © Corbis/Vol. 127; (tennis): © PhotoDisc/OS25; (cards): The McGraw-Hill Companies, Inc./Jacques Cornell photographer; (baseball): © PhotoDisc/OS25; Table 2-9 (breakfast): Mitch Hrdlicka/Getty Images RF; (lunch): Getty Images/Jonelle Weaver RF; (study snack): Getty Images/Jonelle Weaver RF; (dinner): Royalty Free/Corbis; (late snack): Royalty Free/Corbis; p. 63: © PhotoDisc/Vol. 67; Table 2-10(green): © Stockdisc/PunchStock RF; (orange): © Ingram Publishing/Alamy RF; (beans): C Squared Studios/Getty Images RF; (corn & celery): © Stockdisc/PunchStock RF; p. 64: Reproduction with permission. © Culinary Hearts Kitchen, 1982; p. 65: United States Department of Agriculture

Chapter 3

Opener: L. Hobbs/PhotoLink/Getty Images RF; (inset): © Christopher Kerrigan RF; p. 72: © PhotoDisc Website; p. 73(top): © Comstock/PunchStock RF; (bottom): USDA photo by Peter Manzelli; p. 75(top): USDA photo by Ken Hammond; (bottom): © Royalty Free/Corbis; p. 76(top): RF/Corbis; (bottom): © Royalty Free/Corbis; p. 77: C Squared Studios/Getty Images; p. 78: David Buffington/Getty Images; p. 79: Sandra Ivany/Brand X Pictures/Getty Images; p. 80: Photo by Lynn Betts, USDA Natural Resources Conservation Service; p. 81: © The McGraw-Hill Companies, Inc./Barry Barker, photographer; p. 82: © The McGraw-Hill Companies, Inc./Jill Braaten, photographer; p. 83: © Corbis/Vol. 83; p. 85: Burke/Triolo Productions/Getty Images; p. 86: © Object Series 36/PhotoDisc; p. 86a: © Corbis/Vol. 130; p. 86b: The McGraw-Hill Companies, Inc./Bob Coyle, photographer; p. 87(top): The McGraw-Hill Companies, Inc./Andrew Resek, photographer; (bottom): © The Ohio State University Communications Photo Service; p. 88(top): © Burke Tiolo Productions/Getty Images; (bottom): CDC; Table 3-3(salmonella): © Photodisc/Getty Images; (Campylobacter): © I. Rozenbaum/F. Cirou/Photo Alto; (E Coli): John A. Rizzo/Getty Images; (Shigella): © Comstock Images/PictureQuest; (Staphylococcus): Michael Lamotte/Cole Group/Getty Images; (Clostridium): © Ingram Publishing/Fotosearch; (Listeria): Digital Vision/Getty Images; (Clostridium): © Jarden Home Brands; (Vibrio): © I. Rozenbaum/F. Cirou/Photo Alto; (Yersinia): © Foodcollection/Getty Images; p. 92: © Image Source/Corbis; p. 93(left): National Pork Producers Council; (right): CDC; Table 3-5(Trichinella): © Ingram Publishing/Alamy; (Anisakis): © Image Source/Corbis; (tapeworms): © I. Rozenbaum/F. Cirou/Photo Alto; (Toxoplasma): © The Ohio State University Communcations Photo Service; (Cyclospora): © Don Farrall/Getty Images; (Cryptosporidium): © John A. Rizzo/Getty Images/RF; Table 3-6(Mycotoxins): C Squared Studios/Getty Images; (Ergot): © Brand X Pictures/PunchStock; (algae): Digital Vision/Getty Images; (shellfish): © BananaStock/PunchStock; (Scombroid): Photodisc/Getty Images; (Tetrodotoxin): Digital Vision/Getty Images; (Safrole): © Comstock/PunchStock; (Solanine): The McGraw-Hill Companies, Inc./Jill Braaten, photographer; (Mushroom): Photodisc Collection/Getty Images; (herbal): © Mitch Hrdlicka/Getty Images RF; (lectins): C Squared Studios/Getty Images RF; p. 98: © Brand X Pictures/PunchStock RF; p. 99: Corbis/Vol. 83; p. 100: RF/Corbis; p. 102 © Comstock Images/PictureQuest RF; p. 104: Digital Vision/Getty Images RF; p. 105: © BananaStock/PunchStock; p. 106: © Royalty Free/Corbis; p. 107: Object Series 36/PhotoDisc

Chapter 4

Opener: Michael Lamotte/Cole Group/Getty Images RF; p. 118: © PhotoDisc/Vol. 36; p. 126: © Ingram Publishing/Alamy RF; p. 127: © Ingram Publishing/Alamy RF; 4-10a,b: CNRI/SPL/Photo Researchers, Inc.; p. 128: © Comstock/Alamy RF; p. 130: © PhotoDisc; 4-15a: © Dr. Richard Kessel & Dr. Gene Shih/Visuals Unlimited; 4.15b: © Dr. David M. Phillips/Visuals Unlimited; p. 133: © BananaStock/PunchStock RF; p. 135: © PhotoDisc Website; p. 137: CNRI/Science Photo Library/Photo Researchers, Inc.; p. 139(top): © Corbis/Eat Natural; (bottom): © Burke Triolo Productions/Getty Images RF; 4.22: © J. James/Photo Researchers, Inc.; 4.23: © Gladden Willis, M.D./Visuals Unlimited; Table 4-6(cabbage): C Squared Studios/Getty Images RF; (milk): © Ingram Publishing/Fotosearch RF; (artichoke): © Burke Tiolo Production/Getty Images RF; (apple): C Squared Studios/Getty Images RF; (corn): © Ingram Publishing/Alamy RF; (beans): C Squared Studios/Getty Images RF; p. 144: © Ingram Publishing/Alamy RF; p. 145: The McGraw-Hill Companies, Inc./Jacques Cornell, photographer; p. 147: Royalty Free/Corbis

Chapter 5

Opener: Courtesy of The National Human Genome Research Institute RF; p. 157: Beano is a registered trademark of AkPharma, Inc.; p. 158: Greg Kidd & Joanne Scott; p. 159: © Image Source/Corbis RF; 5-7(strawberries & oats): Burke/Tiolo/Getty Images RF; (oats) & (beans): PhotoLink/Getty Images RF;

(celery): © Ingram Publishing/Alamy RF; (bread): Getty Images RF; (kiwi): © Ingram Publishing/Alamy RF; p. 161: © Jupiterimages/ImageSource RF; 5-8(cake): Jules Frazier/Getty Images RF; p. 162: C Squared Studios/Getty Images RF; Table 5-2(sugar): Royalty Free/Corbis; p. 163(top): Steve Allen/Getty Images RF; (bottom): Nancy R. Cohen/Getty Images RF; p. 164: © The McGraw-Hill Companies, Inc./Jill Braaten, photographer; Table 5-3(breakfast): © Image Source/Corbis RF; (lunch): © BananaStock/PunchStock RF; (dinner): © Getty Images/Jonelle Weaver RF; p. 167(top): Getty Images/Digital Vision RF; Table 5-4(cart): © Photodisc/Getty Images RF; (utensils): © CMCD/Getty Images RF; (silverware): © The McGraw-Hill Companies, Inc./Jack Holtel, photographer; p. 169: © Stockbyte/PunchStock RF; p. 172: John A. Rizzo/RF Getty Images; p. 175: © Creatas/PictureQuest RF; p. 176(top): © PhotoDisc/Vol. 49; (bottom): Getty Images/Eyewire; p. 179: © Corbis/Vol. 106; p. 180: © Royalty Free/Corbis; p. 181: CMCD/Getty Images; p. 183: © Lawrence Lawry/Getty Images RF

Chapter 6

Opener: © Jupiterimages/ImageSource RF; p. 190(left): The McGraw-Hill Companies Inc./Ken Cavanagh, photographer; (right): Burke/Triolo Productions/Getty Images RF; p. 194: The McGraw-Hill Companies, Inc./Jill Braaten, photographer; p. 195(left): www.istockphoto; (right): © blickwinkel/Alamy; p. 197(cone): © Ingram Publishing/Alamy RF; (doughnut): © Jules Frazier/Getty Images RF; (bagel): © Ingram Publishing/Alamy RF; p. 198: Royalty Free/Corbis; p. 201: Burke/Tiolo Production/Getty Images RF; p. 203(top): © Mark Kempf; (bottom): © Peter M. Wilson/Alamy; p. 204(top): Bryan and Cherry Alexander Photography; (bottom): © D. Hurst/Alamy RF; 6-16(left): Royalty Free/Corbis; (right): © BananaStock/Punchstock; p. 205(salmon): Corbis/Modern Cuisine; p. 205(students): BananaStock/Jupiterimages RF; p. 211: Getty Images/Digital Vision RF; p. 213: © William Wardlaw; p. 214: © Getty Images; p. 217: © PhotoDisc/Vol. 66; p. 218: Getty Images RF; p. 220: Royalty Free/Corbis

Chapter 7

Opener: © IT Stock Free/Alamy RF; p. 228: © Royalty Free/Corbis; Table 7-2(all): The McGraw-Hill Companies, Inc./Jacques Cornell, photographer; p. 229: Getty Images/Jonelle Weaver RF; p. 231: © Comstock/Jupiterimages RF; 7-6a,b: © Dr. Stanley Flegler/Visuals Unlimited; Table 7-4(breakfast): © Image Source/Corbis; (lunch): John A. Rizzo/Getty Images; (dinner): Kevin Sanchez/Cole Group/Getty Images; (snack): © Comstock/PunchStock; p. 234(bottom): © Don Farrall/Getty Images/RF; p. 235(beans): © Corbis/Vol. 83; p. 236(top): Digital Vision/Getty Images RF; (bottom): RF/Getty Images; p. 237: Greg Kidd & Joanne Scott; p. 238(top): © Createas/PictureQuest; (bottom): David Buffington/Getty Images RF; 7-14c(left): © Mediscan/Visuals

Unlimited; (right): SPL/Photo Researchers, Inc.; p. 244: © BananaStock/PictureQuest/RF; 7-15(Kwashiorkor): © Kevin Fleming/Corbis; (Marasmus): © Peter Turnley/Corbis; p. 247: © Corbis/Vol. 52; p. 248: PhotoLink/Getty Images; 7-16(all): Photos courtesy of Dennis Gottlieb; p. 250: C Squared Studios/Getty Images; p. 251(top): Getty Images/Jonelle Weaver; (bottom): © Ingram Publishing/Alamy; p. 252: © Tony Anderson/Getty Images/RF; p. 253: The McGraw-Hill Companies, Inc./Jacques Cornell, photographer

Chapter 8

Opener (potatoe): © Stockdisc/PunchStock; (corn): © Stockdisc/PunchStock; (apple): © Ingram Publishing/Alamy; (grapes): © Photodisc/PunchStock RF; (rice): The McGraw-Hill Companies, Inc./Jacques Cornell, photographer; (sugarcane): © Burke/Triolo Productions/Getty Images; (agave) & (rye & wheat): © Brand X Pictures/PunchStock RF; p. 258(wine): Getty Images/Jonelle Weaver RF; (martini): Photodisc Collection/Getty Images RF; (beer): Burke/Triolo Productions/Getty Images RF; Table 8-1(beer): © Photodisc/PunchStock RF; (spirits): C Squared Studios/Getty Images RF; (wine): © Photodisc/PunchStock RF; (mixed drinks): © Ingram Publishing/Alamy RF; p. 259: © Brand X Pictures/PunchStock RF; (bottom): © Stockdisc/Getty Images RF; p. 260(top): © Photodisc/PunchStock RF; (bottom): © Purstock/PunchStock RF; p. 261: Brand X Pictures RF; p. 262: Ryan McVay/Getty Images; 8-1(both): RubberBall Productions RF; p. 264: Dynamic Graphics/Jupiterimages RF; p. 265(top): Getty Images RF; (bottom): © PhotoAlto/PunchStock RF; p. 266(left): © Burke/Triolo Productions/Getty Images RF: (right): C Squared Studios/Getty Images RF; p. 268: © PhotoDisc Website; p. 269: Jack Star/PhotoLink/Getty Images/RF; p. 271: Jack Hollingsworth/Getty Images RF; p. 272: © Dynamic Graphics/Jupiterimages/RF; p. 273: © BananaStock/Punchstock/RF; p. 275: Royalty Free/Corbis; p. 276: Scott T. Baxter/Getty Images RF; p. 277: © Burke/Triolo Productions/Getty Images RF

Chapter 9

Opener: © Brand X Pictures/PunchStock RF; p. 282: John A. Rizzo/Getty Images RF; p. 291(top): Getty Images RF; (bottom): © Comstock/Alamy RF; p. 303: © Creatas/PunchStock RF; p. 304: © Royalty Free/Corbis; p. 305: Photodisc Collection/Getty Images RF; p. 306: Digital Vision/Getty Images RF; p. 307: Photodisc Collection/Getty Images RF; p. 308: © Comstock/Alamy RF

Chapter 10

Opener: © BananaStock/PunchStock RF; p. 317: © Stockbyte/PunchStock RF; p. 319: © Samuel Ashfield/SPL/Photo Researchers, Inc.; p. 320: PhotoDisc/Getty Images RF; 10-5: Penoyar/Getty Images RF; p. 321: Burke/Triolo Productions/Getty Images RF; 10-9: Rich O'Quinn, University

of Georgia; 10-10: Courtesy of Life Measurement Instruments; p. 325: FotoSearch Stock Photography; 10-12: Maltron International Ltd.; 10-13: DEXA; p. 328(top): © The Ohio State University Communications Photo Service, Jodi Miller; (bottom): © PhotoDisc/Vol. 82; p. 330: © PhotoDisc/Vol. 20; 10-16(energy intake) © Digital Vision; (problem behaviors): Jupiterimages; (exercise): Ryan McVay/Getty Images; p. 331: PhotoDisc/Vol. 76; p. 332: Royalty Free/Corbis; p. 334: Pando Hall/Getty Images; p. 336: PhotoDisc/Vol. 67; p. 338: Michael Lamotte/Cole Group/Getty Images RF; p. 341: The McGraw-Hill Companies, Inc./Lars A. Niki, photographer; p. 344: Ryan McVay/Getty Images; p. 345(top): Dave J. Anthony/Getty Images RF; (bottom): © PhotoDisc Website; p. 346: © Royalty Free/Corbis; p. 347: © PhotoDisc/Vol. 83; p. 348: © PhotoDisc/Vol. 95; p. 350: © PhotoDisc/EP047; 10-24: © PhotoDisc/EP047; p. 351(bottom): © Paul Casamassimo, DDS, MS; p. 352(top)Royalty Free/Corbis; (bottom): Jack Star/PhotoLink/Getty Images RF; p. 353: © PhotoDisc Website; p. 354: © RF/Corbis; p. 355: Doug Menuez/Getty Images RF; p. 356: © Photodisc Inc/Getty Images RF

Chapter 11

Opener: photo by John Van Winkle RF; 11-1: The McGraw-Hill Companies, Inc./Lars A. Niki, photographer; p. 363: Dynamic Graphics/Jupiterimages; p. 365: © PhotoDisc/EP040; 11-4(computer use): © Stockdisc/PunchStock; (roller blading): © Ingram Publishing/Fotosearch; (biking): © Photodisc/Getty Images; (flexibility & strength training): © Ingram Publishing/Fotosearch; (gardening): © Stockdisc/PunchStock; (stroller): © Ingram Publishing/Fotosearch; p. 367(left): Getty Images RF; (middle): © Corbis/Vol. 223; (right): Karl Weatherly/Getty Images; p. 368: PhotoLink/Getty Images; p. 371: © Stockdisc/PunchStock RF; 11-8(steak): © Comstock/Jupiterimages RF; (muffin): John A. Rizzo/Getty Images RF; (oil): The McGraw-Hill Companies, Inc./Jacques Cornell, photographer; (guy): Royalty Free/Corbis; p. 374: Digital Vision/Getty Images; p. 376: Ryan McVay/Getty Images RF; Table 11-3 (golfer): © Ingram Publishing/Alamy RF; (basketball): © Ingram Publishing/AGE Fotostock RF; (runner): © Photodisc Inc./Getty Images RF; (starting block): © Photodisc Inc./Getty Images RF; p. 377: © Photodisc Inc./Getty Images RF; p. 378: © Royalty Free/Corbis; 11-11: © Sean Thompson/Photodisc/Getty Images RF; p. 379: Sean Thompson/Photodisc/Getty Images RF; Table 11-5(rice): © Photodisc/PunchStock RF; (peppers): Jules Frazier/Getty Images RF; (grapes): © Ingram Publishing/Alamy RF; (milk): Royalty Free/Corbis; (cookie): © Jules Frazier/Getty Images RF; p. 382: © Comstock/Jupiterimages RF; p. 383: Stockbyte/PunchStock RF; p. 384: Imagebroker/Alamy; p. 385(top): © PhotoDisc/Vol. 51; (bottom): © Comstock/Jupiterimages RF; p. 387: © Corbis/Vol. 103; Table 11-9(cereal): © Stockbyte/PunchStock RF; (spaghetti): © Comstock/Jupiterimages RF; p. 390: The McGraw-Hill Companies, Inc./Gary He, photographer; Table 11-10(all): © Burke/Triolo Productions/Getty Images

Chapter 12

Opener: © Digital Vision; p. 400: © Corbis Website; 12-3: © Ingram Publishing/Alamy RF; p. 404(bottom): Getty Images RF; 12-6: National Eye Institute, National Institutes of Health; 12-7: A Colour Atlas and Text of Nutritional Disorders by Dr. Donald D. McLaren/Mosby-Wolfe Europe Ltd.; p. 411: Creatas/PicturesQuest RF; p. 412: Courtesy of the Golden Rice Humanitarian Board; p. 413: Royalty Free/Corbis; 12-10(soy milk): The McGraw-Hill Companies, Inc./Andrew Resek, photographer; (seafood): Digital Vision/Getty Images RF; p. 415(left): © Goodshoot/Alamy RF; (right): Hisham F. Ibrahim/Getty Images; (bottom): © Greg Kidd & Joanne Scott; 12-14: © Jeffrey L. Rotman/Corbis; p. 419: C Squared Studios/Getty Images RF; 12-15(bread): Burke/Triolo/Getty Images RF; (peanut butter): The McGraw-Hill Companies, Inc./Jacques Cornell, photographer; 12-18: Visuals Unlimited; 12-19: © Burke Triolo Productions/Getty Images RF; p. 423: C Squared Studios/Getty Images RF; p. 425: Digital Vision/Getty Images RF; p. 427: Photodisc Collection/Getty Images RF; p. 429: © PhotoDisc/Vol. 67

Chapter 13

Opener: © Digital Archive Japan/Alamy; 13-1: © Digital Vision; p. 440: C Squared Studios/Getty Images RF; 13-6: © Foodcollection/Getty Images RF; p. 441: Ernie Friedlander/Cole Group/Getty Images RF; 13-7: Getty Images/Jonelle Weaver RF; p. 445: © The McGraw-Hill Companies, Inc./Ken Cavanagh, photographer; 13-8a: A Colour Atlas and Text of Nutritional Disorders by Dr. Donald D. McLaren/Mosby-Wolfe Europe Ltd.; 13-8b: Dr. P. Marazzi/Science Photo Library; 13-9: G.K. & Vikki Hart/Getty Images RF; p. 447: Getty Images/Jonelle Weaver RF; 13-11a: Dr. M.A. Ansary/Photo Researchers, Inc.; 13-11b: © Lester V. Bergman/Corbis; p. 450: © Comstock/PunchStock RF; 13-12: The McGraw-Hill Companies, Inc.; 13-13: The McGraw-Hill Companies, Inc./Ken Cavanagh, photographer; p. 453: © Comstock/PunchStock RF; p. 455: © Image Club RF; 13-14: © Stockdisc/PunchStock/RF; 13-16: John A. Rizzo/Getty Images RF; p. 459: C Squared Studios/Getty Images RF; 13-18(top): Abbey/Photo Researchers, Inc.; (bottom): Biophoto Associates/SPL/Photo Researchers, Inc.; p. 463: © Royalty Free/Corbis; 13.19: Isabelle Rozenbaum & Frederic Cirou/PhotoAlto/PunchStock RF; p. 464: © Royalty Free/Corbis; p. 467: © Steve Mason/Getty Images/RF; 13-22: Burke/Triolo Productions/Getty Images RF; p. 469: Jupiterimages/Dynamic Graphics RF; 13-24: © Ingram Publishing/Alamy RF; p. 471: © Ingram Publishing/Alamy RF; 13-25(both): Dr. P. Marazzi/Photo Researchers, Inc.; p. 474: Michael Matisse/Getty Images RF; p. 476: © D. Fischer & P. Lyons/Cole Group/Getty Images/RF; p. 477: © Photodisc/PunchStock RF

Chapter 14

Opener: Digital Vision/Getty Images RF; 14-1: Ryan McVay/Getty Images; 14-5: © Ingram Publishing/Alamy RF; p. 489: Digital Vision/Getty Images RF; p. 490(juice): © Ingram Publishing/Alamy RF; (margarita): John A. Rizzo/Getty Images RF; (milkshake): Burke/Triolo Productions/Getty Images

RF; p. 491: Getty Images RF; p. 495: © Hugh Sitton/zefa/Corbis; p. 496: © The McGraw-Hill Companies, Inc./John Flournoy, photographer; p. 497: MHHE Image Library; p. 498: © Image Source/RF; 14-11(pickle): Burke/Tiolo Productions/Getty Images RF; (salt shaker): © Image Club RF; p. 500: C Squared Studios/Getty Images RF; p. 503: © Corbis/Vol. 552; 14-12: Brand X/RF; p. 504: © liquidlibrary/PictureQuest; p. 505: © Image Club RF; p. 507: © PhotoDisc/Vol. 40; p. 508: Nancy R. Cohen/Getty Images RF; p. 509: C Squared Studios/Getty Images RF; p. 510: Fred Lyons/Cole Group/Getty Images RF; p. 511: © Steven Mark Needham/Envision/Corbis; 14-13: © Stockdisc/PunchStock RF; 14-14(spinach): © Burke/Triolo Productions/Getty Images RF; (beans): © Comstock/Jupiterimages RF; (milk, bok choy): C Squared Studios/Getty Images RF; (cauliflower head): © Burke/Triolo Productions/Getty Images RF; p. 513: MHHE Image Library; p. 517: The McGraw-Hill Companies, Inc./Andrew Resek, photographer; p. 519: © Digital Vision/PunchStock RF; 14-20(a): © Michael Klein/Peter Arnold, Inc.; (b): © Dr. P. Marazzi/Photo Researchers, Inc.; (c): © Yoav Levy/Phototake; p. 523: © Don Mason/Blend Images/Corbis; 14-23: Burke/Tiolo Productions/Getty Images; p. 524: Chris Shorten/Cole Group/Getty Images; 14-24: C Squared Studios/Getty Images; p. 526: C Squared Studios/Getty Images; p. 528: © Comstock/Jupiterimages

Chapter 15

Opener: PhotoLink/Getty Images; p. 536(top): © IT Stock/PunchStock;(bottom): Ohio State University Extension/Malcolm W. Emmons; 15-1(clam): © Comstock/Jupiterimages RF; p. 537: C Squared Studios/Getty Images; p. 539: © Photo Disc/Vol. 48; 15-4 & 15-6a: SPL/Photo Researchers, Inc.; 15-6b: Omikron/Photo Researchers, Inc.; 15-7(both): Martyn F. Chillmaid/Photo Researchers, Inc.; p. 542: Dr. P. Marazzi/Photo Researchers, Inc.; 15-8: C Squared Studios/Getty Images RF; 15-9: Photo courtesy of Harold H. Sandstead, M.D.; p. 545: © Comstock/PunchStock RF; 15-10: Photo courtesy of Stephanie A. Atkinson, Ph.D.; p. 547(top): BananaStock/Jupiterimages RF; (bottom): Gordon Wardlaw; 15-11(lobster): C Squared Studios/Getty Images RF; 15-12: © Medical-on-Line/Alamy; 15-13: C Squared Studios/Getty Images RF; p. 550(bottom): C Squared Studios/Getty Images RF; 15-14: The McGraw-Hill Companies, Inc./Jacques Cornell, photographer; p. 552: RF/Corbis; p. 555(top): © PhotoDisc/Vol. 70; (bottom): © Corbis/Vol. 43; 15-17: Burke/Triolo Productions/Getty Images RF; p. 558: C Squared Studios/Getty Images RF; 15-19: © Paul Casamassimo, DDS, MS; p. 560: PhotoDisc/Vol. 02; p. 562: © Comstock Images/PictureQuest RF; p. 563: © Dennis Sabangan/epa/Corbis; p. 567: © Ricardo Elkind/Getty Images RF

Chapter 16

Opener: © Brand X/Corbis RF; p. 574(top): © Corbis/Vol. 19; (bottom): Don Tremain/Getty Images; p. 578: © Brand X Pictures/PunchStock RF; p. 580: PhotoDisc/Getty Images RF; p. 581: Blend Images/Getty

Images; 16-6b: © MedicalRF.com/Corbis; p. 585(top): Ryan McVay/Getty Images; (bottom): Brand X Pictures/Jupiterimages; p. 586: © Brand X Pictures/Jupiterimages; p. 587(top): Getty Images/Jonelle Weaver; (bottom): © Brand X Pictures/Jupiterimages; p. 588(top)Keith Brofsky/Getty Images; (bottom): Connie Coleman/Getty Images; p. 590: Smith/Getty Images; p. 591: X Pictures/Punchstock; p. 592: RF/Corbis; p. 593: Royalty Free/Corbis; p. 597: © Royalty Free/Corbis; p. 599: © Corbis/Vol. 83; p. 600: Images; p. 604: USDA; p. 606(top): © PhotoDisc/EP039; (bottom): © Royalty Free/Corbis; p. 608: Brand X Pictures/Jupiterimages

Chapter 17

Opener: Royalty Free/Corbis; p. 614 & 618(top): Courtesy of seca weighing and measuring; (bottom). © PhotoDisc/Vol. 61; p. 622: USDA Photo by: Ken Hammond; 17-4: The McGraw-Hill Companies, Inc./Jill Braaten, photographer; p. 625: © Creatas/PictureQuest; p. 626: Getty Images; p. 627: E. Dygas/Getty Images; Table 17-2(Birth to 4 months): Barbara Penoyar/Getty Images; (4 to 6 months): © Ingram Publishing/Alamy; (7 to 9 months): © Stockbyte/PunchStock; (10 to 12 months): © Creatas/PictureQuest; (12 to 24 months): © Brand X Pictures/PunchStock; p. 629: © PhotoDisc/Vol. 113; p. 630: © Brand X Pictures/Jupiterimages; p. 631(top): © Greg Kidd and Joanne Scott; (bottom): © PhotoDisc/Vol. 113; p. 632: © BananaStock/PunchStock; p. 633(top): Corbis/Vol. 552; (bottom): © D. Hurst/Alamy; p. 634: Ryan McVay/Getty Images; p. 635: Bronwyn Kidd/Getty Images; p. 636: © Jamie Grill Corbis; 17-6: USDA; p. 638: © Tim Pannell/Corbis; p. 639(top): White Rock/Getty Images; (bottom): RF/Corbis; p. 640(top): Getty Images/SW Productions; (bottom): BananaStock/Jupiterimages; p. 641: Stockbyte; p. 643(pizza): Brand X Pictures; (hamburger): Burke/Triolo Productions/Getty Images; p. 644: © Bananastock/PictureQuest; 17-7: © Paul Casamassimo, DD, MS; p. 646: © image 100 Ltd; 17-8: USDA; p. 647: PhotoDisc/Vol. 95; p. 648: © Corbis/Vol. 124

Chapter 18

Opener: © Dynamic Graphics Group/Creatas/Alamy; p. 656: © Stockbyte/PunchStock; p. 658(top): © Royalty Free/Corbis; (bottom): © Stockbyte/PunchStock; p. 659: Keith Thomas Productions/Brand X Pictures/PictureQuest; p. 660(top): Nick Koudis/Getty Images; (bottom): © Corbis/Vol. 81; p. 661: © Corbis/EP038; p. 662: C Squared Studios/Getty Images; p. 664: Mason/Getty Images; p. 665: © Jupiterimages; p. 671: © Getty Images/Digital Vision; p. 675(top): © PhotoDisc/Vol. 58; (bottom): © PhotoDisc Website; p. 676: © Corbis/Vol. 81; p. 678: Kevin Peterson/Getty Images; p. 679: Don Farrall/Getty Images; p. 680(top): Mitch Hrdlicka/Getty Images; (bottom): Royalty Free/Corbis; p. 682: © Comstock

Appendix

Fig A-1: K.G. Murti/Visuals Unlimited; E-1(all): © Greg Kidd & Joanne Scott

Dietary Reference Intakes (DRIs): Recommended Intakes for Individuals, Vitamins

Food and Nutrition Board, Institute of Medicine, National Academies

Life Stage Group	Vitamin A (μg/d)[a]	Vitamin C (mg/d)	Vitamin D (μg/d)[b,c]	Vitamin E (mg/d)[d]	Vitamin K (μg/d)	Thiamin (mg/d)	Riboflavin (mg/d)	Niacin (mg/d)[e]	Vitamin B_6 (mg/d)	Folate (μg/d)[f]	Vitamin B-12 (μg/d)	Pantothenic Acid (mg/d)	Biotin (μg/d)	Choline (mg/d)[g]
Infants														
0–6 mo	400*	40*	5*	4*	2.0*	0.2*	0.3*	2*	0.1*	65*	0.4*	1.7*	5*	125*
7–12 mo	500*	50*	5*	5*	2.5*	0.3*	0.4*	4*	0.3*	80*	0.5*	1.8*	6*	150*
Children														
1–3 y	300	15	5*	6	30*	0.5	0.5	6	0.5	150	0.9	2*	8*	200*
4–8 y	400	25	5*	7	55*	0.6	0.6	8	0.6	200	1.2	3*	12*	250*
Males														
9–13 y	600	45	5*	11	60*	0.9	0.9	12	1.0	300	1.8	4*	20*	375*
14–18 y	900	75	5*	15	75*	1.2	1.3	16	1.3	400	2.4	5*	25*	550*
19–30 y	900	90	5*	15	120*	1.2	1.3	16	1.3	400	2.4	5*	30*	550*
31–50 y	900	90	5*	15	120*	1.2	1.3	16	1.3	400	2.4	5*	30*	550*
51–70 y	900	90	10*	15	120*	1.2	1.3	16	1.7	400	2.4[h]	5*	30*	550*
>70 y	900	90	15*	15	120*	1.2	1.3	16	1.7	400	2.4[h]	5*	30*	550*
Females														
9–13 y	600	45	5*	11	60*	0.9	0.9	12	1.0	300	1.8	4*	20*	375*
14–18 y	700	65	5*	15	75*	1.0	1.0	14	1.2	400[i]	2.4	5*	25*	400*
19–30 y	700	75	5*	15	90*	1.1	1.1	14	1.3	400[i]	2.4	5*	30*	425*
31–50 y	700	75	5*	15	90*	1.1	1.1	14	1.3	400[i]	2.4	5*	30*	425*
51–70 y	700	75	10*	15	90*	1.1	1.1	14	1.5	400	2.4[h]	5*	30*	425*
>70 y	700	75	15*	15	90*	1.1	1.1	14	1.5	400	2.4[h]	5*	30*	425*
Pregnancy														
≤18 y	750	80	5*	15	75*	1.4	1.4	18	1.9	600[j]	2.6	6*	30*	450*
19–30 y	770	85	5*	15	90*	1.4	1.4	18	1.9	600[j]	2.6	6*	30*	450*
31–50 y	770	85	5*	15	90*	1.4	1.4	18	1.9	600[j]	2.6	6*	30*	450*
Lactation														
≤18 y	1,200	115	5*	19	75*	1.4	1.6	17	2.0	500	2.8	7*	35*	550*
19–30 y	1,300	120	5*	19	90*	1.4	1.6	17	2.0	500	2.8	7*	35*	550*
31–50 y	1,300	120	5*	19	90*	1.4	1.6	17	2.0	500	2.8	7*	35*	550*

mg = milligram, mg = microgram

NOTE: This table (taken from the DRI reports, see www.nap.edu) presents Recommended Dietary Allowances (RDAs) in **bold type** and Adequate Intakes (AIs) in ordinary type followed by an asterisk (*). RDAs and AIs may both be used as goals for individual intake. RDAs are set to meet the needs of almost all (97 to 98 percent) individuals in a group. For healthy breastfed infants, the AI is the mean intake. The AI for other life stage and gender groups is believed to cover needs of all individuals in the group, but lack of data or uncertainty in the data prevent being able to specify with confidence the percentage of individuals covered by this intake.

[a] As retinol activity equivalents (RAEs). 1 RAE = 1 μg retinol, 12 μg β-carotene, 24 μg α-carotene, or 24 μg β-cryptoxanthin. To calculate RAEs from REs of provitamin A carotenoids in foods, divide the REs by 2. For preformed vitamin A in foods or supplements and for provitamin A carotenoids in supplements, 1 RE = 1 RAE.

[b] cholecalciferol. 1 μg cholecalciferol = 40 IU vitamin D.

[c] In the absence of adequate exposure to sunlight.

[d] As α-tocopherol. α-Tocopherol includes RRR-α-tocopherol, the only form of α-tocopherol that occurs naturally in foods, and the 2R-stereoisomeric forms of α-tocopherol (RRR-, RSR-, RRS-, and RSS-α-tocopherol) that occur in fortified foods and supplements. It does not include the 2S-stereoisomeric forms of α-tocopherol (SRR-, SSR-, SRS-, and SSS-α-tocopherol), also found in fortified foods and supplements.

[e] As niacin equivalents (NE). 1 mg of niacin = 60 mg of tryptophan; 0–6 months = preformed niacin (not NE).

[f] As dietary folate equivalents (DFE). 1 DFE = 1 μg food folate = 0.6 μg of folic acid from fortified food or as a supplement consumed with food = 0.5 μg of a supplement taken on an empty stomach.

[g] Although AIs have been set for choline, there are few data to assess whether a dietary supply of choline is needed at all stages of the life cycle, and it may be that the choline requirement can be met by endogenous synthesis at some of these stages.

[h] Because 10 to 30 percent of older people may malabsorb food-bound B-12, it is advisable for those older than 50 years to meet their RDA mainly by consuming foods fortified with B-12 or a supplement containing B-12.

[i] In view of evidence linking folate intake with neural tube defects in the fetus, it is recommended that all women capable of becoming pregnant consume 400 μg from supplements or fortified foods in addition to intake of food folate from a varied diet.

[j] It is assumed that women will continue consuming 400 μg from supplements or fortified food until their pregnancy is confirmed and they enter prenatal care, which ordinarily occurs after the end of the periconceptional period—the critical time for formation of the neural tube.

Adapted from the Dietary Reference Intakes series, National Academies Press. Copyright 1997, 1998, 2000, 2001, by the National Academy of Sciences. The full reports are available from the National Academies Press at www.nap.edu.

Dietary Reference Intakes (DRIs): Recommended Intakes for Individuals, Elements

Food and Nutrition Board, Institute of Medicine, National Academies

Life Stage Group	Calcium (mg/d)	Chromium (μg/d)	Copper (μg/d)	Fluoride (mg/d)	Iodine (μg/d)	Iron (mg/d)	Magnesium (mg/d)	Manganese (mg/d)	Molybdenum (μg/d)	Phosphorus (mg/d)	Selenium (μg/d)	Zinc (mg/d)
Infants												
0–6 mo	210*	0.2*	200*	0.01*	110*	0.27*	30*	0.003*	2*	100*	15*	2*
7–12 mo	270*	5.5*	220*	0.5*	130*	11	75*	0.6*	3*	275*	20*	3
Children												
1–3 y	500*	11*	340	0.7*	90	7	80	1.2*	17	460	20	3
4–8 y	800*	15*	440	1*	90	10	130	1.5*	22	500	30	5
Males												
9–13 y	1,300*	25*	700	2*	120	8	240	1.9*	34	1,250	40	8
14–18 y	1,300*	35*	890	3*	150	11	410	2.2*	43	1,250	55	11
19–30 y	1,000*	35*	900	4*	150	8	400	2.3*	45	700	55	11
31–50 y	1,000*	35*	900	4*	150	8	420	2.3*	45	700	55	11
51–70 y	1,200*	30*	900	4*	150	8	420	2.3*	45	700	55	11
>70 y	1,200*	30*	900	4*	150	8	420	2.3*	45	700	55	11
Females												
9–13 y	1,300*	21*	700	2*	120	8	240	1.6*	34	1,250	40	8
14–18 y	1,300*	24*	890	3*	150	15	360	1.6*	43	1,250	55	9
19–30 y	1,000*	25*	900	3*	150	18	310	1.8*	45	700	55	8
31–50 y	1,000*	25*	900	3*	150	18	320	1.8*	45	700	55	8
51–70 y	1,200*	20*	900	3*	150	8	320	1.8*	45	700	55	8
>70 y	1,200*	20*	900	3*	150	8	320	1.8*	45	700	55	8
Pregnancy												
≤18 y	1,300*	29*	1,000	3*	220	27	400	2.0*	50	1,250	60	12
19–30 y	1,000*	30*	1,000	3*	220	27	350	2.0*	50	700	60	11
31–50 y	1,000*	30*	1,000	3*	220	27	360	2.0*	50	700	60	11
Lactation												
≤18 y	1,300*	44*	1,300	3*	290	10	360	2.6*	50	1,250	70	13
19–30 y	1,000*	45*	1,300	3*	290	9	310	2.6*	50	700	70	12
31–50 y	1,000*	45*	1,300	3*	290	9	320	2.6*	50	700	70	12

NOTE: This table presents Recommended Dietary Allowances (RDAs) in **bold type** and Adequate Intakes (AIs) in ordinary type followed by an asterisk (*). RDAs and AIs may both be used as goals for individual intake. RDAs are set to meet the needs of almost all (97 to 98 percent) individuals in a group. For healthy breastfed infants, the AI is the mean intake. The AI for other life stage and gender groups is believed to cover needs of all individuals in the group, but lack of data or uncertainty in the data prevent being able to specify with confidence the percentage of individuals covered by this intake.

SOURCES: Dietary Reference Intakes for Calcium, Phosphorus, Magnesium, Vitamin D, and Fluoride (1997); Dietary Reference Intakes for Thiamin, Riboflavin, Niacin, Vitamin B-6, Folate, Vitamin B-12, Pantothenic Acid, Biotin, and Choline (1998); Dietary Reference Intakes for Vitamin C, Vitamin E, Selenium, and Carotenoids (2000); and Dietary Reference Intakes for Vitamin A, Vitamin K, Arsenic, Boron, Chromium, Copper, Iodine, Iron, Manganese, Molybdenum, Nickel, Silicon, Vanadium, and Zinc (2001). These reports may be accessed via www.nap.edu.

Adapted from the Dietary Reference Intake series, National Academies Press. Copyright 1997, 1998, 2000, 2001, by the National Academy of Sciences. The full reports are available from the National Academies Press at www.nap.edu.

Dietary Reference Intakes (DRIs): Recommended intakes for Individuals, Macronutrients
Food and Nutrition Board, Institute of Medicine, National Academies

Life Stage Group	Carbohydrate (g/d)	Total Fiber (g/d)	Fat (g/d)	Linoleic Acid (g/d)	α-Linolenic Acid (g/d)	Protein[a] (g/d)
Infants						
0–6 mo	60*	ND	31*	4.4*	0.5*	9.1*
7–12 mo	95*	ND	30*	4.6*	0.5*	13.5
Children						
1–3 y	130	19*	ND[b]	7*	0.7*	13
4–8 y	130	25*	ND	10*	0.9*	19
Males						
9–13 y	130	31*	ND	12*	1.2*	34
14–18 y	130	38*	ND	16*	1.6*	52
19–30 y	130	38*	ND	17*	1.6*	56
31–50 y	130	38*	ND	17*	1.6*	56
51–70 y	130	30*	ND	14*	1.6*	56
>70 y	130	30*	ND	14*	1.6*	56
Females						
9–13 y	130	26*	ND	10*	1.0*	34
14–18 y	130	26*	ND	11*	1.1*	46
19–30 y	130	25*	ND	12*	1.1*	46
31–50 y	130	25*	ND	12*	1.1*	46
51–70 y	130	21*	ND	11*	1.1*	46
>70 y	130	21*	ND	11*	1.1*	46
Pregnancy						
14–18 y	175	28*	ND	13*	1.4*	71
19–30 y	175	28*	ND	13*	1.4*	71
31–50 y	175	28*	ND	13*	1.4*	71
Lactation						
14–18 y	210	29*	ND	13*	1.3*	71
19–30 y	210	29*	ND	13*	1.3*	71
31–50 y	210	29*	ND	13*	1.3*	71

NOTE: This table presents Recommended Dietary Allowances (RDAs) in **bold type** and Adequate Intakes (AIs) in ordinary type followed by an asterisk (*). RDAs and AIs may both be used as goals for individual intake. RDAs are set to meet the needs of almost all (97 to 98 percent) individuals in a group. For healthy breastfed infants, the AI is the mean intake. The AI for other life stage and gender groups is believed to cover needs of all individuals in the group, but lack of data or uncertainty in the data prevent being able to specify with confidence the percentage of individuals covered by this intake.

[a]Based on 0.8g protein/kg body weight for reference body weight.

[b]ND = not determinable at this time

SOURCES: Dietary Reference Intakes for Energy, Carbohydrate, Fiber, Fat, Fatty Acids, Cholesterol, Protein, and Amino Acids (2002). This report may be accessed via www.nap.edu.

Adapted from the Dietary Reference Intake series, National Academies Press. Copyright 1997, 1998, 2000, 2001, by the National Academy of Sciences. The full reports are available from the National Academies Press at www.nap.edu.

Dietary Reference Intakes (DRIs): Recommended Intakes for Individuals, Electrolytes and Water

Food and Nutrition Board, Institute of Medicine, National Academies

Life Stage Group	Sodium (mg/d)	Potassium (mg/d)	Chloride (mg/d)	Water (L/d)
Infants				
0–6 mo	120*	400*	180*	0.7*
7–12 mo	370*	700*	570*	0.8*
Children				
1–3 y	1,000*	3,000*	1,500*	1.3*
4–8 y	1,200*	3,800*	1,900*	1.7*
Males				
9–13 y	1,500*	4,500*	2,300*	2.4*
14–18 y	1,500*	4,700*	2,300*	3.3*
19–30 y	1,500*	4,700*	2,300*	3.7*
31–50 y	1,500*	4,700*	2,300*	3.7*
51–70 y	1,300*	4,700*	2,000*	3.7*
> 70 y	1,200*	4,700*	1,800*	3.7*
Females				
9–13 y	1,500*	4,500*	2,300*	2.1*
14–18 y	1,500*	4,700*	2,300*	2.3*
19–30 y	1,500*	4,700*	2,300*	2.7*
31–50 y	1,500*	4,700*	2,300*	2.7*
51–70 y	1,300*	4,700*	2,000*	2.7*
> 70 y	1,200*	4,700*	1,800*	2.7*
Pregnancy				
14–18 y	1,500*	4,700*	2,300*	3.0*
19–50 y	1,500*	4,700*	2,300*	3.0*
Lactation				
14–18 y	1,500*	5,100*	2,300*	3.8*
19–50 y	1,500*	5,100*	2,300*	3.8*

NOTE: The table is adapted from the DRI reports. See www.nap.edu. Adequate Intakes (AIs) are followed by an asterisk (*). These may be used as a goal for individual intake. For healthy breastfed infants, the AI is the average intake. The AI for other life stage and gender groups is believed to cover the needs of all individuals in the group, but lack of data prevent being able to specify with confidence the percentage of individuals covered by this intake; therefore, no Recommended Dietary Allowance (RDA) was set.

SOURCE: *Dietary Reference Intakes for Water, Potassium, Sodium, Chloride, and Sulfate.* This report may be accessed via www.nap.edu.

Acceptable Macronutrient Distribution Ranges

	Range (percent of energy)		
Macronutrient	**Children, 1–3 y**	**Children, 4–18 y**	**Adults**
Fat	30–40	25–35	20–35
omega-6 polyunsaturated fats (linoleic acid)	5–10	5–10	5–10
omega-3 polyunsaturated fats[a] (α-linolenic acid)	0.6–1.2	0.6–1.2	0.6–1.2
Carbohydrate	45–65	45–65	45–65
Protein	5–20	10–30	10–35

[a]Approximately 10% of the total can come from longer-chain n-3 fatty acids.

SOURCE: *Dietary Reference Intakes for Energy, Carbohydrate, Fiber, Fat, Fatty Acids, Cholesterol, Protein, and Amino Acids (2002).* The report may be accessed via www.nap.edu.

Adapted from the Dietary Reference Intakes series, National Academies Press. Copyright 1997, 1998, 2000, 2001, by the National Academy of Sciences. The full reports are available from the National Academies Press at www.nap.edu.

Dietary Reference Intakes (DRIs): Tolerable Upper Intake Levels (UL[a]), Vitamins
Food and Nutrition Board, Institute of Medicine, National Academies

Life Stage Group	Vitamin A (µg/d)[b]	Vitamin C (mg/d)	Vitamin D (µg/d)	Vitamin E (mg/d)[c,d]	Vitamin K	Thiamin	Riboflavin	Niacin (mg/d)[d]	Vitamin B-6 (mg/d)	Folate (µg/d)[d]	Vitamin B-12	Pantothenic Acid	Biotin	Choline (g/d)	Carotenoids[e]
Infants															
0–6 mo	600	ND	25	ND	ND	ND	ND	ND	ND	ND	ND	ND	ND	ND	ND
7–12 mo	600	ND	25	ND	ND	ND	ND	ND	ND	ND	ND	ND	ND	ND	ND
Children															
1–3 y	600	400	50	200	ND	ND	ND	10	30	300	ND	ND	ND	1.0	ND
4–8 y	900	650	50	300	ND	ND	ND	15	40	400	ND	ND	ND	1.0	ND
Males, Females															
9–13 y	1,700	1,200	50	600	ND	ND	ND	20	60	600	ND	ND	ND	2.0	ND
14–18 y	2,800	1,800	50	800	ND	ND	ND	30	80	800	ND	ND	ND	3.0	ND
19–70 y	3,000	2,000	50	1,000	ND	ND	ND	35	100	1,000	ND	ND	ND	3.5	ND
>70 y	3,000	2,000	50	1,000	ND	ND	ND	35	100	1,000	ND	ND	ND	3.5	ND
Pregnancy															
≤18 y	2,800	1,800	50	800	ND	ND	ND	30	80	800	ND	ND	ND	3.0	ND
19–50 y	3,000	2,000	50	1,000	ND	ND	ND	35	100	1,000	ND	ND	ND	3.5	ND
Lactation															
≤18 y	2,800	1,800	50	800	ND	ND	ND	30	80	800	ND	ND	ND	3.0	ND
19–50 y	3,000	2,000	50	1,000	ND	ND	ND	35	100	1,000	ND	ND	ND	3.5	ND

[a]UL = The maximum level of daily nutrient intake likely to pose no risk of adverse effects. Unless otherwise specified, the UL represents total intake from food, water, and supplements. Due to lack of suitable data, ULs could not be established for vitamin K, thiamin, riboflavin, vitamin B-12, pantothenic acid, biotin, or carotenoids. In the absence of ULs, extra caution may be warranted in consuming levels above recommended intakes.

[b]As preformed vitamin A only.

[c]As α-tocopherol; applies to any form of supplemental α-tocopherol.

[d]The ULs for vitamin E, niacin, and folate apply to synthetic forms obtained from supplements, fortified foods, or a combination of the two.

[e]β-Carotene supplements are advised only to serve as a provitamin A source for individuals at risk of vitamin A deficiency.

[f]ND = Not determinable due to lack of data of adverse effects in this age group and concern with regard to lack of ability to handle excess amounts. Source of intake should be from food only to prevent high levels of intake.

SOURCES: Dietary Reference Intakes for Calcium, Phosphorus, Magnesium, Vitamin D, and Fluoride (1997); Dietary Reference Intakes for Thiamin, Riboflavin, Niacin, Vitamin B-6, Folate, Vitamin B-12, Pantothenic Acid, Biotin, and Chloline (1998); Dietary Reference Intakes for Vitamin C, Vitamin E, Selenium, and Carotenoids (2000); and Dietary Reference Intakes for Vitamin A, Vitamin K, Arsenic, Boron, Chromium, Copper, Iodine, Iron, Manganese, Molybdenum, Nickel, Silicon, Vanadium, and Zinc (2001). These reports may be accessed via www.nap.edu.

Adapted from the Dietary Reference Intakes series, National Academies Press. Copyright 1997, 1998, 2000, 2001, by the National Academy of Sciences. The full reports are available from the National Academies Press at www.nap.edu.